Leadership and Nursing Care Management

evolve

⁝• To access your Instructor Resources, visit:

http://evolve.elsevier.com/Huber/leadership/

Evolve® Student Learning Resources for Huber: *Leadership and Nursing Care Management*, Third Edition, offer the following features:

Student Resources

- **Weblinks**
  This exiciting resource allows you to link to hundreds of websites carefully chosen to supplement the content of the textbook. The WebLinks are regularly updated, with new ones added as they develop.

Leadership and Nursing Care Management

Third Edition

Diane L. Huber, PhD, RN, FAAN, CNAA, BC

Professor
College of Nursing
The University of Iowa
Iowa City, Iowa

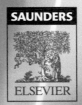

SAUNDERS
ELSEVIER

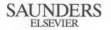

SAUNDERS
ELSEVIER

The Curtis Center
Independence Square West
Philadelphia, Pennsylvania 19106

LEADERSHIP AND NURSING CARE MANAGEMENT

ISBN-13: 978-1-4160-0168-3
ISBN-10: 1-4160-0168-9

NOTICE

Nursing is an ever-changing field. Standard safety precautions must be followed, but as new research and clinical experience broaden our knowledge, changes in treatment and drug therapy may become necessary or appropriate. Readers are advised to check the most current product information provided by the manufacturer of each drug to be administered to verify the recommended dose, the method and duration of administration, and contraindications. It is the responsibility of the licensed prescriber, relying on experience and knowledge of the patient, to determine dosages and the best treatment for each individual patient. Neither the publisher nor the author assumes any liability for any injury and/or damage to persons or property arising from this publication.

Previous editions copyrighted 2000, 1996

International Standard Book Number 13: 978-1-4160-0168-3
International Standard Book Number 10: 1-4160-0168-9

Senior Editor: Yvonne Alexopoulos
Developmental Editor: Kristin Hebberd
Editorial Assistant: Sarah Vales
Publishing Services Manager: John Rogers
Senior Project Manager: Helen Hudlin
Designer: Amy Buxton

Printed in the United States of America

Last digit is print number: 9 8 7 6 5 4 3 2

Contributors

Lecia A. Albright, BS, CPHQ, Certified
   Outcomes Manager
Principal and Owner
LARA Consulting, LLC
Spotsylvania, Virginia

G. Rumay Alexander, EdD, MSN, BSN
Director, Office of Multicultural Affairs
School of Nursing
University of North Carolina at
   Chapel Hill
Chapel Hill, North Carolina

Mary K. Anthony, PhD, RN, CS
Associate Professor
Frances Payne Bolton School of Nursing
Case Western Reserve University
Cleveland, Ohio

Suzanne M. Boyle, RN, DNSc
Vice President, Nursing/Patient Care
   Services
New York Presbyterian Weill Cornell
   Medical Center
New York, New York

Thomas R. Clancy, RN, MA, MBA
Vice-President, Professional Services
Department of Patient Care
Mercy Hospital
Iowa City, Iowa

Robert W. Cooper, PhD
Employers Mutual Distinguished Professor of
   Insurance
College of Business and Public Administration
Drake University
Des Moines, Iowa

Karen S. Cox, PhD, RN, CNAA
Senior Vice President
Patient Care Services
Children's Mercy Hospitals & Clinics
Kansas City, Missouri

Kathleen B. Cox, PhD
Assistant Professor
Department of Adult Health Nursing
School of Nursing
East Carolina University
Greenville, North Carolina

Laura Cullen, MA, RN
Advanced Practice Nurse
Evidence-Based Practice Coordinator
Department of Nursing Services and Patient Care
The University of Iowa Hospitals and Clinics
Iowa City, Iowa

Stacey T. Cyphert, PhD
Investigator
Acute Pain Management in the Elderly
Evidence-Based Practice
The University of Iowa Hospitals and Clinics
Iowa City, Iowa

Amy London Deutschendorf, MS, RN, AOCN
Principal
Clinical Resource Consultants, LLC
Pikesville, Maryland

Karen N. Drenkard, RN, MSN, CNAA, BC
Vice President of Nursing
Chief Nurse Executive
Department of Professional Practice
Inova Health System
Falls Church, Virginia

Harriet Forman, EdD, RN, CNAA
President
Omni Management Consultants, Inc.
New York, New York

Betsy Frank, PhD, RN
Professor
Baccalaureate and Higher Degree Nursing
College of Nursing
Indiana State University
Terre Haute, Indiana

Gregory O. Ginn, PhD, MEd, MBA, CPA, BA
Assistant Professor
Department of Health Care Administration
University of Nevada, Las Vegas
Las Vegas, Nevada

Kimberly Y. Harris-Eaton, RN, MSN
Nurse Manager
MUSC College of Nursing Instructor
Medical Surgical Infant Toddler Unit
Medical University of South Carolina
Charleston, South Carolina

L. Jean Henry, PhD
Associate Professor
Department of Health Promotion
School of Public Health
University of Nevada, Las Vegas
Las Vegas, Nevada

Patricia L. Horstman, RN, MSN, CNAA
Director
Department of Clinical Program Development
West Virginia University Hospitals
Morgantown, West Virginia

Michelle A. Janney, PhD, RN, CNAA
Vice President, Operations
Chief Nurse Executive
Department of Executive Administration
Northwestern Memorial Hospital
Chicago, Illinois

Katherine R. Jones, PhD, RN, FAAN
Acting Dean and Professor
School of Nursing
Yale University
New Haven, Connecticut

JoEllen Koerner, PhD, RN, FAAN
President
Global Nursing Academy
Sioux Falls, South Dakota

Jo Manion, PhD, RN, CNAA, FAAN
Principal Consultant
Manion & Associates
Oviedo, Florida

Maureen T. Marthaler, RN, MS
Assistant Professor
School of Nursing
Purdue University Calumet
Hammond, Indiana

Amelia McCutcheon, PhD, RN
Executive Lead, Professional Practice
Chief Nursing Office
Corporate Offices
Vancouver Coastal Health
Vancouver, British Columbia

Jacqueline Moss, PhD, RN
Assistant Professor
School of Nursing
University of Alabama, Birmingham
Birmingham, Alabama

Mary Ellen Murray, PhD, RN
Associate Professor
School of Nursing
University of Wisconsin–Madison
Madison, Wisconsin

Lynne S. Nemeth, PhD, RN, MS
Director
Care Management, Research, & Evaluation
Medical University of South Carolina
Charleston, South Carolina

Luc R. Pelletier, MSN, APRN, BC, FAAN, FNAHQ
Editor in Chief
Journal for Healthcare Quality
National Association for Healthcare Quality
Glenview, Illinois;
Healthcare Consultant
Self-Employed
San Diego, California;
Project Director
Danya International, Inc.
Silver Spring, Maryland

Belinda E. Puetz, PhD, RN
President and Chief Executive Officer
Puetz & Associates, Inc.
Pensacola, Florida

Richard W. Redman, PhD, RN
Professor and Director
Doctoral and Postdoctoral Programs
School of Nursing
University of Michigan
Ann Arbor, Michigan

Gene S. Rigotti, RN, MSN, CNAA, BC
Director
Department of Professional Practice
Inova Health System
Falls Church, Virginia

Claudia DiSabatino Smith, RN, MSN, CNA, BC
Education Specialist
Department of Nursing and Patient Education
St. Luke's Episcopal Hospital
Houston, Texas

Karen Weaver, RN, MA
Director of Surgery
Women and Infant Services
Medical University of South Carolina
Charleston, South Carolina

Dana Woods, MBA, BA
Director
Department of Marketing & Strategy
    Integration
American Association of Critical-Care Nurses
Aliso Viejo, California

Linda L. Workman, PhD, MSN
Associate Professor
Director of Nursing Education and Professional
    Practice
College of Nursing
University of Cincinnati and The University
    Hospital
Cincinnati, Ohio

Reviewers

Carol B. Allen, PhD, RN
Clinical Associate Professor
College of Nursing
Washington State University
Spokane, Washington

Martha C. Baker, PhD, RN, CCRN, APRN-BC
Director
BSN Program
Associate Professor
St. John's College of Nursing and Health Sciences
Southwest Baptist University
Springfield, Missouri

Karen J. Brasfield, RN, MSN, CMSN
Instructor
Department of Nursing
Everett Community College
Everett, Washington

Kathleen Lamaute, EdD(c), MS, MA, FNP, CNAA
Coordinator and Assistant Professor
Family Nurse Practitioner Graduate Nursing Program
Molloy College
Rockville Center, New York

Thom J. Mansen, PhD, RN
College of Nursing
University of Utah
Salt Lake City, Utah

Preface

There has never been such an urgent need for the twin competencies of leadership and management in nursing practice. Highlighted by a series of reports from the prestigious Institute of Medicine (IOM), it is clear that nurses are a pivotal focal point in health care delivery systems. Yet the United States is in the midst of a severe and continuing nurse shortage. For clients (and their safety), for delivery systems (and their viability), and for payors (and their solvency), strong nurse leaders and administrators are an imperative. Some have called this the *Age of the Nurse*. Yet the pressures to balance cost and quality considerations in a turbulent health care environment remain. Although society's need for excellent nursing care remains the nurse's constant underlying reason for existence, nursing is in reality much more than that. It is the Age of the Nurse precisely because nurses offer cost-effective expertise in solving problems in the coordination and delivery of health care to both individuals and populations in society. What this means is that nurses are well prepared to lead clinical change strategies and effectively manage the coordination and integration of interdisciplinary teams, population needs, and systems of care across the continuum.

It can be argued that nursing is a unique profession in which the primary focus is caring: giving and managing the care that clients need. Thus nurses are both health care providers and health care coordinators; that is, they have both clinical and managerial role components. *Leadership and Nursing Care Management* adopts the philosophy that there are two components to the nurse's managerial role that can be discussed separately but that in fact overlap. Because all nurses are involved in coordinating client care, leadership and management principles are a part of the core competencies needed by nurses to function in a complex health care environment.

The turbulent swirl of change within this country's health care industry has provided challenges and opportunities for nursing. As the nursing environment has changed and become more complex, nurses have needed a stronger background in nursing leadership and client care management to be prepared for contemporary and future nursing practice. As nurses mature in advanced practice roles and as the health care delivery system restructures, nurses will become increasingly key in health care delivery. Leadership and management are crucial skills and abilities for complex, integrated community and regional networks that employ and deploy nurses to provide health care services to clients and communities.

In the present and future of nursing practice, nurses will be expected to be able to lead and manage care across the health care continuum, a radically different approach to the practice of nursing than has been the norm for hospital staff nursing practice. In all settings, including nurse-owned and nurse-run clinics, nursing leadership and management are complementary skills that add value to solid clinical care and client-oriented practice.

Hospital nursing services across the country are recovering from a phase of restructuring, changing staff mix, and vesting staff nurses with the responsibility for decisions previously made by nurse managers. This movement increased the urgent need to advance staff nurses' knowledge about essential precepts of nursing leadership and management. In addition, nurses who are expected to make and implement day-to-day management decisions need to know how these precepts can be practically applied to the organization and delivery of nursing care to clients in a way that conserves scarce resources, reduces costs, and maintains or improves quality of care.

Acute care hospitalization has been eliminated as the primary modality for health care in the United States. As prevention, wellness, and alternative sites for care delivery become more important, nurses will be able to draw on their already rich experiential tradition of practice in these settings. This text reflects this contemporary trend by blending the hospital and nonhospital perspectives when examining and analyzing nursing care, leadership, and management. For example, it adopts the convention of "client" instead of "patient." The reader will notice examples from the wide spectrum of nursing practice settings as specific applications of nursing leadership and care management principles.

PURPOSE AND AUDIENCE

The intent of this text is to provide both a comprehensive introduction to the field and a synthesis of both nursing leadership and nursing management. It is a research-based blend of practice and theory. It breaks new ground by explaining the intersection of nursing care with leading people and managing organizations and systems. It highlights the evidence base for care management. It combines traditional management perspectives and theory with contemporary health care trends and issues and consistently integrates leadership and management concepts. These concepts are illustrated and made relevant by practice-based examples.

The impetus for writing this text comes from teaching both undergraduate and graduate students in nursing leadership and management and from perceiving the need for a comprehensive, practice-based textbook that blends and integrates leadership and management into an understandable and applicable whole.

Therefore the main goal of *Leadership and Nursing Care Management* is twofold: (1) to clearly differentiate traditional leadership and management perspectives and (2) to relate them in an integrated way with contemporary nursing trends and practice applications. This textbook is designed to serve the needs of the nurse who seeks a foundation in the principles of coordinating nursing services. It will serve the nurse's need for these principles, whether in relation to client care, peers, superiors, or subordinates.

ORGANIZATION AND COVERAGE

This third edition is strikingly different from the first two editions specifically with regard to authorship. The first two editions were single-authored texts. For the third edition, 29 of the 40 chapters are authored or co-authored by contributors. This approach draws together the best thinking of experts in the field—both nurses and non-nurses—to enrich and deepen the presentation of core essential knowledge. Their contributions are stellar, a blend of true expertise and dedicated hard work.

The organizational framework of this book groups the 40 chapters into the following seven parts:

- **Part I**, "Leadership and Care Management Overview," provides an orientation to the basic principles of both leadership and management.
- **Part II**, "The Professional's Role," addresses the nurse's role and career development. The reader is prompted to examine the role of the nurse manager in health policy development in what promises to continue to be a health care system in flux. Three core competencies of managing time and stress, critical thinking, and decision making form the foundation for leadership and care management skills.
- **Part III**, "Health Care Organizations and Systems," reviews the changing environment and context of nursing care delivery. The discussion highlights the importance of understanding the health care system and the organizational structures within which nursing care delivery must operate. This section

includes information on traditional organizational theory, such as organizational climate and culture, mission statements, policies, and procedures; and the dynamics of decentralized and shared governance. Building on organizational theory are chapters that demonstrate the importance of integrating organizations and systems with the current technology and theory applications, including data management and informatics, strategic management, and marketing.

- **Part IV**, "Care Management," addresses evolving modes of nursing care delivery. An overview of models of care delivery is followed by case management and disease management as major emerging models for nurses. Communication, persuasion, and negotiation are featured as essential care management skills. New to the third edition are chapters on all-hazards disaster preparedness (sometimes called *bioterrorism*) and evidence-based practice.

- **Part V**, "Human Resources Management," highlights the opportunities and challenges for the nurse manager-leader in dealing with the health care workforce. The wide range of human resource responsibilities of nurse managers is reviewed, and resources for further study are provided. The significant share of scarce organization budgets that is consumed by the human resources of the institution makes this area of management a key challenge requiring intricate skills in leadership and management. Chapters in this section look at some of the important factors in the nursing and health care environment that must be considered by the nurse leader-manager. Cultural diversity is a growing reality in our society, and the make-up of the health care work needs to recognize and reflect the changing cultural mix of force the client population. Legal and ethical issues increase in importance in a dynamic health care environment, and the pace of change requires that nurses know how to manage effectively in the workplace. Among the areas of special focus in this section are chapters on confronting the nursing shortage, cultural and generational workforce diversity, prevention of workplace violence, and collective bargaining.

- **Part VI**, "Fiscal Management," visits the financial resource arena of nursing management and reviews those activities that have become increasingly important, given scarce financial resources and pressures for cost containment.

- Finally, in **Part VII**, "Outcomes Management," change, quality, and outcomes each have separate chapters devoted to key concepts and strategies. Nurse leaders and managers will use change management as a major skill to contain costs, improve quality, and deliver desired outcomes.

Each of the 40 chapters is organized into a consistent format highlighting the following features:

- Concept definitions
- Theoretical and research background
- Leadership and management implications
- Current issues and trends

This format is designed to bridge the gap between theory and practice and to increase the relevance of nursing leadership and management by demonstrating the way in which theory translates into behaviors appropriate to contemporary leadership and nursing care management.

TEXT FEATURES

In addition to the traditional text features—chapter objectives, chapter summary, and references—this book contains other interesting and effective aids to readers' comprehension and application.

Study Questions At the end of every chapter the study questions ask students not only to recall specific information but also to synthesize what they have read. Answers to these questions were prepared by Lori Houghton-Rahrig, MSN, APRN, BC, and appear in the *Study Guide for Leadership and Nursing Care Management*, third edition, by Jean Nagelkerk, PhD, RN, FNP-C.

Critical Thinking Exercises Also at the end of each of the chapters is a situation that is presented along with questions that challenge readers to inquire and reflect and to analyze critically the knowledge they have absorbed and apply it to the situation.

Research Notes These summaries of current research studies are highlighted in every chapter and introduce the reader to the liveliness and applicability of the research literature now available in nursing leadership and management.

Leadership & Management Behaviors This box, one of which is found in every chapter, summarizes the applicable behaviors that fall under either leadership or management and also identifies behaviors that overlap these areas. This listing is designed to help readers reflect back on the chapter content in a way that distinguishes leadership from management and also demonstrates how the two are integrated.

NEW! *Case Studies* New to the third edition are case studies at the end of each chapter. The case studies are vignettes that introduce the reader to the "real world" of nursing leadership and management and demonstrate the ways in which the concepts in the chapter operate in specific situations. These vignettes all show the creativity and energy that characterize expert nurse administrators as they tackle issues in practice.

NEW! *Leading & Managing Defined* Also new to the third edition is this definition box, which appears near the beginning of each chapter. It provides the reader with a quick summary of the key terms and accompanying definitions needed to master each chapter's content. Key terms within this box are also highlighted within the text to allow the reader quick access to a more detailed contextual discussion of each work or phrase.

NEW! *Glossary* The third edition now features a glossary to allow readers easy to access to a compilation of all the key terms within the text. This comprehensive alphabetical listing can be found at the back of the book.

TEACHING/LEARNING AIDS

This innovative text is accompanied by the following two excellent teaching-learning tools:

1. *Evolve Resources for Leadership and Nursing Care Management*, third edition, features a complete Instructor's Resource Manual (IRM) accompanied by Lecture Slides, both of which were prepared by Jean Nagelkerk, PhD, RN, FNP-C, and a Test Bank (TB) prepared by Lori Houghton-Rahrig, MSN, APRN, BC.

   - The IRM guides the instructor through each chapter of the textbook with a chapter focus, key terms, and learning objectives. In addition, it offers critical thinking activities for the classroom (including role-playing and other group activities), both class discussion and essay questions, and a case study with analysis questions that facilitate classroom discussion of how concepts in the textbook relate to realistic situations.

   - **NEW!** The Lecture Slides feature between 15 and 30 PowerPoint slides for each chapter to guide classroom lecture. Slides refer to specific key textual definitions and concepts to highlight the most important points of note.

   - **NEW!** The Test Bank is composed of approximately 400 NCLEX-style questions presented in ExamView. Instructors can download these questions and customize their own exams by adding, deleting, and modifying questions to fit their particular test-assessment needs.

2. *Study Guide for Leadership and Nursing Care Management*, third edition, also prepared by Jean Nagelkerk, follows the textbook chapter by chapter, condensing key terms, information, and concepts into each chapter's study focus. Learning tools such as group activities, self-assessments, and case studies with questions for analysis encourage students to explore different roles, responsibilities, and challenges related to nursing leadership management. Students can test their comprehension of text content at the end of each chapter with short-answer discussion questions and objective exam-preparation questions in multiple-choice, true/false, and matching formats (with answers provided in the back of the book). Each chapter contains a listing of references and supplemental readings and concludes with answers to the text short-answer Study Questions.

Diane L. Huber

Acknowledgments

This book is dedicated to my husband, Bob Huber. He made this book a reality and was the text and graphics support behind it. For his love, caring, and support I am eternally grateful. To my children, Brad Gardner and Lisa Witte, and their spouses, Nonalee Gardner and John Witte, for their enthusiasm and love, I am forever privileged that they are in my life. I thank them for the gifts of Kathryn Anne Gardner (the Princess) and Anthony James Gardner. I love being grandma. Also special are Chris Huber, Beth and Brad Nau, Von and Kirk Danielson, and grandchildren: Brandon, Danielle, Creighton, and Cameron Nau; and Kory, Ryan and Sean Danielson.

To my professional colleagues who inspired me and served as examples of excellence in nursing, I am grateful. To my nursing students, past and future, my thanks for being a source of continual intellectual stimulation and challenge.

This book's first two editions evolved under the tender care of Thomas Eoyang, Editorial Manager at W.B. Saunders Company, whose guidance, support, and caring were invaluable. To Yvonne Alexopoulous and Kristin Hebberd, editors in the Elsevier Nursing Division, who worked so hard to facilitate everything related to the third edition, and to the excellent staff at Elsevier Saunders, a sincere thank you.

Diane L. Huber

Contents

PART VI
FISCAL MANAGEMENT

LEADERSHIP AND CARE MANAGEMENT OVERVIEW

I

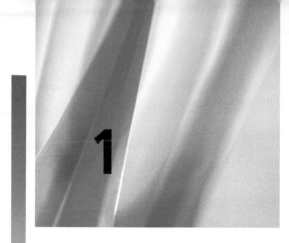

Leadership Principles

Diane L. Huber

CHAPTER OBJECTIVES

- Define and describe leadership
- Formulate the process of leadership
- Critique the qualities of leadership
- Analyze leadership styles
- Distinguish among theories of leadership
- Specify the linkage between followership and leadership
- Apply leadership to nursing practice
- Exercise critical thinking to conceptualize and analyze possible solutions to a practice exercise

An enduring question persists about why leadership is important to study, learn, and practice. After all, there are critical, pressing needs for nurses to focus on in taking care of patients. However, today's health care work environment is characterized by complexity, continuous and rapid change, turbulence, and chaos. Such an environment generates threats to the nurse's identity, coping skills, and the ability to work with others in harmony. It also presents the opportunity to lead, challenge assumptions, consolidate a purpose, and move a vision forward. An inescapable need exists for nurses to possess knowledge and skill in the art and science of solving problems in work groups, systems of care, and the environment of care delivery. The effectiveness of an individual staff nurse depends partly on individual competence and partly on the creation of a facilitating environment and the gaining of sufficient resources to accomplish goals. The nurse leader combines clinical, administrative, financial, and operational skills to solve problems in the care environment so that staff nurses can provide cost-effective care in a way that is satisfying and health promoting for clients. Such an environment does not simply happen; it requires special skills. Thus the study of nursing leadership and care management focuses critical thinking on what it takes to be a nursing "environment architect", transition leader, and manager of care delivery.

Nursing is a service profession whose core mission is the care and nurturing of human beings in their experiences of health and illness. Nurses have two basic roles: care providers and care managers. The first role is more often the role envisioned or emphasized. In the United States the acute care medical model in hospitals over time came to be the primary focus of attention and jobs for nurses. In this illness-focused model, the nurse's care provider or "doing" role was the most important and valued aspect of nursing. Little reward came from the "thinking" and integrating skills nurses were capable of. With a shift to managed care, the nurse's care management role has become more prominent, needed, and valued. The delivery of nursing services involves the organization and coordination of complex activities. Nurses use managerial and leadership skills to facilitate delivery of quality nursing care.

Leadership is an activity of human engagement and a relationship experience founded in trust, communication, inspiration, action, and "servanthood." The leadership role is so important because it embodies commitment and forward-reaching action. Arising from a drive to make things better, leaders use their power to bring teams together, spark innovation, create positive communication, and drive forward toward group goals. Leadership has been described by others in many ways:

Great necessities call forth great leaders.

Abigail Adams

Leadership: the art of getting someone else to do something you want done because he wants to do it.

Dwight D. Eisenhower

Leadership is the special quality which enables people to stand up and pull the rest of us over the horizon.

James L. Fisher

Leadership and learning are indispensable to each other.

John F. Kennedy

Leadership is lifting a person's vision to higher sights, the raising of a person's performance to a higher standard, the building of a personality beyond its normal limitations.

Peter F. Drucker

The first step to leadership is servanthood.

John Maxwell

The first responsibility of a leader is to define reality.

Max DePree

Leadership has a harder job to do than just choose sides. It must bring sides together.

Jesse Jackson

The only test of leadership is that somebody follows.

Robert K. Greenleaf

Leadership is getting people to work for you when they are not obligated.

Fred Smith

The main characteristics of effective leadership are intelligence, integrity or loyalty, mystique, humor, discipline, courage, self sufficiency and confidence.

James L. Fisher

Leadership is a unique function. It can be part of a formal organizational managerial position, or it can arise spontaneously in any group. Certain characteristics, such as being motivated by challenge, commitment, and autonomy, are thought to be associated with leadership. Effectiveness is a key outcome of leadership efforts in health care. It has been suggested that there is a scarcity of leaders and a crisis in leadership in nursing. This is crucial, because in times of chaos, complexity, and change, leadership is absolutely essential to provide the guidance, direction, and sense of stability needed to ensure followers' effectiveness and satisfaction.

The focus on leadership as a crucial need arises from the impact of significant changes that have occurred in the organization, delivery, and financing of health care in the past 10 years. This period has been characterized as "turbulent" and "tumultuous" because of "waves of chaos." Under such circumstances, nursing is challenged to respond with leadership. Although health professionals are experiencing a degree of trauma, they need to respond by adapting to the changes forced on them, seeking new tools for dealing with the new health care environment, and leading the way with client-centered strategies (Sherwood, 1997).

Both nurses and the health care delivery systems in which they practice need leaders to arise and address the complex chaotic environment of care delivery. The current health care environment is seen as a period of profound transition characterized by competition, conflict, consumer orientation, rapid communication, and chaos (Hagenow, 2001). Potential health care leaders likely will possess "a passion to make things better, a commitment to values, a focus on creativity and innovation, and the knowledge and skills necessary to identify health care needs and then to mobilize and array the human and other resources necessary to achieve goals and effect outcomes" (Huber & Watson, 2001, p. 29). These leaders can emerge from a foundation of quiet but respected competence. A leader may be the "wise" or "go-to" person within the group, a superior problem solver, a strategic communicator, or someone who is emotionally intelligent and strong in interpersonal relationship skills. Leaders may grow gradually out of a smoldering issue or erupt through a crisis event. Clearly, "something changes as leadership blossoms" (Huber & Watson, 2001, p. 29).

LEADERSHIP OVERVIEW

Leadership is a natural element of nursing practice because the majority of nurses practice in work groups or units. Possessing the license of an RN implies certain leadership skills and requires the ability to delegate and supervise the work of others. Leadership can be seen as the ability to inspire confidence and support among followers, especially in organizations where leadership is focused toward those whose competence and commitment produce performance.

Leadership is an important issue related to how nurses integrate the various elements of nursing practice to ensure the highest quality of care for clients. There are two critical skills that every nurse needs to possess to enhance professional practice. One is a skill at interpersonal relationships. This is fundamental to leadership and the work of nursing. The second is the skill of applying the problem-solving process. This involves the ability to think critically, to identify problems, and to develop objectivity and a degree of maturity or judgment. Leadership skills build on professional and clinical skills. Hersey and colleagues (2001) identified the following three skills needed for leading or influencing:

1. *Diagnosing:* Diagnosing involves being able to understand the situation and the problem to be solved or resolved. This is a cognitive competency.

2. *Adapting:* Adapting involves being able to adapt behaviors and other resources to match the situation. This is a behavioral competency.
3. *Communicating:* Communicating is employed to advance the process in a way that individuals can understand and accept. This is a process competency.

Among the important personal leadership skills is emotional intelligence. Based on the work of Goleman (1997, 2000), relational and emotional integrity are hallmarks of good leaders. This is because the leader operates in a crucial cultural and contextual influencing mode. The leader's behavior, patterns of actions, attitude, and performance have a special impact on the team's attitude and behaviors and on the context and character of work life. Followers need to be able to depend on role consistency, balance, and behavioral integrity from the leader. The four skill sets needed by good leaders are as follows:

1. *Self-awareness:* Ability to read one's own emotional state and be aware of one's own mood and how this affects staff relationships
2. *Self-management:* Ability to take corrective action so as not to transfer negative moods to staff relationships
3. *Social awareness:* An intuitive skill of empathy and expressiveness in being sensitive and aware of the emotions and moods of others
4. *Relationship management:* Effective communication with others that disarms conflict and the ability to develop the emotional maturity of team members

These interpersonal relationship skills are crucial to the work of leadership. The chaos and complexity of the seismic shifts in health care structure, delivery, form, technology, and content have made visible the urgent need for leaders to emerge, mobilize, and encourage followers. Leaders are key to bridging the efforts of followers with the goals of organizations. This is both tricky and risky and may be overwhelming (Porter-O'Grady, 2003). However, good leaders are anchors to the vision and the larger goal, guides to coping and being productive, and champions of energy and enthusiasm for the work.

Leadership content in nursing is studied as a way of increasing the skills and abilities needed to facilitate working with people across a variety of situations and to increase understanding and control of the professional work setting. Bennis (1994) made a strong argument for leadership, stating that quality of life depends on the quality of the leaders. He noted three reasons why leaders are important: the character of change in society, the deemphasis on integrity in institutions, and the responsibility for the effectiveness of organizations. Fiedler and Garcia (1987) argued that leadership is one of the most important factors that determine the survival and success of groups and organizations. Effective leadership is important in nursing for those same reasons, specifically because of its impact on the quality of nurses' work lives, being a stabilizing influence during constant change, and for nurses' productivity and quality of care.

Leadership theory often is discussed separately from management theory. Their area of overlap may not be clear or explained. The premise of this textbook is that leadership and management are not identical ideas. They are distinct, and yet they overlap. Both leadership and management will be explored separately in this chapter and in Chapter 2, and their intersection will be developed within each of the chapters in order to better integrate the two concepts with nursing practice.

Nurses need to have a solid foundation of knowledge in leadership and care management. This applies at all levels: nurse care provider, nurse manager, and nurse executive. However, the depth and focus of care management roles and skills may vary by level. For example, the nurse care provider concentrates on the coordination of nursing care to individuals or groups. This may include such activities as access to services, direct care provision, referrals, and family support. In contrast, the nurse manager concentrates on the day-to-day administration of services provided by a group of nurses. The nurse executive's role and function concentrates on long-term administration of an institution or program that delivers nursing services.

If the delivery of nursing services involves the organization and coordination of complex activities in the human services realm, then both leadership and management are important elements. The definitions of these two concepts indicate that they are not identical to each other. Bennis (1994) noted that the leader focuses on people; the manager focuses on systems and structure. Thus while both are processes used to accomplish goals, each focus is different. For example, a nurse may use leadership strategies or management strategies to motivate others. However, the desired outcome of the motivation is likely to be different. There are, however, similarities between leadership and management in an area of overlap. In this area of overlap, the processes and strategies look similar and may be employed for a similar outcome or blended together to accomplish a goal.

DEFINITIONS

There are a variety of definitions of leadership. **Leadership** is defined here as the process of influencing people to accomplish goals. Key concepts related to leadership are influence, communication, group process, goal attainment, and motivation. Hersey and colleagues (2001) defined leadership as a process of influencing the behavior of either an individual or a group, regardless of the reason, in an effort to achieve goals in a given situation. Burns (1978) noted that leadership occurs when human beings with motives and purposes mobilize in competition or conflict with others so as to arouse, engage, and satisfy motives.

All leadership definitions incorporate the two components of an interaction among people and the process of influencing. Thus leadership is a social exchange phenomenon. Leadership is influencing people. In contrast, management involves influencing employees toward the organization's goals and is focused primarily on organizational goals and objectives. Bennis (1994) listed a number of distinctions between leadership and management. He noted that the leader focuses on people, whereas the manager focuses on systems and structures. Another distinction is that a leader innovates,

⚠ LEADING & MANAGING **DEFINED**

Leadership

The process of influencing people to accomplish goals.

Management

The coordination and integration of resources through planning, organizing, coordinating, directing, and controlling to accomplish specific institutional goals and objectives.

Leadership Styles

Different combinations of task and relationship behaviors used to influence others to accomplish goals.

Followership

An interpersonal process of participation.

Empowerment

The act of giving people the authority, responsibility, and freedom to act on what they know.

---

whereas a manager administers. Kotter (2001) noted that managers cope with complexity while leaders cope with change.

Management is defined as the coordination and integration of resources through planning, organizing, coordinating, directing, and controlling to accomplish specific institutional goals and objectives. Hersey and colleagues (2001) defined management as the "process of working with and through individuals and groups and other resources (such as equipment, capital, and technology) to accomplish organizational goals" (p. 9). They identified management as a special kind of leadership that concentrates on the achievement of organizational goals. If this idea were visualized, it would be in concentric circles, not as overlapping separate circles.

Leadership is a broad concept and a process that can be related to any group. Grant (1994) noted that leadership, management, and professionalism have different but related meanings, as follows:

- *Leadership:* Guiding, directing, teaching, and motivating to set goals and for achievement
- *Management:* Resource coordination and integration to accomplish specific goals
- *Professionalism:* An approach to an occupation that distinguishes it from being merely a job, focuses on service as the highest ideal, follows

a code of ethics, and is seen as a lifetime commitment.

A distinction can be made between leadership and management roles. Management relates to managing the resources of an organization. Managers derive power from their position and title (Trott & Windsor, 1999). The idea of management can generate a negative reaction when it is equated with the "command and control" concept of bureaucratic organizations. Old models of management do not fit well with an environment experiencing constant change. Some pressures influencing the role of the manager and demanding new skill sets to facilitate clinical work include the pace of technology out-running clinicians' ability to learn and the phenomenon of managing temporary workers employed by others. It appears that the manager is called away from a unit or service more frequently to address systems issues, leaving less time to plan and focus on unit management. The demands of management work are increasing in amount, scope, complexity, and intensity and thus causing increased role stress (Porter-O'Grady, 2003). However, the principles of management endure and have relevance to managing systems. Porter-O'Grady (1997) noted that process leadership is needed to replace the former role of the manager. He suggested a need for two levels of leadership: one that integrates the system and one that coordinates the service. Leader/managers will need to provide overwhelming evidence that they facilitate the development of effective support systems and generate efficiencies directed to improving processes.

Leadership is considered key to the success of health care organizations. Nurses are pressed to demonstrate the outcomes of their care and provide evidence of the effectiveness of their service delivery. The link between leadership style and staff satisfaction highlights the importance of leadership in times of chaos. A nurse leader needs to be dynamic, show interpersonal skills, and be a visionary for the organization and the profession. The ability to inspire and motivate followers to carry out the vision contributes to organizational survival (Trott & Windsor, 1999). Leaders need to be agents of change, work with teams of people, develop relationships for productivity, and pioneer new cultures (Drenkard, 1997).

A key point to remember about leadership and management is that these two concepts are not exactly the same thing, although they are related, can be integrated, and may be the same at an area of overlap. Related leadership terms are *leadership styles, followership,* and *empowerment*. **Leadership styles** are defined as different combinations of task and relationship behaviors used to influence others to accomplish goals. **Followership** is defined as an interpersonal process of participation. **Empowerment** means giving people the authority, responsibility, and freedom to act on what they know; it involves instilling in people belief and confidence in their own ability to achieve and succeed (Kramer & Schmalenberg, 1990).

BACKGROUND

Leadership can be best understood as a process. Much attention has been focused on leadership as an organizational process. For example, transformational leadership is one aspect of organizational change that is influenced by the context or environment (Pawar & Eastman, 1997). Leadership also can be viewed as being exercised on three different levels: individual, group, and

organizational. At the individual level, leaders mentor, coach, and motivate. At the group level, leaders build teams and resolve conflicts. At the organizational level, leaders build a culture (Mintzberg, 1998). In all cases there appear to be five interwoven elements fundamental to understanding what occurs in the leadership process.

LEADERSHIP: FIVE INTERWOVEN ASPECTS

Hersey and colleagues (2001) noted that the leadership process is a function of the leader, the followers, and other situational variables. The leadership process includes five interwoven aspects: (1) the leader, (2) the follower, (3) the situation, (4) the communication process, and (5) the goals (Kison, 1989). Figure 1.1 shows how these components relate to one another. All five elements interact within any given leadership moment.

Process Part 1: The Leader

The values, skills, and style of leaders are important. Their internalized pattern of basic behaviors influences actions and the ability to lead. Leaders' perceptions of themselves and their roles also make a difference in the leadership situation.

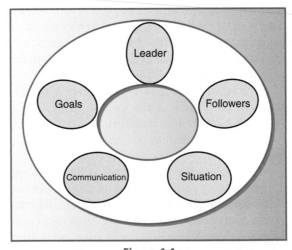

Figure 1.1
Components of a leadership moment.

Their expectations have an impact on their followers. Internal forces in leaders that impinge on leadership style are values, confidence in employees, leadership inclinations, and sense of security in uncertainty (Tannenbaum & Schmidt, 1973). Interpersonal and emotional intelligence skills also contribute to the effective leadership of knowledge workers (Goleman, 1997, 2000; Porter-O'Grady, 2003).

Process Part 2: The Follower

Followership is the flip side of leadership. Followers are vital because they accept or reject the leader and determine the leader's personal power (Hersey et al., 2001). If the leader needs self-awareness, then the followers also must know themselves in reference to their expectations. Situations in which the group is not accustomed to working together or does not hold shared expectations frequently lead to conflict. Groups have personalities that include a discernible level of trust. The leader must assess the readiness level of the group. The leadership situation in a group that is knowledgeable and experienced in solving problems is very different from the leadership situation in a group that is not experienced at the task or at working together.

Process Part 3: The Situation

The specific circumstances surrounding any given leadership situation will vary. Elements such as work demands, control systems, amount of task structure, degree of interaction, amount of time available for decision making, and external environment shape the differences among situations (Hersey et al., 2001). Organizational culture and ethos also are important factors in the situation. For example, in one setting the culture may resemble one big happy family, in which every occasion includes a morale-boosting event. The cultural aspects of that leadership situation are different from those of an organization in which everyone marches to a fast tempo and people seem very busy. Environmental or cultural differences also cause the leadership situation to vary. The personality styles of both superiors and subordinates have an influence on the situation, the work demands, and the amount of time and resources available.

Process Part 4: Communication

Communication processes vary among groups as to the patterns and channels used and in regard to how open or closed the communication flow is. Communicating is basic to the process of influencing. Through communication the leader's vision and message are received by the followers. After choosing a channel, the sender transmits a message. However, the message is filtered through the receiver's perception. Communication is transmitted through both verbal and nonverbal modes. Organizations include a variety of communication structures and flows. These may be downward, upward, horizontal, grapevines, or communication networks. Communication may be formal or informal (Hersey et al., 2001). Certain acts performed by leaders have positive effects and make people feel more respected; listening and informal chatting are prime examples (Alvesson & Sveningsson, 2003).

Process Part 5: Goals

Organizations have goals, and individuals working in organizations also have goals. These goals may or may not be congruent. For example, the goal of the organization may be to decrease costs. In contrast, the goal of the individual nurse may be to spend time counseling and teaching clients because that is what is seen by the nurse as the most important activity. Goals may thus be in conflict, in which case there is tension and a need for leadership.

Clearly, leadership is a complex and multidimensional process. Nurses need to be aware of the interacting elements in any leadership situation. Critical thinking can be applied to diagnosing and analyzing the five elements, adapting to the situation, and communicating for effectiveness. For example, if a nurse works in a situation in which there is a high level of frustration, it may be time to step back and analyze the five interwoven elements. Doing so sets the stage for better decision making about change strategies.

LEADERSHIP THEORIES

The three basic approaches recognized in leadership theory can be grouped as trait, attitudinal, and situational (Hersey et al., 2001). The trait approach focuses on identifying specific characteristics of leaders. The attitudinal approach measures attitudes toward leader behavior. The situational approach focuses on observed behaviors of leaders and how leadership styles can be matched to situations. Research and theory about leadership has a long history. Leadership theories have evolved away from an early focus on the traits or characteristics of the leader as a person because it was found that it is not possible to predict leadership from clusters of traits. However, several authors have developed lists of traits common to good leaders (Bass, 1982; Bennis & Nanus, 1985; Yukl, 1981), and interest still remains in the characteristics to look for in good leaders. Further background on the history of leadership research can be found online (e.g., *www.sedl.org/change/leadership/history.html*).

CHARACTERISTICS OF LEADERSHIP: TRAIT THEORIES

In the trait approach, theorists have sought to understand leadership by examining the characteristics of leaders. The trait approach has generated multiple lists of traits proposed to be essential to leadership. Bennis (1994) identified a recipe for leadership that contained six ingredients: a guiding vision, passion, integrity (including self-knowledge, candor, and maturity), trust, curiosity, and daring. Leaders arise in a context, and they are said to be "made," not "born." They appear to learn leadership skills in stages (Bennis, 2004). Thus leadership skills can be both taught and learned. It is important for nurses to recognize that they can learn, practice, and improve their personal leadership competencies.

Drucker (1996) noted that effective leaders know the following four things:

1. The only definition of a leader is someone who has followers.

2. Popularity is not leadership; results are.
3. Leaders are visible and set examples.
4. Leadership is not rank but responsibility.

Leaders ask questions such as these: What needs to be done? What can I do to make a difference? What are the goals? What constitutes performance and results? Thus leaders do not need to know all the answers, but they do need to ask the right questions (Heifetz & Laurie, 1997).

Leaders are active, not passive. The risk-taking element of leadership involves taking action. Leaders engage their environment with behaviors of doing, influencing, and moving. These are action terms. Pagonis (1992) noted that to lead successfully a leader must demonstrate two active, essential, and interrelated traits: expertise and empathy. Leaders are those who talk about adventures into new territory and take the risks inherent in innovation (Kouzes & Posner, 1987). Leadership means giving guidance and using a focused vision.

A leader may see the need to chart a course that is new or unknown, unpopular, or risky because it challenges vested interests who have much to lose. In a way, nursing's struggle for greater economic parity in health care is courageous and risky. Clancy (2003) noted that leaders need to "consistently find the courage to hold true to their beliefs and convictions" (p. 128). Both ethical fitness and moral courage form the backbone of making necessary and hard—but right and unpopular—decisions. Cost containment, patient's rights, safe staffing, stress and anger, and ethical dilemmas all challenge the leader to identify right from wrong and act from their sense of conviction. The leadership courage continuum runs from "good coward" (cannot muster courage to make tough choices) to "reckless courage" (shoot from the hip). Leaders need to be willing to make tough choices plus overcome the fear associated with them (Clancy, 2003).

Research by Bennis and Thomas (2002) indicated that extraordinary leaders possess skills required to overcome adversity and emerge stronger and more committed. They suggest that "one of the most reliable indicators and predictors of true leadership is an individual's ability to find meaning in negative events and to learn from even the most trying circumstances" (2002, p. 39). "Crucible" experiences shape leaders. These are trials, tests, and transformative experiences that force leaders to questions themselves and what matters and to hone their judgment. Consequently, leaders come to a new or altered sense of identity. "Crucible" experiences can occur from positive or negative triggers, but leaders see them as opportunities for reinvention. Great leaders possess the following four essential skills:

1. The ability to engage others in shared meaning
2. A distinctive and compelling vocal tone
3. A sense of integrity

4. A combination of hardiness and ability to grasp context, called "adaptive capacity"

Starting with whatever natural talent a nurse possesses, essential leadership skills can be practiced over time for greater effectiveness.

Effective leadership uses empowerment. Empowering in nursing leadership means transferring power over clinical practice decisions to staff nurses and enabling them to do what they do best. This process is similar to nurses empowering clients. Leadership also is forward thinking or visionary. A leader needs to articulate a vision as a way to motivate people. Leadership involves

---

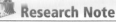 **Research Note**

Source: Upenieks, V. (2003). Nurse leaders' perceptions of what compromises successful leadership in today's acute inpatient environment. *Nursing Administration Quarterly, 27*(2), 140-152.

Purpose

The purpose of this research was to explore nurse leaders' perceptions of the value of their roles and their beliefs about how power and gender interface with leadership success. Data were gathered via interviews with 16 nurse leaders: 7 from magnet institutions and 9 from nonmagnet designated hospitals. Qualitative content analysis techniques were used. The theoretical framework guiding the study was Kanter's Structural Theory of Organizational Behavior.

Discussion

The results showed that 83% of the nurse leaders validated that access to power, opportunity, information, and resources created an empowered environment and fostered leadership success and aided job satisfaction of nurses. In addition, four other factors contributed to leadership success and role worth: supportive organizational culture committed to the professional expertise of nurses, leadership qualities of the nurse leader, teamwork among physicians and other providers, and compensation reflecting the value of nursing. Leadership traits deemed essential were being visible, accessible, influential, visionary, credible, honest, articulate, knowledgeable, and supportive of advancement and educational opportunities.

Application to Practice

Leadership, particularly when coupled with organizational position, is an opportunity for nurses to accomplish group goals. Certain organizational structural characteristics predispose nurse leadership success. Nurse leaders need to seek to develop, acquire, or elicit access to power, opportunity, information, and resources. Once this foundation is laid, nurse leaders need to mobilize their personal leadership skills and abilities, such as visibility, responsiveness, passion, and business astuteness to create and nurture a supportive organizational culture, collaborative interdisciplinary teamwork, and a meaningful compensation structure for nurses. To do so should affect nurse satisfaction and retention. Magnet research studies support the transformational leadership style as the most often reported type used in magnet hospitals and a work environment that fosters professional nursing practice as an essential element for increasing nurse job satisfaction. Strategic leadership applications make a difference.

elements of vigor and vision and can be understood as a dynamic combination of competence, willingness to take responsibility, and strength of character to do what is right because it is the right thing to do.

Characteristics such as knowledge, motivating people to work harder, trust, communication, enthusiasm, vision, courage, being able to see the big picture, and the ability to take risks are associated with important leadership qualities in research findings. For example, Bennis and Nanus (1985) studied 90 chief executives from 1978 to 1983 and found that there were two key leadership traits. One is a guiding set of concepts, and the other is the ability to communicate a vision. Kouzes and Posner (1987) defined the following five behaviors that correlated with leadership excellence:

1. *Challenging the process:* Leaders go beyond the status quo to search for opportunities, experiment, and take risks to achieve lofty goals.
2. *Inspiring shared vision:* Leaders envision the future and enlist others in sharing the dream.
3. *Enabling others to act:* Leaders foster collaboration and develop and strengthen others so that the whole team performs well.
4. *Modeling the way:* Leaders set an example and structure events so that incremental progress is celebrated as small wins.
5. *Encouraging the heart:* Leaders appreciate and recognize individual contributions and formally celebrate accomplishments.

These five practices identified by Kouzes and Posner can be seen as the way leaders get extraordinary things done through people in an organization. The practices and qualities of leadership help nurses to enrich their own style and contribute to a more productive workplace. The following list identifies qualities that people say they want to see in their leaders (Curtin, 1989):

- *Visibility:* People want to see their leaders and have frequent, casual contacts with them.
- *Flexibility:* People learn from leaders who can "roll with the punches," tolerate ambiguity, and have a sense of personal empowerment.
- *Authority:* This is the right to make decisions, give direction, and accept/administer criticism. Authority is recognition granted from below.

- *Assistance:* This occurs by serving those who serve, create, or produce and by creating the environment and resources necessary to do the job.
- *Feedback:* People want their leaders to listen to them and give them quality feedback as they go about their particular work.

The following eight competencies of leaders are synthesized from the literature by Murphy and DeBack (1991):

1. Managing the dream
2. Mastery of change
3. Organizational design
4. Anticipatory learning
5. Taking the initiative
6. Mastery of interdependence
7. Holding high standards of integrity
8. Exercising broad-perspective decision making

One research-based nursing model (Mathena, 2002) identified the following six core behaviors critical for nursing leadership success:

1. Visioning
2. Interdisciplinary team building
3. Workload complexity analysis
4. Work process analysis
5. Stakeholder analysis
6. Interactive planning

Although the lists of leadership characteristics and competencies vary somewhat, the functions of visioning, setting the direction, inspiration, motivation, and enabling systems and followers are at the core of leadership activity.

Leadership is founded on trust: "Trust is the emotional glue that binds leaders and employees together and is a measure of the legitimacy of leadership" (Malloch, 2002, p. 14). Organizations that focus on sustaining a healing culture rebuild organizational trust by focusing on building trust in relationships with employees. Behaviors that build trust include sharing relevant information, reducing controls, and meeting expectations. Trust-destroying behaviors including being insensitive to beliefs and values, avoiding discussion of sensitive issues, and encouraging competition via winners and losers. Nurses can be aware of the crucial nature of trust in the leadership and management relationship. Trust goes both ways and must be nurtured. Nurses can start by examining their own behaviors and then taking deliberative actions to strengthen trust in the environment.

Followers expect that leaders will provide a sense of vision and a sense of direction with standards for achieving the group's goals. Leaders can create an environment that is positively charged for productivity or allow the followers to languish without direction or mission. It is possible that leaders can create a negative climate that becomes destructive to the group. If the leader plays a major role in creating a group's culture and ethos, then closing down communication, breeding distrust and competition, and neglecting positive motivation can sow the seeds of group disintegration. Thus the characteristics possessed and used by the leader can make a crucial difference in the functioning and effectiveness of any group.

Attitudinal Leadership Theories

As leadership theories evolved, leadership came to be viewed as a dynamic process and an interaction among the leader, the followers, and the situation. Leadership theory began to highlight the concept of leadership styles. Leadership styles will be discussed next, followed by a discussion of attitudinal leadership theories.

LEADERSHIP STYLES

Leadership styles are defined as different combinations of task and relationship behaviors used to influence others to accomplish goals. They are sets or clusters of behaviors used in the process of effecting leadership. Leaders need to be concerned about both tasks to be accomplished and human relationships in groups and organizations. Hersey and colleagues (2001) said that leadership styles are the consistent behavior patterns exhibited in influencing the activities of others by working with and through them, as perceived by those others. There are different styles that evoke variable responses in different situations. The way people influence others through actions taken and the perspectives of other people is related to leadership

efforts and constitutes leadership style. The two major leadership terms are *task behavior* and *relationship behavior;* thus a leader's leadership style is some combination of task and relationship behavior. Hersey and colleagues (2001) defined these terms as follows:

- *Task behavior:* The extent to which leaders organize and define roles, explain activities, determine when, where, and how tasks are to be accomplished, and endeavor to get work accomplished
- *Relationship behavior:* The extent to which leaders maintain personal relationships by opening communication and providing psychoemotional support and facilitating behaviors

Tannenbaum and Schmidt (1973) suggested that a leader might select one of seven behavior styles arrayed along a continuum. The continuum ranges from democratic to authoritarian (or subordinate-centered to leader-centered). Their work suggested that there is a variety of leadership styles (Figure 1.2). Essentially, however, there are three distinct leadership styles or points along the continuum: authoritarian, democratic, or laissez-faire (Tannenbaum & Schmidt, 1958, 1973; White & Lippitt, 1968), although some individuals are able to integrate all three styles and flexibly match to the situation at hand.

Authoritarian

This style is reflected in primarily directive behaviors. Techniques and activity procedures are determined by the leader and dictated to the followers. Decisions of policy are made solely by the leader. Leaders tell the followers what to do and how to do it. This style emphasizes a concern for task. Authoritarian leaders are characterized by giving orders. Their style can create hostility and dependency among followers. It may also stifle creativity and innovation. On the other hand, this style can be very efficient, especially in a crisis.

Democratic

This approach implies a relationship and person orientation. Policies are a matter of group discussion and decision. The leader encourages and

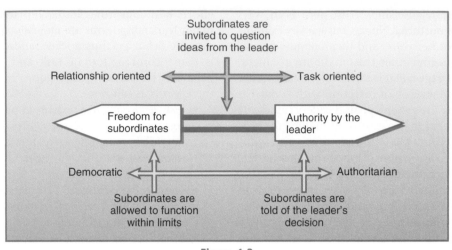

Figure 1.2
Continuum of leader behavior.

assists discussion and group decision making. Human relations and teamwork are the focus. The leader shares responsibility with the followers by involving them in decision making. The current nursing literature emphasizes how important teamwork is in nursing. For example, continuous quality improvement implies interdisciplinary teamwork. The democratic style moves slower and is thought to take longer than an authoritarian style. Group consensus needs to be considered. Furthermore, the needs of disenfranchised minority groups must be balanced. Intergroup cohesion is needed with this style. The challenge of the democratic style is to get people with different professional backgrounds, personal biases, and psychological needs together to focus on what the problem is and how can it be fixed.

Laissez-Faire

This style promotes complete freedom for group or individual decisions. There is a minimum of leader participation. This style, as defined, may seem apathetic to some. Because the style is based on noninterference, there may never be a clear decision formulated. The laissez-faire style is a decision, conscious or otherwise, to avoid interference and let events take their own course.

The leader is either permissive to foster freedom or is inept at guiding a group. Despite its potential drawbacks, this style has advantages with groups of independent care providers or professionals working together.

One style is not necessarily better than another. Each has advantages and disadvantages. The styles should vary according to the appropriateness of the situation with reference to an evaluation of effectiveness. Flexibility is important to effectiveness. For example, one nurse prefers to operate in a democratic style. Suddenly, however, a code situation occurs. The nurse must rapidly switch from a democratic to an authoritarian style. Some democratic leaders cannot vary their style sufficiently to handle crisis situations. On the other hand, in a staff meeting, an authoritarian leader may be ineffective with a group of professionals and would need to be flexible enough to switch to a democratic or laissez-faire style, depending on the circumstances. The basic need is for leader self-awareness and to know the group's ability and willingness levels before examining the situational elements and choosing a leadership style.

In summary, to be effective, leadership styles need to match the situation. Styles of leadership range from authoritarian to permissive to democratic and from transactional to transformational. The individual nurse's task is to determine in which environments he or she functions best and is most comfortable with or where he or she most likely will succeed. This facilitates placement for success and a better match between leader and follower.

ATTITUDINAL THEORIES

Hersey and colleagues (2001) identified a second approach to leadership research that focused on the measurement of attitudes or predispositions toward leader behavior. Occurring mainly between 1945 and the mid-1960s, the attitudinal approaches began with the Ohio State Leadership Studies and included the Michigan Leadership Studies, Group Dynamics Studies, Likert's Management Systems, and Blake and McCanse's Leadership Grid.

Leader behavior was described as having two separate dimensions, as follows:

1. Initiating structure and consideration in the Ohio State Leadership Studies
2. Employee-orientation and production-orientation in the Michigan Leadership Studies

These dimensions are similar to the authoritarian (or task) and democratic (or relationship) ideas of the leader behavior continuum. The Group Dynamics Studies highlighted goal achievement (similar to task) and group maintenance (similar to relationship) elements of leadership behavior (Cartwright & Zander, 1960). Likert (1961) studied high-performance managers to develop an understanding of a general pattern of management. He found that close supervision was less associated with high productivity. High productivity was associated with clear objectives and transmitting an idea about what is to be accomplished to the subordinates, then giving them the freedom to do the job. He described a continuum of management styles, called System 1 through System 4, from no trust in subordinates through condescending confidence, substantial but not complete confidence, to complete trust and confidence in subordinates. This parallels the task-to-relationship continuum.

Blake and Mouton (1964) used task and relationship concepts in their grid, which was later modified by Blake and McCanse (1991). The following five types of leadership or management styles, based on concern for production (task) and concern for people (relationship), emerged:

1. *Impoverished:* This style uses minimal effort to get the work done.
2. *Country club:* This approach emphasizes attention to the needs of people to effect satisfying relationships.
3. *Authority-obedience:* This style strives for efficiency in operations.
4. *Organizational man:* This approach works on balancing the necessity to accomplish the task with maintaining morale.
5. *Team:* This style promotes work accomplishment from committed people and interdependence through a common stake, leading to trust and respect.

Hersey and colleagues (2001) noted that Blake and Mouton's (1964) conceptualization tended to be an attitudinal model that measured the values and feelings of managers, whereas the Ohio State model included both attitudes and behaviors and focused on leadership. Both the leadership style (task versus relationship) and the attitude of the leader about leadership behaviors are important. However, they still did not fully capture the leadership experience because the environment was not factored in.

SITUATIONAL THEORIES

A third phase of leadership theories grew out of contingency theories postulating that organizational behavior is contingent on the situation or environment. Situational leadership theories focus on the frequency of observed behaviors to make predictions. What is needed by the leader is diagnostic ability. The leader observes abilities and motives in the followers. With sensitivity, cues in the environment can be identified and fed into choices made regarding leadership style. What is key to understand is that people make choices. One choice a leader has is to alter his or her own behavior and the leadership style used. A leader would choose to alter his or her behavior and style if the needs and motives of the followers varied. Personal flexibility and leadership skills are needed to vary one's style when the followers' needs and motives are different. The ability to diagnose, choose, and alter behavior to implement a leadership style best matched to the situation is a critical skill needed for leadership for effectiveness. Thus no one leadership style is optimal in all situations. The nature of the situation needs to be considered. Styles can be chosen to match the situation (Hersey et al., 2001).

Fiedler's Contingency Theory

As situations become more complex, leadership becomes more difficult. Fiedler (1967) developed a Leadership Contingency Model. He classified group situational variables of leader-member relations, task structure, and position power into eight possible combinations, ranging from high to low on the three major variables. *Leader-member relations* refers to the type and quality of the leader's personal relationships with followers. *Task structure* means how structured the group's assigned task is. *Position power* refers to that power conferred on the leader by the organization as an integral component of the assigned job. Fiedler examined the favorableness of the situation from the perspective of the leader's influence over the group. The most favorable situation occurs with good leader-member relations, high task structure, and high position power. The least favorable situation occurs when the leader is disliked, has an unstructured task, and has little position power. With Fiedler's model, group situations can be analyzed to determine the most effective leadership style.

Fiedler (1967) examined which style (task-oriented versus relationship-oriented) would be most effective for each of eight situations. A key general principle is that the need for task-oriented leaders occurs when the situation is either highly favorable or very unfavorable. A task-oriented style is needed for the situations on the extremes, whereas a relationship-oriented style is needed when the situation is moderately favorable.

For example, a staff nurse goes into a nursing unit meeting not wanting any extra assignments but hoping that some of the ongoing problems will be solved. If the nurse has a reasonably good relationship with the leader, the leader should use a high-relationship style with the nurse. The leader should use selling, convincing, encouraging, and motivating strategies. The leader should make the nurse feel good about his or her ability to accomplish a task, to provide something of quality, and to work with other people. If, however, the staff nurse's mind is closed about any changes, or if passive-aggressive or subversive actions occur, then the leader needs be more directive. A possible reaction might be to give the nurse an assigned task. On the extremes of highly favorable or highly unfavorable situations, leaders need to use task-oriented behavior to get the work moving. In the middle of the continuum, a high-relationship style is needed.

In situational leadership theory, leadership in groups is never a static circumstance. The situation is subject to change. In a very difficult situation, relationships may be the leader's preferred emphasis. However, if interpersonal relationships are not an immediate problem or if the group is on the verge of collapse, then what is needed is strong authoritative direction to get the group moving and accomplishing. For this situation the task-oriented leader is a more effective match between leader and job. However, groups do not remain static; they move back and forth through stages. When the problem no longer is the need to just get the group moving but includes solving numerous interpersonal conflicts, a relationship-oriented leader is better matched to the situation. Eventually, as the situation progresses, a relationship-oriented leader can become less effective. This occurs because once the group has less conflict, individuals may begin to coast, and positive motivation may be lost as individuals become apathetic. Once again, a task-oriented style is called for—challenging individuals with the continuing motivation that they need to continue to produce. Because of the factor of constant change, maintaining good leadership is complicated for any group. One way to foster effective leadership is to evaluate leaders according to Fiedler's contingency model

(1967) and then use this information to increase leaders' awareness of their natural style tendency: relationship-oriented or task-oriented. Fiedler's measure for leadership style is the Least Preferred Coworker (LPC) scale (Fiedler & Chemers, 1984). The LPC is an 18-item semantic differential scale that is the personality measure of Fiedler's contingency model (Fiedler & Garcia, 1987).

Favorable or unfavorable situations are determined in part by the receptivity of the followers, but they are also determined by whether the larger environment is positive or negative. Here is an example of an unfavorable situation in nursing: A nurse's job is to lead and manage a hospital's critical care area, which has serious morale problems. The nurse has a master's degree but soon discovers that a majority of the followers have a diploma from the School of Nursing, which was run by that hospital for many years but is now defunct. In this example, both educational and experiential backgrounds are likely to differ, and there may be clashes between the leader and the followers. The task is to change the environment, but the nurse discovers that this work group has maintained its traditions over a long period. This is an unfavorable situation and a leadership challenge. Fiedler's theory (1967) suggested that the best leadership style under unfavorable circumstances is task-oriented.

Hersey and Blanchard's Tri-Dimensional Leader Effectiveness Model

Hersey and colleagues (2001) described the Tri-Dimensional Leader Effectiveness Model first developed by Hersey and Blanchard. First, a two-dimensional model was constructed, in which task behavior and relationship behavior were displayed on a grid from high to low and were divided into four quadrants: (1) high task, low relationship; (2) high task, high relationship; (3) high relationship, low task; and (4) low task, low relationship (Figure 1.3). These quadrants represent four basic leadership styles: telling, selling, participating, and delegating. As applied to the continuum of authoritarian versus democratic styles, telling would be authoritarian and delegating would be democratic. In the middle are the

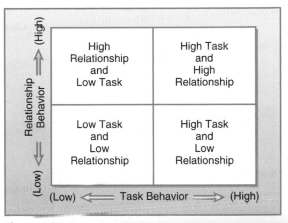

Figure 1.3
Hersey-Blanchard two-dimensional model of leadership. (From Hersey, P., Blanchard, K.H., & Johnson, D.E. [2001]. *Management of organizational behavior: Leading human resources* [8th ed.; p. 118]. Upper Saddle River, NJ: Prentice-Hall, with permission from the Center for Leadership Studies.)

two styles that draw from both—the selling and the participating leadership styles. Selling is a little more authoritarian than participating, and participating is a little more democratic than authoritarian, but both are mixed styles.

To choose an appropriate style, the leader needs to be knowledgeable about the readiness of the followers. This leads to the third dimension of effectiveness (Figure 1.4). *Effectiveness* is defined as how appropriately a given leader's style interrelates with a given situation. The third dimension is the environment in which a leader operates and that interacts with the leader's style.

Overlaid on the basic grid is a continuum of readiness ranging from low to high. Readiness has two aspects: ability and willingness. Job *ability* is predicated on the amount of past job experience, job knowledge, problem-solving ability, ability to take responsibility, and ability to meet deadlines. This forms a composite of the ability to do the job. The other part of readiness is psychological *willingness*. Psychological willingness means being willing to take responsibility and have a positive attitude toward accepting the obligation to complete a task. Psychological readiness is manifested by willingness

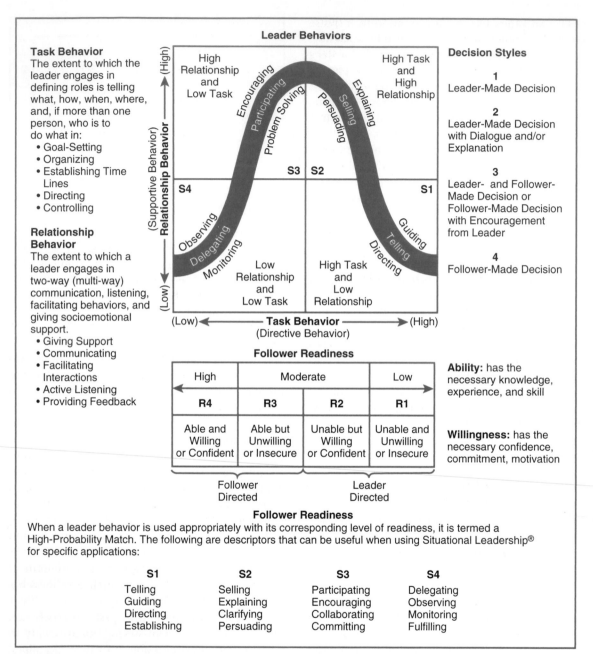

Task Behavior
The extent to which the leader engages in defining roles is telling what, how, when, where, and, if more than one person, who is to do what in:
- Goal-Setting
- Organizing
- Establishing Time Lines
- Directing
- Controlling

Relationship Behavior
The extent to which a leader engages in two-way (multi-way) communication, listening, facilitating behaviors, and giving socioemotional support.
- Giving Support
- Communicating
- Facilitating Interactions
- Active Listening
- Providing Feedback

Leader Behaviors

High Relationship and Low Task

High Task and High Relationship

S3 S2

S4   S1

Low Relationship and Low Task

High Task and Low Relationship

(Low) ← **Task Behavior** → (High)
(Directive Behavior)

Encouraging Participating Problem Solving

Explaining Selling Persuading

Observing Delegating Monitoring

Guiding Telling Directing

Decision Styles

1
Leader-Made Decision

2
Leader-Made Decision with Dialogue and/or Explanation

3
Leader- and Follower-Made Decision or Follower-Made Decision with Encouragement from Leader

4
Follower-Made Decision

Follower Readiness

	High	Moderate		Low
	R4	**R3**	**R2**	**R1**
	Able and Willing or Confident	Able but Unwilling or Insecure	Unable but Willing or Confident	Unable and Unwilling or Insecure

Follower Directed   Leader Directed

Ability: has the necessary knowledge, experience, and skill

Willingness: has the necessary confidence, commitment, motivation

Follower Readiness
When a leader behavior is used appropriately with its corresponding level of readiness, it is termed a High-Probability Match. The following are descriptors that can be useful when using Situational Leadership® for specific applications:

S1	S2	S3	S4
Telling	Selling	Participating	Delegating
Guiding	Explaining	Encouraging	Observing
Directing	Clarifying	Collaborating	Monitoring
Establishing	Persuading	Committing	Fulfilling

Figure 1.4
Expanded Situational Leadership® Model. (Modified from Hersey, P. [1985]. *Situational selling* [p. 35]. Escondido, CA: Center for Leadership Studies. Copyright 1998 by Center for Leadership Studies.)

to take some risk and by accepting the job requirements. It includes achievement motivation, wanting to do well, persistence, a work attitude, and a sense of independence. These factors create a willingness to take on and complete a job. Hersey and colleagues (2001) combined ability and willingness into four levels of readiness. Level 1 is unable and unwilling or insecure. Level 2 is unable but willing or confident. Level 3 is able but unwilling or insecure. Level 4 is able and willing or confident. These readiness levels can be matched with the corresponding leadership styles of level 1 with telling, level 2 with selling, level 3 with participating, and level 4 with delegating. Thus readiness assessment can help predict appropriate leadership style selection.

Hersey and colleagues (2001) emphasized the readiness of followers. Readiness can be applied to a work group. Have the members worked together for a long time in the job, or are they new employees? The culture is more solidified in a work group that has worked together for many years on a particular unit. The leader's leadership style would have to take into account where the followers are in terms of their readiness as a critical factor for determining the style to choose. Using leadership theory, leaders assess themselves, look at the followers' readiness, and assess the situation to determine whether it is favorable or unfavorable. Then a telling, selling, participating, or delegating style is selected.

For example, telling is an appropriate leadership style to use with followers who are at the novice level, as well as in other situations in which the followers are not able or willing. For example, a nurse is appointed as chair of a committee. First, the nurse might undertake a leadership analysis to determine whether this group needs high-relationship behaviors. If they do not know each other and the situation is politically charged, the nurse leader needs to help people become comfortable with each other. If the nurse leader is a task-oriented person, a high-relationship person may need to be called on to assist the group process so that it is facilitated and becomes effective.

One currently accepted view of organizational behavior describes leadership as situational or contingent and concerned with what produces effectiveness. Hersey and colleagues (2001) noted that the common themes include the following: the leader needs to be flexible in behavior, able to diagnose the leadership style appropriate to the situation, and able to apply the appropriate style. Thus there is no one best way to influence others or one best style. Situational Leadership® is a synthesis of the interplay among task behavior, relationship behavior, and the readiness of the followers.

Transactional and Transformational Leadership

Following the eras of trait, attitudinal, and situational leadership theories, an interest arose in how leaders produced quantum results. Burns (1978) and Dunham and Klafehn (1990) broadened the concept of leadership styles to include two types of leaders: the transactional leader and the transformational leader.

A *transactional leader* is defined as a leader or manager who functions in a caretaker role and is focused on day-to-day operations. Such leaders survey their followers' needs and set goals for them based on what can be expected from the followers. A transactional leader is focused on the maintenance and management of ongoing and routine work.

A *transformational leader* is defined as a leader who motivates followers to perform to their full potential over time by influencing a change in perceptions and by providing a sense of direction. Transformational leaders use charisma, individualized consideration, and intellectual stimulation to produce greater effort, effectiveness, and satisfaction in followers (Bass & Avolio, 1990). Figure 1.5 distinguishes between transactional and transformational leadership.

The transactional leader is more common. This type of leader approaches followers in an exchange posture, with the purpose of exchanging one thing for another, such as a politician who promises jobs for votes. Burns (1978) said that transactional leadership occurs when the leader takes the initiative in contacting others for the exchange of valued things. Therefore transactional leadership is comparable to a bargain or contract for mutual benefits that

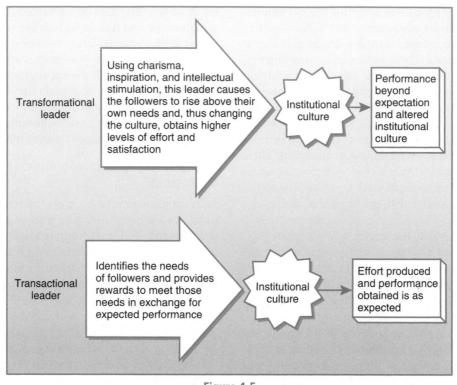

Figure 1.5
Transactional and transformational leadership.

aids the individual differences of both the leader and the follower. Key characteristics are contingent rewards and management-by-exception. Expected effort and expected performance are the outcomes. The transactional leader works within the existing organizational culture and is an essential component of effective leadership (Bass & Avolio, 1990). In nursing an example would be the exchange of a salary for the services of a nurse to provide care (Barker, 1991). Another example occurs when a leader offers release time to entice staff members to do quality monitoring or committee work. Continuous or incremental change, the first order of change, can be handled well at the transactional level.

Transformational leadership occurs when persons engage with others so that leaders and followers raise each other to higher levels of motivation and ethical decision making (Burns, 1978).

Instead of emphasizing differences between the leader and the followers, transformational leadership focuses on collective purpose and mutual growth and development. Transformational leadership augments transactional leadership by being committed, having a vision, and empowering others to heighten motivation in a way that attains extra effort beyond performance expectations. Transformational leadership is used for higher-order change and to change the organization's culture. Circumstances of growth, change, and crisis call forth transformational leaders (Bass & Avolio, 1990). In nursing an example would be "magnet hospitals," where the nursing organizations facilitate the best effort in their staff. Based on the original work by McClure and colleagues (1983), the American Nurses Credentialing Center now has a magnet recognition program. The affiliated website has a helpful checklist for self-assessment prior to beginning an application *(www.nursingworld. org/ancc/magnet.html)*.

Transformational leadership is a concept that is useful and applicable to nursing. The finding that leadership quality is a key element in developing a culture of excellence among magnet hospitals is important for nursing management (Kramer, 1990). Organizations with a transformational leader would exhibit characteristics such as pride and satisfaction in the work, enthusiasm, team spirit, a sense of accomplishment, and satisfaction (Barker, 1990). Bennis and Nanus (1985) identified the following four activities for transformational leadership:

1. Creating a vision
2. Building a social architecture that provides meaning for employees
3. Sustaining organizational trust
4. Recognizing the importance of building self-esteem

Three factors underlie effectiveness as a transformational leader: individual consideration, charisma, and intellectual stimulation (Bass et al., 1987; McDaniel & Wolf, 1992). In one comparative study, nurse executives' transformational scores were found to be higher than those of general managers (Bass, 1985; Dunham & Klafehn, 1990). Other research has been done to test transformational leadership theory in nursing (McDaniel & Wolf, 1992). Transformational leadership was the type of leadership most often reported in magnet research studies (Upenieks, 2003). Transformational leadership qualities appear to be better suited to the work of professionals. Nurses can experiment with transformational leadership and work to set up structures to facilitate this in practice.

CONTEMPORARY LEADERSHIP RESEARCH

Society has moved into the information age, and there has been a metamorphosis in organizations as they transform into knowledge or learning organizations. Nurses are knowledge workers who use expertise and specialized knowledge in the care of patients. They need matching organizations that will value, nurture, and foster the acquisition of the data, information, and knowledge needed for effectiveness. Today's health care environments demand that front-line workers such as nurses have and maintain the expertise and the information necessary to take action to solve problems (Drucker, 1994). In this milieu, leadership is interactional, relational, and needed at all levels. Contemporary leadership theories emphasize these characteristics (Helgesen, 1995a, 1995b; Wheatley, 1992).

Arising in conjunction with the application of complexity theory and chaos theory (see Chapters 2 and 7 for more background and application of these theories), the new view of leadership was described by Wheatley (1992) as being simpler, less stressful and more appropriate to complex organizations in the midst of chaos. Her view of leadership emphasized the importance of connectedness and relationships within self-organizing systems. Nursing has a natural niche within interactional and relationship leadership theories. Optimal health care delivery is truly interdisciplinary and holistic. When connections and relationships are strong, patients benefit.

New definitions of leadership describe leadership as the result of a relationship between leaders and followers where a distinct set of competencies is used to allow the relationship to achieve shared goals (Wilson & Porter-O'Grady, 1999). This is complex and requires nurses to have creativity and flexibility. Old ways of leading and managing are insufficient to present circumstances. Thus it is proposed that quantum leadership is needed to produce results in today's health care environment. Quantum leadership is about discovering: an ongoing process of exploration, curiosity, and asking questions (McCauley, 2004). The elements of quantum leadership are discovering, authenticity, passion, creating, relationship, inquiry, and fiscal astuteness. Driven by organizational stress and the feeling that there is a need for something more and different in work life, quantum leadership is one type of leadership strategy that helps nurses focus on the future, stretch and break boundaries, and encourage breakthrough thinking in order to solve problems in a complex care environment.

Another popular new leadership concept is called servant leadership. Greenleaf (2002) used the term to describe leaders who choose first to serve others and then to be a leader, as opposed to those who are leaders first (often because of a power drive or need to acquire material possessions) and later choose to serve. Servant-leaders put others first. They choose to make sure that other people's highest-priority needs are being served in a way that promotes personal growth and help others to become freer and more autonomous. When applied to health care, servant leadership is an attractive alternative to the traditional bureaucratic environment experienced by nurses. A new model is needed that enhances the personal growth of nurses, improves the quality of care, values teamwork, and promotes personal involvement and caring behavior. The servant leadership model draws attention to the necessity for leaders to be attentive to the needs of others.

Leadership styles appear to have a gender component. The feminist perspective on leadership was presented by Helgeson (1995a, 1995b). She identified female leadership as a weblike structure—dynamic and continuously expanding and contracting. It is characterized by a concern for family, community, and culture. The inclination is for a democratic power style, and the emphasis is on the importance of establishing relationships, maintaining connections with others, and deriving strength from empowering others. By contrast, leadership approaches taken by men tend to be influenced by the military and participating in team sports. Men tend to spend their time on meetings and tasks requiring immediate attention, focusing on completion of tasks and achievement of goals. Women tend to focus on process, men on achievement and closure. Women tend to be more flexible and value cooperation, connectedness, and relationships. The value of exploring the feminist perspective on leadership is that it provides food for thought as health care organizations, and the nurses working in them, struggle with not wanting to let go of the familiar hierarchy management style yet needing to reconfigure to the circular or web structure in order to be effective.

In the business world, leadership is important for building and maintaining companies that return investment to stockholders. Interesting research was done by Collins (2001) to study the leaders of eleven companies who followed a "good-to-great" growth pattern of cumulative stock returns. He found that the behaviors and competencies of leaders settled into one of five hierarchical levels. Individuals can move among levels, but results in the business world appeared to differ according to the level of leadership exhibited by the leader. The five levels of leadership are as follows:

1. Highly capable individual
2. Contributing team member
3. Competent manager
4. Effective leader
5. Executive

The level 5 leader builds enduring greatness and is characterized as having a paradoxical blend of personal humility and professional will. The level 5 leader first addresses "who" by getting the right people in the right jobs and then addressing the "what" by figuring out the best path to greatness. By contrast, the level 4 leader first addresses the "what" by setting a vision and developing a plan and then addresses the "who." Level 5 leaders also confronted brutal facts without losing faith, transcended the curse of competence, created a culture of discipline, and pioneered the application of carefully selected technology. It is not known whether or how Collins' (2001) work applies to nursing and health care, but the emphasis on people as assets is also important to nursing services.

Leadership research in nursing has revealed the following factors central to successful nursing leadership (Upenieks, 2003):

- Formal and informal power
- Access to information and resources
- Opportunity to grow from new challenges
- Supportive organizational cultures in which nurses are valued for their expertise
- Visibility, responsiveness, a passion for nursing, and business astuteness shown by nurse leaders
- Respectful and collaborative teamwork
- Adequate compensation representing value

▨ Research Note

Source: Vance, C., & Larson, E. (2002). Leadership research in business and health care. *Journal of Nursing Scholarship, 34*(2), 165-171.

Purpose

The purpose of this study was to profile and summarize health care and business literature on leadership and identify leadership outcomes on individuals, groups, and organizations. A computerized literature search from years 1970-1999 was conducted. Articles were screened and categorized based on data-based research or nonresearch, type of participants, research design, primary topic area, and effects or outcomes measured. Only 4.4% ($n = 290$) of 6,628 articles were data-based. Most were anecdotal or theoretical discussions. Data were analyzed using chi-square to examine trends and compare health care with business literature.

Discussion

The concept of leadership receives a lot of attention in the literature. In this study, 4.4% ($n = 290$) of all articles were data-based, 41.4% ($n = 120$) of the 4.4% were purely descriptive of demographic characteristics or personality traits of leaders, and only 5.2% ($n = 15$) included correlations of characteristics or styles with measurable outcomes in recipients or positive changes in organizations. Health care citations were 155 of the 290 total research reports. Of these 155, 36.1% ($n = 56$) included measurement of the effect of leadership on outcomes such as satisfaction, retention, or performance. Studies published after 1990 were significantly more likely to measure effects.

Application to Practice

Leadership is an important variable related to professional nursing practice. Although it has received much attention in the business and health care literature, little actual research can be found. This makes it a challenge to determine the evidence base for practice. Much research is descriptive, and limited research on health care outcomes exists to guide changes in patient care or organizational improvements. In a complex and chaotic organizational environment in health care, leadership research about its declared substantial effects on people and organizational outcomes is urgently needed. This article also displays a listing of the 15 studies from business and health care literature in which changes in outcomes were measured, which is a useful summary of the known evidence base.

Many of the factors crucial to successful nursing leadership are similar to those in the business world. Leadership effectiveness can be examined for guidance for nurses seeking to use and improve their leadership competency.

EFFECTIVE LEADERSHIP

Effective leadership is an integrated blend of leadership principles and characteristics with management principles and techniques. Longest (1998) identified six core management competencies needed to manage an integrated health system: conceptual, technical managerial/clinical, interpersonal/collaborative, political, commercial, and governance. Using this model, Tornabeni (2001) outlined practical leadership techniques for the nurse leader. Table 1.1 displays practical actions for nurses to take to improve leadership skills. Nurses can grow such skills by knowledge and awareness (such as through assessment tools) and then putting knowledge and skills to work through guided exercises and mentored experiences.

Leadership effectiveness is based on the ability to adapt in a complex and chaotic environment. Adaptive problems arise from change and chaos and often are systems problems that affect people, planning, institutional operations or work processes. Adaptive solutions engage followers in confronting the issue and the situation. Effective leadership for

Table 1.1

Tornabeni's Practical Advice	
Longest's Category	Tornabeni's Advice
Conceptual	Have a vision
	Gather information
	Broaden your scope
	Take risks
Technical managerial/ clinical	Devise a step-by-step approach and plan
	Generate buy-in
	Delegate tasks
	Motivate continuously by recruiting competent people; developing them; giving them appropriate tools, authority and resources; holding them accountable; and rewarding "right" behavior
Interpersonal/ collaborative	Build your team
	Look for talent within
	Pick the cream of the crop
	Establish a sense of collegiality
	Help your people cope with change
Political	Understand the politics
	Build an internal network
Commercial	Build an external network
	Exchange ideas and challenges with outside colleagues
Governance	Trust your intuition
	Have a sense of purpose
	Do the hard work (perspiration)
	Have passion

Data from Tornabeni, J. (2001). The competency game: My take on what it really takes to lead. *Nursing Administration Quarterly, 25*(4), 1-13.

adaptive problems includes the following types of behaviors (Heifetz & Laurie, 1997):

- Giving direction to identify the issue, key questions, and appropriate discussion
- Protecting the group by regulating distress
- Maintaining disciplined attention
- Managing conflict
- Shaping norms and group adaptation through learning

Effective leaders have a grasp of themselves, their team, their goals, nursing and health care, and evaluative data. They use their personal style, vision, and energy to focus on goal attainment.

Followership

Pagonis (1992) noted that by definition leaders do not operate in isolation. Instead, leadership involves cooperation and collaboration. The basic nature of leadership is interactive; it is involved with the interpersonal relationships among leaders and followers. Therefore cooperation and collaboration between leader and followers and between followers and leader enhance the group's effectiveness.

Followership is an interpersonal process of participation. It implies an engagement of the follower with the leader, and possibly a group, by which the follower takes guidance and direction from the leader in order to accomplish group goals. The importance of followership is emphasized because leadership requires the presence of followers. The relationship between the leader and the followers defines leadership. The corollary to leadership is followership, or helping to get the job done. A good leader clearly needs good followers (Brakey, 1991). Bennis (1994) noted that there are three things that followers need from leaders: direction, trust, and hope. With these three elements in place, followers are empowered in their participation efforts.

It may be that as nurse leadership becomes recognized as a vital element in meeting future challenges, nurse followership will assume a greater importance in practice. At one level the nurse functions as a leader within the nurse-patient relationship and within the framework of care management. However, within nursing the staff nurse often is viewed as being at the level of a follower in the nursing organizational hierarchy.

There are different degrees of followership engagement. Murphy (1990) reviewed Kelley's (1988) model of five categories of followers and applied them to nursing. "Sheep" are followers who lack initiative, sense of responsibility, and critical thinking. "Yes-people" lack enterprise and yield to the opinions, will, or decisions of others. "Alienated" followers are capable of independence and critical thinking but appear passive because they resist open opposition; the result is frustration and disillusionment. "Survivors" never make waves or take risks; they check which way the wind is blowing. "Effective" followers have initiative and think for themselves. They manage themselves well and are responsible and well balanced. They are competent and committed. Effective followers are an asset to be nurtured, developed, and valued. Effective followers contribute to success in organizations. Nurses can and should examine their own behavior and ask themselves, In this situation, what kind of follower am I?

Guidera and Gilmore (1988) stated that the enlightened follower incorporates the cohesiveness of collective group thought without being afraid to be candid or to criticize objectively. Self-awareness is an important aspect of both leadership and followership. This means that nurses can assess themselves to better understand their own style and leadership characteristics. Self-assessment tools are available to assist nurses in awareness of leadership and followership behaviors. One example is the LEAD instruments developed by Hersey and colleagues (2001). Leadership self-assessment instruments can be found online (e.g., *www.nwlink.com/~donclark/leader/survlead.html*). Other instruments include the Leader Behavior Description Questionnaire, or LBDQ-12 (Stodgill, 1963), the Least Preferred Coworker Scale (Fiedler & Chemers, 1984; Fiedler & Garcia, 1987), the Leadership Practices Inventory (Kouzes & Posner, 1988), the Multifactor Leadership Questionnaire (MLQ) (Bass & Avolio, 1990), the Self-Assessment Leadership Instrument (Smola, 1988), and multiple

training instruments. Leadership-related research instruments were identified, compared, and evaluated by Huber and colleagues (2000). Some instruments are useful for research and others for leadership training or self-diagnosis. There is a wide variety of tools available. Individuals can increase their effectiveness through greater awareness and subsequent nurturing of both their leadership and followership skills.

A related leadership-followership concept is a psychological idea called the Pygmalion effect or self-fulfilling prophecy. It is related to theories about expectations. If the leader holds and communicates clearly an expectation that the group will perform well, that group members are bright and motivated, and that they will work in positive ways, those expectations are likely to be fulfilled. If the leader holds and communicates an expectation that the group is incapable and unmotivated, the leader is likely to get the kind of response that was expected. Therefore leaders should have positive assumptions about followers' potential (Hersey et al., 2001). This self-fulfilling prophecy is manifested through leadership styles and in the communication of the leader's attitudes. Leader expectations are thought to interact with leadership styles to result in managerial behavior (Getzels & Guba, 1957). The value system, confidence in subordinates, leadership inclination, and feelings of security of managers influence their leadership style (Tannenbaum & Schmidt, 1973) and are transmitted to the followers in both verbal and nonverbal ways. It is through the dynamic interaction between leaders and followers that leadership results in productivity and other outcomes.

LEADERSHIP AND MANAGEMENT IMPLICATIONS

Leadership is a key element in operating successful groups and organizations. It is a key resource for the improvement of nursing services. The following five practices are common to most exceptional leadership achievements (Kouzes & Posner, 1990):

1. Challenging the process by searching for opportunities, experimenting, and taking risks

◢ LEADERSHIP & MANAGEMENT **BEHAVIORS**

Leadership Behaviors

- Shows followers how to think about old problems in new ways
- Treats followers as unique individuals
- Stimulates critical thinking
- Inspires followers
- Demonstrates expertise and empathy
- Is visible to followers
- Is flexible
- Provides assistance and feedback (coaching)
- Communicates a vision
- Establishes trust
- Motivates the group to achieve goals
- Promotes innovation and risk taking
- Empowers followers
- Masters change

- Mentors followers
- Is creative and innovative

Management Behaviors

- Makes decisions
- Communicates
- Plans and organizes
- Manages changes
- Motivates followers

Overlap Areas

- Exercises broad-perspective decision making
- Communicates with followers
- Motivates followers

2. Inspiring a shared vision by envisioning the future and enlisting the support of others
3. Enabling others to act by fostering collaboration and strengthening others
4. Modeling the way by setting an example and planning small successes
5. Encouraging the heart by recognizing contributions and celebrating accomplishments

Nurse leaders can read, learn, and practice leadership skills. For example, the five practices identified through research as being associated with exceptional leadership can serve as an assessment guide for leadership situations. Furthermore, they can form the basis for strategic plans and activities to improve a given nursing work environment. Individuals can use this information for self-assessment.

As nurses work in a rapidly changing practice environment, leadership is important because it affects the climate and work environment of the organization. It affects how nurses feel about themselves at work and about their jobs. By extension, leadership is thought to affect organizational and individual productivity. For example, if nurses feel goal-directed and think that their contributions

are important, they are more motivated to do the work. Important for the professional practice of nurses is how they feel about themselves and how satisfied they are with their jobs. Both aspects have implications for how well nurses are retained and recruited. Leadership cannot be overlooked because leaders function as problem finders and problem solvers. They are people who help everyone else overcome obstacles. The leadership role is one of bridging, integrating, motivating, and creating organizational "glue."

Leadership in nursing is a key element to the profession because of a number of factors. *First,* it is important to nurses because of the size of the profession. Nurses comprise the largest single health care occupation and one that is experiencing critical shortages. Pressures, including costs, in the health care environment are rapidly thrusting nurses into leadership roles in highly complex and stressful work situations.

Second, nursing's work is complex, often conducted in complex settings. Tremendous changes in nursing have occurred in the last 25 years. These are changes in philosophy, knowledge base, technological complexity, ethical dilemmas, and impacts from constant change and societal pressures. Thus leadership is needed to guide and motivate the nurses and health care delivery systems toward positive achievements for better patient care.

Third, nurses enter the practice of nursing by licensure, but they come from a variety of educational backgrounds. A baccalaureate degree does not automatically confer advanced leadership skills. However, without this academic degree at minimum, nursing as a profession is disadvantaged when compared with other professions whose preparation is baccalaureate or above. Thus nurses will need strong leadership to resolve the interprofessional dilemmas derived from educational diversity and the related issues of professionalization and being attractive providers to clients. For example, each nurse will need to develop leadership skills in relating to peers who have different educational backgrounds and value systems. Nursing needs strong leadership for public policy advocacy on behalf of nursing as a profession and for its own growth and advancement in the provision of cost-effective patient care.

Nursing's leadership challenge includes developing strategies that help followers cope with change and develop the ability to adapt in positive and productive ways. Indeed, "one of the future leader's most important functions is to cultivate the human capital of their organization" (Anderson, 1997, p. 334). Leaders help to create an environment for followers to be able to use innovation, creativity, and collective problem solving. An important role for the leader is to instill confidence in followers. The leader needs to be able to encourage, coach, and question in order to increase the learning and growth of followers (Anderson, 1997).

Nurses are knowledge workers in an information age. Knowledge workers respond to inspiration, not supervision. Although professionals require little direction and supervision, what they do need is protection and support (Mintzberg, 1998). This is best manifested in the covert leadership of the unobtrusive actions that permeate all the things the leader does. Inspiration also can come from a focus on results. Leaders need to model what they want. Positive leadership outcomes are balanced, strategic, lasting, and selfless (Ulrich et al., 1999).

CURRENT ISSUES AND TRENDS

There are four current issues and trends that have significance for leadership in nursing. The first is the U.S. demographic data related to the aging of the "Baby Boom" generation. Next is the demographic profile of nursing in the United States. Also important are issues of collective action and ethical leadership in nursing.

Awareness of a major societal and public policy issue related to the aging of a large demographic bulge (commonly known as the "Baby Boom" generation) is just beginning to reach the U.S. general public. Called the "2030 problem" (Knickman & Snell, 2002), this socioeconomic and demographic phenomenon is real, looming, urgent, and fraught with health care challenges. The current status shows approximately 35.6 million Americans aged 65 and older, representing 12.4% of the population, or 1 in 8 Americans (AOA, 2003). The percentage of Americans 65 and older has tripled since 1900. Characteristic of older adults are issues related to health burdens and chronic illness. In fact, persons 85 and older may spend up to half of their remaining lives inactive or dependent.

U.S. population and health trends are assessed and monitored by governmental agencies such as the U.S. Census Bureau, Centers for Disease Control and Prevention, Bureau of Labor Statistics, and Health Resources and Services Administration. The statistics related to the Baby Boom generation are impressive. In 2000 Baby Boomers represented 28% of the U.S. population (U.S. Census Bureau, 2001). Born between 1946 and 1964, Baby Boomers in 2030 will be between the ages of 66 and 84 and are projected to number 61 million people. In addition to Baby Boomers, the U.S. population in 2030 is projected to also include 9 million people born before 1946. This predictable tidal wave will make chronic illness and long-term care a huge economic burden. Knickman and Snell (2002) suggested that there are four key "aging shocks": (1) uncovered costs of prescription medications, (2) uncovered medical care costs, (3) private insurance costs for the "Medi-gap," and (4) costs of long-term care. They projected that there will be an overwhelming economic burden if tax rates need to be raised dramatically, economic growth is retarded due to high service costs, or future generations of workers have worse general well-being due to service costs or income transfers. Nurses will be challenged to find evidence-based care delivery and service systems models to address the projected growth industry in chronic illness.

Examining the demographic profile of nursing in the United States offers a clue about nursing followership. The average age of a licensed, registered professional nurse in the United States was 43 in 1992 (Rosenfeld, 1994). This figure rose to 44.3 years in 1996 as the federal government's RN sample surveys documented the aging of the RN population (USDHHS, 1997). The Seventh National Sample Survey of Registered Nurses was conducted in 2000 and published in 2002 (USDHHS, 2002). There were an estimated 2,714,671 licensed RNs in the United States, and 81.7% were employed in nursing. The RN population is continuing to age. The average age of the total RN population was 45.2 years in 2000. Only 9.1% were under age 30, with 18.3% under age 35 and 31.7% under age 40. The profile of RNs reveals fewer young nurses entering the workforce, large cohorts of the RN population moving into their 50s and 60s, few minorities entering the profession (12%), and even fewer men (5.4%). The basic educational preparation for the largest proportion of RNs (40%) is the associate degree. Diploma program and baccalaureate program educational preparation were equal in proportion (30% each). However, a look at just the recent (past 5 years) graduates shows a dramatically different profile: 56% associate degree, 38% baccalaureate degree, and 6% diploma. Hospitals remain the major employer of nurses (59%), down from a peak of 68% in 1984. Public and community health, ambulatory care, and other noninstitutional settings had the largest percentage gain in

RN employment from 1980 to 2000. The average actual annual earnings of full-time RNs was $46,782 (USDHHS, 2002). This implies that nurses are going to need to look at how nursing is structured and organized, since nursing is no longer a young person's profession, on average. The bulk of nursing's population is advancing each year in average age. Therefore roles, deployment, and workforce utilization in nursing may need to shift to accommodate nursing demographics.

The direction of current trends indicates that there will be major changes in nursing practice demographics occurring in the twenty-first century. The number of diploma nurses is decreasing, there are fluctuating enrollments in nursing schools, and there are only small increases in the number of men (4.3% to 5.4% from 1992 to 1996 and 2000) and minorities (about 10% in 1996 to 12% in 2000) in nursing. There are more advanced practice nurses being prepared as nurse practitioner programs increase and as primary care becomes emphasized. Practice is increasingly complex, and practice settings are evolving.

The strength of a profession lies in its internal unity and ability to mobilize collective action. Yet only about 5% of all RNs belong to the American Nurses Association (ANA), which is the organization that represents nursing at the national level. This is a problem for leadership and followership in nursing. The fact that there are more than 2.7 million RNs, but that few belong to the major organization that speaks for nursing, reflects a potential dilution of the power of the profession. Individual nurses who are not members are cut off from participation in the collective and from information that can help them in their practice. However, there are many specialty groups in the nursing profession. These groups have organized into a national organization of specialty groups in nursing, the Nursing Organizations Liaison Forum (NOLF), and are linked with the ANA through the Tri-Council for Nursing. At the national level the many nursing groups have banded together so that when there are issues that are relevant to all nurses with a need to act from one position, nursing can speak with a united voice.

Under conditions of health care reform, turbulence, pressures for cost containment and better management of care, and constant change, ethical leadership becomes crucial. For instance, there are consequences to the changes being undertaken to achieve the goal of containing costs. The downsizing of nursing personnel in the 1990s led to an awareness of medical errors and patient safety issues. Yet solutions were costly and sometimes prohibitive. Nurses will find themselves in positions of both formal and informal leadership when ethical issues arise. There may be questions of advocacy for both patients and nurses. For example, must nursing services be targeted for downsizing? When downsizing occurs, how are justice, fairness, respect for persons, and prevention of harm handled? How are scarce nursing resources allocated and advocated? What institutional mechanisms help or hinder ethical decision making (Aroskar, 1994)? How can hospitals and other institutions remain financially viable with intense reimbursement reductions? Remarkably parallel issues arise over the management of scarce resources in long-term care, ambulatory care, home health care, and other nursing care settings. How nurses incorporate ethics into their leadership styles and decision making affects nurses, nursing, and the delivery of patient care.

Summary

- Effective leadership is important in nursing.
- Leadership principles can be learned through education and practice.
- Leaders must know themselves and their followers, the situation, the communication process, and goals, and they must be flexible enough to make necessary adaptations.
- Leaders are those who innovate and take the risks inherent in new approaches.
- Effectiveness means matching leadership behaviors to the environment and then adapting within that environment.
- Leaders who never vary their style are probably ineffective some of the time.

- Leadership involves a concern for task and a concern for people.
- Good leaders need good followers.

Study Questions

1. How would you describe a leader? Identify one person who personifies leadership.
2. What are the important qualities of leadership?
3. What tools are available to assess leadership skills?
4. Who are the leaders in nursing?
5. Can you be a leader in nursing?
6. What are some examples of leadership opportunities or challenges that you have faced? How did you handle them?
7. What is a good follower?
8. What is your favored leadership style? Followership style?

CASE STUDY

Nurse Kathryn Gardner has worked for 5 years as a staff nurse providing care to patients with developmental disabilities. She now has the opportunity to apply for her "ideal" job as the director of an innovative program funded by a local charity. Nurse Gardner has obtained the job description and related application forms. The request to write a description of her philosophy of leadership and management has her stuck. She believes in patient empowerment for self-care management. Unsure of how to translate this into a leadership statement, Nurse Gardner consults the literature. As she reads, she comes across a leadership style assessment instrument. Using this tool, she identifies herself as higher on task than relationship style. With further reading, she begins to formulate the germ of an idea: her leadership style uses activities of bridging, integrating, motivating, and creating organizational "glue" in order to empower nurses to help patients achieve self-management skills. She writes several drafts. When she believes that the document is polished, she completes the rest of the paperwork to apply for the job. She now feels more confident about presenting herself well in a job interview.

CRITICAL THINKING EXERCISE

Nurse Victoria Munoz has been reading leadership theory. She had hoped to be inspired by this new knowledge and discover better ways to solve some problems in the nursing work environment. Instead, Nurse Munoz is puzzled. The real work environment is dramatically different from what the theory says it should be. Many articles call for strong, motivating leadership in nursing with shared leadership and empowerment of staff nurses. However, in the health care environment in which Nurse Munoz works, nursing units have been consolidated and reorganized. The inpatient nurse managers are now responsible for multiple nursing units. The nurse managers of the ambulatory clinics have been realigned to report to a physician Director of Clinics. Everyone has a new role, position, boss, and followers.

Furthermore, the nurses of the inpatient clinical departments have been exhausted from work overload and now feel angry and devalued because of the effects on the Department of Nursing. The final straw comes when they realize that the new directors of the nonclinical departments have been promoted within 3 months of the organizational changes while the nurse managers remain at their previous level.

1. What is the problem?
2. What are the key issues?
3. How should Nurse Munoz handle the situation?
4. What should Nurse Munoz do first to demonstrate leadership?
5. What leadership style would be most appropriate in this situation?
6. What leadership and management strategies might be helpful?

REFERENCES

Administration on Aging. (AOA). (2003). *A profile of older Americans: 2002.* Washington, DC: U.S. Department of Health and Human Services. Retrieved July 5, 2004, from *www.aoa.gov/prof/statistics/profile/profiles2002%5Fpf.asp*

Alvesson, M., & Sveningsson, S. (2003). Managers doing leadership: The extra-ordinarization of the mundane. *Human Relations, 56*(12), 1435-1459.

Anderson, R. (1997). Future organizational leadership. *Journal of Professional Nursing, 13*(6), 334.

Aroskar, M. (1994). The challenge of ethical leadership in nursing. *Journal of Professional Nursing, 10*(5), 270.

Barker, A. (1990). *Transformational nursing leadership: A vision for the future.* Baltimore: Williams & Wilkins.

Barker, A. (1991). An emerging leadership paradigm: Transformational leadership. *Nursing & Health Care, 12*(4), 204-207.

Bass, B. (1982). *Stogdill's handbook of leadership.* New York: The Free Press.

Bass, B. (1985). *Leadership and performance beyond expectations.* New York: The Free Press.

Bass, B., & Avolio, B. (1990). *Transformational leadership development: Manual for the Multifactor Leadership Questionnaire.* Palo Alto, CA: Consulting Psychologists Press.

Bass, B., Waldman, D., Avolio, B., & Bibb, M. (1987). Transformational leadership and the falling dominos effect. *Group and Organizational Studies, 12*(1), 73-87.

Bennis, W. (1994). *On becoming a leader.* Reading, MA: Addison-Wesley.

Bennis, W., & Nanus, B. (1985). *Leaders: The strategies for taking charge.* New York: Harper & Row.

Bennis, W.G. (2004). The seven ages of the leader. *Harvard Business Review, 82*(1), 46-53.

Bennis, W.G., & Thomas, R.J. (2002). Crucibles of leadership. *Harvard Business Review, 80*(9), 39-45.

Blake, R., & Mouton, J. (1964). *The managerial grid.* Houston: Gulf Publishing.

Blake, R.R., & McCanse, A.A. (1991). *Leadership dilemmas—Grid solutions.* Houston: Gulf Publishing.

Brakey, M. (1991). Are you a good follower? *Nursing 91, 21*(12), 78-81.

Burns, J. (1978). *Leadership.* New York: Harper & Row.

Cartwright, D., & Zander, A. (Eds.). (1960). *Group dynamics: Research and theory* (2nd ed.). Evanston, IL: Row, Peterson.

Clancy, T.R. (2003). Courage and today's nurse leader. *Nursing Administration Quarterly, 27*(2), 128-132.

Collins, J. (2001). *Good to great.* New York: HarperCollins, Publishers.

Curtin, L. (1989). Things unattempted yet. *Nursing Management, 20*(7), 7-8.

Drenkard, K. (1997). Executive journey: From 1,300 FTEs to none. *Nursing Administration Quarterly, 22*(1), 57-63.

Drucker, P.F. (1994). *The post-capitalist society.* New York: Harper & Row.

Drucker, P.F. (1996). Foreword. In F. Hesselbein, M. Goldsmith, & R. Beckhard (Eds.), *The leader of the future: New visions, strategies, and practices for the next era.* San Francisco: Jossey-Bass.

Dunham, J., & Klafehn, K. (1990). Transformational leadership and the nurse executive. *Journal of Nursing Administration, 20*(4), 28-34.

Fiedler, F. (1967). *A theory of leadership effectiveness.* New York: McGraw-Hill.

Fiedler, F., & Chemers, M. (1984). *Improving leadership effectiveness: The leader match concept* (2nd ed.). New York: John Wiley & Sons.

Fiedler, F., & Garcia, J. (1987). *New approaches to effective leadership: Cognitive resources and organizational performance.* New York: John Wiley & Sons.

Getzels, J., & Guba, E. (1957). Social behavior and the administrative process. *The School Review, 65*(4), 423-441.

Goleman, D. (1997). *Emotional intelligence.* New York: Bantam Books.

Goleman, D. (2000). *Working with emotional intelligence.* New York: Bantam Books.

Grant, A. (1994). *The professional nurse: Issues and actions.* Springhouse, PA: Springhouse.

Greenleaf, R.K. (2002). *Servant leadership: A journey into the nature of legitimate power and greatness* (25th anniversary ed.). Mahwah, NJ: Paulist Press.

Guidera, M., & Gilmore, C. (1988). In defense of followership. *American Journal of Nursing, 88*(7), 1017.

Hagenow, N.R. (2001). Care executives: Organizational intelligence for these times. *Nursing Administration Quarterly, 25*(4), 30-35.

Heifetz, R.A., & Laurie, D.L. (1997). The work of leadership. *Harvard Business Review, 75*(1), 124-134.

Helgeson, S. (1995a). *The web of inclusion: A new architecture for building organizations.* New York: Doubleday.

Helgeson, S. (1995b). *The female advantage: Women's ways of leadership* (2nd ed.). New York: Doubleday.

Hersey, P., Blanchard, K.H., & Johnson, D.E. (2001). *Management of organizational behavior: Utilizing human resources* (8th ed.). Upper Saddle River, NJ: Prentice-Hall.

Huber, D.L., Maas, M., McCloskey, J., Scherb, C.A., Goode, C.J., & Watson, C. (2000). Evaluating nursing administration instruments. *Journal of Nursing Administration, 30*(5), 251-272.

Huber, D.L., & Watson, C.A. (2001). *Effective leadership in health care organizations.* Indianapolis: The College Network.

Kelley, R. (1988). In praise of followers. *Harvard Business Review, 66*, 142-148.

Kison, C. (1989). Leadership: How, who and what? *Nursing Management, 20*(11), 72-74.

Knickman, J.R., & Snell, E.K. (2002). The 2030 problem: Caring for aging baby boomers. *Health Services Research, 37*(4), 849-884.

Kotter, J. (2001). What leaders really do. *Harvard Business Review, 79*(11), 85-96.

Kouzes, J., & Posner, B. (1987). *The leadership challenge.* San Francisco: Jossey-Bass.

Kouzes, J., & Posner, B. (1988). *The leadership practices inventory.* San Diego: Pfeiffer & Company.

Kouzes, J., & Posner, B. (1990). *Leadership practices inventory (LPI): A self-assessment and analysis.* San Diego: Pfeiffer & Company.

Kramer, M. (1990). The magnet hospitals: Excellence revisited. *Journal of Nursing Administration, 20*(9), 35-44.

Kramer, M., & Schmalenberg, C. (1990). Fundamental lessons in leadership. In E. Simendinger, T. Moore, & M. Kramer (Eds.), *The successful nurse executive: A guide for every nurse manager* (pp. 5-21). Ann Arbor, MI: Health Administration Press.

Likert, R. (1961). *New patterns of management.* New York: McGraw-Hill.

Longest, B.B. Jr. (1998). Managerial competence at senior levels of integrated delivery systems. *Journal of Healthcare Management, 43*(2), 115-133.

Malloch, K. (2002). Trusting organizations: Describing and measuring employee-to-employee relationships. *Nursing Administration Quarterly, 26*(3), 12-19.

Mathena, K.A. (2002). Nursing manager leadership skills. *Journal of Nursing Administration, 32*(3), 136-142.

McCauley, G. (2004). *Leadership in a quantum age.* Ottawa, Ontario, Canada: ProGenerations, a division of the WEL Systems Institute. Retrieved September 6, 2004, from *www.progenerations.com/articles/Leadership.htm*

McClure, M., Poulin, M., Sovie, M., & Wandelt, M. (1983). *Magnet hospitals. Attraction and retention of professional nurses.* Kansas City, MO: American Nurses Association.

McDaniel, C., & Wolf, G. (1992). Transformational leadership in nursing service: A test of theory. *Journal of Nursing Administration, 22*(2), 60-65.

Mintzberg, H. (1998). Covert leadership: Notes on managing professionals. *Harvard Business Review, 76*(6), 140-147.

Murphy, D. (1990). Followers for a new era. *Nursing Management, 21*(7), 68-69.

Murphy, M., & DeBack, V. (1991). Today's nursing leaders: Creating the vision. *Nursing Administration Quarterly, 16*(1), 71-80.

Pagonis, W. (1992). The work of the leader. *Harvard Business Review, 70*(6), 118-126.

Pawar, B.S., & Eastman, K.K. (1997). The nature and implications of contextual influences on transformational leadership: A conceptual examination. *Academy of Management Review, 22*(1), 80-109.

Porter-O'Grady, T. (1997). Process leadership and the death of management. *Nursing Economic$, 15*(6), 286-293.

Porter-O'Grady, T. (2003). A different age for leadership, Part 1. *Journal of Nursing Administration, 33*(2), 105-110.

Rosenfeld, P. (1994). *Profiles of the newly licensed nurse: Historical trends and future implications* (2nd ed.) (Publ. No. 19-2530). New York: National League for Nursing Press.

Sherwood, T.A. (1997). Is nursing under new management or is it a matter of semantics? *Nursing Administration Quarterly, 22*(1), 72-75.

Smola, B. (1988). Refinement and validation of a tool measuring leadership characteristics of baccalaureate nursing students. In O. Strickland & C. Waltz (Eds.), *Measurement of nursing outcomes* (Vol. 2; pp. 314-366). New York: Springer.

Stodgill, R. (1963). *Manual for the Leader Behavior Description Questionnaire—Form XII: An experimental revision.* Columbus, OH: Ohio State University.

Tannenbaum, R., & Schmidt, W. (1958). How to choose a leadership pattern. *Harvard Business Review, 36,* 95-101.

Tannenbaum, R., & Schmidt, W. (1973). How to choose a leadership pattern. *Harvard Business Review, 51*(3), 162-180.

Tornabeni, J. (2001). The competency game: My take on what it really takes to lead. *Nursing Administration Quarterly, 25*(4), 1-13.

Trott, M.C., & Windsor, K. (1999). Leadership effectiveness: How do you measure up? *Nursing Economic$, 17*(3), 127-130.

Ulrich, D., Zenger, J., & Smallwood, N. (1999). *Results-oriented leadership.* Boston: Harvard Business School Press.

Upenieks, V. (2003). Nurse leaders' perceptions of what compromises successful leadership in today's acute inpatient environment. *Nursing Administration Quarterly, 27*(2), 140-152.

U.S. Census Bureau. (2001). *Age: 2000. Census 2000 brief.* Washington, DC: U.S. Census Bureau.

U.S. Department of Health and Human Services (USDHHS). (1997). *The registered nurse population.* Rockville, MD: USDHHS.

U.S. Department of Health and Human Services (USDHHS). (2002). *The registered nurse population, March 2000: Findings from the national sample survey of registered nurses.* Rockville, MD: USDHHS. Retrieved July 5, 2004, from *www.bhpr.hrsa.gov/healthworkforce/reports/rnsurvey/rnss1.htm*

Wheatley, M.J. (1992). *Leadership and the new science: Learning about organization from an orderly universe.* San Francisco: Berrett-Koehler.

White, R., & Lippitt, R. (1968). Leader behavior and member reaction in three social climates. In D. Cartwright & A. Zander (Eds.), *Group dynamics: Research and theory* (3rd ed.) (pp. 318-335). New York: Harper & Row.

Wilson, C.K., & Porter-O'Grady, T. (1999). *Leading the revolution in health care: Advancing systems, igniting performance* (2nd ed.). Gaithersburg, MD: Aspen.

Yukl, G. (1981). *Leadership in organizations.* Englewood Cliffs, NJ: Prentice-Hall.

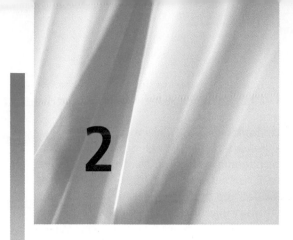

2

Management Principles

Diane L. Huber

CHAPTER OBJECTIVES

- Define and describe management and nursing management
- Formulate the management process
- Critique the nature of managerial work
- Analyze the roles a manager plays
- Distinguish classic management thought from contemporary theories
- Relate management concepts to nursing leadership and management
- Review legal aspects of management
- Exercise critical thinking to conceptualize and analyze possible solutions to a practice exercise

The global information age has arrived, bringing with it new challenges to health care management. Along with a whole array of opportunities, such as instantaneous communication across vast distances, health care organizations and the people in them face struggles with an ever-accelerating rate of change, knowledge explosion, and information flow. The context for management is embedded within a nurse shortage and fierce competition, doing more with less and less, waves of technology revisions, information proliferation, consumerism, generational values differences, and cultural diversity. The recruitment, development, deployment, motivation and leveraging of human capital as scarce resources and prime assets is a critical management issue for service industries in general, and nursing and health care specifically.

At the core, managers manage people and organizations. People's time and effort, as well as organizations' money, facilities, and supplies, need to be directed in a coordinated effort to achieve best results and meet objectives. Following are some thoughts about management:

The conventional definition of management is getting work done through people, but real management is developing people through work.

Agha Hasan Abedi

My main job was developing talent. I was a gardener providing water and other nourishment to our top 750 people. Of course, I had to pull out some weeds, too.

Jack Welch

I mean, there's no arguing. There is no anything. There is no beating around the bush. "You're fired" is a very strong term.

Donald Trump

Executives owe it to the organization and their fellow workers not to tolerate nonperforming people in important jobs.

Peter Drucker

Never tell people how to do things. Tell them what to do and they will surprise you with their ingenuity.

George S. Patton

The best executive is the one who has sense enough to pick good men to do what he wants done, and self-restraint enough to keep from meddling with them while they do it.

Teddy Roosevelt

Things may come to those who wait, but only the things left by those who hustle.

Abraham Lincoln

LEADERSHIP AND MANAGEMENT DIFFERENTIATED

Leadership and management are equally important processes. Since their focus is different, their importance varies according to what is needed in a specific situation. They are overlapping but distinct ideas. However, some have viewed them as almost identical or very similar. For example, Hersey and colleagues (2001) felt that leadership was a broader concept than management. They described management as a special kind of leadership. This view would pose management as a subpart of leadership, not as a distinct concept. According to their definitions, characteristics, and processes, leadership and management are different. However, at the area of overlap, they look similar. For example, directing occurs in both leadership and management activities (the area of overlap), whereas inspiring a vision is clearly a leadership function. Both leadership and management are necessary, although some propose the death of management altogether (Porter-O'Grady, 1997) and a shift to process leadership. This may be similar to Mintzberg's (1994) idea of

nursing management occurring in an interactive model rather than following a step-by-step list approach.

In a similar fashion, Bass and Avolio (1990) distinguished transactional leadership from transformational leadership. They noted that there is a similarity between what they called *transactional leaders* and traditional descriptions of managers. Transformational leaders, however, reflected the "strong forces" of leadership. Transactional leaders, or in this case, managers, focus on maintenance of the quality and quantity of performance, reduction in resistance to change, and the implementation of decisions in a specific situation. By contrast, increasing effort, making leaps in performance, changing group values and needs, creating innovative ideas, and improving quality are the activities of transformational leaders. In this model the transactional process occurs first and appears to be essential to effective leadership in that it provides the traditional management functions. It would appear that transactional leadership is another name for management functions and that this theory sees management as a process leading to expected outcomes. The area of overlap with leadership is not addressed, but there is presumed to be some overlap along this continuum. Distinctions between leadership and management are important for choosing an effective style that is matched to the situation.

Under conditions of maintenance and stability, transactional management appears to be needed. For growth, crisis, or change, transformational leadership is a component of effectiveness. Thus management and leadership do not appear to be identical. The focus of each is different. It is possible that management is focused on task accomplishment and leadership is focused on human relationship aspects. They may be sequential, and they are interrelated. Clearly, a balance of the two is necessary. There is a "gray area" in which the foci of their outcomes overlap. This overlap occurs where the two processes are integrated or synthesized to accomplish goals and where the same strategies are employed even though the goals may differ.

DEFINITIONS

Management is defined here as the process of coordination and integration of resources through planning, organizing, coordinating, directing, and controlling to accomplish specific institutional goals and objectives. Management has been viewed as an art and a science related to planning and directing human effort and scarce resources to attain established objectives. Management has been viewed in a variety of ways. Another definition of management is a process by which organizational goals are met through the application of skills and the use of resources. Hersey and colleagues (2001) defined management as "the process of working with and through individuals and groups and other resources (such as equipment, capital, and technology) to accomplish organizational goals" (p. 9).

Management, then, applies to organizations. The definition of leadership emphasizes actions that influence toward group goals; the definition of management focuses on organizational goals. The achievement of organizational goals through leadership and manipulation of the environment is management. In a systems approach to management, the inputs would be represented by human resources and physical and technical resources. The outputs would be the realization of goals (Figure 2.1). Koontz (1961) concluded that management is the art of the following:

- Getting things done through and with people in formally organized groups
- Creating an environment in an organized group in which people can perform as individuals yet cooperate to attain group goals
- Removing blocks to performance
- Optimizing efficiency in effectively reaching goals

Thus management is a separate function with a specific purpose and related roles but one that is focused on organizations. To achieve organizational goals, managers are involved in activities such as analyzing issues, establishing goals and objectives, mapping out work plans, organizing assets and supplies, developing and motivating people, communicating, managing technology, handling change and conflict, measurement, analysis, and evaluation. Without talent and attention to these functions, effectiveness and morale drop.

Effective managers are thought to be those who can weave strategy, execution, discipline, inspiration,

⚠ LEADING & MANAGING **DEFINED**

Management

The coordination and integration of resources through planning, organizing, coordinating or directing, and controlling to accomplish specific institutional goals and objectives.

Nursing Management

The coordination and integration of nursing resources by applying the management process to accomplish nursing care and service goals and objectives.

Planning

Determining the long- and short-term objectives and the corresponding actions that must be taken to achieve these objectives.

Organizing

Mobilizing the human and material resources of the institution to achieve organizational objectives.

Coordinating

Motivating and leading personnel to carry out the desired actions

Controlling

Comparing the results of work with predetermined standards of performance and taking corrective action when needed.

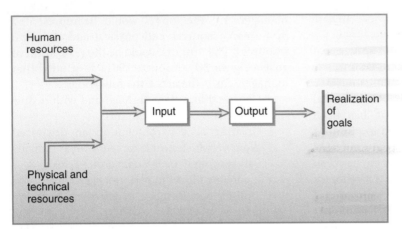

Figure 2.1
Systems view of management.

and leadership together as they unite an organization toward achieving its goals. Sull (2003) found that successful managers may vary in personal attributes but all excel at managing commitments. Managerial commitments may be capital investments, hiring or firing decisions, public statements, or other strategy decisions. A commitment is defined as "any action taken in the present that binds an organization to a future course of action" (Sull, 2003, p. 84). Commitments give employees a clear sense of focus for prioritization and motivation; however, they limit flexibility. The most enduring commitments tend to be strategic frames, resources, processes, relationships, and values.

Drucker (2004) also noted that effective executives do not need to be leaders. "Great managers may be charismatic or dull, generous or tightfisted, visionary or numbers oriented. But every effective executive follows eight simple practices" (Drucker, 2004, p. 59). These eight practices are divided into three categories:

Practices That Give Executives the Knowledge They Need

1. They asked: "What needs to be done?"
2. They asked: "What is right for the enterprise?"

Practices That Help Executives Convert Knowledge to Action

1. They developed action plans.

2. They took responsibility for decisions.
3. They took responsibility for communicating.
4. They were focused on opportunities, not problems.

Practices That Ensure That the Whole Organization Feels Responsible and Accountable

1. They ran productive meetings.
2. They thought and said "we" not "I."

Effective management also appears to be a result of artful balancing. Managers need to function at the point at which reflective thinking combines with practical doing (Gosling & Mintzberg, 2003). Described as managerial mind-sets within the bounds of management, managers interpret and deal with their world from the following five perspectives (Gosling & Mintzberg, 2003):

1. *Reflective mind-set:* managing self
2. *Analytic mind-set:* managing organizations
3. *Worldly mind-set:* managing context
4. *Collaborative mind-set:* managing relationships
5. *Action mind-set:* managing change

The five mind-sets were described as being like threads for the manager to weave. The process is as follows: analyze, act, reflect, act, collaborate, reanalyze, articulate new insights, and act again.

Management is central to the work of nursing. **Nursing management** is defined as the coordination and integration of nursing resources by applying the management process to accomplish nursing care and service goals and objectives.

BACKGROUND: THE MANAGEMENT PROCESS

An organization can be any institution, agency or facility. Working to achieve an organization's goals involves the process of management. The principles that guide the process of management need to be identified in order to be useful for greater effectiveness. A Frenchman named Henri Fayol (1949) reasoned that management could not be taught because of the lack of basic principles, whereas physics could be taught because of Newton, and geometry could be taught because of Euclid. To explain the management process, Fayol formulated the principles that created a basis for management practice. He said that managers perform unique and discrete functions: they plan, organize, coordinate, and control. Fayol's ideas were revolutionary in that, for the first time, management was seen as a unique and separate activity form the work of producing a product. Workers labor to produce the product; managers labor to manage organizations toward goal achievement. Someone needs to monitor financial indicators, hire, train and evaluate personnel; improve quality; coordinate work and effort; fix systems problems and ensure that goals are met. In nursing, this

means that nurses do the work of nursing while nurse managers coordinate and integrate the work of individual nurses with the larger system.

The four steps of the management process are as follows (Fayol, 1949; Figure 2.2):

1. Planning
2. Organizing
3. Coordinating or directing
4. Controlling

These functions comprise the scope of a manager's major effort. Planning involves determining the long- and short-term objectives and the corresponding actions that must be taken. Organizing means mobilizing human and material resources to accomplish what is needed. Directing relates to methods of motivating, guiding, and leading people through work processes. Controlling has a specific meaning closer to the monitoring and evaluating actions that are familiar to nurses. The management process can be compared to performing an orchestra concert or playing a football game. There is a plan and an organized group of players. A director manages the performance and controls the outcome by making corrections and adjustments along the way. The management process is a rational, logical process based on problem-solving principles (see Figure 2.2). Fayol's classic management process idea remains the core framework around discussions about what management is and does.

Figure 2.2
Four steps of the management process.

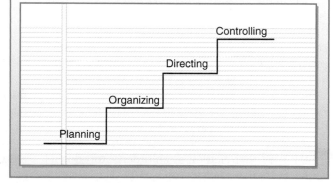

Planning

Planning is the managerial function of selecting priorities, results, and methods to achieve results (McNamara, 1999a). It is setting the direction for a system and then guiding the system to follow the direction (McNamara, 1999b). Planning is defined as determining the long- and short-term objectives and the corresponding actions that must be taken to achieve these objectives. Steiner (1962, p. 28) described planning as "the conscious determination of courses of action to achieve preconceived objectives." Planning can be detailed, specific, and rigid, or it can be broad, general, and flexible. Planning is deciding in advance what is to be done and when, by whom, and how it is to be done. Hersey and colleagues (2001) described planning as involving the setting of goals and objectives and developing "work maps" to show how they are to be accomplished. Planning activities include identifying goals, objectives, methods, resources, responsible parties, and due dates.

The two types of planning are as follows (Levenstein, 1985):

- *Strategic planning:* More broad-ranged, this approach means determining the overall purposes and directions of the organization. This is often focused on mission, vision, and major goal identification. Scenario planning may be used in the strategic planning process to help participants see the "big picture" and analyze multiple chaotic influences (see Chapters 6 and 7 for more information on scenario planning).
- *Tactical planning:* More short-ranged, this type means determining the specific details of implementing broader goals. Examples are project planning, staffing planning, and marketing plans.

Levenstein (1985) identified three errors that can create planning flaws: (1) errors of fact: the plan is based on misinformation, (2) errors in assumption: the plan is based on incorrect assumptions, and (3) errors of logic: the plan is based on faulty reasoning. Planning flaws carry over into organizing, directing, and controlling activities.

An alternative conceptualization to the model of planning that views it as an orderly, top-down sequence is the model proposed by Hayes-Roth and Hayes-Roth (1979). Their idea was that opportunistic planning approaches are used to face complex planning tasks. Planners, under conditions of complexity, pursue whatever seems opportune or promising at the time. A plan becomes multidirectional and develops by increments. This approach may appear chaotic compared with systematic planning, but it leads to better plans in complex task situations. Similar to the interactive planning that nurses do with patients, interactive planning between nurses and nurse managers also is the best strategy for effective planning.

Planning is a process that is heavily dependent on the decision-making process. Part of planning is choosing among a certain number of alternatives. Thus in nursing the manager often must balance the needs of clients, staff, administrators, and physicians. Since resources are limited, planning involves an analysis of how to best proceed under the given constraints (Kepler, 1980).

Planning involves considering systems inputs, processes, outputs, and outcomes. The process of planning in its larger context means that planners work backwards through the system. Starting with the results, outcomes, or outputs desired, they then identify the processes needed to produce the results and then identify the inputs or resources needed to carry out the processes (McNamara, 1999b). Typical planning phases include the following:

- Identify the mission
- Conduct an environmental scan
- Analyze the situation (e.g., SWOT analysis of strengths, weaknesses, opportunities, and threats)
- Establish goals
- Identify strategies to reach goals
- Set objectives to achieve goals
- Assign responsibilities and timelines
- Write a planning document
- Celebrate success and completion

Many plans fail as a result of incompletion; thus it is important to focus on ensuring that the plan is carried out or that deviations are recognized and managed. Recommended guidelines are as follows (McNamara, 1999b):

- Involve the right people in planning
- Do a written plan and communicate it widely

- Establish goals and objectives that are specific, measurable, acceptable, placed in a time frame, stretching, and rewarding
- Build in accountability (regular review)
- Note deviations and replan
- Evaluate the planning process and the plan
- Conduct ongoing communications
- Make the planning process compatible with the preferences of the planners
- Acknowledge and celebrate results

The planning process is intimately involved with establishing objectives. Fayol (1949) identified planning as examining the future and drawing up a plan of action. Activities involved include the laying out of the work to be done, determining the use of resources, and establishing the standards for evaluation. Levenstein (1985) argued that the role of the nurse manager as planner is critical to the successful functioning of the institution and the care of clients. This is because the plan of care is shaped and reshaped with nursing input and then implemented by the nursing staff. Thomas (1983) noted that the institution is held or glued together by the nurses, enabling it to function. The nurse is engaged in a constant mental planning operation when deciding what specific things are to be accomplished for the client. The same is true for the nurse manager who is deciding how to accomplish a positive and productive work environment for nurses.

Planning is a function that assumes stability and the ability to predict and project into the future. Yet the current environment is turbulent, making planning difficult. Learning and adapting are important abilities in a changeable environment. Interactive planning has been suggested as an approach to planning in complex situations and changing environments (Ackoff, 1981; Foust, 1994). Interactive planning takes a developmental approach. Problems are viewed as interrelated. Interactive planning principles emphasize the importance of participation among participants, a nonlinear view of relationships called systems thinking, and a focus on creating a desired future outcome. Interactive planning can contribute to effective care planning and to effective care management by nurses (Foust, 1994).

Organizing

Organizing is a management function related to allocating and configuring resources to accomplish preferred goals and objectives. It is the activities done to collect and configure resources to effectively and efficiently implement plans (McNamara 1999a, 1999c). Organizing can be defined as mobilizing the human and material resources of the institution to achieve organizational objectives. Fayol (1949) noted that organizing was building up the material and human structures. Authority, power, and structure are used for influence. The goal is to get the human, equipment, and material resources mobilized, organized, and working. Organizing so that the goals and objectives can be accomplished includes establishing some relationship between the workers and the environment. The first step is to organize the work; then the people are organized; finally the environment is organized.

Organizing closely follows the planning process. In fact, these terms are often referred to together: planning and organizing. Organizing encompasses activities designed to bring together an array of various resources including personnel, money, and equipment in a manner that is the most effective for accomplishing organizational goals. Therefore the essence of organizing is the integration and coordination of resources (Hersey et al., 2001).

There are a wide variety of topics related to organizing, which is considered to be one of the major functions of management. Lack of organization can be a major source of stress. McNamara (1999a, 1999c) identified the following categories under managerial organizing:

- Organizing yourself, your office, your files
- Organizing a task, job, or role through task and job analysis, job descriptions, and time management
- Organizing various groups of people such as staff, committees, meetings, and teams
- Organizing human resources through benefits, compensation, staffing and deployment, and training and development
- Organizing facilities and technology

Organizing also can be thought of as a process of identifying roles in relationship to one another. Thus organizing involves activities related to establishing a structure and hierarchy of jobs and positions within a unit or department. Responsibilities are assigned to each job. The complexity of this aspect of organizing is related to the size of the organization and the number of employees and jobs. For nurse managers the activities of budget management, staffing, and scheduling are all organizing activities that are interrelated and tied to role relationships (Kepler, 1980). Organizing in nursing also relates to other human resources and personnel functions such as orientation and staff in-service development. Examples of how nurses organize nursing include developing committees and bylaws. Organizations organize by establishing a structure, such as a hierarchy with divisions or departments, and by developing some method for division of labor and subsequent coordination among subunits.

Directing

Directing is the managerial function of establishing direction and then influencing people to follow that direction. Directing can also be called leading (McNamara, 1999a) or coordinating. **Coordinating** or directing is defined as motivating and leading personnel to carry out the desired actions. Fayol (1949) identified activities of binding together, unifying, and harmonizing the activity and effort of various personnel as part of coordinating or directing.

Motivation often is included with the description of the activities of directing others, along with communicating and leading. Motivating is a major strategy related to determining the followers' level of performance and thereby to influencing how effectively the goals of the organization will be met. The amount of employee effort that can be influenced by motivation is thought to be from 20% to 30% at the low end and as high as 80% to 90% for highly motivated people (Hersey et al., 2001). This is a wide range of effort that can be influenced through motivation. Motivation is a complex activity, but it is a critical managerial function. (See Chapter 23 for more information on management theories related to motivation.)

On a day-to-day basis, coaching is used as a technique to direct and motivate followers. While working through assigned staff members, the manager delegates activities and responsibilities. The function of directing involves actions of supervising and guiding others within their assigned duties. The use of interpersonal skills is required to delicately balance the need to direct and supervise with the need to create and maintain a motivational climate (Kepler, 1980). Nurses with disabilities have become a special case of managerial directing. Federal laws now apply (i.e., Americans with Disabilities Act), and managers have to manage accommodations and the responses of other staff.

Within nursing there is a legal element to the managerial directing function. In some state licensing laws, supervision is a defined legal element of nursing practice. Delegation and supervision are viewed legally as a part of the practice of nursing. Thus nurses have a specific need to know and understand this area of nursing responsibility within their scope of practice. Nurses carry responsibility and accountability for the quality and quantity of their supervision, as well as for the quality and quantity of their own actions in regard to care provision. Nurses also are being tapped for their important role as a care coordinator. Nurse managers carry the added responsibility and accountability for the coordination of groups of nurse providers and assistive or ancillary personnel. Nurse managers also have an overall responsibility to monitor and provide surveillance or vigilance regarding situations that can lead to failure to rescue, patient safety errors, or negligence. Too many hours worked, nurse fatigue from stress, too heavy a patient work-load, and other systems problems are situations to monitor.

Controlling

Controlling is the management function of monitoring and adjusting the plan, processes, and resources to effectively and efficiently achieve goals.

It is a way of coordinating organizations by systematically figuring out whether what is occurring is what is wanted (McNamara, 1999a, 1999d). The controlling aspect of the managerial process may seem at first to carry a negative connotation. However, when used in reference to management, the word *control* does not mean being negatively manipulative toward others. Managerial controlling means ensuring that the proper processes are followed. Fayol (1949) called this the activity of seeing that everything occurs in conformity with established rules. In nursing the term *evaluation* is used to refer to similar actions and activities. Control or evaluation means ensuring that the flow and processes of work, as well as goal accomplishment, proceed as planned. *Controlling* is defined as comparing the results of work with predetermined standards of performance and taking corrective action when needed. This means ensuring that the results are as desired, and if they are not up to standards, then taking some action to modify, remediate, or reverse the variances.

Coordination of elements of a system is one aspect of managerial control to reach effective outcomes. Other managerial control elements are financial management, compliance, quality and risk management, feedback mechanisms, performance management, policies and procedures, and research and trend analysis. These elements are used by managers to communicate to reach a goal, track activities toward the goal, guide behaviors, and coordinate efforts and decide what to do. Managerial coordination and control are important to the success of any organization (McNamara, 1999a, 1999d). Ongoing, careful review using standardized documents, informatics systems, and standardized measures avoids drift and the waste of time and resources that occur when direction is vague. Well-exercised, managerial control is flexible enough to allow innovation yet present enough to effectively structure groups and organizations toward goal attainment.

The management function of controlling involves the feeding back of information about the results and outcomes of work activities, combined with activities to follow up and compare outcomes with plans. Appropriate adjustments need to be made wherever outcomes vary or deviate from expectations (Hersey et al., 2001). In nursing, when a critical path is used to track client care, the variances are analyzed and corrected as a function of managerial control. The controlling function of management has been described as a constant process of reevaluation to see whether what is currently occurring meets needs, plans, and standards, as well as to identify where improvements might be a benefit (Kepler, 1980).

In summary, by using the four steps of the management process, goals can be accomplished by and through other people. These managerial functions primarily are aimed at the productivity element of an organization. For nursing, within a human services industry, managerial skills are employed to enhance the utilization of human resources (Kepler, 1980).

MANAGEMENT IN NURSING PRACTICE

Nurses have two major components to their role: care provider and care integrator. McClure (1991) called these the caregiver and integrator roles. The image of the "bedside nurse" emphasizes the care provider aspect of nursing. The integrator role is a complementary function that arises from nursing's central positioning in the day-to-day coordination of service delivery and central location at the hub of information flow regarding care and service delivery. This linkage relationship is depicted visually in Figure 2.3. Coordination of care has always been a key nursing function. It is becoming more visible and valued in health care and as nurses assume case management roles that focus on integrating clinical care. However, the relative proportion of the nurse's role that is devoted to management and coordination functions varies within nursing according to the job category. One useful way to analyze nursing jobs is to assess the relative balance of the two role components in any job.

At the lowest levels of an organization, employees are hired for some technical or professional skill. In highly technical, constantly

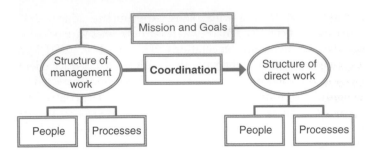

Figure 2.3
Linkage of clinical and management domains.

changing fields such as nursing, it takes nearly all of a nurse's time to be technically competent. Yet for a middle manager, only a part of the work time can be spent being technically competent. The other part is spent doing management: planning, organizing, coordinating or directing, and controlling the work of nursing and other personnel. With advancement to the highest nurse executive level, the job change inevitably results in the nurse executive becoming the least competent technician because the job demands an increasing focus on management and leadership activities. These are normal organizational dynamics. They occur because management is a discrete function. Part of the task is to link the top of the organization to the bottom and vice versa in a two-way street. The bottom also has to know what the top is doing and recognize the fact that managers do management while technicians do their work; together the group accomplishes individual and organizational goals (Organizational Dynamics, 1975). This view highlights the value of investing in infrastructure that organizes and supports the work that nurses do. Managers in nursing perform discrete and important functions that provide an environment to facilitate delivery of client services. Mintzberg (1994) described this managing as blended care.

Mintzberg (1994) compared management as cure, which is intermittent and interventionist, with management as care, which is continuous and involved. Management as care is thought to be more effective. In this modality, nurses are postulated to be able to move more easily and naturally into management because of nursing's roots in caring. Mintzberg noted that in this sense

nursing is management, as contrasted to medicine with its focus on cure. Mintzberg's ideas (1994) coincide with a contemporary view of organizations and their management. Organizations are living entities composed of people in relationships. Management becomes a view of work as being accomplished through relationships and people who are self-organizing. Skill at facilitation becomes a major management role (Crowell, 1998). Porter-O'Grady (1997) called this process *leadership*.

In nursing the management process is primarily directed toward the human element, or the management of human resources. It is through this dynamic and interactive process that the work of nursing is accomplished. Nurse managers balance two competing needs: the needs of the staff related to growth, efficiency, motivation, morale, and accomplishment and the needs of the employer for productivity, quality, and cost-effectiveness. Desired outcomes include staff satisfaction and productivity (Kepler, 1980).

MANAGEMENT IN ORGANIZATIONS

The Nature of Managerial Work

Lewin (1947) said that the behavior of human beings is a function of individual psychology, the needs patterns of people, and the environment in which they work. Behavioral theory and its applications to the management of people focuses on organizing and processing work and accomplishing organizational objectives at a targeted minimum cost and minimum waste. The responsibility for doing that lies with management. Managers manage people and the environment.

One view of management suggests that the manager's behavior, the role, and the situation created for people to work in causes the followers' behavior. Thus the manager's role is distinct and important for individual and organizational outcomes.

Mintzberg (1973, 1975) reformulated Fayol's ideas about the nature of managerial work. Mintzberg's synthesis of research findings about managers in general revealed the following:

- Managers work at an unrelenting pace at activities characterized by brevity, variety, and discontinuity. Managers are strongly action-oriented.
- Managers handle exceptions and perform regular work, such as ritual and ceremonial duties, negotiation, and processing of soft information linking the organization to its environment.
- Managers prefer oral communication, especially telephone calls and meetings.
- "Judgment" and "intuition" describe the procedures managers use to schedule time, process information, and make decisions.

Zaleznik (1992) noted that managerial culture emphasizes rationality and control—a manager is a problem solver. He noted that it takes neither genius nor heroism to be a manager. What is needed is persistence, tough-mindedness, hard work, intelligence, analytical ability, tolerance, and goodwill. Some would suggest that positive interpersonal relationship skills also are necessary for success. Drucker (1954) suggested that the three jobs of management are to manage a business enterprise, manage managers, and manage workers and work. The skills needed by nurse managers include conceptual or thinking skills, technical skills in nursing methods and techniques, and group and human relations skills (Katz, 1955).

Mintzberg (1975) described the manager's job in terms of ten roles or sets of behaviors. Derived from the formal authority and status of the position are three interpersonal roles: figurehead, leader, and liaison. As the nerve center of the organizational unit, information processing is a key part of the role. Informational roles are monitor, disseminator, and spokesperson. Information is the basic input to decision making. The decisional roles are entrepreneur, disturbance handler, resource allocator, and negotiator (Figure 2.4). Mintzberg suggested a number of important managerial skills, as follows:

- Developing peer relationships
- Carrying out negotiations

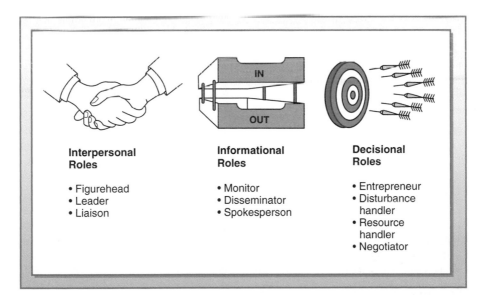

Figure 2.4
Mintzberg's ten managerial roles. (Data from Mintzberg, H. [1975]. The manager's job: Folklore and fact. In M. Matteson, & J. Ivancevich [Eds.], *Management classics* [3rd ed.; pp. 63-85]. Plano, TX: Business Publications.)

- Motivating subordinates
- Resolving conflicts
- Establishing information networks and disseminating information
- Making decisions in conditions of extreme ambiguity
- Allocating resources

If management is important to achieving organizational goals, then the skills, abilities, functions, actions, and strategies used by managers to manage are important to know and understand. Kepler (1980) suggested that the managerial skills to be mastered are processes of understanding, communication, and effective use and manipulation (through selective use of rewards and punishment) of personnel.

Mintzberg (1994) elaborated his earlier work on the nature of managerial work by expanding it to an interactive model of managerial work (Figure 2.5). The model uses concentric circles. At the core is a person who is in a job. The person has some unique set of values, experiences, knowledge, and competencies. The combination of the person and the job creates a frame composed of the job's purpose, the person's perspective about what needs to be done, and selected strategies for doing the job. The frame can range across two continua: from vague to very specific and from

Research Note

Source: Mintzberg, H. (1994). Managing as blended care. *Journal of Nursing Administration, 24*(9), 29-36.

Purpose

The purpose of this research is to develop and enhance a new model of managerial work. The new model is based on a review and integration of identified managerial work roles, visualized in concentric circles. The model was tested in a research project on managerial work. Using a case study research design approach, one head nurse of a hospital unit in Canada was intensively observed and described and her activities were analyzed during one working day. Roles of leading, linking, controlling, and doing were analyzed and reported. Conclusions were drawn about effective management styles.

Discussion

Mintzberg's classic work on management roles appeared in 1973 with *The Nature of Managerial Work*. This new model advanced his thinking from a list approach to an interactive model approach. At the center of the model is a person in a job who creates a frame. The frame is manifested by an agenda of issues and work schedules. Above this core are three levels through which work can take place: information, people, and action. Roles pervade the levels, which are depicted by circles. The research methodology was participant observation, designed to assess the usefulness of the model and identify role behaviors and styles. "Caring" management described this head nurse's management style. It is a kind of blended care that is practiced by being out on the unit and visible to workers. It resembles a craft style of management.

Application to Practice

This female head nurse administered continuous care. There was a natural rhythm, flow, and blending of the component parts of the Mintzberg model. Thus the doing activities are interwoven with the leading and communicating activities. Mintzberg comments on gender and style research and his observations in health care. He distinguishes the differing perspectives of physicians and nurses regarding good care management. The two professions care differently and in complementary ways; yet they need to work out ways to collaborate to the client's benefit. This article emphasizes how management, like nursing, can be a caring type of work. In a sense, nursing is management.

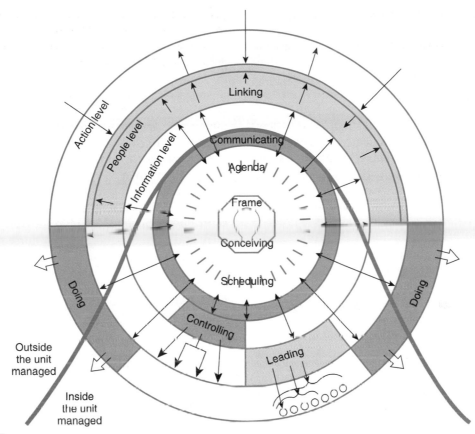

Figure 2.5
Mintzberg's **Model of Managerial Work.** (Redrawn from Mintzberg, H. [1994]. Managing as blended care. *Journal of Nursing Administration, 24*[9], 30.)

person-selected to externally imposed. The frame results in an agenda of work issues and time scheduling. Placed at the center of the figure, these elements form the core of the job of a manager. Managerial roles and behaviors at this level include conceiving the frame and scheduling the agenda.

Growing out of the core are three concentric circles—from abstract to concrete. These are called the information, people, and action levels of managerial work. At the most abstract level the manager processes information and uses it to drive the action. At the next level the manager works with people to encourage work activities. At the most concrete level the manager manages the action.

At the information level the associated managerial roles are communicating information and controlling by using information to control the work of others. At the people level the managerial roles are leading and linking. Leading involves encouraging and enabling individuals (by mentoring and rewarding), groups (by team building and conflict resolution), and the whole organization (by building a culture). Linking roles have the manager relating to the external environment by building networks of contacts and acquiring information from the environment to transmit back to the unit. At the action level the associated managerial role is called doing or supervising. Behaviors include doing, handling disturbances, and negotiating (Mintzberg, 1994).

Mintzberg's (1994) interactive model provides a visual display of a way of thinking about managerial work and associated roles and activities. The model could be used as a basis for self-assessment and can be applied to specific managerial jobs. Nurses who strive to apply the concepts to their managerial work could use the model to examine and analyze managerial styles, behaviors, and roles. As managers, nurses manage both people (clients, themselves, and other staff or providers) and the environment of client care delivery. An understanding of the management process and the roles related to the work of a manager can assist nurses to improve their personal effectiveness and their organization's productivity.

Contemporary Management Theories

Human organizations are complex in nature. It is tricky to provide overall direction for an organization in times of rapid environmental change. The recent focus of leadership theory has been on interactional, relational, and transformational leadership to guide organizations through successful change and chaos. However, less attention has been focused on how to advise managers who are working toward the organization's goals and trying to use resources effectively and efficiently under conditions of change and complexity. It is thought that the nature of how the four managerial functions of planning, organizing, coordinating or directing, and controlling are carried out needs to change to accommodate a new management paradigm. Although the four functions recur throughout organizations and are highly integrated, organizations are morphing and changing rapidly. Because of forces such as technology, the Internet, increasing diversity, and a global marketplace, organizations have been pressured to be more sensitive, flexible, and adaptable to stakeholders' expectations and demands (McNamara, 1999e, 1999f).

The result has been a reconfiguration or restructuring of many organizations from the classic hierarchical, top-down, rigid form to a more fluid, organic, team-based, collaborative structure. This has had an impact on how managers manage. Managers cannot control continued rapid change. Old familiar plans and behaviors no longer provide clear direction for the future. Managers now need to focus on two major aspects of management: managing change through constant assessment, guidance, and adaptation and managing employees through worker-centered teams and other self-organizing and self-designing group structures (McNamara, 1999f). Bureaucratic management is out; organic and virtual management is in.

A variety of contemporary theories of management have arisen to help organize management thought. Four major management theories now predominate: contingency theory, systems theory, complexity theory, and chaos theory. Each one contributes principles useful for nursing management and administration and for nurse managers working to coordinate and integrate health care delivery.

Contingency Theory

Contingency theory is discussed under leadership theories but also applies to management. The basic principle is that managers need to take into account the situation and all its elements when making a decision. Managers need to act on the key situational aspects with which they are confronted. Sometimes described as "it all depends" decision making, contingency theory is most often used for choosing a leadership or management style. The "best" style depends on the situation (McNamara, 1999g).

Systems Theory

Systems theory has helped managers to recognize their work as being embedded within a system and to better understand what a system is. Managers have learned that changing one part of a system inevitably affects the whole system. General systems theory was derived from the work of Ludwig von Bertalanffy (1968) as a way of thinking about studying organizational wholes. General systems theory uses the following concepts:
- Organization
- Wholeness
- Control
- Self-regulation
- Purposiveness

Table **2.1**

Open System and Health Care Elements	
Open System Elements	Health Care Elements
Inputs to the system (resources)	Money, people, technology
Transforming processes and interactions (throughputs)	Nursing services, management
Outputs of the system	Clinical outcomes, better quality of life
Feedback	Customer and nurse satisfaction, government regulation, accreditation, lawsuits

- Environment
- Boundaries
- Equilibrium
- Steady state
- Feedback

A system is a set of interrelated and interdependent parts that are designed to achieve common goals. Systems contain a collection of elements that interact with each other in some environment. The elements of an open system and related examples in health care are shown in Table 2.1.

A key principle of systems theory is that changes in one part of the system affect other parts, creating a ripple effect within the whole. Using systems theory implies a rational approach to common goals, a global view of the whole, and an emphasis on order rather than chaos. The input-throughput-output model exemplifies this linear thinking aspect of general systems theory.

Systems theory is easy to understand but difficult to apply in bureaucratic systems or organizations with strong departmental "silos." This is because coordinators and integrators with sufficient organizational power to cross the system are needed but often not deployed. Without integrators, systems parts tend to make changes without consideration of the whole system. Shifting to systems theory thinking helps managers view, analyze, and interpret patterns and events through the lens of interrelationships of the parts and coordination of the whole (McNamara, 1999g).

In health care, concepts such as interrelatedness and interdependence fit well with multidisciplinary teamwork and shared governance professional models. However, concepts of attaining a steady state and equilibrium are difficult to reconcile with the reality of uncertainty, risk, change, and ambiguity that characterize the turbulence of change that characterize the health care delivery environment. Previously, managers were advised to draw up five- and even ten-year plans; managers today have seriously shortened their strategic planning and other related time lines in response to the rapidity of change. An example of the use of systems theory is basing an analysis of a planned change, such as implementing a new program, on systems concepts by identifying inputs, throughputs, outputs, and feedback loops in order to more effectively plan how the new program fits into the existing system.

Complexity Theory

Arising in scientific fields such as astronomy, chemistry, biology, geology, and meteorology and involving disciplines such as engineering, mathematics, physics, psychology, and economics, there is growing literature since the late 1980s on the behavior of complex adaptive systems (Rosenhead, 1998). Complexity theory is the more general category under which chaos theory is a more specific focus on a particular type of behavior. The focus of complexity theory is the behavior over time of certain complex systems. These are dynamic systems capable of changing over time. The concern is about the predictability of their behavior. The systems of interest in complexity theory are systems that under certain conditions perform in regular and predictable ways; yet in other conditions they change in irregular and unpredictable ways, are unstable, and move further away from the starting conditions unless stopped by an overriding constraint. What is most intriguing is that almost undetectable differences in initial conditions will lead to diverging reactions in these systems until the evolution of their behavior is highly dissimilar. Thus stable and unstable behavior is the focus of interest (Rosenhead, 1998).

Stable and unstable behavior can be thought of as two zones. In the stable zone a disturbed system returns to its initial state. In the unstable zone a small disturbance leads to movement away from the starting point and further divergence. Which type of behavior occurs depends on the conditions. The area between them is called chaotic behavior. This refers to systems that have behavior with certain regularity yet defy prediction based on that regularity. The classic example of this is weather prediction (Rosenhead, 1998).

Prior to complexity theory, the unpredictability of systems was attributed to randomness that was measured by statistical probability. Now it is understood that a small difference in starting conditions

Research Note

Source: Ebright, P.R., Patterson, E.S., Chalko, B.A., & Render, M.L. (2003). Understanding the complexity of registered nurse work in acute care settings. *Journal of Nursing Administration, 33*(12), 630-638.

Purpose

Complexity in nursing comes from multiple goals, obstacles, hazards, missing data, and behaviors surrounding care situations. To keep things from going wrong, nurses make decisions to adapt and manage complexity in the midst of a changing environment. The purpose of this research was to investigate RN work complexity in an acute care setting using a human performance framework. Field observations followed by semistructured interviews were the methods used with a purposive sample of eight expert RNs. The research question was this: "What human and environmental factors affect decision making by expert RNs on medical-surgical acute care units?"

Discussion

Content analysis resulted in the emergence of 22 patterns across participants that were grouped into the following three main categories:

1. Patterns of work complexity ($n = 8$) that are human and environmental factors affecting work, such as disjointed supply sources, repetitive travel, and interruptions
2. Patterns of cognitive factors driving performance and decisions ($n = 8$), such as maintaining patient safety and knowing unit routines and work flow
3. Patterns of care management strategies ($n = 6$), such as stacking and stabilizing and moving on

The results revealed multiple patterns that characterize RN work on medical/surgical acute care units and how RNs cope and adapt to manage workload demands.

Application to Practice

This study examined the actual work of RNs in the context of patient assignments within conditions of unpredictability, missing information, and unreliable access to resources and processes. The rich data suggested ways to redesign systems to decrease or better manage work complexity. The human performance framework helped to uncover routine aspects of the daily management of work that came to be seen as a series of gaps and discontinuities that serve to distract RNs from focusing on critical role functions such as clinical reasoning about patient care. Managerial actions to fix these systems gaps support the work of nursing and avoid wasting large amounts of valuable time.

can result in apparently random, quite different trajectories that are highly irregular but not without some form. Plotted over time, apparently random meanderings of these systems show a pattern to the movements. Variation stays within a pattern that repeats itself (Rosenhead, 1998).

Complexity theory has been applied to management theory. Previous management theories heavily emphasized rationality, predictability, stability, setting a mission, determining strategy, and eliminating deviation. Discoveries from complexity and chaos theories include the fact that the natural world does not operate like clockwork machinery. Key findings of complexity theory are the "effective unknowability" of the future and the understanding of the role of creative disorder. Managers need to alter their reflex behaviors, put an emphasis on "double-loop learning" that also examines appropriateness of assumptions, foster diversity, be open to strategy based on serendipity, welcome disorder as a partner, use instability positively, provoke a controlled ferment of ideas, release creativity, and seek the edge of chaos in the complex interactions that occur among people. Change management takes on a very different form when complexity theory is used (Rosenhead, 1998).

The selection of a management theory and related managerial activities may be seen as more appropriately based on ordinary versus extraordinary management needs (Stacey, 1993). Ordinary management would be selected for day-to-day operations and problem solving. It would use classic, rational management theory and Fayol's (1949) framework for planning and management, with control at the center. To deliver cost-effective performance, competent basic management is necessary (Rosenhead, 1998). Extraordinary management would be used to transform organizations under conditions of open-ended change. This form of management seeks to unlock and activate the hidden knowledge and the creativity that is potentially available. Informal groups and self-organizing teams are used. The focus is on learning and adapting. Both ordinary and extraordinary management are needed and have to be enabled to coexist for maximum effectiveness (Rosenhead, 1998; Stacey, 1993).

Chaos Theory

Chaos is seen as a particular mode of behavior within the more general field of complexity theory (Rosenhead, 1998). Sometimes the two are used together: chaos and complexity. Chaos, as used in complexity theory, is not utter confusion and disorder, but rather a system that defies prediction despite certain regularities. Chaos is the boundary zone between stability and instability, and systems in chaos exhibit bounded instability and unpredictability of specific behavior within a predictable general structure of behavior. They may pass through randomness to evolve to a higher order of self-organized complex adaptive structures (Rosenhead, 1998).

As many health care organizations move away from bureaucratic models and recognize organizations as whole systems, more organic and fluid structures are replacing the older ones. Sometimes referred to as "learning organizations," these structures are tapping into the inherent capacity for individuals to exhibit self-organization. In the transition, experiences of change, information overload, entrenched behaviors, and chaos reflect human reactions to organizations as living systems that are adapting and growing (Wheatley, 1999). Complexity and a sense of things being beyond one's control create a search for a simpler way of understanding and leading organizations.

Randomness and complexity are two principal characteristics of chaos. There is a paradox in the fact that even in the simplest of systems, it is extraordinarily difficult to accurately predict the course of events; yet some order arises spontaneously even in these simple systems. Patterns form in nature—some are orderly, and some are not orderly. Concepts of nonlinearity and feedback help to explain situations of complexity without randomness (with order). Chaos theory suggests that simple systems may give rise to complex behavior, and complex systems may exhibit simple behavior. At the essence of chaos is a fine balance between forces of stability and those of instability. Two examples are snowflake formation and the behavior of the weather.

It is difficult for minds trained in linear thinking to grasp chaos theory. In the past, the effects of nonlinearity were discounted. Much of scientific thought was based on assumptions of linearity and beliefs that small differences averaged out, slight variances converged toward a point, and approximations could give a relatively accurate picture of what could happen. It was assumed that predictability would come from learning how to account for all variables and a greater level of detail. However, the wholeness of systems resists being studied in parts. Both chaos and order are important elements in the powerful and unpredictable effects created by iteration in nonlinear systems (Wheatley, 1999). An example of chaos theory in action is when a seemingly small change, such as using assistive personnel instead of professionals, in effect creates ripples and larger impacts on the system than preplanning would seem to indicate.

There are many implications of chaos theory for health care delivery systems. The slightest variation can have enormous results in a dynamic and changing system. What is important is the quality of the system, its complexity, its distinguishing shapes, how it develops and changes, and how it differs from or compares with another system.

A search for ever-finer measures for discrete parts of the system probably is futile. Looking for themes or patterns rather than isolated causes is encouraged. Clearly, predictability still exists. However, for nonlinear variables and systems, randomness plays a key role in the creation of patterns of complexity and harmony of form (Wheatley 1999).

Chaos theory can be applied to management in health care organizations. Viewing the organization as similar to a living organism, taking a holistic approach, and trusting in a natural organizing phenomenon, the manager combines expressed expectations of acceptable behavior and the grant of the freedom to individuals to assert themselves in nondeterministic ways. Guiding principles or values create powerful motivation. The manager's job is to reveal and handle the mostly hidden dynamics of the system and forge a direction for the organization as a complex adaptive system. The goal is for a self-managed system with people capable of engaging in cooperative behavior, using feedback to learn and adapt, self-organizing, and operating with flexibility.

LEADERSHIP AND MANAGEMENT IMPLICATIONS

It can be argued that all nurses are managers. Staff nurses are the employees at the most critical point in fulfilling the purpose of health care organizations: they are in close and frequent contact with the client, and they coordinate the delivery of health care services.

The administration of nursing services is divided into two basic levels: the nurse manager and the nurse executive. Both have the responsibility to create a work environment that facilitates and encourages nursing staff and nursing practice. The nurse manager manages one or more defined areas of nursing services and is responsible to a nurse executive. Nurse managers allocate available resources, coordinate activities, facilitate interactive management, and have major responsibility for implementing the vision, mission, philosophy, goals, plans, and standards of the organization and nursing services (ANA, 2004; ANCC, 2004).

The nurse executive is responsible for managing organized nursing services from the perspective of the organization as a whole and to transform values into daily operations to produce an efficient, effective and caring organization. The nurse executive is accountable for the environment in which clinical nursing practice occurs. The nurse executive provides leadership and direction (ANA, 2004; ANCC, 2004).

The work of nursing is complex, and the role of the nurse manager is influenced by human and environmental factors in complex organizations. Being on the front lines of health care, nurse managers collaborate with others and carry out activities such as the following:

- Managing clinical nursing practice and care delivery on assigned areas

⚠ LEADERSHIP & MANAGEMENT **BEHAVIORS**

Leadership Behaviors

- Is visible
- Communicates a vision
- Motivates followers
- Seeks out new resources
- Evaluates outcomes

Management Behaviors

- Coordinates client care
- Plans daily operations
- Makes assignments
- Sets goals for subordinates
- Hires staff
- Responds to needs/desires of subordinates as long as the work is accomplished

- Exchanges rewards for work effort
- Manages resource allocation
- Monitors work and quality processes
- Takes corrective actions
- Counsels subordinates
- Manages change
- Handles conflict situations
- Communicates among levels

Overlap Areas

- Exercises broad-perspective decision making
- Communicates
- Motivates subordinates
- Evaluates process and outcomes

- Coordinating care with other disciplines to integrate services
- Managing the budget
- Managing human resources
- Being responsible for staffing and scheduling
- Evaluating the quality and appropriateness of care
- Orienting and developing employees
- Ensuring compliance with regulatory and professional standards
- Maintaining patient safety

Because of chaos, complexity, and change, client care management has needed new structures and managerial behaviors. Predicated on trust and cooperation in human relations, managers are challenged to promote consistency and stability and be anchors in an unstable world. Curtin (2000) suggested the following 10 ethical principles that might help managers to reconcile perspectives and interests while centering on mission and core values:

1. Frugality and sophisticated therapeutic skill (doing the most with the least resource expenditure)
2. Clinical credibility through organizational competence

3. Presence (visibility)
4. Responsible representation at highest levels
5. Loyal service
6. Deliberate delegation
7. Responsible innovation
8. Fiduciary accountability
9. Self-discipline
10. Continuous learning

Clearly, nurse managers and executives both need a background and ability in the day-to-day fundamentals of management to achieve goals. Beyond this, skill and ability in "extraordinary management" will serve to enhance individual and collective competence. Balancing day-to-day operations with transformative management and leadership is a creative synthesis of the best of the "old" with the best of the "new" management theories.

Management has been described as a discipline that uses a set of tools to achieve desired outcomes. It becomes nursing management when the desired outcomes are nursing goals. If management occurs at all levels of nursing, the nursing profession needs methods for assisting nurses to develop competence in management (Genovich-Richards & Carissimi, 1986). One beginning step is to measure and evaluate managerial behavior. For example, a measurement instrument was developed by Morse and Wagner (1978) to identify specific behavior and activities characteristic of managerial work. Built around Mintzberg's nine managerial roles (1973), the final instrument contained 51 items tapping six role factors. Although managerial roles are somewhat distinct, testing this instrument revealed that the factors are interrelated to a moderate degree. The final six role factors are (1) managing the organization's environment and resources, (2) organizing and coordinating, (3) information handling, (4) providing for growth and development, (5) motivating and conflict handling, and (6) strategic problem solving. This instrument can be used to measure and evaluate similarities and differences in managerial work, such as before and after restructuring occurs.

Using a conceptual framework of three domains of nursing management behaviors—client care management, operational management, and human resources management—Genovich-Richards and Carissimi (1986) described the use of a management assessment center technique for nursing. Seven key areas—(1) leadership ability; (2) decision-making skill; (3) analytical ability; (4) organizational ability; (5) group performance skill; (6) personal characteristics such as sensitivity, flexibility, and competitiveness; and (7) self-awareness—were the focus of an intensive 1-day session using exercises, simulations, and management activities for practice. A management assessment center technique is one tool that nurses can use to develop individuals and enhance their managerial skills and abilities. It could become a staff development or in-service program. This tool could be used for growth and self-assessment for staff who desire or contemplate advancement along a nursing administration career track. Management skills also need to be taught to baccalaureate nursing students (O'Halloran, 1996). A combination of simulated and practice-based experiences that apply management content can be created by using a flexible assignment plan and clinical resources.

Legal Aspects of Management

The managers of any health care organization are responsible to the policy-making body of the organization. The managers also have an obligation to comply with the laws of society at local, state, and national levels. Managers are responsible for ensuring that laws are adhered to—both in the actions of management itself and in the actions of those employees who assist the managers in carrying out the mission of the organization. Concern for the law involves three general areas: personal negligence in clinical practice, liability for delegation and supervision, and organizational liability related to employment issues.

Activities of clinical client care involve corresponding legal accountability and risk. Errors do happen. Some lead to injury to a client. At minimum, nurses have an ethical obligation to nonmaleficence (to do no harm to clients). This duty is discharged in part by remaining competent in knowledge and skills and the standards of practice. Nursing negligence occurs when nurses' actions are unreasonable given the circumstances or fail to meet the standard of care or when the nurse fails to act and causes harm. Harm can arise from acts that are unintentional, such as omissions or negligence, or it can result from acts that are intentional, such as defamation, invasion of privacy, assault and battery, false imprisonment, or intentional infliction of emotional distress (Aiken, 1994).

Four elements of negligence are required for malpractice: a duty owed to the client (e.g., to render nursing care), breach of duty, proximate cause or causal connection to the nurse, and damages. Common clinical practice areas of negligence or liability include the general areas of treatment, communication, medication, and monitoring/observing/supervising/surveillance. Examples of common negligence allegations in nursing malpractice suits include client falls, use of restraints, medication errors, burns, equipment injuries, retained foreign objects, failure to monitor, failure to ensure safety, failure to take appropriate nursing action, failure to confirm accuracy of physician's orders, improper technique or performance of treatments, failure to respond to a client, failure to follow hospital procedure, and failure to supervise treatment (Aiken, 1994).

Beyond personal liability for clinical practice, nurses and nurse managers have accountability and liability for their acts of delegation and supervision. Nurses and nurse managers both carry an obligation to report incompetent practice that occurs at any point in the care delivery process. Nurse managers have a duty to train, orient, and evaluate the ability of nursing staff to perform specific functions and tasks. Health care organizations have a duty to monitor the competence and ability of nursing and medical professionals and to inquire about their credentials (Aiken, 1994). Both nurses and nurse managers have a duty to follow policies and procedures when reasonable. Nurse managers are advised to review policies and procedures carefully, including the language used, to adhere to legal and ethical parameters more closely. Clearly, management in nursing practice means that nurses must fulfill obligations and duties both to clients and to the organization. This means using knowledge, skill, and decision making abilities to reduce the incidence of negligence and malpractice by employees as a way to reduce harm to clients and legal risk to the organization. As the primary care coordinators, nurses need to manage the environment of care delivery. Ensuring staff competence and reporting incompetent practice are key activities. For example, in nursing, legal and ethical issues arise when a nurse is impaired by substance abuse. The overall consideration is protecting the client from harm. Confronting a staff member suspected of substance abuse must be done carefully. However, when an incident occurs, the nurse manager has a responsibility to intervene.

Organizations are constrained by specific laws related to employment issues. Although the various health care providers and their employing organizations have specific legal and ethical obligations to clients, such as informed consent and preserving patients' rights as outlined in the Patient Self-Determination Act of 1990,

organizations carry specific legal and ethical obligations toward employees. The employer has an obligation to provide a safe and secure care delivery environment (Aiken, 1994). For example, the Occupational Safety and Health Administration's (OSHA's) rules and regulations must be followed. As a branch of the U.S. Department of Labor, OSHA has become involved with issues related to protecting health care workers from exposure to blood and body fluid-borne pathogens such as hepatitis B (HBV) and the virus that causes acquired immunodeficiency syndrome (AIDS), human immunodeficiency virus (HIV). By enforcement of universal precautions among health care workers, the principal idea is to prevent the transmission of the pathogens from worker to client or client to worker, thus providing a safer work environment. Guidelines from the Centers for Disease Control and Prevention (CDC) were adopted by OSHA. The mandates include use of universal precautions, employer provision of protective equipment, inspection procedures, and risk management of potentially exposed employees. The employer incurs the costs of HBV vaccine, protective equipment and supplies, and exposure prevention and management. OSHA uses the mechanisms of surprise inspections and steep fines to enlist compliance.

Employment decisions are subject to liability for wrongful failure to hire, wrongful failure to advance, and wrongful discharge. Title VII of the U.S. Civil Rights Act of 1964, the Age Discrimination and Employment Act (ADEA) of 1967, and the Americans with Disabilities Act (ADA) of 1990 are some specific pieces of federal legislation that affect hiring and employment. In addition, there are other federal statutes, governmental mandates, and state and municipal laws that prescribe and proscribe various actions that are part of or relate to the employment process.

The Equal Employment Opportunity Commission (EEOC) is a federal agency that enforces many of the federal mandates concerning discrimination. There are other federal agencies, including funding agencies, that also have enforcement responsibilities in this area. Most states and many municipalities also have antidiscrimination enforcement agencies, and some laws provide the individual employee with the opportunity to bring private litigation through the courts.

The antidiscrimination statutes, in general, were designed to protect employees from discrimination in the workplace when it is based on race, color, sexual orientation, religion, gender, pregnancy, national origin, age, or physical or mental disability. In some cases discrimination based on some of these characteristics is legally acceptable if it is based on what the law describes as a bona fide occupational qualification (BFOQ). The use of BFOQs to justify discrimination is usually defined in very narrow fashion. Two examples of gender discrimination in employment that can be justified as BFOQs are "wet nurse" and "sperm donor."

Management policies and procedures must be in compliance in the areas of hiring, performance appraisal, management of employees with problems, and termination (Aiken, 1994). Lawsuits also have formed the basis for the standards to be met for the termination of employees. Discharges may occur for lack of adherence to employer-established policies or standards, "good cause" per institutional policy, illegal activity, assault, insubordination, or excessive absenteeism. Written notice and the reasons for termination avoid misunderstandings and show justice through due-process procedures. Careful documentation is important. If the employee is a member of a protected group, the employer may be required to submit formal justification for the termination (Aiken, 1994).

The various legal and ethical considerations of nursing management span client, provider, and employer rights and obligations. Both nurses and their employing organizations are responsible for knowing and following the various applicable laws and regulations. In-service education can increase knowledge and awareness. Nurse managers need to manage the environment of nursing care to ensure client safety, provider justice and safety, and organizational compliance with the law.

CURRENT ISSUES AND TRENDS

The classic notions of management and managerial work were developed in a sociopolitical era of industrialization and bureaucratization. Currently in business and industry, competitive pressures and economic forces are compelling corporations to adopt new flexible strategies and structures. Organizations are being urged to become leaner, more entrepreneurial, and less bureaucratic. This trend has created levels of complexity and interdependency.

The result has altered conventional ideas and realities of managerial work, including shifts in roles and tasks. Traditional sources of power are eroding, and some motivational tools are less effective. The erosion of power from hierarchical positions is perceived as a loss of authority and may create confusion about how to mobilize and motivate staff (Kanter, 1989). Kanter noted that in a leaner and flatter corporation there are many more channels for action, and managers need to work synergistically with other departments. Managers' strategic and collaborative roles become more important as they serve as integrators and facilitators, not as watchdogs and interventionists.

Current and emerging issues in health care are complex and ethically challenging for managers. The "big three" issues of access, cost, and quality continue to be organizing themes that affect any organization's internal operations. Insurance coverage is an issue of access, as is the geographic location of facilities, providers, and services. Increased complexity and technology prompt provider specialization and affect cost. Consumer preferences and increased health care awareness levels affect both cost and quality. Critical medical errors and patient safety issues create pressure related to the need for quality. Complexity, randomness, and chaos created by change all call for new management and leadership strategies.

Within health care delivery systems, issues and trends facing today's managers include the following:

- Management of populations with chronic illnesses
- Resources to acquire technology on an ongoing basis
- The need for primary and preventive services and programs, including complementary and alternative programs
- Integration and seamlessness of clinical and financial services and information
- Protection of consumers' privacy
- Shortages of key personnel, especially registered nurses
- Financing structures such as capitation and managed care
- Care delivery and process management
- Management of knowledge workers and personal accountability
- Pressures for quality and sustainable outcomes
- Leadership skills related to change management

Herzliner (1998) predicted a managerial revolution in the U.S. health care sector. He critiqued vertically integrated systems and managed care organizations and noted that they cannot provide the convenient, supportive, moderate cost health care that is desired by the U.S. public. It is likely that "focused factories" will arise in response to the "everything-for-everybody" current situation. In health care, these focused organizations would consist of a multidisciplinary team of health care providers who have frequent interaction to achieve focused goals such as delivering services for complex medical problems. Other foci might include care for a chronic disease, handling a high volume of diagnoses, or providing information and support. This phenomenon has been manifested in the rise of case management and disease management processes and programs. These structures will proliferate if there is sufficient market pressure for them.

Drucker (1988) used the hospital, the university, and a symphony orchestra as models for organizations evolving in today's society. As health care reconfigures, health care delivery settings will likely be knowledge-based organizations composed primarily of specialists whose performance is directed by organized feedback from colleagues, clients, and headquarters. Nurses are positioned at the care coordination intersection and have needed skills for facilitating flow and integrating care delivery. Nurses' roles may change, but their need for managerial competence will remain. Nurses are well prepared to serve as integrators and facilitators of client care. Thus nurses appear to move easily into management and blend care into management for effectiveness (Mintzberg, 1994).

Summary

- A manager's job is to coordinate and integrate resources.
- Classical management theory defined the management process as planning, organizing, coordinating or directing, and controlling.
- Mintzberg described ten roles that managers play.
- Mintzberg developed a model of managerial work that elaborated on managerial roles.
- New managerial theories emphasize contingency, complexity, and chaos.
- All nurses are managers; they coordinate and deliver health services to clients.
- As institutions adopt new flexible strategies and structures, managerial roles and tasks are being reconfigured.
- Nurses have valuable related skills of coordination and integration.

Study Questions

1. Which concept is more important: leadership or management? Why?
2. Why is management important to a nurse?
3. Describe a scenario in which middle managers become obsolete.
4. How do Mintzberg's ten roles differ for nurses at different positions in a hierarchical bureaucracy?

5. Why is it easier for nurses to change to a new managerial role than it is for other types of health care workers?

6. In what way is case management a managerial role? How can the clinical focus be described as management?

CASE STUDY

Nurse Anthony Kaufman is the director of Ambulatory Clinic A. Last year he participated in strategic planning for all the ambulatory clinics. A plan for Clinic A also was developed and approved. This year Nurse Kaufman concentrated on fine-tuning the management of the clinic. He developed a data tracking system, and trend data are now in. One disturbing trend is the rise in visit cancellations. Although the rate of cancellations is not a threat to clinic management, the increase needs to be evaluated. He does further analysis and discovers that the increase has been occurring mostly among adult females of the Muslim religion. Nurse Kaufman needs to determine the root cause: Is this an issue of individual staff cultural sensitivity, a systems problem, or some other cause?

The data are shared with the staff, and a brainstorming session occurs. One of the staff has a terrific idea: to use community contacts and internal group leaders to help inform the clinic staff as to the problem(s). The marketing and social services departments are enlisted to help. They set up round-table gatherings, championed by the local leaders among Muslim women. One major concern emerges from these meetings: the traditional hospital gown is too revealing, unacceptable, and embarrassing. Many Muslim women had cancelled appointments for this very reason. The information is eye-opening for Nurse Kaufman. First, he is glad that it was not a staff performance issue. Second, it had never occurred to him. Hospital gowns have been the same for a very long time, and no one questions them. He calls another meeting, explores the results with staff, and asks for creative solutions. This seems like a simple managerial move. However, as the mostly female staff members begin to analyze the issue, they become excited about the possibility of a needed change. Nurse Kaufman is afraid that things might spin out of control as nurses discuss hospital gown redesign options, such as contacting New York name-brand designers. Eventually the process is worked through, using multidisciplinary collaboration, and a new gown design with extra coverage is approved and ordered.

CRITICAL THINKING EXERCISE

Nurse Su-lin Zhang sits down to the computer and opens up a new document file. It is time to put some thoughts down in writing. The long-term care facility where she works recently merged with a private, for-profit integrated delivery system dominated by administrators from the acute care hospital. In the aftermath of the merger, a form of program or product-line management was instituted that uses interdisciplinary teams. In addition, her long-term care facility will be competing against the other ones in the network based on "best practices" benchmarks that have not yet been specified. Nurse Zhang wants to be sure that her facility comes out in first place.

1. What problem(s) do you see in this scenario?
2. Why is this a problem?
3. What are the issues involved?
4. How might Nurse Zhang handle the situation?
5. What should Nurse Zhang do with her text when it is completed?
6. What management role would be best suited to this situation?
7. What management strategy might be most effective?

REFERENCES

Ackoff, R. (1981). *Creating the corporate future.* New York: John Wiley & Sons.

Aiken, T. (1994). *Legal, ethical, and political issues in nursing.* Philadelphia: F.A. Davis.

American Nurses Association (ANA). (2004). *Scope and standards for nurse administrators.* (2nd ed.). Washington, DC: ANA.

American Nurses Credentialing Center (ANCC). (2004). *ANCC certification: Specialty nursing, nursing administration (basic, advanced) clinical nurse specialist (community health and home health).* Washington, DC: ANA.

Bass, B., & Avolio, B. (1990). *Transformational leadership development: Manual for the Multifactor Leadership Questionnaire.* Palo Alto, CA: Consulting Psychologists Press.

Crowell, D.M. (1998). Organizations are relationships: A new view of management. *Nursing Management, 29*(5), 28-29.

Curtin, L.L. (2000). The first ten principles for the ethical administration of nursing services. *Nursing Administration Quarterly, 25*(1), 7-13.

Drucker, P.F. (1954). *The practice of management.* New York: Harper & Row.

Drucker, P.F. (1988). The coming of the new organization. *Harvard Business Review, 68*(1), 45-53.

Drucker, P.F. (2004). What makes an effective executive. *Harvard Business Review, 82*(6), 58-63.

Fayol, H. (1949). *General and industrial management.* London: Pitman & Sons.

Foust, J. (1994). Creating a future for nursing through interactive planning at the bedside. *Image, 26*(2), 129-131.

Genovich-Richards, J., & Carissimi, D. (1986). Developing nurses' managerial competence. *Nursing Management, 17*(3), 36-38.

Gosling, J., & Mintzberg, H. (2003). The five minds of a manager. *Harvard Business Review, 81*(11), 54-63.

Hayes-Roth, B., & Hayes-Roth, F. (1979). A cognitive model of planning. *Cognitive Science, 3,* 275-310.

Hersey, P., Blanchard, K.H., & Johnson, D.E. (2001). *Management of organizational behavior: Leading human resources* (8th ed.). Upper Saddle River, NJ: Prentice-Hall.

Herzliner, R.E. (1998). The managerial revolution in the U.S. health care sector: Lessons from the U.S. economy. *Health Care Management Review, 23*(3), 19-29.

Kanter, R.M. (1989). The new managerial work. *Harvard Business Review, 69*(6), 85-92.

Katz, R. (1955). Skills of an effective administrator. *Harvard Business Review, 33*(1), 33-42.

Kepler, T. (1980). Mastering the people skills. *Journal of Nursing Administration, 10*(11), 15-20.

Koontz, H. (1961). The management theory jungle. *Academy of Management Journal, December,* 174-188.

Levenstein, A. (1985). Planning. *Nursing Management, 16*(9), 54-55.

Lewin, K. (1947). Frontiers in group dynamics: Concept, method, and reality in social science; social equilibria and social change. *Human Relations, 1*(1), 5-41.

McClure, M. (1991). Introduction. In I. Goertzen (Ed.), *Differentiating nursing practice: Into the twenty-first century* (pp. 1-11). Kansas City, MO: American Academy of Nursing.

McNamara, C. (1999a). *Skills and practices in organizational management.* Minneapolis, MN: Carter McNamara. Retrieved July 6, 2004, from *www.managementhelp.org/mgmnt/skills.htm*

McNamara, C. (1999b). *Basic guidelines for successful planning process.* Minneapolis, MN: Carter McNamara. Retrieved July 6, 2004, from *www.managementhelp.org/plan_dec/gen_plan/gen_plan.htm*

McNamara, C. (1999c). *Management function of organizing: Overview of methods.* Minneapolis, MN: Authenticity Consulting, LLC. Retrieved July 6, 2004, from *www.mapnp.org/library/orgnzing/orgnzing.htm*

McNamara, C. (1999d). *Management function of coordinating/controlling: Overview of basic methods.* Minneapolis, MN: Authenticity Consulting, LLC. Retrieved July 6, 2004, from *www.mapnp.org/library/cntrllng/cntrllng.htm*

McNamara, C. (1999e). *Introduction to management.* Minneapolis, MN: Authenticity Consulting, LLC. Retrieved July 6, 2004, from *www.managementhelp.org/mng_thry/mng_thry.htm*

McNamara, C. (1999f). *New paradigm in management.* Minneapolis, MN: Carter McNamara. Retrieved July 6, 2004, from *www.managementhelp.org/mgmnt/paradigm.htm*

McNamara, C. (1999g). *Brief overview of contemporary theories in management.* Minneapolis, MN: Authenticity Consulting, LLC. Retrieved July 6, 2004, from *www.managementhelp.org/mgmnt/cntmpory.htm*

Mintzberg, H. (1973). *The nature of managerial work.* New York: Harper & Row.

Mintzberg, H. (1975). The manager's job: Folklore and fact. In M. Matteson, & J. Ivancevich (Eds.), *Management classics* (3rd ed.) (pp. 63-85). Plano, TX: Business Publications.

Mintzberg, H. (1994). Managing as blended care. *Journal of Nursing Administration, 24*(9), 29-36.

Morse, J.J., & Wagner, F.R. (1978). Measuring the process of managerial effectiveness. *Academy of Management Journal, 21*(1), 23-35.

O'Halloran, V.E. (1996). Teaching management skills in the clinical setting: An essential curriculum component. *Journal of New York State Nurses Association, 27*(4), 7-9.

Organizational Dynamics. (1975). *The evolution of management theory: Part I* [Videotape]. Burlington, MA: Organizational Dynamics.

Porter-O'Grady, T. (1997). Process leadership and the death of management. *Nursing Economic$, 15*(6), 286-293.

Rosenhead, J. (1998). Complexity theory and management practice. *The Human Nature Daily Review.* Retrieved July 6,

2004, from *www.human-nature.com/science-as-culture/ rosenhead.html*

Stacey, R.D. (1993). *Strategic management and organizational dynamics.* London: Pitman.

Steiner, G. (1962). Making long-range company planning pay off. *California Management Review, 4*(2), 28-41.

Sull, D.N. (2003). Managing by commitments. *Harvard Business Review, 81*(6), 82-91.

Thomas, L. (1983). *The youngest science: Notes of a medicine watcher.* New York: Viking Press.

von Bertalanffy, L. (1968). *General systems theory.* New York: George Braziller.

Wheatley, M.J. (1999). *Leadership and the new science: Discovering order in a chaotic world* (2nd ed.). San Francisco: Berrett-Koehler Publishers

Zaleznik, A. (1992). Managers and leaders: Are they different? *Harvard Business Review, 70*(2), 126-135.

II

THE PROFESSIONAL'S ROLE

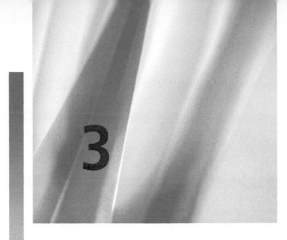

Professional Practice and Career Development

Mary K. Anthony

3

CHAPTER OBJECTIVES

- Overview professional nursing practice
- Analyze factors that influence nursing as a profession
- Formulate an understanding of the role of the nurse
- Define and describe a profession
- Analyze aspects of careers in nursing
- Exercise critical thinking to conceptualize and analyze possible solutions to a practice experience

At some point, each nurse made the decision to enter the profession of nursing. This decision may have been made for a variety of reasons, including a desire to help people, a motivation toward healing, the role modeling of a significant person, or job security. For some, nursing was an attractive occupation offering a variety of jobs. For other nurses, there was a strong motivation toward life-long work in a career. Each nurse responds to a unique composite of values, goals, interests, and aspirations on the path of work chosen over an adult life span. Examining these elements helps the nurse to better understand the work of nursing and his or her own career path.

The work of a professional extends over an anticipated lifetime of occupational service, encompassing activity, employment, and productivity. Career commitment is a nurse's attitude toward nursing as a profession or vocation and is the motivation to work in a chosen career role. Commitment to a career is different from commitment to a job or to an organization. Commitment to a career is important in nursing because of its relationship to the attraction, development, satisfaction, and retention of staff nurses in organizations and to the overall profession.

Nurses play an important role in providing care and contributing to the health of society. Nursing has had a long history of establishing itself as a profession with a unique perspective. Contemporary nursing is a complex practice profession that reflects an evolutionary composite of influences coming from the profession of nursing, society at large, changes in health care economics, care delivery systems, management of exploding health information, and changing population demographics. These influences have shaped and will continue to shape the past, present, and future of nursing. These powerful influences have contributed to, or in some cases hindered, the practice of profession of nursing. Specifically, the role of the professional nurse has been influenced by legal, professional, and organizational forces.

The first influence comes from a legal perspective. The practice of nursing is a regulated profession, meaning that the scope of practice for nurses is defined through governmental laws at the state level. The intention behind regulation comes from governmental mandates to provide oversight for the health, welfare, and safety of the public. There are four approaches to regulation: designation/recognition, registration, certification, and licensure (NCSBN, 1999). Designation/recognition is the least restrictive approach to regulation and provides the public with information about special credentials. Registration is the second level of regulation and involves having the person's name on an official roster maintained by a particular agency that can provide services. Persons who are registered and meet certain requirements are permitted to use titles that go along with being registered. Certification is the third level of regulation. It imposes a more stringent form of regulation and is given when identified requirements are met. Those who meet the requirements are then permitted to use an associated title that recognizes their professional competence. Both professional organizations and regulatory boards use various processes of certification. Specialty certification implies that certain standards have been met that often require taking a certifying exam. For example, the practice of advanced practice nurses is governed by certification and is required for third-party reimbursement and prescriptive authority. Licensure occurs when the "agency of the state government grants permission to an individual to engage in a given profession upon a finding that the applicant has attained the minimal degree of competency necessary to perform a unique scope of practice" (NCSBN, 1999, p. 17). This regulatory method is used when regulated activities are complex and require specialized knowledge and skill and independent decision making. In each of the 50 states, licensure laws define the legal boundaries and scope of professional nursing practice and are passed in the state legislature. State Boards of Nursing are regulatory agencies that are given the authority by the legislature to enact those laws.

Licensure of nurses is more than 100 years old. New Zealand was the first country to license nurses in 1901, and the state of North Carolina was the first state to enact a registration law in 1903. New York was the first state to adopt a mandatory licensure law in 1938 (NCSBN, 1999). By the 1970s licensing of all registered nurses, regardless of educational preparation, became mandatory in all states and U.S. jurisdictions, and by 1996, advanced practice nursing also became regulated in 49 of 50 states (NCSBN, 1999).

The second influence on professional nursing practice comes from professional organizations. Professional organizations provide nurses with an avenue for a collective voice to shape standards of practice and address health care issues to shape policy (Logan et al., 2004). Numerous professional organizations exist, representing the professional interests of nurses who work in a variety of settings such as critical care, home care, long-term care, and schools, as well as in a variety of specialties such as orthopedics and neurology. In addition to these specialized organizations, the American Nurses Association (ANA) is the professional organization that represents all of the 2.7 million American registered nurses. The distinction between the ANA and the multiple other nursing professional and specialty organizations is that the ANA is nursing's referent professional organization for the practice of nursing. As such, it has promulgated the standardized definition of nursing, standards of practice for nursing, and nursing's code of ethics. These documents reflect nursing's professionalism and are the documents looked to in legal cases regarding the scope and practice of nursing. The ANA also represents nursing in the health policy arena as the collective voice of nursing.

The ANA is more than 100 years old, having first been established in 1896 as the Nurses Associated Alumnae of the United States. It began drafting bylaws and a constitution for its first meeting in 1897 (ANA, 2002a). The mission of ANA is to promote nursing practice by defining and supporting ethical and practice standards consistent with high-quality nursing practice, promoting the economic and noneconomic rights of nurses in the work place, promoting an image of professional nursing practice that realistically reflects the breadth and scope of practice, and lobbying Congress and other regulatory bodies on health care issues that affect both nurses and the public (ANA, 1997). Although the ANA represents all nurses, only 5% of U.S. nurses belong (Stierle, 2003). This has a powerful effect on the relative influence that nurses have in shaping health policy and in mobilizing collective power. Because a hallmark of a profession is its collective self-representation, nurses bear a responsibility to belong to their professional organization.

The third influence on professional nursing practice arises from the workplace. Most nurses work in a formalized health care organization, such as a long-term care facility, home care agency, or a hospital. An organization influences nursing practice by defining the structural and contextual environment in which nurses practice. For instance, the structural dimensions of organizations shape nursing practice by having policies related to nurses' roles, workload, and working environment, while the contextual aspects of the organization shape the amount of control over practice. As a result of organizational influences, nurses' roles and the environment in which they practice are changing. For instance, as the health care labor force becomes more diverse in job roles, nurses spend less time providing direct care and more time delegating and supervising persons with lower skill and knowledge. Nurses' workloads also are changing as a consequence of an aging population and related social forces. In some cases, such as in California, the legislatures have passed mandatory nurse-patient ratios. On the other hand, for financial viability reasons in health care, organizations have imposed constraints on how nurses practice by encouraging shorter lengths of stay or fewer visits that allow less time for nurses' interventions such as patient teaching.

To address these and other issues, many work places such as hospitals are working toward achieving Magnet status. Magnet recognition is an award of achievement conferred by the ANA's credentialing body, the American Nurses Credentialing

Center (ANCC), to recognize facilities that provide quality nursing care and create a work environment that recognizes, rewards, and promotes professional nursing and positive patient outcomes (ANCC, 2003a). Dating back to 1982, studies have been conducted to define the best places for nurses to work. These were characterized as places where nurses have autonomy, control over practice, and collaborative relationships with physicians, other nurses, and administrators. The ideal work environment had adequate numbers of staff and good support services (McClure et al., 1982). Today there are renewed efforts by hospitals to achieve Magnet recognition, a designation developed in 1994 by the ANCC. Because the Magnet Recognition Program™ is based on evaluation of quality indicators and ANA's standards, Magnet designation is seen as a "seal of approval" regarding the quality of nursing care in that institution. Evidence of upholding professional nursing practice is central to the basis for magnet recognition. Institutions seek Magnet status for its prestige and evidence of quality. Nurses seek employment in Magnet hospitals for the prestige and evidence of a desirable work environment. Magnet hospitals have demonstrated evidence of having programs that attract and retain registered nurses.

DEFINITIONS

Profession

A **profession** is defined as an occupational group. There are general professions (e.g., professional plumbers) and learned professions (e.g., law and medicine). A **professional** is an individual engaged in a profession by virtue of meeting and

⚠ LEADING & MANAGING **DEFINED**

Profession	**Professionalism**
An occupational group.	*Individual:* extent to which the member adheres to standards and ethics and identifies with a profession; *group:* degree to which a group defines, standardizes, and directs its own practice.
Professional	
Individual engaged in a profession.	

conforming to standards and sometimes licensure. **Professionalism** of an **individual** is the extent to which the person adheres to standards, practices ethically, and identifies with the profession. In the collective **group,** professionalism refers to the degree to which a group defines the profession, establishes standards and an ethical code, and directs its own practice and evolution.

Nursing Roles

The practice of nursing occurs in a variety of settings with a diverse set of roles than can be interdependent, simultaneous, or overlapping. A role is defined as both the expected and actual behaviors of an individual in a specific position. The enactment of a role depends on being in relationship with another person and provides guidance for appropriate behaviors that are unique to that role (Cresia, 1996). Roles in nursing can be broadly thought of as falling into one of two categories: provider of services or coordinator of care. McClure (1991) described the nurse's twofold role as caregiver and integrator. The caregiver role is more closely identified with basic nursing practice. It includes functions such as dependency care, comfort, education, therapeutic treatments, and monitoring. The caregiver role is most closely aligned with the concept of the traditional bedside staff nurse.

The integrator role is one of performing a coordinative function in complex organizations and work groups. The function of monitoring links the caregiver and integrator roles. The integrator role has become central to complex health care and is seen as vital to continuity of care. Because all clients need care management, the coordination and integration of client and family care needs to be linked into the services of specialized care providers and across settings and sites of service. Because today nurses are so well positioned as care integrators, some have called this the "age of the nurse." The scope and functions of professional nursing practice are changing and evolving. Yet the basic roles of caregiver and integrator endure. They undergird what nursing is and does to meet its societal mission.

There are numerous roles for nurses. Clinicians who provide one-to-one care to patients to meet their physical, emotional, and psychological needs are usually thought of as bedside nurses, but this role also includes nurses who provide care in clinics, in the home, or in schools. Administrators have primary responsibility for managing the work environment. They may be responsible for budgeting, personnel, productivity, and setting goals. In managing the environment, administrators are responsible for the care given to a group of patients and to promote an optimum and safe work environment. Administrators are found in all levels of the organization. In a hospital, they are first line unit managers, supervisors, or senior executives. In each of these administrative roles, the scope of responsibility for guiding patient care and managing the work environment varies.

Education is another role of the professional nurse. It is divided into subroles that differ in purpose and function. Educator roles can be informal or formal. Bedside nurses often assume a simultaneous role as an educator when they provide teaching to patients. However, there are formal educator roles that exist in the clinical practice setting and in academia. In the clinical setting, educators often assume the function of managing a centralized orientation and provide continuing education for nurses. Some educators in the clinical arena are exclusively hired to teach patients how to maintain wellness in light of their physical disease, such as in the role of a diabetic educator. Advanced practice nurses who are clinical nurse specialists also have roles as educators that can include education for nurses or patients. In academia, educators provide the structure for conveying and generating knowledge and for teaching and learning about nursing. They may teach in associate degree programs, diploma programs, or at the college and university level. Educators are responsible for the didactic and clinical aspects of nursing education and for developing and disseminating nursing's knowledge base.

Regardless of whether the nurse is a clinician, administrator, or educator, nurses have an ethical and social responsibility to advocate for patients.

Advocacy permeates whatever role a nurse assumes. Advocacy is at the heart of nursing's value system and means that the nurse works on behalf of patients to promote autonomous decision making and to protect patients' rights (Oermann, 1997).

Other roles of the professional nurse have evolved as a consequence of societal developments, growth in health care's technological complexity, and knowledge expansion. For instance, case managers oversee the care given to a group of patients. This role is designed to control costs while maintaining quality. Advanced practice nurses such as nurse practitioners, nurse midwives and nurse anesthetists assume blended medical and nursing roles for diagnosis, management and care of specific patient populations. Nurse researchers have important roles in generating a body of knowledge that is specific to nursing practice and that advances the science. Whatever the individual role of the nurse, nurses view themselves as professionals. But what does that mean?

NURSING AS A PROFESSION

Whether nursing is a profession or an occupation has been debated for decades. An occupation is defined as on-the-job training, a job that usually does not include specialized knowledge, a set of values, beliefs, and ethics, or a lasting commitment (Larisey, 1996). In contrast, a profession has distinctive characteristics. Numerous authors have listed criteria necessary for a profession. Perhaps the most noted author is Flexner (1910, 1915), who identified a profession as one that has intellectual activities, is learned, is practical and can be taught through education, and has a strong internal organization of members who have a desire to help others. Greenwood (1957) characterized professions as having skills that flow from a systematic body of theory, a distinctive culture, community sanction of its power and privileges, a code of ethics, and authority. Hall (1968) described a profession by its structure and attitudinal characteristics: a formalized use of professional associations, belief in self-regulation and service to the public, a sense of being called to the

profession, and a sense of commitment and autonomy in which the professional is free to exercise judgment and decision making. Bixler and Bixler (1959) translated these criteria for nurses and identified characteristics of a nursing profession as having specialized knowledge gained through scientific investigations, knowledge learned in institutions of higher education, knowledge applied to improve and to benefit human and social welfare, autonomy, attraction to individuals who are motivated to serve others, and providing opportunities for continuous learning and economic security. Despite variation in the number of criteria, four common themes emerge in the definition of a profession: a specialized body of knowledge, service, autonomy, and a professional code of ethics.

Knowledge

In the past, nursing had been criticized for not having its own body of specialized knowledge. Specialized knowledge is knowledge that is viewed from a unique disciplinary perspective. In nursing this has focused around four main concepts: nursing, person, environment, and health (Fitzpatrick & Whall, 2005). With the advent of more nurses with doctoral degrees, the development of an organized and unique body of knowledge in nursing is emerging through the work of nurse researchers and theorists. Specialized knowledge is obtained from basic nursing education and through continuing education. It is especially important for nurses to have access to the evidence base for practice and be able to use this to improve care and services.

Licensure is the process by which an agency of state government grants permission to an individual to engage in a given profession upon finding that the applicant has attained the essential degree of competency necessary to perform a unique scope of practice (NCSBN, 2004, p. 1).

Obtaining a license from a state to become a registered nurse generally requires that the individual must have completed a certain level of education.

There are three major educational paths to registered nursing: a bachelor's of science degree in nursing (BSN), an associate degree in nursing (ADN), and a diploma. BSN programs, offered by colleges and universities, take about 4 years to complete. In 2002, 678 nursing programs offered degrees at the bachelor's level. ADN programs, offered by community and junior colleges, take about 2 to 3 years to complete. About 700 RN programs in 2002 were at the ADN level. Diploma programs, administered in hospitals, last about 3 years. Only a small and declining number of programs offer diplomas. Generally, licensed graduates of any of the three types of educational programs qualify for entry-level positions as staff nurses (U.S. Department of Labor, Bureau of Labor Statistics, 2004, p. 1).

Traditional nursing education programs in the United States prepare an individual to sit for the basic licensure examination as a registered nurse. A new type of educational program that has developed to prepare individuals for licensure as an RN is the second degree program for individuals who already have a baccalaureate degree in another field. More specialty programs have emerged, such as RN to BSN, RN to MSN, and RN to DSN or ND, to accelerate educational attainment.

The flexibility in the educational programs available for preparation for entry to nursing practice is an advantage to meet the personal circumstances of many individuals and provide a more open door to the profession. However, such diversity also is a disadvantage because of the resulting lack of a standardized "product" of nursing education and subsequent dissonance in practice and image issues.

The lack of a requirement for a baccalaureate degree as the minimum entry into the practice of nursing has placed nursing at a disadvantage in the workplace. Power and respect are more difficult to obtain when nurses with less than a baccalaureate degree are compared with other professions with master's or other graduate degrees.

These options for entry-level education have generated a significant debate and dissension within the profession since 1965, when the ANA recommended that the basic entry into the profession should be a baccalaureate degree. Currently, nurses take the same licensing exam regardless of whether they attend a 2-, 3-, or 4-year program. There are many stakeholders involved in this decision, as well as issues of cost, equity, loyalty, and professional identity. Thus 40 years later, nursing has not yet reached the goal of a baccalaureate minimum. Recently, the Association of California Nurse Leaders developed an initiative to upgrade the entry level of nurses into nursing by recommending that by 2010, the entry level of all California nurses be a baccalaureate degree (Barter & McFarland, 2001). Until the profession takes a stand and requires a baccalaureate education, nursing will be plagued with the notion of being undereducated and not meeting the criteria to be accepted as a full profession. Unfortunately, baccalaureate education as the entry level into nursing is not likely to become a widespread reality in the foreseeable future, especially with the current projected nurse shortage.

A second aspect to acquiring specialized knowledge is the need for lifelong learning achieved through ongoing continuing education. As the world in general and health care specifically changes, knowledge is needed to grow and keep pace with updated information. The usefulness of existing knowledge changes more rapidly than ever before. To this end, many states have continuing education requirements as a prerequisite to license renewal. Nurses are knowledge workers who are human capital assets to their organizations. Thus investment in continuing education is an organizational imperative for effectiveness.

Service

Service is a universally accepted criterion for a profession and one that nurses meet by virtue of providing service to society. The service of nursing is the work of providing personalized care in meeting the health needs of those who are ill and those who are well. It is the work of providing physical, psychological, and emotional care. Nursing service provides teaching and comfort. It is the work that goes into improving a person's quality of life. The values and beliefs of a service orientation have a relationship with how that service is organized and delivered. For example, the religious origins of nursing have led to a conceptualization of service that includes self-sacrifice. This view that service equates to personal self-sacrifice has not served the profession well. For instance, nurses' pay was held low for many years, with a prevailing assumption that nurses should be motivated by a self-sacrificing service orientation. Today there is a different view of service in nursing. The nursing service orientation includes the following three characteristics (Logan et al., 2004):

- Commitment to the standards of practice and lifelong learning
- Commitment to the community of nurses that share common goals
- Commitment to civility (nurse to nurse) despite individual differences (p. 55)

The medium in which nurses have typically delivered service to society has been through face-to-face interactions. As health care becomes more complex and the supply of nurses drops, technology will play a more prominent role in how service is delivered. Various forms of telehealth have already redefined the methods by which service is provided, and this trend is projected to continue.

Autonomy

Society grants professionals, by virtue of their specialized body of knowledge, the right to control their own activities and thus to regulate their own practice (Greenwood, 1957). Autonomy in nursing includes both knowledge and competence in exercising the freedom and the authority to act independently and to control one's practice; it applies to both decisions and actions within one's scope of practice (Ballou, 1998; Larisey, 1996). However, the degree to which nurses can exercise their autonomy is limited by several factors. First, each state has a nurse practice act that defines the scope of nursing practice. It sets the boundaries over which nurses can exercise their autonomy. Second, most nurses work in organizations with policies and procedures that place limits on the degree to which nurses can exercise their autonomy. Even though autonomy is characteristic of a profession, the practice of nursing requires a dependent, interdependent, and independent role that is part of a collaborative framework. Providing quality care is an interdisciplinary effort, and research has shown that better outcomes are achieved when care is delivered within a collaborative framework (Mitchell et al., 1989). In this sense, the nurse's role is as an interdependent team member, but autonomy as a unique professional is maintained.

Ethics

Ethical codes are guidelines for professional groups for decision making based on values and standards for ethical conduct. Ethical decision making includes six primary principles that nurses balance: principles of justice (*fairness*), autonomy (*freedom to decide and act*), fidelity (*accountability*), beneficence (*to do good*), nonmalfeasance (*to avoid harm*), and veracity (*truthfulness*). The historical traditions of nursing have been concerned with the rights of persons and the ethical standards of professionals who serve those persons. In response to these concerns, the ANA defined a nursing Code of Ethics in 1950 with revisions in 1985 and 2001. The Code of Ethics consists of nine statements with subprovisions that mandate the standards of conduct for its practitioners (ANA, 2001).

In summary, nursing clearly meets some of the criteria for full status as a profession but not others. Debate exists among professional leaders and scholars as to whether and where on a continuum of professionalization nursing exists. Organizations such as the ANA identify nursing as a profession (ANA, 1997). Etzioni (1969), however, distinguished between semiprofessional and professional occupations. Semiprofessionals were seen as having less education, less specialized body of knowledge, less autonomy, and less status than fully professional groups. Etzioni labeled nursing as a semiprofession. Thus it is unclear whether or not nursing is a full or mature profession.

PROFESSIONALIZATION

Professionalism is important to nurses because it affects the way nurses think about themselves and their work. However, historical and contemporary issues have affected nursing's travels on the road to becoming a fully accepted profession. The image of nursing has not historically been one that has promoted the social value of nursing as a profession. In the pre-Nightingale era, nursing was affiliated with the religious who nursed within the context of selflessness, altruism, obedience, and passivity. During these early ages, nursing was often conducted in the home and thus thought of as being intuitive, as mothering, and as the work of an "angel of mercy" (Strodtman, 1997). Images began to change with Florence Nightingale, who during the Crimean War demonstrated the benefits of an organized, knowledge-based approach to caring for patients. Nightingale's notable contributions included recognizing the influence of the environment on health, identifying the need for research in building the base for nursing knowledge, and establishing a school of nursing (Strodtman, 1997).

Long-standing images of nurses have been difficult to overcome in light of the need to be autonomous decision makers. In more contemporary times, the image of nursing has paralleled the changes in social roles for women that reflect independence and autonomy, but the image of nurses portrayed by the media has not followed this social movement. In general, the media image of nursing has yet to adequately inform the public of what nurses do. "Television nurses" often are portrayed as a being in a technical career that is tangential to physician work, doing less important tasks, and only advancing professionally by going to medical school (Summers & Summers, 2004). This image of nursing does not reflect the critical thinking, judgment, and expertise that are hallmarks of contemporary nursing practice.

Gender has been a deterrent to the image of nursing as a profession as well. With nearly 94% of the workforce being female, nursing is characterized as a women's profession that has not been legitimized for men (Evans, 1997). Thus carryover effects from women's roles in society in general are often seen in nursing. These include issues related to power, authority, and influence. At least in part because nursing is a predominately female profession and is rooted in subservient historical traditions, nurses often speak and act as an oppressed group. Furthermore, myths exist that have limited or diminished the presence and voice of nurses in important health care matters. These myths include the idea of nurses being "born to be nurses" because they are nurturing, gentle, and womanly, as well as women becoming nurses to improve their marriage prospects or to be physicians' helpers (Hughes, 2001). On the other hand, men are a minority in nursing and have been criticized for separating themselves from their female colleagues by occupying roles and positions of power and prestige (Evans, 1997).

Despite these barriers, some important initiatives are occurring that enhance the image of nursing and support its acceptance as a profession. For instance, in 2002, the Johnson and Johnson company invested in a multimillion-dollar nationwide effort to address the nursing shortage. "The Campaign for Nursing's Future" included television ads to recruit and retain nurses. The recent emphasis by the ANCC for Magnet status has paralleled industry efforts to highlight excellent organizations. There is also a growing emphasis on recognizing professional achievement through certification. More than 150,000 nurses are certified in one of the 40 specialty areas offered by the ANCC (2003b). Certification recognizes personal achievement in expertise. Certifications are often recognized by employing institutions for rewards, increased pay, and status. In 1993, the status of the Nursing Center within the National Institute of Health (NIH) was raised to the level of an Institute, creating the National Institute for Nursing Research (NINR) and thus recognizing the important contributions of nursing research to the health of the American public. NINR's yearly budgets, although small in comparison to those of other NIH institutes, have increased, providing another signal of the importance of nursing research (NIH, 2003). The recent research by Aiken and colleagues (2002) that demonstrated the effects of staffing on mortality has been a critical contribution to the image of nurses and their work. These and other movements can provide the beginning of a groundswell that enhances the external view of nursing as a profession.

CAREERS

For professionals, there is a difference between a job and a career (Brink, 1988). A job is defined as an offered position, a contract with an employer for day-to-day work that is performed for pay. A career is an investment in a chosen path, made with the self for a satisfying pattern of professional contributions. A career encompasses a practical, self-directed lifelong plan for personal and professional growth that includes investment and involvement in a chosen field. Having a career means having a professional trajectory over a lifetime of employment that may include organizational advancement, making multiple lateral career moves, or assuming entrepreneurial or intrapreneurial opportunities.

As people grow and mature, they transcend different phases of adulthood based on their needs, values, and changing circumstances. Henderson and McGettigan (1994) identified the following eight stages of adulthood:

1. Transition to adulthood (18-22 years)
2. Young adulthood (23-30 years)
3. Adulthood (31-37 years)
4. Transition to mid-adulthood (38-45 years)
5. Mid-adulthood (46-53 years)
6. Transition to later adulthood (54-61 years)
7. Later adulthood (62-69 years)
8. Senior adulthood (70+ years)

Typical activities correspond to adult developmental stages and range from exploring identity (18 to 22), to balancing one's life (46 to 53), to doing what one is able and remembering (70+).

Clearly, as adults progress through predictable development stages, their needs, values, and inclinations will vary over time and in degree or strength. Thus for nurses, growth and development changes affect the balance among work, self, and family needs and roles. This inevitably impacts individuals' work and career needs and decisions. It can be predicted that needs related to

a career will vary throughout the course of an adult's life. Changing career needs that parallel changing adult developmental stages appear to be normal and natural dynamics. However, many view careers as static, not dynamic.

Nurses can enhance their career development efforts through periodic self-analysis of their needs and goals. Centering within a career trajectory is enhanced by self-awareness and self-assessment activities (Figure 3.1). Self-assessment can be applied to career decision points, such as decisions about accepting a job, moving to a new job location, returning to school, sitting for certification in a specialization, or moving from full-time to part-time work. Nurses can explore and analyze the stage they are currently in and then project where they want to advance toward. One way to do this is to examine the individual talents, value, and motives as they apply to an individual who has unique needs and talents and is in a specific developmental stage.

Adult developmental cycle has two implications for nurses. First, as the professional status of nursing improves, nursing as a career becomes more desirable to people in adulthood and beyond. More nurses are entering nursing either after they have already obtained a baccalaureate degree or as a second career. In either case, the needs for employment circumstances change as persons integrate their nursing career with parallel changes in family situations. Second, persons who enter the nursing profession as more mature adults with varied life experiences will seek out different opportunities and approach them with different skills.

Nursing as a Career

Nursing as a career offers many interesting possibilities for nurses. Nursing provides significantly more interesting part-time opportunities than most other occupations. For any individual, a career is a choice; a career can be structured, or it may just happen without preplanning and is recognized in hindsight.

Opportunities do arise in nursing. Therefore contemplation and planning steers an individual toward a pattern that is woven from among work,

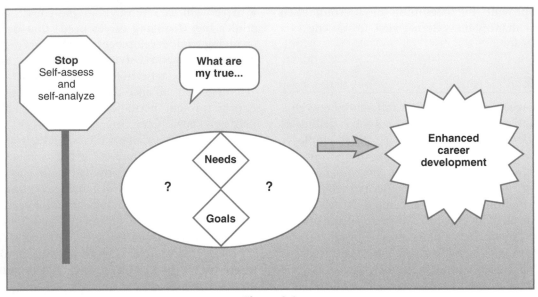

Figure 3.1
Centering within a career trajectory.

self, and family roles into a coherent whole with individual meaning. Planning for a career may be tough to do, but it is essential for helping the individual to capitalize on opportunities. For example, nurses can reflect on what they want to be doing at different points in their lives or where they want to be in 2, 5, or 10 years. Analysis of goals is based on techniques of self-analysis. Numerous books and self-help guides are available to help nurses in identifying their unique talents and strengths. Analysis of experiences is another technique. For example, those nursing situations in which the individual feels the most comfortable and productive may indicate talents and abilities useful on which to build a career. Some people enjoy the high stimulation, fast pace, and quick decision making of an ICU setting. Others may feel the most comfortable helping the elderly or counseling oncology clients.

Certain information is helpful to know in planning a career (Table 3.1). First, building self-awareness as a strategy for career growth suggests

Table 3.1

Influences on Career Planning			
Self	Real World	Workplace Change	Goals
Personal goals	Available options	Trends and issues in health care	Personal goals
Strengths and needs	Available opportunities	Trends and issues in nursing	Family goals
Anchors			Career goals
Desires for contribution to a practice area			

the discovery of such information about an individual as personal goals, strengths, needs, anchors, and desires for contribution to an area of practice. Second, the options and opportunities realistically available will color a career. They need to be evaluated. Third, trends and issues in health care and nursing might contribute to a career trajectory. For example, research has demonstrated that nurse practitioners are cost-effective, and legislation has been enacted to allow third-party reimbursement for specialist nursing services. As opportunities within a reconfigured health care system open up for advanced practice nurses, this becomes an attractive career path to many nurses. Changes occurring as a result of health care reform provide opportunities for nurses in new and creative career directions. Finally, nurses face issues of the relative timing of personal and family goals with career goals. Goals may mesh or create tension.

Thriving and making a success of a career is based on planning and making positive changes. The pace of change, the explosive growth of technology, and organizational restructuring may appear to create barriers to nurses' careers. However, strategies are available to overcome barriers to career success. A key strategy is enhancing an individual's capacity to accept change and adapt. Finding a coach to give guidance, healthy self-care practices, self-nurturing, and self-empowerment, and updating or reframing expectations help reduce internal barriers to success.

Nursing is a career that fits with changing career goals and changing life situations. Nursing is exciting because of the number of unlimited

Research Note

Source: Fagerberg, I. (2004). Registered nurses' work experiences: Personal accounts integrated with professional identity. *Journal of Advanced Nursing, 46,* 284-291.

Purpose

The purpose of this study was to examine how nurses viewed their work 5 years after their graduation from nursing school. During the study, 16 Swedish nurses working in acute care and in the community were interviewed.

Discussion

After nurses were interviewed, their comments were analyzed using a qualitative method to discover what they believed nursing is about. The data analysis uncovered three themes that were about caring for the patient, working within an organization, and individual characteristics of the nurse. Care of the patient meant that nurses had a holistic perspective of caring for patients in which trust was established between the nurse and the patient. The meaning of organization had to do with having enough qualified staff and resources and being able to make decisions about how to organize their work. Finally, a nurse's level of self-esteem was important to being a nurse, and nurses with low self-esteem were less likely to advocate for their patients.

Application to Practice

This study identified the complexity of three intersecting factors in identifying what nursing is about. According to Benner's model, nurses at 5 years represent the advanced stage of skill acquisition, and they are considered as candidates for burnout. However, given the findings of this study, managers have the opportunity to focus on another side of burnout, which is supporting the commitment of nurses. By addressing the challenges of how nurses perceive providing care in an environment that supports holistic care and addressing nurses' personal characteristics, managers can develop strategies to support nurses' commitment to nursing. The findings from this study can provide the basis for flipping our thinking from burnout and failure to thriving and renewal in commitment.

opportunities to practice that exist on a full-time or part-time basis. Nurses can practice as generalists or a specialists in almost every place health care is delivered. With the almost constant changes in health care, new and parallel opportunities continually arise.

CAREER GOALS

A basic human need related to having a job is the desire for that job to be satisfying. Thoughtful career planning provides an ongoing mechanism to achieve a satisfying professional career. For nurses, satisfaction in their job is associated with being able to practice as a professional with autonomy, peer commitment and support (Blegen, 1993), opportunity for growth (Yoder, 1995), and responsibility (Crose, 1999). Nurses also obtain satisfaction from the organization in which they are employed (Hinshaw et al., 1987). When a nurse seeks a job, finding a fit between the nurse's goals, the role, and the organization is essential for job satisfaction. Vogel (1990) identified the following six steps in career planning:

1. Self-analysis is identifying what is important to you based on values and goals.
2. Career analysis includes identifying what you want to achieve and deciding how your priorities are set.
3. Integration is assessing whether your goals need to be revised.
4. Planning is matching goals for achievement to what is actually happening.
5. Implementing is assessing whether you are actively pursuing goals.
6. Evaluation is assessing progress toward goals.

Transition points occur periodically in any career trajectory. Evaluating these transitions means conducting a thorough assessment of internal and external factors and to reidentify directional strategies that address long-term goals based on vision and values. In evaluating transitions, adaptive strategies are identified, including whether the nurse wants to expand, contract, or maintain the scope of the practice role. This may include seeking job opportunities, decreasing commitments,

or staying in the present environment (Ginter et al., 2002; O'Connor, 2004).

SOCIALIZATION

As nurses graduate from school and move from the academic environment to the work environment, they undergo several processes to integrate the realities of the work environment into being a practicing professional. Work transitions have to do with changes in employment, job content, or a passage in status involving a professional identity in which attitudes, behaviors, and skills change (Ibarra, 1999; Nicholson, 1984). Kramer (1974) recognized that nurses experience "reality shock" as they make this transition from student nurse in an academic environment to a practicing professional in a health care organization. Reality shock consists of four phases (honeymoon, shock, recovery, and resolution) that result in conflict between student roles and roles prescribed in a bureaucratic institution.

To minimize reality shock, successful work transitions require nurses to be socialized into the professional role as well as to the organization. Socialization has been described as the process by which information, values, and ideals are transmitted to the individual (van Maanen & Schein, 1979). Nurses new to the field undergo several processes as a newcomer. First, newcomers experience change, often a change in role and professional identity. Second, a letting-go of old roles occurs. The third process is surprise, which constitutes the reality between expectations and experiences (Louis, 1980).

Socialization is a way of making sense of these phases and experiencing them in both a professional and organizational perspective (Brohm, 2003). Professional socialization takes place as the nurse learns and understands how to use the skills learned in school. Nurses may experience different ideologies of other nurses with whom they work, and the socialization process may not occur smoothly. If the ideological expectations of the nurse cannot become congruent with the rest of the group, the nurse may experience conflict and dissatisfaction and leave that group. Organizational socialization is the second type of socialization that nurses experience. Here the organization's culture will guide the socialization. Visible and invisible symbols of the culture guide the nurse as to what is acceptable behavior. Visible symbols may include the organization's policy and procedure book, whereas the invisible symbols include values, beliefs, and assumptions, such as how nurses address patients. Professional and organizational socialization determines how the individual "learns the ropes" (van Maanen & Schein, 1979). The formation of professional and organizational roles has been reported to differ based on the type of nurses' educational preparation. Corwin (1961) reported that diploma-schooled nurses have higher organizational and lower professional conceptions of their role, whereas this is the opposite for nurses with an academic degree. This may have implications for how nurses are socialized into their roles and how workplace conflict is managed.

The processes by which nurses are socialized vary. The socialization of the nurse into the profession begins in nursing school and continues throughout the nurse's career. Nurses, whether beginning a first job or starting a subsequent job or different role, will experience a period of orientation. The purpose of orientation to a job is to expose the nurse to the requirement of the role, position, or organization and allows for a short on-the-job training period. A simultaneous method for professional socialization is to establish a mentorship program in which a mentor is identified for each new nurse. A mentor is usually an experienced nurse who has developed expertise and can be a strong force in shaping a nurse's identity as a professional. Mentors show their mentees "the ropes" by providing them with information, advice, support, ideas on how to navigate the organization, and tips for how to succeed (Restifo & Yoder, 2004). Although organizations frequently use preceptors to help a new nurse during orientation, their relationship with the new nurse is short-term. Mentors, on the other hand, have a long-lasting relationship and commitment with their junior colleagues. Mentors are defined by their long-term commitment to the development of a nurse (Restifo & Yoder, 2004). Personal, professional,

and interpersonal characteristics of mentors have been identified by Restifo and Yoder (2004). Ideal characteristics of mentors include having a positive outlook on life and a caring approach to others. Mentors should strive to have a personal chemistry with their mentees. As professionals, mentors have experience and have reached a level of expertise; they model professional behavior, and value ongoing learning. The ideal interpersonal characteristics of mentors include being a good communicator and listener and being trusted, respected, and admired. Mentors usually have been mentees themselves. Because the opportunities for nurses are so varied, having both lifelong and multiple mentors is useful.

Using the Dreyfus model of skill acquisition, Benner (1982) identified a continuum of skill-based performance that has traditionally been associated with nurses' entry into the profession. The development of nurses' skill is based on a combination of experience and education. Benner characterizes proficiency as consisting of five stages. These stages are *novice* (beginners with no experience), *advanced beginner* (some real world experiences to perform acceptably), *competent* (been on the job for 2-3 years), *proficient* (perceives situations as whole rather than as fragmented part; performance is guided by maxims) and *expert* (experiences have moved to having an intuitive understanding of situations). Although this categorization scheme originally was intended to describe nurses' entry into the profession, it may also be appropriate to recognize these transitions as nurses make other career choices. A nurse who has achieved a level of competence in critical care and transitions into home care will not initially exhibit his or her previous level of performance. However, the nurse who transitions into another role or specialty may pass through the skill performance phases more quickly.

JOB TENURE

Organizations invest resources into new employees and have a stake in the success of the socialization process. Seyboldt (1983) conducted a theory-based study that described five phases of tenure in an organization and identified work and role design needs within each stage.

The *entry period,* from job entry to less than 6 months, occurs when new employees are beginning to understand the nature of the work and are transitioning through the orientation period. Feedback is an important activity to establish how well they are doing. Conflict may occur when expectations about the role and the work are different from what is experienced.

The *early period,* from 6 months to 1 year, occurs when employees have learned the basics of the job and are ready to move on if they are dissatisfied. During this vulnerable stage, they have finished with orientation but have not yet passed being a novice. Unless they are strongly mentored, they may be left to struggle alone.

The *middle period,* from 1 to 3 years, is characterized by relatively stable performers who need to have enough freedom to make decisions and work independently. Validating expectations of the job is important.

The *advanced period* is 3 to 6 years. This is a time when employees need validation that their work and contributions are meaningful.

The *later period,* over 6 years, may be where the employee emerges as an informal leader. They are the "pillars" of the organization and contribute to creating the work environment. These professionals are particularly attuned to relationships with the formal leadership.

The length of tenure in an organization has implications for the nurse and the organization. The first year in a job is critical because expectations and experiences either converge or diverge. For instance, job satisfaction, organizational commitment, and professionalism have been shown to decrease during the first year of work (McCloskey & McCain, 1987), suggesting the need for a more intensive approach to reconciling expectations and experiences. When nurses feel a sense of commitment, research has shown that this has been positively related to more satisfaction and less turnover (Blegen, 1993; Mueller & Price, 1989).

Other factors that are influenced by a nurse's tenure are related to costs and productivity. When a nurse leaves a medical-surgical unit, the reported cost to replace that nurse can be as high as $42,000 (Kerfoot, 2000). Yet these visible costs of turnover account for only 10% to 15% of total costs (McConnell, 1999). When nurses leave their workgroup, it has an effect on the remaining group's ability to function effectively coupled with a diminished efficiency for the nurse who is in the process of leaving (McConnell, 1999). It has been reported that it takes 18 to 24 months for an organization to realize its return on investment from hiring a new nurse (Mann, 1989). Organizations that recognize nurses as their most important asset will likely be those organizations in which there is a high level of commitment and satisfaction.

LEADERSHIP AND MANAGEMENT IMPLICATIONS

The beginning of the twenty-first century finds a changing health care delivery system, workplace, and nurse—all of which have implications for nurse leadership and management. Social, environmental, technological, and economic forces are driving changes in the ways that health care is delivered and have a profound impact on the professional role and practice of nurses.

In times of nursing shortages, recruitment and retention of nurses is brought into the forefront. The average age of the nursing workforce is 45.2 years (National Sample Survey, 2000), which means that the numbers of those expected to retire within the next decade is increasing. Paradoxically, as the workforce gets older, sociocultural trends, such as an aging population, a growing health care system, science and technology explosion, diversity, and globalization, are increasing the need for nurses. Those in managerial and leadership positions must find a way to utilize the expertise of aging nurses. The physical demands in the work of nursing may not be tolerated by the aging nurse. However, with the diversity of roles that exists for nurses, creative exploration of how to utilize the older nurse's expertise is needed.

▲ LEADERSHIP & MANAGEMENT BEHAVIORS

Leadership Behaviors

- Envisions nursing as a full profession
- Communicates with nurses about professional attributes in nursing and related issues
- Influences nurses to be professional
- Guides changes in research, education, and practice that improve nursing's professional status
- Opens a dialogue to promote nursing as a profession
- Promotes nursing as a viable career choice
- Influences followers to develop a professional career
- Envisions a mentoring environment
- Enables followers to pursue career opportunities
- Communicates career values
- Mentors new nurses
- Is a role model of professionalism in nursing
- Creates career growth opportunities
- Challenges the system to promote opportunities for nurses

Management Behaviors

- Plans for workforce diversity
- Organizes nursing practice to best utilize professional registered nurses
- Directs the work of nurses as professional employees
- Manages professional-bureaucratic conflicts
- Influences employees to develop skills and abilities
- Manages employees with diverse career patterns
- Plans for a career-diverse skill mix of staff
- Organizes the work environment to facilitate career and professional development
- Assists employees to develop elements of career portfolios

Overlap Areas

- Delivers professional nursing practice
- Balances professional and bureaucratic role demands
- Influences others in career development
- Encourages professionalism in nursing

Attention to the work environment is particularly important for managers. The configuration of most health care organizations is typically hierarchical and bureaucratic, which is philosophically at odds with the professional ideal of autonomy. In a hierarchical structure, decisions are made at a specified position within the organization, so decision making is typically slowed and autonomy stifled. Successful organizations in the twenty-first century are being labeled as learning organizations and are characterized in part by authority that is decentralized to the point of where the service occurs (Daft, 2004). A similar transition in level of authority must occur in health care. Historically, professionalization has differed with bureaucratization on at least three dimensions: the degree to which tasks are standardized, the degree of authority allowed, and the degree to which there are competing goals of efficiency and quality (Corwin, 1961). Nurses have been particularly vulnerable to increased bureaucratization because of the uncertainty of where they are on the occupation-professional continuum. Mintzberg (1993) tried to reconcile this discrepancy by describing an organizational structure called the "professional bureaucracy." Here professionals at the bottom of the hierarchy control their work with their clients and have considerable amount of power by virtue of their expertise, education, and experience (Mintzberg, 1993). Contemporary views assert that as professionals, nurses need to make decisions at the point of service (Porter-O'Grady, 1996). This has implications for the nurse who is providing one-to one care and is in the best position to understand the needs of the patients.

Another issue related to nursing's position on the occupation-professional continuum involves collective bargaining/unionization and mandatory payment of overtime for nurses. While these two issues continue to be challenged in the courts, the U.S. Department of Labor, Employment Standards Administration (2004), reiterated its view that RNs are exempt from claims for overtime pay: "The Department's long-standing position is that RNs satisfy the duties test for exempt learned professionals... The Department did not and does not have any intention of changing the current law regarding RNs..." (p. 22153).

One of the chief roles of the manager is to provide the interface between the interests of the professional and the administrative needs of the organization, as well as external forces that define the boundaries for health care (Mintzberg, 1993). In a professional bureaucracy, first-line managers have a particularly important role in shaping the structure and processes of practice that promote nurses' autonomy and retention. First-line managers have a key role in promoting teamwork, communication, and flexibility. Coaching and advocacy are important to retention because they assist nurses to fulfill their roles. Constructing socialization practices such as good orientations, precepting, and mentorship is also important to retaining nurses (Anthony et al., 2005).

Furthermore, managers are managing multiple generations of employees, each with different values and priorities in approaching work and life. For example, Baby Boomers represent the older segment of the workforce, those nurses who were born between 1946 and 1964. They are very different from GenXers, who were born between 1963 and 1977 (Wieck et al., 2002). Each of these generations is influenced by existing societal and technical forces. Baby Boomers have group characteristics that include a strong work ethic, loyalty to their employers, and reliability. They have a strong commitment to quality, are customer-oriented, and command respect in the workplace. Because they have greater job and life experiences, they can serve as mentors to younger employees (Raines, 1997).

On the other hand, GenXers seek change and challenges to avoid boredom. They want autonomy, empowering positions, and independence, and they expect managers to set a good example. GenXers want constant feedback and are willing to work assigned hours that are flexible. However, they are generally not interested in overtime and want to balance work with other priorities. For GenXers, quality of life is a driving force (Raines, 1997). Managers of GenXers need to provide opportunities, diversity, and fun in a dynamic learning environment that tolerates a "learn as you go" approach to risk taking and failure. Unlike Baby Boomers, who prefer to work independently, GenXers like to work in teams but manage their own time (Hays, 1999). Finally, GenXers regard companies as a place to grow, not to grow old (Billingsley, 2000), so managers will need to attend to their needs in a dynamic way to avoid turnover. These examples suggest how important it is to balance multiple diversities in nursing professional practice.

The nursing shortage and changes in health care systems have brought about a need for reexamination of the nurse's role as a provider of direct patient care. As the number of RN vacancies increases and the use of nurses from short-term agencies increases, the traditional notions of how to establish effective teams to deliver quality care are challenged. At the same time, lengths of stay in a variety of settings are being shortened, limiting the available time to develop a meaningful relationship with patients. In both of these cases there is a need to rethink the processes needed for patient care delivery. Meyerson and colleagues (1996) introduced a concept called *swift trust*. In a fluid, flexible, constantly changing environment, professionals need to be able to quickly and efficiently establish trust-based working relationships. These authors suggest that, among other characteristics, the formation of trust is necessary in temporary teams where people have worked together for only a limited amount of time and where team members are dependent on one another to accomplish complex tasks. For example, for nurses working in a team with a number of float personnel and temporary agency nurses, as well as providing care to sick patients with short lengths of hospital stay, the formation of trust needs to develop quickly.

Economic and professional issues are on the cusp of shaping the future of nursing as a profession. Salary and compensation structures are one area in which changes can lead to opportunities to enhance the professional status of nursing. Historically, nurses' wages have been low and not commensurate with their scope of responsibility or comparable to the vital role they play in the health and wellness of persons. Their wages tend to rise when there is a shortage and wage readjustments are made. Nurses' wages flatten out early in their career, with experience salary scales capping on average at 7 to 10 years. Therefore nurses' wages do not keep pace with the salary growth seen in other professions (Colosi, 2002). The future of nursing depends, in part, on a compensation structure that reflects the value of this profession to health and health care.

Another economic concern is that nursing is not typically a revenue-generating cost center. In contrast to the medical model of care, physician skills and intensity of service are recognized by variations in their compensation. Unlike the physician revenue-generating model of care, nurses' wage and benefits are tightly integrated into other bundled services such as hospital room rates. Under this system, the intensity of nursing service and care goes unrecognized. In unbundling nursing care, and consistent with an income-generating model, there is an explicit recognition of the professional nurse's distinctive expertise and competence that is brought to patient care. Health care organizations can revamp the compensation structure by setting a strategic goal that recognizes and rewards nurses' contribution to quality and the financial well-being of the hospital. Creative models are needed that move the current compensation structure to one that breaks the presumption that nursing is only a cost. To this end, investigation is needed into what unbundled services lead to good outcomes. Then nurses can be at least partially compensated on a merit basis that represents quality.

CURRENT ISSUES AND TRENDS

In 2001, the American Nurses Association convened a committee representing 19 professional organizations to identify what nursing should look like and where it should be by 2010 (ANA, 2002b). The following 10 key areas were identified:

1. *Leadership and planning:* Nursing organizations will be unified in achieving a systematic plan for the future state of nursing. Leadership behavior will be evidence-driven.

2. *Delivery systems:* Models for delivery of care are developed as integrated models that are achieved through strategic partnerships and that enhance the image of nursing.

3. *Legislation/regulation/policy:* Nurses support a unified standard toward nursing education and practice. Nurses are instrumental in developing evidence-based policy that ensures access to safe and quality nursing care.

4. *Professional/nursing culture:* Nurses are recognized as equal partners in health care delivery, and as such they embrace their accountability and responsibility in upholding high practice, professional, and ethical standards.

5. *Recruitment and retention:* Recruitment initiatives will address the image, the diversification of individuals into the profession, and the provision of adequate sources of economic support in pursuit of nursing education. Retention strategies will address funding, practice models, work environments, and professional development.

6. *Economic value:* Nurses are recognized as providers of cost-effective quality care and are compensated accordingly.

7. *Work environment:* The attention provided to the work environment of nurses is gaining momentum. The work environment provides nurses the opportunity to use their specialized knowledge and skills and promotes shared decision making, collaboration, and professional growth.

8. *Public relations/communication:* Various public constituencies are aware of the unique contributions nurses make in the quality of people's lives. Their image as respected professional should be commensurate with that contribution.

9. *Education:* As the needs of society change, nurses must be prepared educationally to meet those needs. Thus nursing education needs to be clear about the roles, scope of practice, and image portrayed to the public as having excellence within the enterprise. Nurses are attracted to roles as faculty in order to create dynamic learning environments.

10. *Diversity:* The population's economic, ethnic, and social landscape is changing. Nurses will need to recognize this diversity and be culturally competent in the delivery of care. Valuing diversity among the workforce creates parallel opportunities for both nurses and for the patients for whom they care.

Summary

- The practice of professional nursing is shaped by governmental regulations, professional organizations, and employing institutions.
- There are many roles for the professional nurse, including caregiver, administrator, educator, and advanced practice nurse. In each of these roles, nurses also have a patient advocacy role.
- Professions have four characteristics: specialized knowledge, service, autonomy, and ethics.
- Nurses' image and educational entry into practice are barriers to being recognized as a full profession.
- Nursing provides opportunities for a lifetime career.
- Professional and organizational socialization is necessary for nurses to transition from student to practicing nurse and to minimize reality shock.
- A nurse's tenure in an organization goes through several stages in which the nurse is more or less likely to leave.

Study Questions

1. On what basis can nursing argue that it is a profession?
2. Do nurses need to act and look professional to give a professional impression?
3. Should nurses care about image and appearance? If so, why?
4. What is the most prevalent media stereotype of nurses today? How could this be changed?
5. Can you design the "ideal" nursing uniform—one that nurses like and find comfortable and practical and yet clients can identify?
6. Why should nurses plan a career? Why not just follow the available jobs?
7. Why are you motivated for a job or a career in nursing?
8. What developmental stage are you in? How does that affect your career planning?
9. How much should your employer contribute to your career development?
10. Is career planning encouraged in your employment setting? Why or why not?

CASE STUDY

Louise Sutton has been the head nurse on her unit for 10 years, and most of her staff have been there about 8 years. Because of a change in acuity, Nurse Sutton has hired five new nurses who are considerably younger than her "older crew." Nurse Sutton is finding she now must manage two different kinds of nurses. One area that is particularly difficult is the use of a new information system that has been installed. The older nurses who work for have difficulty in adopting and do not feel comfortable using the technology. The new younger nurses, however, readily embrace it and find innovative ways to use it to simplify their work. Nurse Sutton identifies that she needs to utilize the strengths of both age generations of nurses and decides to implement a "reverse" preceptor program. In this program each technologically advanced nurse is responsible for being the

CRITICAL THINKING EXERCISE

Cheryl Numo has just graduated from a BSN program and has been hired onto a medical-surgical unit. She is very excited about starting her first job and has always done well in her clinical rotations. She is not expecting any problems with this job.

Nurse Numo has been assigned a preceptor during her 6-week orientation program. Her new unit is short-staffed, and her preceptor is teaching her to do "her job." She is having trouble integrating all the new experiences and is surprised to find out how many things there are to take care of in completing her patient assignment. Because the unit is short-staffed, Nurse Numo's preceptor has her own patient load, seems to listen only while "on the run," and does not have time to find out much about her new trainee. Nurse Numo

had expected her preceptor to be like her clinical instructor during her school years; she is becoming more dissatisfied and is thinking about talking over this situation with her nurse manager.

1. What is the problem?
2. How might Nurse Numo respond proactively to her situation?
3. What are the professional and organizational issues?
4. Is Nurse Numo's preceptor serving in a mentoring relationship?
5. What are the conflicts for Nurse Numo's preceptor?
6. What are the possible ways for the nurse manager to respond that may keep Nurse Numo from leaving the unit?

resource for a nurse who is not comfortable with computerized technology, and the older nurses serve as resources for helping the newer nurses with other areas in which they are less comfortable. How might Nurse Sutton use this strategy to enhance the professionalism of all the nurses?

REFERENCES

Aiken, L.H., Clarke, S.P., Sloane, D.M., Sochalski, J., & Silber, J. (2002). Hospital nurse staffing and patient mortality, nurse burnout, and job dissatisfaction. *Journal of American Medical Association, 288*(16), 1987-1993.

American Nurses Association (ANA). (1997). *Mission Statement.* Silver Spring, MD: ANA. Retrieved May 10, 2004, from *www.nursingworld.org/about/mission1.htm*

American Nurses Association (ANA). (2001). *The center for ethics and human rights. Code of ethics for nurses—Provisions.* Silver Spring, MD: ANA. Retrieved May 10, 2004, from *www.nursingworld.org/ethics/chcode.htm*

American Nurses Association (ANA). (2002a). *Ensuring nursing's future: 2002 annual stakeholders report.* Silver Spring, MD: ANA. Retrieved May 6, 2004, from *www.nursingworld.org/about/lately/stkhld02.pdf*

American Nurses Association (ANA). (2002b). *Nursing's agenda for the future: A call to the nation.* Silver Spring, MD: ANA. Retrieved May 10, 2004, from *www.nursingworld.org/naf/*

American Nurses Credentialing Center. (2003a). *American Nurses Credentialing Center: Certified nursing excellence. ANCC magnet program—Recognizing excellence in nursing services.* Silver Spring, MD: ANCC. Retrieved May 25, 2004, from *www.nursingworld.org/ancc/magnet.html*

American Nurses Credentialing Center (ANCC). (2003b). *American Nurses Credentialing Center: Certified nursing excellence.* Silver Spring, MD: ANCC. Retrieved May 25, 2004, from *www.nursingworld.org/ancc/inside.html*

Anthony, M.K., Standing, T.S., Glick, J., Duffy, M., Paschall, F., Sauer, M., et al. (2005). Leadership and nurse retention: The pivotal role of nurse managers. *Journal of Nursing Administration, 35*(3), 146-154.

Ballou, K. (1998). A concept analysis of autonomy. *Journal of Professional Nursing, 14,* 102-110.

Barter, M., & McFarland, P. (2001). BSN by 2010: A California initiative. *Journal of Nursing Administration, 31,* 141-144.

Benner, P. (1982). From Novice to expert. *American Journal of Nursing, 82,* 402-407.

Billingsley, M. (2000). Satisfying GenX: Can we do it? *Nursing Connection 13*(1), 72-74.

Bixler, G., & Bixler, R. (1959). The professional status of nursing. *American Journal of Nursing, 59,* 1142-1147.

Blegen, M. (1993). Nurses' job satisfaction: A meta analysis of related variables. *Nursing Research, 42,* 36-41.

Brink, P. (1988). The difference between a job and a career. *Western Journal of Nursing Research 10*(1), 5-6.

Brohm, L. (2003). *The nursing debut: The work entry transition.* Unpublished paper, Case Western Reserve University, Cleveland.

Colosi, M.L. (2002). Rules of engagement for the nursing shortage. *JONA's Healthcare Law, Ethics and Regulation,* 4, 50-54.

Corwin, R. (1961). The professional employee: A study of conflict in nursing roles. *American Journal of Sociology,* 66, 604-615.

Cresia, J. (1996). Professional nursing roles. In J.L. Cresia & B. Parker (Eds.), *Conceptual foundations of professional practice* (pp. 67-91). St Louis: Mosby.

Crose, P. (1999). Job characteristics related to job satisfaction in rehabilitation nursing. *Rehabilitation Nurse,* 24, 95-102.

Daft, R.L. (2004). *Organization theory and design* (8th ed.). Mason, OH: Thompson South- Western Publishing.

Etzioni, A. (1969). *The semi-professions and their organizations.* New York: The Free Press.

Evans, J. (1997). Men in nursing: issues of gender segregation and hidden advantage. *Journal of Advanced Nursing,* 26, 226-231.

Fagerberg, I. (2004). Registered nurses' work experiences: Personal accounts integrated with professional identity. *Journal of Advanced Nursing,* 46, 284-291.

Fitzpatrick, J.J., & Whall, A.L. (2005). *Conceptual models of nursing: Analysis and application* (4th ed.). Upper Saddle River, NJ: Pearson Prentice Hall.

Flexner, A. (1910). *Medical education in the United States and Canada.* Boston: Merymount Press.

Flexner, A. (1915). Is social work a profession? *School and Society,* 1(26), 901-911.

Ginter, P.M., Swayne, L.E., & Duncan, W.J. (2002). *Strategic management of health care organizations* (4th ed.). Oxford: Blackwell Publishers Ltd.

Greenwood, E. (1957). Attributes of a profession. *Social Work,* 2(3), 45-55.

Hall, R.L. (1968). Professionalization and bureaucratization. *American Sociological Review,* 33, 92-104.

Hays, S. (1999). Generation X and the art of reward. *Workforce,* 78, 44-48.

Henderson, F.C., & McGettigan, B.O. (1994). *Managing your career in nursing* (2nd ed.). New York: National League for Nursing Press.

Hughes, L. (2001). The public image of the nurse. In E. Hein (Ed.), *Nursing issues in the 21st century* (pp. 55-73). Philadelphia: Lippincott.

Hinshaw, A.S., Smeltzer, C.H., & Atwood, J.R. (1987). Innovative retention strategies for nursing staff. *Journal of Nursing Administration,* 17(6), 8-16.

Ibarra, H. (1999). Provisional selves: Experimenting with image and identity in professional adaptation. *Administrative Science Quarterly,* 44, 764-791.

Kerfoot, K. (2000). The leader as a retention specialist. *Nursing Economic$,* 18, 216-218.

Kramer, M. (1974). *Reality shock: Why nurses leave nursing.* St Louis: Mosby.

Larisey, M. (1996). Socialization to professional nursing. In J.L. Cresia & B. Parker (Eds.), *Conceptual foundations of professional nursing practice* (pp. 46-66). St Louis: Mosby.

Logan, J., Franzen, D., Pauling, C., & Butcher, H. (2004). Achieving professionhood through participation in professional organizations. In L. Haynes, T. Boese, & H. Butcher (Eds.), *Nursing in contemporary society* (pp. 52-70). Upper Saddle River, NJ: Pearson Prentiss Hall.

Louis, M.R. (1980). Surprise and sense making: What newcomers experience in entering unfamiliar organizational settings. *Administrative Science Quarterly,* 25, 226-251.

Mann, E. (1989). A human capital approach: *Journal of Nursing Administration,* 19(10), 8-16.

McCloskey, J., & McCain, B. (1987). Satisfaction, commitment, and professionalism of newly employed nurses. *Image Journal of Nursing Scholarsh,* 19, 20-24.

McClure, M., Poulin, M., Sovie, M., & Wandelt, M. (1982). *Magnet hospitals: Attraction and retention of professional nurses.* Kansas City, MO: American Nurses Association.

McClure, M.L. (1991). Introduction. In I.E. Goertzen (Ed.), *Differentiating nursing practice into the twenty-first century* (pp. 1-9). Kansas City, MO: American Academy of Nursing.

McConnell, C.R. (1999). Staff turnover: Occasional friend, frequent foe, and continuing frustration. *Health Care Manager,* 18(1), 1-13.

Meyerson, D., Weick, K., & Kramer, R. (1996). Swift trust in temporary groups. In R. Kramer & T. Tyler (Eds), *Trust in organizations: Frontiers of theory and research* (pp. 166-196). Thousand Oaks, CA: Sage.

Mintzberg, H. (1993). *Structure in fives: Designing effective organizations.* Englewood Cliffs: NJ: Simon & Schuster.

Mitchell, P., Armstrong, S., Simpson, T., & Lentz, M. (1989). American Association of Critical-Care Nurses demonstration project: Profile of excellence in critical care nursing. *Heart and Lung,* 18, 219-237.

Mueller, C.W., & Price, J.L. (1989). Some consequences of turnover: A work unit analysis. *Human Relations,* 42, 389-402.

National Council of State Boards of Nursing (NCSBN). (1999). *Uniform core licensure requirements: A supporting paper National Council Paper.* Chicago: NCSBN. Retrieved May 6, 2004, from *www.ncsbn.org/regulation/nursing-practice_nursing_practice_licensing.asp*

National Council of State Boards of Nursing (NCSBN). (2004). *Nursing regulation: Nursing licensure & certification.* Chicago: NCSBN. Retrieved August 5, 2004, from *www.ncsbn.org/regulation/nlc.asp*

National Institutes of Health (NIH). (2003). *Estimates of funding for various diseases, conditions, research areas.* Bethesda, MD: NIH, U.S. Department of Health and Human Services. Retrieved May 31, 2004, from *www.nih.gov/news/fundingresearchareas.htm*

National Sample Survey. (2000). *Findings from the National Sample Survey of Registered Nurses*. Washington, DC: Report of the Division of Nursing, U.S. Department of Health and Human Services.

Nicholson, N. (1984). A theory of work role transition. *Administrative Science Quarterly, 29*, 172-191.

O'Connor, M. (2004). Strategic planning for career development. *Journal of Nursing Administration, 34*, 1-3.

Oermann, M.H. (1997). Professional nursing practice. In M.H. Oermann (Ed.), *Professional nursing practice* (pp 1-31). Stamford: CT: Appleton & Lange.

Porter-O'Grady, T (1996). More thoughts on shared governance. *Nursing Economic$, 14*(4), 254-255.

Raines, C. (1997). *Beyond Generation X; A practical guide for managers*. Menlo Park, CA: Crisp Publications.

Restifo, V., & Yoder, L. (2004). CETPOC Partnership. Making the most of mentoring [Midwestern edition]. *Nursing Spectrum, 5*(5), 20-23. (Available: 2353 Hassell Road, Suite 110, Hoffman Estates, IL 60195-2102).

Seyboldt, J. (1983). Dealing with premature employee turnover. *California Management Review, 25*(3), 107-117.

Stierle, L. (2003). *ANA—Advancing the profession through practice, policy, and governmental affairs*. Silver Spring, MD: American Nurses Association. Retrieved May 6, 2004, from *www.nursingworld.org/about/lately/2002/ca02.pdf*

Strodtman, L. (1997). The historical evolution of nursing as a profession. In M.H. Oermann (Ed.), *Professional nursing practice* (pp. 33-59). Stamford: CT: Appleton & Lange.

Summers, S.J., & Summers, H.J. (2004). Media "nursing" retiring the handmaiden. *American Journal of Nursing, 104*(2), 13.

U.S. Department of Labor, Bureau of Labor Statistics. (2004). *Registered nurses*. Washington, DC: Bureau of Labor Statistics. Retrieved August 5, 2004, from *www.stats.bls.gov/oco/ocos083.htm*

U.S. Department of Labor, Employment Standards Administration. (2004). *ESA final rule* (p. 22153). Washington, DC: U.S. Department of Labor. Retrieved August 5, 2004, from *www.dol.gov/esa/regs/fedreg/final/20040009016.htm*

van Maanen, J., & Schein, E.H. (1979). Toward of theory of organizational socialization. *Research in Organizational Behavior, 1*, 209-264.

Vogel, G. (1990). Career development: An integrated process. *Holistic Nursing Practice, 4*(4), 46-53.

Wieck, K., Prydun, M., & Walsh, T. (2002). What the emerging workforce wants in its leaders. *Journal of Nursing Scholarship, 34*, 283-288.

Yoder, L. (1995). Staff nurses career development relationships and self-report of professionalism, job satisfaction and intent to stay. *Nursing Research, 44*, 290-297.

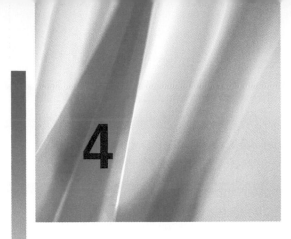

Managing Time and Stress

Karen S. Cox   Diane L. Huber

CHAPTER OBJECTIVES

- Create a recognition of time management issues and possibilities
- Define time management
- Examine time management processes
- Construct an array of time management strategies and techniques
- Define and describe stress, job stress, and burnout
- Illustrate a general model of stress
- Compare stress mediators
- Analyze sources of stress in nursing
- Analyze coping and adaptation in nursing
- Exercise critical thinking to conceptualize and analyze possible solutions to a practice exercise

TIME MANAGEMENT

Time may be the most precious resource to manage. There is an old saying that time is money. In health care, time affects both money and quality (Severance & Cervantes, 1996). For each nurse there is a finite and identifiable limit to the hours and minutes available to do the work. With the same 60 seconds in every minute, nurses need to find ways to stretch the time available to meet the needs that arise. Time pressures are a key source of stress and an area in which nurses have the most to gain by learning management techniques.

Many nurses complain about needing more time. They are stressed and frustrated. At any point in time nurses juggle work and other roles such as student, partner, parent, child, or friend. As work places are restructured for efficiency and employ fewer people, personal work-role stress rises. Effective time management is needed.

There is a strong temptation to apply superficial slogans and gimmicky solutions to the issue of time management. It is easy to suggest that nurses learn to work smarter, not harder. However, quick fixes result in temporary solutions, since the problem of time management is pervasive and the solutions often appear elusive (Ferner, 1995). Nurses can relate to Covey and colleagues' (1994) description of feeling caught between what they have to do (the clock) and what they believe is right to do (the compass). For example, paperwork and scheduled tasks are clock aspects of work. Developing a relationship with patients and meeting their spontaneously arising needs are compass aspects of nursing (Severance & Cervantes, 1996). Somehow the balance needs to be found and the increasing scarcity of time brought under control. As Ferner (1995) stated, "Time controls and limits how we use our other resources. Thus, it is often referred to as our most valuable resource" (p. 8).

Definition

For all of us there are 24 hours in a day and 168 hours in a week. In that time, certain activities are conducted by necessity and to fulfill commitments and goals. Typical activities include personal time (to eat, sleep, get dressed, and do personal maintenance), job or work time, free time, and time for personal growth, leisure, and family (Ferner, 1995). When competing demands create a time conflict, time management becomes important.

Time management is defined as the accomplishment of specified activities during the time available. It is the process of managing the things an individual does with his or her time block. In reality, time management is self-management (Ferner, 1995).

Background

The goal of time management is the efficient use of time resources in order to be effective in achieving goals. Principles of analysis and planning need to be used. This may be difficult because time management is personal, cultural, and a matter of individual style and circumstances. However, success in time management is tied to analysis, planning, and the commitment to a course of action. It must be internalized and become a habit. Difficult as it may be, successful time managers control interruptions, say no, and delegate (Ferner, 1995).

Time management has been linked to success and the achievement of goals. The perception of being successful is linked to the perception of how time is spent (Noreiko, 1996). Awareness and analysis of goals and objectives is a beginning step. Goals and objectives may be short (1 week to 3 months), medium (3 months to 1 year), or long-term (1 to 5 years). They should be specific, measurable, achievable, realistic, and defined in terms of time (Noreiko, 1996). Overall, serious attempts to improve time management require commitment to new habits, analysis based on data, planning effort, and follow-up reanalysis (Ferner, 1995).

The Time Management Process

Time management is a deliberative process of identifying and focusing on the activities needed to accomplish tasks and goals. This is important to nurses and nurse managers, who need to organize and be productive in personal time and also need to manage and coordinate the work of others. Individuals cannot control time itself; therefore they need to learn to manage the available time more efficiently. This can be learned, but it may not be easy. The very first step is to mobilize willingness and determination to examine personal characteristics and habits and then to make changes toward greater strength in being in charge of what actually occurs with the time available.

Improved ability to manage time can come from the following (Arnold & Pulich, 2004):

- Examining attitudes toward time
- Analyzing time wasting behaviors
- Developing better time management skills

The place to start is in self-awareness. Time management habits are embedded in personal preferences, childhood experiences, and cultural influences that may be unconscious or rarely consciously examined. For example, individuals have personal work and management styles that may be based in gender, culture, or personal preferences. One example is the monochromic/polychromic continuum (Innovations International, 2004).

Monochronic or Polychronic Continuum

Individuals vary according to how they prefer and choose to approach work task organization. This preference appears to be mediated by cultural and gender influences. As a result of this cultural diversity, discord or conflict may arise if opposites are assigned together and not assisted to understand these differences and how to harmonize style preferences. These preferences array across a continuum.

At one end is the monochromic style. This style is characterized by working through each part of a project in an orderly fashion and completing one task before starting on the next. Orderly, sequential, and logical, persons using this style approach work with specific and detailed plans and schedules to which they are highly committed (highly monochromic) or with an organized approach that addresses tasks in an analytical and prioritized way (moderately monochromic). They tend to be individualistic and prefer an isolated and uninterrupted work place (Innovations International, 2004). Because this is a linear model, it may have disadvantages in work environments of chaos and complexity, such as in nursing.

At the opposite end is the polychromic work style, in which people tend to do multiple tasks simultaneously. They approach work projects multidimensionally, with flexible and adjustable plans and shared responsibilities. They work on many different parts of a project at the same time and are flexible, spontaneous, and adaptable (highly polychromic). If moderately polychromic, individuals prefer performing many activities at the same time, working in teams and within a general competition timeframe, flexibly approaching project implementation (Innovations International, 2004). If not skillfully managed, however, the polychromic style can deteriorate into chaos.

Awareness of individual work and task style enhances personal effectiveness planning and decision making about personal choices and team harmony. Self-tests are available, such as one that can be found on the Innovations International (2004) website (*www.innovint.com/downloads/mono_poly_test.asp*). Illustrated in Figure 4.1, this test is a set of 16 items, each rated on an anchored descriptor scale from A through E.

Analyzing and Managing Time

Time management is like any general management endeavor. It involves the skills of planning, organizing, implementing, and controlling. The time management process is continuous and ongoing and involves a cycle of analyzing, planning, reanalyzing, and replanning with the following eight steps (Ferner, 1995):

1. Analysis of current time use with time logs
2. Analysis of time logs to identify time problems, causes, and solutions
3. Self-assessment
4. Setting goals and establishing priorities
5. Developing action plans that define tasks, resource needs, and time frames
6. Implementing action plans via planning guides, schedules, and to-do lists
7. Developing techniques and solutions to improve time management problems
8. Follow-up and reanalysis

The first step in getting started with planning, prioritizing, and organizing is to analyze how time is currently being spent by keeping a time log. This is a running account of what was actually done. Include things as you do them, such as open mail, chat with coworkers, or make coffee. This log can be analyzed by day, week, month, or year, depending on the circumstances. For example, if the focus is on a work shift, it might be most useful to analyze by the hour for a week. If the focus is on implementing a new project, an overview may be by the month for a year. Figure 4.2 p. 91 shows a sample activity log for the start of a hospital-based RN's work shift. Recording time use makes the abstract idea of time become a concrete reality and identifies time wasters (Pagana, 1994) and specifically where time is lost. Time wasters keep an individual from doing other things that have more value or importance. There are two general categories of time wasters: (1) external ones, such as phone calls and drop-in visitors, and (2) internal, or self-generated, ones. Lack of self-discipline, failure to delegate, procrastination, indecision, and personal disorganization are examples of self-generated time wasters that are within an individual's power to solve. The goal is to control the cause of wasting time by strategies such as deferring a task when there is something more important to do, diminishing the time spent on the task, or eliminating selected parts of the task (Ferner, 1995). Diaries, calendars, organizers, PDAs, and integrated software scheduling tools are all devices to help manage time.

Keeping track of everything that is done and starting a daily planner to log everything that needs to be done initially focuses an individual on personal time management reality. After this comes self-assessment regarding why time is lost or not used effectively. Effective time management is blocked by procrastination, perfectionism, and an inability to prioritize (Rocchiccioli & Tilbury, 1998). Procrastination may occur because of any of the following (BusinessTown.com, 2004):

- You are not really committed to doing the job.
- You are afraid of the job.
- You do not place a high-enough priority on the activity.

Text continued on p. 91

A Monochronic/Polychronic Self Test

This instrument is designed to assist you in understanding your personal cultural preferences, with respect to both work style and management style. It may serve as an indicator of how you might adapt in certain organizations and global regions.

Pick the letter that best describes your preferred opinion or behavior in an organizational situation. The letters A through E are a scale with C representing the midpoint between the two extremes. As best you can, determine where your opinion or behavior would occur most consistently on the scale for each of the situations below.

1. When working on a project, you find it most effective to:

A	B	C	D	E
Work through each part of the project in an orderly fashion.				Work on many different parts of the project at the same time.

2. You work most effectively in an organization when:

A	B	C	D	E
You are seldom interrupted by and rarely interact with other employees.				You are constantly interacting with and interrupted for discussions by other employees.

3. When you are assigned a project that is due at a specific time, you:

A	B	C	D	E
Establish a specific plan for achieving the project by the deadline, if not before.				Create a flexible plan which may or may not accomplish the project by the exact deadline.

Figure 4.1

A monochronic/polychronic self test. (From Innovations International. [2004]. *A monochronic/polychronic self test.* Salt Lake City, UT: Innovations International. Retrieved August 5, 2004, from *www.innovint.com/downloads/mono_poly_test.asp/*)

4. Organizational information is most efficiently shared and disseminated through:

A	B	C	D	E
Detailed or written memos or internal communication systems.				Informal interoffice verbal communication among employees.

5. To be successful, an organization must focus most on:

A	B	C	D	E
Reaching projected goals and accomplishing task objectives.				Developing each worker and establishing quality relationships among employees.

6. The best project results are produced when everyone agrees:

A	B	C	D	E
To a detailed plan which is executed and completed according to the original design.				To an informal plan that is adjusted as the project proceeds.

7. When you want to discuss something with a co-worker whose office door is closed, you would probably:

A	B	C	D	E
Walk away, assuming he or she does not want to be disturbed.				Knock, open the door, and ask for a few minutes to discuss your concern.

Figure 4.1 cont'd

Continued

8. With respect to your valued possessions, you:

A	B	C	D	E
Almost never lend them to anyone.				Lend them often and easily.

9. When you are late for a scheduled appointment, you feel that:

A	B	C	D	E
You should apologize for being late.				You should not apologize, assuming that he/she will understand that something important came up.

10. In general, after you no longer serve a valued client, you tend to:

A	B	C	D	E
Lose contact with him/her because of your busy schedule and/or you no longer work with him/her directly.				Stay in communication to know how his/her life is progressing.

11. A sign of a good manager is her or his ability to:

A	B	C	D	E
Solicit employee input, but use executive decision making where vital business and policy issues are concerned.				Extensively involve employees in deciding vitally important business and policy-making issues.

Figure 4.1 cont'd

12. Your business presentation style tends to be:

A	B	C	D	E
Orderly, sequential, and logical.				Flexible, spontaneous, and adaptable.

13. Businesses run best when job responsibilities are:

A	B	C	D	E
Fixed and uniquely adapted to each employee.				Constantly changing and overlapping between employees.

14. In a fast-paced, decentralized, information-oriented society, important business matters:

A	B	C	D	E
Require immediate and decisive decision making.				Demand sufficient time for discussion, consensus, and deliberation.

15. The most successful business ventures are dependent upon:

A	B	C	D	E
An in-depth analysis and thorough discussion of all information relevant to the transaction.				The people involved and their ability to work together effectively.

Figure 4.1 cont'd

Continued

16. The most effective way to contribute to an organization is to:

A	B	C	D	E
Specialize in one area and become an expert on a subject.				Accumulate cross-disciplinary knowledge in as many areas as possible.

Scoring Instructions

For each letter chosen, A, B, C, D, or E, write the number of times it was circled next to the appropriate letter in the spaces below, and multiply this number by the figure shown. For example, if B was circled five (5) times, write "5" in the blank space beside B and complete the multiplication, "5" × 2 = "10". Finally, add the products in this column to obtain a total numerical score.

A _____ × 0 = _____

B _____ × 2 = _____

C _____ × 5 = _____

D _____ × 8 = _____

E _____ × 10 = _____

TOTAL _____

Interpretation of Scores

0-40 Highly Monochronic = A to B range on the scale.

These individuals approach work with specific and detailed plans and schedules, to which they are highly committed. The realization of business objectives is their highest priority, and personal relationships are one dimension among many toward this end. These individuals prefer specialized and unique work responsibilities, private working conditions, and short-term, formal work relationships. They are inclined to communicate impersonally and in low context. Their decision making tends to be individualistic, timely, and based on their position of influence within the organization. The essence of leadership is the individualistic vision of the future.

41-80 Moderately Monochronic = B to C range on the scale.

These individuals demonstrate an organized approach to projects and are committed to their completion on time. They ultimately prioritize the successful completion of projects, and tend to address tasks in an analytical and information-oriented manner. These individuals tend to prefer an isolated and uninterrupted work environment; social interaction has its appropriate time and place. Their significant communications are usually to the point, logical and written. Though group input is an important element in these individuals' decision-making process, they ultimately rely on personal judgment to make important final decisions.

Figure 4.1 cont'd

81-120 Moderately Polychronic = C to D range on the scale.

These individuals tend to assign work projects into a general time frame for completion, flexibly approaching project implementation and readily adjusting its execution when something more important comes along. They prefer performing many activities at the same time and working in teams. These individuals develop many informal, long-term working relationships as their means to realizing goals. Their communication of information tends to be personal and informal, rather than through official channels. They solicit and rely heavily on employee input for most decision making.

121-160 Highly Polychronic = D to E range on the scale.

These individuals multi-dimensionally approach work projects with flexible, adjustable plans and shared responsibilities. They tend to believe success of business transactions is ultimately determined by the individuals involved and their cohesiveness as a team. Work is founded upon quality interpersonal interaction and long-term investment in community, which takes precedence over all forms of activity. Communication tends to be spontaneous and high context. Decision making is based on extensive group involvement, discussion, and consensus. The essence of leadership is the subtle balance of group consensus and personal vision.

Figure 4.1 cont'd

- You do not know enough to do the task.
- You just plain do not want to do the job.

The following strategies can help to overcome the above reasons:

- Examine motivation and personal benefit; then either do what needs to be done to get out of it or do it anyway for your own reasons.
- Identify and confront the fear and act despite the fear.

- Recast it in positive motivation and act or resign yourself to living with the consequences of inaction.
- Gather the information you need and plunge into the task.
- Tough it out or farm it out.

In summary, overcoming procrastination is a combination of identifying the reasons, confronting attitudes and fears, and weighing

Time	Activity	Notes
7:00 AM	Arrived on unit, changed into scrubs	
7:15 AM	Joined report	
7:35 AM	Conference with nurse manager	
7:45 AM	Phone call from patient's family	
7:55 AM	Began initial assessments	
8:10 AM	Responded to request from physician	
8:15 AM	Medication rounds	

Figure 4.2
Activity log for the beginning of an RN shift.

the consequences. Then mobilization to action is required.

Perfectionism is the need to do everything exactly right—to be perfect. It can lead to procrastination over the fear of making a mistake. The antidote to perfectionism is to set acceptable and realistic standards for goal achievement.

Prioritization is a key aspect of time management. After analysis of personal characteristics, attitudes, and behaviors that may block time management effectiveness comes setting goals and establishing priorities. One way to approach this is to analyze what needs to be done immediately and what can wait. Goals and activities can fall into one of the following four categories (Rocchiccioli & Tilbury, 1998):

1. Important and urgent
2. Important but not urgent
3. Not important but urgent
4. Not important and not urgent

Analyzing and managing time takes concentrated effort and an openness to rethinking habits and routines. Many times a small amount of effort yields large returns, so changes are important. Reframing situations also helps. For example, establishing an approximate hourly cost for your time (hourly salary figure plus benefits, for example) and then multiplying this by the number of hours spent in meetings helps to clarify why actions might be taken to make meetings more efficient and effective. A personal strengths and weaknesses assessment might help focus personal choices for projects or job duties, such as joining a team. Fundamental motivation, such as doing what you enjoy, also helps time management decisions. Balance is a final consideration. Setting realistic goals, preserving contingency-for-the-unexpected time, and carefully identifying essential tasks in the right order help to achieve balanced time management.

Time Management Strategies

Closing the gap between how an individual would like to be spending time versus how the time is actually spent depends on the deployment of an array of time management strategies.

Two fundamental strategies universally recommended are analyzing the workday and prioritizing the workload. In nursing, care needs and work assignments can fluctuate daily, making organizing the workday quite a challenge (Sherry, 1996). Some general strategies can be identified. Their use depends on the individual situation, available resources, and safety considerations, as follows:

- Take control of your calendar by analysis and prioritization.
- Minimize time spent in the office in nonproductive behavior or away from client care.
- Tame the telephone through effective clerical support.
- Simplify documentation using technology.
- Plan ahead.
- Save time for others.

Pagana (1994) created a list of time management techniques useful for nursing students, including the following:

- Omission by decision: deciding what not to do
- Learning to say no: refusal because of time constraints and prioritization
- Blocking interruptions, especially by visitors and phone calls
- Guarding an individual's best or prime time
- Programming blocks of time, especially for large projects
- Organizing work space
- Managing committee meetings
- Delegating
- Planning the use of time

Inpatient nursing is challenging. The shortened lengths of stay have resulted in higher overall activity. The first and last days of a hospital stay are traditionally the most labor-intensive. However, given shortened lengths of stay, every day of a patient's stay is now likely to be labor-intensive.

When confronted with a workload that is overwhelming, a nurse can try several beneficial strategies. First, it is crucial to take 15 to 20 minutes to plan the day. Skipping this will cost time throughout the shift because of the downtime to do extra steps that could have been economized or the rework time of doing things over. The things that must be accomplished need to be prioritized at the outset. As the day progresses and priorities change, the high-priority items will be the guide for making the best decisions under time limits. Often when a person is overwhelmed, it is tempting to focus on less important tasks like making a bed when those 10 minutes could best be served reviewing home care planning with a family.

Asking for help is an important time management strategy. Often, nurses see this as a sign of inadequate performance and thus may wait far too long to engage others. What specifically would be most helpful for someone else to do needs to be thought through before asking for help.

Nurse managers face multiple and competing priorities on a daily basis. It is not unusual to feel overwhelmed and unsure about what to do first. Not unlike in a direct care role, planning is key. What are the things that are critical to accomplish today? Keeping these goals in the forefront will help throughout the day when the unexpected occurs and new things end up on the to-do list.

Keeping a close handle on how the unit staff members are doing can pay off in time management. By building in opportunities for daily communication, many issues can be addressed before they become major problems. There is no substitute for the nurse manager being available, especially for staff members who work off-shifts and frequently feel neglected by administration.

Many time management strategies surround the analysis, setting of priorities, motivation, and planning and follow-up structure of effective time management. Analysis is a detailed and honest look at what actually occurs during an allotted period of time versus what is productive. Deciding priorities based on the importance and urgency of goals and then developing action plans and schedules can help to better align time use with desired outcomes. Motivation is an internal strategy to overcome potential barriers and delays. It takes planning and follow-up to ensure that goals get met within the set timeframes.

Often when individuals feel that there is too much to do and they cannot handle it all, it is difficult to focus on the fact that it is presumably possible to organize the time in a way that gets it all done. For instance, many students find the requirements of a class overwhelming until they break them down into manageable segments. RNs often have a sense of being overwhelmed by the rapid-fire needs and wants of patients, families, coworkers, and bosses until they impose analysis, prioritization, organization, and delegation on the chaos. Some time management tips and strategies are as follows:

- Continually analyze and examine how time is spent. What can be dropped or delegated?
- Keep a time log, calendar, or other scheduling device.
- Develop a specific statement of major goals: short-term, intermediate, and long-term. Focus on goal attainment.
- Focus on getting yourself started and keeping yourself motivated.
- Keep daily to-do lists and continually reprioritize them.
- Aim to keep a balanced lifestyle. Take breaks. Find your productive time and maximize this.
- Learn when and how to decline to participate in time-wasting activities. Instead, ask others to cooperate with you in productive activities.
- Anticipate unexpected events and be realistic but stay organized.
- Capitalize on technology to assist time management.
- Work to conduct and keep meetings effective.
- End the work day as close to on-time as possible.

Many projects can be more successfully time-managed by the use of checklists, division into smaller tasks or steps, tracking progress, using Gantt charts, and managing group meetings (Figure 4.3). Control over time empowers individuals and frees up energy to handle multiple competing demands (Pagana, 1994). The practice and improvement of time management habits can increase successful goal achievement and reduce stress.

STRESS MANAGEMENT

Nurses are healers. They focus on activities related to caring in the diagnosis and treatment of human responses to health and illness phenomena.

Activities	Days of the Month															
	1-2	3-4	5-6	7-8	9-10	11-12	13-14	15-16	17-18	19-20	21-22	23-24	25-26	27-28	29-30	31
Activity #1	X	X														
Activity #2		X	X													
Activity #3						X	X									

Figure 4.3
Gantt Chart project tracking sheet.

However, inherent in this caring occupation are numerous sources of built-in stress that become occupational hazards for nurses. For example, dealing with human illness and suffering, life-and-death situations, clients who are demanding or in pain, making critical judgments about interventions and treatments, and balancing work and family commitments become forces that realistically generate stress in nurses (Aurelio, 1993). Furthermore, the organizations that employ nurses may become stressful environments in which to practice nursing. For example, organizational cultures may devalue nurses, policies and deployment practices may prevent nurses from using their knowledge and skills, and job and professional autonomy may be restricted (Aurelio, 1993). Empowerment of staff nurses has been significantly related to lower burnout and higher work satisfaction (Laschinger et al., 2001a, 2001b). Clearly, for nurses, it is important to have work-related empowerment strategies in place.

Under conditions of restructuring and reengineering, layoffs and downsizing, nurses feel threatened and concerned about the personal security of their employment. Furthermore, perceived short-staffing and increasing workloads raise concerns about client safety and the nurse's ability to cope and deliver adequate service to clients (Sovie & Jawad, 2001). As with the level of conflict, the level of stress needs to be neither too high nor too low. Moderate levels should be the target. At stress levels that are too low, nurses may become apathetic or nonproductive. At too high a stress level, energy is absorbed in trying to deal with stress and is therefore diverted from productivity. Performance drops as stress reaches high levels.

Clearly, both nurses and their employers have a stake in managing stress and stressful environments.

Definitions

Stress is one concept that links and examines the effects of behavior on health (Fagin, 1987). **Stress** is defined as "a physical, mental, psychological, or spiritual response to a stressor" (Narasi, 1994, p. 73). A **stressor** is defined as an experience in a person-environment relationship that is evaluated by a person as taxing or exceeding resources and threatening the sense of well-being (Dietz, 1991; Lazarus & Folkman, 1984). Stress has been seen as a stimulus, a response, or a transaction (Lyon & Werner, 1987) that is either internal or external.

Selye's (1965) general stress theory forms the theoretical background for understanding stress. According to Selye (1965, 1976), stress is a nonspecific state composed of a variety of induced changes in the human biological system. Thus stress is a syndrome with a characteristic set of symptoms. It can lead to acute and chronic health problems. Stress also is described as a personal response and a phenomenon that occurs inside a body as a reaction to the stimulus of a stressor. The body's emotional and physical response is a result of a "fight-or-flight" syndrome (Woodhouse, 1993).

The concept of stress has been applied from Selye's (1965, 1976) biophysiology framework to psychosocial states in individuals. For example, stress has been viewed as something that occurs

when individuals interact with their environment in such a way that they are presented with a demand, a constraint, or an opportunity for behavior (McGrath, 1976).

Occupational or job stress is defined as a tension arising in a person that is related to the demands of the person's role or job (McVicar, 2003). Job stress, or "disquieting influences," can accumulate into levels that are too high and reach the point of burnout (Hinshaw & Atwood, 1983). **Burnout** is defined as "a response to chronic emotional stress with three components: (a) emotional and/or physical exhaustion, (b) lowered job productivity, and (c) overdepersonalization" (Perlman & Hartman, 1982, p. 293). Burnout in nursing is described as being the terminal phase of the individual's failure to resolve work stress or the accumulated inability to cope with day-to-day job stresses (Smythe, 1984). Levels of job stress that are too low or too high decrease individual productivity (Benson & Allen, 1980; Hinshaw & Atwood, 1983).

Background

Stress is a pervasive part of everyday life and a common theme in nursing. Many of the effects of stress are personal and individual. It is necessary for nurses to understand stress both on a personal level and in relation to their work (Schwab, 1996).

From the work of Selye (1965, 1976), stress is known to have biophysiological effects on humans. However, in nursing practice, stress is most often

---

⚠ LEADING & MANAGING **DEFINED**

Stress	**Occupational or Job Stress**
Physical, mental, psychological, and spiritual responses to any stressor.	A tension arising in a person that is related to the demands of the role or job.
Stressor	**Burnout**
An experience in a person-environment relationship that is evaluated by a person as taxing or exceeding resources and threatening the sense of well-being.	Responses to chronic emotional stress that have three components: (1) emotional or physical exhaustion, (2) lowered job productivity, and (3) overdepersonalization.

applied to a discussion of the psychosocial state of persons as they interact with their environment. Demands, constraints, and opportunities occur that trigger stress (McGrath, 1976).

One general model of stress portrays stress along a continuum from potential stressor to consequences or outcomes (Elliott & Eisdorfer, 1982). At one end is a potential stressor, such as a demanding client. Then come mediators, such as social support, coping behaviors, or defense mechanisms; the individual's psychological reactions, such as emotional states of anxiety or fear; and biological reactions, such as an increase in catecholamines. Finally, there are consequences or outcomes, such as physical illness, burnout, or coping. In this model, stress is pictured as a dynamic process across a continuum and the result of an interaction between an individual and the environment (Lowery, 1987; Figure 4.4).

In general, there appear to be two important processes that mediate the person-environment relationship: coping and cognitive appraisal. Coping is the individual's actions and activities

for adapting to the situation as presented. Coping relates to the means or methods used to deal with or manage a perceived stressful event (Dietz, 1991). The other major mediator is cognitive appraisal. This is the individual's assessment or interpretation of the stressor or potential stressor. Cognitive appraisal relates to the individual's evaluation or perception of whether and to what degree any event or transaction is stressful (Dietz, 1991; Lowery, 1987). Coping strategies can be either active or inactive. Active strategies work toward resolving or reducing the stress. Inactive strategies are focused on avoiding the stress (Simoni & Paterson, 1997).

Stress responses vary widely from one person to another. Lazarus (1966) suggested that perception and cognitive appraisal of the stress factor is key to understanding the psychological stress response. Thus psychological stress is based on a relationship between the person and the environment that is appraised by the person as taxing or exceeding coping resources (Lazarus & Folkman, 1984). The stress phenomenon includes the

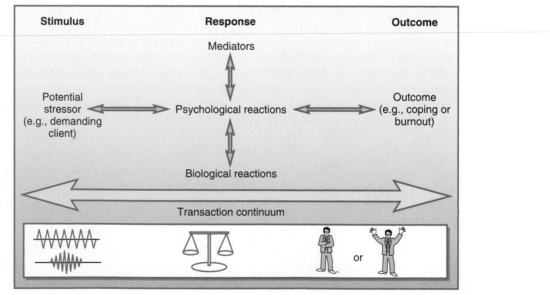

Figure 4.4
General model of stress. (Data from Elliott, G., & Eisdorfer, C. [1982]. *Stress and human health.* New York: Springer; Lowery, B. [1987]. Stress research: Some theoretical and methodological issues. *Image, 19*(1), 42-46; and Lyon, B.L., & Werner, J.S. [1987]. Stress. *Annual Review of Nursing Research, 5,* 3-22.)

objective stressor, the person's perception, the context of the situation, intervening processes, residual stimuli, and the manifestations of the stress response (Pollock, 1984). What this means is that a stress event is a complex interaction and that the psychological response is under the individual's control via his or her cognitive framing or interpretation. Theoretically, changing the cognitive interpretation could change the stress response and increase coping and adaptation ability.

Nurses have studied a variety of stress reactions that occur as emotional and psychological manifestations of failed defense and coping. Chief among these are anxiety and depression. Often overlooked in research are the consequences or outcomes of exposure to stress. The outcomes can be either positive or negative. It is not known whether exposure to stress helps to immunize the individual against severe reactions to future stressors or whether the individual becomes worn down and more susceptible to being overwhelmed by the next stressor. Mastery of stress is advocated but is not easily translated into simple techniques (Lowery, 1987). In nursing, hardiness and burnout have been investigated as stress outcomes.

Sources of Stress in Nursing

Stress is associated with the work of nursing. Individual nurses may experience internal tension, conflict, or stress. Occupational or job stress derives from the jobs and organizations that employ nurses. Stress in nursing is an occupational and managerial concern (Huber, 1994). Individual nurses' health, job satisfaction, absenteeism, and turnover, along with client welfare, are thought to be affected by high levels of work-related stress (Norbeck, 1985). For an in-depth background on stress in nursing, there are at least three articles that extensively analyze the theoretical and research literature (Hardy & Conway, 1988; Hinshaw & Atwood, 1983; Lyon & Werner, 1987).

It is important to recognize that stress is subjective and a person's level of eustress, stress, or distress is an interaction within an individual in the entirety of his or her environment. This includes both the personal and professional environments. A person's perception of his or her stress level is in large part a reflection on his or her perception about being equipped to handle it. A stressful event today may be viewed differently a month from now (McVicar, 2003).

Individual Sources of Stress

Sources of stress that arise from the individual nurse can be either internal or external in origin. For example, the individual nurse may bring to work internal personal emotional conflicts or the need to balance work and family roles. Similar to intrapersonal conflict and tensions in women's careers, the pressure to balance multiple roles in life may create an internal tension that is manifested by personal stress (Huber, 1994). Stress on the individual nurse from an external source may be derived from the characteristics of an individual's personality. For example, the individual's personality may not fit in or match a given work situation (Getzels, 1958). This is an external stress source in that the external work situation impinges on the individual.

Potential outcomes or consequences of the sources of stress that arise from the individual nurse include hardiness (McCranie et al., 1987; Rich & Rich, 1987; Wagnild & Young, 1991), burnout (Bailey, 1980; Stehle, 1981), and reality shock (Kramer, 1974; Kramer & Schmalenberg, 1977; Schmalenberg & Kramer, 1979). Hardiness is a personality characteristic composed of commitment, control, and challenge. This outcome of withstanding high job stress is a variable that may reduce or buffer burnout. Buffering occurs because the higher the personal hardiness, the lower the burnout (Simoni & Paterson, 1997).

Burnout has been described as a syndrome of emotional exhaustion, negative attitudes, and cynicism toward clients that afflicts individuals in the helping professions (Maslach & Jackson, 1981). Apathy, alienation, job dissatisfaction, and depersonalization of clients are associated with burnout (Tarolli-Jager, 1994). In the new graduate the movement from school to active practice can create an incongruence or conflict in the values and behaviors of the two subcultures in nursing, termed "reality shock." Reality shock can create feelings of helplessness, powerlessness, frustration, and dissatisfaction. This crisis of role transformation may be resolved by adopting organizational values, returning to school, limiting personal involvement or commitment, becoming burned out, hopping among jobs, abandoning nursing, or becoming bicultural and working with the best of both worlds (Schmalenberg & Kramer, 1979). Burnout is a condition that develops from continuous job-related stress, but not all nurses under stress develop burnout (Schwab, 1996). Mediation or stress-resistance resources include hardiness and the use of social resources (Sawatzky, 1998). A person's self-esteem may be the most important personal factor predicting burnout potential (Schwab, 1996).

Organizational Sources of Stress

In contrast to the sources of stress generated within or from an individual, nurses experience stress that comes from the nature of nursing and the organizations that typically employ nurses. Sources of stress that arise from the job or occupational environment relate either to the intrinsic nature of the work or to a specific work environment. The intrinsic nature of nursing's work is recognized as stressful. This includes bedside nursing care delivery to ill or hospitalized clients (Laschinger et al., 2001a).

Work environments and organizations that employ nurses also generate stress for nurses. For example, the role of the nurse can be a source of stress and strain (Dewe, 1987). Organizations can and do generate multiple and conflicting demands on nurses, resulting in a job experience that generates numerous stressful situations. Energy and coping resources are devoted to the

Research Note

Source: Santos, S.R., & Cox, K.S. (2000). Workplace adjustment and intergenerational differences between Matures, Boomers and Xers. *Nursing Economic$, 18*(1), 7-13.

Purpose

Stress in the nursing work environment is inherent and complex. Previous studies have concluded that how individuals cope with stress often affects their response to it. The purpose of this study was to assess occupational stress, strain, and coping of inpatient registered nurses ($n = 413$) at a large pediatric hospital.

Discussion

This mixed-methods study used an instrument that measured occupational stress, strain, and coping skills. The results indicated significant differences in these scales between three age groups of nurses (those born 1909-1945, 1946-1964, and 1965-1981) using the Occupational Stress Inventory* and focus group confirmation. Baby Boomers had significantly higher mean scores on the stress subscales of role overload, role boundary, and physical environment. Boomers also had the most negative scores on the four coping scales of self-care, recreation, cognitive, and social support. Generational themes of orientation to work, length of service, and work place behavior were identified.

Application to Practice

It is important to address ways nurses use coping skills to ensure design of the most effective ways to decrease and or mitigate stress. This study utilized focus groups to clarify quantitative survey results. This allowed for more specific information, which ultimately helped to design improvement strategies. Also, generational differences exist and must be considered in all aspects of the work environment.

*Osipow, S.H., & Spokane, A.R. (1981). *Occupational stress inventory manual.* Odessa, TX: Psychological Assessment Resources, Inc.

task of adapting and mastering the stress of role pressures and competing role expectations.

Role stress and strain has been an important leadership and management topic for many years. Hardy (1978) developed a typology of seven sources of role stress: role ambiguity, role conflict, role incongruity, role overload, role underload, role overqualification, and role underqualification. Role theory (Thomas & Biddle, 1966) is a collection of concepts and hypotheses that predict how an individual will perform in a given role. It indicates the circumstances under which certain types of behavior can be expected (Conway, 1988).

Role stress and role strain have been linked to stress in social systems (Hardy, 1978; Miller, 1971). Role expectations, location of the role in the social structure, inadequate resources, and the social context create role difficulties and stressors. Role stress arises from sources external to the role occupant. It is a social structural condition generated from role obligations that are vague, irritating, difficult, conflicting, or impossible to meet. Role strain is a subjective state of emotional arousal that occurs in response to external conditions of social stress (Charnley, 1999; Hardy & Hardy, 1988; Huber, 1994). The organizations that employ nurses can create role ambiguity when role expectations are unclear, role conflict when role expectations are incompatible, role incongruity when the nurse's professional values conflict with role expectations, role overload when too much is expected in the time available, or role underload when advanced practice nurses are underutilized. Thus role stress and strain are common to nursing practice.

Specific work environments also generate stress in nursing. Specific characteristics present in health care organizations create stress. For example, the physical and technical environment, patterns of interpersonal relationships, professional-bureaucratic role conflict, multiple expectations, management, leadership style, communication patterns, staffing and workload, negative client outcomes, relationships with physicians, lack of participation in policy decisions, and inadequate knowledge and skills for role functions each can

be a source of stress (Hinshaw & Atwood, 1983; McGrath, 1976). Clearly, the dynamics between nurses and physicians contribute to nurses' satisfaction with their jobs (Mills & Blaesing, 2000). Leatt and Schneck (1980) categorized the organizational sources of stress as derived from either role-based or task-based situations. Huckabay and Jagla (1979) categorized intensive care unit (ICU) nursing stressors into the four categories of interpersonal communication problems, knowledge-base stressors, environmental stressors, and patient care situations.

Hospitals and health care organizations have environmental contexts with elements that may help or hinder the work of nurses (McClure et al., 1983). Structural, procedural, and contextual factors cause stress and conflict (Landstrom et al., 1989). Stress interrelates with other organizational variables, such as organizational climate, group cohesion, job satisfaction, turnover, productivity, conflict, change, and organizational restructuring (Hinshaw & Atwood, 1983; Hinshaw et al., 1987; Huber, 1994). Job strain has increased in many nursing environments because of increased workload and higher acuity (Laschinger et al., 2001b).

Job satisfaction and turnover have been the major outcome variables of organizational stress that have been studied (Hinshaw et al., 1987; Irvine & Evans, 1995; Landstrom et al., 1989; McCloskey & McCain, 1987; Price & Mueller, 1981; Weisman et al., 1981). Job satisfaction is a major predictor of anticipated turnover or intent to stay or leave. Anticipated turnover is a major predictor of actual turnover (Hinshaw, 1989). Job stress is an individual factor that influences job satisfaction, thereby having an indirect effect on anticipated turnover (Hinshaw et al., 1987). In critical care environments, perceived stress is related to job satisfaction and psychological symptoms (Bratt et al., 2000).

Turbulence and organizational change create stress. Regionalization and integration transform simple organizations into complex networks of community health care systems. As health care organizations change in response to social, consumer-related, governance, technology, and economic pressures, chaos and opportunities arise (Schumacher & Larson, 1993). With dramatic changes in the structures and functions of health care organizations, stress has become an ongoing reality for staff (Santos & Cox, 2000).

A new concept described in the nursing literature is operational failures (Tucker, 2004). Operational failures are defined as disruptions or errors in the supply of needed information or materials. These failures are frustrating; however, nurses tend to learn how to compensate for them as opposed to bringing them to the attention of managers.

A sense of perceived control over related work pressures is critical to perceived stress and stress outcomes. External forces beyond a nurse's control that interfere with the ability to deliver quality care increase occupational stress. For example, some nursing stressors are lack of control over staffing patterns and staff mix, lack of resource availability such as supplies and equipment, and lack of autonomy (McVicar, 2003). Furthermore, as organizations create and deploy work teams to deliver quality care, interpersonal stressors from the group dynamics of teams may create stress for both staff and managers (AHA, 2002). Implementing strategies and structures for empowerment is a major technique for organizational innovations designed to increase participation and decrease burnout as evidenced by the research in Magnet-designated environments (Laschinger et al., 2003).

Coping and Adaptation

Stressors are demands or threatening experiences either from an individual's internal or external environment that create disequilibrium. Restoration and balance are sought as a result of stressors (Keenan et al., 1993). Excessive occupational stress can lead to the undesirable outcome of burnout. Burnout in nurses undermines the nurse's helping relationship. Therefore it is counterproductive for organizations to allow occupational stress to flourish without checks and balances. A preferable outcome goal is for nurses to function as self-dependent innovators who operate

within realistic expectations and exercise control within a stressful work environment (Grant, 1993).

The array of coping strategies is vast, but not all coping strategies elicit an adaptive response. Generalized resistance resources include personality characteristics, predispositions, social supports, and health practices. Each can function as a buffer. Consequently, some individuals who experience high stress levels do not become ill and may actually thrive on stress (Sawatzky, 1998). Social support and the personality characteristic of hardiness were key mechanisms of Pollock's 1984 Adaptation Nursing Model.

The concept of hardiness grew out of the observation that high stress does not create illness in all people and that there is a modest relationship between stressful life events and illness symptoms (Kobasa et al., 1982). Hardiness is a personality style that contains elements of commitment, control, and challenge and that affects coping by buffering the stress-illness relationship. It also appears to affect adaptation by influencing the individual's perception of the stressful event and strategies and resources chosen (Sawatzky, 1998).

An individual's coping ability is the major variable modulating stress and its outcome. Coping strategies are key elements of nurses' stress reactions. The coping process is composed of the perception of stress, conditions and situational factors affecting cognitive appraisal, assessment of coping mechanisms, and the selection of a coping strategy (Harris, 1989). Nurses need to learn to manage or cope effectively with daily work stressors by evaluating and moderating response patterns. For example, attitudes and skills, habits or typical approaches to problems, and specific actions for stress management all can be used to intervene between stress and the outcome. Effective coping actions reduce emotional distress, resolve or diminish problems, and maintain or enhance the sense of self (Woodhouse, 1993).

There have been various recommendations for nurses for coping with and managing stress. For example, the development of an internal warning system to alert the individual to stress and provide a choice of responses has been recommended (Hartl, 1989). Nurses need to test the subjective and objective boundaries of stress and be willing to look after their own best interests. This may be a competing value to the concept of altruistic, unselfish service to others. However, guilt may be used by organizations to induce nurses to respond in ways that primarily serve the interests of the institution (Woodhouse, 1993). The updated Code of Ethics developed by the American Nurses Association (2001) makes it clear that nurses must consider their own needs as well as those of the patients they serve. The fifth principle of the Code of Ethics states that the nurse owes the same duty to self as to others, and this includes the responsibility to preserve integrity and patient safety.

Stress management techniques range from those focused on the individual to those focused on the organization. Some coping strategies used by nurse executives include spending time on nonwork-related interests, using a personal support network, being active in the larger professional arena, identifying resources for problem solving, manifesting somatic symptoms, walking away from situations to gain perspective, considering resigning, rigid adherence to rules, complying, and participating in dysfunctional competition (Scalzi, 1988). Humor in communication can also be used as a mechanism for coping with stress and thereby enhancing morale and productivity (Woodhouse, 1993).

A comprehensive stress management plan may be needed for organizations. It begins with a baseline stress assessment to determine the levels and types of occupational stress. Interactions of departments and availability of support systems can be analyzed in relationship to nursing stress levels. Educational programs can be developed around universal stress and coping themes, such as work overload, time management, decision making, prioritization skills, and change management. Assessments of nurses' perception of their workload may help target changes where the most impact will be felt (Cox, 2002).

Other methods of personal or organizational strategies for coping with stress include physical activity; nutritional control; environmental control; psychological strategies to improve attitudes, self-esteem, and self-mastery; and interpersonal strategies related to social support. Exercise, sports, hobbies, meditation, relaxation, and spiritual exercises are advocated. Stress audits can be personal assessments or organization-wide reports. Balancing an increase in personal control with coping with what is beyond control is a key strategy. Monitoring the effects of caffeine, nicotine, and sleep/rest are advocated to increase coping. Intervention techniques can be focused on filtering, buffering, and adapting to stress.

LEADERSHIP AND MANAGEMENT IMPLICATIONS

Time management is a central strategy for reducing stress and improving coping ability. Stress is an important concern for leaders and managers in nursing. It is a pervasive fact of organizational operations. Both personal and occupational stresses create consequences for leaders and managers that also may have an effect on meeting goals and levels of productivity. The list of work- and nonwork-related stressors is long. Leaders and managers will need to assess the levels and types of stress in individuals and in the environment to begin to moderate stress toward useful levels.

Stress at too high a level reduces nurses' coping and adaptive abilities and is counterproductive. Nurse leaders and managers may have a role to play in caring for the psychological needs of the staff. Identifying and addressing prevalent operational failures at the department level can decrease many daily frustrations. Personal hardiness may be augmented by increased awareness. Leaders and managers can provide counseling, support groups, team-building activities, and stress management programs. Generational differences should be considered in developing targeted interventions (Santos & Cox, 2000).

Nurse leaders and managers have a stake in assessing and diagnosing the sources of nursing

◢ LEADERSHIP & MANAGEMENT **BEHAVIORS**

Leadership Behaviors

- Role-models workload prioritization
- Enables followers to cope with stress
- Models personal stress management
- Uses humor
- Encourages adaptation and growth
- Mentors and provides social support
- Communicates ways of coping
- Envisions the future
- Inspires hope
- Influences greater personal and group control

Management Behaviors

- Uses humor

- Manages personal stress
- Plans for stress assessment
- Organizes the environment to decrease stress
- Evaluates individual and occupational stress
- Influences followers to manage time and cope with stress
- Plans goals and activities within time targets
- Organizes work space for efficiency

Overlap Areas

- Uses humor
- Manages personal stress
- Creates ways to constructively manage time

occupational stress. As much as possible, nurse leaders should use psychometrically sound instruments to conduct evaluations in both developing and assessing the impact of interventions (Huber et al., 2000). This becomes the foundation for planning, implementing, and evaluating strategies to manage job stress. Within organizations, nurse productivity, job satisfaction, and retention are improved when occupational stress is managed. Some stressors can be modified, improved, or reduced by making structural or organizational changes. Adequate staffing, correcting problems in the physical environment, and facilitating positive communication are suggested strategies for nurse leaders and managers. Internal organizational systems may be malfunctioning and need correction. For example, organizational structures, client care variables, availability of support services, and nursing care delivery modalities may create stress and be amenable to modification for stress reduction. Organizational remedies should be founded on staff input and be directly related to improving the system (Huber, 1994; Norbeck, 1985).

Nurse leaders and managers may need to find strategies for nurses coping with an environment that creates stress because of the threat of personal danger. For example, nurses who work in abortion clinics may be personally threatened with harm. Instances arise in which infants are kidnapped from hospital nurseries. Clients may physically assault caregivers. Caregivers may be involved in fistfights or throwing objects. Policies and procedures need to be in place for the protection of nurses and clients from physical injury and bodily harm.

Leaders can inspire hope and a vision for the future. They must role-model the ability to balance personally and professionally. They can communicate with humor and inspire others to adapt to stress. Managers can plan and organize the environment to modulate organizational stress. This includes restructuring to increase nurses' access to formal and informal power and to information, resources, and support (Kanter, 1993; Laschinger et al., 2003). Leaders and managers can manage personal stress and influence others toward enhanced coping and support of one another. Thus both individual and occupational stress can be managed.

CURRENT ISSUES AND TRENDS

Health care reform and economics are creating stress and pressure for nurses both directly and indirectly. The turbulence and change that occur

Research Note

Source: Shader, K., Broome, M.E., Broome, C.D., West, M.E., & Nash, M. (2001). Factors influencing satisfaction and anticipated turnover for nurses in an academic medical center. *Journal of Nursing Administration, 31*(4), 210-216.

Purpose

This quantitative study examined the relationship between work satisfaction, stress, age, cohesion, work schedule, and anticipated turnover. Determining the impact of these relationships on intent to leave could provide nurse leaders with the knowledge to design interventions to improve work environment and retention.

Discussion

In one academic medical center a variety of factors believed to influence satisfaction and anticipated turnover were studied using a cross-sectional survey of nurses using three self-report instruments. Job stress, work satisfaction, group cohesion, and weekend overtime were all individually predictive of anticipated turnover. However, there were differences in these predictors based on age of the nurse. Also, the more job stress, lower group cohesion and work satisfaction, the higher the anticipated turnover. Many of the findings are supportive of previous work environment research.

Application to Practice

This study considered a number of important aspects in the nursing work environment. However, some key issues embedded in the surveys as discrete concepts such as manager support, workload, and nurse-physician relationships were not analyzed. Regardless of this, important relationships were confirmed. It is important to assess nurses' perceptions of the work environment to make significant changes. Without pre- and post-intervention assessments, nurse leaders won't know the actual impact of changes.

---

as health delivery systems merge, integrate, regionalize, and restructure in turn cause uncertainty, anxiety, role ambiguity, and stress. Pervasive stress is inevitable with such large-scale reforming processes of systems. Nurses must cope with new ways of thinking and delivering care. Individual stress responses, turf battles, and conflicts occur as the friction surfaces among individuals. For example, teamwork and collaboration may ultimately provide a fertile ground for systems improvement, but teamwork may be a new mode of operating and therefore a source of stress. Individuals are likely to feel helpless, anxious, and out of control when faced with massive systems changes (Huber, 1994).

Leaders and managers may themselves be under sufficient stress and thereby have less energy to devote to helping their staff through difficult psychological transitions. Cost-containment pressures may result in decisions to eliminate staff

education for stress management. Institutional remedies may be substantially diminished.

It is difficult to prescribe methods for work-related stress management during periods of high environmental turbulence. Educating and supporting staff nurses, reducing paperwork, changing organizational climates, enhancing nurses' participation in decision making, and reducing workloads—positive strategies for reducing nurses' stress—may not be implemented by organizations during unstable environmental conditions. Furthermore, under health care reform initiatives there have been major redesigns of roles and tasks in nursing and health care. Role ambiguity has become a major source of stress, directly related to both advanced practice nurses and to unlicensed assistive personnel. With so many focal points for stress, nursing as a profession is challenged to create a vision for the future and strategies for today.

Stress and conflict also may create opportunities for nursing. Clarity of direction for the profession in carving out key nursing roles and responsibilities in a community-based, managed care environment is a key stress and coping strategy. For example, case management has become a growth area for nursing as payers begin to value and pay for cost-effective care coordination and management. Changes prompt the need to adapt. Building and nurturing teams, managing change, and providing strong leadership can create a climate for innovation and creativity as one productive response to uncertainty and stress. Conflicts and changes generate stress. Positive and proactive responses help nurses to cope and adapt to stress in a way that produces growth and productivity.

Summary

- Time is a scarce and valuable resource.
- Time management is self-management of activities.
- Time management strategies are aimed at organizing and mobilizing effective activities.
- Planning, analysis, and prioritization are key elements of time management.
- The current health care environment is turbulent and stressful.
- Stress is built into healing occupations.
- Stress needs to be neither too high nor too low.
- Stress is an individual response to a stressor.
- A stressor is an experience that is taxing or threatening.
- Occupational stress is a tension related to the job or role.
- Burnout is a response to chronic stress.
- Stress moves from potential stressor to outcomes and consequences.
- Coping and cognitive appraisal mediate stress.
- Stress consequences are either positive or negative.
- Sources of stress are individual or organizational.
- Multiple factors cause stress in nursing.
- Stress outcomes take different forms—from positive to negative.

- Coping modulates stress and its outcome.
- There are both individual and organizational stress-management techniques.
- Leaders and managers can influence stress and stress management.

Study Questions

1. Why is self-management so important to time management?
2. What strategies of time management work best for nurses?
3. What sources of stress do you find to be the most important in your life and work?
4. What coping strategies are most useful for stress reduction? Why are they helpful?
5. To what extent should employers pay for stress management programs for nurses?
6. Why should nurses manage their own stress?
7. Why should nurses promote reality shock support for new graduates?
8. What can nurses do to manage stress in work teams?

CASE STUDY

Nurse Maria Vasquez is thrilled with the results of the time management training she recently received. A year ago, when she became the new nurse manager for both the operating rooms and the trauma center, she felt that everything was crashing in on her. She would arrive for work to find 15 to 20 phone messages to return, a 5-inch stack of mail to open, and 50 e-mail messages waiting on the computer. Nurse Vasquez found that on most days her attention was diverted by numerous "brush fires" that kept cropping up. In addition to the daily complaints from her staff about the normal employee concerns, there had been rumors that some nurses were talking about forming a collective bargaining unit as protection against short staffing and layoffs.

Nurse Vasquez went to her nursing director and asked for help. The director suggested that she take a couple of days and attend a time

CRITICAL THINKING EXERCISE

Nurse Whitney Gould was initially very excited about her recent promotion to nurse manager of a 50-bed regional intensive care nursery. Before this promotion, she had been a charge nurse for 5 years on the unit. She felt this had prepared her for the position, but things have not fallen smoothly into place for her. Every time she enters her office she is greeted with 50 e-mails, a stack of mail, and several voice messages. Each day she thinks this will be the day she finally has time to regroup and get organized.

Today was a good example of how that just never works out. Nurse Gould arrived at 6:30 AM to find the night charge nurse and nursing supervisor in a disagreement about day staffing. The charge nurse also told her several night nurses were taking a patient care concern to the ethics committee if she did not intervene. A surgeon called and voiced issues about a specific nurse that required immediate investigation. A recently hired graduate nurse called in

tears because she failed boards. Staffing was short for the upcoming night shift. The chief nursing officer called and requested that Nurse Gould not only give a tour for some potential donors in the unit, but also complete her staffing variance report before the end of the day. It is now 6:00 PM and she is heading out the door physically and emotionally exhausted wondering whether tomorrow will just be more of the same.

1. What problem(s) do you see in this scenario?
2. Why is this a problem?
3. What should Nurse Gould do first?
4. What factors should Nurse Gould assess and analyze?
5. What sources of stress are present?
6. How does Nurse Gould's stress affect the stress of nurses in the unit?
7. What strategies could be employed to control stress and enhance coping?

---

management class to see if it would give her any ideas to help in organizing her work and improve her efficiency.

Once she completed the class, Nurse Vasquez was excited about the idea of using an activity log to record her daily activities as a first step towards increasing her efficiency. She discussed the idea with the nursing supervisors that report to her, and they were interested in using the activity log idea themselves. Since then, Nurse Vasquez and her supervisors have found that by using the activity logs and identifying what is consuming their time, they have been better able to organize and have increased their efficiency as a result.

REFERENCES

American Hospital Association (AHA). (2002, April). *In our hands: How hospital leaders can build a thriving workforce.* Chicago: AHA.

American Nurses Association (ANA). (2001). *Code of ethics for nurses with interpretive statements.* Silver Spring, MD: ANA. Retrieved August 4, 2004, from *www.nursingworld.org/ethics/ecode.htm*

Arnold, E., & Pulich, M. (2004). Improving productivity through more effective time management. *Health Care Manager, 23*(1), 65-70.

Aurelio, J. (1993). An organizational culture that optimizes stress: Acceptable stress in nursing. *Nursing Administration Quarterly, 18*(1), 1-10.

Bailey, J.T. (1980). Stress and stress management: An overview. *Journal of Nursing Education, 19*(6), 5-8.

Benson, H., & Allen, R.L. (1980). How much stress is too much? *Harvard Business Review, 58*(5), 86-92.

Bratt, M.M., Broome, M., Kelber, S., & Lostocco, L. (2000). Influence of stress and nursing leadership on job satisfaction of pediatric intensive care unit nurses. *American Journal of Critical Care, 9*(5), 307-317.

BusinessTown.com. (2004). *Five reasons why we procrastinate and five strategies to put off putting off.* Retrieved August 4, 2004, from *www.businesstown.com/time/time-5reasons.asp*

Charnley E. (1999). Occupational stress in the newly qualified staff nurse. *Nursing Standard, 13*(29), 32-37.

Conway, M. (1988). Theoretical approaches to the study of roles. In M.E. Hardy & M.E. Conway (Eds.), *Role theory: Perspectives for health professionals* (2nd ed.) (pp. 63-72). Norwalk, CT: Appleton & Lange.

Covey, S., Merrill, A., & Merrill, R. (1994). *First things first.* New York: Simon & Schuster.

Cox, K.S. (2002). Inpatient nurses and their work environment. *Nursing Leadership Forum 7*(1), 34-37.

Dewe, P.J. (1987). Identifying the causes of nurses' stress: A survey of New Zealand nurses. *Work & Stress, 1*(1), 15-24.

Dietz, M. (1991). Stressors and coping mechanisms of older rural women. In A. Bushy (Ed.), *Rural nursing* (Vol. 1) (pp. 267-280). Newbury Park, CA: Sage.

Elliott, G., & Eisdorfer, C. (1982). *Stress and human health.* New York: Springer.

Fagin, C. (1987). Stress: Implications for nursing research. *Image, 19*(1), 38-41.

Ferner, J.D. (1995). *Successful time management: A self-teaching guide* (2nd ed.). New York: John Wiley & Sons.

Getzels, J.W. (1958). Administration as a social process. In A.W. Halpin (Ed.), *Administrative theory in education* (pp. 150-165). Chicago: University of Chicago Press.

Grant, P. (1993). Manage nurse stress and increase potential at the bedside. *Nursing Administration Quarterly, 18*(1), 16-22.

Hardy, M.E. (1978). Role stress and role strain. In M.E. Hardy & M.E. Conway (Eds.), *Role theory: Perspectives for health professionals* (2nd ed.). Norwalk, CT: Appleton-Century-Crofts.

Hardy, M.E., & Conway, M.E. (1988). *Role theory: Perspectives for health professionals* (2nd ed.). Norwalk, CT: Appleton & Lange.

Hardy, M.E., & Hardy, W.L. (1988). Role stress and role strain. In M.E. Hardy & M.E. Conway (Eds.), *Role theory: Perspectives for health professionals* (2nd ed.) (pp. 159-239). Norwalk, CT: Appleton & Lange.

Harris, R. (1989). Review of nursing stress according to a proposed coping adaptation framework. *Advances in Nursing Science, 11*(2), 12-28.

Hartl, D. (1989). Stress management and the nurse. *Advances in Nursing Science, 11*(2), 91-100.

Hinshaw, A.S. (1989). Programs of nursing research for nursing administration. In B. Henry, C. Arndt, M. Di Vincenti, & A. Marriner-Tomey (Eds.), *Dimensions of nursing administration* (pp. 251-266). Boston: Blackwell.

Hinshaw, A.S., & Atwood, J.R. (1983). Nursing staff turnover, stress, and satisfaction: Models, measures, and management. *Annual Review of Nursing Research, 1*, 133-153.

Hinshaw, A.S., Smeltzer, C.H., & Atwood, J.R. (1987). Innovative retention strategies for nursing staff. *Journal of Nursing Administration, 17*(6), 8-16.

Huber, D., Maas, M., McCloskey, J. Scherb, C.A., Goode, C.J., & Watson, C. (2000). Evaluating nursing administration instruments. *Journal of Nursing Administration, 30*(5), 251-272.

Huber, D. (1994). What are the sources of stress for nurses? In J. McCloskey & H. Grace (Eds.), *Current issues in nursing* (4th ed.) (pp. 623-631). St Louis: Mosby.

Huckabay, L.M.D., & Jagla, B. (1979). Nurses' stress factors in the intensive care unit. *Journal of Nursing Administration, 9*(2), 21-26.

Innovations International. (2004). *A monochronic/polychronic self test.* Salt Lake City, UT: Innovations International. Retrieved August 5, 2004 from *www.innovint. com/downloads/mono_poly_test.asp*

Irvine, D.M., & Evans, M.G. (1995). Job satisfaction and turnover among nurses: Integrating research findings across studies. *Nursing Research, 44*(4), 246-253.

Kanter, R.M. (1993). *Men and women of the corporation* (2nd ed.). New York: Basic Books.

Keenan, M., Hurst, J., & Olnhausen, K. (1993). Polarity management for quality care: Self-direction and manager direction. *Nursing Administration Quarterly, 18*(1), 23-29.

Kobasa, S.C, Maddi, S.R, & Kahn, S. (1982). Hardiness and health: A prospective study. *Journal of Personality & Social Psychology, 42*(1), 168-177.

Kramer, M. (1974). *Reality shock: Why nurses leave nursing.* St Louis: Mosby.

Kramer, M., & Schmalenberg, C. (1977). *Path to biculturalism.* Wakefield, MA: Contemporary Publishing.

Landstrom, G.L., Biordi, D.L., & Gillies, D.A. (1989). The emotional and behavioral process of staff nurse turnover. *Journal of Nursing Administration, 19*(9), 23-28.

Laschinger, H.K., Almost, J., & Tuer-Hodes, D. (2003). Workplace empowerment and Magnet hospital characteristics. *Journal of Nursing Administration, 33*(7/8), 410-422.

Laschinger, H.K., Finegan, J., & Shamian, J. (2001a). Promoting nurses' health: Effect of empowerment on job strain and work satisfaction. *Nursing Economic$, 19*(2), 42-52.

Laschinger, H.K., Finegan, J., Shamian, J., & Almost J. (2001b). Testing Karasek's demands-control model in restructured healthcare settings. Effects of job strain on staff nurses' quality of work life. *Journal of Nursing Administration, 31*(5), 233-243.

Lazarus, R. (1966). *Psychological stress and the coping process.* New York: McGraw-Hill.

Lazarus, R., & Folkman, S. (1984). *Stress, appraisal and coping.* New York: Springer.

Leatt, P., & Schneck, R. (1980). Differences in stress perceived by head nurses across nursing specialties in hospitals. *Journal of Advanced Nursing, 5*, 31-46.

Lowery, B. (1987). Stress research: Some theoretical and methodological issues. *Image, 19*(1), 42-46.

Lyon, B.L., & Werner, J.S. (1987). Stress. *Annual Review of Nursing Research, 5*, 3-22.

Maslach, C., & Jackson, S. (1981). The measurement of experienced burnout. *Journal of Occupational Behaviour, 2*, 99-113.

McCloskey, J.C., & McCain, B.E. (1987). Satisfaction, commitment, and professionalism of newly employed nurses. *Image, 19*, 20-24.

McClure, M., Poulin, M., Sovie, M., & Wandelt, M. (1983). *Magnet hospitals: Attraction and retention of professional nurses.* Kansas City, MO: American Nurses Association.

McCranie, E., Lambert, V., & Lambert, C. (1987). Work stress, hardiness, and burnout among hospital staff nurses. *Nursing Research, 36,* 374-378.

McGrath, J.E. (1976). Stress and behavior in organizations. In M.D. Dunnette (Ed.), *Handbook of industrial and organizational psychology* (pp. 1351-1395). Chicago: Rand McNally.

McVicar, A. (2003). Workplace stress in nursing: A literature review. Integrative literature reviews and meta-analyses. *Journal of Advanced Nursing, 44*(6), 633-642.

Miller, J. (1971). The nature of living systems. *Behavioral Science, 16,* 278.

Mills, A.C., & Blaesing, S.L. (2000). A lesson from the last nursing shortage: The influence of work values on career satisfaction with nursing. *Journal of Nursing Administration, 6,* 309-315.

Narasi, B. (1994). A tool for living through stress. *Nursing Management, 25*(9), 73-75.

Norbeck, J.S. (1985). Perceived job stress, job satisfaction, and psychological symptoms in critical care nursing. *Research in Nursing & Health, 8,* 253-259.

Noreiko, P. (1996). Time management: Getting the most out of the day. *Occupational Health: A Journal for Occupational Health Nurses, 48*(5), 172-174.

Pagana, K.D. (1994). Teaching students time management strategies. *Journal of Nursing Education, 33*(8), 381-383.

Perlman, B., & Hartman, E. (1982). Burnout: Summary and future research. *Human Relations, 35*(4), 283-305.

Pollock, S. (1984). The stress response. *Critical Care Quarterly, 3,* 1-13.

Price, J.L., & Mueller, C.W. (1981). *Professional turnover: The case of nurses.* New York: Spectrum.

Rich, V.L., & Rich, A.R. (1987). Personality hardiness and burnout in female staff nurses. *Image, 19,* 63-66.

Rocchiccioli, J.T., & Tilbury, M.S. (1998). *Clinical leadership in nursing.* Philadelphia: Saunders.

Santos, S.R, & Cox, K. (2000). Workplace adjustment and intergenerational differences between Matures, Boomers and Xers. *Nursing Economic$, 18*(1), 7-13.

Sawatzky, J.V. (1998). Understanding nursing students' stress: A proposed framework. *Nurse Education Today, 18*(2), 108-115.

Scalzi, C. (1988). Role stress and coping strategies of nurse executives. *Journal of Nursing Administration, 18*(3), 34-38.

Schmalenberg, C., & Kramer, M. (1979). *Coping with reality shock: The voices of experience.* Wakefield, MA: Nursing Resources.

Schumacher, L., & Larson, K. (1993). Thriving and striving on the turbulence of rural health care. *Nursing Administration Quarterly, 18*(1), 11-15.

Schwab, L. (1996). Individual hardiness and staff satisfaction. *Nursing Economic$, 14*(3), 171-173.

Selye, H. (1965). *The stress of life.* Toronto: McGraw-Hill.

Selye, H. (1976). *Stress in health and disease.* Boston: Butterworth.

Severance, J.S., & Cervantes, E. (1996). Time management training for home care workers. *Caring, 15*(5), 58-61.

Sherry, D. (1996). Time management strategies for the new home care nurse. *Home Healthcare Nurse, 11*(9), 710-720.

Simoni, P.S. & Paterson, J.J. (1997). Hardiness, coping, and burnout in the nursing workplace. *Journal of Professional Nursing, 13*(3), 178-185.

Smythe, E. (1984). Burn-out: From caring to apathy. In E. Smythe (Ed.), *Surviving nursing* (pp. 46-57). Menlo Park, CA: Addison-Wesley.

Sovie M.D., & Jawad, A. F. (2001). Hospital restructuring and its impact on outcomes. *Journal of Nursing Administration, 31*(12), 588-600.

Stehle, J.L. (1981). Critical care nursing stress: The findings revisited. *Nursing Research, 30,* 182-186.

Tarolli-Jager, K. (1994). Personal hardiness: Your buffer against burnout. *American Journal of Nursing, 94*(2), 71-72.

Thomas, E.J., & Biddle, B.J. (1966). Basic concepts for classifying the phenomena of role. In B.J. Biddle & E.J. Thomas (Eds.), *Role theory: Concepts and research* (pp. 23-45). New York: John Wiley & Sons.

Tucker, A.L. (2004). The impact of operational failures on hospital nurses and their patients. *Journal of Operations Management, 22,* 151-169.

Wagnild, G., & Young, H.M. (1991). Another look at hardiness. *Image, 23*(4), 257-259.

Weisman, C.S., Alexander, C.S., & Chase, G. (1981). Determinants of hospital staff nurse turnover. *Medical Care, 19*(4), 431-443.

Woodhouse, D. (1993). The aspects of humor in dealing with stress. *Nursing Administration Quarterly, 18*(1), 80-89.

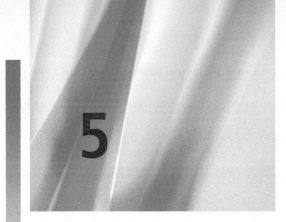

5

Health Policy, Health, and Nursing

Katherine R. Jones

CHAPTER OBJECTIVES

- Define and describe policy and politics
- Define and describe health policy
- Overview the policy-making process
- Compare policy formulation models
- Contrast interest group strategies
- Describe the legislative process
- Analyze health policy
- Exercise critical thinking to conceptualize and analyze possible solutions to a practice exercise

Policy is a field of study that few nurses pursue formally, but most or all nurses experience the influence of policy throughout their careers. Nurses, nursing, and policy intersect in multiple ways. After graduation from nursing school, regulatory policies dictate that the graduate must pass a licensing examination in order to use the initials *RN* and to practice as a registered nurse. On the job, nurses must comply with institutional policies that spell out such things as dress code, overtime and floating requirements, and performance review criteria and procedures. Thus nurses are influenced by policies at the state and national level (e.g., RN licensure or Medicare reimbursement for nurse practitioners) and at the local level (institutional policies at the work site). Nurses also have a role to play in influencing health policy via political action. Nurses need to be visible and vocal.

As members of a professional association, nurses may contribute money to political action committees (PACs) and contribute to the creation of policy agendas. If greater involvement in policy is desired, nurses may serve in a governmental relations capacity (e.g., as lobbyists), or work on a political campaign to help officials with specific political beliefs be elected to office. At the local level, many nurses play important policy roles as they serve on boards of directors of nonprofit agencies, where they must carefully distinguish policy from day-to-day operations. Finally, nurses may run for office themselves and develop a political agenda that includes health and nursing issues or become policy analysts for an organization or association, evaluating the impact of proposed or newly created policies on various stakeholder groups. In short, given the pervasiveness of policy influences on their everyday lives, nurses should be well informed about policy and the policy-making process.

As nursing has matured as a profession, nurses have become more aware of the need for activism in health policy and politics at all levels. As the largest health care provider group, nurses need to be a visible and vocal presence in the debate about health policy directions. Nurses hold individual, personal perspectives as citizens and consumers of health care. They exercise their voices when they vote. Nurses as a professional group are integral to the delivery of health care services and need to be active as client advocates. Nurses as a provider group are a special interest lobby with identifiable skills, abilities, potential, and turf area. In order to have influence over legislation and other health policy decisions, nurses can organize, lobby, coordinate grassroots activities, serve on legislative staffs, or become elected officials. Involvement in policy and politics is important for nurses because it is the right thing to do and because if nurses are not visible and active, others will make decisions affecting nursing.

DEFINITIONS

Because the terms *policy* and *politics* carry different meanings, it is important to distinguish between these two concepts. **Policy** is the formulation of value statements, the "shoulds" and "oughts" of larger and more important issues. Policy is defined as a plan, direction, or goal for action. It is a result of setting goals and determining directions. In authoritative decision making, policy is a course of action or inaction, consciously chosen. Policies are choices made about goals, priorities, and ways of allocating resources. Thus policies reflect the values of the decision makers (Mason et al., 2002). Policy decisions are, therefore, meant to direct or influence the actions, behaviors, or decisions of others (Longest, 1997). Public policies are authoritative decisions made in the legislative, executive, and judicial branches of government (Longest, 2002). Public policy encompasses anything a government chooses to do or not to do (Dye, 1987). Health policies are public policies that pertain to health or the pursuit of health by the public; the defining purpose of the governmental health policy is to support the public in its quest for health (Longest, 1997; 2002). Health policy decisions usually influence a category of providers (physicians, nurses, pharmacists), organizations (hospitals, clinics, managed care organizations, health plans, medical schools), or care recipients (elderly, children, the poor).

Policies tend to change in small increments. Policies are generated at institutional levels (e.g., personnel policies in a long-term care facility) and at local, state, and national levels (e.g., public health sanitation policies or meat inspection rules). Institutional policies are developed by a discrete employer to govern its operations. Organizational policies are promulgated by professional organizations or other official entities and function as position statements, guidelines, or rules (Mason et al., 2002).

Politics, on the other hand, is the process of influencing the allocation of scarce resources or the use of power for change. Politics occurs within the arenas of competition and conflicting values. However, politics is a fundamental aspect of operating where multiple interest groups compete for scarce resources. Nurses can have an effect on change in four major spheres of political influence: in the workplace, government, organizations, and the larger community (Mason et al., 2002).

Health policy is the entire set of public policies that are related to or influence health and illness. The federal, state, and local levels of government all are involved in formulating health policy and making decisions to promote the health of individual citizens (Mason et al., 2002). Health policy can be general (Do all citizens have a right to

---

▲ LEADING & MANAGING **DEFINED**

Policy
A plan, direction, or action goal.

Politics
The process of influencing the allocation of scarce resources or the use of power for change.

Health Policy
The entire set of public policies that are related to or influence health and illness.

health care?) or specific (Do all health care providers have to be tested for HIV/AIDS or submit urine samples for drug screening?). Health policy decisions set an overall tone for how a society decides to solve recurring issues in the health care needs of the people.

Public Policy Making

Policy making goes on in many settings. It is an activity that has been described as complex, multidimensional, and dynamic (Mason et al., 2002). At issue are values. Public policy occurs through the acts of government or governmental agencies, such as by national commissions, by legislation, by the judicial system, by state and local governments, in the private sector, and by regulatory agencies. In some countries, a centralized ministry of health is the major health policy agency. In the United States the process is more complex, decentralized, and layered. The absence of one identifiable decision maker creates greater influence possibilities for nurses; yet the system can appear confusing and formidable.

Policy making is dependent on both values and analysis. This is because choices come from both values and analysis, and policy making implies choice. For example, within the health policy arena there are numerous conflicts over values. One example is the issue of which criteria are used to judge the health care system and thereby make resource allocation decisions. A feminist perspective on power, politics, and policy making indicates that nurses, as members of a predominantly female occupation, may hold values that conflict with the predominant values of society. Nursing values caring, collaboration, and collectivity, whereas the dominant values in U.S. society include individuality and competition (Backer et al., 1998; Mason et al., 2002).

Analyses are done to provide data input into policy-making decisions. For example, detailed economic analyses or predictive modeling may be done. The selection of which analyses are done and the interpretation of the results also reflect decision makers' values and perspectives. As a structured approach to decision making, Hanley (2002)

recommended the following five-step policy analysis framework:

1. Establish the context, definition of the problem, and objectives.
2. Identify policy options and alternatives.
3. Project consequences for each option.
4. Specify criteria to evaluate each option.
5. Recommend the optimal solution.

This framework can be used as the general outline of a policy analysis or white paper or for addressing the discussion and analysis of many issues. For example, analyzing the outcomes of care is important for making informed decisions and influencing health policy. Research findings need to be translated into policy-relevant recommendations (Jones et al., 1997). Cost-effectiveness analysis (CEA) is one strategy to inform decision makers about how much health improvement can be achieved per dollar invested (Allred et al., 1998). It also has been proposed as appropriate for resource allocation decisions in the delivery of care and for improving clinical care overall (Stone, 1998). CEA uses a decision analysis technique derived from operations research and game theory to evaluate the outcomes and costs of health interventions. A CEA cost-effectiveness ratio is calculated, with the health outcome measured in health units and cost of treatment measured in dollars. A problem and alternative options are identified, modeled, and analyzed. The CEA can assist with determining which policies should be followed or which programs should be funded (Buerhaus, 1998; Stone, 1998).

Policy makers in the public sector face the challenge of deciding how to allocate public resources. These resources are limited, so it is usually possible to promote one desired objective only at the expense of another worthy objective. At the state level, this means that enhanced funding for prisons and tourism may come at the expense of funding for higher education and programs to promote the arts. At the federal level, higher expenditures for defense and Medicare may translate into lower or flat budgets for highways and biomedical research. Moreover, specific policy choices will result in some winners and some losers in terms of achieved benefits. For example, the discount drug cards made available in 2004 under a new Medicare drug benefit may help some Medicare beneficiaries cover their drug costs, but at the same time they may exert significant financial pressure on small pharmacies that traditionally operate with lean operating margins.

Public policies may take one of several different forms. Laws are perhaps the best known form of public policy. They may have extensive impact on the health care field. For example, the Health Insurance Portability and Accountability Act of 1996 (HIPAA), administered by the Centers for Medicare and Medicaid Services (CMS), has multiple unrelated provisions. The health insurance reform aspect of the Act provides for the portability of health insurance coverage and may be extremely important at times of job loss. The administrative simplification component of the Act calls for national standards for electronic health care transactions; national identifiers for providers, health plans, and employers; and security and privacy of health data. These new requirements have had a major impact on health care providers, as well as researchers and educators.

Rules and regulations are another aspect of policy. These are established to guide the implementation of laws (Longest, 2001). Such rule-making may generate hundreds or thousands of pages of text. Operational decisions by agencies within the executive branch also represent policies (Longest, 2001). An example is the decision by the FDA not to allow the "morning-after" pill to be available over the counter. Policies may also be derived from judicial decisions. Several courts have ruled on Congress' attempt to ban partial-birth abortions, overturning the legislation and, in effect, allowing existing policies to stay in place.

FACTORS DRIVING PUBLIC POLICY MAKING

Market Failures

Public policy making occurs when the marketplace fails to allocate resources efficiently. In a freely competitive market, the following five conditions are said to exist (Longest, 1997; 2001):

1. Both buyers and sellers of services or products have sufficient information to make informed choices.
2. A large number of buyers and sellers participate in the market; no one buyer or seller dominates the market.
3. More sellers of the service or product can easily enter the market.
4. Each seller's products or services can be substituted for those of competitors.
5. The quantity of products or services available in the market does not unduly influence the balance of power toward either buyers or sellers.

To address market failures, the government has a choice of the following actions:

- Do nothing.
- Attempt to improve the working of the market.
- Require people to behave in specified ways.
- Provide incentives that influence the decisions of individuals and organizations.
- Engage directly in the provision of goods and services.

Health Policy and Market Failure

In the United States, it has long been presumed that private markets (capitalism) best determine the production and consumption of goods and services, including those produced by the health care system (Longest, 1997). However, private markets sometimes fail to achieve desirable social objectives, and the government may choose to intervene to correct or address the market failure using one or more of the strategies described above. The health care industry is one example of a situation in which markets are not able to function effectively to allocate goods and services. Longest (1997) has described how the health care marketplace violates the assumptions of a freely competitive market: consumers in general do not have the information necessary to make informed decisions but instead must rely on information and guidance provided by the supplier of those services; sellers of health care services do not easily enter the market but are instead confronted by an extensive array of regulations and certification and licensing requirements; and health insurance alters consumer decisions to obtain health care services because the buyer is shielded from the actual costs of purchasing those services. To address these and other market failures, the government generates policies relevant to the health care marketplace. The policies have ranged from "do nothing" to direct engagement in the provision of goods and services. For example, as a nation, the Unites States has done little toward establishing a comprehensive long-term care service delivery and financing program. On the other hand, the government provides comprehensive health care services directly to the nation's veterans through the national Veterans Administration health care system.

PUBLIC POLICY-MAKING PROCESS

Public policies are made within the public policy-making framework (Longest, 2001). The public policy-making process is dominated by three major players: interest groups that are affected by or concerned with a particular policy area; the executive agency that has administrative responsibility over the related policy area; and the congressional committees and subcommittees that have legislative authority in these policy areas (Block, 2004). These three players have been termed the "Iron Triangle" because of their lock on policy development (Kronenfeld et al., 1984).

In the United States the public policy-making process occurs in a multidimensional fashion. It is an ongoing process and one in which virtually all decisions are subject to modification or reversion. Thus there are numerous influences, often external from special interest groups and stakeholders that buffet or impact the process. Clearly, policy making resembles an open system, by virtue of the sensitive impact of the external environment (Longest, 2002).

Interest Group Politics

Interest Groups and Lobbying

Most problems get placed on the policy agenda through the efforts of organized interest groups.

In general, organizations have a significant advantage over individuals in the political marketplace (Longest, 2002). Organizations have more resources and tend to have more concentrated interests. The most effective advocates for health policy are the organized interest groups. An interest group is an organization of people with similar policy goals who enter the political process to try to achieve those aims (Lineberry et al., 1995). Interest group politics refers to the efforts of these organized groups to influence government policy. Through combining and concentrating their resources, interest groups can have a large impact in political markets (Longest, 2002). Some of the most effective interest groups, based on their size and resources, are the American Medical Association (AMA), American Hospital Association (AHA), American Association for Retired Persons (AARP), American Association of Health Plans (AAHP), and the Pharmaceutical Research and Manufacturers of America (PhRMA). In nursing, the American Nurses Association (ANA) has been an active and effective interest group, but the ANA does not speak alone for nurses. The American Association of Nurse Anesthetists (AANA), American College of Nurse Midwives (ACNM), American Association of Colleges of Nursing (AACN), National League for Nursing (NLN), American Organization of Nurse Executives (AONE), and other nursing groups are also active; but the many nursing interest groups tend to fragment the profession and might diminish the overall influence of nursing in public policy making. Box 5.1 provides a list of many of the health-related interest groups. Longest (1997) described four strategies that interest groups use to influence the public policy-making process: lobbying, electioneering, litigation, and influencing public opinion.

Lobbying

Interest groups attempt to influence the views of individual representatives and senators or key members of the executive branch on specific issues. The exertion of influence in public policy making is the process by which people successfully persuade others to follow their advice, suggestions,

Health Care Interest Groups

American Academy of Pediatrics
American Association for Homes and Services
   for the Aging
American Association of Colleges of Nurses
American Association of Health Plans
American Association of Retired Persons
American Cancer Society
American College of Healthcare Executives
American College of Surgeons
American Dental Association
American Federation of Home Health Agencies
American Health Care Association
American Heart Association
American Hospital Association
American Medical Association
American Nurses Association
Association of American Medical Colleges
Association of University Programs in Health
   Administration
BlueCross BlueShield Association
Group Health Association of America
Health Insurance Association of America
Hospice Association of America
National Council for Senior Citizens
National Association for Home Care
National Association of Medical Equipment
   Suppliers
National Association of Social Workers
National League for Nursing
Pharmaceutical Research and Manufacturers
   of America

or orders (Keys & Case, 1990). Interest groups hire lobbyists (also called *governmental relations officers* or *specialists*), who communicate with policy makers for the purpose of influencing their decisions to be more favorable to, or consistent with, the preferences of those doing the lobbying (Buchholz, 1994). Some interest groups are more effective than others. Milio (1984) identified the

following guidelines for effectively influencing policy: organize; do your homework; frame your arguments to appeal to the specific audience you want to persuade; concentrate your finite organizational energies; act in a timely fashion at the right points in the policy-making process; and always obtain or develop the best data available on your policy position.

Electioneering

This strategy involves working to elect or retain in office policy makers who are sympathetic to the interests of the group's members (Longest, 1997). One very popular way to do this is to direct money into PACs. Another approach is direct involvement with political campaigns, including fund raising, participation in phone banks, and canvassing neighborhoods.

Litigation

This strategy involves the use of lawsuits to challenge existing policies, stimulate new policies, or alter specific aspects of the implementation of policies (Longest, 1997). Litigation may be used at both the state and federal levels; this is an increasingly popular way to exert influence in the policy arena. A recent example is the case brought by the California Hospital Association to challenge the implementation of the minimum staffing ratios in California hospitals.

Shaping public opinion

Policy makers are influenced by public opinion, so interest groups may be able to achieve their objectives by helping to shape these opinions. One current policy area in which public opinion is a major target is the new Medicare Drug Benefit. Television and newspaper ads are being financed by various groups in an attempt to inform and influence the public's response to the new Medicare drug cards and other aspects of the complex new law.

Policy Development

Health policies are created within the dynamic public policy-making process that takes place at the federal, state, or local levels of government. Health policies are also created in the private sector. For example, health plans have policies related to the required procedures for accessing medical specialists; hospitals have policies related to mandatory overtime or floating staff to other units. These policies, similar to those in the public sector, are also authoritative decisions that influence the actions, behaviors, or decisions of others (Longest, 2002). The development of any kind of policy is a process that reflects the values of the individuals or groups supporting that policy position. These individuals or groups identify a problem for which a policy solution is sought. Longest (1997, 2002) has identified the following

three interconnected phases of the public policy-making process (Figure 5.1):

1. *Formulation phase:* Incorporates activities associated with agenda setting and the subsequent development and adoption of the legislation

2. *Implementation phase:* Incorporates activities associated with rule making and policy operation; mobilization of human and financial resources to comply with the policy (Longest, 2002)

3. *Modification phase:* As a result of policy assessment, addresses whether the implemented policy is in compliance with its statutory requirements and achieving its objectives in regard to the policy problem (Dunn, 1994)

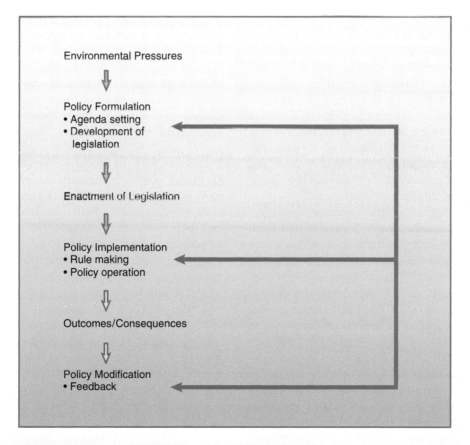

Figure 5.1
Public policy-making process. (Modified from Longest, B.B., Jr. [2002]. *Health policymaking in the United States* [3rd ed.]. Chicago: Health Administration Press.)

POLICY FORMULATION

A window of opportunity is created for an issue to emerge on the public policy agenda when problems, possible solutions, and political circumstances come together in a favorable configuration. Problems may be serious but not emerge into policy issues. When they reach an unacceptable level, they may emerge into the public consciousness. For example, the number of people with AIDS and the number of people without health care coverage (uninsured) are national health problems. Problems tend to be noticed when they are widespread and affect large numbers of people, when they affect a small but powerful group, when they attract the attention of the nation via media coverage, or when they are linked closely to other well-accepted policy issues (Longest, 2002).

When a problem comes to the forefront, possible solutions help to trigger policy formulation. Differences or conflict may arise over the criteria to be used in evaluating alternative solutions to the problem. Policy making may be slowed by the time it takes to critique and debate the relative merits of competing alternatives. Arguments may be generated over the likelihood of a solution to solve the problem, implementation timelines and feasibility, costs, benefits, and political considerations (Longest, 2002).

The political circumstances surrounding policy making relate to the power necessary to launch substantive legislation initiatives. A political force may arise from a variety of sources. For example, public opinion or concern about an issue may initiate political forces. Special interest groups, key political leaders, and any other policy issues currently in focus may be powerful enough to create the window of policy-making opportunity (Longest, 2002).

Research and concept analysis are important tools for the formulation phase of the policy-making process. By analyzing data, providing documentation, providing an issues synthesis, or recommending a course of action (prescription), research can influence public policy (Brown, 1991). Sometimes a large and diverse set of policies results from the offering of solutions by multiple special interest groups armed with data (Longest, 2002). Research can be used to help define a problem, although timing may be crucial. Data on advanced practice nursing may be useful to turn a challenge around (Diers, 1998).

Agenda setting means getting the identified problem to the attention of the government or policy makers. Survival on the policy agenda depends on the following five factors (Milstead, 1999):

1. Technical feasibility
2. Value acceptability within the policy community
3. Tolerable cost
4. Anticipated public agreement
5. Reasonable chance that elected officials will be receptive to it

The policy-making process is more of a political process than a rational decision-making process. The preferences and influences of interest groups, political bargaining, vote trading, and ideological biases may come into play at any point in the public policy-making process. Several useful models of the public policy process have been developed for doing analyses.

Kingdon Model of Policy Formulation

Kingdon's (1995) framework described the constant interaction that occurs between participants in the process and the policy problem, its politics, and policy solution. Kingdon described three streams of activities that must line up in order for a particular problem to make it to the policy agenda, as follows (Figure 5.2):

1. The problem stream
2. The policy solution stream
3. The political circumstances stream

An essential step in the policy formulation process is to figure out how to convince a policy maker to put a particular problem on the policy agenda. At least one possible solution must be available for any problem to be placed on the agenda. Multiple alternative solutions may be available, which will slow down the policy development process as each of the possible solutions is reviewed and considered. Alternative policy

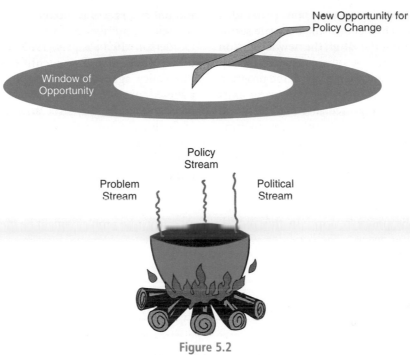

Figure 5.2
A depiction of how Kingdon's model of public policy formation might look.

solutions come from the many subsystems of policy making, including congressional staff, researchers, interest group members, and bureaucrats. The goal, as described in Kingdon's model, is to match a possible solution to a problem that is floating around the policy space. However, a problem and a possible solution are not the only elements necessary for generating policy development. There must also be the political will to make it happen. The political stream considers other factors in the environment that influence the policy agenda, such as the economy, size of the federal deficit, public attitudes and opinions, positions of key political leaders, and the presence of other competing items on the policy agenda (Longest, 1997). The coupling of problems and policy streams allows for the creation of policy change only when the political stream is favorable as well; this "window of opportunity" occurs on an infrequent basis.

Policy proposals that receive serious consideration must meet several criteria, including technical feasibility, fit with the dominant values and the national priorities of the day, and budget feasibility (Kingdon, 1995). A recent example of the confluence of a policy problem and solution with a positive political stream was the passage of the Medicare Prescription Drug, Improvement, and Modernization Act of 2003. Pressure to do something about the high cost of prescription medicine and lack of a drug benefit in the Medicare program was mounting. The media reported stories of elderly individuals doing without food or heat in order to pay for their prescription medications. States were setting up programs that were not consistent with the ideology of the federal administration (e.g., state-level negotiation with drug companies to lower drug prices; importation of drugs from Canada). Possible policy solutions at the federal level included adding a new benefit to the current Medicare program (expanded government entitlement) or using a private sector approach. Choosing the latter, the new legislation has created a government-subsidized prescription benefit as part of Medicare but opens the program to price competition through a premium support model. The Centers for Medicare and Medicaid Services (CMS) have the task of implementing this complex law.

Stage-Sequential Model of Policy Formulation

The stage-sequential model is another model explaining public policy making. In this model,

the policy process is viewed as a series of stages in which a number of functional activities occur (Anderson, 1990; Ripley, 1985, 1996). A group's policy problem is first identified and placed on the policy agenda. Next, a policy is developed, adopted, implemented, and evaluated. The stages are dynamic and cyclical and include a policy evaluation and oversight stage to identify whether the program is functioning well or might require revision or even generation of an entirely new policy. The specific steps in the stage-sequential model are as follows:

- *Stage 1:* Identification of the policy problem (e.g., the problem might be identified as safety

Research Note

Source: Laraway, A.S., & Jennings, C.P. (2002). Health insurance flexibility and accountability demonstration initiative (HIFA): A policy analysis using Kingdon's policy streams model. *Policy, Politics, & Nursing Practice, 3*(4), 358-366.

Purpose

Laraway and Jennings used the policy formulation model developed by Kingdon to analyze how and why the Health Insurance Flexibility and Accountability Demonstration Initiative (HIFA) was implemented by the (George W.) Bush administration. The problem stream was characterized as the lack of access to health insurance by low-income individuals. The magnitude of the uninsured problem was informed by several studies and reports. These reports demonstrated significant growth in the number of uninsured in the U.S. These "indicators" helped point to the uninsured as a problem that needed to be addressed by policy makers.

Discussion

Expanding insurance coverage to cover the unemployed can be linked to many potential policy solutions. The options contained in the policy stream included allocating additional federal funds to the states and encouraging them to expand coverage; expansion of the state SCHIP programs; extending Medicaid and SCHIP coverage to parents of children enrolled in these programs; and expanding coverage to the uninsured through a HIFA waiver. The political stream was described as being made up of three major components: the national mood, organized political forces, and events occurring within the government. The national mood was generally positive at the time the discussions were taking place; interest groups were putting pressure on the President to do something about the growing problem of the uninsured; the media was publishing stories about the problem as well as the high cost of health care and health insurance; and the waiver approach fit with the Republican emphasis on federalism, giving greater responsibilities to the states.

Application to Practice

Laraway and Jennings concluded that HIFA was born because the idea of expansion of health services and coverage of previously uninsured persons through state empowerment and action was seen by policy makers as a viable and politically acceptable solution to a pressing problem. This article demonstrates how nurses can use policy models to analyze the various factors surrounding a policy issue. Armed with analysis, nurses are in a more powerful position to mobilize political action at the most opportune time and in the most strategic manner.

and quality issues in hospitals; the problem could then be restated as a policy problem or issue—that of inadequate numbers of RNs staffing hospital units)

- *Stage 2:* Policy formulation (e.g., the establishment of laws requiring hospitals to meet minimum staffing ratios for RNs, as done in California)
- *Stage 3:* Program implementation (e.g., the California Department of Health was charged with establishing the minimum staffing ratios for different types of units within hospitals)
- *Stage 4:* Policy evaluation (e.g., the implementation, performance, and impact of the policy solution [minimum staffing ratios] are evaluated to determine how well the new policy is meeting its stated goals and objectives)

Political Process

The policy formulation phase concludes with the development of legislation. Formal enactment of legislation bridges the policy-making process into the next phase of policy implementation. The complexity of the legislative process in the United States is a reminder to nurses that getting a law passed is arduous and tricky.

Legislative process

At the federal level, bills are introduced in the U.S. House of Representatives or the Senate and then assigned to a committee with jurisdiction over the substance of the bill. A number of committees in the House and Senate are involved with health legislation. In the House, a health-related bill is usually considered by the Energy and Commerce Committee or its Subcommittee on Health and Environment, the Ways and Means Committee or its Subcommittee on Health, the Committee on Veteran's Affairs, the Committee on Education and Labor, or the Select Committee on Aging. In the Senate, a bill may be heard by the Health, Education, Labor and Pensions Committee or its Subcommittee on Public Health, the Senate Finance Committee or its Subcommittee on Health Care, the Committee on Finance, the

Committee on Labor and Human Resources, the Committee on Veteran's Affairs, or the Select Committee on Indian Affairs. Appropriations are decided by the Appropriations Subcommittee on Labor, Health, and Human Services, Education, and Related Agencies in both the Senate and the House.

There are three types of committees in Congress, as follows (Wakefield, 1999):

1. Oversight committees that monitor issues related to the committee focus
2. Appropriation committees that allocate funding on a fiscal year basis to support specific programs (The appropriations levels cannot exceed the ceilings established by the authorizing legislation, but they can fund at a significantly lower level.)
3. Authorization committees that establish or change federal programs and set limits on the amount of federal funding that can be spent to implement a particular program

The chair of the authorization committee determines which bills will be considered by the committee during a legislative session. During the deliberations, hearings are held and oral or written testimony presented. After the hearings are done, a bill is next "reported out" or sent to the floor of the House or Senate for a vote. Both chambers must act on a bill before it can become a law. Successful bills are sent to conference committees composed of members from both the House and Senate to negotiate any differences in the respective bills. Finally, the negotiated final version of the bill is reported out for a final vote by both chambers and, if passed, forwarded on to the President for signature and enactment into law or vetoed. Re-authorization of programs occurs every 3 to 5 years.

POLICY IMPLEMENTATION PHASE

After a law is enacted, the focus shifts from the policy formulation phase to the policy implementation phase. Policy implementation is the process of putting a policy into effect to accomplish its policy goals and objectives. The new policy may direct change in the actions or behaviors of individuals or organizations, or it may rearrange existing behavior patterns to comply with the policy decision (Wilken, 1999). Executive agencies must create the rules and regulations that are necessary for a newly enacted program to become functional (Milstead, 1999). The organization or agency that is responsible for implementing the new law must publish in the *Federal Register* a Notice of Proposed Rule Making (NPRM) (Longest, 2002). Once the rule is drafted, the public is able to review and comment on the proposed rules for implementing the law. This often results in changes in the proposed rules. This is one of the most active points of involvement for individuals and organizations seeking to influence the policy-making process (Longest, 1997). Rules and regulations established through the formal rulemaking process have legal standing and are, in effect, policies. These policies are codified in the Code of Federal Regulations (CFR) and are available to the public to read and review (Longest, 2002).

Stages of implementation proceed from the implementation decisions made by the responsible agency to the subsequent compliance of target groups with these decisions. The actual impact of the new law (both intended and unintended consequences) is evaluated, and revisions or attempted revisions frequently are made (Wilken, 1999). Because of the continued involvement of different interest groups, it is important to constantly monitor the implementation of a new program or law. The following three issues are critical to address (Wilken, 1999):

1. To what extent are the policy results or outcomes consistent with the officially stated objectives?
2. To what extent have the original objectives been modified during the implementation process?
3. What principal factors have affected the degree of change and modifications that have occurred in the new program?

Policies must be effectively implemented in order to have a chance of achieving their intended effect (Longest, 1997). Although laws are implemented primarily in the executive branch of government, within departments such as Health and Human Services, Labor, Education, and Commerce, the Legislative branch does maintain oversight responsibility of policy implementation through funding appropriations, hearings, and agencies such as the General Accounting Office (GAO) and Congressional Budget Office (CBO) (Longest, 1997). Wilken (1999) has concluded that policy implementation is inherently unpredictable. During this phase various forces will try to change the policy, including interest groups, opposition parties, affected individuals and organizations, and the bureaucracy that has the responsibility for implementation (Wilken, 1999). More important, however, members of the nursing community, from individual nurses to national nursing organizations, can also affect implementation of new policy programs and laws. This may be one area where nurses can have a strategic impact to benefit patients and society.

POLICY MODIFICATION PHASE

In this phase of the public policy-making process, individuals and organizations provide feedback to the policy makers and policy implementers regarding the impact of the new law or program. Actual experiences in the implementation phase are presented to the lawmakers, the courts, or the legislative branch. Portions of the new programs might be struck down or modified, or the entire bill may be vacated, as happened with Medicare Catastrophic Coverage. The Medicare Catastrophic Coverage Act, passed in 1988, was a major reform initiative, but it was short-lived. Angry senior citizens were quick to let their congressional representatives know their displeasure with the law, and it was repealed in 1989. In short, policy modification is an important phase of the policy-making process. Individuals will seek changes that provide more benefits or protect existing ones; those who are affected negatively by a policy will seek to modify it and reduce the negative consequences; those who formulate or implement policies will seek changes when the policies fail to measure up to their preferences and objectives (Longest, 2002). Longest (2002) pointed out that the policy modification phase makes the public policy-making process both dynamic and continuously evolving. In addition, some policies are made obsolete because of biological, social, cultural, demographic, ecological, economic, ethical, legal, psychological, and technological changes (Longest, 1997).

Allocative and Regulatory Health Policies

Health policy is a subset of public policy. It includes those public policies that are related to or influence health and illness. Health policies generally affect either a group of individuals or certain types of organizations. A complex and large number of decisions go into health policy formulation. Health policies emerge in the forms of laws, rules and regulations, judicial decisions, resource allocations, and broad "macro" policies such as global health care budgets.

Health policy is important to nursing in multiple ways, from the regulation of practice to the structure of the practice environment and professional practices (Algase et al., 2004). Health policy decision making influences what nurses and other clinicians can do in practice and determines what professional services will be reimbursed by government and third-party payers and for how much (Algase et al., 2004).

Health policies fall within two broad categories: allocative and regulatory (Block, 2004). Allocative policies are designed to provide benefits to one group of individuals or organizations at the expense of others in order to meet specific policy objectives (Longest, 2002). Some allocative policies are meant to address imbalances in supply and demand of certain products or services. Other allocative policies are used to make sure certain segments of the population have access to health care services (Longest, 1997). The funding of graduate medical education programs under the Medicare program is an example of an allocative policy. Given the expense of medical education, it was believed that a sufficient supply of physicians

would not be produced without this public subsidy of medical education. Regulatory policies, on the other hand, are meant to influence the actions, behaviors, and decisions of others through a directive approach. State practice acts that dictate what activities are within a health professional's scope of practice are an example of a regulatory policy. Longest (1997) has identified the following five categories of regulatory health policies:

1. Market-entry restrictions
2. Rate or price-setting controls on health service providers
3. Quality controls on the provision of health services
4. Market-preserving controls
5. Social regulation

The first four types of health policies are focused on economic issues; the fifth, however, seeks to achieve socially desired ends (Longest, 1997). Market-entry regulations include the state policies related to licensing of practitioners or organizations, including advanced practice nursing certification and prescriptive authority. Rate-setting regulations include the Medicare program's imposition of the prospective payment system (PPS) using diagnosis-related groups (DRGs), and the resource-based relative value scale (RBRVS) payment system for physicians under Medicare. Regulations related to quality controls includes the stringent safety and efficacy standards that must be met before a new drug is approved by the FDA. Another example is the recent requirement by Medicare for public reporting of performance data by both nursing homes and home health agencies (Nursing Home Compare and Home Health Compare). Market-preserving regulations are those that seek to retain competitiveness among providers and organizations by restricting the formation of monopolies through enforcement of the Sherman Antitrust Act, the Clayton Act, and the Robinson-Patman Act (Longest, 2001). Socially desirable regulations include rules for workplace safety (OSHA) or rules that prevent age or sex discrimination in hiring (Longest, 2002).

Unintended Consequences of Public Policy

Analysis may reveal that policies intended to have one outcome may have unintended consequences that totally overwhelm the intended outcomes. An example of this is what happened as a result of a state Medicaid drug cost-containment policy for the chronically mentally ill (Soumerai, 2003). The intent of the policy was to reduce Medicaid expenditures for drugs used to manage chronic mental illness. In New Hampshire, the state Medicaid program introduced a drug-payment "cap" that set a limit of three reimbursable medications a person could receive per month. A structured policy analysis revealed that the drug cap did indeed reduce the use of prescription drugs among the elderly and mentally ill but at the same time increased hospital and nursing home admissions, partial hospitalizations, distribution of psychoactive medications by community mental health centers, and use of emergency mental health services. The analysis showed that vulnerable populations are likely to experience adverse effects from hastily applied drug cost-containment policies, and the resulting compensatory measures may create more expenses than the policy removes (Soumerai, 2003).

Policy Analysis

Policy analysis is the systematic study of the content and anticipated or actual effects of existing or proposed policies. It is primarily concerned with explanations rather than with prescriptions (Block, 2004). Policy analysis is carried out by individuals from multiple disciplinary backgrounds and professional groups (Block, 2004), including nursing. Policy analysts may take either a technical or a political approach. The technical approach consists of an objective examination of the operations of the new program and its consequences on the intended and unintended targets. Program monitoring techniques include direct observations, program records, surveys of participants and community surveys. The political approach involves functioning as an advocate for a specific issue or group. It is important to remember that even objective analyses of

policy-related data will be filtered through the ideological lens of the individual or group conducting the analysis (Block, 2004). In fact, the same data may be evaluated by different groups and used to support divergent positions. Stokey and Zeckhauser (1978) developed a useful, comprehensive framework for conducting an objective, structured policy analysis.

LEADERSHIP AND MANAGEMENT IMPLICATIONS

Power

The ability to influence in any realm, including policy making, requires power. Sources of power include (French & Raven, 1959; Longest, 1997) the following:

- *Legitimate or positional power* is derived from an individual's position in a social system or in an organization; also called formal power or authority (Longest, 2002). Executives and union leaders tend to have more power than supervisors or rank-and-file employees.
- *Reward power and coercive power* are based on an individual's ability to reward compliance or to punish noncompliance, with the preferred decisions, actions, and behaviors that are sought from others (Longest, 1997). Reward and coercive powers are derived from the ability to provide or withhold from any person something of value to that person. For example, supervisors and managers usually have the power to determine pay increases and nominate individuals for promotion.
- *Expert power* is derived from possessing expertise or information that is valued by others (Longest, 1997). Expert power might include the ability to solve problems or perform critical tasks. It may also be vested in trusted advisers or associates. In the health care field, physicians are often viewed as the professional group possessing expertise related to health care issues.
- *Referent power* refers to a circumstance in which persons, organizations, or interest groups engender admiration, loyalty, and emulation

⚠ LEADERSHIP & MANAGEMENT BEHAVIORS

Leadership Behaviors	Management Behaviors
• Envisions directions for health policy initiatives	• Communicates about health policy needs
• Communicates about health policy issues	• Gives testimony
• Acts to influence health policy and legislation	• Writes letters to support a policy direction
• Enables followers to influence health policy	• Bargains for scarce resources
• Lobbies influential decision makers	• Implements laws and regulations affecting nursing practice
• Models supportive networking for information and influence	**Overlap Areas**
• Drafts legislation	• Communicates about health policies
• Encourages followers to be politically aware and active	• Takes action to influence and acquire scarce resources

from others to such an extent that they gain the power to exert influence as a result (Longest, 2002). This is also called charismatic power. Some recent examples include the ability of the actor Michael J. Fox to garner support for increased funding for Parkinson's disease research. Nurses have referent power to some extent because of their position of trust with the general public.

Hersey and colleagues (1979) added two additional sources of power to this list: (1) information power—when one individual has special information that another individual desires—and (2) connection power—granted to those perceived to have privileged connections with individuals or organizations. Power is translated into influence through interpersonal and political skills (Longest, 1997). Nurses as a group tend to have fewer resources and less cohesion than other powerful groups in health care. Nurses on the whole also tend to lack prowess in the public arena and visibility in the political process; as a group, nurses generally lack the knowledge, skills, and sophistication to influence health policy (Algase et al., 2004). However, this has been changing in recent years, as the associations representing nurses become more politically active

and engage the services of experienced and effective lobbyists.

Becoming Active in Policy

The discipline of nursing has identified the importance of policy advocacy as a strategy to enhance population health, as well as the need for nurses to become more knowledgeable about the policy process (ICN, 2001). The ICN has published guidelines for shaping effective health policy and identified nurses' essential roles in influencing health policy and understanding the policy process (Reutter & Duncan, 2002). Several authors have gone further and called for nurses to expand their policy focus from health policy to complex social problems such as poverty, homelessness, and violence (Morgan & Marsh, 1998; Reutter, 2000; Reutter & Williamson, 2000). The American Nurses Association's Social Policy Statement (Cohen & Milone-Nuzzo, 2001) asserted that social policies are under the purview of nursing care and research.

Public policy is a process as well as a product, requiring choices about valuing aspects of life (Malone, 1999; Stone, 1997). Specific skills and knowledge are required for policy work (Reutter & Duncan, 2002). Critical elements of the policy process include problem framing and definition, creation of policy agendas, policy instruments and their implementation, policy network and community analyses, and evaluation of policy impacts (Reutter & Duncan, 2002). Nurses must be aware that political, economic, and social contexts determine which policy problems, agendas, and strategies are enacted. Cramer (2002) found that greater participation of nurses in political activity occurred when individuals possessed the values of political interest, political information, personal efficacy, and civic skills. She believed that instilling these values is a deliberate process that begins early in a nurse's education and continues through graduation. She suggested that professional associations partner with schools to ensure a future cadre of nurses who possess at least a minimum level of information and interest in policy and the political process.

To become politically active and participate in public policy making, the practicing nurse can do the following:

- Establish a base of contact with elected officials, community leaders, and public policy makers
- Work with professional associations—keep eyes and ears open to activities that bear upon legislative priorities
- Become members of grassroots networks, to stay informed and work within a framework for participation in public policy process

To prepare nurses to become politically active and effective, schools can do the following:

- Provide educational preparation in policy advocacy
- Require course work in sociology, economics, and political science
- Assign students to monitor and report on state and national legislation potentially affecting nurses or patients
- Encourage or require students and faculty members to attend a Legislative Day at their state capital

It is also crucial that nurse researchers translate their findings into policy-relevant recommendations (Jones et al., 1997). To use research and data to influence policy and policy making, reports of nursing research should consider the following questions (Wakefield, 2001):

- Is the linkage between the topic and specific public policies or programs explicit?
- Is the topic related to a current or emerging health policy concern?
- Is the research framed in the context of health care access, costs, and/or quality?
- Are populations important to policy makers identified?
- Is the language understandable to policy makers and the general public?
- Do research reports include policy-relevant content in the literature review and in the discussion of findings?
- Can the manuscript content be used at all stages of the policy-making process?
- Is the content useful to advocacy groups?

Decisions are made that influence the context in which care is delivered and affect the occupation and practice of nursing. These decisions may restrict or enable payment for care services or affect rules governing licensure and the work environment. The decisions are made with or without nursing's involvement and goals. Therefore nurses will be drawn into politics and need to refine their political skills and power bases. It is vital that nurses become involved in both politics and health policy. Nurses provide the caring element in the health care system and uphold a long and distinguished tradition in health promotion, wellness, and public health advocacy. They remind the public that health care is more than medically-focused disease treatment and surgery. For example, nurses have taken the leadership to pressure state legislatures to pass motorcycle helmet laws for the purpose of primary prevention of head injuries.

Nurses also can take a leadership role at the local, state, and federal levels of health policy activities. For example, nurses can use their expertise to develop white papers and policy analysis data for key decision makers. Nurses can vote, lobby, campaign, and protest as activism methods to influence health care policy. Nurses can be locally active in communities by being involved on boards and commissions and by communicating about health policy issues. Buresh and Gordon's (2000) book is an excellent resource guide.

Nurses can become involved in leadership and management roles within the politics of organizations. For example, professional nursing organizations such as the ANA develop position papers, debate health policy issues, and support candidates and positions. Nurses also may lobby or contribute money to lobbying efforts of PACs. Nurses may even choose to provide testimony to support a health policy effort.

At the individual level, nurses' leadership and management roles in client care management involve the use of influence at multiple levels. Nurses need to take the responsibility to keep informed about health policy and political issues. Awareness may be triggered and enhanced by sources such as professional organizations' position papers, reading professional journals, newspapers and other public media, or networking with colleagues in person or electronically. Nurses may contact their elected representatives for information or to express an opinion. Clearly, nurses need to be informed and aware of health policy issues. They need to be active in their efforts to influence. They need to communicate their positions to others and to support and lobby in conjunction with others as a group strategic action team. By taking these leadership actions, nurses can influence others to make changes needed to positively affect health care policy and politics.

CURRENT ISSUES AND TRENDS

Current Policy Issues

Several issues are currently at the top of the nursing policy agenda. The nursing shortage, including the shortage of nurse faculty members, is of high concern, because it relates to patient safety and quality of care. State legislators are taking the nursing shortage very seriously (Cooksey et al., 2004). In 2002, the shortage was ranked as a "high priority" by 39 states and a "priority" by another 7 states (NCSL, 2001). Some states have reported

substantial growth in total applicant pools in nursing schools as a result of different recruitment initiatives; yet not all of these applicants can be accommodated because of faculty shortages and insufficient numbers of new clinical educational sites. The high number of nursing vacancies requires new policies for nurse recruitment and nurse retention. One policy issue is the recruitment of foreign nurses, a practice that has global implications. Another is organizational policies to promote retention of experienced nurses. Currently, policies favor retirement rather than retention of the older nurse. A major piece of federal legislation was the Nurse Reinvestment Act. Although successful in getting the issue on the policy agenda and the enactment of a new law, the Nurse Reinvestment Act has subsequently suffered from inadequate and static federal appropriations (Sochalski, 2003). The amount being allocated by the federal government falls far short of what is needed to maintain even the current level of funding for nursing education.

A related policy issue is the quality of care being delivered in health care institutions and the safety of patients being cared for within these facilities. States have taken the lead in this policy arena and have passed or are considering the imposition of minimum staffing ratios and the outlawing of mandatory overtime. Judicial attempts to modify these new laws are common. For example, the minimum staffing ratios passed in California were challenged by the California Hospital Association (CHA), in particular the requirement that the minimum ratios be met at all times (including staff meal and break times). The CHA felt this was an unreasonable interpretation of the law. A court recently rejected the hospital association's case, so the law will not be modified at this point in time as a result of judicial decision making.

Nursing Organizations' Policy Agenda

Most, if not all, professional nursing associations develop an annual list of policy issues pertinent to their association members. These associations

Research Note

Source: Glaessel-Brown, E.E. (1998). Use of immigration policy to manage nursing shortages. *Image, 30*(4), 323-327.

Purpose

One solution to labor shortages in the United States is to modify immigration policy to allow nurses from other countries to work with temporary, nonimmigrant visas. The purpose of this article was to explore the long-term implications of using such temporary, nonimmigrant nurse programs to manage fluctuations in the demand for registered nurses.

Discussion

This article used a policy analysis of theories, concepts, and perspectives on nurse migration to review the literature and existing studies on international migration. The Immigration Nursing Relief Act (INRA) of 1952 was discussed. Local labor market impact studies were carried out in five major metropolitan areas to evaluate the INRA's effectiveness. There were no adverse effects on wages, benefits, or working conditions. Foreign nurses did not take jobs from experienced, licensed RNs. The U.S. nurses felt more threatened by the use of unlicensed assistive personnel than by the foreign nurses. Employers sought foreign nurses to avoid the cost of agency nurses. Despite significant concentration in a few metropolitan areas, foreign-educated nurses have never represented more than 1% of nurses working in the United States.

Application to Practice

In the United States, the use of foreign nurses tends to be a complement to, rather than a substitute for, local labor. Thus there is no direct threat to RN jobs. However, policy analysis revealed foreign nurse recruitment to be a short-term solution whose long-term consequences turn out not to be in nursing's best interest. A vulnerable workforce is created. A pattern of dependency is created in the sending country, and a delay in long-range solutions to domestic labor problems occurs in the host country. Exchanges of skilled nurses stimulate energy, ideas, cultural sensitivity, and opportunity. Yet ethical considerations arise over transferring education costs to other countries while delaying investment in nontraditional U.S. candidates. Other issues arise over whether separate immigration legislation for RNs is justified, whether foreign RNs are guests or immigrants, and whether recurring nonimmigrant worker programs are in the best interest of U.S. nursing.

also have on their professional staffs one or more governmental relations experts who monitor state and federal policy initiatives that could affect their association members either positively or negatively. For example, the Association of Operating Room Nurses (AORN) published their 2003 legislative and regulatory priorities in their official journal (Franko, 2003). Every year this association develops and recommends legislative priorities at both the state and national levels. The AORN Board of Directors reviews and approves the list, which then steers the organization's public policy activities. The four priorities for 2003 were as follows:

1. *Patient safety:* Support federal legislation to improve patient safety; identify, monitor, support, and introduce state and federal legislation to address the needs of perioperative nursing safety—e.g., correct surgery site, reducing medical errors, smoke evacuation, needle sticks.

2. *Scope of practice:* Require RNs in the circulating nurse position; support basic educational standards for assistive personnel such

as surgical technologists and surgical assistants; oppose licensure of surgical technologists and surgical assistants (bills introduced in Illinois and Oregon; rules issued in New York State).

3. *Support the Nurse Reinvestment Act:* Affirm that the minimum nurse-to-patient ratio is one professional nurse dedicated to each patient undergoing an invasive procedure during the entire intraoperative experience.

4. *Reimbursement:* Support the Medicare Certified RN First Assistant Direct Reimbursement Act; support third-party reimbursement for RN first assistants in the states (close to 20% of the states already passed this legislation).

For the fourth priority, reimbursement, AORN set a political strategy. The political strategy for the reimbursement policy proposal called for either a stand-alone bill or an attachment to a larger bill that had good prospects of passing through Congress. The association was successful in getting a Senator to amend a pilot study onto the Senate version of the Medicare bill, to establish a 3-year, five-state pilot project for direct Medicare reimbursement for Certified Registered Nurse First Assistants. At the state level, the association was successful in achieving direct reimbursement for RN first assistants, most recently in Louisiana. However, they were not successful in Missouri, where this bill has been introduced in the last five sessions but defeated each time. The keys to legislative success are persistence and dedication to the issue (Franko, 2003). It is important to determine the reason why a piece of legislation does not pass so that a new strategy can be devised (Franko, 2003). Lack of success in getting a particular policy enacted may relate to other issues having more salience to the lawmakers and thus being higher on their policy agendas. The following year might be better timing for the policy makers.

There is a strong linkage between health policy and health. All health care professionals, therefore, have a vested interest in understanding the health care policy-making process (Longest, 2001). Nurses' political development has been described

as moving through four stages. The first was "buy-in," through beginning participation in politics and policy. The second was "self-interest," or the leading of collective efforts for nursing's self-interest. The third was "political sophistication" by participating in coalitions targeted to broader health issues. Nursing is now said to be moving to the fourth stage of "leading the way," which is characterized by taking the lead in mobilizing constituencies to action related to issues outside of nursing (Cohen et al., 1996; Mason et al., 2002). For nurses, a higher degree of political competence would translate into a greater ability to assess the influence of public policy on nursing practice and a greater ability to exert influence in the public policy-making process (Longest, 1997; Longest, 2001). Essential competencies in this domain of practice include knowing how and where to exert influence by knowing how public policies are formulated, implemented, and modified (Longest, 1997). As described by Kingdon (1995), nurses can influence health policy in the formulation phase, by helping to define the problems that are placed on the policy agenda; in the implementation phase, by monitoring the rules and regulations that guide the implementation of new laws and providing formal comments on proposed rules and regulations; and in the modification phase, by providing data related to the intended and unintended consequences of a policy. Development of political competency needs to occur as part of the basic educational preparation of nurses. There also is a need for specialization in health policy making at the graduate level, especially through interdisciplinary training programs.

Summary

- Nurses need to be visible and vocal in public policy and health policy debates.
- Policy is the formulation of value statements.
- Politics is the influencing of the allocation of scarce resources.
- Health policies are a set of public policies influencing health and illness.

- The public policy-making process follows stages of formulation, implementation, and modification.
- The Kingdon and stage-sequential models are two policy formulation models.
- There are four strategies used by interest groups.
- Health policies may be allocative or regulatory.
- Nurses have a leadership and management role in public and health policy.

Study Questions

1. What are nursing's major health care values?
2. What role do consumers play?
3. Is caring a health care policy? Why or why not?
4. What kind of public policies govern your life? Govern nursing practice?
5. Which level of government is responsible for the health of the citizens?
6. Should illegal aliens be included in health care policy and benefits?
7. Why are nursing's professional issues important enough to be on the public policy agenda? Which ones are?
8. Why is politics useful to nurses? What strategies are most successful?
9. Why can nurses be influential in policy and politics? How does this happen?

CASE STUDY

Nurse Diane Kiplinger has always been politically active. She has volunteered in numerous presidential campaigns and has been the local county Republican Party chair. She has been active with the League of Women Voters. Now there is a pressing nursing and health care issue on the forefront: mental health parity. Nurse Kiplinger knows just what to do. She begins networking with state and local nursing groups to build support. She starts outreach efforts to align with other interest groups. She enlists faculty and students from the nearby university to write letters, develop fact sheets and position papers, and hold seminars. She hosts gatherings with legislators and organized media events, using Buresh and Gordon's (2000) book as a guide. When the tragic death of a child occurs as a result of a lack of mental health funding, she works with the distraught parents to lobby for Medicaid reforms and other insurance legislation. As a result, mental health parity becomes a state health policy agenda issue and a compromise bill is enacted.

CRITICAL THINKING EXERCISE

Nurse Kelly Murrell works with the organ donation team of the tertiary care hospital. She has been active in efforts to increase public knowledge about signing donor cards and the need for organ donation. Currently, there is debate over whether the allocation priority of organs should go to the local area where the organ is donated or to the person at the top of the national list of the most ill transplant-eligible patients. The issue is controversial, confounded with stakeholder interests, and emotionally charged. Nurse Murrell feels the decision will directly affect her patients and the viability of this transplant program. However, in the past, Nurse Murrell has felt that politics do not belong in health care delivery and has concentrated only on quality clinical care and consumer education.

1. What is (are) the problem(s)?
2. Why is (are) it (they) a problem(s)?
3. What should Nurse Murrell do?
4. What public policy issues are involved?
5. What politics are involved?
6. What health policy issues are involved?
7. What actions can Nurse Murrell take to affect public health policy?

REFERENCES

Algase, D.L., Beel-Bates, C., & Ziemba, R. (2004). Lead, link, and learn: A policy/research fellowship program in aging. *Policy, Politics, & Nursing Practice, 5*(2), 116-124.

Allred, C.A., Arford, P.H., Mauldin, P.D., & Goodwin, L.K. (1998). Cost-effectiveness analysis in the nursing literature, 1992-1996. *Image, 30*(3), 235-242.

Anderson, J.E. (1990). *Public policymaking.* Boston: Houghton-Mifflin.

Backer, B.A., Costello-Nickitas, D.M., Mason, D.J., McBride, A.B., & Vance, C. (1998). Feminist perspectives on policy and politics. In D.J. Mason & J.K. Leavitt (Eds.), *Policy and politics in nursing and health care* (3rd ed.) (pp. 18-28). Philadelphia: Saunders.

Block, L.E. (2004). Health policy: What it is and how it works. In C. Harrington & C.L. Estes (Eds.), *Health policy: Crisis and reform in the U.S. health care delivery system* (4th ed.) (pp. 4-14). Boston: Jones and Bartlett Publishers.

Brown, L. (1991). Knowledge and power: Health services research as a political resource. In E. Ginsberg (Ed.), *Health services research: Key to health policy* (pp. 20-45). Cambridge, MA: Harvard University Press.

Buchholz, R.A. (1994). *Business environment and public policy: Implications for management and strategy formulation* (5th ed.). Englewood Cliffs, NJ: Prentice Hall.

Buerhaus, P.I. (1998). Milton Weinstein's insights on the development, use, and methodologic problems in cost-effectiveness analysis. *Image, 30*(3), 223-228.

Buresh, B., & Gordon, S. (2000). *From silence to voice: What nurses know and must communicate to the public.* Ottawa, Ontario, Canada: Canadian Nurses Association.

Cohen, S., Mason, D., Kovner, C., Leavitt, J., Pulcini, J, & Sochalski, J. (1996). Stages of nursing's political development: Where we've been and where we ought to go. *Nursing Outlook, 44*(6), 259-266.

Cohen, S., & Milone-Nuzzo, P. (2001). Advancing health policy in nursing education through service learning. *Advances in Nursing Science, 23*(3), 28-40.

Cooksey, J.A., McLaughlin, W., Russinof, H., Martinez, L.I., & Gordon, C. (2004). Active state-level engagement with the nursing shortage: A study of five Midwestern states. *Policy, Politics, & Nursing Practice, 5*(2), 102-122.

Cramer, M.E. (2002). Factors influencing organized political participation in nursing. *Policy, Politics, & Nursing Practice, 3*(2), 97-107.

Diers, D. (1998). Research as a policy/political tool. In D.J. Mason & J.K. Leavett (Eds.), *Policy and politics in nursing and health care* (3rd ed.) (pp. 191-207). Philadelphia: Saunders.

Dunn, W.N. (1994). *Public policy analysis: An introduction.* Englewood Cliffs, NJ: Prentice-Hall.

Dye, T.R. (1987). *Understanding public policy.* Englewood Cliffs, NJ: Prentice-Hall.

Franko, F.P. (2003). Health policy issues: 2003 legislative and regulatory update. *AORN Journal, 78*(5), 846-851.

French, J.R.P., & Raven, B. (1959). The basis of social power. In D. Cartwright (Ed.), *Studies in social power* (pp. 150-167) Ann Arbor, MI: The University of Michigan.

Hanley, B.E. (2002). Policy development and analysis. In D.J. Mason, J.K. Leavitt, & M.W. Chaffee (Eds.), *Policy and politics in nursing and health care* (4th ed.) (pp. 55-69). Philadelphia: Saunders.

Hersey, P., Blanchard, K.H., & Natemeyer, W.E. (1979). Situational leadership, perception, and impact of power. *Group Organizational Studies, 4,* 418-428.

International Council of Nurses (ICN). (2001). *Guidelines on shaping effective health policy.* Geneva, Switzerland: ICN.

Jones, K.R., Jennings, B.W., Moritz, P., & Moss, M.T. (1997). Policy issues associated with analyzing the outcomes of care. *Image: Journal of Nursing Scholarship, 29*(3), 261-267.

Keys, B., & Case, T. (1990). How to become an influential manager. *The Executive, 4,* 38-51.

Kingdon, J.W. (1995). *Agendas, alternatives and public policies* (2nd ed.). New York: Addison-Wesley Longman.

Kronenfeld, J., Whicker, J., & Lynn, M. (1984). *U.S. national health policy: An analysis of the federal role.* New York: Praeger.

Lineberry, R.L., Edwards, G.C., & Wattenberg, M.P. (1995). *Government in America* (2nd ed.). New York: HarperCollins College Publishers.

Longest, B.B., Jr. (1997). *Seeking strategic advantage through health policy analysis.* Chicago: Health Administration Press.

Longest, B.B., Jr. (2001). *Contemporary health policy.* Chicago: Health Administration Press.

Longest, B.B., Jr. (2002). *Health policy making in the United States* (3rd ed.). Chicago: Health Administration Press.

Malone, R. (1999). Policy as product: Morality and metaphor in health policy discourse. *Hastings Center Report, 29,* 16-22.

Mason, D.J., Leavitt, J.K., & Chaffee, M.W. (2002). Policy and politics: A framework for action. In D.J. Mason, J.K. Leavitt, & M.W. Chaffee (Eds.), *Policy and politics in nursing and health care* (4th ed.) (pp. 1-18). Philadelphia: Saunders.

Milio, N. (1984). The realities of policymaking: Can nurses have an impact? *Journal of Nursing Administration, 14*(3), 18-23.

Milstead, J.A. (1999). *Health policy and politics: A nurses' guide.* Gaithersburg, MD: Aspen.

Morgan, I., & Marsh, G. (1998). Historic and future health promotion contexts for nursing. *Image: Journal of Nursing Scholarship, 30,* 379-383.

National Conference of State Legislatures (NCSL). (2001). *State health priorities survey.* Washington, DC: NCSL.

Reutter, L. (2000). Socioeconomic determinants of health. In M.J. Stewart (Ed.), *Community nursing: Promoting Canadians' health* (2nd ed.) (pp. 174-193). Toronto, Ontario, Canada: Harcourt Canada.

Reutter, L., & Duncan, S. (2002). Preparing nurses to promote health-enhancing public policies. *Policy, Politics, & Nursing Practice, 3*(4), 294-305.

Reutter, L., & Williamson, D.L. (2000). Advocating healthy public policy: Implications for baccalaureate nursing education. *Journal of Nursing Education, 39*, 21-26.

Ripley, R.B. (1985). *Policy analysis in political science.* Chicago: Nelson-Hall.

Ripley, R.B. (1996). Stages of the policy process. In D.C. McCool (Ed.), *Public policy theories, models, and concepts: An anthology* (pp. 157-162). Englewood Cliffs, NJ: Prentice-Hall.

Sochalski, J. (2003). Investing in the nurse reinvestment act. *Journal of Professional Nursing, 19*(4), 182-183.

Soumerai, S. (2003). Unintended outcomes of Medicaid drug cost-containment policies on the chronically mentally ill. *Journal of Clinical Psychiatry, 64*(Suppl 17), 19-22.

Stokey, E., & Zeckhauser, R. (1978). *A primer for policy analysis.* New York: Norton.

Stone, D.A. (1997). *Policy paradox: The art of political decision-making.* New York: Norton.

Stone, P.W. (1998). Methods for conducting and reporting cost-effectiveness analysis in nursing. *Image, 30*(3), 229-234.

Wakefield, M. (2001). Linking health policy to nursing and health care scholarship: Points to consider. *Nursing Outlook, 49*(4), 111-113.

Wakefield, M. (1999). Government response: Legislation. In J.A. Milstead (Ed.), *Health policy and politics: A nurse's guide* (pp. 77-103). Gaithersberg, MD: Aspen.

Wilken, M. (1999). Policy implementation. In J.A. Milstead (Ed.), *Health policy and politics: A nurse's guide* (pp. 187-218). Gaithersberg, MD: Aspen.

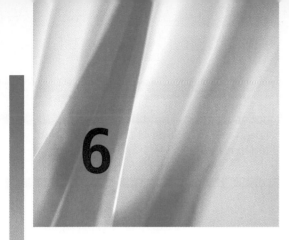

6

Critical Thinking Skills

Betsy Frank

CHAPTER OBJECTIVES

- Understand the role critical thinking plays in nursing practice
- Explore the relationship between critical thinking and problem solving
- Describe a method for good problem solving
- Apply the problem-solving process to nursing management practice
- Discover the role that critical thinking plays in leadership and management roles
- Use critical thinking to conceptualize and analyze possible solutions to a practice exercise

Nurses are a cadre of knowledge workers within the health care system. As such, they need information, resources, and support from their environment. The environment surrounding this system has moved from a process-oriented system characterized by a reliance on procedures and controlled by the providers to a system that is outcome-driven, best practice–oriented and controlled by the user (Porter-O'Grady, 2003). The emergence of managed care as a dominant form of health care financing and delivery has created upheaval in clinical practice. However, the savings from managed care have disappeared as health insurance premiums have experienced double-digit inflation (Emanuel, 2002). In acute care hospitals and other health care delivery settings, complexity, change, and unpredictability in the environment have left nurses with increased uncertainty and a perception that critical information for decision making has been lacking. In addition, nurses often have been regarded as having little impact on the policies that influence or drive spending for health care (Peters, 2002).

Such environmental stressors make creative problem solving and high-quality decision making crucial skills for all nurses to survive and thrive in any setting where health care is delivered. These skills have many uses and applications. They can be refined and practiced until they become a systematic way of thinking.

Critical thinking is both an attitude toward handling issues and a reasoning process. Critical thinking is not synonymous with problem solving and decision making (Figure 6.1), but certainly effective problem solving and concurrent decision making cannot occur without critical thinking (Lemire, 2002a). Figure 6.2 illustrates the way obstacles such as poor judgment or biased thinking create detours to good judgment. Critical thinking helps to overcome these obstacles. Critical thinking skills may not come naturally. The nurse who is a critical thinker has to be open-minded and have the ability to reflect on present and past actions and to analyze complex information.

Nurses make decisions and choices all the time. Assessment, diagnosis, planning, intervention, and evaluation of outcomes constitute activities of clinical problem solving and decision making. Nurses are in a human service profession that requires decisions in response to client problems,

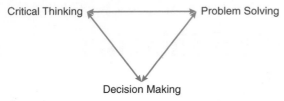

Figure 6.1
Differences and interactions among critical thinking, problem solving, and decision making.

such as determining what treatments or actions are to be performed. The quality of these decisions is based on skills in clinical performance, situational appraisal, and clinical reasoning. Benner (1984) said that nurses go through five stages of skill acquisition. The five levels are novice, advanced beginner, competent, proficient, and expert. As the nurse moves to a higher level of competence, the nurse develops more expertise in critical thinking that is exhibited in a higher level of clinical problem-solving abilities. Benner, as well as Finkelman (2001), acknowledged the strong role that intuition plays in clinical problem

solving. What this means is that at stage 5, or expert level, the nurse has a large background of experience and exhibits an intuitive grasp of situations, a deep understanding of the total situation, and a fluid and flexible style. It may be difficult to describe the critical thinking chain, because it is more holistic. This is often attributed to relying on intuition; yet it is actually expert reasoning.

DEFINITIONS

Critical thinking is a skill that can be used to reflect analytically, to reconceptualize events, and to avoid the tendency to act hastily or on the basis of inadequate information. Various definitions of this concept exist. **Critical thinking** has been defined as an intellectual process involving a reflective dimension to identify and challenge assumptions and explore and imagine alternatives (Brookfield, 1991). Facione and Facione (1996) pointed out that critical thinking is not only a skill but also a disposition. They noted that the critical thinker is honest and continually seeks out knowledge and reconsiders issues if needed.

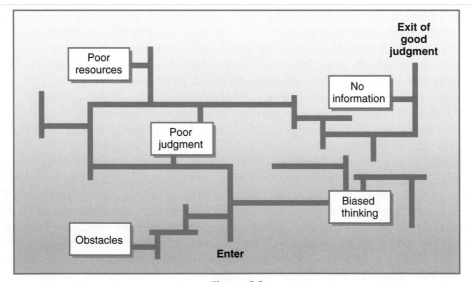

Figure 6.2
The problem-solving maze.

◭ LEADING & MANAGING **DEFINED**

Critical Thinking	Problem
A cognitive process that is rational thinking process and includes knowledge acquisition, analysis, problem solving behaviors, reflection, and intuition.	A deficit or surplus of something or a situation that is perplexing.
	Problem Solving
	Identification of obstacles to outcome or goal achievement.

Lemire (2002a) stated that "critical thinking involves the acquisition of knowledge, reasoning and rational appraisal skills, analytical problem solving behaviors, and reflective thinking" (p. 51). Thus critical thinking represents cognitive thought processes of assessing and evaluating ideas and situations in an unbiased and objective manner (Polge, 1995).

Critical thinking in nursing can be defined as:
… an essential component of professional account-ability and nursing care. Critical thinkers in nursing exhibit these habits of the mind: confidence, contextual perspective, creativity, flexibility, inquisitiveness, intellectual integrity, intuition, open-mindedness, perseverance, and reflection. Critical thinkers in nursing practice the cognitive skills of analyzing, applying standards, discriminating, information seeking, logical reasoning, predicting and transforming knowledge (Scheffer & Rubenfeld, 2000, p. 357).

Another way of viewing critical thinking in nursing is as a "complex mental process by which data are synthesized to make accurate nursing decisions" (O'Sullivan et al., 1997, p. 25). Clearly, "making clinical nursing judgments is central to the practice of nursing, and critical thinking skills are essential to making clinical judgments" (Polge, 1995, p. 4). Lemire (2002a) emphasized that critical thinking is a higher order thinking skill. And, as Tanner (2000) has pointed out, critical thinking is much more than just the five steps of the nursing process.

A **problem** is defined as a deficit or surplus of something that is necessary to achieve one's goals.

It can be thought of as a difference or gap between what exists and a goal. Thus a problem is a deficiency or undesirable current state (Le Storti et al., 1999). Paul (1992) noted that a problem is a "question, matter, situation, or person that is perplexing or difficult to figure out, handle, or resolve" (p. 663). Given this broad definition, no wonder Le Storti and colleagues (1999) stated that all nursing practice is problem solving: "The main focus of nursing is problem solving of one kind or another" (p. 63). Luft (1970) defined **problem solving** as the process that attempts to identify obstacles that inhibit accomplishment of a specific goal. Ackoff (1974) noted that successful problem solving requires finding the right solution to the right problem. The specific problems selected for solution, as well as the way they are formulated as problems, appear to be related to an individual's philosophy and world view more than to science and technology.

Problems exist where outcomes need to be achieved (Pesut & Herman, 1999). Finkelman (2001) stated that problems present opportunities for decision making and change and require critical thinking in order to arrive at the best solution. The logical extension of this would be that problem solving is the process of fixing something that needs to be fixed. In nursing, problem solving occurs within the context of direct client care, team leadership, case management, and client advocacy. Nurses are challenged to supplement traditional problem-solving techniques with creative thinking (Cohen, 2002; Kalischuk & Thorpe, 2002; Le Storti et al., 1999).

BACKGROUND

Critical Thinking

Critical thinking is a skill that is developed for clarity of thought and improvement in problem-solving effectiveness. The roots of the concept of critical thinking can be traced to Socrates, who developed a method of probing questioning as a way of thinking more clearly and with greater logical consistency. He demonstrated that people often cannot rationally justify confident claims to knowledge. Confused meanings, inadequate evidence, or self-contradictory beliefs may lie below the surface of rhetoric. Therefore it is important to ask deep questions and probe into thinking sequences, seek evidence, closely examine reasoning and assumptions, analyze basic concepts, and trace out implications. Other thinkers, such as Plato, Aristotle, Thomas Aquinas, Francis Bacon, and Descartes, emphasized the importance of systematic critical thinking and the need for a systematic disciplining of the mind to guide it in clarity and precision of thinking. In the early 1900s Dewey equated critical thinking with reflective thought (El Paso Community College, 2004).

All reasoning occurs within points of view or frames of reference, proceeds from some goals and objectives, has an information base, uses data that must be interpreted using concepts and assumptions, and results in inferences that have implications. Two common approaches to reasoning are inductive and deductive. In deductive reasoning, the movement is from the general to the specific; with inductive reasoning movement is in the opposite direction or from a specific case to a generalization (El Paso Community College, 2004). Implicit in both forms of reasoning is the idea that reaching a conclusion involves questioning.

Some critical thinking questions include the following (El Paso Community College, 2004):

- Why?
- How?
- What is the most fundamental issue?
- What can I infer from these data?
- Is this a credible source of information?
- How could I check the accuracy of this?
- Are these two things consistent?
- What might happen if …?

Critical Thinking in Nursing

Nurses in clinical practice continually make judgments and decisions based on the assessment and diagnosis of client needs and practice problems or situations. Clinical judgment is a complex skill grounded in critical thinking. Clinical judgment results in nursing actions directed toward achieving health outcomes (Pesut & Herman, 1999). The two cognitive processes used in critical thinking for nursing judgments are analytical and intuitive (Polge, 1995). Emphasizing the value of expert experience and holistic judgment ability, Benner (2003) cautioned that clinical judgments must not rely too heavily on technology and the economic incentives to use technology at the expense of human critical thinking and reasoning in individual cases.

Critical thinkers have been distinguished from traditional thinkers in nursing. A traditional thinker, thought to be the norm in nursing, preserves the norm or status quo. A critical thinker challenges and questions the norm. Traditional thinkers do use problem solving, but they choose a solution within the realm of their immediate clinical knowledge. Critical thinkers ask the *why* question and challenge routine practice. The advantage of critical thinking is the increase in the choice of possible solutions (Stark, 1996).

Both the individual nurse and the organization have accountability for developing critical thinking (Hansten & Washburn, 1999). Bulman & Schutz (2004) contended that reflection during care delivery and after a clinical practice incident is a key element of critical thinking. Therefore, the individual practitioner who reflects on mistakes and learns from them helps to deepen critical thinking skills. Hansten and Washburn also asserted that asking the right questions fosters a systematic approach to critical thinking. Questions include what is right and wrong about a situation and what can be done about a situation. Organizations also have accountability for critical thinking in that a climate that fosters critical thinking also encourages individuals to ask those important questions (Hansten & Washburn, 1999). A climate that promotes critical thinking stresses the role of the nurse-patient relationship (Benner, 2003).

Critical thinking also has been associated with creative thinking (Buhler, 2004; Cohen, 2002). Creative thinking is oriented to the formation and production of a novel idea or product. Creativity is what contributes to the intuitive component of critical thinking (Kalischuk & Thorpe, 2002). Critical thinking is oriented to the determination of the authenticity, accuracy, or value of an idea or product (Le Storti et al., 1999). Creative thinking is making judgments based on insight, intuition, "gut reactions," and right-brain thinking. Creative thinking is described by three attributes: (1) knowledge is received as a whole; (2) awareness of knowledge is immediate; and (3) knowledge is acquired independent of linear reasoning (Benner & Tanner, 1987; Polge, 1995). Creative thinking and critical thinking are complementary modes of thought that can be used to deal proactively with problems rather than waiting for problems to occur (Alfaro-LeFevre, 1997). Use of critical pathways can foster a proactive approach to management of clinical problems, and critical thinking helps the nurse to evaluate the appropriateness of care delivered within the critical pathway framework.

PROBLEM SOLVING

Creativity and problem solving are inextricably linked. **Creative problem solving** is defined as "thinking directed toward the achievement of a goal by means of a novel and appropriate idea or product" (Le Storti et al., 1999). Although traditionally problem-solving has emphasized rational-logical thought, creativity is essential if the best clinical outcomes are to be achieved.

Creative problem solving rests on two principles called deferred judgment and divergent-convergent thinking sequences. Deferred judgment means the temporary suspension of criticism or evaluation. This is important for the generation of unique and useful ideas. Deferring judgment

helps eliminate bias and jumping to quick conclusions (Le Storti et al., 1999). Divergent-convergent thinking sequences are an opening up to possibilities, followed by the subsequent selection of the most promising possibilities. What this means is that several alternative problem statements are generated in such a way as to offer different perspectives and different senses of direction as to solving a problem. The divergent questions are then evaluated, and selection converges on one path to take (Le Storti et al., 1999). The goal is to develop innovative problem-solving strategies that are productive and useful. One strategy to promote creative problem solving is to encourage brainstorming (Colwell, 2001), an activity that can be used in groups wherein the manager facilitates the generation of multiple solutions to a problem. Brainstorming can help groups to see connections between seemingly unrelated ideas (Buhler, 2004).

Problem-solving activity has been conceptualized from two points of view: (1) individual or clinical problem solving and (2) managerial problem solving. At the level of an individual, problem solving is viewed as intimately related to how the individual processes information. In health care, a concern about accuracy and effectiveness has placed an emphasis on diagnostic reasoning and clinical decision making. Problem solving becomes more complex for managers in organizations because of multiple stakeholders and the dynamic state in which it occurs (see Figure 6.2); thus managerial problem solving rests on an understanding of general systems theory (Lemire, 2002a). As noted in Chapter 2, general systems theory postulates that a change in one part of a system affects all other parts of the system. Because of these dynamic effects, problem-solving effectiveness requires the incorporation of systems effects from a decision. Frequently, groups are involved in problem solving, so there is a greater need for interaction, a slower process, and a need for consensus. Problems may be solved at the best possible level, as opposed to an ideal level.

Problem solving as a process can be linked to the delivery of nursing care and the organizational change process. A problem-solving model has been proposed by deChesnay (1983). Within the arena of problem solving and decision making, some situations produce problems (a difficulty), others create problems in which conflicts arise (a dilemma), and yet others become problems in which the solution appears not to have a logical path (a paradox). The complexity of decision making and its psychological impact increase as the situation moves along a hierarchy from difficulty to paradox. Thus problems can be categorized by their level of complexity. Once categorized, the nursing process and the change process can then be applied to strategically enhance problem solving. The problem can be framed as either an individual's problem or a system's problem. The evaluation of the outcome of problem solving involves an assessment of effectiveness. If the problem is resolved, the problem-solving process would be judged as effective. It would be judged ineffective if the problem stayed the same or worsened (deChesnay, 1983).

Because each situation is different in complexity, managing a difficulty, dilemma, or paradox may require different strategies depending on the situation. A difficulty is only a minor problem and may need only a straightforward solution. For example, a minor problem occurs when two competing values arise, such as valuing time off and valuing having a job. A dilemma results from the combination of a difficulty plus conflict. One example occurs with cultural differences, such as when professional values clash with the values of the client. In this case, critical thinking is needed to balance difficulty plus conflict. A paradox is a situation in which there is no logical solution to the problem (deChesnay, 1983). In practice, paradoxes are found commonly within ethical issues, in which ethical principles would be applied in critical thinking and decision making with no clear right answer.

Newell and Simon (1972) defined human problem solving as information processing. Information-processing behavior is dependent on the characteristics of the problem solver and the task. In nursing, the concepts of clinical decision making and nursing informatics are discussed in relation to problem solving as information processing.

The nursing process also is a generic problem-solving strategy widely applicable in nursing practice, but delivery of nursing care grounded solely on the step-by-step nursing process has been called into question by some (Tanner, 2000). Redding (2001) has conceptualized critical clinical judgment as much more than nursing process. She determined that clinical judgment consists of five processes: problem solving, caring, unbiased inquiry, intuition, and reflection-in-action.

Hurst and colleagues (1991) found that nurses do not always problem-solve according to a step-by-step process. Moreover, Taylor (1997) showed that novice nurses differed from more expert nurses in their diagnostic reasoning abilities used in clinical problem solving. In some instances novice nurses did not independently problem-solve but rather copied a more expert nurse's performance. Kennedy (2002) found that nurses use cue interpretation from data presented before a patient encounter in order to begin to define the problem at hand.

Many organizational interactions occur around the need to identify, define, and solve problems. Individuals appear to have a relatively stable personality-related problem-solving style. It appears that problem-solving styles have an influence on how well people are able to work together. Furthermore, the personality style relates to how an individual acquires, stores, retrieves, and transforms information (Kirton, 1994). Thus there may be a relationship between problem-solving style and effectiveness in any given situation. As with leadership style, no one style is optimum. The effectiveness of a style is situational, determined by what is appropriate to the circumstances. The Kirton Adaption-Innovation Theory (Kirton, 1994) identified two types of problem solvers: adaptors and innovators. Adaptors seek solutions to problems in tried and accepted ways. They are focused on resolving problems rather than finding them. They rarely challenge rules and are methodical, reliable, and efficient. Innovators are the opposite. They seek solutions to problems in original, creative, and challenging ways. They discover problems and avenues for resolution. Innovators question current practices and promote changes. Kirton's theory resembles the distinction between traditional thinkers versus critical thinkers (Stark, 1996).

Organizations in a stable steady state of maintenance tend to prefer adaptors. Organizations in a growth state or undergoing a rapid rate of change or crisis tend to prefer innovators (Adams, 1994). Problem-solving style can be measured by either the Kirton Adaption-Innovation Inventory (KAI) (Kirton, 1976, 1991) or by Hersey and Natemeyer's (1988) Problem-Solving and Decision-Making Style Inventory, which measures the extent to which an individual engages in directive or supportive behavior. Although there are different ways of thinking about problem-solving styles, an analysis of personal style increases a nurse's self-awareness and knowledge about alternative ways of acting on problems.

Steps in the Problem-Solving Process

The steps of the problem-solving process are listed somewhat differently in various literature sources. Box 6.1 provides a seven-step general framework for problem solving drawn from various sources (Davidhizer & Bowen, 1999; Finkelman, 2001). In no way, however, is it implied that the process is linear or assumed to occur in a straight-line fashion from step 1 to step 7. In fact, the process is iterative. This means that information and activities of one step feed back into the dynamic process, and the cycle of steps may start over again before completing all steps. For example, as information is gathered, a problem might have to be redefined; as solutions are generated, new information may come to light that, in turn, may yet again redefine the problem. The seven steps can be interpreted as follows:

1. *Define the problem.* Does a problem really exist that requires an investment in time and resources to solve? Perhaps an already existing protocol can be used to deal with the issue at hand. On the other hand, perhaps the problem in question really consists of more than one problem, or perhaps what appears to be a problem may not require action at all (Davidhizer & Bowen, 1999). Clearly formulating the problem may be helped by refining a written statement of the problem (e.g., "The problem is …").

2. *Gather information.* The problem solver cannot overestimate the critical importance of this step. Too often people start the problem-solving process without having spent enough time gathering information about the problem. It is important to start by gathering as much input and information as possible from a variety of sources. Shortening the information-gathering process to save time may cause difficulty later. The information must be analyzed by separating important from peripheral information, and timetables of prior events may need to be determined in order to gain a full understanding of the problem (Finkelman, 2001).

3. *Determine the overall goal or desired outcome.* This step guides decision making and actions toward the desired outcome. An outcomes focus aids the effectiveness of chosen activities. In fact, determining the over-all goal can illuminate the need for more information as well as facilitate the generation of possible solutions (Pesut & Herman, 1999).

4. *Develop solutions.* Notice that the word *solutions* is plural. A problem suggests more than one alternative solution (Davidhizer & Bowen, 1999;

Box **6.1**

Seven Steps of Problem Solving

1. Define the problem
2. Gather information
3. Determine desired outcome
4. Develop solutions
5. Consider consequences
6. Make decisions
7. Implement and evaluate solutions

Finkelman, 2001). One basic idea is that people have choices, and therefore problems have solutions. It may be that in the whole array of multiple solutions to any problem, none of them are particularly enticing. However, solutions or multiple options to any given problem situation always exist. Expanding the ability to look at problems as always having a potential for multiple solutions is a key conceptual element in dealing with problems. It helps to avoid knee-jerk reactions that occur when the problem is identified without careful deliberation or critical thinking. It may be seductive to short-cut the time and energy involved with careful problem analysis and take an easily available solution.

5. *Consider the consequences.* This step should be done carefully for each alternative solution. The first action is to list the potential consequences. This is a critical thinking strategy. It requires a broad perspective that includes all potential consequences. The problem solver's values will play a role in the analysis and evaluation of the consequences. For example, a consequence seen as very negative by one person may be perceived as less so by another.

6. *Make a decision.* This is the decisive action stage. At some point analysis needs to be brought to closure and a decision made. There are various techniques useful for driving decision making to one selected choice.

7. *Implement and evaluate the solution.* This is the action and feedback stage. The results of the problem-analysis and decision-making cognitive processes now culminate in the direct action determined as necessary to be taken. This step may require risk and courage. Periodic checks on effectiveness need to be made and then fed back into the problem-solving process. Some people can never seem to get to this stage. They cannot seem to generate solutions. Observe your colleagues. Are they problem identifiers? Some people have great difficulty clearly identifying the problem. Others can easily figure out what the problem

is but then cannot get beyond problem identification. Are individuals solution generators? Or are they locked into preformed ideas, a type of "hardening of the concepts"? If they are able to generate solutions, can they then move into the risk-taking steps of making a decision and implementing a solution?

Some questions to ask during problem solving include the following:

- What specifically is the problem?
- Why, how, and to whom is it a problem?
- Why should anything be done about it?
- What are the facts, and what do they mean?
- What are the possible solutions?
- Which solutions are acceptable?
- What is the ideal or preferred solution?
- What is the best solution?
- Will it work? Is it worth doing?
- Is it the right thing to do?

Problem solving starts with an awareness of a problem. Perhaps a nurse announces that there is a problem. The above questions might be asked of the nurse as a clarification process. For example, what are the facts, what do the facts mean, and what kind of solution should be sought? Is the optimum or ideal solution desired, or is it best to look for a solution that is just adequate? Is any solution that comes along acceptable? What are the possible solutions? Which one is the best solution? Will it work, and is it worth doing? This process of critical thinking aids careful deliberations.

When diagnosing a problem, the nurse needs to ferret out all the facts, then separate the fact from fiction and interpretation (Davidhizer & Bowen, 1999). A deliberate effort needs to be made to separate facts from interpretation, since the two are not always consonant. Facts can have multiple interpretations because of the phenomenon of human perceptions. One person's interpretation of facts may or may not be consonant with the known facts, and it may or may not be an appropriate interpretation. Therefore the nurse needs to determine the facts in detail.

Another danger during problem diagnosis is the human tendency to jump to conclusions.

Jumping to conclusions without clearly defining the problem and considering multiple alternatives can lead to errors of faulty decision making. For example, a common mistake of novice nurse managers may occur when one employee comes to complain about behaviors or actions of another employee. The nurse manager may promise to "take care of it," assuming the story was complete and accurate. Upon further investigation, however, another side of the story emerges, suggesting that the complaining employee was actually the instigator. It is better to take all matters under advisement pending a full investigation.

Finally, the magnitude and scope of the problem needs to be established. For example, problems may have an urgency difference that distinguishes one from another and allows for prioritization. The problem can be assessed according to how urgent and how immediate it is, according to the following guidelines:

- A potential problem can emerge at any time. It is just sitting there like a time bomb and can emerge spontaneously.
- An actual problem is occurring in real time and needs prompt action. It is unfolding in the moment.
- A critical problem is highly urgent and needs crisis intervention.

The continuum of time ranges from "the problem is not happening, but it could" to "an immediate crisis is unfolding." The urgency and the importance of action can be two variables plotted against each other and displayed on a grid (Covey, 1990). This is useful as an analysis tool. The first consideration is to decide whether the problem is important. The problem then can be analyzed as to its urgency. The problem may be important but not urgent, or it may be urgent but not important. When this activity is applied to nursing situations, it can give some guidance in terms of the prioritization of time, especially when competing demands are made on an individual regarding the immediacy and impact of a problem (Figure 6.3).

Managers use urgency and importance assessments when they attempt to manage their scarce time resources. This is a time management technique. For example, a typical morning might bring many requests that arrive simultaneously to the nurse manager. The following demands might need to be prioritized: committee minutes to be prepared, phone or e-mail messages to be returned, staffing schedule to be finalized, a replacement to be made for a sick call-in, and a report about a client or family complaint to handle. A similar phenomenon occurs when staff nurses have multiple requests for their time and attention from their many clients. A time and urgency rating schema can be used as a way of sorting out competing demands and planning and organizing for effectiveness.

Strategies for Problem Solving

The fourth basic problem-solving step is to develop solutions. It is helpful to think of all problems as having multiple potential solutions and to consider all available options or strategies systematically. It is also wise to consider both the intended and possible unintended consequences of each solution or action. There are a number of different strategies for resolving problems. Strategies used by nurses and nurse managers for problem resolution are shown in Figure 6.4.

Direct Intervention

This is carrying out some direct physical or verbal activity to intervene in a situation and resolve a problem. Problem solvers themselves are directly involved in the actions taken to implement a resolution when they use direct intervention. This is a strategy of personally doing or taking action.

Indirect Intervention

Being at the center of a communications and operations network, the nurse manager may use interpersonal skills to work around the sides of the problem: for example, getting disputants to talk to each other as a way of indirectly intervening. Negotiation, conflict resolution, persuasion, and confrontation are all examples of indirect intervention in which interpersonal skills are used to work through other people to help them solve

Nursing Situation	Urgency					Importance				
	Low				High	Low				High
A Hospital Floor Nurse finds that a cleaning person just finished vacuuming a room and the cord is stretched across a walkway in a(n):										
• **empty office at night**	①1	2	3	4	5	1	2	③3	4	5
• **nursing station during a weekday**	1	2	3	4	⑤5	1	2	③3	4	5
• **ambulatory outpatient geriatric clinic**	1	2	3	4	⑤5	1	2	3	4	⑤5

Setting	Immediacy					Impact				
	Low				High	Low				High
A Community Health Nurse Manager reviews a pile of new mail, including:										
• **a memo about Information Services' daily news summary sheet**	①1	2	3	4	5	①1	2	3	4	5
• **a letter from a sales representative announcing a sale of needed equipment**	1	2	③3	4	5	1	2	3	④4	5
• **a client's complaint letter alleging negligent care**	1	2	3	4	⑤5	1	2	3	4	⑤5

Figure 6.3
Activity prioritization.

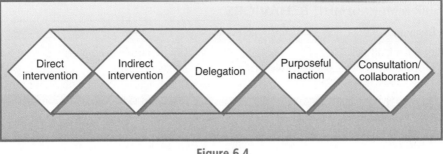

Figure 6.4
Strategies for problem solving.

their own problems. The nurse manager does not carry out the actions of resolution; rather, action is taken to influence others to resolve the problem. Nurses use this strategy with clients and their families.

Delegation

Delegation is assigning certain responsibilities and tasks to others. It is used to solve the problem of workload distribution. Delegation occurs frequently in nursing and is associated with care delivery systems, the use of nurse extenders, and differentiated practice.

Purposeful Inaction

Some problems will go away—with time—if little attention or emphasis is given to them. Purposeful inaction is a conscious decision *not* to act. It may be thought of as "watchful waiting." Deciding when intervention is absolutely necessary and when purposeful inaction or benign neglect is more likely to allow a problem to go away is sometimes complex. Inaction may be advantageous in certain situations (Davidhizer & Bowen, 1999). An example of purposeful inaction occurs when a nurse manager begins to hear complaints about a new process or procedure. While still maintaining open communication and freedom of expression, the nurse manager is unable to diagnose a specific problem beyond staff discontent, which may work itself out naturally with time as the comfort level of the staff rises after time to try things out.

Consultation or Collaboration

This strategy involves finding a peer and exchanging information and ideas. It increases the available knowledge resources as input for analysis in problem solving. This approach is associated with strategies related to networking and coordinating with others. Davidhizer and Bowen (1999) noted that involving staff in problem solving helps to decrease blaming and helps staff to feel vested in the outcome.

If there are multiple potential solutions to problems, then a review and analysis of the possible strategies for problem solving can be helpful in identifying options. Leaders and managers may want to try out new strategies to increase their personal and professional effectiveness.

LEADERSHIP AND MANAGEMENT IMPLICATIONS

Critical thinking skills enhance the quality of clinical judgment, problem solving, and decision making. Nursing problems may be complex and high-risk, necessitating thorough deliberation and some creativity. In one study, acute care environments were found to be turbulent and uncertain for nurses because of workload, loss of workplace identity, and reengineering for new skill mix and other changes (Geddes et al., 1999). Critical thinking is one skill applicable to making delegation decisions (Davidson et al., 1999). Furthermore, critical thinking has been identified as one of the top skills needed for competent practice as a nurse leader/ manager (Connelly et al., 2003; Lemire, 2002b).

▲ LEADERSHIP & MANAGEMENT **BEHAVIORS**

Leadership Behaviors

- Enables critical thinking skills
- Influences group and individual problem-solving activity
- Inspires others to solve problems
- Envisions creative alternatives to problems
- Motivates the group to innovate in response to identified problems
- Models good problem-solving behavior
- Networks with nurse colleagues

Management Behaviors

- Acts to resolve problems
- Plans for projected organizational deficits and surpluses

- Organizes the environment to decrease problems
- Directs individuals in problem resolution
- Delegates tasks and responsibilities
- Controls levels of conflict

Overlap Areas

- Uses problem-solving processes and critical thinking techniques to accomplish goals
- Motivates individuals and groups to problem-solve

▨ Research Note

Source: Connelly, L.M., Yoder, L.H., & Miner-Williams, D. (2003). A qualitative study of charge nurse competencies. *MEDSURG Nursing, 12*(5), 298-305.

Purpose

One of the first leadership/management roles a nurse may take on is that of a charge nurse on an inpatient unit. The purpose of this article is to describe the results of a qualitative research study that sought to uncover the competencies necessary for being an effective charge nurse.

Discussion

Charge nurses are the first-line managers on a nursing care unit. If they are not effective in their role, the quality of patient care can suffer. Using Katz's (1974) three categories of management competencies (technical, human, and conceptual) as a guide, 42 participants were interviewed in order to identify charge nurse competencies. The sample included military staff nurses, charge nurses, head nurses, and other nursing supervisory personnel. Results were categorized according to a modification of Katz's original schema. Categories of identified competencies critical to the nurse role were clinical/technical competencies, human relations competencies, organizational competencies, and critical thinking competencies. Included within critical thinking competencies were decision making, prioritization and time management, problem solving and dealing with change.

Application to Practice

A high level of critical thinking is essential for a nurse to function effectively in the charge nurse role. Connelly and colleagues suggest that educational programs could include patient care scenarios in order to help new nurses' critical thinking abilities. Head nurses could mentor new charge nurses by helping them to reflect on their practice. All nurses can benefit from learning to question and to reflect on their practice.

A key role for the nurse leader or manager is to promote critical thinking and good problem solving among care teams. Although traditional theoretical depictions of managerial functions stress planning, directing, organizing, and controlling, problem-solving is in fact one of the top activities in which managers engage (Timmreck, 2000). Strategies that nurse leaders/managers can use to encourage critical thinking and problem solving are questioning and brainstorming (Colwell, 2001). They can use change-of-shift reports to promote critical thinking and subsequent problem solving by asking such questions as "What nursing interventions have been effective?" or "What will happen if this course of action is chosen?" (Oermann, 1999). Another strategy for promoting critical thinking is to create a climate wherein mistakes can be made and then analyzed, without fear of punishment, for why the mistake occurred (Cohen, 2002).

In practice, nurses find that they are solving many types of problems, including large, small, explosive, political, fun, sad, and ordinary day-to-day problems. Think about problems faced by the typical adult: planning a wedding, handling a difficult roommate, paying debts, or finding adequate child care. Individuals are faced with many problems, both in the personal and professional arenas. The fact that problems are a common phenomenon means that most of us have some experience base for managing them. Despite this experience, workplace and nursing care problems take on a unique character.

In their professional work, nurses use a level of expertise in problem solving that goes beyond common knowledge and home remedies. They use a complex and sophisticated level of knowledge and skill in providing and coordinating health care and illness care. The essence of professional practice is the utilization of expertise to solve problems for *clients*. Nurses need to be licensed, considered professional, and have autonomy for practice because they make decisions based on nursing expertise. Clients report that an expert nurse makes all the difference in their therapy, care, and psychosocial well-being. What nurses do in decision making involves applying specialized expertise in solving problems for clients.

Nurse managers, as an extension of nursing care, also find themselves faced with problems calling for decisions. Some problems must be solved in a short turnaround time and without the benefit of much contemplation: for example, how to staff the next shift. In their budget process, nurse managers solve problems and make decisions about capital equipment, staffing, and allocation of scarce resources. The nurse manager's job, then, involves the utilization of expertise to solve problems in the work environment. Leadership and management in nursing practice are intimately involved with setting up a work environment, including the climate, the culture, the leadership style, and the task structure that allow nurses to function at the highest possible levels. Decisions made by nurses include the structuring of the work environment and the allocation of scarce resources. Both are challenges to problem-solving skills. With an emphasis on participatory decision making and shared governance in nursing, the ability and willingness of staff nurses to participate in problem solving is a leadership and management issue.

Experience and skill in problem solving, like competence with interpersonal relationships, are elemental skills for nurses. For leadership and management in nursing, success depends on developing both interpersonal and problem-solving skills.

CURRENT ISSUES AND TRENDS

Critical thinking is a key skill for all nurses and has been identified as a core component of knowledge development, professional practice, and education for all the health professions (Pew Health Professions Commission, 1998) and the development of an educated public. The National League for Nursing Accrediting Commission (NLNAC) supported the competencies as outlined in the Pew Health Commission report as a basis for curriculum development (NLNAC, 2003). A number of teaching strategies have been used to promote critical thinking, but their effectiveness has been primarily anecdotal (Staib, 2003). Some standardized measurement instruments are available, such as the Watson-Glaser Critical Thinking Appraisal (Watson & Glaser, 1980), the California Critical Thinking Skills Test, and the California Reasoning Appraisal (Insight Assessment, 2004). In one integrative review of 20 research studies from 1977 to 1995 on the critical thinking abilities of professional nursing students, the Watson-Glaser Critical Thinking Appraisal was used in 18 of the studies. Results were mixed about whether critical thinking skills increased during nursing education (Adams, 1999). Clearly, more research needs to be done. Nevertheless, nurturing, developing, and demonstrating evidence of critical thinking skills remain important issues in nursing education and practice.

In the leadership and management of nursing practice, problems can arise spontaneously, be chronic, or recur in cycles. For example, two recurring management problems in nursing practice are (1) cycles of nursing shortage and surplus and (2) concern over alleged unsafe patient care resulting from low staffing of registered nurses (RNs) (Aiken et al., 2002). The strategies adopted to solve these problems vary from individual to group action. Economic interests are at the heart of the clash between nurses who feel stretched thinner and thinner and health care institutions that are responding to reimbursement pressures. Despite the chronic nature of this tension, nursing has not resolved its staffing issues. The cycles continue. However, research evidence on nursing effectiveness and outcomes is beginning to be compiled. The linkage to staffing issues is an ongoing challenge.

Problem-Solving Teams

Current nursing literature emphasizes the use of problem-solving teams as a leadership and management strategy designed to improve productivity and effectiveness. A team-based problem-solving method is designed to improve the participation and empowerment of key decision implementers. Davidhizer and Bowen (1999) noted that it is essential for managers to enlist staff in problem solving

as a way to generate more possible solutions. One question is, Does good problem solving have a positive impact on patient care? In problem solving with patients, the nurse needs to start with the patient's goals. Then the problem-solving process is applied. Shaw and colleagues (2003) studied registered nurse case managers who had undergone training in problem-solving techniques. Results showed that those who had undergone training were better able to work collaboratively with patients to identify barriers to recovery and return to work. Case managers used the following six-step process:

1. Work with patient to identify and select a problem interfering with return to work.
2. Analyze the problem using such strategies as active listening.
3. Generate possible solutions.
4. Select and plan solution taking into account costs, benefits, and feasibility.
5. Implement the solution by setting a timetable and involving all interested parties, including the employee's manager.
6. Evaluate the solution.

A related approach to using systematic tools and teamwork to solve problems is the use of an affinity map and a relationship diagram. Problem solving begins with analysis of the gap, the difference between the ideal and the real situation. However, some problems are complex, urgent in severity, have no easy solution, and require time and participation to resolve. Affinity maps and relationship diagrams can guide teams in moving toward consensus resolution of such problems (Lepley, 1998).

Summary

- Critical thinking is the basis for good problem solving.
- All nurses, including nurse leaders/managers, need skills in critical thinking and problem solving.
- A problem is a situation in need of resolution.
- Problem solving is a process of coming to a solution for the problem.

- The steps of the problem-solving process lead to logical analysis and strategy selection.
- There are multiple strategies for solving problems.

Study Questions

1. How can critical thinking and problem solving be used in nursing practice?
2. Identify a problem you are dealing with now. What approaches might you use to solve this problem?
3. How do you tend to respond to a problem? Emotionally? Logically? Why is it important to identify your habitual responses to problems?
4. What strategy do you tend to use for problem solving? What are other strategies you would like to use?
5. How do leaders/managers facilitate critical thinking and problem solving?

CASE STUDY

Mannee Upona, Mike McCan, and Lily Pond are three nurse colleagues chosen for a leadership development intensive experience. They have worked together on several committees and share a desire to improve client care in the Visiting Nurses Association (VNA) where they work. They are all experts at home visits and community health nursing. However, they have been unable to "mesh" as a team, often "agreeing to disagree" and going their own ways.

Their first assignment is to self-administer and analyze standardized instruments such as a leadership style survey, conflict mode instrument, critical thinking appraisal, and a problem solving style measure. Each of the nurses completes the instruments and analyzes himself or herself.

Next they are asked to participate in a facilitated discussion about how individuals vary. The topic of facts, interpretations, and feelings is enlightening. Nurses Upona, McCan, and Pond begin to recognize and compare patterns and discuss what this means for teamwork and synergy. They begin to outline individual strengths and weaknesses and how these can be blended to capitalize on their collective strengths. Later, the new insight is put to the test as they tackle a group-identified problem as a team.

CRITICAL THINKING EXERCISE

Nurse Brad Flint works the 12-hour evening shift on a busy surgical unit in a 200-bed community hospital. He has been employed on this same unit for 5 years. During this past year he has been late six times and he often receives several calls per shift from his children. Unit manager Susan Smith has verbally counseled Nurse Flint and placed a disciplinary warning in his personnel file. If Nurse Flint doesn't consistently arrive on time for his shift for the next 3 months, he will be suspended without pay and perhaps lose his job.

1. What is the problem?
2. Why is it a problem?
3. What are the key issues?
4. What should the unit manager do first when dealing with Nurse Flint?
5. How should critical thinking be used?
6. What problem-solving strategies should unit manager Smith use with Nurse Flint?

REFERENCES

Ackoff, R. (1974). *Redesigning the future.* New York: John Wiley & Sons.

Adams, B.L. (1999). Nursing education for critical thinking: An integrative review. *Journal of Nursing Education, 38*(3), 111-119.

Adams, C. (1994). The impact of problem-solving styles of NE-CEO pairs on nurse executive effectiveness. *Journal of Nursing Administration, 24*(11), 17-22.

Aiken, L.H., Clarke, S.P., Sloane, D.M., Solchaski, J., & Silber, J.H. (2002). Hospital nurse staffing and patient mortality, nurse burnout and job satisfaction. *Journal of the American Medical Association, 288,* 1987-1993.

Alfaro-LeFevre, R. (1997). *Improving your ability to think critically.* Hoffman Estates, IL: Nursing Spectrum. Retrieved May 25, 2004, from *www.nsweb.nursingspectrum. com/ce/ce168.htm*

Benner, P. (2003). Beware of technological imperatives and commercial interests that prevent best practices! *American Journal of Critical Care, 12*(5), 469-471.

Benner, P. (1984). *From novice to expert: Excellence and power in clinical practice.* Menlo Park, CA: Addison-Wesley.

Benner, P., & Tanner, C. (1987). Clinical judgment: How expert nurses use intuition. *American Journal of Nursing, 87*(1), 23-31.

Brookfield, S.D. (1991). *Developing critical thinkers: Challenging adults to explore alternative ways of thinking and acting.* San Francisco: Jossey-Bass.

Buhler, P. M. (2004). Managing in the new millennium: The talent search: Every manager's responsibility. *Supervision, 65*(4), 20-22.

Bulman, C., & Schutz, S. (Eds.) (2004). *Reflective practice in nursing* (3rd ed.). Oxford, UK: Blackwell Publishing.

Cohen, S. (2002). Don't overlook creative thinking. *Nursing Management, 33*(8), 9-10.

Colwell, J.L. (2001). Beyond brainstorming: How managers can cultivate creativity and problem solving in employees. *Supervision, 62*(8), 6-9.

Connelly, L.M., Yoder, L.H., & Miner-Williams, D. (2003). A qualitative study of charge nurse competencies. *MEDSURG Nursing, 12*(5), 298-305.

Covey, S. (1990). *The seven habits of highly effective people: Restoring the character ethic.* New York: Simon & Schuster.

Davidhizer, R.E., & Bowen, M. (1999). There are solutions to problems. *Health Care Manager, 18*(1), 14-19.

Davidson, S.B., Scott, R., & Minarik, P. (1999). Thinking critically about delegation. *American Journal of Nursing, 99*(6), 61-62.

deChesnay, M. (1983). Problem solving in nursing. *Image, 15*(1), 8-11.

Emanuel, E. (2002). Health care reform: Still possible. *Hastings Center Report, 32*(2), 33-34.

El Paso Community College. (2004). *Think bank.* El Paso, TX: El Paso Community College/The Texas Collaborative for Teaching Excellence. Retrieved May 27, 2004, from *www.epcc.edu/Special/Critical/home.htm*

Facione, N.C., & Facione, P.A. (1996). Externalizing the critical thinking in knowledge development and clinical judgment. *Nursing Outlook, 44*(3), 129-136.

Finkelman, A.W. (2001). Problem-solving, decision-making, and critical thinking: How do they mix and why bother? *Home Care Provider, 6*(6), 194-197.

Geddes, N., Salyer, J., & Mark, B.A. (1999). Nursing in the nineties: Managing the uncertainty. *Journal of Nursing Administration, 29*(5), 40-48.

Hansten, R.I., & Washburn, M.J. (1999). Individual and organizational accountability for development of critical thinking. *Journal of Nursing Administration, 29*(11), 39-45.

Hersey, P., & Natemeyer, W. (1988). *Problem-Solving and Decision-Making Style Inventory: Perception of self.* Escondido, CA: Leadership Studies, Inc.

Hurst, K., Dean, A., & Trickey, S. (1991). The recognition and non-recognition of problem-solving stages. *Journal of Advanced Nursing, 16,* 1444-1455.

Insight Assessment. (2004). *Testing tools and assessment services: Critical thinking skills and reasoning tests.* Millbrae, CA: Insight Assessment/California Academic Press, LLC. Retrieved August 18, 2004, from *www.insightassessment. com/tests.html*

Kalischuk, R.G., & Thorpe, K. (2002). Thinking creatively: From nursing education to practice. *The Journal of Continuing Education in Nursing, 33*(4), 155-163.

Katz, R. (1974). Skills of effective administrators. *Harvard Business Review, 52*(5), 90-102.

Kennedy, C. (2002). The decision making process in a district nursing assessment. *British Journal of Community Nursing, 7*(10), 505-513.

Kirton, M. (1976). Adaptors and innovators: A description and measure. *Journal of Applied Psychology, 61,* 622-629.

Kirton, M. (1994). *Adaptors and innovators: Styles of creativity and problem solving.* London: Routledge.

Lemire. J.A. (2002a). Leader as critical thinker. *Nursing Leadership Forum, 7*(2), 69-76.

Lemire, J.A. (2002b). Preparing nurse leaders: A leadership education model. *Nursing Leadership Forum, 7*(2), 47-52.

Lepley, C.J. (1998). Problem-solving tools for analyzing system problems: The affinity map and the relationship diagram. *Journal of Nursing Administration, 28*(12), 44-50.

Le Storti, A.J., Cullen, P.A., Hanzlik, E.M., Michiels, J.M., Piano, L.A., Ryan, P.L., et al (1999). Creative thinking in nursing education: Preparing for tomorrow's challenges. *Nursing Outlook, 47*(2), 62-66.

Luft, J. (1970). *Group process.* Palo Alto, CA: Mayfield Publishing.

National League for Nursing Accrediting Commission (NLNAC). (2003). *NLNAC 2003 Interpretive guidelines by program type: Core competencies adapted by NLNAC.* New York, NLNAC. Retrieved May 27, 2004, from *www.nlnac.org/Manual%20&%20IG/2003Edition/Guidelines_General.pdf*

Newell, A., & Simon, H. (1972). *Human problem solving.* Englewood Cliffs, NJ: Prentice-Hall.

Oermann, M.H. (1999). Two-way talks: Get the most from your clinical discussions with staff. *Nursing Management, 30*(6), 56-58.

O'Sullivan, P.S., Blevins-Stephens, W.L., Smith, F.M., & Vaughan-Wrobel, B. (1997). Addressing the National League for nursing critical-thinking outcome. *Nursing Educator, 22*(1), 23-29.

Paul, R. (1992). *Critical thinking: What every person needs to survive in a rapidly changing world* (2nd ed.). Santa Rosa, CA: Foundation for Critical Thinking.

Pesut, D.J., & Herman, J. (1999). *Clinical reasoning: The art and science of critical and creative thinking.* Albany, NY: Delmar Publishers.

Peters, R.M. (2002). Nurse administrators' role in health policy: Teaching the elephant to dance. *Nursing Administration Quarterly, 26*(4), 1-8.

Pew Health Professions Commission. (1998). *Twenty-one competencies for the twenty-first century.* San Francisco: Center for the Health Professions. Retrieved May 28, 2004, from *www.futurehealth.ucsf.edu/pewcomm/competen.html*

Polge, J. (1995). Critical thinking: The use of intuition in making clinical nursing judgments. *Journal of the New York State Nurses Association, 26*(2), 4-9.

Porter-O'Grady, T. (2003). A different age for leadership: Part 2. *Journal of Nursing Administration, 33*(3), 173-178.

Redding, D.A. (2001). The development of critical thinking among students in baccalaureate nursing education. *Holistic Nursing Practice, 15*(4), 57-64.

Scheffer, B.K., & Rubenfeld, M.G. (2000). A consensus statement on critical thinking in nursing. *Journal of Nursing Education, 39*(8), 352-359.

Shaw, W.S., Feuerstein, M., Miller, V.I., & Wood, P.M. (2003). Identifying barriers to recovery from work related upper extremity disorders: Use of a collaborative problem solving technique. *AAOHN Journal, 51*(8), 337-346.

Staib, S. (2003). Teaching and measuring critical thinking. *Journal of Nursing Education, 42*(11), 498-508.

Stark, J. (1996). Critical thinking for outcomes-based practice. *Seminars for Nurse Managers, 4*(3), 168-171.

Tanner, C.A. (2000). Critical thinking: Beyond nursing process. *Journal of Nursing Education, 39*(8), 338-339.

Taylor, C. (1997). Problem solving in clinical nursing practice. *Journal of Advanced Nursing, 26,* 329-336.

Timmreck, T.C. (2000). Use of classical functions of management by health services midmanagers. *Health Care Manager, 19*(2), 50-67.

Watson, G., & Glaser, E. (1980). *Watson-Glaser Critical Thinking Appraisal manual.* New York: Macmillan.

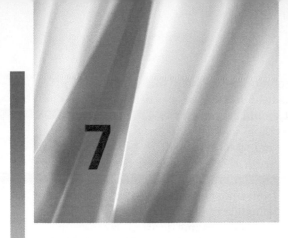

7

Decision-Making Skills

Thomas R. Clancy

CHAPTER OBJECTIVES

- Connect decision making to problem solving
- Define and describe decision making
- Outline 10 steps to follow for decision making
- Illustrate decision-making situations
- Examine administrative decision-making models
- Analyze decision-making strategies
- Relate perception, creativity, and innovation to decision making
- Translate decision making to leadership and management
- Exercise critical thinking to conceptualize and analyze possible solutions to a practice exercise

ecision making is the essence of leadership and management. It is what leaders and managers are expected to do. Thus decisions are visible outcomes of the leadership and management process. The effectiveness of decision making is one criterion for evaluating a leader or manager: "Organizational performance is largely dependent upon the decision making processes that a particular organization uses. In every organization, decisions have to be made on a daily basis" (Lahti, 1996, p. 1). Therefore both individual and group decisions need to be as efficient and effective as is possible.

Making decisions may be the most important component of any nurse's job. It is also the most difficult and riskiest aspect (Hammond et al., 1998). Poor decisions can impede progress, waste resources, cause harm or damage, and affect a career. The results of poor decisions may be subtle and not appear until years later. Take, for instance, a decision to reduce expenses by decreasing the ratio of registered nurses to nurse's aides. There may be a short-term cost savings, but if not implemented appropriately, this tactic may result in the gradual erosion of patient care over time. Unintended effects may include higher turnover of experienced nurses, increased adverse events such as medication errors, decreased staff morale, and lower patient satisfaction scores. The long-term outcome of this decision may actually result in the exact opposite of the original objective—that of reducing expenses. Thus it is vitally important for nurses to understand decision making and explore styles and strategies to enhance decision-making skills.

Decision making is a vital component of problem solving. It is important to recognize that *decision making* is not a passive concept; rather it is a behavior—the critical mental action that is taken. For any problem-solving process, there may be a time separation between the problem solving and the decision making. Decision making may or may not be the result of an immediate problem. Identifying a course of action is the purpose of decision making. Ideally, what is desired is a high level of effectiveness, meaning that more decisions will turn out to be good than bad. The quality of decision making relates to "vigilant information processing" (Janis & Mann, 1977).

Decision making can be thought of as a process with identifiable steps. Nurses make decisions in personal, clinical, and organizational situations and under conditions of certainty, uncertainty, and risk. There are various decision-making models and strategies. Nurses' control over decision making may vary as to amount of control and where in the process they can influence decisions. Awareness of the components, process, and strategies of decision making contributes to effectiveness in nursing leadership and management decision making.

DEFINITIONS

A *decision* is a choice among alternatives. Grainger (1990) called decision making the act of choosing. Veninga (1982) described it as the process of converting information into action. **Decision making** can also be defined as a behavior exhibited in making a selection and implementing a course of action from among alternative courses of action for dealing with a situation or problem. It may or may not be the result of an immediate problem. The problem-solving process is initiated as the result of an immediate problem. Decision making, however, may occur some time later. **Problem solving** and decision making both use information and draw conclusions about information. Both require critical thinking. Values, life experiences, and individual thinking preferences create variability in these processes. However, decision making differs from problem solving in that it is influenced by emotions and intuition, it is purposeful and goal-directed, it involves a choice among options, and it does not always start with an immediate problem. Problem solving includes

a decision-making step but is focused on an immediate problem or gap between what is and what should be (Saulo, 1996).

Decision making also may be the result of opportunities, challenges, or leadership initiatives as opposed to being triggered by an immediate problem. The process of selecting one course of action from among alternatives forms the basic core of the definition of decision making. As a corollary to responsibility, making decisions means realizing the consequences in advance (McKenzie, 1985). In any decision the conscious presence of both the end to be accomplished and the means to be used are involved (Barnard, 1982).

There are five core elements to decision making, as follows:

1. Identification of a problem, issue, or situation
2. Establishment of the criteria to be used to evaluate potential solutions
3. Search for alternative solutions or actions
4. Evaluation of the alternatives
5. Selection of a specific alternative

These elements can be summarized as the three phases of deliberation, judgment, and choice (Schaefer, 1974). Nurses use deliberation, judgment, and choice in managing client care. Nurse managers use these three phases in managing resources and the environment of care delivery. Management of decision making involves an evaluation of the effectiveness of the outcomes that result from the decision-making process (Figure 7.1).

Another way of looking at problems to determine the appropriate decision strategy is to ask the following questions: Who owns the problem? Is it an individual's problem, or is it a system's problem? This is a process of framing the problem.

▲ LEADING & MANAGING **DEFINED**

Decision Making	**Problem Solving**
A behavior exhibited in making a selection and implementing a course of action from alternatives; it may or may not be the result of an immediate problem.	The process that attempts to identify obstacles that inhibit accomplishment of a specific goal.

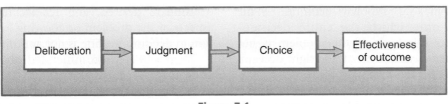

Figure 7.1
Core elements of decision making.

The determination of where ownership of a problem lies indicates whether to approach the problem individually with the person or by a group strategy (e.g., problem-solving or creativity techniques) (deChesnay, 1983). Nurse administrators need to recognize the different analogies individual executives and managers may use to view problems. The chief executive officer may frame issues as a competitive struggle not unlike a sports event. The marketing staff may interpret problems as military battles that need to be won. Nurse executives may view concerns from a care or family frame that emphasize collaboration and working together. Regardless of the individual, learning and understanding which frames and analogies offer the best view of a problem is vital to effective decision making. It may be necessary for nurse managers to expand their frame boundaries and be willing to consider even the most outlandish ideas. Obviously, it is important to begin the problem definition phase with staff members who are closest to the problem. However, it is wise to then consider adding individuals who have no connection with the issue whatsoever. Often it is these "unconnected" staff members who bring new decision frames to the meeting and have the most unbiased view of the problem.

In nursing and health care, quality improvement techniques emphasize the framing of problems as systems problems and the subsequent use of group problem-resolution strategies. For example, nurses may encounter a "difficult" client. Framing this as a system's problem would lead the nurse to decide to use intervention strategies such as increased care coordination, assignment to an interdisciplinary team, staffing adjustments,

environmental restructuring, and teaching or counseling the family. Framing the same problem as an individual's problem would lead to a decision to counsel the nurse to change his or her attitude, habits, or approaches toward the client.

BACKGROUND

The basic elements of problem solving and decision making can be summarized into the following two parts (1) identifying the problem and (2) making the decision.

Identifying the Problem

The antecedent activities of decision making are those of problem solving and are directed at gathering facts. Decision making assumes that problem-solving activity has been taking place. However, it is still vital to identify specifically the nature of the problem that the decision making is to address. There is a tendency when decision making to bypass a thorough analysis of the problem and move quickly into solutions. The American business culture has a long tradition of emphasizing action and decisiveness. Much of this comes from a rich history of rugged individualism in a free market system. In contrast, the Japanese place a much greater emphasis on building consensus on what the problem is and what decision needs to be made (Drucker, 1974). A Japanese strategic planning team may spend up to 50% of the decision-making process on problem definition alone. However, once the problem is defined and a decision is made, the Japanese move to implementation at lightening speed. What lessons can be learned from the Japanese in terms of decision making? Problem definition is the foundation onto which the entire decision-making process is built. If the problem is not clearly defined from the onset, the right decision may be made for the wrong problem.

Capturing the essence of a problem can also be elusive. Most problems reside somewhere along a continuum of interrelated issues. For example, a typical problem continuum may resemble the following:

- Decreased patient satisfaction scores are the result of …
- High overall nurse vacancy rates resulting from …
- Difficulty in recruiting and retaining nurses as a result of …
- Low staff morale and high stress levels as a result of …
- A perceived poor work environment resulting from …
- A perception of poor follow-up by management on staff problems as a result of …

Just where to begin problem analysis along the continuum is the most common challenge managers face. In the above example, assuming that the root cause of decreased patient satisfaction scores is high nurse vacancy rates ignores the deeper problem of poor follow-up by managers. Defining the problem at its optimum point along the continuum takes patience and thoughtful analysis. Before moving to the next phase in the decision-making process, nurse leaders need to build consensus among all stakeholders about just where the problem lies.

Making the Decision

Once the situation is identified, the next activity is to determine what outcome is desired and what criteria need to be met when a solution is generated. The desired outcome may vary—from an ideal or short-term resolution to covering up the situation. What is desired may be (1) for the problem to go away forever, (2) to make sure that all involved in this problem are satisfied with the solution and gain some benefit from it, or (3) to obtain an ideal solution. Sometimes a quick

decision is desired, and researching different aspects of the problem or allowing for participation in decision making is not appropriate.

Wren (1974) recommended the following 10 steps in decision making:

1. Become aware of the situation.
2. Investigate the nature of the situation.
3. Determine the objective of the solution.
4. Determine alternative solutions.
5. Weigh the consequences and relative efficiency of each alternative solution.
6. Evaluate or pilot-test various alternatives.
7. Select the best alternative solution.
8. Implement the decision. Communicate it and train those who will carry out the solution.
9. Evaluate the solution at intervals to determine if it was the best solution and if it is still solving the problem.
10. Correct, change, or withdraw the solution if evaluation indicates that it is no longer appropriate.

Thus decision-making steps are similar to those of the problem-solving process. However, they form a specific subset. Decision making itself is a critical process and thus is examined separately. Nurses exhibit leadership in care delivery and management when they use expertise to make decisions on behalf of clients' care needs.

Desired decisions can be categorized into two end points: minimal and optimal. A minimal decision results in an outcome that is sufficient, satisfies basic requirements, and minimally meets desired objectives. This is sometimes called a *"satisficing" decision.* An *optimizing decision* includes comparing all possible solutions against desired objectives and then selecting the optimal solution that best meets objectives. The two factors of quality and acceptance are factored into evaluating the effectiveness of a decision (Janis & Mann, 1977; Saulo, 1996).

Flaws in thinking can create hidden traps in decision making. These are common psychological tendencies that create barriers or biases in cognitive reflection and appraisal. Six common distortions are as follows (Hammond et al., 1998):

1. *Anchoring trap:* When a decision is being considered, the mind gives a disproportionate

weight to the first information it receives. Trends and old numbers may become anchors, giving too much weight to past events. It is human nature to focus on an event that leaves a memorable or strong impression. All individuals have preconceived notions and biases that influence decisions in a variety of ways. Ignoring the "base rate" is one example of the tendency to disregard or discount the overall odds in a given situation as a result of preconceived notions (Hammond et al., 1999). For instance the Institute of Medicine (IOM, 2001) endorsed the use of computerized physician order entry (CPOE) as one solution to reduce medication errors. Following close on the heels of the IOM's report, the Leapfrog Group, a consortium of Fortune 500 companies, announced that use of a CPOE would be included as one of three criteria used to evaluate a health system's quality practices. Since both the IOM and Leapfrog Group's announcement, the number of orders from health systems for purchase of CPOE systems has significantly increased. However, the base rate for installation of CPOE systems nationwide is fewer than 3 per 100 hospitals (California HealthCare Foundation, 2000). Although CPOE systems show great promise, the primary reason for the low base rate is the enormous cost and complexity of installing them. Nurse executives should consider the base rate carefully when evaluating new technology.

2. *Status-quo trap:* Decision makers display a strong bias toward alternatives that perpetuate the status quo. Often this is the result of accelerating change in the work environment. Past practices that exhibit any sense of permanence provide managers with a feeling of security. Maintaining the status quo thus holds a magnetic attraction.

3. *Sunk-cost trap:* Past decisions become sunk costs, and new choices are often made in a way that justifies past choices. This may result in becoming trapped by an escalation of commitment. All too often managers allow past investments to influence current decisions when they should have little bearing on them (Russo & Schoemaker, 1989). Because of rapid, ongoing advances in medical technology, managers are frequently pressured to replace existing equipment before it is fully depreciated. If the new equipment provides a higher level of quality at a lower cost, the sunk cost of the existing equipment is irrelevant to the decision-making process. However, managers may delay purchasing new equipment and forgo subsequent savings because the equipment has yet to reach the end of its useful life.

4. *Confirming-evidence trap:* This bias leads people to seek out information that supports an existing instinct or point of view while avoiding contradictory evidence. A typical example includes favoring new technology over less glamorous alternatives. A decision maker may become so enamored by technological solutions (and slick vendor demonstrations) that she or he may unconsciously decide in favor of these systems even though there is strong evidence that supports implementing less costly solutions first.

5. *Framing trap:* The way a problem is initially framed profoundly influences the choices made. Different framing of the same problem can lead to different decision responses. A decision frame can be viewed as a window into the many and varied reasons a problem exists. As implied by the word *frame,* individuals may perceive problems only within the boundaries of their own frame. The human resources director may perceive a staffing shortage as a compensation problem, the chief financial officer as an insurance reimbursement issue, the director of education as a training issue, and the chief nursing officer as a work environment problem. It is obvious that all issues may contribute, in part, to the problem; however, each person, in looking through his or her individual frame, sees only that portion with which he or she is most familiar.

6. *Estimating and forecasting traps:* People make estimates or forecasts about uncertain events, but their minds are not calibrated for making

estimates in the face of uncertainty. The notion that experience is the father of wisdom suggests that mature managers, over the course of their careers, learn from their mistakes. It is reasonable to assume that the knowledge gained from a manager's failed projects would be applied to future decisions. As logical as this sounds, there is a tendency in human behavior to disregard negative outcomes and remember the positive ones (Belsky & Gilovich, 1999). Whether right or wrong, humans tend to take credit for successful projects and find ways to blame external factors on failed ones. Unfortunately, this form of overconfidence often results in overly optimistic projections in project planning. This optimism is usually buried in the analysis done before ranking alternatives and recommendations. Conversely, excessive cautiousness or prudence may also result in faulty decisions. Dramatic events may overly influence decisions because of recall and memory exaggerating the probability of rare but catastrophic occurrences. It is important that managers objectively examine project planning assumptions in the decision-making process to ensure accurate projections. Because misperceptions, biases, and flaws in thinking can influence choices, actions related to awareness, testing, and mental discipline can be employed to ferret out errors in thinking before the stage of decision making (Hammond et al., 1998).

DECISION-MAKING SITUATIONS

The situations in which decisions are made may be personal, clinical, or organizational (Figure 7.2). Personal decision making is a familiar part of everyday life. Personal decisions range from multiple small daily choices to time management and career or life choices.

Clinical decision making in nursing relates to quality of care and competency issues. Also called clinical problem solving, clinical reasoning, clinical judgment, or the nursing process, it is defined as a series of decisions made by the nurse

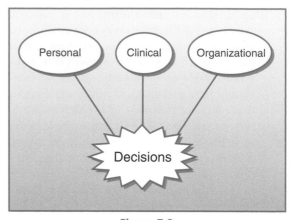

Figure 7.2
Decision-making situations.

in interaction with the client (Tanner, 1987). In nursing, clinical decision making is made difficult because of unclear, changing, and overlapping areas of practice in medicine and nursing, increasing complexity of clinical practice, and multidisciplinary (joint or team) approaches to decision making (Prescott et al., 1987). The process of diagnostic reasoning used in medicine has been refined into a general four-step model and applied to nursing: (1) attending to initially available clues (signs and symptoms), (2) activating hypotheses that may explain the initial cues, (3) gathering data to rule in or out hypotheses, and (4) evaluating hypotheses in light of each new clue until a diagnosis is accepted (Elstein et al., 1978; Tanner et al., 1987).

The major nursing practice decisions are judgments about a client problem (diagnosis) and nursing actions (interventions) for the selected diagnosis (Grier, 1984). Clinical decision making is the foundation of nursing practice, the criterion used to judge expertise, and the differentiation between professional and technical nursing personnel (Hughes & Young, 1992). Clinical decision making was defined in one model as choosing nursing actions (Pesut & Herman, 1998). In this model, reflection and decision making about interventions, alternatives, and consequences help clients make a transition from the initial (present) state to a desired outcome state. Thus clinical decision making is founded on clinical reasoning processes. Two methods for studying nurses' clinical decision making are (1) protocol analysis, in which participants are asked to think out loud as they make decisions in situations, and (2) line of reasoning, in which an argument or set of arguments leading to a conclusion is examined to determine how knowledge is used to make a decision. Line of reasoning is consistent with information processing theory, in which problem solving and decision making are seen as cognitive tasks. Decision-making behavior is described as person-task interaction (Narayan & Corcoran-Perry, 1997).

Nurses manage care and make decisions under conditions of certainty, uncertainty, and risk. For example, if research has shown that under prescribed conditions, selection of a specific nursing intervention is highly likely to produce a certain outcome, then the nurse in that situation faces a condition of certainty. An example would be the prevention of decubitus ulcers by frequent repositioning. If little knowledge is available or if the specific situation is more complex or variant from the usual, then the nurse faces uncertainty. Risk situations occur when there is a threat of harm to clients. Conditions of risk also occur commonly in relationship to the administration of medications, crisis events, infection control, invasive procedures, and the use of technology in nursing practice. Furthermore, these conditions also apply to the administration of nursing care delivery, in which decision making is a critical function.

Research Note

Source: Anderson, R.A., & McDaniel, R.R., Jr. (1999). RN participation in organizational decision making and improvements in resident outcomes. *Health Care Management Review, 24*(1), 7-16.

Purpose

Participation in decision making (PDM) is suggested as a way for nursing homes to improve performance. However, the allocation of scarce registered nurse (RN) time needs to be directed at activities that demonstrate effectiveness. The purpose of this article was to discuss the results of a study relating PDM by RNs to improvement in resident outcomes and suggest guidelines.

Discussion

Complexity theory served as the framework of this study. Organizations are considered to be complex adaptive systems existing in either stability, instability, or chaos. Complex adaptive systems can be moved from state to state by manipulating control parameters of information flow, connectivity, and information models. PDM is a strategy for managing control parameters. The decision context includes both strategic decisions (operations and marketing) and tactical decisions (resident and nonresident care). A descriptive survey design was used to send questionnaires to directors of nursing in 566 nursing homes in Texas. PDM was measured by using the Nursing Participation in Decision Making Instrument. The results indicated that nursing homes with the most improvements in residents' outcomes had greater RN participation in decision making than did homes with the least improvements.

Application to Practice

Under increasing pressure to improve residents' outcomes in a resource-constrained environment, nursing home directors of nursing traditionally decided to focus on enhancing clinical processes and improving care providers' skill levels. To compete on quality of care, additional organizational processes may be tapped to influence improvements in outcomes. PDM in tactical resident and nonresident care by RNs was associated with a significant difference in outcomes. It can help manipulate system control parameters of information and linkage. PDM does not need to be a costly innovation. It can be targeted to selected aspects of decision activities, especially those related to clinical care.

Conditions of uncertainty and complexity are common in nursing care management. Over time, the complexity of health care processes has increased as a natural outgrowth of innovation and new technology. Each new innovation acts as a building block for later innovations (Johnson, 2001; Waldrop, 1992). For example, the earlier technology developed for department-based pharmacy, radiology, lab, billing, registration, and decision support information systems are today's building blocks for integrated computerized physician ordering systems (California HealthCare Foundation, 2000). Although new technology streamlines processes, the additive effect of combining older technology to create new technological innovation may actually increase complexity (Perrow, 1984). Today's computerized hospital information systems have multiple common mode interdependencies with other departments. Because one common mode enables order entry for lab, radiology, and medications, subtle failures in any one system can go unnoticed and result in catastrophic outcomes (Perrow, 1984).

Complexity is also increased by the sheer scope of new information. The recent "information revolution" fueled by growth in the Internet has dramatically reduced both the production and transmission costs of information. On the Internet the amount of available information is doubled every 2.8 years (Harris, 2002). As a result, information is now more widely accessible and dispersed among the population than ever before. Unfortunately, improved access to information comes with a price. Wading through the vast amounts of data can be literally overwhelming to managers. In fact, terms such as "data smog" and "information overload" are creeping into the literature in response to the onslaught of mounting information (Shenk, 1997).

It is important for nurse leaders to understand that innovation and new technology are the driving force behind the discovery of new knowledge and improvements in patient care. However, because earlier technology acts as the foundation for newer technology, future processes within the health care system will continue to show increasing

complexity. Overlapping, unclear, and changing roles for nurses as a result of new technology and services create complex decision-making situations. In addition, the use of multidisciplinary and interdisciplinary teams to make client care decisions increases the complexity of clinical decision making for nurses (Prescott et al., 1987).

ADMINISTRATIVE AND ORGANIZATIONAL DECISION MAKING

Organizational decision making is choosing options directed toward the resolution of organizational problems and the achievement of organizational goals (Kerrigan, 1991). For example, the purpose of decision making in nursing might be to coordinate nursing care to deliver optimal client outcomes while controlling cost. Etzioni (1989) noted that the traditional model for business decisions was rationalism; however, he further asserted that as information flow became more complex and faster-paced, a new decision-making model based on the use of partial information not fully analyzed had begun to evolve. He called this model "humble decision making."

This approach arises in response to the need to make a decision when there is too much data and too little time. For instance, predicting the outcome of clinical and administrative decisions in health care is problematic because such processes are collectively defined as complex adaptive systems (CAS). A CAS is characterized by "nonlinear interactive components, emergent phenomena, continuous and discontinuous change, and unpredictable outcomes" (Zimmerman et al., 1998, p. 263). Complex adaptive systems are ubiquitous, occurring in such phenomena as weather patterns (Lorenz, 1963a, 1963b, 1964, 1979), cell formation (Kauffman, 1993, 1995), animal schooling or flocking behavior (Camazine et al., 2001), economic markets (Arthur, 1990), and human social networks (Carley & Prietula, 1994; Johnson, 2001).

In CASs, use of traditional planning tools, such as regressing system behavior in a linear manner, often results in inaccurate predictions (Perrow, 1984). The consequences of such forecasts can result in serious adverse outcomes. Consider the decision by the executive team at Cedars-Sinai Medical Center in 2003 to implement a computerized physician order entry system at its flagship hospital in Los Angeles (Langberg, 2003). After planning for over 2 years, the high-profile, multimillion dollar system was suspended amid mounting physician complaints only 3 months after its implementation.

Another decision consequence is noted in the 175% increase in registered nurse (RN) union petitions since 1995, at least partly the result of decisions by nurse administrators to reengineer nursing processes and reduce staffing (Van Drake, 2003). Furthermore, the adverse effects of reduced RN staffing on patient safety has recently been substantiated by the 2003 report by the Institute of Medicine (IOM) entitled *Keeping Patients Safe: Transforming the Work Environment of Nurses.* In their report, the IOM wrote "leaner nurse staffing is associated with increased length of stay, nosocomial infection (urinary tract infection, postoperative infection, and pneumonia, and pressure ulcers. … These studies … taken together, provide substantial evidence that richer nurse staffing is associated with better patient outcomes." (IOM, 2003, p. 3). Clearly, the outcomes associated with prior decisions by nurse administrators in these examples are not reflective of their original intent. However, even with the best laid plans, unexpected and often negative results occur.

Janis and Mann (1977) described four types of administrative decision-making strategies. These include "satisficing," incrementalism, mixed scanning, and optimizing. *Satisficing* has the goal of selecting a course of action that is "good enough." *Incrementalism* is slow progress toward an optimal course of action. *Mixed scanning* combines the stringent rationalism of optimizing with the "muddling through" approach of incrementalism to form substrategies. *Optimizing* has the goal of selecting the course of action with the highest payoff (maximization). Limitations of time, money, or people may prevent the decision maker from selecting the more deliberative and slower process of optimizing. Still, the decision maker needs to focus on techniques that will enhance effectiveness in decision-making situations.

DECISION STYLES

Vroom and Yetton (1973) proposed a managerial decision-making model that identified five managerial decision styles on a continuum from minimal subordinate involvement to delegation. Their model is a contingency approach, which assumes that situational variables and personal attributes of the leader influence leader behavior and thus can affect organizational effectiveness. To diagnose the situation, the decision maker examines the following seven problem attributes:

1. The importance of the quality of the decision
2. Whether there is sufficient information/expertise
3. The amount of structure to the problem
4. The extent to which acceptance/commitment of followers is critical to implementation
5. The probability that an autocratic decision will be accepted
6. The motivation of followers to achieve the organizational goals
7. The extent to which conflict over preferred solutions is likely

Diagnostic questions guide the decision process. This process is arrayed on a decision tree. The decision maker uses the diagnostic questions to work through the decision tree to the end result of one of five decision styles (Hersey et al., 2001).

The decision styles range from autocratic to delegatory/participative. With individual decisions, the leader acts alone by making the decision alone. For consultative decisions, advice, information, or opinions are sought by the leader before making the decision. For group decisions a group is consulted by the leader, who asks for assistance in making the decision or delegates decision making to the group. The advantages of group decisions are increased understanding and acceptance of the final decision. Decision-making styles are as follows (Hersey et al., 2001):

- *Authoritative* or *autocratic:* The leader makes the decision without seeking assistance.

- *Consultative* or *collective-participative:* The leader seeks input before making the decision yet makes the final decision.
- *Facilitative:* The leader and followers work together to reach a shared decision.
- *Delegative:* Only the group is involved in the decision, and the leader gives up control over the decision.

Thus there is a range of decision-making styles available. The choice of style is dependent on the situation for effectiveness. The use of a range of decision styles matched to situational needs increases the probability of effective decision making.

THE DECISION PROCESS

Decisions can be thought of as resulting in action. This action occurs after a series of sequential steps are taken (Figure 7.3). The five steps of the decision-to-action process are as follows:

1. Collect information.
2. Process information into advice.
3. Make the choice.
4. Authorize the implementation.
5. Execute what is to be done.

The end result, action, is controlled by more than simply making a choice. It is useful to recognize that a decision does not guarantee desired actions. Outside influences can exert power or control over any of the steps of the decision process, thereby exerting power over the whole process (Mintzberg, 1983; Paterson, 1969). This idea is helpful to keep in mind as nurses use decision making with their clients (e.g., in managing care) and with situations in their work setting (e.g., in coordinating nursing services delivery). Essentially what this means is that those charged with implementation can exert power and influence through the multiple small implementation-related actions that occur, possibly changing the character of the final result. As the questions outside the boxes in Figure 7.3 show, after each step a critical question can be asked in order to focus activity for moving effectively through the next step. This framework also guides decision making evaluation and feedback.

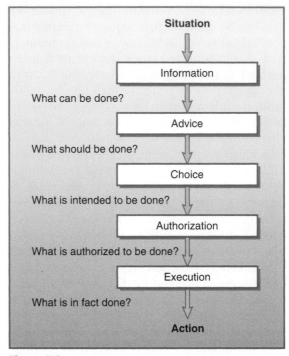

Figure 7.3
Continuum of control over the decision process. (Modified from Mintzberg, H. [1983]. *Structure in fives: Designing effective organizations* [p. 100]. Englewood Cliffs, NJ: Prentice-Hall.)

Nurses can improve personal decision making by expanding their perspective about what determines their choices and how they make decisions. To improve this understanding, they can review recent decisions in their own lives. One example is deciding among financial alternatives. In considering some of the decisions that seem, in retrospect, to have been good decisions, individuals can analyze the process that was followed to arrive at the decision. What decision style was used? Was it fast and impulsive or slow, methodical, and analytical? Was much time spent in gathering information? Did the decision maker follow a gut feeling or use rationality and logic? Was a specific, logically structured decision process used? The greater the number of possible choices within a range of behavior and thinking, the more likely a good decision will be made

(Grainger, 1990). Personal decision making also can be improved by an examination of which steps in the decision-making process are subject to the influence, power, or control of the individual.

DECISION-MAKING STRATEGIES

Various strategies are used for problem solving and decision making. These strategies reflect time and mental structure variations—for example, fast, slow, impulsive, intuitive, or logical. The following are some formal decision-making strategies.

Trial and Error

This method means that a shoot-from-the-hip or dart-throw type of solution is put into effect. A solution that seems attractive is chosen and simply tried out. Those managers who use trial and error as the usual strategy for decision making often are seen as ineffective. They are perceived as poor problem solvers.

Pilot Projects

This strategy involves experimentation with limited trials. Pilot projects or limited trials are used to experiment by trying out a solution alternative on a limited basis to see whether major problems will occur and to reduce risk. Pilot project strategies may resemble research projects.

Problem Critique

This approach occurs in a one-on-one situation, in which, for example, a nurse manager sits down with a staff person and the two people dialogue about the problem. The purpose is to critique the problem and thereby determine what the facts are, what the problem is, and what potential solutions might be used.

Creativity Techniques

These include brainstorming sessions, the Delphi process, and nominal group techniques, in which a group gathers for free thinking exercises (Van de Ven & Delbecq, 1974). They are especially suited to a complex problem that appears to have no good solution. Creativity techniques are used as a way to generate solutions, ideas, and thoughts by approaching the problem with freedom from preformed bias. Such techniques often are team-based strategies.

Decision Tree

A decision tree is a graphic model that visually displays the options, outcomes, and risks to be anticipated (see the Case Study at the end of this chapter). A decision tree starts to the left and flows to the right. A question or problem is posed, and the possible options become branching nodes. Thus decision paths can be traced through option points and beyond. For example, a very simple decision tree might start with the question, "Are you committed to becoming a nurse?"

The answer to that question is *yes* or *no*. Depending on the answer, the corresponding path is followed as mapped out on the decision tree. The tree enables visualization of the alternatives and their consequences. It helps with decision making through analysis and clarity (Hamilton & Kiefer, 1986).

Decision trees and algorithms are used as protocols for therapy administration. The advantage is to be able to analyze mapped alternatives, both positive and negative. For example, Aucott and colleagues (1994) developed algorithms for outpatient management of cardiovascular disorders. Willey (1989) designed a decision tree model of high technology beds and mattress overlays for clients who are immobilized. The initial question was, "Can the client be turned?" Different paths are selected if that answer is *no* as opposed to *yes*. The tree leads to an analysis of which beds and mattresses would be best for a given immobility diagnosis. Jensen and colleagues (1998) developed a decision tree for siderail use as a part of a restraint reduction program.

Critical paths are similar to decision trees and algorithms. Critical pathways are descriptions of the protocol for critical or key incidents that must occur in a predictable or timely order to keep the expected outcomes, length of stay, and overall costs appropriate and within diagnosis-related group (DRG) allotted time frames (Thompson et al., 1991). They are developed as a part of managed care or case management nursing care models (Mosher et al., 1992; Thompson et al., 1991). Critical pathways are designed to incorporate multidisciplinary perspectives to display and track the client's entire expected course of treatment and expected outcomes. Variances are identified immediately and managed by the case manager.

As nursing evolves in sophistication and knowledge base, with better identification of nursing diagnoses and the array of matching nursing interventions, the use of decision trees may provide a useful way to display the linkages of interventions to diagnoses.

Fish Bone or Cause-and-Effect Chart

Fish bone charts are graphic figures used to help identify the possible causes of production problems. They resemble the figures used to diagram sentences. These charts are used in business and industry to clarify the production process and indicate possible points for improvement. The figures flow from left to right, with a horizontal line through the middle that ends with the outcome, product, or end result indicated at the far right. On the horizontal line is placed the main process. Diagonals above and below flow into the main horizontal line. All feeder processes are indicated by the diagonals. The diagonals also have branching lines that indicate other processes that feed into each diagonal. Flow charts, control charts, and fish bone diagrams have been popularized in Deming's approach to quality management (Aguayo, 1990).

Group Problem Solving and Decision Making

In this technique the leader calls the group together to discuss and participate in solving a problem. The leader invites participation, either in the problem identification or the problem resolution part of the decision-making process. Personality and type style appear to influence the effectiveness of group or team problem solving and decision making (Saulo, 1996). There are

a number of models of group decision making. The four general models are as follows:

1. The rational model, based on an economic perspective of decision making and maximum utility
2. The political model, based on power, influence, negotiation, bargaining, and interest group influence
3. The process model, which uses standard operating procedures and guidelines
4. The "garbage can" model, characterized by difficult problem identification and difficult problem solution under circumstances of ambiguity, complexity, and nonrationality

Analysis of the cognitive flow of group decision making is valuable to aid insight and understanding of the rationale for judgments (Lahti, 1996). See Chapter 26 for further description of models of group decision making.

Cost-Benefit Analysis

This method is a formal balancing of driving and restraining forces. A list is made of the benefits or positive factors supporting an affirmative decision. Likewise, a list of the detriments or negative factors supporting a negative decision is compiled. These lists should be written so that they can be arrayed visually (Figure 7.4).

The process of writing out the elements helps to organize decision making. Counselors use this technique to help people with difficult personal life decisions. In the nursing practice setting, when the nurse needs to balance the use of scarce resources, a pro-con or cost-benefit analysis helps to clarify the elements inherently related to the problem and to facilitate subsequent decision making. Cost-benefit analysis and cost-effectiveness analysis are gaining popularity in nursing as ways for nurses to demonstrate their value. For example, Gift (1995) recommended designing cost effectiveness research to evaluate products or interventions. Cost-effectiveness analysis was described and critiqued in a series of articles in *Image* in 1997 and 1998 (Allred et al., 1998; Buerhaus, 1998; Jones et al., 1997; Stone, 1998).

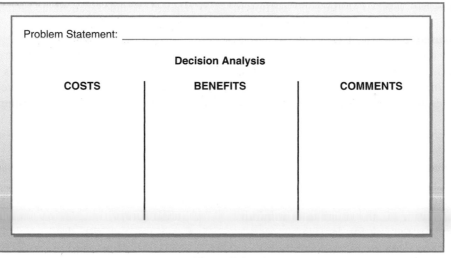

Problem Statement: _____

Decision Analysis

COSTS	BENEFITS	COMMENTS

Figure 7.4
Cost-benefit form.

In cost-benefit analysis, it is most effective to quantify the various alternatives through a standardized method. For example, calculating the "net present value" and "internal rate of return" of each alternative's cash flow is an excellent method for comparing the financial impact of alternatives. A simple definition of net present value is the present worth of a future sum of money. Present value calculations are ideal because they consider an alternative's start-up costs, periodic one-time capital expenses, operating revenues, and expenses and compare them with a discount rate or level of risk (see this chapter's Case Study). Most commercial computerized spreadsheets contain present value and internal rate of return functions to allow easy calculation. An excellent summary of present value calculations can be found in *Analysis for Financial Management* by Higgins (1992).

SCENARIO PLANNING

Scenario planning is a problem-solving and decision-making strategy given an uncertain and changing future. It is a group process strategy that encourages group participants to create "possible future" stories. Thus it is forward-looking and appropriate for fluid and changing environments, where there are many possible futures. This technique asks the questions "what if . . . ?"; then different stories of the future are described (scenarios). In this way, a wide array of perspectives is gathered, and the entrenched mindset is overcome. Stories of the future are constructed in a way that highlights pathways, driving forces, turning points, and deep behavioral forces. Scenario planning helps to illuminate early warning signs, trigger new opportunity ideas, and may protect from some risks.

Worst-Case Scenario

This technique is especially helpful in making decisions that involve risk. Risky decisions frequently, but not always, relate to the use of money or prestige. In this technique the "worst case" (i.e., everything that could go wrong does go wrong) is determined. The worst case is outlined for each known alternative. Then the alternative with the best result—when, or if, everything possible does go wrong—is selected. So if money or reputation is on the line, the "least of all the evils" is chosen. For instance, computerized physician order entry systems, if used correctly, have been shown to significantly reduce medication errors. However, because of the enormous cost and social change required to implement such systems, it has been difficult to establish an adequate return on the investment. Unfortunately, documented savings from avoidable and unavoidable adverse drug events may be thought of as "soft" numbers and open to speculation. By determining the absolute worst that could happen and working backward from that scenario, the decision maker chooses the best alternative for the situation to minimize potential anticipated risk for damage.

In their book *Smart Choices*, Hammond and colleagues (1999) recommend creating a "consequences table" for addressing multiple alternatives. To develop such a table, list the problem consequences objectives along the left side of a page and the various alternatives along the top. To rate the ability of each alternative to meet the desired objective, create a standardized key that ranks each alternative.

Consider the following problem statement regarding medication errors:

The rate of adverse drug events has exceeded the benchmark rate for three consecutive quarters. This has coincided with two sentinel events that required extended patient hospitalization and potential litigation.

After a period of analysis, a cross-functional team lists the following alternatives as potential solutions to the medication error problem:
- Develop an automated medication administration system that includes bar coding, automated storage and control units on the floors and robot technology.
- Implement computerized physician order entry with decision support.
- Standardize all medication abbreviations on order sheets.
- Remove high-risk drugs such as potassium chloride from ward stock and place pharmacists on the floor to assist with medication orders.

Table 7.1 displays the desired objectives and a standardized key to analyze and rank them.

By ranking the various alternatives through a standardized key, a fair comparison among alternatives can assist managers in eliminating undesirable choices. When developing a consequences table, it is important to view the long-term or downstream effects of implementing specific alternatives. Make sure to "play out" different scenarios and the tactics needed to overcome them. For instance, in evaluating whether or not to implement computerized physician order entry

Table 7.1

Desired Objectives Analysis				
Objective	Alternative A	Alternative B	Alternative C	Alternative D
1. Reduces the number of med transactions	5	4	2	3
2. Enables med administration through automation	5	4	2	2
3. Meets or exceeds net present value target	3	2	5	3
4. Meets regulatory standards	3	3	3	3
5. Improves accuracy	4	4	5	4
TOTAL SCORE	20	17	17	15

1, Does not meet objective; *2,* meets some aspects of objective; *3,* meets objective; *4,* exceeds objective; *5,* significantly exceeds objective.

Table 7.2

Scenario Analysis: Implement CPOE on All Inpatient Units by a Given Date		
Result Period #1	Result Period #2	Result Period #3
Physician response to training is poor, resulting in …	Difficulty in operating the system, resulting in …	The nursing staff having to use both a paper and an online record …
There are many computer interface problems, resulting in …	A slow, unreliable and cumbersome system, leading to …	Refusal of the staff to use the system, leading to …
Physicians have to change their med ordering practice, leading to …	Longer patient rounding time, resulting in …	A perception of less physician productivity, leading to …

(CPOE), several scenarios may result and need to be evaluated in planning and management. As shown in Table 7.2, identifying how one action can lead to another makes it possible to preempt significant barriers to implementation.

COMPUTERIZED DECISION MAKING

In the arena of decision-making strategies and analytical tools, there are also sophisticated and computerized forecasting techniques, such as linear programming models and mathematical techniques that assign a probability to each possible outcome. These are elaborations of decision tree models and are used for decision analysis (Grier, 1976). A computation of the statistical probabilities from certain "knowns" can be performed. These forecasting models use computers to calculate outcomes. They are used in forecasting and in sophisticated policy analyses (Baumann & Deber, 1989). For example, the Multiattribute Utility Model is "a graphical or mathematical model used to estimate the utility of an item based on the analysis of its attributes or qualities" (Gokenbach, 1995, p. 198). It is used in group decision making for vendor/project selection.

Traditional analytic methods fail to capture the dynamic and nonlinear aspects of complex systems such as hospitals (Effken et al., 2003).

All too often as the number of variables and stochastic (i.e., containing random variables) cross-level interactions increase (as in human organizations), the computer time to solve the problem rises exponentially. As a result, complex system problems quickly become intractable using standard statistical analysis tools. One tactic suggested in the IOM report to overcome this problem was to increase the use of simulation (computational modeling) as a decision tool in designing safer processes within complex hospital systems (IOM, 2001).

Computational Modeling

A computational modeling approach views organizations (hospitals) as a collection of computer-simulated agents that are both intelligent and adaptive. By conducting "virtual experiments" computational models can provide a "what-if" analysis of various tactics aimed at decision making. Although a variety of methods may be used, the general process for computational modeling begins with encoding a series of statements in propositional calculus or "if … then …" format into a computer program. Through a series of computer algorithms these statements can represent various theories and produce output that simulates corresponding social behavior. The resulting output (behavior) of the simulation can then be compared with similar elements in real-world systems (Ilgen & Hulin, 2000; Weiss, 1999). Modeling benefits the study of complex systems by translating metaphor into the language of mathematics and links theory with data. Simulation is particularly well suited for modeling complex systems because (1) unanticipated emergent properties may be discovered, (2) studies can be run over many (simulated) years, (3) problems often become computationally intractable using traditional statistical methods and, (4) simulation can be much less expensive than real-world studies.

Information Processing

The core of professional nursing practice is nursing expertise applied to problem solving and decision making about client care and care management. Nursing decisions are based on data; therefore the process of collecting, classifying, storing, retrieving, and analyzing data (called *information processing*) is an area of knowledge related to both problem solving and decision making. Clearly, nurses need to acquire and use data for decision making. For example, requests for funding or policy change need to be accompanied by hard data.

Nursing's data have been described as being "invisible" since they are not clearly identified, defined, collected, or used (Grier, 1984). This is especially true in large national databases. Lack of standardized definitions and measures decreases the comparability of data and ultimately the quality of administrative decisions. Standardized data sets, including one for nursing management, have been proposed to alleviate this gap in nursing's data (Huber et al., 1992; Huber et al., 1997). Although there is no shortage of information in health care, decision support tools enabled by automation are needed to standardize and customize performance measures and quality outcomes data (Ward, 1999). In one model the clinical, fiscal, quality, productivity, and care provider variables served as data categories for a decision support database (Urden, 1996). Improvements in access to critical management information across an organization come from health enterprise data warehousing and health

care–specific decision support applications (Waldo, 1998).

The recent emergence of the "information revolution," coupled with development of a global information infrastructure, has dramatically reduced both the production and transmission costs of information. As a result, information is now more widely accessible and dispersed among the population than ever before. The information revolution is rapidly narrowing the gap between consumers' and providers' knowledge of disease diagnosis, treatment, and prevention. As a result of improved access to medical information, the relationship between patients and providers is changing. For example, the asymmetry of information between physicians and their patients is narrowing or, at least, being challenged. Armed with the latest information from the Internet, consumers often arrive at their physician appointment prepared to discuss the latest research on their illness (Dev et al., 2001). In many cases, this has increased the workload on providers who must now sift through reams of articles and reports with well-intentioned patients. Provider roles are transforming into those of mentors who provide patients a range of treatment alternatives based on more accessible clinical outcome data (Dev et al., 2001). As a result, the unique differences between non–health care and health care market models are diminishing. Future health care market behavior will reflect more of the competitive characteristics seen in today's non–health care markets.

As technology dramatically improves access to health care information, nurses will experience greater volatility in health care markets. The expanded flow of information between health care providers, businesses, and consumers will decrease new product cycle times and transaction costs and drive an increasingly faster rate of change. To successfully compete in a rapidly evolving environment, health care systems need to become adaptive, and nurses will play a key role in this transformation.

An adaptive organization has the capacity to respond quickly to changing market conditions in an effort to remain competitive. Evolving market conditions may require nurse administrators to quickly analyze and decide on new services, practices, and technology. Conversely, rigid and inflexible organizations will suffer a competitive disadvantage in future health care markets. The inability to respond rapidly to changes in market conditions may result in missed opportunities and erosion of market share.

Information in the new economy will be ubiquitous. Nursing staff will need to be connected to this vast information network both internal and external to the institution. Those nurse administrators who successfully manage both tacit and explicit knowledge within their organizations will emerge as leaders among their peer hospitals. Knowledge management in this context means capturing, storing, accessing, and using information to leverage the talents and skills of a health system's own workforce. Nursing staff will need to be proficient in the use of e-mail, online clinical documentation, decision support, expert systems, and telehealth applications. Otherwise, institutions will be unable to provide staff with quick access to valuable information or capture data important to the health system.

By understanding the fundamental economic principles driving today's health care markets, nurse administrators can appreciate the importance of sound decision making. Embracing technology through enabling information technology such as the Internet, telehealth, computerized provider order entry, online clinical documentation, bar coding, decision support, and expert systems, nurse administrators will position nursing for health care markets of the future.

Perception and Innovation: Tools for Decision Making

Perception is a powerful influence on problem solving and decision making. *Perception* is defined as an individual's filtering and interpretation of events. It is how the person sees what is happening (Kramer, 1994). Perception is influenced by such elements as culture, values, and biases. An individual's perception can cloud objectivity and rationality in decision making. Perception can diminish creativity and the range of options identified for decision making, or it can trigger routine or automatic decision responses.

Perception affects how problems are viewed and what actions are determined to be the "best" solutions. There have been many problems that have been defined as unsolvable or for which only one solution path has been identified. However, creative solutions can be an outcome of changing the perception of what is a failure. One example is the development of Post-it Notes by 3-M. Post-it Notes were the result of an inspiration by Art Fry in 1974. Fry was sitting in his church with a hymnal book, and he kept flipping back and forth between pages. He started thinking about how wonderful it would be if there was some paper with nonpermanent glue that could be used to mark the hymnal pages. Meanwhile, a scientist in research and development at 3-M had been experimenting with glues in the research laboratory and had come up with a glue that did not stick permanently. The scientist had considered this glue a total failure, and the experiment was shelved. Fry came to the laboratory with his idea for something that would work if there were a type of glue that did not permanently stick. Thus the concept for Post-it Notes was developed. It took Fry some time to convince 3-M to manufacture these notes, but they became overwhelmingly successful (Post-It Notes, 1990), and today it is difficult to imagine doing clerical work without them.

The need for creativity and innovation in health care is clear, and it is an urgent need. Creativity and innovation can be used as modes of decision making to expand available courses of action. Drucker (1986) urged that innovation be a purposeful, systematic activity. He noted that systematic innovation means monitoring seven sources of innovative opportunity: (1) the unexpected, (2) incongruity, (3) innovation based on process need, (4) changes in the industry structure or market structure, (5) demographics (population changes), (6) changes in perception, mood, or meaning, and (7) new knowledge. Health care in the United States will benefit from nurses who take basic knowledge, employ critical thinking, refuse to see abnormal or different paths as failure, and apply creativity to nursing's needs. Currently, one pressing need is for people who can adapt technology to nursing's productivity gaps. For example, wireless devices, bar coding, robotics, and communications technology are areas that could be creatively engineered to make technology work for nurses.

In one situation a nurse at a tertiary hospital was caring for a 69-year-old female client who refused to accept a bandage. The woman said she was tired of fooling with bandages since it was hard to get them off when they had to be picked at with fingernails, which hurt her skin. Thinking about bandages and skin care for older adults, the nurse developed and patented a bandage designed for ease of pull from the end. Her innovation was generated from a genuine and practical client concern (Anderson, 1989). Clearly, creativity can be fostered in nursing. Reframing problems and encouraging inventors are key strategies. Nurse managers play an important leadership role in stimulating innovation instead of accepting the status quo. Creating an environment that is "safe"—one in which mistakes are viewed as learning experiences—enables and encourages creativity and innovation.

LEADERSHIP AND MANAGEMENT IMPLICATIONS

Decision making is a central component of leadership and management activity. Leadership decision making focuses on choices made to advance the group's goals. Management decision making centers on coordinating, integrating, and allocating scarce resources to accomplish organizational goals. Therefore the focus of leadership and management decision making is more closely related to the nurse's role as care coordinator than to the role of caregiver.

Decision-making skill is valued in nursing practice, as evidenced by the construction of RN licensure examination questions related to decision-making skills of the nurse. What would the nurse do first? How much would the nurse do, versus sharing the decision with the client or vesting the decision totally with the client? Clinical decision-making skills can be focused and enhanced by the use of critical thinking. Nurses can and do use decision making in all aspects of care management.

Nurse managers face decisions about budgeting, future planning, buying equipment, staffing implementation, and day-to-day tactical management of the nursing service unit. Nagelkerk and

⚠ LEADERSHIP & MANAGEMENT **BEHAVIORS**

Leadership Behaviors

- Inspires followers to make decisions
- Communicates desired values for decisions
- Motivates followers to be creative and innovative
- Models decisive actions
- Develops strategic plans
- Influences followers to make autonomous decisions
- Monitors feedback about the acceptability and effectiveness of decisions

Management Behaviors

- Makes decisions about resource allocation
- Motivates subordinates to come to consensus

- Plans day-to-day operations
- Resolves selected problems
- Organizes the work
- Evaluates productivity
- Takes corrective action

Overlap Areas

- Uses decision-making strategies to accomplish goals
- Assists individuals and groups to make decisions
- Makes decisions

Henry (1990) identified two types of executive decisions: (1) routine and operational and (2) nonroutine and strategic. Routine decisions about daily operations are made most often and carry minimal to moderate risk. Step-by-step rational approaches can be used. Nonroutine decisions about novel situations or complex problems involve high risk and a dynamic set of decision activities using intuition and political knowledge. One approach to management decision making in nursing is to use nursing management diagnoses as a standardized language for description. A nursing management diagnosis is a judgment about nursing management problems that is essential to effective management decision making. For example, a rise in staff conflict that results from development of a new procedure can be analyzed using nursing management diagnoses and interventions. The diagnoses form the basis for nurse manager interventions. In one study, 71 management diagnoses were validated for nursing management (Morrison, 1995). Using the nursing management evidence base in practice is one recommendation of the IOM (2003).

An important activity related to managerial decision making is the setting of priorities. This is done for time management purposes and to ensure that the most important activities are completed. For example, delegation is a tool that is used to distribute the workload. As more decisions are made at the work unit level, nurses will need to delegate care to others. In one study the Nursing Assessment Decision Grid provided RNs with a tool to enhance delegation decision making (Parsons, 1997).

Prioritization is an important part of decision making. Manthey (1988) discussed the issue of who owns a staff nurse's time. Her premise was that nursing resources are insufficient for the existing workload, making the time of an RN one of the scarcest resources in health care. Workload factors are not under the control of the nursing department, which results in uncontrollable fluctuations. Furthermore, multiple influences are brought to bear: hospital and health care administrators desire greater productivity to take better care of more clients with less cost; clients desire more nursing time and attention; physicians desire flexibility with their schedules to ease their job; and nurse managers desire nursing time to be spent when scheduled and dedicated to the work assigned. Since nearly everyone lays claim to staff nurses' time, the answer to the question of what to do when there is more work than time available is prioritize. Manthey (1988) noted that "the concept of autonomy in a service profession involves decision making about the kind and degree of service a client will receive" (p. 24). The decision uses a complex professional reasoning process about the need and the resources available. Autonomous decision making includes deciding what will and will not be done if there is more work than time available. Empowerment results from nurses being enabled to control the use of their time to meet clients' needs.

Complexity and Chaos

Complexity and chaos theory have application to leadership and management decision making. The behavior of nurses is governed, to some extent, by the rules (formal and informal), information flow, diversity, and interconnectedness of the organization (Chu et al., 2003). This complex web of interdependence and mutual causality among nurses, physicians, and support staff results in emergent phenomena; continuous and discontinuous change; and nonlinear, unpredictable system behavior. Organizational performance often appears as macro, emergent phenomena resulting from the seemingly invisible interactions occurring at micro levels.

Complex systems yearn for order and readily adapt to changing environments as a means of survival (Kauffman, 1995). Over time, a highly effective set or rules may evolve to create the emergence of order without centralized control. For example, the human brain has billions of interacting neurons that are continuously receiving inputs and generating outputs to other neurons. Without centralized control, the multiple interactions of these neurons create the collective emergence of consciousness and thought in humans

(Holland, 1998; Wilson, 1996). Even cities maintain their coherence in a constantly changing population as new physical structures are created and old ones are destroyed. In all theses examples, order has emerged as multiple "agents" have "self-organized" to adapt in a constantly shifting environment.

Emergence can be defined as the sudden generation of unpredicted phenomena resulting from the interaction and self-organization of multiple agents adapting to the current environment (Johnson, 2001; Stacey, 1996; Zimmerman et al., 1998). The term *agent* is used to represent some type of entity that interacts, such as a neuron or even a staff nurse. Examples of emergence abound in complex systems such as hospitals. The development of information clusters after the introduction of e-mail on nursing units is one example of emergence. Another example is a sudden, unexpected pattern of medication errors that emerges as a result of invisible interactions deep within the medication administration system. Even the difference in cultures from nursing unit to nursing unit emerges from the complex interactions among the unit's patients, nurses, physicians, and manager.

Understanding the significance of emergence is important for today's nurse managers. Emergence is often the result of "self-organization" by the nursing staff as the unit attempts to transition out of an unstable environment. The term *self-organization* in this context means the emergence of new structures, patterns, or processes regardless of influence by a central or external authority (Zimmerman et al., 1998). A typical example may be the so-called "work-around" in which staff find an alternate process to work-around a recent change. The use of bar code technology, for instance, requires nurses to scan a patient's identification band before administering medication. However, if not properly implemented, bar code technology can increase the time it takes to pass medications. If expectations by the manager are for staff to complete all assignments in the same time period, a "work-around" may emerge. For example, staff may copy the patient's bar codes and place them in the medication room, where

they can swipe two or three of them at once to expedite passing medications. In this case the work-around defeats the objective of providing safer medication delivery through the use of bar code technology.

A more global form of self-organization and emergence is the attempt by staff to be represented by a labor union. The emergence of a unionized staff often occurs after a period of instability within the organization in which the staff members self-organize to achieve certain objectives. These objectives may include more participation in decision making, better recognition through pay and benefits, and job security.

The "good old days," when life was more predictable and less chaotic, appear to be gone. History has shown that past technological innovations combine to form new technological innovations, and with each iteration, complexity increases (Waldrop, 1992). Because change is occurring so rapidly, past practices that exhibit any sense of permanence may provide managers with a feeling of security. Leading in a world of complexity does not necessarily require a new set of management tools. Rather, nurse leaders must first learn to recognize complex, nonlinear systems and then assess which management strategies are most effective in dealing with them.

Pattern Recognition

Complex social organizations, like hospitals, produce patterns that can be difficult to recognize (Wheatley, 1999). Patterns known as *attractors* keep complex social organizations stable in the face of constant change. Attractors *emerge* as the result of many factors, including an organization's formal and informal rules, degree of management control, flow of information, and system constraints (Stacey, 1996; Wheatley, 1999). In the broadest sense, attractors in hospitals may include the organization's overall culture. Repeating patterns may take form in the manner in which staff members respond to questions regarding the hospital's mission, values, and vision. If there is a consistent, positive commitment by staff to the hospital's overall goals and objectives, then the underlying culture acts as an attractor for this pattern (Wheatley, 1999).

Unfortunately, attractors can also be negative. If a repeating pattern of negativity pervades throughout an organization or even in one unit, then something in the underlying culture is attracting this kind of response. Whether the system's rules are inconsistent, the flow of information is limited, or the constraints are too tight, it is important for nurse managers to recognize when negative patterns are emerging. If unchecked, negative patterns can suddenly degenerate into a period of randomness and instability. It is at these times that staff morale plummets and a sense chaos ensues.

Tuning Parameters

Nonlinear complex systems are sensitive to initial conditions, especially during periods of instability (Kauffman, 1995; Waldrop, 1992; Wolfram, 2002). At these times small perturbations in the environment can result in enormous reactions. Instability may be a transition state between order and chaos in which the system remains stable but is open to change. A nursing unit exhibiting unstable behavior is tense, like a rubber band pulled taught and ready to snap. This energy can be channeled into either positive or negative change, depending on how the manager adjusts rules, constraints, information flow, and centralized control (Stacey, 1996). For example, after being informed of the need to reduce expenses on a unit, staff may begin to exhibit unstable behavior. Tension is high, rumors abound, and there are numerous opinions on how the reductions should be implemented. The confluence of tension (motivation), rumors (information flow), and opinions (diversity of ideas) in a complex nonlinear system may eventually lead to self-organization and emergence. What emerges, however, may be unanticipated as well as undesirable.

Although the outcomes of complex nonlinear systems cannot be predicted, managers can "tune" system parameters to increase the probability of acceptable ones. Parameters may include information flow (memos, e-mail, verbal communication), rules (policies and procedures, objectives, expectations), diversity of ideas (brainstorming sessions), control (centralized versus decentralized), and constraints (external regulations, physical space, job descriptions). Rather than attempting to control outcomes, managers should strive for the optimum balance of system parameters. This will expedite the natural occurrence of staff self-organization and the emergence of an acceptable range of solutions.

By tuning system parameters, managers may be able to prevent unstable behavior from degenerating into chaos. For example, Kauffman (1995) has shown that within networks, order emerges spontaneously if there is a bias for a specific outcome. In other words, if the network rules result in a high percentage of one outcome over another, then the system is considered biased. The same logic can be applied in social organizations going through a transition from an unstable environment to a stable one. If information flow is considered a network input, then tuning this variable to build consensus around specific issues will spontaneously create order within a complex system. That is why communication and consensus building are so important during periods of transition—because together they create spontaneous order and prevent chaos.

Mistakes

When is a mistake a failure? Nurses make decisions under conditions of uncertainty and risk. It is part of the human condition to make mistakes. Sometimes an error in judgment results in harm or death. However, when a mistake has been made, the nurse manager makes a decision about how to approach corrective action. Some adopt the attitude that it is wrong or bad to make mistakes. The person may be labeled as "at fault" and subjected to negative or punitive corrective action. The natural response to this is to avoid, deny, or become defensive. The person may experience anger, lowered self-esteem, and blocks to positive learning (Kowalski, 1992).

A serious concern with mistakes in health care is their impact on patient safety and whether a nurse should be disciplined or fired for a serious error.

Some think that using serious consequences is the only way an employee will learn and not make the mistake again. Clearly, concern about health care error and patient safety are substantial quality problems in the U.S. health care system (IOM, 2001, 2003). In fact, strategies to reduce errors and enhance safety have moved into the public policy–making arena.

An alternative view of errors in health care is to see them as system failures. Described as "moving from whodunit to what happened," seeing errors as occurring because the *system* failed helps a manager to move from using discipline to searching for a solution in the system itself (Greene, 1999, p. 50). For example, the system of providing medications to patients is a complex one with multiple subprocesses interacting with numerous agents. The subprocesses of the medication use system can be described as prescribing, dispensing, administering, monitoring, and management control (IOM, 2000). The agents interacting in the medication use system include physicians, nurses, pharmacists, patients, and other support staff. The inherent complexity of the medication use system makes it prone to a variety of accidents. Strategies to reduce medication errors must take into consideration the characteristics and complexity of such systems. Attributes of systems with complex interactions (Perrow, 1984) typically are characterized by the following:

- Proximity of parts or units that are not in a production sequence
- Many common mode connections among components
- Unfamiliar or unintended feedback loops
- Many control parameters with potential interactions
- Indirect or inferential information sources
- Limited understanding of some processes

The interactions within complex systems can lead to unexpected, nonlinear outcomes. The response of complex system events is not necessarily equal to the stimulus. Thus an apparently simple medication error can lead to a chain reaction of seemingly unrelated events that could result in a catastrophic outcome. On the other hand, linear systems are characterized by sequential, segregated, and dedicated single-purpose interactions with fewer feedback loops, more information, and extensive understanding. The outcomes in a linear system tend to be more predictable. A manufacturing production line is one example of a linear system. Strategies aimed at reducing medication errors should focus on tactics that move the medication use process closer toward a more reliable or linear system in order to better manage for consistent quality outcomes.

Nurse managers should thus aim decision-making strategies at improving the medication use process by focusing tactics on those solutions that incorporate appropriate design components, provide the greatest impact at reducing errors, are supported by research, and are practical from a cost and implementation standpoint. For example, in its report, the IOM (2000) specifically listed the following 14 tactics to reduce medication errors that meet this criteria:

1. Adopt a system-oriented approach to medication error reduction.
2. Implement standard processes for medication doses and dose timing.
3. Standardize prescription writing and prescription rules.
4. Limit the number of different kinds of common equipment.
5. Implement physician order entry.
6. Use pharmaceutical software.
7. Implement unit dosing.
8. Have the central pharmacy supply high-risk intravenous medications.
9. Use special procedures and written protocols for the use of high-risk medications.
10. Do not store concentrated solutions of hazardous medications on patient care units.
11. Ensure the availability of pharmaceutical decision support.
12. Include pharmacists during rounds of patient care units.
13. Make relevant patient information available at the point of patient care.
14. Improve patients' knowledge about their own treatment.

The sentinel events policy of the Joint Commission on Accreditation of Healthcare Organizations (JCAHO) encourages the system failure viewpoint by requiring a thorough and credible study of the organization's systems via root cause analysis. Based on this view, the "fix" for a sentinel event is not employee firing but employee participation in the root cause analysis, including assessment of the organization's culture and communication (Berman, 1998; Kobs, 1999).

Research in nursing has shown a correlation between workload and error rate (Petroff, 1999). Thus the analysis of mistakes needs to consider all possibilities: a good employee who made a mistake, a problem employee, an educational deficit, and a process that creates barriers to performance or makes it easier to do things wrong than to do them right. Making subsequent decisions on corrective actions taps into the root cause analysis.

For some managers, mistakes are viewed as learning experiences. The focus is on what was learned and what corrections need to be made. If the manager asks what could be done differently next time and characterizes the error as a component of learning, a sense of responsibility and learning from the experience is instilled in the person who made the error (Kowalski, 1992). Some view this as a humanistic approach to mistakes, one that fosters growth of the knowledge worker.

CURRENT ISSUES AND TRENDS

Decision-making activities in nursing include standardization of care and improving quality and safety through evidence-based protocols. The standardization of care is one strategy nurse administrators can use to reduce the complexity of care and enable nurses to make better decisions. Complex systems are created through a rich network of interacting agents that can produce a near infinite "state space." The term *state space* refers to the range of alternative states a process may exhibit (Kauffman, 1995). The size of a state space is driven by the number of variables within

the system. The higher the number of variables within the system, the greater the state space. The larger the state space, the more unpredictable a system becomes. Thus limiting the number of system variables should reduce the degree of complexity within the system. The documentation of nursing diagnoses during the assessment process is an example. Without the aid of a standardized nursing language, such as that of the North American Nursing Diagnosis Association (NANDA), the vocabulary of terms used to describe a diagnosis, intervention, or outcome would be confusing and significantly error-prone. For example, three frequently seen NANDA nursing diagnoses—Knowledge Deficit Related to Cognitive Impairment, Gas Exchange Impairment Related to Altered Oxygen Supply, and Fluid Volume Deficit Related to Excessive Loss of Fluids—can be combined to define eight different states. Suppose, however, that a standardized language is not used, and two terms are routinely interchanged to describe the same diagnosis. In other words, there are now six terms used to describe three diagnoses. The combination of terms to describe a nursing diagnosis has now jumped from a state space of 8 to a state space of 64. By using two terms to define the same diagnosis, complexity has increased nearly 8-fold. One can only imagine the degree of complexity when all nursing diagnoses are considered in an organization not using a standardized nursing language. Standardization should not be limited to only nursing languages. Policies, procedures, supplies, and equipment should all be evaluated for their degree of variation. The complexity in an organization can be significantly decreased as a result of standardization across multiple areas.

The development of national standards and guidelines has been stimulated by quality improvement and effectiveness initiatives in health care. Regulatory agencies have established programs to promote the development of national standards and guidelines as a way of enhancing decision making related to quality of care and reducing variance in professional practice patterns. The JCAHO's Agenda for Change has promoted the identification and use of appropriate, measurable clinical indicators in nursing. These indicators are quantitative measures to monitor and evaluate the quality of care. They may include the occurrence of medication errors, self-extubations of clients on ventilators, or well-prepared clients at discharge—all of which can be quantified. For example, the number of medication errors can be divided by the number of doses dispensed (Scholz, 1990; Williams, 1991).

Disciplines and specialties promulgate standards and guidelines for their own practice. When there is overlap between and among specialties, a multidisciplinary approach results in a comprehensive way to meld divergent practices and intertwined policies. In some cases, such as the work done by the Agency for Healthcare Research and Quality (AHRQ), formerly the Agency for Health Care Policy and Research (AHCPR), multidisciplinary evidence-based clinical practice guidelines have been developed for selected significant and broadly applicable problems that have a wide variation in decision strategies, research base, and cost implications of care (Cole & Houston, 1999). For example, there are clinical practice guidelines on management of acute pain, urinary incontinence, pressure ulcers, cataracts, and depression that are disseminated via a website called the National Guideline Clearinghouse (*www.guideline.gov*). Nurses have been actively involved in the development of some of these guidelines. It is suggested that, in the future, unsubstantiated deviation from these extensively developed and research-based guidelines may be considered failure to act as a reasonable and prudent nurse. The use of research knowledge to formulate evidence-based nursing practice is a key current issue. Although it is a current and future imperative, implementing evidence-based practice requires time, resources, organizational commitment, and a considerable educational effort (Stetler et al., 1998). Thus knowledge about problem-solving methods and decision-making tools is essential for nurses.

Other trends and issues related to decision making are deciding the preferred future for nursing and evaluating the effectiveness of decision making in practice. Both are aimed at making careful projections about what decisions to make, given uncertainty, to improve organizational and system performance.

The question for the future of nursing is what decisions must be made as nursing and health care evolve. In times of change, nursing has an opportunity to make decisions that proactively direct the future. The future can be analyzed as possible, plausible, probable, and preferable (Korniewicz & Palmer, 1997). To anticipate the future, nurses must engage in future think, mobilize energy and resources, anticipate trends, and plan accordingly (Pesut, 1997).

The efficiency, efficacy, and effectiveness of health care decisions will continue to enjoy a strong focus, with shifts toward outcomes specification. As performance improvement specialists, nurses will be challenged to make decisions that directly affect quality, access, cost, productivity, and the "bottom line." Effective approaches to decision making are needed when multiple stakeholders need to be served, time is constrained, and there is an overwhelming amount of information. Both performance measures and productivity measures need to be evaluated. Malloch (1999) recommended seven steps to reach a decision about an optimal course of action: (1) clarify the situation, (2) identify goals, (3) select measures, (4) identify options, (5) consider trade-offs, (6) select the most congruent option for the goals, and (7) evaluate the choice. A systematic process helps to improve the quality of decision making.

Summary

- Decision making is a key aspect of leadership and management.
- Decision making involves the act of choosing and implementing a course of action from among alternatives.
- Decision making may or may not be the result of an immediate problem.

- The core phases of decision making are deliberation, judgment, and evaluation.
- Decision making is a process with identifiable steps.
- Decision-making situations are personal, clinical, or organizational.
- There are various administrative decision-making models.
- There are different decision styles and strategies.
- Perception and innovation are influences on, as well as tools for, decision making.
- The essence of professional practice is the application of expertise to solve problems for clients.
- Nurses make decisions all the time.
- Professional autonomy includes decision making about what will and will not be done for clients.

Study Questions

1. What is your typical or preferred decision style?
2. How does clinical decision making differ from managerial decision making?
3. How are problem solving and decision making related in nursing?
4. What important decisions do nurses make? On which ones do they collaborate?
5. What strategies work best for clinical decision making? For managerial decision making?
6. How can information processing help nurse decision making?
7. What resources are available to assist with decision making?
8. What creative or innovative ideas do you have?
9. What if ... (describe an innovative strategy)?

CASE STUDY

Effective decision making relies, in part, on analyzing alternative levels of uncertainty or risk. In addition to making "apples to apples"

comparisons through such tools as present value calculations, estimating the probability that each alternative will actually occur can be helpful. For instance, a hospital interested in improving nurse vacancy rates analyzed nursing salaries under the following four scenarios: (1) no change over current rates, (2) adjusting rates to the local market, (3) adjusting rates slightly above the local market, or (4) adjusting rates well above the market. For each alternative, the net present value of the savings from decreased recruitment costs offset by the increased salary expense over 5 years was calculated. Utilizing studies from similar markets, the probability that each alternative would achieve the desired vacancy rate was estimated. The hypothetical results of the four alternatives are summarized in Figure 7.5.

As noted on Figure 7.5, alternative 2 (matching the nurse's salaries to the current market rate) has the highest estimated savings (adjusted by its probability) of the four alternatives. It is important to note that relying on just the net present value without taking into consideration its probability can be misleading. Alternative 1 (doing nothing) actually has the highest present value, but the probability of achieving the desired outcome is only 25%. Thus alternative 1's estimated total savings are actually the lowest of the four alternatives.

Figure 7.5 is an example of a "decision tree." Diagrams such as decision trees can be invaluable in understanding complicated alternative solutions. New research into knowledge representation has shown that human cognition is more effective through visualization rather than text. Decision trees, fishbone diagrams, problem continuums, and flow charts are frequently used as visualization tools in problem analysis. To assist in visualization techniques, managers should consider placing a large "grease board," dry-erase board, or flip chart in their office to quickly map out various alternatives.

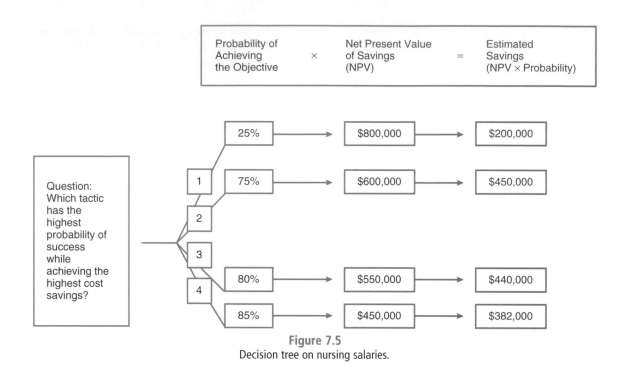

Figure 7.5
Decision tree on nursing salaries.

CRITICAL THINKING EXERCISE

The process of nurse staffing within a hospital meets many of the characteristics of a complex adaptive system. Numerous agents (nurses) interact in a diverse social network (patients, physicians, therapists) that overlaps multiple hospital systems (admission, care, treatment, evaluation, discharge) to safely provide the appropriate number of trained staff throughout the hospital. The staffing system, constrained by rules (policies and procedures), is managed through the hierarchal management structure of the hospital.

Floating, a subprocess of the staffing system, is often used to redistribute nursing staff from overstaffed to understaffed units. In a stable environment, floating process behavior may settle into a reoccurring pattern of (1) the daily assignment of float staff to units, (2) communication to individual nurses about their assignments, and (3) a productive feedback loop between nurses and management regarding patient assignments. However, in an unstable environment, floating process behavior may take on an entirely different form. For instance,

if float nurses are routinely expected to manage unfamiliar patients on unfriendly, foreign units without appropriate orientation and training, a reoccurring pattern of negative behavior may develop (a reinforcing positive feedback loop). In this case the pattern may be characterized by (1) the daily assignment of float staff to units, (2) communication to individual nurses of their assignments, (3) resistance by staff to float, and (4) a daily feedback loop of escalating conflict between management and float staff.

In complex systems such as staffing, any small disturbance in a positively reinforcing feedback loop may amplify in a "nonlinear" fashion throughout the system. Examples of a small disturbance may include changes in floating policies, miscommunication between management and staff, or even one nurse having a particularly negative floating experience. The cascading effect of disturbances within the complex social network of staff may result in unanticipated outcomes. For example, the pattern may manifest itself as staff refusing to float or demands for premium pay when floating. Regardless of its pattern, the emergence of new staff behavior is the result of multiple agents (staff) spontaneously self-organizing in an effort to adapt to the current environment.

Complex systems are nonlinear and unpredictable. However, by altering or "tuning" system parameters, managers may be able to "steer" system behavior in such a way that staff self-organize in a desired direction (Carley, 2003). For instance, if done correctly, the implementation of simple rules can create positively reinforcing feedback loops that allow self-organization and emergence to occur.

In the floating example, nurse administrators could allow staff to develop "a code of floating conduct" that requires all nurses to adhere to the following five simple rules:

1. Treat float staff cordially when on a unit.
2. All float staff are assigned a resource nurse from the floor.
3. The resource person must orient the float nurse using a standardized form.
4. The resource nurse must regularly check on the float nurse.
5. Both the float and resource nurse must fill out an evaluation form at the end of the shift.

To reinforce behavior, nurse administrators would review all evaluation forms daily. If a negative floating experience is noted, the nurse administrator would follow up with the float nurse, resource nurse, and manager of the unit within 24 hours. In addition, all evaluation forms would be trended for problems and presented to a committee of staff nurses on a monthly basis. If a particular unit showed a problem trend, the data would be shared with the manager and unit staff and follow-up action to alleviate the problem would be required. Data also would be shared with units that consistently scored high on float evaluations as a reward.

By tuning the rules, information flow, and communication parameters, nurse administrators can steer the system toward a positively reinforcing feedback loop and a new attractor that incorporates the five rules. The result, demonstrated in Figure 7.6, is a self-policing float system. Units that consistently score poorly on float evaluations self-organize to improve their image and prevent being labeled an unfriendly area. Eventually a new culture will "emerge" throughout the organization as units naturally compete among themselves to improve.

Although seemingly simple, the float example illustrates an alternative strategy for managing in a CAS environment. Rather than using management strategies that concentrate on enforcing top-down complicated policies and procedures, the CAS uses simple rules to enable naturally occurring, bottom-up self-organization and emergence. Instead of attempts to force system elements directionally, emphasis is on creating a climate for positive change but with an understanding that the final outcome remains uncertain.

Application Questions

1. What undesirable patterns should managers be on the alert for when implementing change in a complex process such as floating?
2. What key parameters within the floating process can managers "tune" to move the system in a desirable direction?
3. Describe examples of tactics that could be employed to control parameters surrounding the floating process.
4. How might managers create positively reinforcing feedback loops that enable staff to "self-organize" around attractive solutions?

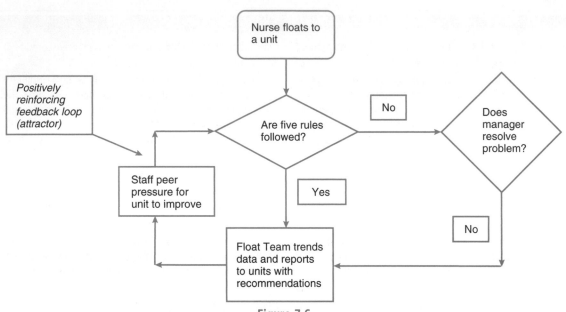

Figure 7.6
Tuning system parameters to steer the float system toward a new attractor.

REFERENCES

Aguayo, R. (1990). *Dr. Deming: The American who taught the Japanese about quality.* New York: Carol Publishing Group.

Allred, C.A., Arford, P.H., Mauldin, P.D., & Goodwin, L.K. (1998). Cost-effectiveness analysis in the nursing literature, 1992-1996. *Image, 30*(3), 235-242.

Anderson, C. (1989, July 29). Little invention avoids big ouch. *The Iowa City Press-Citizen,* p. 1.

Arthur, W.B. (1990). Positive feedbacks in the economy. *Scientific American, 262,* 92-99.

Aucott, J.N., Taylor, A.L., Wright, J.T., Jr, Ganz, M.B., Landefeld, C.S., Pelecanos, E.I., Carrol, A.M., Dombrowski, R.C., Van Why, K.J., & Lederman, R. (1994). Developing guidelines for local use: Algorithms for cost-efficient outpatient management of cardiovascular disorders in a VA medical center. *The Joint Commission Journal on Quality Improvement, 20*(1), 17-32.

Barnard, C. (1982). The environment of decision. *Journal of Nursing Administration, 12*(3), 25-29.

Baumann, A., & Deber, R. (1989). The limits of decision analysis for rapid decision making in ICU nursing. *Image, 21*(2), 69-71.

Belsky, G., & Gilovich, T. (1999). *Why smart people make big money mistakes and how to correct them.* New York: Simon & Schuster.

Berman, S. (1998). Identifying and addressing sentinel events: An interview with Richard Croteau. *The Joint Commission Journal on Quality Improvement, 24*(8), 426-434.

Buerhaus, P.I. (1998). Milton Weinstein's insights on the development, use, and methodologic problems in cost-effectiveness analysis. *Image, 30*(3), 223-228.

California HealthCare Foundation (2000). *A primer on physician order entry.* Oakland, CA: California HealthCare Foundation.

Camazine, S., Deneubourg, J., Franks, N., Sneyd, J., Theraulaz, G., & Bonabeau, E. (2001). *Self-organization in biological systems.* Princeton, NJ: Princeton University Press.

Carley, K., & Prietula, M. (1994). *Computational organizational theory.* Hillsdale, NJ: Larwence Erbaum Assoc.

Carley, K. (2003). *Intra-organizational computation and complexity* (United States Navy Grant No. N00014-97-1-0037 and the National Science Foundation, Grant, No. IRI9633662). Pittsburgh, PA: Carnegie Mellon University at Pittsburgh.

Chu, D., Strand, R., & Fjelland, R. (2003). Theories of complexity. *Complexity, 8*(3), 19-30.

Cole, L., & Houston, S. (1999). Structured care methodologies: Evolution and use in patient care delivery. *Outcomes Management for Nursing Practice, 3*(2), 53-59.

deChesnay, M. (1983). Problem solving in nursing. *Image, 15*(1), 8-11.

Dev, P., Hoffer, E.P., & Barnett, G.O. (2001). Computers in medical education. In E.H. Shortliffe, L.E. Perreault, G. Wiederhold, & L.M. Fagan (Eds.), *Medical informatics: Computer applications in health care and biomedicine* (2nd ed.) (pp. 610-637). New York: Springer-Verlag.

Drucker, P.F. (1974). *Management: Tasks, responsibilities, practices.* New York: Harper & Row.

Drucker, P.F. (1986). *Innovation and entrepreneurship: Practice and principles.* New York: Harper & Row.

Effken, J., Brewer, B., Patil, A., Lamb, G., Verran, J., & Carley, K. (2003). Using computational modeling to transform nursing data into actionable information, *Journal of Biomedical Informatics 36,* 351-361.

Elstein, A., Schulman, L., & Sprafka, S. (1978). *Medical problem-solving: An analysis of clinical reasoning.* Cambridge, MA: Harvard University Press.

Etzioni, A. (1989). Humble decision making. *Harvard Business Review, 67*(4), 122-126.

Gift, A.G. (1995). Cost effectiveness: Designing research for product evaluation. *Clinical Nurse Specialist, 9*(4), 204-206.

Gokenbach, V. (1995). Better decision making: A practical model for nurse managers. *Nursing Economic$, 13*(4), 197-202.

Grainger, R. (1990). Making better decisions. *American Journal of Nursing, 90*(6), 15-16.

Greene, J. (1999). From whodunit to what happened. *Hospitals and Health Networks, 73*(4), 50-54.

Grier, M. (1976). Decision making about patient care. *Nursing Research, 25*(2), 105-110.

Grier, M. (1984). Information processing in nursing practice. *Annual Review of Nursing Research, 2,* 265-287.

Hamilton, J., & Kiefer, M. (1986). *Survival skills for the new nurse.* Philadelphia: J.B. Lippincott.

Hammond, J.S., Keeney, R.L., & Raiffa, H. (1998). The hidden traps in decision making. *Harvard Business Review, 76*(5), 47-58.

Hammond, J.S., Keeney, R.L., & Raiffa, H. (1999). *Smart choices: A practical guide to making better decisions.* Boston, MA: Harvard Business School Press.

Harris, J. (2002). Blindsided, how to spot the next breakthrough that will change your business forever. *Audio-Tech Business Book Summaries, 11,* 5-6.

Hersey, P., Blanchard, K.H., & Johnson, D.E. (2001). *Management of organizational behavior: Leading human resources* (8th ed.). Upper Saddle River, NJ: Prentice-Hall.

Higgins, R.C. (1992). *Analysis for financial management* (3rd ed.). Homewood, IL: Business One.

Holland J.H. (1998). *Emergence.* New York: Perseus Books.

Huber, D.G., Delaney, C., Crossley, J., Mehmert, P., & Ellerbe, S. (1992). A nursing management minimum data set: Significance and development. *Journal of Nursing Administration, 22*(7/8), 35-40.

Huber, D., Schumacher, L., & Delaney, C. (1997). Nursing management minimum data set (NMMDS). *Journal of Nursing Administration, 27*(4), 42-48.

Hughes, K., & Young, W. (1992). Decision making: Stability of clinical decisions. *Nurse Educator, 17*(3), 12-16.

Ilgen, D., & Hulin, C. (Eds.) (2000). *Computational modeling of behavior in organizations.* Washington, DC: American Psychological Association.

Institute of Medicine (IOM). (2000). *To err is human: Building a safer health system.* Washington DC: National Academies Press.

Institute of Medicine (IOM). (2001). *Crossing the quality chasm: A new health system for the 21st century.* Washington, DC: National Academies Press.

Institute of Medicine (IOM). (2003). *Keeping patients safe: Transforming nurses work environment.* Washington DC: National Academies Press.

Janis, I., & Mann, L. (1977). *Decision making: A psychological analysis of conflict, choice, and commitment.* New York: Free Press.

Jensen, B., Hess-Zak, A., Johnston, S.K., Otto, D.C., Tebbe, L., Russell, C.L., & Waller, A.S. (1998). Restraint reduction: A new philosophy for a new millennium. *Journal of Nursing Administration, 28*(7/8), 32-38.

Johnson S. (2001). *Emergence: The connected lives of ants.* New York. Simon & Schuster.

Jones, K.R., Jennings, B.M., Moritz, P., & Moss, M.T. (1997). Policy issues associated with analyzing outcomes of care. *Image, 29*(3), 261-267.

Kauffman, S. (1993). *Origins of order: Self-organization and selection in evolution.* Oxford, UK: Oxford University Press.

Kauffman, S. (1995). *At home in the universe.* Oxford, UK: Oxford University Press.

Kerrigan, K. (1991). Decision making in today's complex environment. *Nursing Administration Quarterly, 15*(4), 1-5.

Kobs, A. (1999). "Closet" incidents. *Nursing Management, 30*(3), 48-49.

Korniewicz, D.M., & Palmer, M.H. (1997). The preferable future for nursing. *Nursing Outlook, 45*(3), 108-113.

Kowalski, K. (1992). From failures to major learning experiences. *MCN, 17*(1), 9-10.

Kramer, M. (1994). Perception and community: Seeing what we need to see. *Change, 26*(5), 50-51.

Lahti, R.K. (1996). *Group decision making within the organization: Can models help?* Denton, TX: Center for the Study of Work Teams, University of North Texas. Retrieved August 19, 2004, from *www.workteams.unt.edu/reports/lahti.htm*

Langberg, M.L. (2003, 1 February). Challenges to implementing CPOE: A case study of a work in progress at Cedars-Sinai. *Modern Physician.* Retrieved August 19, 2004, from *www.modernphysician.com*

Lorenz, E. (1963a). Deterministic, nonperiodic flow. *Journal of the Atmospheric Sciences, 20,* 130-141.

Lorenz, E. (1963b). The mechanics of vacillation. *Journal of the Atmospheric Sciences, 20,* 448-64.

Lorenz, E. (1964). The problems of deducing the climate from the governing equations, *Tellus, 16,* 1-11.

Lorenz, E. (1979). *On the prevalence of aperiodicity in simple systems in global analysis.* New York: Springer-Verlag.

Malloch, K. (1999). The performance measurement matrix: A framework to optimize decision making. *Journal of Nursing Care Quality, 13*(3), 1-12.

Manthey, M. (1988). Who owns a staff nurse's time? *Nursing Management, 19*(9), 22-23.

McKenzie, M. (1985). Decisions: How you reach them makes the difference. *Nursing Management, 16*(6), 48-49.

Mintzberg, H. (1983). *Structure in fives: Designing effective organizations.* Englewood Cliffs, NJ: Prentice-Hall.

Morrison, R.S. (1995). Validation of nursing management diagnoses. *Image, 27*(4), 267-271.

Mosher, C., Cronk, P., Kidd, A., McCormick, P., Stockton, S., & Sulla, C. (1992). Upgrading practice with critical pathways. *American Journal of Nursing, 92*(1), 41-43.

Nagelkerk, J., & Henry, B. (1990). Strategic decision making. *Journal of Nursing Administration, 20*(7/8), 18-23.

Narayan, S.M., & Corcoran-Perry, S. (1997). Line of reasoning as a representation of nurses' clinical decision making. *Research in Nursing and Health, 20,* 353-364.

Parsons, L.C. (1997). Delegation decision making: Evaluation of a teaching strategy. *Journal of Nursing Administration, 27*(2), 47-52.

Paterson, T. (1969). *Management theory.* London: Business Publications, Ltd.

Perrow, C. (1984). *Normal accidents.* New York: Basis Books.

Pesut, D.J. (1997). Future think. *Nursing Outlook, 45*(3), 107.

Pesut, D.J., & Herman, J. (1998). OPT: Transformation of nursing process for contemporary practice. *Nursing Outlook, 46*(1), 29-36.

Petroff, B. (1999). Correlation of error rate and workload in a home infusion company. *Home Health Care Consultant, 6*(6), 29-30.

Post-It Notes: A product that's stuck for 10 years. (1990, February 11). *The Des Moines Register,* p. 12X.

Prescott, P., Dennis, K., & Jacox, A. (1987). Clinical decision making of staff nurses. *Image, 19*(2), 56-62.

Russo, J.E., & Schoemaker, P.J.H. (1989). *Decision traps: The ten barriers to brilliant decision-making and how to overcome them.* New York: Simon & Schuster.

Saulo, M. (1996). Quality problem-solving, decision-making, type theory, and case managers. *Nursing Case Management, 1*(5), 201-208.

Schaefer, J. (1974). The interrelatedness of decision making and the nursing process. *American Journal of Nursing, 74*(10), 1852-1855.

Scholz, D. (1990). Establishing and monitoring an endemic medication error rate. *Journal of Nursing Quality Assurance, 4*(2), 71-74.

Shenk, D. (1997). *Data smog: Surviving the information glut.* San Francisco: Harper.

Stacey, R.D. (1996). *Complexity and creativity in organizations.* San Francisco: Bennett-Koehler Publishers.

Stetler, C.B., Brunell, M., Giuliano, K.K., Morsi, D., Prince, L., & Newell-Stokes, V. (1998). Evidence-based practice and the role of nursing leadership. *Journal of Nursing Administration, 28*(7/8), 45-53.

Stone, P.W. (1998). Methods for conducting and reporting cost-effectiveness analysis in nursing. *Image, 30*(3), 229-234.

Tanner, C. (1987). Teaching clinical judgment. *Annual Review of Nursing Research, 5,* 153-173.

Tanner, C., Padrick, K., Westfall, U., & Putzier, D. (1987). Diagnostic reasoning strategies of nurses and nursing students. *Nursing Research, 36*(6), 358-363.

Thompson, K.S., Caddick, K., Mathie, J., Newlon, B., & Abraham, T. (1991). Building a critical path for ventilator dependency. *American Journal of Nursing, 91*(7), 28-31.

Urden, L.D. (1996). Development of a nurse executive decision support database: A model for outcomes evaluation. *Journal of Nursing Administration, 26*(10), 15-21.

Van de Ven, A., & Delbecq, A. (1974). The effectiveness of nominal, Delphi, and interacting group decision making processes. *Academy of Management Journal, 17*(4), 605-621.

Van Drake, S. (2003, September 19). Nurses treat staffing issue with union. *South Florida Business Journal.* Retrieved September 22, 2003, from *www.bizjournals.com/southflorida/stories/2003/09/22/story3.html*

Veninga, R. (1982). *The human side of health administration: A guide for hospital, nursing, and public health administrators.* Englewood Cliffs, NJ: Prentice-Hall.

Vroom, V., & Yetton, P. (1973). *Leadership and decision making.* Pittsburgh, PA: University of Pittsburgh Press.

Waldo, B.H. (1998). Decision support and data warehousing tools boost competitive advantage. *Nursing Economic$, 16*(2), 91-93.

Waldrop, M. (1992). *Complexity, the emerging science at the edge of order and chaos.* New York: Simon & Schuster.

Ward, M.D. (1999). Decision support information for health care delivery and management. *Inside Case Management, 6*(1), 9-11.

Weiss, G. (1999). *Multi-Agent Systems: A modern approach to distributed artificial intelligence,* Cambridge, MA: MIT Press.

Wheatley, M. (1999). *Leadership and the new science.* San Francisco: Bennett-Koehler Publishers.

Willey, T. (1989). High-tech beds and mattress overlays: A decision guide. *American Journal of Nursing, 89*(9), 1142-1146.

Williams, A. (1991). Development and application of clinical indicators for nursing. *Journal of Nursing Care Quality, 6*(1), 1-5.

Wilson, E.O. (1996). *Consilience.* New York: Vintage Books.

Wolfram, S. (2002). *A new kind of science.* Champaign, IL: Wolfram Media, Inc.

Wren, G. (1974). *Modern health administration.* Athens, GA: University of Georgia Press.

Zimmerman, B., Lindberg, C., & Plsek, P. (1998). *Edgeware.* Irving, TX: VHA Inc.

III

HEALTH CARE ORGANIZATIONS AND SYSTEMS

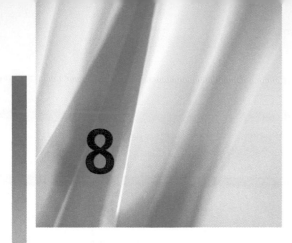

8

The Health Care System

Stacey T. Cyphert

CHAPTER OBJECTIVES

- Define and describe the U.S. health care system
- Trace the historical background of changes to the U.S. health care system over time
- Identify organizations, agencies, and components related to the health care system
- Analyze current challenges and trends
- Exercise critical thinking to conceptualize and analyze possible solutions to a practice experience

The health care system in the United States has evolved into a unique patchwork of diverse components. It is not a true "system" in the strict sense of the word. There is no central oversight agency to coordinate operations to achieve efficiency or fairness. Rather, the U.S. health care system is fragmented and complex, composed of a multitude of players with different objectives, some of whom may be functioning in isolation from or in conflict with others. It operates under a complicated variety of rules and regulations. Utilization of health care services varies widely by geographic region, with much of the variation attributable to differences in resources and capacity to provide care. Considered as a whole, it is also a large employer with a huge economic impact nationally, at the state level, and in many local communities. Although the U.S. health care system is frequently sought out by citizens of other countries for its health professions educational programs and its care is touted by some as the best in the world, varying degrees of access and quality exist.

DEFINITIONS

Basic health and medical care is a pervasive social need. Taken as a whole, the collective subsystems of health care form a unique system. In a broad sense, the health care delivery system refers to the major components of the system and the process that enables individuals to receive health care (Shi & Singh, 2001). The **health care system** is defined as all of the structures, organizations, and services designed to deliver professional health and wellness services to consumers.

Traditionally, U.S. health care has been organized around the physician and the acute care hospital. A triad of client, nurse, and physician became the basis of health care delivery, although not all members had equal status. Today, health care is increasingly more complex, and care frequently is delivered by a multidisciplinary team of providers across a continuum of care. Nursing personnel constitute the largest group of health care providers in the United States. They are the health care personnel who both deliver and coordinate care for clients. Therefore nurses are poised to be the care providers most prepared for population health and care coordination roles. As health care

▲ LEADING & MANAGING **DEFINED**

Health Care System	**Medicaid**
All (1) structures, (2) organizations, and (3) services designed to deliver professional health and wellness to consumers.	A joint federal and state program designed to pay for medical long-term care assistance for individuals and families with low incomes and limited resources.
Medicare	
The national health insurance program for persons age 65 and older, some disabled persons, and persons with end-stage renal disease.	

becomes coordinated and integrated across settings and sites, nurses will need to better understand the larger health care system.

EVOLUTION OF THE HEALTH CARE SYSTEM

Today's health care system is much different from health care in the early history of this country. It has been transformed from a relatively weak and minor enterprise into a vast and sprawling empire. Advancements in science played an important part in this transformation, but social and other factors, including the growing involvement of government, were instrumental as well.

Government today plays a pervasive role in the financing and delivery of services in the U.S. health care system (Feldstein, 1994), and its influence is exercised at the federal, state, and local levels. This pervasiveness was not always the case, however; the government's role has evolved over time (Litman, 1997). Justification of the role of government in health care is often made along the lines that health care is not like other goods. It truly can be a matter of life and death, and the absence of personal health and medical knowledge forces many people to rely on advice from the field. Furthermore, it is known that private enterprise may not have the incentive to adequately address the health issues that society deems necessary. For example, it may make good sense from a business perspective to focus only on areas where

money can be made. This, unfortunately, might preclude access to costly life-saving services or pharmaceuticals. Funding for medical education and research, which can be viewed as public goods, would also likely be significantly less without government participation. On the other hand, the involvement of government in the health care system at multiple levels sometimes leads to confusing, conflicting and cumbersome regulations. In fact, regulatory paperwork now requires at least 30 minutes for every hour of patient care provided in hospitals—in many cases, much more (AHA, 2002).

First 150 Years

As eloquently described in *The Social Transformation of American Medicine* (Starr, 1982), in the early stages of this country the family was the locus of most care for the sick. Many held the belief that ordinary people were capable of treating illness. In fact, guides to domestic medicine were popular and used to spread medical knowledge. Early hospitals were primarily charitable organizations. The people who used them tended to be poor, without access to family, or in need of isolation. Because of the spread of infection, early hospitals were also places that people were well advised to avoid.

Advances in medical knowledge and technological progress during the latter half of the nineteenth century led to greater reliance on hospitals as locations for the delivery of care and the dissemination of new knowledge. Important factors in this development included the ability to control pain through drugs such as morphine; to anesthetize patients with ether, chloroform, or other options; and to control the spread of infection with antiseptic procedures. Also instrumental were the establishment of laboratories and the use of x-rays to facilitate diagnosis. Eventually, hospitals became regarded as necessary for the delivery of care because of the superior services they could provide. This success enabled hospitals to attract paying patients, which encouraged the growth of health insurance.

Although health insurance was already in existence, the beginning of modern private health insurance can be attributed to the creation of a Blue Cross plan in 1929, whereby an arrangement for hospital services was struck between a group of teachers and the Baylor Hospital in Dallas, Texas (Whitted, 1999). Coverage for physician services came about later with the establishment of Blue Shield plans. The growth and development of hospitals also facilitated increases in both the number and specialization of the health care system's workforce. By 1929, the number of hospitals had grown to 6,665, up from only 178 in 1872 (Raffel & Barsukiewicz, 2002; Shi & Singh, 2001).

The skill set of early doctors varied widely since there were no significant barriers to becoming a doctor and most were trained under an apprenticeship system (Raffel & Barsukiewicz, 2002). For instance, of the 3,500 to 4,000 doctors at the time of the American Revolution, only about 400 had formal medical training. Many people counted being a doctor as among their multiple occupations. The first medical school in this country was chartered in Philadelphia in 1765. Medical schools multiplied after the war of 1812, growing to 42 schools by 1850, but many were of dubious quality (Starr, 1982). The Association of American Medical Colleges, organized in 1876, sought to improve the quality of medical education. In 1891 it supported a 3-year training period and in 1894 was persuaded to support a 4-year curriculum. By 1900, there were 160 medical schools, although the American Medical Association, which was founded in 1847, deemed only 82 acceptable, 46 doubtful, and 32 unacceptable (Raffel & Barsukiewicz, 2002).

The Carnegie Foundation for the Advancement of Teaching was invited by the American Medical Association to conduct an independent assessment of the nation's medical schools. Abraham Flexner performed the work on behalf of the Foundation. His report of 1910 had a profound effect on modern medicine. The Flexner report concluded that there was an oversupply of poorly trained physicians produced by a number of educationally deficient medical schools. By 1915, the number of medical schools had decreased by 36, or by slightly more than one-third, although some of this decrease was the result of mergers. Flexner had actually recommended a greater decrease, but state legislatures frequently sought to keep at least one medical school in their state. Changes brought about as a result of Flexner's report led to significant improvements in the physician education process (Raffel & Barsukiewicz, 2002; Starr, 1982).

Like physicians, the abilities of early nurses also varied widely. Physicians gave lectures to nurses intermittently during the early and mid-1800s, but this did not constitute formal courses of instruction. Private duty nursing was the main form of employment for early nurses. In the 1870s, the formation of nursing schools in Connecticut, Massachusetts and New York marked the beginning of formal training of nurses in the United States. Growth of hospital training schools for nurses followed, with student nurses providing a low-cost source of labor. By 1900, there were more than 400 schools of nursing, and more than 1700 by 1920. Quality concerns existed, however, and shortly after the 1926 creation of the Committee on the Grading of Nursing Schools, the committee produced a report concluding that there were too many inadequately prepared nurses and that improvements were necessary. Enhancements to educational programs were made in the 1930s, including changes in coursework and a shift of focus in the primary function of nursing schools as places to educate nurses, not simply to provide services to hospitalized patients. After the 1930s, hospital staff nursing replaced private duty nursing as the major form of nursing employment (Kalisch & Kalisch, 2004; Schorr & Kennedy, 1999).

Rise of the Modern System

In answer to a shortage of hospital beds, due in part to a standstill in civilian construction during World War II, the Hill-Burton Act of 1946 was passed to create a federal-state matching program to fund the construction of hospitals. This program proved extremely successful, and the number of nonfederal, short-term general and specialty hospitals grew from 4,444 with 473,000 beds in 1946 to 5,407 hospitals and 639,000 beds by 1960 (AHA, 2004a). The expansion of acute bed capacity under Hill-Burton enabled an increase in hospital utilization to occur. Admissions alone jumped from 13.7 million in 1946 to 23.0 million in 1960. This contributed to a need for more health care providers, as did factors such as greater expectations from a more affluent public and pressures from underserved areas.

The 1959 publication of the Surgeon General's Consultant Group on Medical Education report (the Bane report), which predicted a physician shortage of 40,000 by 1975, played an important role in expanding the physician supply (Blumenthal, 2004). The Health Professions Educational Assistance Act of 1963 provided federal funds for construction and modernization of medical and health science schools and inducements to expand enrollments. Medical school enrollments, for example, grew from 32,000 in 1963 to over 50,000 by 1973 (Jolly & Hudley, 1998), and new technicians, paraprofessionals, and allied health occupations began to arise around this time (Thomas, 2003). The Nurse Training Acts of 1964 and 1971 are examples of legislation passed during this time period that specifically provided federal funds for nursing education (Sultz & Young, 2004).

With increases in buildings and human resources necessary to deliver health care addressed, facilitating patient access represented the next challenge. Employer-based health insurance did exist, but it was more available in larger, urban-based companies than in rural parts of the country (Geyman, 2002). For most people, the only way to obtain and keep health insurance was to work for an employer that provided it. Although not comprehensive in nature, Titles 18 and 19 of the Social Security Act created the Medicare and Medicaid programs, respectively, in 1965. **Medicare** was designed as a federal program to provide access to health care for the elderly, and **Medicaid** was designed as a combination federal/state program to provide access to health care for the poor. Medicaid's dual-program status has resulted in each state customizing the program to fit its needs within general parameters established by the federal government, whereas Medicare is more uniform. Both programs have grown substantially since their inception, and their escalating costs are currently significant challenges to be addressed. In fact, Medicaid expenditures are now approximately 21% of all state spending (National Governors Association, 2004), and in 2003 Medicare spending totaled $6,880 per enrollee, or about $272 billion (MedPAC, 2004). Table 8.1 provides a list of terms related to the health care system.

The increasing complexity of hospitals and the environment in which they operated resulted in the need for more of a business orientation, and professional administrators began to arise as leaders. Nurses and physicians had previously occupied this role. Government became increasingly concerned about cost control and accountability as it expanded its involvement in health care. In the 1970s, health system agencies and certificates of need (CON) were implemented as strategies to alleviate these concerns. These initiatives sought to address cost and accountability issues through planning and regulating the supply of services. After it was clear that they failed to stem rising costs, prospective payment was introduced in the Medicare program in 1983 with the implementation of diagnosis-related groups (DRGs).

The idea behind DRGs was to encourage efficiency in the inpatient hospital setting by fixing payment for categories of similar patients in advance. Before the implementation of DRGs,

Table 8.1

Glossary of Acronyms	
Acronym	Full Name
AHA	American Hospital Association
AHRQ	Agency for Healthcare Research and Quality
BBA	Balanced Budget Act of 1997
BBRA	Balanced Budget Refinement Act of 1999
BIPA	Benefits Improvement Protection Act of 2000
CDC	Centers for Disease Control and Prevention
COGME	Council on Graduate Medical Education
DHHS	U.S. Department of Health and Human Services
DRGs	Diagnosis-Related Groups
EMTALA	Emergency Medical Treatment and Active Labor Act
ERISA	Employee Retirement Income Security Act
GAO	General Accounting Office
HEDIS	Health Plan Employer Data and Information Act
HIPAA	Health Insurance Portability and Accountability Act of 1996
HMO	Health Maintenance Organization
HRSA	Health Resources and Services Administration
JCAHO	Joint Commission on the Accreditation of Healthcare Organizations
MedPAC	Medicare Payment Advisory Commission
MMA	Medicare Prescription Drug Improvement and Modernization Act of 2003
NCQA	National Committee for Quality Assurance
NIH	National Institutes of Health
OECD	Organization for Economic Cooperation and Development
PhRMA	Pharmaceutical Research and Manufacturers of America
PPO	Preferred Provider Organization

hospitals received cost-based reimbursement, whereby the more they did, the greater the reimbursement, so there were few incentives to control costs. The implementation of DRGs also helped facilitate a shift in the delivery of care from the inpatient to the outpatient setting. The concept of fixing payment for like categories of care was subsequently adopted by other payers, and even expanded to the outpatient side. However, this strategy is still vulnerable to increases in volume or enhanced coding of the health problems used to assign a DRG.

Managed care systems, such as health maintenance organizations (HMOs) and preferred provider organizations (PPOs), were yet another development in the quest to contain costs. Managed care represents a shift in the power relationship between payers and providers. Managed care refers to linkages between the financing and delivery of services in such a way as to permit payers to exercise control over the delivery of services. Common elements include provider panels, limited choice, gatekeeping, risk sharing, and quality management and utilization review (Sultz & Young, 2004). The premise is that costs can be controlled by constraining beneficiary choice of providers while simultaneously supplying providers with an incentive for efficient practice.

Managed care has been successful in stemming the rise of health care costs, although public reaction to gatekeeping and restrictive networks has been negative in many cases. The number of people enrolled in HMOs actually peaked in 1999 at 81.3 million and has since dropped to 76.1 million in 2002 (NCHS, 2003). Still, all but 5% of employees covered by employer health benefits in 2003 were enrolled in some form of managed care (Sultz & Young, 2004).

Patients were not the only group to react to managed care. Providers also expressed concerns and many sought "any willing provider" laws to prohibit closed panels that would have denied them business. Individual states' ability to address concerns across the spectrum of managed care plans was limited, however, by the Employee Retirement Income Security Act (ERISA) of 1974. Although ERISA was primarily intended to keep employees from losing their pensions and to free employers from differing state regulations, it also had the effect of limiting the ability of states to regulate health plans covered by ERISA. This latter provision preempted a state's ability to mandate benefits for managed care plans covered by ERISA and necessitated, for example, federal action to address coverage limitations related to areas such as postnatal hospitalization (Mariner, 1996).

The Balanced Budget Act of 1997 (BBA) was a major reform that called for savings in excess of $125 billion in Medicare and Medicaid spending over 5 years. Among the many changes, including the creation of Medicare + Choice plans, which offered broader choices to Medicare beneficiaries, were reductions in Medicare and Medicaid payments to providers. Teaching hospitals were particularly hard-hit, experiencing both care-related payment changes and cuts in medical education payments (Dickler & Shaw, 2000). When Congress created the prospective payment system for Medicare in 1983, it included graduate medical education payments that increased with the number of trainees. Although the number of U.S. medical school graduates increased only modestly in the years since DRGs were implemented, the number of trainees in hospitals increased significantly as a result of an influx of international medical school graduates (Blumenthal, 2004). The BBA capped the number of residency positions eligible for federal support at each hospital and phased in a reduction of indirect medical education payments.

Several pieces of legislation—including the Balanced Budget Refinement Act of 1999 (BBRA); the Medicare, Medicaid, and State Children's Health Insurance Program Benefits Improvement and Protection Act of 2000 (BIPA); and the Medicare Prescription Drug, Improvement, and Modernization Act of 2003 (MMA)—helped restore some funding that had been cut by BBA and expand access to health insurance for children. The MMA bill also contained language that significantly changed the Medicare program by calling for the creation of a prescription drug benefit for Medicare beneficiaries. An interim prescription drug discount card program began June 1, 2004, and is the first step toward realizing this benefit. Medicare coverage of prescription drugs is slated to be implemented in 2006. Highly controversial during debate, the MMA has received even greater attention since its passage and the revelation that its projected costs are $534 billion over the next 10 years, rather than the approximately $400 billion Congress was told.

In summary, the evolution of the modern health care system has been described as encompassing four phases. The institutionalization of health care phase occurred from about 1850 to 1900, with the establishment of large hospitals and the clustering and coordination of services and personnel. The second phase, occurring from 1900 to World War II, was associated with the introduction of the scientific method into medicine and the subsequent recognition of medicine as having a solid scientific base. The third phase, from World War II until the 1980s, is characterized by the growing interest in the social and organizational structure of health care with the growing involvement of the federal government and the increased attention toward financing. Finally, the fourth and current phase is described as an era of limited resources, restrictions on growth, and reorganization of the methods of financing and delivery of care (Torrens, 2002).

COMPONENTS OF THE HEALTH CARE SYSTEM

Health care has been defined as "the total societal effort, undertaken in the private and public sectors, focused on pursuing health" (Longest et al., 2000, p. 4). The U.S. health care system is composed of a diverse collection of organizations and individuals that address specific needs in ways that are sometimes separate, coordinated, or overlapping. These needs include such tasks as the production and delivery of services and supplies, financing, and oversight. A broad continuum of health care services exists over which components may interact, including preventive care, primary care, specialized care, chronic care, long-term care, subacute care, acute care, rehabilitative care, and end-of-life care (Shi & Singh, 2001). Patients can become involved with the health care system at any of these points. Because changes in one component can have an impact on others, it is important to have an awareness of environmental trends.

Providers

There are more than 200 occupations and professions among the health care workforce (Sultz & Young, 2004), encompassing a diverse range of provider roles, including physicians, nurses, dentists, pharmacists, and allied health professions, such as physical and occupational therapists, laboratory technologists, and dietitians, to name but a few. Different services tend to be rendered by these providers, depending on their training and scope of practice. One can also classify providers by type of organization, such as community health centers, hospitals, or nursing homes. The major characteristics differentiating institutional providers include services offered (such as primary, secondary, tertiary, or quartenary), length of direct service provision (i.e., short-term, long-term), ownership (public or private), financial provisions (for-profit, not-for-profit), teaching status, geographic location, and accreditation and licensure status (Brooks, 2003).

Physicians

Physicians are the highest-paid professionals in the United States (Weinberg, 2004) and occupy the dominant role in the provider hierarchy. This is related to their training and knowledge, as well as requirements that care be delivered under their orders (Raffel & Barsukiewicz, 2002). They are independent practitioners who primarily hold a Doctor of Medicine (MD) or a Doctor of Osteopathy (DO) degree. Although graduates from foreign countries also practice here, most U.S. physicians received their degree from one of this country's 126 allopathic medical schools or 20 colleges of osteopathic medicine. The number of allopathic medical school graduates remained relatively stable each year between 1995 and 2001 at approximately 15,800, whereas the number of osteopathic medical graduates increased from approximately 1800 to 2600 (NCHS, 2003). Approximately 25% of the physicians currently in the United States are international medical graduates, and this represents a growing trend (McMahon, 2004). The number of physicians per 1,000 population grew from 2.4 in 1990 to 2.8 in 2000. This ratio was equal to the median of the industrialized counties that are members of the Organization for Economic Cooperation and Development (OECD) in 1990 but is lower than the 3.1 median reported for 2000 (Anderson et al., 2003).

Earning a degree does not constitute the final step in the process before a physician is able to receive a permanent license. Although state laws vary, the minimum requirement is at least a 1-year graduate medical education experience, and many states require more. Most physicians complete residencies lasting several years, specializing in areas including, but not limited to, anesthesiology, dermatology, emergency medicine, family practice, general surgery, internal medicine, neurology, obstetrics-gynecology, ophthalmology, orthopedics, pathology, pediatrics, psychiatry, radiology, and urology. The National Resident Matching

Program is a computerized service used to match residency positions with physicians, based on the interests of both parties. Most physicians in the United States are specialists rather than primary care physicians. A growing number are becoming hospitalists, which is a relatively new role in which they care for the patients of office-based physicians when these patients require inpatient hospital care.

Nurses

Nurses are the largest group of health care professionals. Most currently work in hospitals, although opportunities exist in a number of settings such as physician offices, nursing homes, schools, insurance and pharmaceutical companies, occupational health or home health care, or as independent practitioners (Raffel & Barsukiewicz, 2002). Approximately 90% of registered nurses are female (Weinberg, 2004). The nursing workforce is aging, with most nurses currently in the 35- to 49-year-old age range. Projections are for nearly half of the nursing workforce to be greater than 50 years old by 2010 (Buerhaus et al., 2003). Differences exist with respect to the means by which registered nurses enter the field. Hospital diploma, associate degree, and baccalaureate degree programs constitute the major pathways, with diploma programs on the decline and the profession's preference for baccalaureate preparation. Only 2,310 nurses graduated from diploma programs in 2001, compared with 41,567 from associate degree programs and 24,832 from baccalaureate programs (NCHS, 2003). Master's and doctoral level preparation also exist. Licensed practical nurses, certified nurse midwives, certified registered nurse anesthetists, and advanced registered nurse practitioners are additional nursing-related designations.

Hospitals

Hospitals represent one of the most recognizable components of the health care system. The total number of hospitals in the United States in 2002 was 5,794. These hospitals contained some 976,000 beds, admitted more than 36 million patients, and provided more than 640 million outpatient visits.

The majority of these were general, community hospitals. Only 323 hospitals (5.6%) had more than 500 beds, and only 375 hospitals (6.5%) had between 6 and 24 beds. The largest percentage of hospitals had 100 to 199 beds (23.9%), followed by 23.2% with 50 to 99, 18.0% with 25 to 49, 12.3% with 200 to 299, 7.0% with 300 to 399, and 3.5% with 400 to 499. Hospitals employ more than 4.6 million full-time equivalent personnel, including 99,829 physicians and dentists, 1,073,468 registered nurses, and 155,863 licensed practical nurses (AHA, 2004a).

Insurers and Payers

Insurers and third-party payers represent yet another component involved in the U.S. health care system. They are important in facilitating access to and payment for services. Unlike countries with a single-payer system, multiple payers are common in the United States. Commercial insurers, Blue Cross Blue Shield plans, Medicare, and Medicaid are examples as are businesses that choose to self-insure. More than 900 health and medical insurance firms existed in the United States in 1997 (Sultz & Young, 2004). Insurance companies are regulated by the states, although self-insured plans are exempt from state regulation under ERISA. In 2002, approximately 85% of the U.S. population was covered by private or government health insurance, with slightly more than a quarter of the population enrolled in an HMO (U.S. Census Bureau, 2003, Chart 151). Private payers accounted for 54% of spending on personal health care in 2002, which can be broken down as private insurance accounting for 35%, out-of-pocket spending 14%, and other private payments accounting for 5%. Public spending on health included Medicare at 17%, Medicaid and the State Children's Health Insurance Program spending at 16%, with other public spending accounting for 12% (MedPAC, 2004).

Education and Research

Although payment and delivery are important components, without organizations and individuals involved in education and research, the human resources and skills necessary for the health care system would not exist. Medical, nursing, and allied health provider schools and programs are part of the educational system that is needed. They also contribute to the knowledge base. Academic health centers are the principal sites for educating and training health personnel, as well as important sites for the conduct of research (Sultz & Young, 2004). A disproportionate amount of indigent care is also provided in this setting.

Funding from, and the conduct of research by, public and private foundations and government agencies are also imperative for the advancement of the field. The magnitude of government funding on research has expanded over time, even though the total percentage of dollars expended on health research and development by the federal government has been declining. It is estimated that approximately 6 cents of every health dollar spent in 2002 was for research. Of this approximately $92 billion, 54% came from industry, 34% came from the federal government, and 12% came from other sources (Thompson & Propst, 2004). The Pharmaceutical Research and Manufacturers of America (PhRMA) reported that its members alone spent an estimated $33.2 billion on research for new disease treatments in 2003 (PhRMA, 2004).

One of the primary ways in which government is involved in the funding of research is through the National Institutes of Health (NIH). The NIH is part of the U.S. Department of Health and Human Services. It both conducts and supports medical research using a competitive peer review process. The NIH's budget was recently doubled over the course of 5 years. With a 2004 budget of approximately $28 billion, more than 80% of the budget is competitively awarded to external investigators. A portion is also dedicated for internal scientists conducting research, primarily on the NIH campus in Bethesda, Maryland. The new director of the NIH, Elias Zerhouni, MD, recently crafted a "roadmap" to provide a framework for the priorities that NIH will address and to hasten the movement of discoveries from the bench to the bedside. The three themes of the "roadmap" include (1) new pathways to discovery, (2) research teams of the future, and (3) reengineering the clinical research enterprise (NIH, 2004).

Suppliers

Suppliers also comprise a significant piece of the health care system. A huge assortment of medical supplies and products must be continuously provided in a timely fashion, along with routine items such as paper, pens, and food. New diagnostic, therapeutic, or monitoring technologies must also be developed, installed, and maintained. The pharmaceutical industry, in particular, is a major supplier in the health care system with the distribution and development of new, more-effective drugs a key goal. Information technology suppliers are also playing an increasingly important role.

Supply management is critical for health care providers. If a provider holds too much inventory, there are implications for cash flow and storage costs, as well as obsolescence. Too little inventory can result in shortages of critical items. Arrangements are often made with suppliers for maintaining just-in-time inventories. Providers also seek to join group purchasing organizations to enhance their buying power.

Professional Associations

Professional associations exist in almost every field. They are organized to promote a profession's mission to society, provide collective action, and to enhance and protect the interests of its members. Local, state, and national chapters may exist. A professional association may engage in a number of activities, including, but not limited to, promoting the field, developing standards, communicating news, providing educational programming, honoring achievements, and lobbying on behalf of the profession. Several health-related groups are among the most powerful lobbyists in Washington, D.C. Among them are the American Medical Association, the American Hospital Association, the Health Insurance Association of America (which merged with the American Association of Health Plans in October 2003 to form America's Health Insurance Plans), and the

Pharmaceutical Research and Manufacturers Association (Birnbaum, 2001). The American Dental Association, American Public Health Association, and the American Nurses Association also play important roles.

Regulatory Bodies

A number of entities at the national, state, and local level are involved in the regulation of the health care system. Congress, as well as state legislatures and local officials, pass laws governing the operation of the health care system. As might be suspected, these laws cover a broad spectrum, from what constitutes the practice of a particular occupation to how health insurance plans may operate. Numerous health occupations are subject to regulation via licensure, certification, or registration. Health facilities, health products, and educational institutions are regulated as well. The regulations are made and enforced by various licensing boards and state and federal agencies, including the Centers for Medicare and Medicaid Services, the Office of the Inspector General, the Food and Drug Administration, and the Occupational Safety and Health Administration, to name but a few. Although many regulatory bodies have a government connection, private entities, such as the Joint Commission on the Accreditation of Healthcare Organizations (JCAHO) and the National Committee for Quality Assurance (NCQA), also play significant roles.

The JCAHO is an independent, not-for-profit organization that engages in the accreditation of various health care organizations, including home care organizations, ambulatory care organizations, assisted living facilities, long-term care facilities, clinical laboratories, and hospitals. More than 16,000 organizations are accredited by JCAHO, including more than 4,700 hospitals. Accreditation is voluntarily sought for many purposes, including fulfillment of state licensure requirements and certain third-party payer requirements, including Medicare certification requirements (JCAHO, 2004).

The National Committee for Quality Assurance is another private, not-for-profit organization. Among the reasons managed care plans voluntarily seek NCQA accreditation is to demonstrate compliance with state requirements. More than half the states currently recognize NCQA accreditation as meeting this purpose (NCQA, 2003a).

LEADERSHIP AND MANAGEMENT IMPLICATIONS

Health care forecasters predict that soon the principal point of care delivery will no longer be at the acute care hospital. Care will move toward being community-based. As the health care delivery system is reformed in this dramatic way, the roles and functions of the nurse will undergo a simultaneous dramatic change. A deemphasis on acute medical care will increase the demand for nursing skills.

The complexity of the nursing role is increasing with technological advancements and the greater overall acuity of hospitalized patients as more and more care delivery shifts to the ambulatory setting. Changes in accepted standards of practice are occurring such that health care teams are becoming more involved in treatment decisions and health care providers other than physicians, such as physician assistants and nurse practitioners, are assuming greater roles. There is also an increasing movement toward the practice of evidence-based medicine and health care. Nurses are contributing to the outcomes research on which that is based. Additionally, the growing emphasis on prevention and management of chronic conditions has implications for the skill sets nurses require, including the ability to educate patients under conditions of multiculturalism and short interaction times.

The need for coordination of care internally within a setting, as well as across settings, serves as an important reason for nurses to know how the health care system functions. Horizontal and vertical integration provide increased opportunities for managing a continuum of care, and the nursing profession plays important roles across this continuum.

◢ LEADERSHIP & MANAGEMENT **BEHAVIORS**

Leadership Behaviors

- Understands the health care system
- Is knowledgeable about health care economics and finance
- Provides planning and direction for salary equity and workforce skill mix
- Guides the organization's human resources policies
- Fosters creativity and innovation

Management Behaviors

- Understands the health care system
- Is knowledgeable about health care costs/charges

- Administers the salary structure and position control plan
- Implements human resources policies
- Manages resources and reduces costs

Overlap Areas

- Understands the system
- Understands the impact of economic and health care policies on nursing service delivery

📋 Research Note

Source: Steele, S., Rocchiccioli, J., & Porche, D. (2003). Analyzing and promoting issues in health policy: Nurse manager's perspective. *Nursing Economic$, 21*(2), 80-83.

Purpose

The clinical knowledge and advocacy orientation of nurses form the basis of the pivotal role nurses play in the health care system. Nearly 2.7 million strong, nurses have a unique opportunity to influence health care and policy. Involvement in policy can be enhanced by a user-friendly framework for health policy analysis. The purpose of this article was to display and discuss the policy analysis model (PAM).

Discussion

The PAM uses the following five-step analysis framework to begin:

1. Define the problem.
2. Identify policy options and alternatives.
3. Project consequences for each option.
4. Specify criteria to evaluate each option.
5. Recommend the optimal solution.

    Several forces are important to consider in step 1 while defining the problem: social factors, financial constraints, ethical/legal constraints, political constraints, and stakeholders. After the background of a problem is fully analyzed, the nurse can move on more easily to steps 2 through 5. This article displays two useful figures to present the PAM. One is the core model; the second is the concept of nursing shortage as an example of how the PAM can be applied to a real-world practice problem in the health care system. The article discusses each of the five steps and each of the important forces.

Application to Practice

The PAM is useful as a cognitive map to guide nurses through an analysis model. Nurse managers can use this model to mentor the learning of their staff and to facilitate the involvement of staff in health system and policy issues. A streamlined and clear policy analysis framework, such as the PAM, aids nurses in their efforts for patient and professional advocacy and for safe and competent care.

These recent and anticipated changes in the U.S. health care delivery system appear to offer exciting opportunities for the value of nursing to more fully emerge and be recognized. Since nurses manage and coordinate the environment in which all providers deliver client care, as well as directly providing some of that care, managed care programs rely heavily on the expertise and actions of nurses. As health care delivery changes to emphasize primary care, nursing is poised to become a mainstay of the health care delivery system. Nurses in advanced practice have a special set of abilities to offer the health care system. New roles for NPs, such as primary care and case and disease management jobs, capitalize on nurses' skills. This trend is being identified as the "age of the nurse."

Leadership in nursing means knowing the group's goals and how to get to the "preferred future." Innovation in the form of fostering creativity and the implementation of new ideas is a key strategy. Nurses have the skills to focus on the care of special populations, such as the elderly, and on community and preventive population-based services. Nursing will need to make strides in solving internal problems such as diverse educational levels and in generating research to demonstrate effectiveness. Clearly, however, nurses' unique preparation in leadership and management ability and coordination and integration roles appear to be a good "fit" with the direction of change in health care.

CURRENT ISSUES AND TRENDS

There are many challenges facing the health care system. Costs are high and increasing, new technologies continue to drive up costs, too many people lack access to health care, and aging Baby Boomers will increase health care demand at a time when human resources may not be sufficient. Quality is inconsistent, error rates are too high, and not enough attention is directed toward prevention. In addition to health care, providers must also contend with issues related to homeland security and information privacy.

Financial Issues

Health care spending in the United States was $1.6 trillion in 2002, which represented 14.9% of the gross domestic product. This is more than double the share of the GDP in 1970 and equates to spending of $5,440 per person. Private funds, such as insurance and out-of-pocket expenses, accounted for $839.6 billion, or approximately 54% of the spending. The bulk of the public spending occurred through Medicare and Medicaid. Hospitals accounted for 31% of total spending, physicians 22%, and prescription drugs 11%, while dental and other professional services, home health, nursing homes, durable medical equipment, and all other spending combined comprised 36% (Levit et al., 2004).

The economic and social impact of the U.S. health care system on communities, states, and the nation as a whole is huge. Even disregarding the benefit of improved health status, the ripple effect of spending on employees, supplies, buildings, and equipment helps to support the economy and generate taxes. In addition, spending by patients and visitors also contributes to the economy. The Association of American Medical Colleges, which represents the nation's 126 accredited allopathic medical schools and some 400 major teaching hospitals and their faculty, has estimated the combined economic impact of its member institutions in 2002 totaled more than $326 billion (Tripp Umbach Healthcare Consulting, 2003). Nationally, each hospital job supports approximately two additional jobs, and hospitals directly or indirectly support one of every nine jobs in the United States. Combined, community hospitals had a $1.3 trillion impact on the U.S. economy in 2002 (AHA, 2004b).

Growth in per capita health care spending decelerated in 2003 relative to previous years, increasing by only 7.4%. This growth rate is down from 9.5% in 2002 and 10.0% in 2001. In spite of this trend, these growth rates are still faster than the overall economy (Strunk & Ginsburg, 2004). Early data for 2005 HMO rates indicated a likely increase averaging 13.7%, which also represents a moderation from the previous year. Increases of this magnitude, however, still provide employers with an incentive to reduce costs through health plan design changes and greater employee cost sharing (Hewitt Associates, 2004). In an attempt to control premiums for employers while meeting patient desires for flexibility in access, health plans are developing products that shift more financial responsibility to patients and enhancing their management of high-using patients. Disease management programs, focusing on conditions such as asthma, diabetes, and hypertension, along with intensive case management of high users of health care, are examples of approaches being considered (Draper & Claxton, 2004). Instituting tiered copayments within HMO networks is also gaining momentum as HMOs seek to permit choice while encouraging prudent behavior (Steinbrook, 2004).

Health spending is, and historically has been, highly concentrated on a small percentage of people. The top 1% of the population accounted for 27% of aggregate expenditures in 1996, with the top 5% accounting for 55%, and the top 50% of the population accounting for 97%. The lower 50% of the population collectively accounted for only about 3% of total health expenditures. It is interesting to note that the majority of people in the top 1% are not elderly, nor do they consider themselves to be in fair or poor health (Berk & Monheit, 2001). During the last year of their lives, the nearly 5% of Medicare beneficiaries who die each year account for approximately one quarter of Medicare outlays (MedPAC, 2004).

The rising cost of medical malpractice insurance is also a growing challenge to the health care system. Many health care providers are experiencing decreased availability of malpractice insurance and higher prices for the options that exist. Physicians in Illinois, Pennsylvania, Nevada, New Jersey, New York, and West Virginia, among other states, have walked off the job or threatened to do so (Haugh, 2003), and some hospitals are no longer providing normal newborn care. Some providers are also choosing to retire or relocate to areas where malpractice insurance is more available and affordable. Although losses on malpractice

claims appear to be the largest driver of increased premium costs, falling investment income for insurers has also contributed (GAO, 2003). Arguments have been advanced that the increases in the frequency of claims and size of payouts are attributable to increased public awareness of medical errors, lower levels of trust in the health care system, advances in medical innovation and intensity, rising patient expectations, and increasing reluctance of attorneys to settle cases for amounts that sufficed in the past (Studdert et al., 2004). One consequence of this challenge is the increasing adoption of defensive medicine practices, such as declining high-risk cases or the ordering of extra tests.

Technology is also a major driver of increasing health care costs. Types of medical technology include those related to diagnosis (MRI), survival (intensive care units), illness management (pacemaker), cure (organ transplant), prevention (vaccines), and systems management (information systems) (Longest et al., 2000). Spending more for technology does not guarantee health improvements for a population (Blank, 1997). While new technologies may replace older versions and improve efficiency, it is not uncommon for a new technology to be provided in addition to, rather than in place of, an older technology. Nor is it uncommon for a new technology to result in more services being provided, particularly as patients demand the latest and providers seek to distinguish themselves from competitors, which causes costs overall to increase.

Some advances in technology require highly trained technicians to operate them and/or necessitate special construction to house them. Although greater knowledge of the cost-effectiveness of a new technology is useful, the advances being made in many areas, such as robotic surgery, are undeniably impressive. Relative to other countries, the availability of advanced medical technology in the United States is fairly high. For example, compared with other OECD industrialized countries, the U.S. had 8.1 MRI units per million population in 2000 versus the median of 4.7 and had 13.6 CT scanners per million population compared with the median of 12.2 (Anderson et al., 2003).

Pharmaceuticals, with price increases many times the rate of inflation, present a particular financial strain on those without prescription drug coverage. Prices among the top 30 brand-name drugs dispensed to senior citizens rose, on average, by 4.3 times the rate of inflation from January 2003 to January 2004 (Families USA, 2004a).

The fragmentation of the health care system contributes to the difficulty in sharing information among providers. Uneven information system distribution and lack of coordination contribute to the challenge. It is estimated that 20% of laboratory tests and x-rays are performed because prior results are unavailable and that net efficiency gains of more than $131 billion per year could be achieved through greater information technology use in health care. On April 27, 2004, a presidential executive order created the position of a national health information technology coordinator within the Department of Health and Human Services to coordinate efforts toward a national health information infrastructure (Fyffe, 2004).

Access

The view of many in the United States that health care is "a right" remains in conflict with the reality of access. The United States is rare among the industrialized countries of the world in that it does not guarantee access to health care. Instead, most people in the United States tend to obtain health insurance through an employer, or via a spouse or parent who is employed and has access to health insurance, although the percentage of workers covered by employee-based health insurance has been declining in recent years. Nearly 175 million Americans are covered by employer-based insurance (Gabel et al., 2003), and there are tax and competitive reasons why many employers provide access to this benefit. Not all employers are financially able or willing to provide access to health insurance for their employees, however, and even when an employer offers health insurance,

there are still many employees unable to afford its cost. For those who have health insurance through their employer or their spouse's employer, the loss of a job, a change in jobs, a divorce, or the death of the spouse may result in a disruption in their health insurance coverage. Furthermore, not all health insurance is the same; high copayments, high deductibles, or coverage limitations, such as those for mental health services, may impinge on access to care. A market for individual insurance exists but tends to be expensive. Consequently, many people are unable to afford health insurance.

Government programs such as Medicare, Medicaid, and the State Children's Health Insurance Program were designed to help address the problem of a lack of affordable health insurance, although not all people without health insurance qualify for these programs. The number of people served by Medicare and Medicaid combined is now approximately 80 million. The costs of these programs continue to grow. Recent estimates are that approximately 82 million Americans were without health insurance for all or part of 2002 and 2003 (Families USA, 2004b), and many more are underinsured. Hospitals have recently started to consider possible modifications to their billing and collection practices related to those with a limited ability to pay in order to lessen such patients' financial burden.

A consequence of being without insurance is poorer health (IOM, 2004a). Uninsured people are more likely to go without needed care and to be in worse condition when they do present for care. Differences exist by race with respect to lack of health insurance. For example, working Hispanic and black adults are more likely to be uninsured than working white adults (States Health Access Data Assistance Center, 2004). Hospital emergency rooms often serve as the safety net for the uninsured. The Emergency Medical Treatment and Active Labor Act (EMTALA), passed as part of the Consolidated Omnibus Budget Reconciliation Act of 1986, ensured that people who present to an emergency room will be seen. Care delivered in the emergency room setting, however, tends to be the most expensive.

Workforce

A sizable number of people are employed in the health sector. In 2002, more than 4.6 million people were employed in ambulatory health care settings, such as offices of physicians, dentists, and other health practitioners, as well as in medical and diagnostic laboratories and home health care services. Another 4.2 million were employed in hospitals, and 2.7 million were employed in nursing and residential care facilities (U.S. Census Bureau, 2003, Chart 160). When considered by occupation, these totals included approximately 825,000 physicians, 180,000 dentists, and 2.3 million registered nurses employed in 2002 (U.S. Census Bureau, 2003, Chart 615). Of course, the health sector can be thought of in broader terms than this. The numbers grow substantially when considering people employed in the insurance, pharmaceutical, and medical supply professions, for example.

Workforce shortages represent a cyclical challenge in the U.S. health care system. When key players are in short supply, access to and quality of care may be compromised and costs may increase. The aging of the U.S. population is anticipated to have important implications for the health care workforce. Assuming constant consumption and productivity over time, the aging population is anticipated to increase demand for physicians from 2.8 per thousand population in 2000 to 3.1 in 2020, and the demand for full-time-equivalent nurses from 7.0 to 7.5. Concerns also exist that many in the aging health workforce itself may be retiring as demand grows and that it may be difficult to attract sufficient numbers of new health workers (National Center for Health Workforce Analysis, 2003).

Shortages of nurses are nothing new, although the current nursing shortage that began in 1998 has lasted longer than most. A number of factors likely contributed to the shortage and relate to economic, workplace, social and demographic forces (Buerhaus et al., 2003). Multiple strategies have been attempted to alleviate this shortage, including increasing wages, enhancing recruitment and retention programs through signing bonuses and work environment improvements, using agency nurses, hiring foreign nurses, and recruiting more

men and women into nursing through scholarship and loan repayment programs and accelerated degree programs. Despite these measures, women have more career options than ever before, hospital environments and nursing work shifts are often unattractive, pay rates are flat over time, and the lack of nursing faculty has limited enrollment gains that could have occurred. Without substantial change, the difficulty in filling nursing positions may continue into the future. The National Center for Health Workforce Analysis, using a baseline scenario, indicated that a 41% increase in the demand for full-time equivalent registered nurses will occur between 2000 and 2020 (National Center for Health Workforce Analysis, 2003).

Although predictions of physician supply were, until recently, tending toward a projected surplus, Richard Cooper, former dean of the Medical College of Wisconsin, and his colleagues estimated that demand for physicians will exceed supply by 200,000 in 2020. Analyses undertaken for the Council on Graduate Medical Education (COGME) by Edward Salsberg of the University of Albany have also predicted a physician shortage, but in the range of 85,000 by 2020 (Blumenthal, 2004). In 2004, the COGME report concluded that there is likely to be a significant shortage of physicians over the next 15 years, and there should be an increase in medical school capacity (COGME, 2004). Major professional associations such as the Association of American Medical Colleges and the American Medical Association are no longer projecting surpluses, although neither of these organizations has endorsed the shortage estimates. The costs of educating a surplus of physicians must be weighed against the price of a shortage. The challenge of addressing this country's future physician needs is complicated by the lag time typically associated with policy change and implementation, in addition to the long production cycle to produce each new physician.

Quality, Safety, and Satisfaction

Wide variations in the use of and expenditures for health care services occur across the United States.

What may come as a surprise to some is that this is not necessarily explained by differences in medical diagnosis. Rather, research by Dr. Jack Wennberg and others attributed much of the variation to differences in the resources and capacity of an area to provide health care, implying in some cases that supply drives demand (GAO, 2004). States with higher Medicare spending have actually been found to have lower-quality care, with the additional spending occurring on expensive care that does not change health outcomes (Baicker & Chandra, 2004).

Per-capita spending for health care in the United States is higher than other industrialized nations (Anderson et al., 2003), but arguments can be made that this has not necessarily resulted in the best health results. Many countries currently have longer life expectancies at birth than does the United States (NCHS, 2003). Japan, Sweden, Canada, France, Australia, Spain, Finland, the Netherlands, the United Kingdom, Denmark, and Belgium have all been reported to have higher average rankings on health indicators than the United States in various studies of industrialized countries. The United States' low ranking on infant mortality is frequently among several measures cited to support this conclusion. Possible explanations regarding the reasons for these findings are complex and in need of further study. Among the explanations proposed are differences in public behavior, income inequality, primary care infrastructure, effects from the health system itself, and combinations of these factors (Starfield, 2000).

Various takes on the public's perspective of the U.S. health care system have been reported. Lavizzo-Mourey (2003) asserted that an overwhelming percentage would assign a grade of D, citing an enormous and growing gap between expectations and the quality being delivered. The first annual National Healthcare Quality Report acknowledged that "high quality health care is not yet a universal reality" and that "greater improvement is possible" (USDHHS, 2003, p. 1). The Joint Canada/U.S. Survey of Health, however, found Americans were generally satisfied with the quality of health care received and were more likely than Canadians to report the quality of their health care services was excellent (Sanmartin et al., 2004). According to the Joint Survey, approximately 42% of Americans rated the quality of care they received as excellent, and 47% rated it as good. Only 2% of Americans thought the quality of care they received was poor. More than 53% of Americans also reported that they were very satisfied with any health service received, 37% were somewhat satisfied, and 4% were neither satisfied nor dissatisfied. Less than 2% were very dissatisfied with the care received (Sanmartin et al., 2004).

There are severe financial and human consequences of the inconsistency of performance of the health care system. Approximately 1,000 needless deaths occur each week because of failures to deliver appropriate care. In addition, more than $11 billion in lost productivity could be avoided if best practices were adopted (NCQA, 2003b). Patient safety events associated with hospitalized children have alone been estimated to have contributed to more than $1 billion in additional hospital charges in 2000 (Miller & Zhan, 2004).

A growing consensus is emerging today that the U.S. health care system fails to deliver its potential benefits and, in fact, harms too frequently (IOM, 2001). Estimates have been reported that as many as 98,000 hospitalized Americans die each year as a result of errors in their care (IOM, 2000). Much of the blame has been directed at the outmoded systems of work. New information technologies are seen as a critical component for moving the country toward care that is evidence-based, patient-centered, and systems-oriented so that the best knowledge can be applied across providers and settings.

Created in June of 1998, the Committee on the Quality of Health Care in America was charged with devising a strategy to improve quality of the U.S. health care system over the next decade. It proposed that all health care organizations, professional groups, and public and private purchasers should pursue six major aims—that health care be safe, effective, patient-centered, timely, efficient, and equitable (IOM, 2001).

Educational aspects related to quality improvement are also being addressed. The Committee on Health Professions Education has developed a new vision for clinical education. This vision includes five core competencies and indicates that "all health professionals should be educated to deliver patient-centered care as members of an inter-disciplinary team, emphasizing evidence-based practice, quality improvement approaches, and informatics" (IOM, 2004b, p. 3).

Posting of quality and cost data on websites for consumers is a growing phenomenon. *U.S. News and World Report* has provided ratings of top hospitals and medical specialties for years, and the National Committee on Quality Assurance's (NCQA, 2003b) Health Plan Employer Data and Information Set (HEDIS) has been in existence for some time. Still more and more sources of quality information are becoming available every day. For example, HealthGrades.com was founded in 1999, and the Leapfrog group launched a national quality and safety measurement and reporting effort in 2000. Insurance companies and employers are joining the trend. Concerns exist, however, on the part of providers as to the validity of some of the information presented (Lee et al., 2004). Controversy continues about whether process or outcomes data are better measures. Donabedian argued that the most direct route to assessing quality of care is by examination of the process, with assessment of the structure and the outcome being less direct methods (Donabedian, 1980).

In 2003, a national voluntary effort known as *The Quality Initiative* to compile public information on hospital quality was announced. The Medicare Prescription Drug, Improvement, and Modernization Act of 2003 actually required hospitals to submit data for a set of ten quality indicators established by the Secretary of Health and Human Services in order to avoid a deduction in their Medicare market basket percentage increase. "Pay for performance" strategies are currently in their infancy, but they are anticipated to develop as a means of fostering quality improvement.

Population Changes and Care Demands

The population of the U.S. is aging. During the course of the last century, an increase of more than 12 years occurred in the median age as the population went from half being younger than 22.9 years old in 1988 to half the population being only younger than 35.3 years in 2000. The size of the population over age 65 increased more than tenfold during this period, and rapid growth in this age bracket is expected to continue once the leading edge of the Baby Boom generation reaches age 65 in 2011 (Hobbs & Stoops, 2002). This has implications for the U.S. health care system in general, as care needs for this age group are higher than for younger people, and providers with expertise in caring for the elderly will be in demand. It also has implications for the Medicare and Medicaid programs in particular, because many in this age group will be eligible for services covered by these programs. As the ratio of active workers to beneficiaries is expected to decline from approximately 4.0 today to 2.4 by 2030 (MedPAC, 2004), questions are being raised about whether the funding support for the Medicare program from the payroll and income taxes paid by active workers will be sufficient.

Three broad categories are commonly used to classify medical care: preventive, curative, and restorative (Shi & Singh, 2001). Nearly 95% of U.S. health care expenditures go to direct medical services, whereas only about 5% are allocated to prevention and health promotion (USDHHS, 2003). An increasing call to establish a greater preventive orientation in the health care system has occurred with the rise in chronic conditions, which have come to affect almost half of the U.S. population, are the leading cause of illness, disability and death, and account for the majority of health care expenditures (IOM, 2001). Half of the deaths in the United States in 2000 have been attributed to a number of preventable behaviors and exposures. Among the most common preventable behaviors and exposures were tobacco (associated with 18.1% of the total U.S. deaths in 2000), poor diet and physical inactivity (associated with 16.6%), and alcohol consumption (associated with 3.5%) (Mokdad et al., 2004).

The use of complementary and alternative medicine is growing in the United States. Dissatisfaction with conventional medicine and marketing are among several explanations that have been proposed for this growth. The National Center for Complementary and Alternative Medicine (NCCAM) defined complementary and alternative medicine as "a group of diverse medical and health care systems, practices and products that are not presently considered to be part of conventional medicine" (2004, p. 1). What is considered to be complementary or alternative medicine changes over time as proven therapies are adopted into conventional medicine and new therapies are developed. Complementary medicine is used in conjunction with conventional medicine, whereas alternative medicine is used in place of it.

In 2002, when the definition included prayer for health reasons, nearly two-thirds of adults reported using complementary or alternative medicine. When prayer was excluded, the percentage was approximately one-third. About one-quarter of adult users tried complementary and alternative medicine upon the recommendation of a conventional medical provider, with women tending to use these therapies more frequently than men. Besides prayer for health, use of natural products, deep breathing exercises, meditation, and chiropractic care were among the most common therapies used. The use of complementary and alternative medicine is not without risk, however, since many of its therapies are untested or have the potential to interact with conventional therapies being concurrently delivered (Barnes et al., 2004), especially if all therapies and medicines are not disclosed to the health care provider.

The patient's role in relation to health professionals is changing from one primarily of submission and compliance to being a partner in the decision-making team. Not only has the Internet facilitated patient knowledge about various diseases and treatments, but direct-to-consumer marketing has educated them to some extent as well. Pharmaceutical company direct-to-consumer marketing was only $151 million in 1993 (Findlay, 2001) but increased to $2.6 billion in 2002 and continues to grow (Zaneski, 2004).

Privacy

The Health Insurance Portability and Accountability Act (HIPAA) of 1996 significantly changed the health care system. Among the areas addressed by this legislation was the portability of health insurance, enabling people to change jobs without fear of being denied coverage for preexisting health conditions as long as certain conditions were met. Prior to this, a phenomenon known as "job lock" often caused people to remain with an employer to retain coverage for an existing health condition.

Probably the most widely recognized change brought about by HIPAA was greater privacy protection for health information. HIPAA required the U.S. Department of Health and Human Services (DHHS) to develop a national set of privacy rules (absent action by Congress), which DHHS did (Frank-Stromborg, 2004). The standards established represent a national, federal base of privacy protections, with state laws permitted to provide additional protections. Health care providers are required to protect the privacy of health information and to provide patients with a privacy notice describing various rights, including the right to inspect and amend information, to request restrictions on the release of their information, and to obtain an accounting of disclosures of their protected health information. Business associate agreements governing the sharing of health information with external parties were also required to be developed. Civil and criminal penalties may be imposed on providers who violate the privacy provisions. This has led to costly educational and training efforts and redesign of systems to enhance compliance.

A survey by the American Health Information Management Association found that 91% of respondents felt their institutions were at least 85%

compliant with HIPAA privacy requirements nearly a year after the April 14, 2003, implementation date. The area most frequently identified as problematic was accounting for release of protected information (American Health Information Management Association, 2004). Concerns have also been identified relative to the impact on human subjects research due to such factors as increased time and money required for redacting identifiable information, negative impacts on subject recruitment, and impaired ability to collaborate (Ehringhaus, 2004).

Homeland Security

Although not the first acts of terrorism on U.S. soil, the tragic events of September 11, 2001, which resulted in the destruction of the world trade center towers in New York and damage to the Pentagon in Virginia, served as a wakeup call to most Americans that the world was changing. A new cabinet-level position was created in recognition of the country's vulnerabilities, and Tom Ridge was sworn in as the first Secretary of the Department of Homeland Security (DHS) on January 24, 2003. More than $8.2 billion in grants have subsequently been provided to states and localities by DHS to enhance preparedness since its creation (DHS, 2004). First-responder training and the creation of teams of medical professionals to respond to disasters are two examples of developments.

Concerns have mounted about possible physical, cyber, chemical, biological, or radiological incidents, and emerging new epidemics such as severe acute respiratory syndrome (SARS) have raised questions about the health system's preparedness to respond. Improvements are being sought in a number of areas. Curricular enhancement in health professions schools and continuing education of practitioners are part of the plan, as is integration of hospitals, emergency medical services, public health, and others when responding to emergencies. Improved collaboration and communication, enhanced planning and disaster training, and infrastructure upgrades such as improvements in disease reporting,

surveillance systems, and laboratory capacity are under way as well.

The Department of Health and Human Services (DHHS) announced in May 2004 that it was making $498 million available to states to increase the ability of hospitals and other health care facilities to respond to bioterrorism and other disasters; an additional $849 million was announced in June 2004. Since September 11, 2001, DHHS has invested over $3.7 billion in state preparedness through grants from the Health Resources and Services Administration (HRSA) and Centers for Disease Control and Prevention (CDC) (USDHHS, 2004). The Agency for Healthcare Research and Quality (AHRQ) is also playing a key role in supporting preparedness research and is particularly interested in "surge capacity" to meet large-scale needs in a timely manner. Among the potential strategies to increase hospital surge capacity are discharging patients early, utilizing outpatient areas and hallways for bed space, and partnering with other health care facilities, local schools, and armories (AHRQ, 2004). Challenges with rallying and rotating sufficient staff, managing crowds of worried well, and securing necessary supplies are but a few of the additional issues that must be addressed. It is anticipated that bioterrorism will remain a high-profile issue and that ongoing dedicated funds for building and maintaining preparedness capacity will be required (Staiti et al., 2003).

CONCLUSIONS

The U.S. health care system has evolved and continues to evolve over time in response to a number of social, political, economic, scientific, and environmental issues, among other factors. The specialist-driven biomedical model has been the prevailing paradigm over much of the history of the health care system in this country. Although this system lacks a single central point of coordination for the diverse conglomeration of entities of which it is composed, some degree of interaction does occur among components, and quality health care is frequently provided, although with acknowledged gaps and weaknesses.

The growing costs of the U.S. health care system represent a burden to many, including the federal government, state governments, employers, and patients. Americans are enchanted with medical technology, however, and so far have not been inclined to explicitly ration care as is done in other countries. In truth, though, a lack of health insurance serves to ration care for many. Among the numerous other ethical concerns that exist within the U.S. health care system are the allocation of scarce resources, such as organs for transplantation, emerging capabilities to genetically alter humans, and potential advancements involving stem cells.

Cost challenges and the increased attention on quality provide opportunities for work redesign. This is particularly true given shortages of various health professionals and growth in tiered benefit plans in which high costs without substantiated additional benefit diminish attractiveness. Nurses, as key members of the delivery system, are in an excellent position to assist in addressing these concerns. Of course, nurses may also feel caught in the middle between patient expectations and payer constraints and in trying to provide quality care in such an environment. Although much success has been achieved during the U.S. health care system's brief history, many challenges and opportunities remain. Understanding the system is a first step for nurses on the road to greater effectiveness in health care delivery.

Summary

- The U.S. health care system is fragmented and complex.
- The U.S. health care system has evolved over the last 150 years into a major enterprise.
- Government plays a major role in the financing and delivery of health care services.
- Components of the health care delivery system include providers, hospitals, payers, education,

research, suppliers, professional associations, and regulatory bodies.
- Nurses have key skills for population-based health and illness care coordination.
- There are many issues facing the U.S. health care system.
- Understanding the health care system aids nurses' effectiveness in care delivery.

Study Questions

1. What are several major challenges confronting the U.S. health care system?
2. What role does politics play in the U.S. health care system?
3. How might an emphasis on preventive services affect the U.S. health care system?
4. What role(s) do nurses play in decreasing fragmentation of health care services?
5. How are workforce shortages and quality of care interrelated? Which should be the main focus of resources?

CASE STUDY

Katie Trader is a faculty member at a college of nursing, teaching undergraduate students about leadership and care management. Students are highly focused on gaining clinical technical skills and expertise. Some feel that health policy and care management information distracts from "more clinical" studies. However, Professor Trader knows that nurses will be confronted with a complex health care delivery system to navigate and that a working knowledge of the health care system is important. Following her teaching/ learning philosophy, Professor Trader is determined to teach principles yet make learning fun. To teach this content, she devised a crossword puzzle, using the many acronyms ("alphabet soup") found in health systems terminology. This became a classroom activity enjoyed by the students (see facing page).

		B	B	A		
				H		
	H	I	P	A	A	
	E					
C	D	C				
	I					
	S					

CRITICAL THINKING EXERCISE

The nursing staff of the local Visiting Nurses Association is complaining about their salaries. Salaries for nurses at this VNA are 20% less than salaries for staff nurses at local hospitals. Although the VNA nurses have day shift hours, they do have to use their personal vehicles to go on home visits. They are concerned about the general compensation structure, and grumblings surface from time-to-time. The director of the VNA faces an extremely tight budget as a result of Medicare and Medicaid payment reductions and delays. The director decides to implement an educative strategy. She prepares and gives a PowerPoint presentation that overviews VNA income and expenses. This triggers many more questions from the staff, so she begins to prepare a second phase of educational offerings about the health care system.

1. Is there a problem?
2. What is the problem?
3. What are the key issues?
4. What should the director do to handle this situation?
5. What information would be helpful to the staff?
6. What other strategies should the director try?

REFERENCES

Agency for Healthcare Research and Quality (AHRQ). (2004). Optimizing surge capacity: Hospital assessment and planning. *Bioterrorism and Health System Preparedness Issue Brief*, No. 3. Retrieved June 12, 2004, from *www.ahrq.gov/news/ulp/btbriefs/btbrief3.htm*

American Health Information Management Association. (2004). *The state of HIPAA privacy and security compliance.* Chicago: American Health Information Management Association.

American Hospital Association (AHA) (2002). *Cracks in the foundation: Averting a crisis in America's hospitals.* Chicago: American Hospital Association.

American Hospital Association (AHA). (2004a). *Hospital statistics: 2004 edition.* Chicago: AHA.

American Hospital Association (AHA). (2004b). The economic contributions of hospitals, *TrendWatch, 6*(1), 5.

Anderson, G., Reinhart, U., Hussey, P., & Petrosyan, V. (2003). It's the prices, stupid: Why the United States is so different from other countries, *Health Affairs, 22*(3), 89-105.

Baicker, K., & Chandra, A. (2004, 7 April). Medicare spending, the physician workforce, and beneficiaries' quality of care. *Health Affairs: Web Exclusive*, 184-197. Retrieved August 20, 2004, from *www.content.healthaffairs.org/webexclusives/index.dtl?year=2004*

Barnes, P.M., Powell-Griner, E., McFann, K., & Nahin, R.L. (2004, 27 May). *Complementary and alternative medicine use among adults: United States, 2002. Advance data from vital and health statistics (No. 343).* Washington, DC: Centers for Disease Control and Prevention. Retrieved August 20, 2004, from *www.cdc.gov/nchs/data/ad/ad343.pdf*

Berk, M., & Monheit, A. (2001). The concentration of health care expenditures, revisited. *Health Affairs, 20*(2), 9-18.

Birnbaum, J. (2001). Fat & happy in D.C. *Fortune, 143*(11) 94-97.

Blank, R. (1997). *The price of life—The future of American health care.* New York: Columbia University Press.

Blumenthal, D. (2004). New steam from an old cauldron—The physician supply debate. *The New England Journal of Medicine, 350*(17), 1780-1787.

Brooks, C. (2003). Healthcare organizations. In P. Yoder-Wise (Ed.), *Leading and managing in nursing* (3rd ed.) (pp. 91-105) St Louis: Mosby.

Buerhaus, P., Staiger, D., & Auerbach, D. (2003). Is the current shortage of hospital nurses ending? *Health Affairs, 22*(6), 191-198.

Council on Graduate Medical Education (COGME). (2004). *Physician workforce report.* Rockville, MD: COGME/BHP/HRSA/USDHHS.

Department of Homeland Security (DHS). (2004). *Fact sheet: A better prepared America: A year in review.* Washington, DC: DHS. Retrieved June 12, 2004, from *www.dhs.gov*

Dickler, R., & Shaw, G. (2000). The balanced budget act of 1997: Its impact on U.S. teaching hospitals. *Annals of Internal Medicine, 132*(10), 820-824.

Donabedian, A. (1980). *The definition of quality and approaches to its assessment* (Volume I). Ann Arbor, MI: Health Administration Press.

Draper, D.A., & Claxton, G. (2004). *Managed care redux: Health plans shift responsibilities to consumers.* Issue Brief No. 79. Washington, DC: Center for Studying Health System Change. Retrieved August 20, 2004, from *www.hschange.org/CONTENT/666/?topic=topic03*

Ehringhaus, S. (2004, 8 June). *AAMC project to document the effects of HIPAA on research.* Presentation at the Association of American Medical Colleges Government Relations Representatives meeting, Washington, DC.

Families USA. (2004a). *Sticker shock: Rising prescription drug prices for seniors* (Publ. No. 04-103). Washington, DC: Families USA.

Families USA. (2004b). *One in three: Non-elderly Americans without health insurance, 2002-2003* (Publ. No. 04-104). Washington, DC: Families USA.

Feldstein, P. (1994). *Health policy issues—An economic perspective on health reform.* Ann Arbor, MI: AUPHA Press/Health Administration Press.

Findlay, S. (2001). Direct-to-consumer promotion of prescription drugs. *Pharmacoeconomics, 19*(2), 109-119.

Fyffe, K. (2004, 7 June). *National health information infrastructure (NHII): Overview.* Presentation at the Association of American Medical Colleges Government Relations Representatives meeting, Washington, DC.

Frank-Stromborg, M. (2004). They're real and they're here: The new federally regulated privacy rules under HIPAA. *Dermatology Nursing, 16*(1),13-14, 17-18, 22-24.

Gabel, J., Claxton, G., Holve, E., Pickreign, J., Whitmore, H., Dhont, K., Hawkins, S., & Rowland, D. (2003). Health benefits in 2003: Premiums reach thirteen-year high as employers adopt new forms of cost sharing. *Health Affairs, 22*(5), 117-126.

General Accounting Office (GAO). (2003). *Medical malpractice insurance: Multiple factors have contributed to increased premium rates* (GAO-03-702). Washington, DC: GAO.

General Accounting Office (GAO). (2004). *Health care: Unsustainable trends necessitate comprehensive and fundamental reforms to control spending and improve value* (GAO-04-793SP). Washington, DC: GAO.

Geyman, J. (2002). *Health care in America—Can our ailing system be healed?* Boston: Butterworth/Heinemann.

Haugh, R. (2003). Surviving medical malpractice madness. *Hospitals & Health Networks, 77*(5), 47-50.

Hewitt Associates. (2004). *HMO rates continue double-digit increases, but begin to moderate.* Lincolnshire, IL: Hewitt Associates. Retrieved August 20, 2004, from *www.was4.hewitt.com/hewitt/resource/newsroom/pressrel/2004/06-03-04.htm*

Hobbs, F., & Stoops, N. (2002). *Demographic trends in the 20th century.* Census 2000 Special Reports Series CENSR-4. Washington, DC: U.S. Census Bureau.

Institute of Medicine (IOM). (2000). *To error is human: Building a safer health system.* Washington, DC: National Academies Press.

Institute of Medicine (IOM). (2001). *Crossing the quality chasm: A new health system for the 21st century.* Washington, DC: National Academies Press.

Institute of Medicine. (2004a). *Insuring America's health—Principles and recommendations.* Washington, DC: National Academies Press.

Institute of Medicine. (2004b). *Keeping patients safe—Transforming the work environment of nurses.* Washington, DC: National Academies Press.

Joint Commission on Accreditation of Healthcare Organizations (JCAHO). (2004). *Facts about the Joint Commission on Accreditation of Healthcare Organizations.* Oakbrook Terrace, IL: JCAHO. Retrieved June 12, 2004, from *www.jcaho.org/about+us/index.htm*

Jolly, P., & Hudley, D. (Eds.). (1998). *AAMC data book: Statistical information related to medical education.*

Washington, DC: Association of American Medical Colleges.

Kalisch, P., & Kalisch, B. (2004). *American nursing—A history* (4th ed.). Philadelphia: Lippincott Williams and Wilkins.

Lavizzo-Mourey, R. (2003). President's message. In *The Robert Wood Johnson Foundation Report 2003* (pp. 1-6). Princeton, NJ: Robert Wood Johnson Foundation.

Lee, T., Meyer, G., & Brennan, T. (2004). A middle ground on public accountability. *The New England Journal of Medicine, 350*(23), 2409-2412.

Levit, K., Smith, C., Cowan, C., Sensenig, A., Catlin, A., & the Health Accounts Team. (2004). Health spending rebound continues in 2002. *Health Affairs, 23*(1), 147-159.

Litman, T. (1997). The relationship of government and politics to health care—A sociopolitical overview. In T. Litman, & L. Robins (Eds.). *Health politics and policy* (3rd ed.) (pp. 3-45). Albany, NY: Delmar Publishers.

Longest, B., Rakich, J., & Darr, K. (2000) *Managing health services organizations and systems* (4th ed.). Baltimore: Health Professions Press.

Mariner, W. (1996). State regulation of managed care and the Employee Retirement Income Security Act. *The New England Journal of Medicine, 335*(26), 1986-1990.

McMahon, G. (2004). Coming to America—International medical graduates in the United States. *The New England Journal of Medicine, 350*(24), 2435-2437.

Medicare Payment Advisory Commission (MedPAC). (2004). *Report to the congress—Medicare payment policy, March 2004.* Washington, DC: MedPAC.

Miller, M., & Zhan, C. (2004). Pediatric patient safety in hospitals: A national picture in 2000. *Pediatrics, 113*(6), 1741-1746.

Mokdad, A., Marks, J., Stroup, D., & Gerberding, J. (2004). Actual causes of death in the United States, 2000. *Journal of the American Medical Association, 291*(10), 1238-1245.

National Center for Complimentary and Alternative Medicine (NCCAM). (2004). *The use of complementary and alternative medicine in the United States.* Bethesda, MD: NCCAM. Retrieved August 20, 2004, from *www.nccam.nih.gov/news/camsurvey_fs1.htm*

National Center for Health Statistics (NCHS). (2003). *Health, United States, 2003* (Publ. No. 2003-1232). Hyattsville, MD: U.S. Department of Health and Human Services.

National Center for Health Workforce Analysis. (2003). *Changing demographics: Implications for physicians, nurses, and other health workers.* Washington, DC: U.S. Department of Health and Human Services.

National Committee for Quality Assurance (NCQA). (2003a). *NCQA Overview.* Washington, DC: NCQA. Retrieved June 12, 2003, from *www.ncqa.org/Communications/ Publications/overviewncqa.pdf*

National Committee for Quality Assurance (NCQA). (2003b). *The state of health care quality: 2003.* Washington, DC: NCQA.

National Governors Association. (2004). *The fiscal survey of states.* Washington, DC: National Governors Association and National Association of State Budget Officers.

National Institutes of Health (NIH). (2004). *Overview of the NIH roadmap.* Bethesda, MD: NIH. Retrieved May 31, 2004, from *www.nihroadmap.nih.gov/overview.asp*

Pharmaceutical Research and Manufacturers of America (PhRMA). (2004). *The issues: Research & development.* Washington, DC: PhRMA. Retrieved June 6, 2004, from *www.phrma.org/issues/researchdev/*

Raffel, M., & Barsukiewicz, C. (2002). *The U.S. health system origins and functions* (5th ed.). Australia: Delmar.

Sanmartin, C., Ng, E., Blackwell, D., Gentleman, J., Martinez, M., & Simile, C. (2004). *Joint Canada/United States survey of health, 2002-2003* (Catalogue 82M00220-XIE). Ottawa, Ontario, Canada: Statistics Canada.

Schorr, L., & Kennedy, M. (1999). *100 years of American nursing—Celebrating a century of caring.* Philadelphia: Lippincott.

Shi, L., & Singh, D. (2001). *Delivering health care in America—A systems approach* (2nd ed.). Gaithersburg, MD: Aspen Publishers, Inc.

Staiti, A., Katz, A., & Hoadley, J. (2003). Has bioterrorism preparedness improved public health? *Center for Studying Health System Change Issue Brief,* No. 65.

Starfield, B. (2000). Is U.S. health really the best in the world? *Journal of the American Medical Association, 284*(4), 483-485.

Starr, P. (1982). *The social transformation of American medicine.* New York: Basic Books.

States Health Access Data Assistance Center. (2004). *Characteristics of the uninsured: A view from the states.* Minneapolis, MN: University of Minnesota. Retrieved May 31, 2004, from *www.covertheuninsuredweek.org/ media/research/brffs.pdf*

Steinbrook, R. (2004). The cost of admission—Tiered copayments for hospital use. *The New England Journal of Medicine, 350*(25), 2539-2542.

Strunk, B.C., & Ginsburg, P.B. (2004) Tracking health care costs: Trends turn downward in 2003. *Health Affairs Web Exclusive,* 354-362. Retrieved August 20, 2004, from *www. content.healthaffairs.org/webexclusives/index.dtl?year=2004*

Studdert, D., Mello, M., & Brennan, T. (2004). Medical malpractice. *The New England Journal of Medicine, 350*(3), 283-292.

Sultz, H., & Young, K. (2004). *Health care USA— Understanding its organization and delivery* (4th ed.). Sudbury, MA: Jones and Bartlett Publishers.

Thomas, R. (2003). *Society and health—Sociology for health professionals.* New York: Kluwer Academic/Plenum Publishers.

Thompson, E., & Propst, S. (2004). *2002 Investment in U.S. health research.* Alexandria, VA: Research!America. Retrieved June 1, 2004, from *www.researchamerica.org/ publications/appropriations/healthdollar2002.pdf*

Torrens, P.R. (2002). Historical evolution and overview of health services in the United States. In S. Williams, & G. Torrens (Eds.). *Introduction to health services* (6th ed.) (pp. 2-17). Albany, NY: Delmar Publishers.

Tripp Umbach Healthcare Consulting, Inc. (2003). *The economic impact of medical college and teaching hospital members of the Association of American Medical Colleges (2002).* Washington, DC: Association of American Medical Colleges.

U.S. Census Bureau. (2003). *Statistical abstract of the United States: 2003.* Washington, DC: U.S. Government Printing Office.

U.S. Department of Health and Human Services (USDHHS). (2003). *National healthcare quality report.* Washington, DC: USDHHS. Retrieved August 20, 2004, from *www.qualitytools.ahrq.gov/qualityreport/download_report.aspx*

U.S. Department of Health and Human Services (USDHHS). (2004, 24 May). *HHS awards $498 million to states to improve hospitals' response to bioterror and other diseases* [News release]. Washington, DC: USDHHS. Retrieved August 20, 2004, from *www.hhs.gov/news/press/2004pres/20040524.html*

Weinberg, D. (2004). *Evidence from census 2000 about earnings by detailed occupation for men and women.* Census 2000 Special Reports Series CENSR-15. Washington, DC: U.S. Census Bureau.

Whitted, G. (1999). Private health insurance and employee benefits. In S. Williams, & G. Torrens (Eds.). *Introduction to health services* (5th ed.). Albany, NY: Delmar Publishers.

Zaneski, C.T. (2004, 17 June). Medical sales reps arrive bearing gifts. Pharmaceuticals: The medical profession is taking a closer look at inducements for doctors to prescribe certain drugs. *Baltimore Sun,* p. 1A.

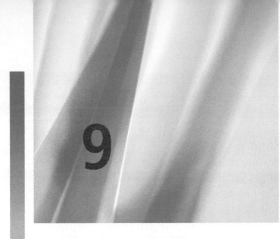

9

Organizational Climate and Culture

Suzanne M. Boyle

CHAPTER OBJECTIVES

- Delineate significance of organizational culture
- Define and differentiate organizational culture and climate
- Evaluate influence of culture on in nursing practice
- Analyze the importance of culture in a new model of care
- Analyze the effect of a culture change
- Exercise critical thinking to conceptualize and analyze possible solutions to a practice exercise

Health care organizations have moved beyond the era of restructuring and now compete in a marketplace based on their ability to demonstrate lean performance, increased efficiency, and safe quality outcomes. The forces of a nurse shortage, lower reimbursement rates, an aging population, increased acuity, and demand for nursing care combine to create a "perfect storm." Nurses are challenged to navigate in these turbulent waters. They may wonder how these factors link with culture and their role as nurses and leaders. This chapter addresses that relationship and focuses on organizational culture.

Culture is not easily defined, but it represents an important phenomenon that has to be understood in order to practice nursing effectively, no matter where the practice environment exists. Nurses must have insight into culture so as to better understand staff behaviors, norms, change processes, expectations and communications. This holds true for all levels of nurses from novice to expert practitioner and manager.

Nurses are positioned as the individuals most able to influence the culture of health care organizations by virtue of their pivotal role in care delivery. Diers (2001) stated, "nursing is two things: the care of the sick (or the potentially sick) and the tending of the entire environment within which care happens" (p. 1). Tending to the environment implies that nurses need to understand the culture of the setting in which they practice. The reason for the existence of the modern hospital is to provide nursing care, although this is not overtly recognized in our culture.

The acute care hospital as an organization affects nursing unit culture, operations, nurses' work, and health care relationships among nurses, doctors, staff, patients, and families. The hospital constitutes one of the most complex organizations in our current social environment. Health care relationships in hospitals are dependent on communication and collaboration between and among caregivers to facilitate intricate processes linked to the delivery of patient care. One way to better understand such relationships is to appreciate how the hospital culture affects nursing units, nursing practice, and patient outcomes.

DEFINITIONS

Hospital can be defined as an organizational structure that exerts a powerful effect on care delivery and quality outcomes; the **nursing unit** will serve as a focus for this discussion of organizational culture. The nursing unit is an example of a small structure embedded within the larger macro hospital organization (Aiken & Sloane, 1998). Such a unit might exist in any setting in which nurses care for patients (e.g., hospitals, home care, nursing homes, communities, etc.) Understanding culture from the unit perspective offers an unprecedented view of nurses' work, the work environment, and the characteristics needed to sustain a positive practice environment, collaborative relationships, and quality outcomes at the unit level. Hospital culture is composed of subcultures that can take the form of departments, nursing units, service groups, or project teams (Deal & Kennedy, 1982). Subcultures develop in nursing units and are designated as "work group culture" when studied at the small-group level (Coeling & Simms, 1993).

For a nurse to function effectively in an organization, whether as a staff nurse or manager, a solid grasp of organizational culture, characteristics, and operations is essential. This means that the explicit and implicit vision, mission, values, priorities, and strategic direction of the organization have to be recognized, understood, and aligned with realities of daily practice and care priorities. This chapter provides an overview of culture and uses the hospital organization to exemplify the effect an organization has on the culture of nursing units, the work of nurses, and patient outcomes.

Culture

Culture can be likened to fog in that it blankets everything, is subtle, and forms an invisible cloud that is so powerful it may obscure vision. Culture is a multifaceted phenomenon, difficult to comprehend and unravel. The study of culture has historically been the domain of anthropologists and sociologists who used methods of ethnography to understand groups of people. Groups and organizations exist within society and develop a culture that has a significant effect on how members think, feel, and act. Culture becomes a learned product of the group experience.

Culture affects the practice of nurses and, consequently, patient outcomes and satisfaction for patients/families and the health care team. Culture is visible in the way an organization structures and supports services for nursing practice as well as the written policies and underlying values that are translated by nurses into the work environment.

BACKGROUND

Organizational culture has been studied as both something an organization *has* and something an organization *is* (Mark, 1996). Peters and Waterman (1982) published a book titled *In Search of Excellence,* which fueled a renewed business focus on culture as the means to achieve organizational success and competitive advantage (Peters &

◢ LEADING & MANAGING **DEFINED**

Nursing Unit
Small structure embedded within a larger macro organization.

Culture
Shared believes and values.

Climate
Perceptions held by individuals about a particular unit or environment.

Waterman, 1982). Industry leaders in the corporate world quickly realized that the philosophy and values of an organization could determine success and secure market advantage (Wooten & Crane, 2003). The health care industry has been slower than the corporate world to embrace culture as a means to optimize organizational performance.

Culture is characterized by complexity and intangibles. It has an effect on nurses as individuals and how they acculturate as members of an organization and unit staff. Nurses have the power to create or change a work culture in order to accomplish a change that may affect productivity, satisfaction, and safe quality patient-centered care. The basic elements that constitute a work culture must be understood prior to any change initiatives. The effect of hospital-level change on the organizational culture is often magnified at the unit level, where the nurse patient relationship transpires (Aiken & Fagin, 1997; Shortell et al., 1994; Wunderlich et al., 1996).

CLIMATE AND CULTURE DIFFERENTIATED

Two common descriptors for organizational environment are climate and culture. Most researchers define these constructs similarly, although there is some disagreement over differences between them (Sleutal, 2000). **Culture** is described as shared beliefs and values, whereas **climate** is defined as the perceptions individuals hold about a particular unit or environment. Some researchers might argue that climate is a result of culture. However, the artificial differences are a matter of semantics or perspective, because the two phenomena are essentially the same and explicitly linked to nurses and practice environments. Climate reflects the employee's perception of organizational culture and is easier to measure, whereas culture is much harder to assess because values and beliefs are not tangible.

Organizational climate describes practices and procedures of an organization or a subunit and influences attitudes and behaviors of individuals. Climate is evident in staff perceptions of policies, practices, and goal achievement. Climate reflects

how things are done and the way they are done in a specific unit or organization. Organizational characteristics provide an alternative way to define climate.

Organizational culture is rooted in anthropology, psychology, sociology, and management theory. The way in which culture is perceived defines the meaning (Thomas et al., 1990). Culture can be viewed from the perspective of effect on behaviors of individuals and teams and consequently on patient outcomes (Fleeger, 1993). Veninga (1982) described organizational culture as an amalgamation of symbols, language, assumptions, and behaviors acquired by an organization. The variables comprise an intricate cluster of interactive components that overtly manifest themselves in a setting, either explicitly through policies, procedures, organizational charts, written vision, and mission statement, or implicitly in unwritten rules and norms that pervade the work environment (most easily missed yet critical to know). Collectively, these variables constitute culture.

One easy way to begin to understand culture would be to observe the recruitment process and entry of students or new staff to the organization and how they are subsequently welcomed and oriented to their assigned unit by the manager and staff members. Is there discussion about organizational commitment to learning, professional career development, a designated preceptor, and a clear individualized orientation plan? Is a mentor assigned? Does the organization allocate resources for staff education and attendance at professional meetings?

The mission statement for an organization offers a snapshot of strategic priorities and is another way to get a sense of organizational values. How does the mission get communicated? Is it evident in organizational decisions?

Schein (1996) is a renowned sociologist who has defined organizational culture as a shared value system developed over time that guides members to problem-solve, adapt to the external environment, and manage relationships. Schein suggests that a deeper understanding of cultural issues in organizations is necessary not only to understand what goes on, but more important, the outcomes.

Organizational culture affects both quality and quantity of nursing care and patient outcomes. Shared meanings, the taken-for-granted practice and assumptions of a work unit group can exert a significant effect on performance and outcomes. The unit work group is where nurses discover, create and use culture. Unit culture can be described as a set of actions devised by a group of nurses to deliver and manage care within a specific unit. Basic underlying assumptions are those that are never questioned and comprise an integral part of the fabric of an organization that extends to the unit work level, such as a commitment to excellence and to the surrounding community. Each organizational unit has cultural norms and values that blend the social realities and features that shape interactions between staff, patients, and families. The manner in which staff perceive organizational culture, manage boundaries, and translate the implied values to a unit level has a direct effect on the production of patient care (Alderfer, 1980).

Measurement of organizational culture and climate is fraught with difficulties, and there is no single best instrument. Qualitative methods are often used for culture, and quantitative measures are used for climate. A range of measurement tools are available; however, all have limitations in terms of scope, ease of use, or scientific properties. The choice of a measurement instrument should be directed by definition, purpose, and context for cultural assessment (Scott et al., 2003).

RESEARCH

There is a growing body of evidence that confirms that the relationship between nurse staffing and patient outcomes is influenced by culture and the organizational characteristics of the structure in which nurses practice (Aiken et al., 1996; Mitchell & Shortell, 1997; Needleman et al., 2001; Seago, 2001; Sovie & Jawad, 2001). Understanding the culture of a unit environment is critical work if professional practice is to evolve fully

(Del Bueno, 1986). Shamian and colleagues (2002) found organizational culture to be a significant predictor of nursing professionalism, underscoring the link between culture and practice.

Magnet Hospitals

Much of the health services organizational research to date has focused on macro structure and culture characteristics at the hospital level such as size, hospital type, and staff (Aiken et al., 1994; Kramer et al., 1987; Silber et al., 1997). Researchers have relied on the hospital as the unit of analysis, ignoring nursing unit culture, operation, and practice. However, the nursing unit is where caregiver relationships and communication intersect to inform care decisions. Thus issues such as patient safety and adverse events are best measured and understood at the nursing unit level.

Magnet hospital research and the organizational framework developed by Aiken, Sochalski, and Lake (1997) provide the means to understand better the link between unit culture characteristics and adverse events. A nursing unit culture that supports and values nurse autonomy and the provision of adequate resources and effective communication among providers most likely constitutes an environment where practice excellence is the norm. Effects of nursing interventions are mediated by such organizational characteristics at the unit level (Aiken & Fagin, 1997). Magnet hospitals are an example of a positive culture that affects nurses and patient outcomes. Magnet designation has become the gold standard for nursing practice work environments and is sought by organizations, nurses, physicians, and the public as the ultimate symbol of excellence.

Change is one certain, constant force in health care that faces every nurse. It is inevitable that changes in the hospital environment affect nursing operations at the unit level, alter care processes, and influence the occurrence of adverse events. Aiken and colleagues (1994) constructed a body of research on a set of hospitals with reputations as good places for nurses to work. The inquiry led to investigation of the relationship between nursing and outcomes measured at the hospital level

Research Note

Source: Boyle, S.M. (2004). Nursing unit characteristics and patient outcomes. *Nursing Economic$, 22*(3), 111-119.

Purpose

Little is known about how nursing unit work characteristics influence the process of nursing care and patient outcomes. The presence of specific unit culture characteristics may support or hinder the ability of nurses to practice safely and effectively.

Discussion

This exploratory cross-sectional study examined how organizational characteristics at the nursing unit level influenced adverse events and failure to rescue. The sample was composed of registered nurses ($n = 390$) and patients ($n = 11,496$) linked to 21 medical or surgical nursing units in one hospital. The Nursing Work Index Revised (NWI-R), administered midway in a 6-month period, measured independent variables. Nurse-sensitive adverse events—falls, pressure ulcers, cardiac arrests, pneumonia, urinary tract infections (UTI), death, and failure to rescue—were dependent variables collected over 6 months. Results suggested significant associations between adverse effects at the unit level and nurse autonomy/collaboration, practice control, nurse manager support, or continuity/specialization as determined by factor analysis. Autonomy/collaboration was associated with pressure ulcers and failure to rescue; practice control with UTIs; and continuity/specialization with death. High autonomy/collaboration factor scores were related to low failure to rescue rates and high pressure ulcer prevalence; high practice control scores with low UTI rates; and continuity/specialization with low death rates. When units were collapsed to high/low NWI-R scores, patterns illustrated the complexity of the relationship between organizational characteristics and adverse events. Exploratory analysis hinted at independent relationships of organizational characteristics and nurse variables (skill mix, experience, vacancy rates) and adverse events. Casemix index and DRG volume by unit emerged as potentially interesting ways to characterize nursing work at the unit level.

Application to Practice

Findings strengthened the premise that effects of nursing interventions are mediated by culture at the unit level. Results validated the power of nurses to prevent adverse events and failure to rescue at the unit level. An immense reservoir of professionalism exists among nurses that deserves to be effectively mobilized in the form of positive work environments that promote the delivery of safe quality care.

and evolved into an organizational change framework. Magnet hospitals were conceptualized as a specific organizational culture with characteristics of autonomy, practice control, and collaboration. Nursing practice was defined as the operant mechanism, and outcomes were measured for nurses and patients (Aiken, Sochalski, & Lake, 1997).

Magnet hospitals have been recognized for excellent patient care, support of strong nursing practice environments, and the ability to attract and retain nurses (ANA, 1997; Kramer & Hafner, 1989). The term *magnet hospital* was derived from

a policy study commissioned in 1982 by the American Academy of Nursing. The study examined the organizational characteristics of U.S. hospitals successful in the recruitment and retention of nurses during a national nursing shortage— hence the name (McClure et al., 1982).

Aiken and colleagues (1994) transformed the initial magnet hospital work into a program of research congruent with quality of care and organizational effectiveness through study of the links between hospital organizational culture and care outcomes. Aiken and colleagues (1994) examined mortality rates in 39 magnet hospitals and 195 control hospitals using multivariate matched control sampling. Magnet hospitals had a significantly lower mortality rate (4.6 % lower) for Medicare patients than did control hospitals. The magnet hospital culture provided higher levels of autonomy and control of practice and fostered stronger professional relationships between nurses and physicians than did nonmagnet hospitals.

Nursing units are enmeshed as part of any health care structure; however; nurses can construct a unit culture and develop a unit reputation for excellent care that differentiates practice and patient outcomes. In fact, variance can be found within organizations in nursing units that care for similar or same patient populations (Aiken, Lake et al., 1997; Czaplinski & Diers, 1998; Flood & Scott, 1987; Flood & Diers, 1988). Specifically, empirical evidence suggests that care in specialized or dedicated units has a positive effect on patient and nurse outcomes (Aiken & Fagin, 1997; Diers & Potter, 1997).

NURSING PRACTICE

Benner and colleagues (1996) described the social embeddedness of clinical care and knowledge within the culture of a nursing unit work group. In nursing, the work unit exists as the geographic site where care is enacted. Conceptually, the unit team forms a social group that holds a collective vision of excellence. In turn, the norm intersects with the notion of good practice and forms a cohesive collaborative unit environment. Expertise is fostered through nurse-to-nurse collaboration and sharing subtleties of warning signs and symptoms related to clinical events. Communication and interactions promote recognition of potential adverse events. Good practice is taken for granted and becomes the standard (Benner et al., 1996). Nursing interventions occur within the dyad of nurse-patient interactions. Implicit in this notion is recognition that the nursing unit work environment reflects a dynamic collective of multi-person actions focused on the common goal of safe quality patient care.

Each nursing unit establishes practice patterns derived from expert knowledge and cultivates a powerful web of experts and a nursing unit identity. Practice patterns establish unit norms for patient care and contribute to the culture of the nursing unit. Knowledge of the patient is derived through subjective, objective, and intuitive observations that are honed as nurses develop a level of expertise in working with specific patient populations. Embedded within the care giving relationship is a core of responsibility and obligation (Benner et al., 1996). The ability of nurses to know the patients and recognize early critical warning signs is a skill derived from knowledge, not a simple task application. Astute recognition of deviations from normal and timely intervention signifies that nurses know their patients and are capable of rescuing them from an adverse event.

A picture of unit culture can be gleaned by listening to shift-to-shift report, that is, the way staff communicate with each other and how they refer to patients and families, identify risk for adverse events, and articulate the plan of care and progress toward discharge goals.

Culture and group norms can have a profound impact on the shared values that are expressed by nursing staff on individual work units in the hospital setting (Koerner, 1996). Socialization can be described as a process used to achieve knowledge, skills, and behaviors of a certain group to belong and participate. Professional socialization is an unconscious means through which occupational identity is gained as values and norms of the profession are internalized. Koerner (1996) conducted research that suggested nurses are sensitive to work group norms and modify their practice accordingly. In effect, cultural and group norms have an impact on the values expressed by nursing staff on units within an organization.

For example, a new nurse may find that documentation is a low priority for unit nursing staff despite the fact that it is the critical evidence of patient care. Peers may comment about a new staff member's comprehensive notes and, in turn, may pressure the nurse to conform to a less-than-optimal unit standard for documentation.

Kramer and Hafner (1989) conducted the early research related to understanding the congruence of a value system with nursing practice in a positive environment. The Nursing Work Index was developed as an instrument by these researchers in an effort to measure nursing work values related to job satisfaction, perceived productivity, and nurse perception of a culture conducive to the delivery of quality nursing care. This instrument has been widely used to measure nurse perceptions of practice environments. Knowledge about how unit culture characteristics may facilitate nurse practice so that patients are rescued from adverse events has significant implications for nurses, patients, and the health care delivery system.

LEADERSHIP AND MANAGEMENT IMPLICATIONS

The role of a nursing leader extends well beyond a formal title into the realm of informal or unauthorized influence in order to affect culture. A primary task of the leader is to create a vision so convincing that the entire team is inspired to engage and move forward. Values drive behaviors. Koerner (1996) asserted, "the extent of the leader's vision, balance and energy is the boundary to which staff will actively migrate" (p. 76). The leader communicates this vision by influencing norms and values through role modeling and ensuring role clarity, accountability, and a work environment that promotes safe patient-centered care. Key areas within the leader's scope of control are recruiting and retaining staff, welcoming new staff, providing orientation, celebrating and recognizing staff accomplishments, facilitating change, and promoting a learning environment. Unit culture is evident in policies, unit norms, dress code and appearance, environment, communication, and teamwork. The nurse manager can articulate the vision, mission, and goals of the organization and work with staff to translate them into unit level values for performance, thus linking the context of the organization to clinical practice.

Values drive the way resources are distributed. They contribute to a general attitude and sense about the quality of working life and reflect the organization's core goals. Clues can be gleaned from organizational documents such as philosophy statements and meeting minutes. Caring values of the organization are reflected in the way the organization treats its staff. Organizational values may not mirror professional values. The leader's role is to bridge such values with the values of individual team members to construct unit culture. Building a culture is based on a framework of support (Figure 9.1). Values support the mission and the related vision, which supports strategies and action plans. The key platform is shared values. A nurse who wants to build a culture would

◭ LEADERSHIP & MANAGEMENT **BEHAVIORS**

Leadership Behaviors

- Envisions a dynamic culture
- Inspires a creative climate
- Models constructive interpersonal relationships
- Enables followers to be productive
- Influences others to work together
- Creates shared values
- Develops stories, rituals, and metaphors

Management Behaviors

- Manages the structure to affect culture positively
- Models constructive interpersonal relationships

- Acts with equity and justice
- Maintains rituals and ceremonies
- Influences employees to work together

Overlap Areas

- Models constructive interpersonal relations
- Influences the group to work together

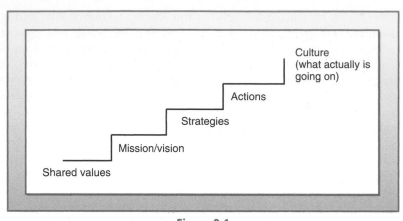

Figure 9.1
Framework of support for building a culture.

(1) identify the desired change, (2) assess current status of the group, (3) create a shared need and group commitment to change, (4) use appropriate communication skills and personal contact to establish open discussion, (5) identify shared values and mission so that the group knows where it is going, (6) determine strategies, and (7) develop an action plan for change.

Transformation and change challenge current cultures in existing structures. Conventional leadership requirements for performance accountability, moral management, and regulatory compliance are now linked with change initiatives such as diversity, service, innovation, continuous improvement, and cost containment.

Leaders are expected to chart a clear course for change and mobilize staff to accomplish organizational goals. This means implementing change effectively. Effective cultural change requires communication, passion, and sense of the whole. The nurse manager can create such opportunities through using focus groups, holding team meetings, coaching and mentoring, posting minutes from staff meetings, consulting communication books, and empowering staff by soliciting their input. The value of communication cannot be overstated. Much of the work is common sense, but the importance of doing this work lies in

carefully attending to the basic change process as a way to avoid the need for damage control later.

Peters and Waterman (1982) stressed that the greatest need for people is to find meaning in their work life. The job of managers is to help better create meaning through the use of stories, slogans, symbols, rituals, legends, and myths that convey the values beliefs and meanings shared among the staff. These managers have to function as passionate leaders in order to motivate staff.

The challenges of leadership belong to every nurse, not just those in formal management roles. Leadership at the staff level may simply take a different form—for example, a staff nurse adapting to a challenging patient assignment, taking initiative to change practice through performance improvement, or challenging the status quo are ways of participating in unit culture construction.

Application to Practice

Culture has evolved as a concept and is taken seriously in both the world of business and management theory (Kanter, 1993; Schein, 1996). The idea of change as a vehicle to excellence is recognized as a factor for success in all industries. Review of the magnet hospital evolution shows that the success of these organizations was linked to change processes and the commitment of leaders within those organizations to support key values and characteristics while trusting the knowledge and skill of their staff. Culture is linked practically and theoretically to commitment and shared understanding, which implies acceptance and integration of values in the culture (Beil-Hildebrand, 2002).

Adverse events impose substantial economic costs and inflict financial and devastating harm to patients and families. Although adverse events serve as the attention-getter, the real issue may be change in a culture that affects the work of nurses and creates an untenable unit work environment with minimal collaboration and practice control. Research findings highlight the importance of creating unit environments with a culture that empowers nurses to practice in ways that effect positive patient outcomes. The challenge is to define and measure nursing unit characteristics that support and transform nursing process into patient outcomes within the context of the nursing unit culture (Boyle, 2004).

In nursing, the work unit exists as the geographic site or floor where culture is enacted. Nursing is a coherent, socially organized practice shaped by a tradition of caring for patients (Benner et al., 1996). The power of social systems and group formation is apparent in the work group culture and nursing practice established on a unit (McCollom, 1995). Organizational culture surfaces as a salient characteristic in the elements of organizational structure. Understanding how hospital organizational culture facilitates quality practice outcomes at the unit level has significant implications for nursing, the delivery of health care, and patient outcomes. A unit work culture can facilitate or hinder the delivery of quality nursing care. Nurse managers or administrators can support or construct organizational and unit cultures that "work." Kanter (1993) suggested that structural conditions for work effectiveness can be created by management practices that support staff capacity and self-efficacy.

Implications

Nurse leaders armed with valid and reliable assessment of current work cultures can identify strategic target areas for change. A thorough understanding of unit and organizational culture is a powerful diagnostic tool that may be used to identify both troubled units and high performance areas. An effective organizational culture empowers nurses to practice fully within the scope of their knowledge and education. This may be seen in failure to rescue rates. Variance in failure-to-rescue rates for adverse events may signal key differences in work cultures within a hospital structure (Aiken et al., 1994). Discrepancies in failure-to-rescue rates may serve as diagnostic markers for identifying effective practice and performance of functioning unit cultures.

Empirical evidence will help delineate how patient outcomes are affected within the context of the unit work culture. The information could provide a method for nurse executives to utilize existing administrative data on adverse events to diagnose a unit work culture. Nurse managers struggle daily to better understand and manage the variances that affect performance and practice outcomes.

The culture of a nursing unit practice environment may exert a significant and independent effect beyond that of staffing and skill mix with patient outcomes by enhancing or impeding interventions once problems are detected. Nurses serve as the surveillance system for early detection of adverse events. The *right* number of nurses may have less influence on patient outcomes than the organization and structure of the work environment itself for nurses, including the perceived level of autonomy, the amount of control over their practice, and effective collaboration with physicians (Aiken et al., 2001; Sochalski et al., 1999; Sovie & Jawad, 2001).

CURRENT ISSUES AND TRENDS

Several recent landmark reports focus on the nursing shortage, crisis in our health care system, and potential strategies to address these challenges. Patient safety has received significant attention in the private and public sector as a result of the Institute of Medicine (IOM) reports *To Err Is Human: Building a Safer Health System* and *Crossing the Quality Chasm* (IOM, 2001; Kohn et al., 2000). The most recent IOM report, *Keeping Patients Safe,* focuses on transforming the work environment of nurses (IOM, 2004). The authors recommend that work processes support nurses through appropriate workspace, work hours, staffing, and organizational cultures that promote safety and quality care solutions.

The Joint Commission on Accreditation of Healthcare Organizations (JCAHO) in *Health Care at the Crossroads: Strategies for Addressing the Evolving Nursing Crisis* (2002) stated "the shortage of registered nurses has the potential to impact the very health and security of our society" (p. 5). A primary recommendation is to transform the work place—that is, to implement organizational culture changes (JCAHO, 2002).

In its 2002 report *HealthCare's Human Crisis: The American Nursing Shortage,* the Robert Wood Johnson Foundation provided a comprehensive overview on the shortage. A core recommendation was the need to reinvent work environments to address and appeal to needs and values of both new and experienced generations of nurses (Kimball & O'Neill, 2002).

The recurrent theme in each of these reports is that a significant level of culture changes must occur if practice settings are going to be able to successfully address the shortage and deliver the desired care system. The current and future workforce shortage is a compelling reality that has relevance for organizations and leaders who must create cultures that promote a positive work environment.

Models of Care

Currently, there is a movement to shift from restructuring toward development of unit level models of care that will transform health care systems. The multiple internal and external forces require financial accountability, competitive posture, and change in the structure of care processes. Ensuring the delivery of safe and effective quality care demands flexibility and engagement of leaders and staff nurses in changing work processes. The term *model of care* surfaces frequently; however, the specifics of how to construct such a model

seem elusive. A direct link exists between this concept and *culture.* Development of a new model must be preceded by assessment of the unit culture, an understanding of who the patient population is, what staff need in order to care for them, and what roles are required to form the unit team. There is no one right model, nor does one size fit all settings. The work entails a deliberative process in order to facilitate change that will produce improved outcomes. Culture development must be an essential component of any new model development.

Summary

- Understanding organizational culture is important for successful functioning.
- Culture gives meaning to behavior and influences decision making.
- Culture is shared values and beliefs.
- There are levels of culture.
- Cultures are both explicit and implicit.
- Cultures have elements that can be identified and measured.
- Culture management is a leadership issue.
- Cultures can and should be built by nurse leaders with staff.
- Culture elements can influence turnover and retention in nursing.

Study Questions

1. What is the relationship between an organization and its values?
2. To what extent does an organization's culture determine job satisfaction?
3. How can you assess an organization's culture?
4. How long does it take to truly perceive the culture?
5. What are the effects of leadership on culture?
6. Does organizational culture reflect an individual's perception of the organization, or is it a relatively enduring characteristic?
7. How can you build a culture?
8. What is the best kind of organizational culture for nursing?

9. What unit cultural values distinguish the nursing environment found in magnet-status institutions? Why are they important?
10. What nursing values create dilemmas?

In response to an anticipated workforce shortage, the patient service leadership team of one organization elected to collaborate with human resources to develop a strategy for future success. It quickly became clear that planning for the shortage translated to a crafting a plan for the future and was far greater than recruitment and retention. The work evolved into a broad initiative with a vision, guiding principles, core strategies, expected outcomes, and development of a leadership infrastructure. This work, called *Striving for Excellence,* was intended to change the culture. The work plan included extensive communication of the vision, identification of key stakeholders, assessment of current and desired future state, gap analysis, and implementation plan. The vision was translated into actionable concrete steps that engaged nurse managers and staff at the unit level in the change process.

A nurse manager identified patient safety as a high-risk issue for the population of children on an inpatient psychiatric unit. A review of the literature substantiated that traumatic sequelae resulted from the use of restraints. Furthermore, regulatory agencies mandated a reduction in the use of restraints.

Challenges facing this manager were cultural resistance, knowledge deficits, and a changing patient population. The *Striving for Excellence* vision served as a unifying concept, and change theory provided the framework for mobilizing staff commitment. Psychodynamic concepts helped ensure that the change was integrated into clinical practice. Use of restraints was viewed as a treatment failure and staff experienced a shift in thinking; that is, interventions moved from stopping aberrant behavior through use of restraints to reflection about what the behavior meant. Outcomes demonstrated a 60% reduction in the use of restraints; this resulted in a sustained change in practice for that nursing unit and has been recognized as a best-practice model. The nurse manager astutely summarized the real work as culture change.

CRITICAL THINKING EXERCISE

Hospital Y made a strategic decision to transform a 12-bed rehabilitation unit that had operated for 30 years and was a recognized leader in excellent multidisciplinary care for patients and families. The experienced nursing staff had low turnover and enjoyed strong partnerships with physicians, social work, physical therapists, and occupational therapists.

The new unit was designed to meet acute care needs of elderly patients with medical diagnoses. The change introduced an entirely new patient population and called for development of a new model of care for acutely ill elder patients who would experience a length of stay that was significantly shorter than a rehabilitation patient population. Subsequently, a new team of caregivers had to be identified to create new processes of care to ensure effective outcomes.

1. What is the problem?
2. Identify challenges faced by manager and staff.
3. What steps would you take to define the new model of care?
4. How will the culture of this unit change?
5. What can the staff do?

REFERENCES

Aiken, L., & Sloane, D. (1998). Advances in hospital outcomes research. *Journal of Health Services Research Policy, 3*, 249-250.

Aiken, L.H., Clarke, S.P., Sloane, D.M., Sochalski, J.A., Busse, R., Clarke, H., Giovannetti, P., Hunt, J., Rafferty, A.M., & Shamian, J. (2001). Nurses' reports on hospital care in five countries. *Health Affairs, 20*(3), 43-53.

Aiken, L.H., & Fagin, C.M. (1997). Evaluating the consequences of hospital restructuring. *Medical Care, 35*, OS1-4.

Aiken, L.H., Lake, E.T., Sochalski, J., & Sloane, D.M. (1997). Design of an outcomes study of the organization of hospital AIDS care. *Research in the Sociology of Health Care, 14*, 3-26.

Aiken, L., Sloane, D., & Lake, E. (1996). Satisfaction with inpatient AIDS care: A national comparison of dedicated and scattered-bed units. *Medical Care, 35*, 948-962.

Aiken, L.H., Smith, H.L., & Lake, E.T. (1994). Lower Medicare mortality among a set of hospitals known for good nursing care. *Medical Care, 32*, 771-785.

Aiken, L.H., Sochalski, J., & Lake, E. (1997). Studying outcomes of organizational change in health services. *Medical Care, 35*, NS6-NS18.

Alderfer, C.P. (1980). *Consulting to underbounded systems.* (Vol. 2). New York: Wiley.

American Nurses Association (ANA). (1997). *Implementing nursing's report card: A study of RN staffing, length of stay and patient outcomes.* Washington DC: American Nurses Publishing.

Beil-Hildebrand, M. (2002). Theorising culture and culture in context: Institutional excellence and control. *Nursing Inquiry, 9*(4), 257-274.

Benner, P.A., Tanner, C.A., & Chesla, C.A. (1996). *Expertise in nursing practice.* New York: Springer Publishing Company.

Boyle, S.M. (2004). Nursing unit characteristics and patient outcomes. *Nursing Economic$, 22*, 111-119.

Coeling, H., & Simms, L. (1993). Facilitating innovation at the nursing unit level through cultural assessment. Part 1. *Journal of Nursing Administration, 23*, 46-52.

Czaplinski, C., & Diers, D. (1998). The effect of staff nursing on length of stay and mortality. *Medical Care, 36*, 1626-1638.

Deal, T.E., & Kennedy, A.A. (1982). *Corporate cultures.* Reading, MA: Addison-Wesley.

Del Bueno, D. (1986). Organizational culture: How important is it? *Journal of Nursing Administration, 16*, 15-20.

Diers, D.K. (2001). *Between practice and . . .* Unpublished dissertation. Sidney, Australia: University of Technology.

Diers, D., & Potter, J. (1997). Understanding the unmanageable nursing unit with casemix data. *Journal of Nursing Administration, 27*, 27-32.

Fleeger, M.E. (1993). Assessing organizational culture: A planning strategy. *Nursing Management, 24*, 39-41.

Flood, A. B., & Scott, W. R. (1987). *Hospital structure and performance.* Baltimore: Johns Hopkins University Press.

Flood, S., & Diers, D. (1988). Nurse staffing, patient outcomes and cost. *Nursing Management, 19*, 34-43.

Institute of Medicine (IOM). (2001). *Crossing the quality chasm.* Washington, DC: National Academies Press.

Institute of Medicine (IOM). (2004). *Keeping patients safe.* Washington, DC: National Academies Press.

Joint Commission on Accreditation of Healthcare Organizations (JCAHO). (2002). *Health care at the crossroads: Strategies for addressing the evolving nursing crisis.* Chicago: JCAHO.

Kanter, R.M. (1993). *Men and women of the corporation* (2nd ed.). New York: Basic Books.

Kimball, B., & O'Neill, E. (2002). *Health care's human crisis: The American nursing shortage.* Princeton, NJ: Robert Wood Johnson Foundation.

Koerner, J.G. (1996). Congruency between nurses' values and job requirements: A call for integrity. *Holistic Nursing Practice, 10*, 69-77.

Kohn, L.T., Corrigan, J.M., & Donaldson, M.S. (Eds.). (2000). *To err is human: Building a safer health system.* Washington, D.C.: National Academies Press.

Kramer, M., & Hafner, L.P. (1989). Shared values: Impact on staff nurse job satisfaction and perceived productivity. *Nursing Research, 38*, 172-177.

Kramer, M., Schmalenbergh, C., & Hafner, L.P. (1987). What causes job satisfaction and productivity of quality nursing care? In T. Moore, & M. Mundinger (Eds.), *Managing the nursing shortage: A guide to recruitment and retention.* (pp. 13-32). Rockville, MD: Aspen.

Mark, B.A. (1996). Organizational culture. In J.J. Fitzpatrick, & J. Norbeck (Eds.), *Annual review of nursing research* (Vol. 14, pp. 145-163.). New York: Springer Publishing Company.

McClure, M., Poulin, M., Sovie, M., & Wandelt, M. (1982). *Magnet hospitals: Attraction and retention of professional nurses.* Kansas City, MO: American Nurses Association.

McCollom, M. (1995). Group formation: boundaries, leadership, and culture. In J. Gillette, & M. McCollom (Eds.), *Groups in context: A new perspective on group dynamics.* Lanham, MD: United Press of America.

Mitchell, P.H., & Shortell, S.M. (1997). Adverse outcomes and variations in organization of care delivery. *Medical Care, 35*, NS19-NS32.

Needleman, J., Buerhaus, P.I., Mattke, S., Stewart, M., & Zelevinsky, K. (2001). *Nurse staffing and patient outcomes in hospitals* (Contract No. 230-99-0021). Boston: Health Resources Services Administration.

Peters, T., & Waterman, R.H. (1982). *In search of excellence.* New York: Warner Communications.

Schein, E.H. (1996). Culture: The missing concept in organization studies. *Administrative Science Quarterly, 41*(2), 220-240.

Scott, T., Mannion, R., Davies, H., & Marshall, M. (2003). The quantitative measurement of organizational culture in health care: A review of the available instruments. *Health Services Research, 38,* 923-945.

Seago, J.A. (2001). Nurse staffing, models of care delivery, and interventions. In K.G. Shojania, B.W. Duncan, K.M. McDonald, & R.M. Wachter (Eds.), *Making health care safer: A critical analysis of patient safety practices* (Vol. 43, pp. 427-450). Rockville, MD: Agency for Healthcare Research and Quality.

Shamian, J., Kerr, M.S., Spence Laschinger, H.K., & Thomson, D. (2002). A hospital-level analysis of the work environment and workforce health indicators for registered nurses in Ontario's acute-care hospitals. *Canadian Journal of Nursing Research, 33,* 35-50.

Shortell, S., Zimmerman, J., Rousseau, D., Gillies, R., Wagner, D., Draper, E., et al. (1994). The performance of intensive care units: Does good management make a difference? *Medical Care, 32,* 508-525.

Silber, J.H., Rosenbaum, P.R., Williams, S.V., Ross, R.N., & Schwartz, J.S. (1997). The relationship between choice of outcome measure and hospital rank in general surgical procedures: Implications for quality assessment. *International Journal of Quality in Health Care, 9,* 193-200.

Sleutal, M.R. (2000). Climate, culture, context, or work environment? Organizational factors that influence nursing practice. *Journal of Nursing Administration, 30,* 53-58.

Sochalski, J., Estabrooks, C.A., & Humphrey, C.K. (1999). Nurse staffing and patient outcomes: Evolution of an international study. *Canadian Journal of Nursing Research, 31,* 69-88.

Sovie, M.D., & Jawad, A.F. (2001). Hospital restructuring and its impact on outcomes. *Journal of Nursing Administration, 31,* 588-600.

Thomas, C., Ward, M., Chorga, C., & Kumiega, A. (1990). Measuring and interpreting organizational culture. *Journal of Nursing Administration, 20,* 17-24.

Veninga, R.L. (1982). *The human side of health administration: A guide for hospital, nursing, and public health administrators.* Englewood Cliffs, NJ: Prentice-Hall.

Wooten, L.P., & Crane, P. (2003). Nurses as implementers of organizational culture. *Nursing Economic$, 21,* 275-279.

Wunderlich, G., Sloan, F., & Davis, C. (1996). *Nursing staff in hospitals and nursing homes: Is it adequate?* Washington, DC: National Academies Press.

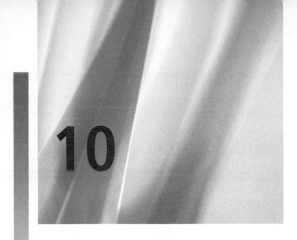

10

Mission Statements, Policies, and Procedures

Diane L. Huber

CHAPTER OBJECTIVES

- Define and describe organizational mission statements, policies, and procedures
- Determine the product of nursing care
- Compare the two dimensions of a social system
- Associate strategic planning with organizational mission statements
- Distinguish among types of organizational purpose statements
- Differentiate policies and procedures
- Relate organizational philosophy to nursing practice
- Exercise critical thinking to conceptualize and analyze possible solutions to a practice exercise

The provision and management of nursing care to clients is a complex endeavor that usually is embedded within the context of an organization. Understanding organizations and how they function is important to nurses who are employed by those organizations because there are practical implications for the work nurses do that arise as a result of the managerial structure imposed by an organization. An organizational structure can be both efficient and effective. However, this situation does not occur by chance. Without specific direction, day-to-day operations fall apart. Thoughtful operational documents form the backbone for managerial planning and direction.

Within an organization there is an established framework for management. For each organization a characteristic collective of power and authority is vested in the managerial hierarchy. This legitimated authority, given by position, is used with the management process, management skills, and whatever resources are available to meet the organization's goals. The elements of management and the resources available combine to form the basic framework for the management and functioning of an organization. Organizations have a mission—to produce a product or service. This goal will be expressed in mission statements and carried through into policies and procedures, all documents that form the basis for guiding standard operations. These documents are generally gathered into an overall strategic plan.

Strategic plans are a collection of written descriptions of organizational values, goals, and vision. They collectively form a conceptual description of an organization and display the framework for an organization's beliefs, intent, desired future, planning, and operations. Underlying mission statements are explicit values that drive organizations and people. Themes in health care mission statements include provision of quality care, customer satisfaction, and continuous improvement (Ehrat, 1994).

Mission, values, and vision are the glue that hold an organization together. They describe what the organization is trying to do, how to go about it, and where it is headed. Knowing these things helps to keep an organization on track. They become yardsticks with which to measure present performance and plans against aspirations. Groups can be brought to crisis by conflicts over basic issues of mission, values, and vision. Without these agreements in place, no organization is truly viable (Adams, 2004). Following are some thoughts about mission, vision, and values:

The mission of the United States is one of benevolent assimilation.

President William McKinley

If your job is to fix trucks, the bottom line is how many trucks you fix. The combat army has a totally different ethic: Accomplish your mission and take care of your men.

Col. Harry Summers, U.S. Army

Where there is no vision, the people perish.

Proverbs 29:18

Your vision will become clear only when you can look into your own heart ... Who looks outside, dreams; who looks inside, awakes.

Carl Jung

The very essence of leadership is that you have a vision.

Rev. Theodore M. Hesburgh, C.S.C.

If you don't know where you're going, any path will get you there.

Synopsis of Alice and the Cheshire Cat from Lewis Carroll's *Alice's Adventures in Wonderland*

Mission, vision, and values statements can be mere words on a page, or they can be "living documents" that unify an organization around a purpose. The process of development needs to bring members into basic agreement and alignment around the statements.

DEFINITIONS

An **organization** is a group of people with specific responsibilities who act together for the achievement of a specific purpose determined by the organization. An organization usually is thought of as an institution, such as a hospital or manufacturing company. All organizations have a purpose, structure, and some collection of people (Figure 10.1). The actual character or nature of any organization is highly variable, depending on the purpose, structure, and collection of people that form the organization.

BACKGROUND

Business management theory has contributed ideas about how to organize a business so that it makes money and runs efficiently. Theories based on business firms do not always apply directly to nursing because nursing is a service industry. Drucker (1973), a prominent business management theorist, said that service institutions are more complex than either businesses or governmental agencies. In a service industry such as nursing, the two key aspects of effectiveness are

◢ LEADING & MANAGING **DEFINED**

Organization

A group of persons with specific responsibilities who are acting together for the achievement of a specific purpose determined by the organization.

Philosophy

An explanation of the systems of beliefs that determine how a mission or a purpose is to be achieved.

Policy

A guideline that has been formalized.

Procedure

A description of how to carry out an activity.

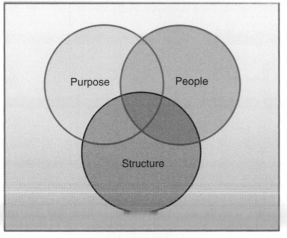

Figure 10.1
Components of an organization.

quality and cost control. Furthermore, service agencies such as hospitals rely on professional staff to accomplish their mission. Thus the relationship of professionals to their employing institutions affects organizational effectiveness in health care. Nurses primarily work in groups, thus making work group functioning and the interactions among people important for effectiveness and mission accomplishment in nursing.

As a service industry, health care has a product. The basic product of health care is client care service, such as disease treatment or health promotion. Health may be the ultimate outcome to be achieved. An interesting question is whether the product of nursing is the same as the product of health care. Quality care is one ideal product of health care. Kramer and Schmalenberg (1988a, 1988b) said that the product of a hospital is a quality, accessible, cost-effective service called client care. In hospitals 90% of client care is delivered by nurses. If the product is "quality care," there needs to be valid and reliable measurement to ensure that "quality care" is delivered and received. The idea has been posed that nursing is not a service composed of tasks, but rather a business with a product of enhanced client outcomes and contained costs (Zander, 1992). This idea takes Drucker's conceptualization and

merges ideas about a service industry with ideas about traditional for-profit businesses. For nursing, the product is derived from the use of expertise to solve problems for clients. Similarly, the product of nursing administration relates to the use of expertise to solve problems for nurses within systems of care.

Organizations are designed to produce goal accomplishment and can be understood as social systems. The Getzels and Guba model (Getzels, 1958) indicated that there are two dimensions to a social system. One part is the environment of the organization. An institution has certain role expectations, a culture, an ethos, and values. If an organization has certain goals—for example, quality client care and cost containment—then individuals have a role in the system with certain expectations related to achieving the goals.

The other part of the social system is the individual person, who has a personality and certain needs. For example, the needs may be for power, achievement, or affiliation. The individual's personality and needs disposition will interact with the institution's need for goal achievement. Somewhere in that dynamic interaction, the behavior seen in organizations is manifested as a result. Sometimes organizations appear to be in total chaos; sometimes they run smoothly and efficiently. The manifested result depends on the dynamic interaction between the organization, with its need to achieve goals, and individual employees, with their own personalities and unique drives and desires (Getzels, 1958) (Figure 10.2). Both organizations and employees have a set of values, personality, and culture. Thus nurses can examine their personal and group "fit" with any organization as one criterion for effectiveness.

For nurses as professional employees, the question is, Whom do they serve? Do they serve the needs of the organization as a business—with pressures for efficiency, mass production, and cost containment? Or do they serve the needs of the client—who may want teaching and counseling time, rehabilitation time, home care planning coordination, and individualized but time-consuming care? There is an underlying dynamic

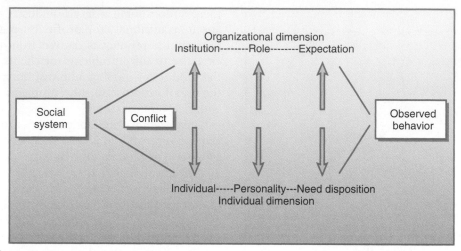

Figure 10.2
Social system and behavior. (Data from Getzels, J. [1958]. Administration as a social process. In A. Halpin (Ed.), *Administrative theory in education* [pp. 150-165]. Chicago: University of Chicago Press.)

tension between bureaucratic and professional values identified as a problem for nurses called "reality shock" (Kramer, 1974). This parallels the organizational-individual tensions that arise in social systems. The behavior of any nurse in a health care organization can be seen as a dynamic interaction and an outcome of the nurse interacting with the specific social system in which the nursing care delivery is embedded.

When a nurse accepts a position in a health care agency, that nurse makes a commitment to the goals and philosophy of the nursing service department within that organization. Likewise, when a nurse assumes a managerial position in an organization, that same commitment is made, as well as a commitment to subscribe to the philosophy of management of that organization. Although an individual may or may not personally believe in or subscribe to the organization's philosophy, taking a position in an organization implies an agreement to accommodate to the organization's philosophy while at work. Therefore an examination of organizational mission statements such as the philosophy, goals, and objectives statements promotes a greater understanding of the specific institution and may promote more

effective organizational participation by nurses. To begin to learn how the organization runs, the first step is to examine the philosophy, structure, and policies. The functional aspects of organizations include the culture, philosophy, purposes, objectives, policies, and procedures related to the work environment. They are key aspects of managerial planning.

ORGANIZATIONAL MISSION STATEMENTS

Strategic Planning

Strategic plans are deliberative organizational documents developed to identify, gain consensus about, and communicate where an organization is going, over what timeframe, how it will get there and how it will decide whether it got there (McNamara, 1999a). The focus for a strategic plan often is the entire organization because these documents need to be unifying and integrated tools for the entire organization. Strategic plans may be developed for specific products, services, or programs, but these would need to be integrated with the total organizational plan. Often a business plan is used instead. Keys to all strategic planning efforts are concentrated attention on the clarity of the meaning of words and on gaining consensus about the final result in order to develop a sense of ownership in the plan.

Factors such as leadership, culture, complexity, size, and internal expertise will have an impact on which model or approach is chosen for strategic planning. Some examples of types of strategic planning models are goals-based, issues-based, organic, and scenario planning (McNamara, 1999a). For example, issues-based strategic planning would start by exploring the issues facing the organization, then identify strategies for those issues, and then move to action plans. The most common form of strategic planning is the goals-based form. This starts with a focus on the organization's mission, followed by vision and values statements. Next, goals are identified, and strategies to achieve the goals and action plans to identify

who is responsible and accountability timeframes are detailed. The timeline (e.g., 1 year, 5 years) into the future and the length of the strategic plan vary. The benefits of strategic planning include the ability to "clearly define the purpose of the organization and to establish realistic goals and objectives consistent with that mission in a defined time frame within the organization's capacity for implementation" (McNamara, 1999a, p. 3). This may require an outside facilitator.

Mission Statements

Using a goals-based strategic planning method, the first step is to develop a mission statement. The mission of any organization is its purpose, function, and reason why it exists. Organizations exist to do something such as produce a product or deliver a service. The founders' intentions for what they wanted to achieve by starting this

---

Research Note

Source: Drenkard, K.N. (2001). Creating a future worth experiencing: Nursing strategic planning in an integrated healthcare delivery system. *Journal of Nursing Administration, 31*(7/8), 364-376.

Purpose

The nurse executive team of a large not-for-profit integrated health care delivery system needed a strategy In order to have nursing care viewed as a competitive advantage in meeting the system's core values of caring for and about people, community responsibility, and innovation. This article describes the planning process, tools, methodology used, and lessons learned.

Discussion

Strategy was seen as a solution to pressing nursing work environment pressures and problems. The strategic planning process was based on an eight-step business planning model. The methodology used a transformational leadership assessment tool, quality planning methods, and large group intervention to engage nurses in implementation strategies. Systems theory formed the foundation for thinking about the process and the application of the results to multiple levels of the organization. Detailed information is given about the following: getting started; the strategic planning process of assessment of the current state, creation of a vision, gap analysis, priority setting using quality tools, engagement of nursing in planning, baseline measurement and target selling; refinement of implementation plans and evaluation of outcomes; application at the unit level; and lessons learned.

Application to Practice

The strategic planning journey is clearly and explicitly detailed in this exemplar on strategic planning. The description is rich in detail and visual displays. Other organizations and nurse executives can use this article as a guide and roadmap to replicate the best parts and avoid or anticipate pitfalls.

organization need to be reexamined and refreshed periodically to keep the organization dynamic (Adams, 2004). For a health care organization, the mission relates to health care services—for example, client care, teaching, and research. For a nursing department's purpose, constraints include the organization's purpose, the state nurse practice act and other legal parameters, the context of the local community, and the directives of regulating agencies. The mission statement should be short, concise, and clear. The mission of the nursing department should mesh with the mission of the institution.

In developing a mission statement, factors such as the organization's products, services, markets, values, public image, and activities for survival need to be considered (McNamara, 1999b). In addition, the intent of the organization's founders and its history are useful to review. Often employees are unaware of historical background. Because the mission statement needs to describe the overall purpose of the organization, the wording needs to be carefully crafted. It needs to be derived by a process that respects the organization's culture. The statement needs to have sufficient description to clearly identify the purpose and scope and suggest some order of priorities (McNamara, 1999b).

Vision Statements

Vision statements are designed to address the preferred future of the organization. They draw on the mission, beliefs, and environment of the organization and are positive and inspiring. Vision statements are crafted to describe the most desirable state at some future point in time. Often, one step in planning is a gap analysis of the difference between the current state and the vision (Drenkard, 2001). The advantage of vision statements are that they transcend bounded thinking; identify direction; challenge and motivate; promote loyalty, focus, and commitment; and encourage creativity. Vision statements are designed to rise above fatigue, tradition, routine, and complacency. Visioning is setting a high-level direction through turbulent times and creating a compelling picture of a desirable future state.

Imagery and stories may be used to sustain the vision. Vision statements need to be vivid enough to keep the organization moving forward.

Values Statements

Core values are strongly held beliefs and priorities that guide organizational decision making. Core values are things that do not change. They are anchors or fundamentals that relate to mission and purpose and hold constant while operations and business strategies change. Values drive how people truly act in organizations. They are the bridge to align how people actually behave with preferred behaviors (McNamara, 1999b). Adams (2004) stated, "articulating values provides everyone with guiding lights, ways of choosing among competing priorities, and guidelines about how people will work together" (p. 2).

One way that core values are expressed are through lists or values statements as part of a strategic plan. Another way to express values as statements is to compose a statement of philosophy. Some organizations have philosophy statements and others use a mix of mission, vision, and values statements as a proxy for their philosophy. Both individuals and organizations can compose a statement of philosophy. For an individual, this would be an expression of personal and professional values, vision, and mission. Although difficult to do, writing a personal professional statement of philosophy is an exercise in clarity and communication.

A statement of **philosophy** is defined as an explanation of the systems of beliefs that determine how a mission or a purpose is to be achieved. An organization's philosophy states the beliefs, concepts, and principles of an organization. It serves as a guide for and an explanation of actions (Poteet & Hill, 1988). The philosophy is abstract: it describes an ideal state and gives direction to achieving the purpose. It often begins with "We believe that … ." For example, the system of beliefs, or philosophy, might be stated in any of the following ways:

- We believe that everyone has a right to the highest quality of client care.

- We believe that we have an obligation to render quality client care at a cost-effective price.
- We believe that any person who walks through the door should receive care, regardless of his or her ability to pay.

The philosophy has implications for a nurse's practice role. If an organization's stated mission includes client care, teaching, and research, then all employees will be expected to be involved in all three aspects of the mission. Part of the nurse's job will be to teach students and be involved in research. The nursing department's philosophy should be congruent with the organization's philosophy. The three vital components that form the core of a nursing department philosophy are the client, the nurse, and nursing practice (Poteet & Hill, 1988).

The organization's philosophy is important to assess as it relates to one's personal philosophy. For example, a potential employee on a job search might compare his or her own philosophy, both of nursing practice and of management, with the philosophy of an organization in which she or he might secure employment. Is there a match? For example, hospitals owned by religious organizations may prefer to hire people who share this same religious faith. If the nurse is not of that religious faith or if she or he has a prejudice or a lack of knowledge about that religious faith, it is advisable to assess personal fit with that particular organization. If there is some part of the philosophy that is personally distasteful, it can have implications for functioning within the practice environment. For example, there may be a specific religious tradition that is still pervasive within the organizational culture, even though the stated philosophy may say that the organization provides care to people of all faiths. That may be bothersome. One example occurs when an organization that is owned and run by a religious group opens each administrative meeting with a prayer. Another example occurs when a nurse believes in providing the total scope of public health services to clients, but the organization is run by for-profit principles that dictate only the provision of services that make a profit. Taking a job in an organization

suggests an implicit agreement to cooperate with the organization's values while at work.

Action Planning

Strategic planning efforts proceed from a focus on mission, vision, and values to the identification of major strategic goals and specific action plans. Establishing goals is an analytical process of deciding what the organization wants to achieve. According to Nickols (2000), actions and decisions are multidimensional in that there are many different kinds of effects that might be sought and created. Furthermore, interventions in complex systems may have a ripple effect when unintended and unforeseen results occur. Nickols recommended using a goals grid: four squares that map out answers to two "Do we want it?" questions and two "Do we have it?" questions. The two "Do we want it?" questions are as follows:

1. What do you want that you do not have (trying to achieve)?
2. What do you want that you already have (trying to preserve)?

The two "Do we have it?" questions are the following:

1. What don't you have that you do not want (trying to avoid)?
2. What do you have now that you do not want (trying to eliminate)?

The goals grid is a useful method for analyzing goals and objectives clearly, in an organized fashion and from four perspectives. Consciously thinking this through is an effort to improve performance.

In the early phase of goal identification, often an environmental analysis is conducted. One common method is called SWOT analysis (strengths, weaknesses, opportunities, and threats). Strengths are positive and internal, weaknesses are negative and internal, opportunities are positive and external, and threats are negative and external factors of the organization's environment. Critical issues are identified and analyzed by a SWOT analysis. This allows the organization to pinpoint and focus in on the critical few issues that have the most impact. As a result of issues analyses, the organization can then set major goals to be achieved.

Sometimes groups doing strategic planning become tired and bored at this point. However, there is one more key phase to accomplish: action planning. Each major goal needs to have objectives, responsibilities, and timelines specified for tracking and evaluation purposes. Without careful action planning and diligent managerial follow-up monitoring, the strategic plan is in danger of drifting away, being ignored, or "collecting dust on a shelf" (McNamara, 1999a, p. 10). Communicating and monitoring the plan are key managerial activities. Managers are aided in this effort by the use of spreadsheet formats and clearly specified objectives to guide actions, decisions, and revisions.

Objectives

Objectives are written, behavior-specific statements of desired outcomes. *Objectives* are defined as the identified outcomes directing activity toward achieving the purpose of the organization or unit (Trexler, 1987). Organizations use written, behavior-specific objectives so that each employee knows what it is that the organization is trying to achieve. Objectives are the fundamental strategy of an institution (Drucker, 1973). The objectives of each work unit are used for establishing priorities, strategies, plans, work assignments, and the allocation of resources (Drucker, 1973; Trexler, 1987). Objectives need to be specific, realistic, attainable, and challenging; they must fit with the organization's goals and emphasize the work of greatest importance.

Policies and Procedures

Policies and procedures are two functional elements of an organization that are extensions of the mission statements. Both are written rules derived from the mission statement. Together they determine the nursing systems of the work unit and the department of nursing. The purpose of policies and procedures is to provide some order and stability so that the unit works as a coordinated group and functions in a coordinated manner within the larger structure of nursing and the institution. Organizations need to integrate the behaviors of the employees to avoid random chaos and maintain some order, function, and structure.

These plans are often referred to as *standard operating policies and procedures.* They guide the personnel in decision making. A **policy** is a guideline that has been formalized. It directs the action for thinking about and solving recurring problems related to the objectives of the organization.

There will be specific times when it is not clear who is supposed to do something, under what circumstances it should be done, or what should be done about unusual circumstances. For example, often there are controversies about the dress code because of disagreements about the definition of what is "appropriate." This occurs, for example, when the dress code says, "Nurses will come to work dressed in appropriate attire."

Policies direct decision making and serve as guides to increase the likelihood of consistency in decisions and actions. Policies should be written, understandable, and general in nature to cover all employees. If written, they should be readily available in the same form to all employees. Policies should be reviewed during employee orientation because they indicate the organization's intentions for goal achievement.

After institutional approval, policies should be placed in a manual, indexed, classified, and noted in the table of contents. Policies so organized can be easily replaced with revised ones, which often become necessary in light of new environmental circumstances. Policy formulation in any organization is an ongoing core process. Hospitals will have a standing committee for the review of policies as a part of the organizational structure. Policies establish broad limits on and provide direction to decision making; yet they permit some initiative and individuality.

Policies can be implied, or unwritten, if they are essentially established by patterns of decisions that have been made. In this situation, the informal policies represent an interpretation of observed behavior. For example, the organization

---

Box **10.1**

Policies

- Serve as guides
- Help coordinate plans
- Control performance
- Increase consistency of action
- Should be written
- Usually are general in nature
- Refer to all employees

---

may expect caring treatment for all clients. This expectation may not be written as a policy of the organization. However, by the decisions and disciplinary actions that occur, an employee can infer that there is a policy that will be enforced even though it is not written. However, the vast majority of policies are and should be written. Informal and unwritten policies are less desirable because they can lead to systematic bias or unfairness in their application and enforcement (Box 10.1).

There are some general areas in nursing that require policy formulation. These are areas in which there is confusion about the locus of responsibility and where lack of guidance might result in the neglect, malpractice, or "malperformance" of an act necessary to the client's welfare. For example, clear policies need to be in place about medication error reporting and follow-up. In those areas in which it is important that all persons adhere to the same pattern of decision making given a certain circumstance, a policy is necessary so that it can be used as a guideline. Also, areas pertaining to the protection of clients' or families' rights should have written policies. For example, the use of restraints to manage difficult clients came under scrutiny as the Omnibus Budget Reconciliation Act of 1987 (OBRA) pushed restraint-reduction strategies and created policy revisions. Another example is the need for policies related to "do not resuscitate" and end-of-life care (Wilson, 1996). Areas involving matters of personnel management and welfare,

such as vacation leave, should have written policies. In such cases, the lack of a uniform policy would be considered unfair. Many conflicts arise about the scheduling of vacations: How many people can be off at any one time? How long in advance must a vacation request be made? How is the priority for granting requests to be determined (e.g., by seniority or by order of request)? The policy is the guideline for determining specific decisions.

Procedures are step-by-step directions and methods for actions to follow in common situations. **Procedures** are descriptions of how to carry out an activity. They are usually written in sufficient detail to provide the information required by all persons engaging in the activity. What this means is that procedures should include a statement of purpose and identify who is to perform the activity. Procedures should include the steps necessary and the list of supplies and equipment needed. A procedure is a more specific guide to action than is a policy statement. Procedures usually are departmental or divisionally specific, so they will vary across an institution. They may be very detailed as to how to perform a specific procedure on a specific unit. They help to achieve regularity. They are a ready reference for all personnel (Box 10.2).

Box **10.2**

Procedures

- Provide step-by-step methods
- Are written in detail
- Provide guidelines for commonly occurring events
- Provide a ready reference
- Guide performance of an activity
- Should include the following:
  - A statement of purpose
  - Identification of who performs activity
  - Steps in the procedure
  - A list of supplies and equipment needed

The similarities between policies and procedures are that both are a means for accomplishing goals and objectives. Both are necessary for the smooth functioning of any work group or organization. The difference between a policy and a procedure is that a policy is a general guideline for decision making about actions, whereas a procedure gives directions for actions. For example, policies about the use of restraints to manage difficult clients would indicate when such restraint use is appropriate. Procedures would cover how to apply specific devices.

There should be a policy written as a guide for the decisions needed in recurrent and anticipated situations. For example, there may be a policy about assisting with an abortion or whether abortions are performed. A policy is a more general guide for decision making; a procedure is more like a cookbook recipe or a how-to guide giving specific directions about how to perform a certain act or function. There are legal implications to the application of policies and procedures. For example, the nurse may be held liable for failing to follow written policies and procedures. Thus it is important for nurses to be informed about the policies and procedures governing practice in an institution.

LEADERSHIP AND MANAGEMENT IMPLICATIONS

Change and competition in health care create circumstances that may drive the need to create or revise an organization's or a department of nursing's strategic plan, vision statement, or statement of philosophy. The philosophy should be a dynamic and vital values statement. Graham and colleagues (1987) described how to implement a new or changed philosophy. They used a marketing-based perspective to transform a traditional philosophy statement into a positioning statement. They articulated a vision and provided a framework for planning to thrive, rather than merely survive, in times of change. This implies that a philosophy may be different from the vision in an organization. Both statements may be required. Graham and colleagues (1987) set a goal of having a philosophy statement that was "unique, concise, measurable, and easy to remember" (p. 15). To accomplish this through group work, a marketing strategy called *positioning* was used as a basis for discussion and communication. A positioning statement about four areas of excellence was developed and integrated into all aspects of the organizational documents and nursing care processes.

⚠ LEADERSHIP & MANAGEMENT **BEHAVIORS**

Leadership Behaviors

- Inspires a vision that is reflected in a philosophy
- Enables followers to accomplish the purpose
- Motivates followers to achieve objectives
- Influences the group to develop the philosophy creatively
- Provides personal consideration
- Guides the development of policies and procedures

Management Behaviors

- Ensures that the nursing department philosophy is meshed with the organization's philosophy

- Measures outcomes
- Reviews and revises policies and procedures
- Directs subordinates to achieve objectives
- Monitors purpose and objectives
- Implements the "philosophy in action"

Overlap Areas

- Develops a philosophy, purpose, and objectives
- Develops policies and procedures

Clearly both the strategic plan and the philosophy need to be reviewed periodically and may need to be revised completely if major changes occur. This is especially true in the case of a merger (Appenzeller, 1993). Normally, the philosophy guides actions. However, in times of rapid change, revision may required so that the strategic plan and the philosophy reflect current practices.

Periodic review is necessary to keep pace with what is or should be occurring in the work environment. With rapid change, it may be easy to overlook the philosophy and mission statements. If the philosophy needs to be revised, who does this? Commitment to a strategic plan or philosophy of nursing is fostered by input from all members and by the participation of the group in its formulation. In one facility this process included task force selection, preparation of the task force, review of strategies to develop a philosophy, details of the process used, and presentation of the resulting document (Cody, 1990).

One implication for leadership and management is the relationship of organizational documents such as strategic plans and goals with the leader/manager's responsibility to create a productive work environment. Brown-Stewart (1987) discussed "thinly disguised contempt," or the translation of managerial decisions into the work environment. The reality of effectiveness in a managerial role is that managers can have a tremendous impact on the work environment by virtue of their basic personality, problem-solving and decision-making strategies, and managerial and leadership style. When the organization's environment promotes contempt, it may affect the availability of competent nurses. Specifically, through the strategic construction of a philosophy and culture, leaders and managers affect the morale and job satisfaction of the nurses. This can be done by a focus on core values.

Behaviors that reflect a lack of concern for people and a contempt for employees create barriers to developing excellence in organizations. Brown-Stewart (1987) listed the following four ways in which contempt for people is demonstrated:

1. Telling clients what they want instead of responding to the client's perceived needs

2. Casting aspersions on or depersonalizing clients

3. Habitual lack of courtesy

4. Contempt for employees

The concept of "thinly disguised contempt" is closely related to the idea of a "philosophy in action." Although there are written mission statements, the implementation of these documents comes through people, especially in managerial decision making and resource allocation. According to Brown-Stewart (1987), some examples of contempt behaviors are a consumptive, as opposed to investment, attitude toward employees; lack of orientation; ambiguity of mission, values, and job requirements; lack of adequate proximate employee parking areas; physicians treated preferentially; ignoring the client's family; lack of attention to client's comfort; amount and type of nursing staff on duty; failure to communicate; and insensitivity when creating an inconvenience. Thus the leadership and management style becomes important at the interface of mission and values with culture and philosophy and any individual nurse in a work environment.

One result of organizational philosophies and cultures that create barriers to quality nursing practice is that nurses manifest a sense of job dissatisfaction, feelings of frustration or powerlessness, a sense of not being a part of the decision-making process, and a feeling that supervisors are not empathetic. Because nurses as professionals work primarily as employees, tension in the relationship with the work environment results in a concern about job satisfaction, commitment, and turnover. There is extensive literature on job satisfaction in nursing. The research on social integration, for example, indicates that nurses feel happy and more satisfied if they are part of a cohesive work group. Thus the philosophy and mission statements may need to be examined to see whether they support work group cohesion. For example, leaders and managers can operationalize values that promote positive resolution of conflict in work groups. Resources can be allocated to work group functioning. Philosophy statements can speak directly to valuing a positive work climate.

It is important to look at the factors in the environment that might impede the functioning of nursing and that therefore could make nurses dissatisfied, unhappy, or at risk for a high degree of turnover. Nurses feel strongly about needing job autonomy and having control over their practice. They feel that they need autonomy to meet legal requirements and client care needs adequately. Generally, nurses want improvements in pay, image, and working conditions (Minnick et al., 1989) (Figure 10.3). These are the three areas in which nurses seek substantial changes. The issues related to working conditions include shift work and rotation, floating, the number of weekends worked, job security, workload, the amount of recognition for the actual work done, the level of legal liability carried, and a sense of autonomy. If nurses are vested with the responsibility to carry out complex client care, they feel the urgency to be free from interference as they make basic decisions

about the care of clients that are necessary to effect outcomes.

Nurse leaders and managers can create and maintain an environment that facilitates the practice of the professional nurse. Leadership is required to bring about a good environment. Three elements form the basis for the creation of a positive professional work environment: fun, hope, and trouble. Nurses can use these elements to support each other, stimulate creativity, and work together successfully (McCloskey, 1991). Another aspect of leadership and management in times of change is the creation of a healthy work environment as a nursing administration core value. Striving for a healthy work environment is a conscious choice. Elements for constructing such an environment include acknowledgment of the reality of the present environment, clear behavioral expectations and standards, systems and structures to ensure that organizational changes

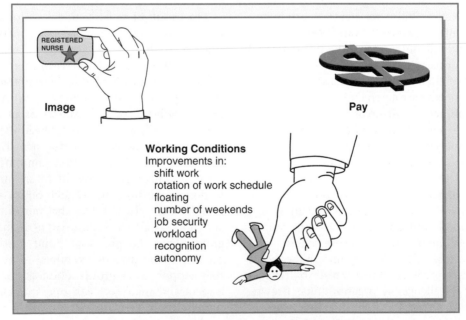

Figure 10.3
What nurses want. (Data from Minnick, A., Roberts, M., Curran, C., & Ginzberg, E. [1989]. What do nurses want? Priorities for action. *Nursing Outlook,* 37, 214-218.)

are enduring, and a means to continually assess the health of the work environment.

Leaders have both the opportunity and the responsibility to preserve concepts of dignity, integrity, honesty, and compassion in the working environment of nursing. In the University of Minnesota Health System, a document listing the characteristics of a healthy work environment was developed and disseminated to describe expectations for the key components of open communication, trust, and mutual respect in effective working relationships. Kreitzer and colleagues (1997) offered this example: "In a healthy work environment: I am viewed as an asset, people call me by name, my contributions and talents are acknowledged and recognized, communication is open, direct and honest" (p. 38).

Nurses are a key and critical component of the functioning of a health care organization. In today's environment, clients come to a hospital for nursing care. As care delivery shifts toward home and community settings, clients still seek nursing care because of needing the assessment, education, and evaluation skills of nurses. Thus, keeping a happy, stable, and satisfied nursing work force is an organizational pressure for hospitals and other health care organizations delivering nursing services. This can be formally expressed as a positive core value in strategic plans.

Caring and Advocacy

Caring is one fundamental philosophical principle of nursing. It has been described as the essence of nursing, and the visibility of caring as an important nursing concept is growing (Pepin, 1992). *Caring* has been interpreted as meaning that persons, events, projects, and things matter to an individual (Benner & Wrubel, 1988). Caring in nursing is seen as related to attention and concern for the client; responsibility for the client; and regard, fondness, or attachment to the client (Gaut, 1983). Swanson (1991) offered the following definition of caring: "a nurturing way of relating to a valued other toward whom one feels a personal sense of commitment and responsibility" (p. 162). The five categories or processes of caring are

knowing, being with, doing for, enabling, and maintaining belief (Swanson, 1991).

As the basis or essence of nursing practice, caring can be seen to be a crucial component of nursing department and unit mission, vision, values and philosophy statements. It then should be explicit in the written documents and obvious in the "philosophy in action." Perhaps, however, not all organizations value caring. If caring is valued by an organization, this will be reflected in decisions, resource allocations, types of power used, handling of conflict, recognition of nurses as professionals, and strategies chosen to motivate nurses. Thus the philosophy of the institution provides a glimpse at the concept of caring and its intersection with leadership and management. If it is a cherished value, then the concept of caring will be incorporated into leadership styles. For example, does caring about employees come through in the day-to-day work situation? Caring can be manifested in resource decisions about personnel, equipment, and supplies. How do organizations respond to a nursing shortage? What strategies are used when there is a need to reduce the size of the workforce? Nurses can examine the written philosophy and the obvious decision patterns to see whether caring is valued and promoted in the organization.

Patient advocacy also is a fundamental philosophical principle of nursing. This core value emphasizes the protection of patients' rights. Patient advocacy is assumed to be an inherent part of clinical practice. Because advocacy is so embedded in nursing practice, it may be invisible and difficult to describe (Foley et al., 2002). Advocacy was initially incorporated into nursing practice when nurses developed a sense of service more to their patients than to physicians. This central role of advocacy was formalized in the 1970s when language changes occurred and the code of ethics published by the American Nurses Association included a definition of patient advocacy (Foley et al., 2002). Research into nurses' advocacy experiences has revealed that learning about advocacy may be haphazard and situationally dependent. Nurses reported that advocacy was part of who they were, that they learned advocacy by watching other nurse-patient interactions, and that they felt more confident in difficult situations that required intervention on behalf of patients when they had strong advocacy skills (Foley et al., 2002).

CURRENT ISSUES AND TRENDS

In times of change, organizational strategic plans, philosophies, policies, and vision statements also may undergo change. What would happen if nurses were the supervisors of physicians—that is, if physicians were employees and the nurses actually managed the work flow? There have been a few organizations where nurses have admitting privileges and physicians do not. Across the country alternative systems of care delivery are being tested, and some of those systems are focused on community-based and nurse-managed centers. There is a persuasive argument that advanced practice nurses are cost-effective providers of primary care. In an era of fiscal constraint, there is an opportunity for nurses to redefine and reposition their roles within the health care delivery system. Strategic plans may need to change in response.

Positive job motivation is an important element in the functioning of human service organizations. It could be assumed that job satisfaction should follow from an environment in which each person's expertise is acknowledged and respected, and nurses go home at the end of their shift feeling good about their work. Thus the influence of philosophy and values on organizational culture may be more visible if it is practiced as well as being written.

Summary

- An organization is a group acting to achieve a goal.
- The two dimensions of a social system are the environment and the individual.
- Behavior in organizations is a function of the dynamic interaction of these two dimensions.

- Service industries, such as nursing and health care, emphasize quality and cost control.
- Strategic plans are developed to clearly communicate the organization's purpose and direction.
- The main parts of a strategic plan are the vision, values, and mission statements and the action plans using goals and objectives statements.
- Policies and procedures are two functional elements of an organization that flow from the mission statements and help to guide decision making and performance.
- Organizational philosophies affect nursing practice through elements related to culture, job satisfaction, and turnover.
- Strategic plans may need to be revised as circumstances change.

Study Questions

1. How do previous employee experiences color perception and attitude? Why do these perceptions linger?
2. Do nurses profess loyalty to the organization/job or to the profession/work of nursing? Can an individual have loyalty to both?
3. How do you use the change process to implement a new philosophy in a preestablished work group?
4. What is the "philosophy in action"? Cite some examples. Describe why this makes a difference.
5. What problems are solved by having policies and procedures?
6. What decisions can nurses make without a written policy?
7. Is caring the central value for nursing? Explain.

CASE STUDY

The executive director (ED) of StayAtHome, a not-for-profit home health care agency, had a problem. He felt that the agency was drifting along aimlessly. The most recent Board of Directors meeting also had been challenging. He had been intensely questioned by the board members about financial and performance outcomes. Action was needed.

CRITICAL THINKING EXERCISE

Nurse Manager Anthony Gardner finds himself in the nurse executive's office. Nurse Gardner has a problem with a staff nurse who was seen yelling at two nursing assistants in the middle of a crowded area. Nurse Gardner is asked to discuss what happened. Nurse Gardner says the staff nurse was irritated by the nursing assistants' loitering and yelled at them to get back to work. Nurse Gardner says he is too busy to spend all his time supervising nurses who have no sense of teamwork. The nurse executive carefully explains that a staff opinion survey has uncovered that a significant proportion of the staff reported experiencing abuse or confrontation in the workplace, leading to conflict, tension, and stress. A major component of the reported abuse on this unit was "being yelled at." The nurse executive explained that the hospital has embarked on a new "healthy work environment" initiative and that there are written behavioral expectations and standards in existence. The nurse executive gives a copy of these standards and the "respect, communicate, and take responsibility" philosophy to Nurse Gardner.

1. Is there a problem?
2. What is the problem?
3. Whose problem is it?
4. What should the nurse manager do?
5. What interactions should have occurred before this point?
6. Whose values are in operation in this situation? Is there a clash of values?
7. If so, how should they be resolved?
8. Are there any legal considerations?

The ED took some time to carefully think through the situation and analyze the organization's status. He realized that goals were unclear and unfocused. Many questions arose, and the ED's objectives seemed to be in conflict with statements made by board members.

To engineer a solution, the ED hit upon a plan: he would prepare an exercise to clarify goals and objectives. First the ED worked through the following questions:

1. What are you trying to achieve?
2. What are you trying to preserve?
3. What are you trying to avoid?
4. What are you trying to eliminate?

Next, he plotted these on the Goals Grid (Nickols, 2000). Then he formulated objectives for each of the goals in the four quadrants.

Armed with his initial Goals Grid exercise, the ED prepared materials (blank forms and the four questions) for the next board meeting. He called the president of the board to discuss the exercise and what he hoped to gain from it. They both agreed that the board would do the exercise "cold" and then compare their results with the ED's.

The exercise was well received at the next board meeting. It generated a lively discussion. Consensus around goals was reached, and further work on specific objectives was delegated to committees. The board decided to hire a consultant to plan and implement formal strategic planning for the agency.

REFERENCES

Adams, D. (2004). *The pillars of planning: Mission values, vision.* Washington, DC: National Endowment for the Arts. Retrieved July 5, 2004, from *www.arts.endow.gov/resources/Lessons/ADAMS.HTML*

Appenzeller, L. (1993). Merging nursing departments: An experience. *Journal of Nursing Administration, 23*(12), 55-60.

Benner, P., & Wrubel, J. (1988). Caring comes first. *American Journal of Nursing, 88*(8), 1072-1075.

Brown-Stewart, P. (1987). Thinly disguised contempt: A barrier to excellence. *Journal of Nursing Administration, 17*(4), 14-18.

Cody, B. (1990). Shaping the future through a philosophy of nursing. *Journal of Nursing Administration, 20*(10), 16-22.

Drenkard, K.N. (2001). Creating a future worth experiencing: Nursing strategic planning in an integrated healthcare delivery system. *Journal of Nursing Administration, 31*(7/8), 364-376.

Drucker, P. (1973). *Management: Tasks, responsibilities, practices.* New York: Harper & Row.

Ehrat, K.S. (1994). Mission statement, goals, and values. In R. Spitzer-Lehmann (Ed.), *Nursing management desk reference: Concepts, skills and strategies* (pp. 37-59). Philadelphia: W.B. Saunders.

Foley, B.J., Minick, M.P., & Kee, C.C. (2002). How nurses learn advocacy. *Journal of Nursing Scholarship, 34*(2), 181-186.

Gaut, D. (1983). Development of a theoretically adequate description of caring. *Western Journal of Nursing Research, 5,* 313-324.

Getzels, J. (1958). Administration as a social process. In A. Halpin (Ed.), *Administrative theory in education* (pp. 150-165). Chicago: University of Chicago Press.

Graham, P., Constantini, S., Balik, B., Bedore, B., Hooke, M., Papin, D., et al. (1987). Operationalizing a nursing philosophy. *Journal of Nursing Administration, 17*(3), 14-18.

Kramer, M. (1974). *Reality shock: Why nurses leave nursing.* St Louis: Mosby.

Kramer, M., & Schmalenberg, C. (1988a). Magnet hospitals: Institutions of excellence: Part 1. *Journal of Nursing Administration, 18*(1), 13-24.

Kramer, M., & Schmalenberg, C. (1988b). Magnet hospitals: Institutions of excellence: Part 2. *Journal of Nursing Administration, 18*(2), 11-19.

Kreitzer, M.J., Wright, D., Hamlin, C., Towey, S., Marko, M., & Disch, J. (1997). Creating a healthy work environment in the midst of organizational change and transition. *Journal of Nursing Administration, 27*(6), 35-41.

McCloskey, J. (1991). Creating an environment for success with fun, hope, and trouble. *Journal of Nursing Administration, 21*(4), 5-6.

McNamara, C. (1999a). *Strategic planning (in nonprofit or for-profit organizations).* St. Paul, MN: Carter McNamara.

Retrieved July 8, 2004, from *www.managementhelp.org/plan_dec/str_plan/str_plan.htm*

McNamara, C. (1999b). *Basics of developing mission, vision and values statements.* St. Paul, MN: Carter McNamara. Retrieved July 5, 2004, from *www.mapnp.org/library/plan_dec/str_plan/stmnts.htm*

Minnick, A., Roberts, M., Curran, C., & Ginzberg, E. (1989). What do nurses want? Priorities for action. *Nursing Outlook, 37,* 214-218.

Nickols, F. (2000). *The goals grid: A tool for clarifying goals and objectives.* Howard, OH: Distance Consulting. Retrieved July 8, 2004, from *www.home.att.net/~nickols/goals_grid.htm*

Pepin, J. (1992). Family caring and caring in nursing. *Image, 24*(2), 127-131.

Poteet, G., & Hill, A. (1988). Identifying the components of a nursing service philosophy. *Journal of Nursing Administration, 18*(10), 29-33.

Swanson, K. (1991). Empirical development of a middle range theory of caring. *Nursing Research, 40*(3), 161-166.

Trexler, B. (1987). Nursing department purpose, philosophy, and objectives: Their use and effectiveness. *Journal of Nursing Administration, 17*(3), 8-12.

Wilson, D.M. (1996). Highlighting the role of policy in nursing practice through a comparison of "DNR" policy influences and "No CPR" decision influences. *Nursing Outlook, 44*(6), 272-279.

Zander, K. (1992). Nursing care delivery methods and quality. *Series on Nursing Administration, 3,* 86-104.

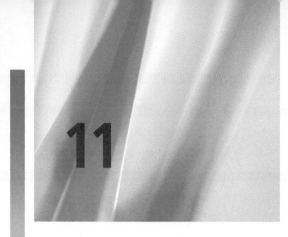

11

Organizational Structure

Patricia L. Horstman   Michelle A. Janney

CHAPTER OBJECTIVES

- Define and describe organizational structure
- Compare and contrast hierarchical, matrix and project team organizational structures
- Analyze organizational types best suited to nursing
- Contrast centralization and decentralization
- Identify current trends in health care and the impact on organizational structure
- Exercise critical thinking to conceptualize and analyze possible solutions to a practice exercise

The structure of an organization is the framework for facilitating the organization's functioning and goal attainment. Organizational structure refers to the linkage of jobs and positions into a coordinated network through which communication, delegation, power, and authority flow. It does not refer to a physical building, or "bricks and mortar." Organizational structure is a part of the infrastructure supporting an organized group of workers gathered to do work. Multiple organizational structure configurations exist. No model is right for all circumstances.

An organization exists for the purpose of achieving a certain goal or set of goals. For example, in health care obvious goals might be higher quality of care, reduction of costs, and increased efficiency. Whether the goals are realized or not may depend heavily on the decisions made by people within the organization.

The general goal of nursing might be described as the delivery of a service that is caring, high-quality, and cost-effective. How nurses' roles intermix with the structure of the organization influences the accomplishment of organizational goals. Cumbey and Alexander (1998) found that organizational structure was one critical variable predicting job satisfaction in a group of public health nurses. "Empirical evidence has shown that the organization of nurse's work is a major determinant of patient and staff welfare" (Havens & Aiken, 1999, p. 19).

DEFINITIONS

Organization Structure

The **structure of an organization** is defined as the total of the ways in which its labor is divided into distinct tasks and the way coordination is achieved among these tasks. Structure is a by-product of two fundamental and opposing needs of every organized human activity: to divide the labor into the specific tasks to be performed and to coordinate these tasks to accomplish the activity or goal. Factors influencing the structural design of an organization include size, age, technical systems

◣ LEADING & MANAGING **DEFINED**

Structure of an Organization

The sum total of the ways an organization's labor is divided into distinct tasks and then the way coordination is achieved among these tasks.

Division of Labor

The way the work is broken up into pieces or tasks and then assigned.

Span of Control

The number of workers supervised by a manager.

Scalar Process

The creation of levels of authority in a hierarchy.

Line and Staff Positions

The array of positions into direct producers and support positions.

Position

A collection of tasks that are configured together for performance, usually by one individual.

Authority

The right to act or command the actions of others.

Responsibility

Allocation and acceptance of a task.

Accountability

The liability for task performance.

Centralization

Power to make decisions concentrated at the top of the organization.

Decentralization

Power to make decisions filtered down toward the individual worker.

---

used, and the environment in which the organization functions (Mintzberg, 1993). In general, organizational structure refers to the mechanisms developed to balance specialization of work roles with a sufficient amount of coordination to accomplish tasks and goals (Mark, 1989) (Figure 11.1).

Nurses typically work within an organizational structure and are employees of an organization. This structure gives the work some kind of order, distinction, and framework. It also serves to control variations in behavior among individuals, avoids chaos, directs the flow of information, determines positions, and provides orderliness to the flow of work.

In organizational theory the idea of management is associated with organizational structure. It is thought that by using the classic concepts of organizational structure such as the division of labor, span of control, scalar process, and line and staff, any human undertaking can be managed and organized.

DIVISION OF LABOR

The **division of labor** is one of the classic elements of management. Because managers cannot do the work by themselves, the work is divided into pieces and assigned or delegated as responsibilities to others. **Span of control** refers to the number of staff nurses and non-nurse personnel reporting to a nurse manager (Pabst, 1993). The **scalar process** is the creation of levels in an organization, or the direct line of command from top to bottom. In nursing, a hierarchical bureaucracy creates layers or scales of positions with differing amounts of power attached to them. **Line positions** are in the direct line of hierarchical authority from top to bottom in an organization. They are central to

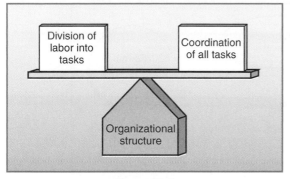

Figure 11.1
Organizational structure.

producing the product of the organization. **Staff positions** are outside the direct hierarchical authority chain. They provide expertise and knowledge to assist the line positions in meeting the organization's goals. The purpose of an organization and its management structure is to convey the vision and directives of the top person down to the bottom level of operations, thereby accomplishing work through delegation.

Influences on Structure

There are four major influences on structure: (1) technology, (2) the social environment, (3) size, and (4) the repetitiveness of the tasks (Mintzberg, 1993). Structures can be highly influenced by the nature of the technology. For example, within nursing and the health care system, technology—including computerization, sophisticated patient care equipment, telecommunications, and technological devices used to deliver nursing care—can and does affect the type of structure that might be effective for nursing.

Like the nature of the technology, the character of the social environment will affect a specific organization and most likely require some changes in the structure. For example, today U.S. health care is affected by the fact that consumers are active and concerned. Furthermore, social change in the larger environment creates financial, psychological, and care delivery implications and drives organizational change within health

care institutions. In addition, generational demographics and age cohorts (e.g., Baby Boomers) influence national financial and political structures and health care delivery because of values, preferences, demands, expectations, and market power.

Structure is further influenced by the size of the organization and how repetitive the work tasks are. There is a different type of structure that works in manufacturing firms such as automobile assembly plants, as compared with the work of nurses in health care. In general, larger organizations are slower to make decisions and more complex to manage. This is partially a function of the greater number of interpersonal interactions that occur and the interrelatedness of roles and functions that are integral to the delivery of care.

Organizations generally appear to show evidence of a life cycle or growth and development changes that occur in spurts and are associated with changes in structure. New organizations start out small, with an organic and nonelaborated structure. As they begin to grow, they shift to an entrepreneurial stage with a powerful chief executive and coordination by direct supervision. Further growth brings a more formalized structure and the eventual shift to a bureaucratic structure and coordination by standardization. As further growth and aging occur, organizations may split into divisional structures that overlay the functional bureaucratic structure. Finally, a matrix structure may develop to rise above the divisional structure (Figure 11.2). A number of forces influence this process, for example, complexity, technical sophistication, stability, competition, hostile environments, and external control (Mintzberg, 1993).

TYPES OF STRUCTURES

Health care delivery systems, as one subset of all organizations, traditionally have used one of three basic types of administrative organizational structure: bureaucracy, matrix, or project team, also referred to as an adhocracy. A *bureaucracy* is an administrative organizational structure that is pyramidal, hierarchical, and centralized. A *matrix*

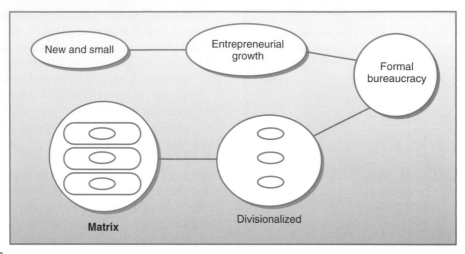

Figure 11.2
Organizational life cycle. (Data from Mintzberg, H. [1993]. *Structure in fives: Designing effective organizations.* Englewood Cliffs, NJ: Prentice-Hall.)

is an administrative organizational structure that is a complex combination or an interweaving of a bureaucratic structure with product and function combined, along with a project team component. A *project team* structure is an administrative organizational structure that is flat and decentralized and uses ad hoc committees or project teams exclusively to produce the work of the organization.

These three types of structures can be thought of as fitting across a continuum from a "giving orders" type of organization (the classic bureaucracy) to a highly delegation-oriented organization that uses sophisticated specialists (project team) (Figure 11.3). An organization's administrative structure can be identified, assessed, and analyzed. For example, in the United States most hospitals have adopted a classic hierarchical bureaucratic form. Some, faced with the need to better use and reward highly trained professional staff, developed a matrix structure. As health care reform drives restructuring, reengineering, and

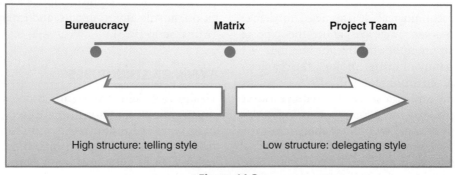

Figure 11.3
Continuum of organizational structures.

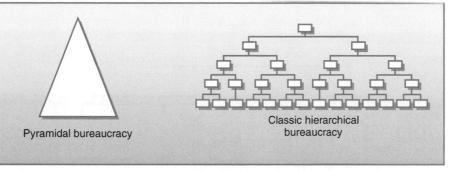

Figure 11.4
Pyramidal and hierarchical structures.

integration efforts, administrative organizational structures will also need to change.

Hierarchical Bureaucratic Structures

The first basic type of organizational structure is the *classic hierarchical bureaucracy* (Figure 11.4). Bureaucracy dates back as far as the ancient Roman army under Julius Caesar and the Roman Catholic Church, two large-sized and geographically dispersed organizations that relied on a bureaucratic structure to expand their scope of influence. This template evolved into one structural form, known as the classic hierarchical bureaucracy. Hospitals have long been organized in the traditional hierarchical pattern of many functional departments grouped into divisions. Each division reports to a vice president, who reports to the CEO.

The bureaucratic structural form, predominant in hospitals and many health care organizations in the United States, is described as being pyramidal. *Pyramidal* literally means shaped like a pyramid, with a wide base and narrow apex (see Figure 11.4). Bureaucracies have a wide base of workers and a narrow apex of decision makers. This model is designed to include a hierarchy of power and authority, arrayed from high to low, among the various organizational positions. Recent models have emerged in response to a new generation of workers desiring great autonomy. These new designs have "flipped" the pyramid

over to place higher authority and enhanced decision making at the staff level, formerly at the bottom of the pyramid; this change has demonstrated positive outcomes.

A *line-and-staff bureaucracy* is a variation of the pyramidal bureaucratic form that emerges when there is a need for technical experts (Figure 11.5). The experts are designated as *staff*. Staff positions rely on expertise and interpersonal power bases and are resource experts who provide expertise to the people who do the core work of the organization. An example of staff positions in nursing is a clinical nurse specialist (CNS) who is hired for knowledge development and expert consultation for selected patient groups. By contrast, line workers are those employees whose positions are in the direct chain of command and are assigned either as the workers producing the product or service or as the supervisors of the workers who produce the organization's output. Line positions have formal authority to make decisions. Common titles include vice president, director, and manager. Staff members serve in an advisory role.

Note that *line* and *staff* are terms used to describe workers' functions (Box 11.1). However, the actual titles given to positions may not correspond to their functions. Thus the designation of a line or staff position is not made based on the title used but rather on the function the position performs in the organization. For example, "staff nurses" in

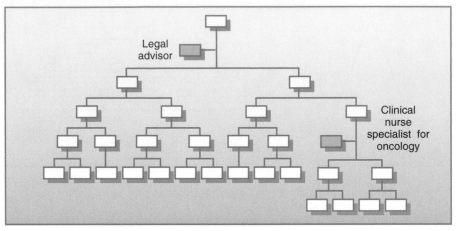

Figure 11.5
Line and staff bureaucracy.

Line and Staff Functions

Line Positions
- Responsible for achievement of organizational objectives
- Indicate lines of authority and accountability

Staff Positions
- Support line positions
- Advisory in nature
- Have no direct authority; use expertise and knowledge

---

a hospital function in a line position because they work directly to produce the product, in this case patient care.

Matrix Structures

Organizations may try to adapt to a turbulent environment by first moving to a matrix structure (Figure 11.6) to enhance operations. The matrix structure is used in environments where the work itself is complex. Essentially, it is a hybrid of bureaucracy and project teams, overlaid and combined.

Thus a matrix is really two structures in one, making it the most complex structure to administer and function within. It is the combination of the two coexisting structures that makes it a matrix form (Mintzberg, 1993).

In a matrix structure the line manager and a project manager function in a collaborative arrangement. In nursing, the nurse manager is the typical example of the line manager. The line manager has responsibility for a functional unit or department with a more narrow scope and focus on departmental outcomes. The rationale behind the approach is the expected gains in efficiency from specialization. The disadvantage is that managers focus on taking care of their particular functional area without adequate consideration of the impact of the combined actions on the overall organizations. A matrix structure combines outcome and function. Project managers help coordinate activities of employees across department lines. Included in the matrix structure are the elements of the classic hierarchical bureaucracy: a boss, intermediate bosses, and workers. For example, in nursing there might be a chief nurse executive, nurse managers, and staff nurses in a line of authority designed to accomplish patient care. Activities are organized according to a product or service and involve grouping

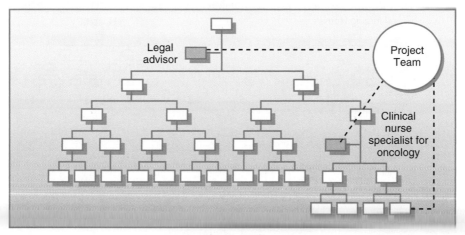

Figure 11.6
Matrix structure within an organization.

diverse functional activities under one administrative unit. The expectation is that the cumulative effect of being able to coordinate all functions for a particular product or service under an administrative unit outweighs any possible efficiency that may have been gained through a functional division. Nursing care in a matrix structure is delivered in a teamwork model or collaborative model that may cut across departments.

With rapidly expanding integration in health care systems, more organizations are moving to matrix structures. Thus interdisciplinary teams or work teams may also cross delivery settings. This situation creates a horizontal expansion of people across units, departments, and other "turf" boundaries. Nurses are natural boundary-spanning personnel because of their integrator role. Interdisciplinary teams need to be interactive within the vertical dimension of the matrix structure. In so doing they assist the health care organization to become more integrated. A matrix organizational structure thus facilitates a fully integrated system that provides a full continuum of health care services (Flarey & Smith, 1999).

A matrix organization is identified and characterized by management responsibilities that are shared between the line manager and the project

---

Box 11.2

Profile of a Matrix Organization

Where management responsibilities are shared between the line manager and the project manager and where both managers share staff and evaluative responsibilities for staff.

---

manager, including the sharing of staff and evaluation of their work (Box 11.2). In this type of combined structure a staff nurse's performance appraisal may have input from multiple sources, based on different work assignments in the organization. Collaborative behavior and an increased need for communication and coordination are important requirements.

In hospitals, especially in larger facilities, liaison roles, task forces, standing committees, and a dual authority structure characterize the matrix structure. As a result the communication becomes more horizontal than vertical. In a bureaucracy, communication goes down and up the chain of authority. In a matrix structure it takes place in a more horizontal fashion as staff talk with peers in other departments across the organization while collaborating on projects.

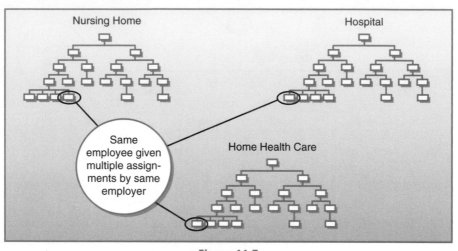

Figure 11.7
Matrix structure in an integrated network.

Matrix structures use connecting links within the organization or across the integrated parts of a large and complex integrated network (Figure 11.7). There are certain liaison roles. For example, in a hospital there may be a nurse liaison for purchasing, radiology, and quality improvement committees. Case managers often fill liaison roles. Matrix organizations are characterized by teamwork, multidisciplinary specialists, and problem-oriented teams. The major disadvantage of a matrix structure is that it requires sophisticated management skills. Furthermore, success is based on having well-educated workers who can handle a complex communication and authority web. For nurses this means an advanced level of interpersonal relationship skills and group and teamwork skills.

One example of a matrix arrangement in hospitals is a cardiopulmonary resuscitation (CPR) team. In a CPR or code team, members from various departments such as respiratory therapy (RT), intensive care unit (ICU) nursing, and electrocardiogram (ECG) staff respond to and run a code. This team forms a matrix group, with its own structure and procedures. Likewise, a renal dialysis or oncology nurse expert might move across the structure to do referrals. Another example is a

psychiatric nurse consultant moving across departments to evaluate a patient who has both a psychiatric and a physical disorder. Multidisciplinary care teams form matrix groups when they pull together personnel from various places to address a concern. For example, developing and implementing critical pathways, evidence-based practices, disease management initiatives, case management projects, or outcomes management efforts all may call forth an interdisciplinary team of specialists in a matrix configuration. Whereas departmentalization creates narrow perspectives and may discourage innovation because of a lack of cross-coordination and cross-fertilization, the benefits of a matrix structure include the organization's ability to be flexible with human resources, to respond to fluctuations in the environment more easily, and to enhance communications among team members.

Project Team Structure

On a continuum of highly structured to loosely structured, the third basic form of organizational structure is an adhocracy, or project team. The word *adhocracy* comes from the term *ad hoc committee.* The latter is an organizational structure that uses teams of specialists who are organized to complete specific jobs (Mintzberg, 1993). This structure is primarily used with highly specialized professional group practices, such as those in accounting, engineering, architecture, or space exploration. The project work comes into the organization, and the expertise of the various members is used according to specialty and needed expertise. Common examples include a research grant team or a National Aeronautics and Space Administration (NASA) project to put a spaceship on the moon or launch a satellite. However, some entrepreneurial nursing businesses or community nursing centers are organized as adhocracies or project teams.

In leadership theory, if the situation contains workers who have job readiness, or both the willingness and the knowledge to do the job, the leader simply delegates to them. The work then is delegated to the member specialists, who join collaborative teams that form and reform in response to the work and the expertise needed.

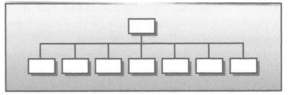

Figure 11.8
Horizontal structure.

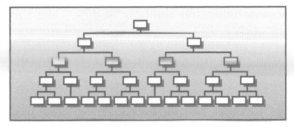

Figure 11.9
Vertical structure.

THE ORGANIZATIONAL CHART

Organizations contain both a *formal structure* and an *informal structure*. The informal structure is simply the network or pattern of social relationships and friendship circles that are outside the formal structure. It is an interconnected web of relationships that operate in and around the formally designated lines of communication. The informal structure does not appear on the formal organizational chart.

The formal structure can be identified on an *organizational chart*. An organizational chart is a visual display of the organization's positions and intentional relationships among positions. The organizational chart reflects the various positions and the formal relationships between and among the positions and, by extension, the people who are a part of the organization. Depending on the chart developer's perspective (one unit versus the whole organization) and the complexity of the chart, all positions may or may not be displayed. For example, in a long-term care facility, each administrative position may be shown, but nursing

aide positions may be categorized together as a job group.

The organizational chart generally presents the line positions, linked together by solid lines to show the flow of authority. Administrative roles are generally shown in vertical and horizontal dimensions. Staff positions or advisory bodies may be depicted on the chart with dotted lines to show consultative relationships. Drawing an organizational chart for a matrix structure presents unique challenges since these charts best suit simple or bureaucratic structures (Figures 11.8 and 11.9). In the process of applying for a job, one of the pieces of information to ask for is the organizational chart. This document can help to describe how the organization is structured— or at least how decision makers think it is structured—as one part of assessing the organization and any individual's place within it.

A *vertical structure* goes from top to bottom and includes multiple layers (see Figure 11.9). Vertical structures are referred to as "tall organizational charts." Tall organizational charts are found in large bureaucratic institutions and typify chain of command, unity of command, and span of control. A tall vertical structure that goes from top to bottom implies a bureaucracy.

In contrast, a *horizontal* or *flat structure* has few administrative layers between management and employees (see Figure 11.8). Flat organizational charts reflect a decentralized approach to structuring the organization. Decentralization diminishes the layers between management and employee, reduces overhead expense, and distributes work accountability and authority to those closest to the work.

Organizational charts help with administrative control, policy making and planning, and evaluating the organization in terms of strengths and weaknesses. They are used to help orient personnel because they show relationships and thus make it clear how people are to interact within the formal organization. For example, an organizational chart of a matrix structure may show dotted lines for the project or interdisciplinary team relationships. Dotted lines mean that there is a relationship to the position or the group that would form for a project (see Figure 11.6).

In health care today, the traditional vertical hierarchies with organized and functional departments and divisions are rapidly being redesigned, reengineered, or reorganized. The challenge remains to design a flatter, more flexible organization whose work forces are capable of delivering "seamless" services or care faster and at lower costs (Sorrels-Jones, 1997).

Empowered work environments are those in which access, support, opportunity, and resources are available to all employees. Kanter's theory of organizational behavior (Kanter, 1977) described three work empowerment structures: opportunity, power, and proportion (Box 11.3) (Upenieks, 2002).

Structure of *opportunity* refers to expectations and future prospects (i.e., opportunities for growth). The structure of *power* stems from gaining information early in the process, plus support and resources. The structure of *proportion* denotes the social arrangement of people who share the same general situation (Upenieks, 2002).

Box 11.3

Kanter's Theory of Organizational Behavior: Three Work Empowerment Structures

Opportunity

Expectations and future prospects

Power

Stems from gaining information early in the process, support, and resources

Proportion

The social arrangement of people who share the same general situation

Data from Kanter, R.M. (1977). *Men and women of the corporation.* New York: Basic Books.

When an organization is structured in such a way that employees feel empowered, the organization is more likely to benefit. The following social structures are important to the growth of empowerment (Manojlovich & Spence Laschinger, 2002):

- Having access to information
- Receiving support
- Having access to resources necessary to the job
- Having the opportunity to learn and grow

Coordination

In designing organizational structures, the division of labor occurs largely in relationship to the job to be done and the technical systems available. Coordination of tasks and jobs is more complex, involving both control and communication mechanisms. Coordination is the element of "glue" holding organizations together. There are five basic coordinating mechanisms or ways in which organizations coordinate their work, as follows (Mintzberg, 1993):

- *Mutual adjustment* coordinates work through simple informal communication. In nursing, mutual adjustment occurs when one nurse consults another nurse about practice issues, such as how to interpret a policy.

- *Direct supervision* coordinates work through the use of a supervisor taking responsibility for the instruction and monitoring of the work of others. In nursing, direct supervision takes place when a nurse supervises the work of unlicensed assistive personnel.
- *Standardization of work processes* coordinates work through specifying or programming content before the work is undertaken. In nursing, standardization of work processes occurs when nurses use standardized critical paths or plans of care.
- *Standardization of work outputs* coordinates work, before the work is undertaken, through the specification of the results, product, or performance desired or expected. In nursing, work outputs are standardized when care is specified as outcome objectives or care is managed for outcomes achievement.
- *Standardization of worker skills* coordinates work by specifying the kind of training or education required to perform the work. It is a more indirect way to control or coordinate work. In nursing, the standardization of worker skills occurs for advanced practice nurses when a master's degree is required or certification is mandated.

It is thought that as work becomes more complex, the means of coordination shifts from mutual adjustment to direct supervision and then to standardization, preferably of work processes. In highly complex environments, coordination may revert to mutual adjustment (Mintzberg, 1993).

Positions, Authority, Responsibility, and Accountability

Structure establishes patterns of authority and collegiality. The pattern results in roles. For example, there are top-level managers, middle managers, and workers in the pattern typical of a bureaucracy. Bureaucracies tend to assume the shape of a pyramid. There is a controlling or policy-making body at the top of the structure, usually called a board (e.g., board of regents, trustees, or directors). The primary function of a board is to control fiscal resources and make policy. A chief executive officer (CEO) manages the organization and reports to the board. Then there are successively larger layers of managers in the middle. At the bottom is a broad base of workers who implement the work tasks. Within organizational structures there are identified jobs with attached titles. A **position** is defined as a collection of tasks configured together for performance, usually by one individual. The terms *position* and *job* are frequently used interchangeably in organizations. A job is a collection of positions that encompasses the same basic configuration of tasks. For example, nurse manager is an organizational job with a job description. Each nurse manager holds a specific position that ideally should have a position description explaining the duties to be performed by the person in that position.

Authority, responsibility, and *accountability* are terms associated with jobs. **Authority** is defined as the right to act or to command the actions of others. It includes the power to issue instructions for others to follow. Authority is granted by the organization to an employee or by a boss to a subordinate. The level of authority is typically based on the placement of the job within the organization, lessening as it flows down the hierarchical organizational chain.

Responsibility is defined as the allocation and acceptance of a task. Responsibility is the obligation to take on and accomplish work. It denotes a duty to secure the desired results. It also is assigned or delegated by a boss to a subordinate and thus flows down the organizational chain. In accepting the obligation of an assigned task, the staff person is accepting responsibility to accomplish the task.

Accountability denotes liability and is defined as the liability for task performance. Accountability means being answerable and liable. It is determined in a retrospective analysis of what occurred. The assignment of responsibility and the granting of authority create accountability. Accountability flows upward or outward: from staff to manager or from provider to client.

Nurses are accountable, answerable, or liable for their own actions, the completion of the assigned task, and their acts of delegation. Each nurse is accountable to both the boss and the patient. Accountability is the one element that cannot be delegated. If the responsibility is great, so is the accountability. Upon taking a job, the nurse accepts the authority and the responsibility for the position. For example, a staff nurse has the authority to perform patient care within the scope of the practice of a professional nurse and accepts the responsibility for completion of the assigned task.

It is important that organizations match the level of authority to the responsibility. Nurses may be responsible for accomplishing the work but may not be given the corresponding authority to carry out the job. For example, nurses carry legal liability for the quality and safety of care delivery; however, they may be unable to influence the dietary department to deliver a tray 15 minutes earlier to avoid interaction with a particular patient's a.m. medications. Nursing's ability to influence systems, processes, and roles to integrate care processes and produce optimal outcomes in the delivery of care is of paramount importance in their scope of responsibility.

Accountability relates to legal aspects and parameters of the practice of a registered nurse (RN). As a part of the role, the professional nurse is assumed to function in the general mode of a leader because there are ancillary workers whom the nurse delegates to and supervises. Leadership skills thus become a useful supplement to clinical skills. Furthermore, RNs are obligated to understand the reality of practice within the parameters of the legal definition of nursing practice. Some resources include The Code for Nurses, state laws and administrative rules, and literature from state and national nurses' associations.

CENTRALIZATION AND DECENTRALIZATION OF POWER

Organizational structuring overlaps with the concept of power. Power can be centralized or decentralized. **Centralization** and **decentralization** refer to the configuration of the organizational structure and the way that power is dispersed throughout the organization.

Centralized power to make decisions is concentrated at the top of the organization and flows down. The person at the top has power by position and uses the power to make decisions. A centralized structure works best when an organization is facing an imminent fiscal threat because there is no time for participative deliberation or making consultative decisions. The leader must make decisions and face the threat.

Decentralized means that power filters down toward the bottom level or point of service. At the individual worker level, people may be empowered—given the authority, responsibility, and autonomy to make decisions about the work and work processes. With decentralization, decision making is diffused down to the lower organizational levels.

Decentralized structures work best when organizations are trying to improve quality and cut costs as a long-term strategy, because the people at the operations level know the work and can provide input about what works best. Once empowered to make decisions and refine the work processes, the whole organization may become more cost-efficient. The result is a higher-quality product, in this case, higher-quality patient care.

Newer trends in organizational structure focus on flexibility, organizational systems, and processes that can adeptly respond to different situations, fewer detailed rules and procedures, greater autonomy and encouragement for initiative due to the differentiated customer needs, increasing diversity in the work place, and an increased pace of change. These trends are supported by flattened structures with fewer levels of management, workers empowered to make decisions, changes in technology that allow less need for communication and control functions of middle managers, and networking, which enhances direct communication across unit boundaries and across unit team structures.

LEADERSHIP AND MANAGEMENT IMPLICATIONS

Leaders and managers can influence the structure in which goals are accomplished. In fact, determining

Research Note

Source: Krairiksh, M., & Anthony, M. (2001). Benefits and outcomes of staff nurses' participation in decision-making. *Journal of Nursing Administration, 31*(1), 16-24.

Purpose

The purpose of this article was to investigate the relationships among the participation of staff nurses in phases of the decision-making process to decisions in nursing practice, nurse manager leadership competency, and nurse-physician collaboration.

Discussion

Decision making is a process that begins with the identification of a problem and ends with the evaluation of the choices and taking a course of action. In this study, phases of decision making were explored: the phase in which problems are identified and clarified; the design phase, in which alternatives are generated, explored, and analyzed; and the selection phase, in which the alternative used in solving the problem is chosen. Nurses make two types of decisions related to practice: patient care decisions that affect direct patient care and condition-of-work decisions that affect the work environment or groups of patients. Although phases of decision making have undergone some empirical evaluation, the extent to which other organizational and professional factors influence specific aspects of decision-making behavior has not been demonstrated.

This study was a cross-sectional correlational descriptive study using a secondary analysis of a primary dataset of the Variations in Nursing Practice Model (VNPM). The sample for the VNPM study consisted of RNs working on 28 adult medical and surgical units in three hospitals. Questionnaires asking 279 nurses about their participation in decision making, their perception of the competency of nurse manager leadership, and their collaboration with physicians were distributed with a response rate of 43%. The findings showed that staff nurses had greater mean scores for participation in decisions about patient care than for participation in decisions about their work environment. Nurse-physician collaboration contributed to greater participation in all phases of both caregiving and condition-of-work decisions. The competency of nurse manager leadership had a small but significant positive correlation with participation in decision making, but it did not have a significant effect on phases of participation in both types of decisions.

Application to Practice

Because nurses are closest to the patients, they encounter greater opportunities in their daily work to participate in decision making. Enhancing their participation in decision making will support effective patient care planning and patient care activities, resulting in not only positive nurse outcomes but also better patient outcomes. The results of this study should serve as a basis for nursing administrators to design systems that support and enhance nurse manager leadership competency for greater nurse participation in decision making. The results also enable nursing administrators and nurse managers to understand the importance of encouraging their staff to collaborate with physicians; this greater collaboration allows staff nurses to be more involved in decision making. The study findings provide evidence to support the relationships among an organizational structure, an organization process, and a provider process of health care. Further research is needed to clarify the relationships of structure, process, and specific outcomes.

▲ LEADERSHIP & MANAGEMENT **BEHAVIORS**

Leadership Behaviors

- Models the acceptance and use of decentralized power
- Inspires the group to restructure when necessary
- Influences the design of the structure
- Enables followers to function within a structure
- Envisions an ideal or desired structure
- Generates an empowering environment within the administrative structure

Management Behaviors

- Develops an organizational chart
- Plans for restructuring to match environmental conditions
- Decides on line and staff positions
- Delegates tasks

- Provides authority to match responsibility
- Monitors accountability
- Plans the structure
- Organizes needed positions
- Decides on number and types of positions and related duties
- Implements structural design
- Evaluates structure for effectiveness
- Monitors stresses and strains created by structure

Overlap Areas

- Influences people to work within a structure
- Plans and develops the structure
- Makes decisions about the administrative structure

the structure is a key responsibility that leaders and managers have in planning an environment that is most conducive to high-quality nursing care. In nursing, determining the structure is a planning and organizing aspect of the management process. As the environment changes, the manager may need to rethink the structure and decide whether a change needs to be made to better match the structure to the work group and its changing environment.

Job structure is one of the organizational factors influencing nursing's work and work excitement (Simms et al., 1990). The effect of structural changes can be seen in the phenomenon of "layoff survivor sickness." In one large hospital the strategic planning process led to the conclusion that the organization needed a greater customer focus. To increase organizational effectiveness and efficiency, foster a culture of commitment to customer-driven service, and flatten the organization to push decision making closer to the point of service, a series of structural changes was implemented that triggered an appreciable, debilitating response among the nursing staff. Pain and loss of productivity were the result of layoff survivor sickness resulting

from the organizational transformation (Triolo et al., 1995).

Although organizational structure is a management decision, it may also be the result of needing to alleviate pressures or solve certain problems of management. For example, as the size of an organization grows, employees need to be able to interact and communicate in an orderly fashion. On the other hand, a small organization may need the creativity and flexibility of a loose structure. As the environment changes, managers may be forced to restructure to survive and thrive. Theory about organizational structures provides a knowledge base with which to gain a greater awareness of options. The research literature may suggest which types of structures are more effective under which conditions. The leader and manager are challenged to assess and use organizational structure and restructuring efforts to ease frictions when the structure, the environment, and the needs of the workers create conflicts or serious threats to organizational effectiveness.

Structural aspects on the job shape a leader's effectiveness. Kanter theorized that nurse leaders who view their jobs as relevant, flexible, and visible

---

Box **11.4**

Forms of Power

Formal Power

Derived from roles that provide recognition and are relevant to key organizational goals

Informal Power

Derived from relationships and key alliances

---

and who have well-established informal alliances perceive that they have access to resources and support and function successfully in their jobs. Kanter's (1977) theory proposed that leadership empowerment evolves from both the formal and informal systems of the organization. Formal power comes from jobs that provide recognition and are relevant to key organizational goals; informal power comes from relationships and alliances with people in the organization. Thus nurse leaders with formal and informal power are in a position to access empowerment structures that enable them to accomplish their work successfully (Upenieks, 2002) (Box 11.4).

The traditional hospital structure was not designed to respond to the needs of patients in a user-friendly manner. The challenge today is for leaders to restructure and reorganize to ensure effective outcomes for patients. Notorious for being fragmented, hospitals have remained organized largely along functional and specialty lines. Despite a decade dedicated to creating integrated delivery models, the hospital remains uniquely fragmented with breakdowns in communications contributing significantly to quality problems and higher costs as noted in the Institute of Medicine's report "Crossing the Quality Chasm" (Dwyer et al., 2003). Structure becomes a central focus for managerial strategies when the environment is turbulent.

Because of the turbulent environment in health care and the rapid change of advancing technology and environmental conditions in society,

decentralized structures are considered to be the structures that are going to work the best for nursing. Organizational theory suggests that a flattened structure and a minimum of layers give nurses job-related decision authority. Unfortunately, this structure also has the consequence of reducing the number of rungs on the career ladder for nurses. Decision autonomy has been equated with professionalism and job satisfaction, although some research indicates that nurses vary in their preferences for decision-making autonomy (Dwyer et al., 1992). Nurses need to be developed so that they achieve the knowledge and expertise level of mature professional experts, in order to be well prepared for patient care decision authority. As organizations grow larger, there is a pull toward bureaucratization and centralization. Nurse leaders and managers will be challenged to analyze organizational structure as health care reform initiatives trigger further structural changes.

For instance, one challenge will be to decide how to integrate and structure nursing within new configurations such as "hospitals without walls." The nurse's role has expanded and broadened as the key coordinator across care settings in the role of case manager. New structures may be necessary for nursing practice. Creating a vision and strategic planning are key activities for nurse leaders. Where restructuring occurs, an analysis of what works for nursing practice may need to be done independently of what works for the health care organization.

Leaders and managers may be involved in revising or changing organizational structures. *Restructuring* means revising or modifying the structure to reshape it or switch to another structural type. Restructuring efforts typically have been geared toward fixing existing operational processes. Reengineering, however, is considered to be a more radical process of rethinking all operational processes. To begin anew, processes are analyzed from the point of view of the customer, as well as the requirement to achieve greater costcontainment, quality, service, and speed. Thus reengineering is a radical redesign of business processes (Hammer & Champy, 1993; Moss et al., 1994).

Curtin (1994) differentiated job redesign from restructuring and reengineering. Job redesign focuses on who does what tasks. Flexibility, cross-training, and productivity become key ideas. Restructuring focuses on the architecture of an organization. Lean, decentralized, self-governing organizations that empower first-line caregivers are the preferred structures to evolve and emerge. The process of reengineering emphasizes renovating the processes used to accomplish goals. User-friendly processes, efficiency, and economy become key ideas.

CURRENT ISSUES AND TRENDS

The decade of the 1990s has been described as a time of turbulent change. In crossing the millennium, the pace of change remained high and difficult to cope with. American hospitals, like their corporate cousins in business and industry, are being forced by rapidly changing economic and competitive forces to seek new, less traditional models of organization. Much attention has been focused on changing organizational structures. Terms like *horizontal networks, functional silos, cross-functional work groups,* and *boundaryless organizations* are considered, as are *downsizing* and *flattening* (Sorrells-Jones, 1997). Part of the current swirl of changes in hospitals and health care organizations includes transforming organizational structures to decentralize, drawing new organizational charts, and instituting collaborative teams to reform bureaucracies and create a structure within an organization to use workers of multiple skill levels. The idea is that flattened, decentralized structures that are highly empowered at the bottom levels will make a difference in terms of effectiveness. Related terms and concepts are case management, use of nurse extenders, professional practice models, contractual models and alternative structures, shared governance, product line management, and outcomes management. What these "new" management ideas really are implying is restructuring in some manner or form.

Porter-O'Grady and Malloch (2003) described the need for "quantum leadership" to advance health care from the brick-and-mortar empires of the twentieth century, in which the focus of work was on performing the right process, to the twenty-first century, in which the focus is on obtaining the right outcomes. With the infrastructure of society becoming increasingly information-based, structures to accommodate an information age are primarily relational and function horizontally, whereas most business structures have functioned vertically. Leading in a horizontal work culture is dramatically different from leading in a predominantly vertical structure. The knowledge needed to get the work done is primarily in the hands of the worker. This causes a shift in power and control to the "knowledge worker" and can cause conflict in traditional structures. Structures need to move away from vertical orientation, hierarchical structures, focus on control, and top-down decision making to a nonlinear structure with a focus on relatedness, center-out decision making, and value-driven actions. Leadership will need to move from managing functions or work to coordinating elements and facilitating relationships at every organizational level.

Beyond restructuring and reengineering is a current trend in health care to integrate different types of organizations across the continuum of care. The idea is for patients to move along the health-illness continuum across settings and sites of care delivery without fragmentation of service delivery. This means coordinating care, a role ideally suited to nurses. From the patient's perspective, a continuum of care exists, but it has not been seamless. Care has not been viewed as a total experience or managed as an ongoing process but rather as an episode needing medical intervention. In fragmented parts, care becomes costly, uncoordinated, and fraught with duplicated effort. Frustrations arise from the effects of fragmentation, but organizing health services around the needs of patients requires new structural arrangements and often means movement to a vertically integrated system (Aikman et al., 1998).

Consumer and payer frustration with rising cost burdens in health care began to drive managed care initiatives. Managed care initiatives began to drive care coordination and a reexamination and transformation of the organizational structures within the entire health care delivery system. New structures emerged. Parts of the health care delivery system began to align into integrated systems as reimbursement incentives began to change from "patient days" to "covered lives." In this process, traditional organizational structures that were vertical and hierarchical began to give way to new structures that were horizontal and organized around processes rather than tasks (Moss et al., 1994).

The rapid advances in information technology will continue to challenge traditional systems and processes. Telecommunication enhances the ability to provide high-quality education to care providers and patients. Telemedicine has had a profound impact on health care. The Internet has provided access to an abundance of health care resources. All of these factors will have to be considered as organizational structures to support a future of health care vastly different from that which has been known for the past many years are explored and reconfigured.

Flannery and Williams (1990) predicted that seven patterns would combine to reconfigure hospital structures in order to create a simpler and more responsive organization. These patterns are flattened organizations, more fluid structures, outcomes (not functions) orientation, redefined staff functions by managers who are better developed and accountable, reduced staff costs, more subcontracting of services, and a refocus on the core business. Where implemented, the result has been a streamlined structure and a fundamental change in jobs and positions.

Certainly structures in health care organizations are changing. Just as pyramidal shapes gave way to internal matrix structures, internal matrix structures are giving way to flat organizations linked via networks of integrated health care organizations. Smaller organizations of providers are configuring as adhocracies or project teams. Work design, defined as changing the actual structure of jobs that people perform by measuring the workload and fitting people into jobs, is one area of high activity in nursing. This approach is the opposite of fitting jobs to people (Tonges, 1992).

Research that investigated the results of hospital restructuring highlighted the difficulties in attributing positive outcomes to restructuring efforts (Bryan et al., 1998). It may be that restructuring does not have a negative impact on patient outcomes; however, it invariably creates an impact on nurses. The question remains as to whether the impact on nursing staff outweighs the gains in other objectives. The nursing leadership and management challenge is to use the best ideas and make them work for nursing. In describing the Transformational Model for Professional Nursing Practice, the authors noted this challenge and offered a "road map" for nursing through major organizational transformation as one solution (Wolf et al., 1994).

Changes in the financial structure of health care, such as competition on price and quality, have triggered restructuring. As the nursing shortage abated in the mid-1990s, the focus shifted from what structure is best suited to attracting and retaining nurses to what structure will help the organization survive under capitated reimbursement. Immediate solutions were implemented to reduce the size of the nursing staff and to substitute assistants in order to ease financial pressures. However, history indicates that these actions set the stage for yet another nursing shortage. Indeed, by the end of the 1990s, another cycle of nursing shortage began to occur.

Reduction-in-force (RIF) and decreasing the nursing staff skill mix to 50% or less RNs were short-term measures that proved to be shortsighted. These decisions brought about other problem issues, such as costs of supervision, appropriate care modality, nurse satisfaction, and low morale. Nurse leaders and managers will continue to be challenged to analyze organizational structuring issues, match them to a specific organization, and lead the nursing staff toward personal adaptation to growth, change, and positive outcomes.

The challenges for nursing in the restructured, reengineered, and integrated organizational structure are many and extensive. Organizational cultures may facilitate or impede nursing's work and the need for nurses to change as the environment changes. For example, the organizational culture may or may not support a seamless continuum of care. Nurses will need to learn new behaviors and new strategies for working across an organization that owns different types of care agencies. The most proactive stance for nursing is to seize the opportunities inherent in nurses' natural care coordination role, reconfigure organizational structures to match care delivery needs and the environment, and advocate for those elements of "what works" for nursing and for patients.

In structuring for the future, it is important to consider how talent is allocated to problems and opportunities, both in the present and in the future. The best talent in an organization should be dedicated to reinventing its work and generating new perspectives. Today, many hospitals, unlike other business enterprises, have no significant infrastructure dedicated to key management resources such as leadership development and training or research and innovation. In order to compete in the future, hospitals will need to be able to make investments in this infrastructure. Those organizations that are able to create an advantage in terms of a better trained work force, better leadership development, new service development, and more consistent innovation, will have a significant strategic advantage (Dwyer et al., 2003).

Summary

- Health care is undergoing a turbulent era of restructuring, reengineering, and integration.
- Organizational structure organizes work, power, and control elements by establishing a framework and pattern of relationships.
- Technology, environment, size, and task repetitiveness influence structure.
- There is no one right way to structure.
- The classic hierarchical bureaucratic structure is one of the major forms of structure found in health care.
- Organizations may try to adapt to a turbulent environment by first moving to a matrix structure as a way to solve some problems.
- Organizational charts show the formal structure; they may be horizontal or vertical in shape.

- Organizational positions carry authority, accountability, and responsibility.
- Power can be structurally centralized or decentralized.

Study Questions

1. What purposes does the structure of an organization serve?
2. What elements of organizational structure are found in nursing organizations?
3. What elements are most important for nursing practice?
4. What factors need to be assessed prior to changing the organizational culture?
5. How do nurses foster or hinder restructuring?
6. What changes are needed in nursing organizations? Why?
7. How are the structures of community agencies the same as or different from hospitals?
8. What coordinating mechanisms are used in nursing and health care organizations?
9. How effective are the coordinating mechanisms used by nursing?
10. How have authority, responsibility, and accountability been used in nursing practice? What feelings do they create?
11. Is power in nursing centralized or decentralized?

CASE STUDY

Bed Turnaround

Between 11:00 A.M. and 8:00 P.M., as many as 17 patients will be discharged and new patients will be admitted on a medical-surgical unit with 34 beds. The responsibility for patient transport and housekeeping duties belongs to the support associate (SA). The SA is pulled away from cleaning a room four or five times per room to transport patients for discharge or to and from ancillary testing. Meanwhile, new admissions are held in the emergency department or outpatient center, awaiting a clean bed. Often, a centralized housekeeping team is STAT-paged to clean the room.

Further analysis identifies that the lack of trust between departments in this facility often results in sending out "spies" to "truly assess" bed status. Lack of teamwork between the SAs and housekeeping personnel exists. The average bed turnaround time from the point of patient discharge to the bed being ready for occupancy is 82 minutes.

As a result, a multidisciplinary team is formed to identify options to reduce bed turnaround and to evaluate the SA role. Team members consist of an administration representative, medical surgical unit manager, three SAs, two housekeeping personnel, a unit clerk, the housewide bed coordinator, and one registered nurse (RN).

Through the work of this team, the reporting relationship of the unit-based housekeeper responsible for cleaning the common areas (e.g., nurses' station, waiting rooms, and hallways) is changed to a matrix reporting structure, in which the housekeeper reports directly to the Director of Environmental Services but also has a dotted-line relationship, reporting to the individual department director. In addition, a centralized support associate STAT team is initiated to work from 1:00 P.M. to 11:30 P.M., Monday through Friday, and 7:00 A.M. to 3:00 P.M. on Saturdays. Dispatch of the STAT team is delegated to the Charge RN via a beeper versus going through the centralized Environmental Services Department. On the off-shift the STAT SA team reports to and is dispatched by the off-shift supervisor. Finally, one SA per unit is assigned to strictly perform discharge room cleaning, which eliminates transport interruptions. As a result of these structure and role changes, the time from discharge of a patient to the time a bed is ready is decreased 53%.

Bed Turnaround Process

Indicator	Baseline July/August/ September, 2003	February 2004
Discharge of patient to bed ready	82 minutes	38 minutes

CRITICAL THINKING EXERCISE

Nurse Caitlin Schultz recently transferred from a director role in an inpatient nursing unit to assume the director role of another department. The previous department director had established a council for recruitment and retention. Composed of three registered nurses and two social workers, this team established a program to fund flowers for any staff member experiencing a family death, wedding or birth, organized holiday activities at the department level, and assisted the director in recognizing staff members during Nurses' Week.

As part of the annual Nurses' Week celebration, each nursing employee was recognized at the department level with an awards luncheon, organizationally through many different scheduled events, and each was given a tote bag with the hospital's logo. Within 1 month of starting the new role, the director attended the first Recruitment & Retention Council meeting, at which the team was discussing preparation for the upcoming week by recognizing one of the nursing specialties practiced in their department.

Staff discussions centered on how to obtain more money from the budget to buy yet another gift for only RN staff members. As the conversation continued, the director became concerned that the focus of the team was centered on recognizing only the RNs (as accomplished during Nurses' Week activities) versus focusing on the work and contributions of the entire department as it pertained to that particular specialty.

1. Is there a problem?
2. What is the problem?
3. How can the director's authority, responsibility, and accountability be explained?
4. What elements of organizational structure could be helpful in this situation? Which could be barriers?
5. What options are there to refocus the team?
6. What problems and decisions face the staff nurses?
7. What challenges face the director?

REFERENCES

Aikman, P., Andress, I., Goodfellow, C., LaBelle, N., & Porter-O'Grady, T. (1998). System integration: A necessity. *Journal of Nursing Administration, 28*(2), 28-34.

Bryan, Y.E., Hitchings, K.S., Fuss, M.A., Fox, M.A., Kinneman, M.T., & Young, M.J. (1998). Measuring and evaluating hospital restructuring efforts: Eighteen-month follow-up and extension to critical care: Part 1. *Journal of Nursing Administration, 28*(9), 21-27.

Cumbey, D.A., & Alexander, J.W. (1998). The relationship of job satisfaction with organizational variables in public health nursing. *Journal of Nursing Administration, 28*(5), 39-46.

Curtin, L. (1994). Restructuring: What works and what does not! *Nursing Management, 25*(10), 7-8.

Dwyer, B., Widner, S., & Beckham, D. (2003). *Hospital of the future: A leaders' perspective.* Abbott Park, IL: Abbott Health Systems.

Dwyer, D., Schwartz, R., & Fox, M. (1992). Decision-making autonomy in nursing. *Journal of Nursing Administration, 22*(2), 17-23.

Flannery, T., & Williams, J. (1990). The shape of things to come: Part 1. *Healthcare Forum Journal, 33*(3), 14-20.

Flarey, D.L., & Smith, S.P. (1999). Management and organizational restructuring: Reforming the corporate system. In S.P. Smith & D.L. Flarey (Eds.), *Process-centered health care organizations* (pp. 141-152). Gaithersburg, MD: Aspen.

Hammer, M., & Champy, J. (1993). *Reengineering the corporation: A manifesto for business revolution.* New York: HarperCollins.

Havens, D.S., & Aiken, L.H. (1999). Shaping systems to promote desired outcomes: The magnet hospital model. *Journal of Nursing Administration, 29*(2), 14-20.

Kanter, R.M. (1977). *Men and women of the corporation.* New York: Basic Books.

Manojlovich, M., & Spence Laschinger, H.K. (2002). The relationship of empowerment and selected personality characteristics to nursing job satisfaction. *Journal of Nursing Administration, 32*(11), 586-595.

Mark, B. (1989). Structural contingency theory. In B. Henry, C. Arndt, M. Di Vincenti, & A. Marriner-Tomey (Eds.), *Dimensions of nursing administration: Theory, research, education, practice* (pp. 175-182). Boston: Blackwell.

Mintzberg, H. (1993). *Structure in fives: Designing effective organizations.* Englewood Cliffs, NJ: Prentice-Hall.

Moss, M., Eagen, M., & Russell, M. (1994). Service integration in the reform era. *Nursing Economic$, 12*(5), 256-260, 286.

Pabst, M. (1993). Span of control on nursing inpatient units. *Nursing Economic$, 11*(2), 87-90.

Porter-O'Grady, T., & Malloch, K. (2003). *Quantum leadership: A textbook of new leadership.* Sudbury, MA: Jones and Bartlett.

Simms, L., Erbin-Roesemann, M., Darga, A., & Coeling, H. (1990). Breaking the burnout barrier: Resurrecting work excitement in nursing. *Nursing Economic$, 8*(3), 177-187.

Sorrells-Jones, J. (1997). The challenge of making it real: Interdisciplinary practice in a "seamless" organization. *Nursing Administration Quarterly, 21*(2), 20-30.

Tonges, M. (1992). Work designs: Sociotechnical systems for patient care delivery. *Nursing Management, 23*(1), 27-32.

Triolo, P.K., Allgeier, P.A., & Schwartz, C.E. (1995). Layoff survivor sickness: Minimizing the sequelae of organizational transformation. *Journal of Nursing Administration, 25*(3), 56-63.

Upenieks, V. (2002). What constitutes successful nurse leadership? A qualitative approach utilizing Kanter's theory of organizational behavior. *Journal of Nursing Administration, 32*(12), 622-632.

Wolf, G., Boland, S., & Aukerman, M. (1994). A transformational model for the practice of professional nursing. *Journal of Nursing Administration, 24*(5), 38-46.

12 Decentralization and Shared Governance

Claudia DiSabatino Smith

CHAPTER OBJECTIVES

- Define and differentiate centralization and decentralization
- Describe examples of centralization and decentralization
- Define and describe shared governance
- Describe one shared governance model
- Evaluate problems associated with implementation of shared governance
- Explore research related to shared governance
- Exercise critical thinking to conceptualize and analyze possible solutions to a practice exercise
- Analyze and identify possible solutions to case study via critical thinking methods

The growing disparity between the supply and demand of registered nurses, along with the coming of age of the generation of Baby Boomers, is leading to a crisis in health care. This widely documented dilemma has been characterized as more complex and of a greater magnitude than any past nursing shortages (The Call to the Nursing Profession, 2002; The Robert Wood Johnson Foundation, 2002). Research studies that link nurse-patient staffing ratios to patient outcomes (Aiken et al., 2002) paint an even bleaker picture in view of the nursing shortage and the focus on patient safety (IOM, 2004).

In response to the technical and social transformation, maturing technology and more educated patients, health care systems are reconfiguring clinical care and service delivery to more mobile, fast-paced, consumer-driven models. Such changes provide additional convenience for patients and less need for inpatient nursing staff. Recommendations to improve the shortage of registered nurses include the application of measures found in Magnet-designated hospitals that appear to improve retention through increased job satisfaction of registered nurses. The implementation of such strategies serve to empower nurses, leading to increased professional autonomy and active participation in decision making on issues of nursing practice and the work environment (AHA Commission on Workforce for Hospitals and Health Systems, 2002; JCAHO, 2002). One strategy for accomplishing this is to radically reconfigure traditional hierarchical organizational structures with multiple levels of managers, which contribute to the frustration of professional registered nurses who complain that they lack autonomy and decision-making authority. With increasing numbers of nurses seeking further education, the traditional organizational structure becomes less adequate to support a professional practice model of nursing. Implementing a shared governance model is one means of empowering nurses to make decisions at the point of care regarding patient care and the practice environment.

DEFINITIONS

Shared governance is a model of organizational decision making premised on a decentralized organizational structure in which staff nurses are empowered through autonomy and accountability. Although it requires an organizational philosophy of belief in the value of shared power and decision making, shared governance is discussed as an aspect of an organization's power structure. Terms related to the concept of shared governance include **centralization, decentralization, horizontal decentralization, organizational chart, selective decentralization, synergy, span of control,** and **vertical decentralization.**

MANAGEMENT AND CENTRALIZATION AND DECENTRALIZATION

Hospitals are organized, and their work structured, around a guiding philosophy. The philosophy serves as the institutional framework that shapes the direction of the acquisition of knowledge and skills and becomes the deciding factor in the long-term development of the institution.

◢ LEADING & MANAGING DEFINED

Shared Governance

An accountability-based model of shared decision making that leads to the empowerment and autonomy of professional nurses; through shared decision making, nurses at the point of service have control over their nursing practice, peer issues, education, quality, and work environment.

Centralization

The extent to which power and authority for decision making rests in top levels of the organization.

Decentralization

The extent to which power and authority for decision making are systematically dispersed to middle and lower levels of the organization; examples include vertical decentralization, horizontal decentralization, and selective decentralization.

Horizontal Decentralization

The decision-making power that flows outside the line authority by which nonmanagement personnel are authorized to effect decision processes.

Organizational Chart

Visual representation of the framework that demonstrates horizontal and vertical reporting relationships within an organization.

Selective Decentralization

A concentration of power for decision-making that resides in functional divisions within the organization; examples include a central sterile processing department, central pharmacy, central human relations department.

Synergy

A condition that exists when parts of an organization interact to produce a joint effect that is greater than the sum of the parts acting alone; the concept that the whole is greater than the sum of its parts (e.g., 1 + 1 = 3).

Span of Control

The number of subordinates who report to one manager.

Vertical Decentralization

The distribution of power down the chain of command, or line of authority, flowing from the top of the organization to the bottom.

Organizations that invest in knowledge that increases the productivity of human capital, or improves the tacit knowledge of their professional staff, will experience productivity increases that are consistent with the growth of the economy (North, 1990). The mission statement, core values, and vision are the instruments that give voice to the organization's philosophy. Likewise, the **organizational chart** is a visual representation of the horizontal and vertical reporting structure of the organization. It illustrates the chain of command, the span of control for managers, and operating relationships. Figure 12.1 illustrates some examples. At a glance, the chart permits the trained observer to make a statement about the organizational philosophy of the organization—whether the authority is primarily centralized or decentralized (Straub & Attner, 1994).

Centralization and decentralization can be viewed as organizational philosophies about power distribution that pertain to the hierarchical level of decision-making authority in the institution. Institutions organize and structure themselves by defining departmental function and authority

relationships in order to achieve a more coordinated effort. An institution's organizational philosophy drives plans and decisions about who reports to whom, as well as who does what. Executives may utilize selective decentralization where power for decision making is concentrated in the functional areas of staffing, purchasing, and operations. Alternatively, they may choose to set limits on purchases at each level of the organization by dollar amounts. A well-organized institution can plan, implement, and evaluate strategies much more effectively than a poorly organized institution.

Centralization and decentralization are relative terms when applied to institutions. Institutions in which the executive leader retains more decision-making authority operate on a more centralized philosophy. Centralized authority allows for rigid control over decision making and power in the institution. However, as institutions have evolved into more complex global operations, it has become extremely difficult for chief executives to manage the information overload that occurs in a highly centralized structure, as well as to stay

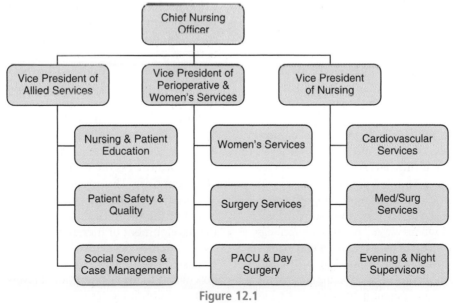

Figure 12.1
Organizational chart.

abreast of new developments. Information asymmetry occurs, bringing about the need for hierarchical development. An institution with centralized decision making is demonstrated in the following example:

> Mary Jones is the nursing director of 2 Main, a medical nursing unit in General Hospital. As such, Nurse Jones interviews nursing applicants to fill the open nursing positions on 2 Main. At the conclusion of the interviews, she offers hiring recommendations to the chief nursing officer (CNO), Sherry Smith. Nurse Smith reviews the file of each applicant interviewed and listens to the recommendation of the nursing director. Nurse Smith most often is in accord with the recommendation of the nursing director, but she holds the final word in the matter. Once the CNO's approval is gained, the nursing director is free to contact the applicant and offer the approved candidate the open position.

Although this is a somewhat simplistic example, the retention of decision-making authority at the nurse executive level is highlighted.

In an organization with a more decentralized approach, decision-making authority rests at lower levels in the organizational framework. Institutions with decentralized decision making encourage and facilitate greater innovation, more input, and faster response times. Decisions are made closer to the point of care, rather than the information passing up through the chain of command to an executive who is far removed from the situation. In the following example, the empowerment of professional staff nurses at lower levels to make the same hiring decision can be observed:

> Charlotte Black is the nursing director of 4 East, a medical nursing unit in City Hospital. With three staff nurse positions vacant, she posts the openings and selects three staff nurses from her unit to serve as the selection committee who will interview candidates for the positions. Based on the needs of the nursing unit and the availability of nursing applicants who match those needs, Nurse Black screens

the files of the applicants. She passes the files of those nurses who meet the requirements for the positions to the selection committee, who then schedules interviews with the applicants. Once the selection committee has interviewed each candidate, it decides on the best candidate for each position. The committee's recommendations, along with the rationale for its choices, are discussed with Nurse Black. Nurse Black meets with the candidates recommended by the selection committee, interviews them, and makes the job offers.

This example illustrates a more decentralized organizational philosophy in action. In this scenario, the CNO does not take an active role in the hiring process of staff nurses. The decision is made based on the input of the staff nurses who will be working side-by-side with the applicant. It is important to note that while the two examples are extremes that would appear on opposite ends of a continuum, institutions may exhibit varying degrees of centralization or decentralization.

It is common to see a more centralized structure in smaller institutions. As institutions become larger and take on more complicated organizational structures, it is not feasible for the CNO to be involved in all of the smaller scale decisions. In the health care arena, where specialized knowledge abounds, information asymmetry occurs between central leaders and those in the specialty care areas. Information asymmetry refers to an imbalance in the level of knowledge about a specific topic or area. For example, nurses in the cardiac catheterization laboratory are highly specialized; and as such, they are better able to make knowledgeable decisions regarding care of patients in the area than is the CNO or the Vice President of Patient Care. This represents a clear example of information asymmetry. Information asymmetry is one of the theoretical justifications that lead to the development of hierarchies (Miller, 1992).

Hierarchies develop when decision making is delegated from the top of the organizational level downward to lower operational levels, where specialized knowledge resides. The degree of decentralization may vary from minimal, in which case decisions are in the hands of one or a few, perhaps at the vice presidential level, to maximal, in which case many employees on the lowest rung of the organizational framework are empowered to make decisions. Managers who delegate authority to subordinates find that they can devote more time to planning and evaluating strategies. A philosophy of centralized decision making results in a narrower span of control and more levels of management. An organization with a philosophy of decentralized decision making generally means that the span of control should be wider for each manager. When subordinates are empowered to make decisions, fewer levels of management will be required, because the staff learn to manage and make decisions about problems at the operational level. However, this requires staff who are empowered and educated in decision-making skills. One effect of decentralization is that staff members are more vulnerable than ever, because there are fewer people above them providing functional supervision. This situation presents a challenge for nurses in executive positions (Beyers, 1999).

Relinquishing decision-making authority to those with the necessary specialized information to make effective decisions allows managers the time to implement strategies to communicate the institutional plan to all employees. Institutions that employ a more decentralized organizational philosophy, emphasize planning and evaluation, and communicate clear goals and objectives can develop synergy. Synergy results when the departments or divisions of an institution work together to accomplish a common goal, and, in so doing, they produce a much greater output than could have occurred by each department working alone (David, 1987).

Nurses provide a unique clinical perspective to policy development and strategic planning. Their focus, along with that of nursing administration, is on the design and management of patient care. Facilitating patients' movement through the maze of the health care system has emerged as one of the primary roles of the nurse. The decade of the 1990s, with its emphasis on organizational redesign and systems thinking, brought about a long-needed change. A vision of a seamless continuity of care that focuses on the welfare of the patient and family came to be recognized as urgently needed. Although the bureaucracy and notions of power continued to be areas of conflict, redesign efforts focused on open communication across disciplines and shared decision making. The traditional view of organizational barriers within hierarchies, caused by the "silo" effect within disciplines, was replaced by a new mindset about multidisciplinary care delivery. Systems theory and total quality management concepts served as change engines during the 1990s, providing the impetus for further development and implementation of interdisciplinary teams for the management of patient care (Beyers, 1999).

SHARED GOVERNANCE

Shared governance has been described as a management strategy to transform the role of nurses from one that was "devalued and subservient to meaningful and autonomous" (Ludemann & Brown, 1989, p. 49). Advocates of shared governance argue that it is a strategy that empowers nurses and leads to accountability, improved quality of care, increased job satisfaction, and commitment to the organization (Minnen et al., 1993; Orsburn et al., 1990; Porter-O'Grady, 2001; Prince, 1997). Research suggests that registered nurses who are empowered through shared governance to make decisions about nursing practice and the workplace have higher levels of job satisfaction and are more likely to remain in the organization (McClure & Hinshaw, 2002). Shared governance exemplifies decentralized decision making.

Decentralization and shared governance were strategies employed in the 1980s to address the acute challenges of the nursing shortage, nurse turnover, and nurse retention. The idea was to empower staff nurses by involving them in client care decision making and in some organizational decision making (Jones et al., 1993). This was seen as a radical departure from the traditional hierarchical hospital management structure in which nurses had little authority, little voice in governance, and low control within the organization (Hess, 1994).

The situation in the health care market of the first decade of the new millennium is not unlike that of the early 1980s. Aside from the looming nursing shortage and an aging population, there are more career choices available for females, a lack of qualified nursing faculty, and little real change in the hierarchical management style of hospitals. Questions have been raised in the literature as to whether the implementation of shared governance, which was first introduced in the late 1970s, represented a true change in hospital management style or merely served as a cosmetic Band-Aid.

Described as an accountability-based model, shared governance is a vehicle through which nurses actively engage in making decisions regarding nursing practice, quality of patient care, education, nursing peer issues, and issues in the work environment. Shared governance promotes involvement, investment, participation, sharing of power, interdependence, cooperation, horizontal relationships and accountability for nursing decisions. Nursing effectiveness is enhanced through the sense of ownership that comes with more active involvement in the leadership of the organization. Shared governance is not a theory, a conceptual framework, an organizational principle, or a structure; shared governance is a concept that leads to the empowerment of nurses and, ultimately, to professional autonomy (Porter-O'Grady, 2003b). It is a journey rather than a single event in time (Porter-O'Grady, 2001; Thompson et al., 2004). Shared governance is seen as a strategy for fostering professional nursing practice through the empowerment of nurses.

Empowerment refers to a process whereby nurses recognize that they have legitimate power and authority to make decisions regarding their practice. There is no transfer of power, but merely a change to an internal locus of control. Authority is not given or taken away. Clinicians at the point of service have the opportunity to be an integral part of the decision-making process. Accountability takes the place of responsibility in clinical practice (Porter-O'Grady, 2001). Empowerment is accomplished through the journey toward shared governance.

The shared governance journey begins with the education of health care executives, administrators, managers, and staff. Research suggests that in order for behavioral change to be sustained in an organization, a supporting structure must be in place (Argyris, 1994). The challenge for administrators is not in creating the structure that supports shared governance, but rather in developing a culture that supports and encourages it. Creating the structure is the easy part of the implementation of shared governance (Brooks, 2004). Perhaps the greater challenge for administrators is justification of the cost in terms of personal time and effort and financial commitment. Evidence supports the value of shared governance in nursing practice (George et al., 2002), but a paucity of direct evidence exists regarding the financial cost and benefits of its implementation (Brooks, 2004; Hess, 2004). The literature reveals indirect cost savings that have been attributed to the implementation of shared governance. Such cost savings have been evidenced in the areas of recruitment and orientation, the utilization of registry nurses, and the number of management staff positions (DeBaca et al., 1993). Furthermore, longitudinal research in the area of financial costs and cost benefits, including the return on investment of shared governance implementation, is warranted (Herrin, 2004).

Shared governance is a dynamic process, one that is constantly changing. It changes as the organization changes, as personnel change, and as the times change. Education should be continually available to employees in the institution that practices shared governance. Programs are needed to instruct new employees and newly elected unit representatives, to continually develop leadership behaviors in nursing staff, and to support and guide nurse managers. Nurse managers are key in determining the degree of shared decision making that will actually occur at the unit level. Those managers who are willing to relinquish control and grant staff members the opportunity to undertake the leadership role for unit activities will find additional time for coaching and mentoring, as well as for planning and strategizing.

Meanwhile, nurse managers will be fostering the development of leadership behaviors in staff nurses, which will ultimately lead to the empowerment and autonomy of the nursing staff.

When governance is restricted to the level of the nursing unit, staff autonomy and participative decision making may increase without affecting the overall organizational structure (Hess, 1994). Shared governance in nursing does not exist unless the authority and accountability for decisions that define and regulate nursing practice and those shared with management are solidified with actual decision-making structures and processes (Maas & Specht, 1990). If an institution employs a shared governance model in which patient care quality is truly the primary focus and bedside clinical staff members are empowered as knowledge workers and decision makers, this should be reflected in both the organizational chart and resource allocations. One example of such an organizational chart is depicted in Figure 12.1.

One obstacle to the implementation of shared governance is the different levels of knowledge that registered nurses bring to the health care setting as a result of the variety of basic educational programs of nursing. Traditionally, nurses have worked in strong, hierarchical institutions with centralized decision making and clear authority structures, rigid approval mechanisms, and extensive policies and procedures. This presents another obstacle in that such conditions constrain peer-based, lateral, and collegial dialogue. As a result, nurses may not have depth of experience in attending committee meetings, setting agendas, developing consensus, dealing with conflict, and conducting meetings. Finally, nurse leaders and managers who rule autocratically present an obstacle to the implementation of shared governance. For the long-time manager, this radical departure from the traditional autocratic management style presents a whole new paradigm, along with the challenges and uncertainty that accompany it.

In shared governance the focus shifts from the skill and expertise with which the nurse manager manages the nursing unit to the skill and innovation of the clinical nursing staff. Staff nurses are viewed as knowledge workers (Drucker, 1999). The responsibility for unit outcomes rests with the whole team, not the individual nurse manager. The clinical credibility of staff nurses on the nursing unit has an impact on the relationships, communications, collegiality, and ultimately, the ability to collaborate with other health care professionals. The nurse manager's role shifts to one of mentoring, coaching, facilitating, enabling and supporting the staff personnel. Modeling adaptation to change, the nurse manager builds a culture of trust and respect, all the while creating an environment in which the care of the patient and family is the central focus. Key elements for successful implementation of shared governance include the following: a client focus, participation in decision making, consensus management, free expression, individual accountability, proper timing, and a sense of cohesion through a common language (Herrick, 1998).

Shared governance models vary as to the degree of nurse participation in decision making, from minimal or informal participation to true sharing of authority and accountability. In his earlier work, Porter-O'Grady (1987) described three approaches to shared governance in nursing: *the councilor model, congressional model,* and *administrative model.* Ten years later, Porter-O'Grady and colleagues (1997) expanded the focus to include shared governance of whole-systems utilizing the councilor model. The councilor model employs committees or councils of elected representatives for structuring staff and managing governance. Each council has defined authority and functions. Primary councils within nursing include practice, quality improvement, education, and management. The congressional model is designed much like the U.S. representative form of government, with elected representatives using the democratic process for decision making. The administrative model has two separate tracks, one with a clinical focus and the other with a management focus. Figure 12.2 displays the councilor model as used in one large teaching hospital in a metropolitan area.

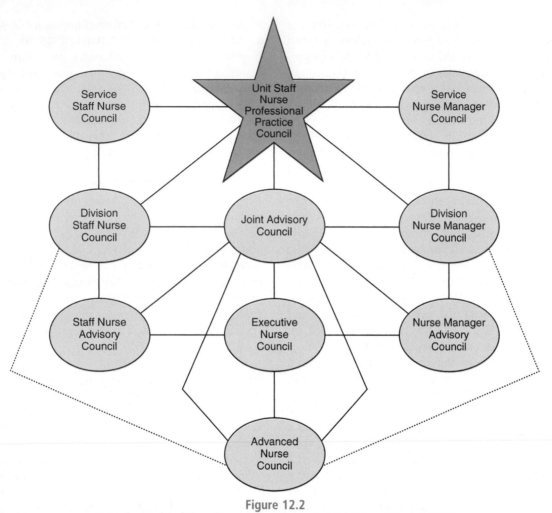

Figure 12.2
Councilor Model of Shared Leadership. (Courtesy St. Luke's Episcopal Hospital, 2000.)

For successful implementation of the shared governance concept, a supporting structure must be designed to fit the individual operating philosophy of the institution or health system. Regardless of the structure, implementation of the shared governance concept establishes the expectation for staff nurse participation and acceptance of personal accountability. The reluctance of some staff nurses to assume such accountability, which is often seen as extra work, is one of the largest sources of frustration for staff nurse advocates of shared governance (D. Thompson, personal communication, June 8, 2004). With the emergence of multidisciplinary teams and new health care systems, nurses will need to analyze and reevaluate the models of shared governance to make way for the developing partnerships. Another level of analysis may become necessary as health care reform and revised payment mechanisms drive changes in health care delivery systems.

As integrated networks form "new organizations," lateral and relational designs are emerging to support community-based health care delivery. These organizations are challenged to create delivery systems that ensure a seamless continuum of care. Clinical accountability and personal "buy-in" will become of paramount importance as partnerships of multidisciplinary players provide service in multisite care environments. Shared governance, with its emphasis on mutual respect and accountability, can form the basis for an integrated delivery care system, something that Porter-O'Grady and colleagues (1997) called *whole-systems shared governance*. This affords nurses the opportunity to take a leadership role in integrated care networks, based on past experiences with decentralization and shared governance.

LEADERSHIP AND MANAGEMENT IMPLICATIONS

Shared governance continues to be one of the many "best practice" options in the nurse leader's toolbox (Herrin, 2004). Although not a new concept to the nursing profession, it remains an illusive dream to some and an exhaustive process to others.

Research Note

Source: George, V., Burke, L.J., Rodgers, B., Duthie, N., Hoffmann, M.L., Koceja, V., et al. (2002). Developing staff nurse shared leadership behavior in professional nursing practice. *Nursing Administration Quarterly, 26*(3), 44-59.

Purpose

The purpose of this research was to demonstrate that implementation of a shared leadership concept educational program in an organized delivery system increases staff use of leadership behaviors, creates professional nursing practice autonomy, and improves patient outcomes. An educational program was offered to professional nurses who wanted to assume greater leadership accountability in the clinical practice environment. Classes consisted of four 8-hour-day modules delivered over a 2-month period to enable participants to practice the concepts on the nursing units. On day 1 the nurses completed a self-assessment with the *Leadership Practices Inventory — Individual Contributor: Self (LPI-IC: Self)* (Kouzes & Posner, 1993). They also distributed the *Leadership Practices Inventory—Individual Contributor: Observer (LPI-IC: Observer)* (Kouzes & Posner, 1993) to five colleagues who work with them in the clinical setting and who would give honest, constructive feedback on the nurse's frequency of leadership behavior use. On the final day the nurses received a summary comparing the observer feedback to their personal self-assessment.

Discussion

Three studies were conducted between 1995 and 1999 to study the process and outcomes of participation in the shared leadership concepts program (SLCP). The first study examined the difference between pre- and postprogram self-perceptions of leadership behavior of nurses who participated in the SLCP versus those who did not participate. The second study compared the pre- and 6-month postprogram changes in leadership behavior and professional nursing practice autonomy. The third study described nurses' perceptions of the processes and outcomes associated with their development and continued use of leadership behaviors in the clinical setting after participation in the SLCP.

Application to Practice

In study 1 there was a statistically significant increase in leadership behaviors between pre-and postprogram for the group who attended the SLCP. In study 2 the nurses showed statistically significant increases in all five self-reported leadership behaviors (i.e., challenging, inspiring, enabling, modeling, and encouraging) and nursing professional practice autonomy. Neither of the two studies established linkages with patient outcomes. In study 3 improvements in patient outcomes were documented and were linked to increased use of leadership behaviors. The studies demonstrated that a shared leadership development educational program and the development of a supportive milieu are effective in improving leadership behaviors in the clinical setting and the respective patient outcomes.

▲ LEADERSHIP & MANAGEMENT **BEHAVIORS**

Leadership Behaviors
- Integrates work effort
- Facilitates communication
- Coordinates plans and actions
- Envisions an empowered decision making environment
- Enables participation
- Liaisons with group members and outside the group

Management Behaviors
- Coaches individual employees
- Teaches others how to handle conflict

- Collaborates with staff
- Consults across units
- Creates a participative governance environment
- Communicates widely
- Coordinates work activities

Overlap Areas
- Communicates
- Coordinates activity
- Enables participation in decision making

Shared governance requires gradual development, continual nurturing and education for many, but the rewards include empowerment, autonomy, commitment, and improved outcomes for both patients and organizations.

New evidence affirms the need to improve workplace partnerships between nurses and their employing institutions (IOM, 2004) in order to ensure the future success of health care. Implementation of shared governance is one strategy to create a culture in which individual professional accountability and autonomy are respected and encouraged. By employing the attributes of accountability, partnership, equity, and ownership (Porter-O'Grady, 2003b), a bond is forged between the nurse and the employing organization. Nurses who enter into such bonds are more committed to the institution and less likely to depart. Evidence suggests that feelings of accountability and ownership by staff lead to improved organizational (DeBaca et al., 1993; Finkler et al., 1994; Jones et al., 1993; Westrope et al., 1995; Zelauskas & Howes, 1992) and patient outcomes (Aiken et al., 1997; Green & Jordan, 2004; Herrin, 2004; Porter-O'Grady, 2003b). Institutions that implement strategies, like "the forces of magnetism" espoused by the Magnet-designated hospitals, demonstrated improved patient outcomes and improved nurse retention

(McClure & Hinshaw, 2002). The forces of magnetism addressed each of the following areas (McClure & Hinshaw, 2002):
- Quality of nursing leadership
- Organizational structure
- Management style
- Personnel policies and programs
- Professional models of care
- Quality of care
- Quality improvement
- Consultation and resources
- Autonomy
- Community and the hospital
- Nurses as teachers
- Image of nursing
- Interdisciplinary relationships
- Professional development

With the focus on more efficacious health care delivery systems that care for patients safely and efficiently, the implementation of shared governance has far-reaching implications for nurse leaders. Involving professionals in the governance of the organizations in which they work is considered pivotal to a positive outcome for costs, coordination of care, and satisfaction (Havens, 1998). Although costs of implementing shared leadership remain uncertain, savings incurred due to treatment efficiency, decreased lengths of hospital stay, reduced nurse turnover, and less orientation time cannot be overlooked. Benefits to nurses include a renewed sense of commitment to the organization, empowerment, increasing autonomy, and training and education in conflict resolution, collaboration, and decision-making processes. Benefits to organizations include increased commitment to the organization; accountability of the nurse; a new level of professional autonomy; a more efficient model for point of service decision-making; more expert involvement at the point of service; a more assured, confident patient advocate; and identified financial benefits. Benefits for the patient include a more efficient model of health care service, more committed health care professionals, quicker responses at the point of service, and a more assured, confident patient advocate.

Nurse leaders stand to realize numerous organizational gains as bedside professional nurses embrace the quest for empowerment and professional autonomy. However, the journey to shared governance is slow and arduous as bedside nurses are groomed for the opportunities of ownership and accountability and taught how to manage these responsibilities. The guiding counsel of the profession's most nurturing leaders will be needed to support nurses in coping with change. Mentoring by clinically credible role models will be an important facet of the transformation toward shared governance.

"The goal is to transfer leadership wisdom not only to aspiring leaders but to all employees. Along this journey, expert leaders provide tools for employees to do their jobs well and to help them feel successful" (Porter-O'Grady & Malloch, 2002, p. 248).

CURRENT ISSUES AND TRENDS

Shared governance continues to be a viable alternative for many health care organizations and systems. Although a relatively recent innovation, it is recognized as an example of a decentralized organizational model. There are as many variations and degrees of shared governance as there are cultures within organizations. Although the concept has been a topic of interest since the early 1970s, the number of average-sized health care systems utilizing this accountability-based model continues to be small in comparison with the number of traditional hierarchical organizational structures.

Models of shared decision making, such as shared governance, make sense in an environment where workers are valued, supported, and respected. Leaders who capitalize on those principles possess the ability to transform the workplace through synergy with the workers. Visionary leaders encourage expert workers at the point of service to question long-time practices in order to establish new, more efficient practice models. Such leaders condone "out of the box" thinking and make allowances for occasional failures. Leaders who cling to traditional management styles instead of embracing a whole different set of leadership skills may find that their organizations cannot compete successfully in the fast-paced, consumer-driven, technologically advanced health care market.

"Whatever defines the contextual framework of success in the past can be temptingly easy to use as the measure of current success, resulting in the wrong measure for the right issue (staffing ratios, more staff, keeping patients longer, more money, etc.)" (Porter O'Grady, 2003a, p. 62).

Both leaders and workers should anticipate continued change. Successful change enhances and improves the worker and the workplace. Reading and discussing the popular book *Who Moved My Cheese?* (Johnson, 1998) is one strategy proactive leaders use to ease the strain of change on workers by helping them to cognitively reframe the idea of change.

In view of the critical nature of the current and forthcoming nursing shortage, nursing leaders are looking at the forces of magnetism (McClure & Hinshaw, 2002) as elements that are likely to contribute to an organizational culture of excellence that will enable them to better recruit and retain registered nurses. Research studies demonstrated that Magnet-designated hospital systems have improved recruitment and retention of professional nursing staff, patient outcomes, and patient satisfaction; nurses in these systems also report higher role autonomy and greater job satisfaction, as well as higher decision-making abilities and control over practice (Scott et al., 1999).

Summary

- Decision-making power is a key element of organizational structure.
- Centralization is the extent to which power and authority for decision making rests at the top of an organizational structure.
- Decentralization is the extent to which power and authority for decision making are systematically dispersed to middle and lower levels of the organization.
- Vertical decentralization is distribution of authority down the chain of command, or line of authority flowing from the top of the organization to the bottom.
- Horizontal decentralization is the flow of power outside the line of authority by which nonmanagement personnel are able to effect decision processes.
- Selective decentralization refers to a concentration of power that resides in functional divisions of an organization.
- *Centralization* and *decentralization* are relative terms on opposite ends of a continuum that indicate levels of decision-making power and authority.
- Shared governance is an accountability-based model of shared decision making that affords professional nurses at the point of service some level of control over their nursing practice.
- Shared governance is a process that leads to the empowerment of professional nurses in the clinical setting.
- Different levels of shared governance exist within health care institutions, just as different cultures exist within different institutions.
- As accountability for nursing practice increases, so do feelings of empowerment and professional autonomy in professional nursing staff.

- Research suggests that hospitals with shared governance have improved nurse retention and improved patient outcomes.
- Some form of the shared governance concept is evidenced in Magnet-designated hospitals.
- Obstacles to implementation of shared governance include the varied levels of skill and knowledge of nurses; the inexperience of nurses in collaboration, conducting meetings, and conflict resolution; and the large number of traditional autocratic nurse leaders and managers.
- Three operating models of shared governance have been identified as councilor, congressional, and administrative. The councilor model is the most common.

Study Questions

1. What is the relationship between decentralization and shared governance?
2. How are shared governance and structure related?
3. What conditions in the facility in which you are a student or employee would facilitate shared governance?
4. Are decentralization and shared governance characteristic of current hospital nursing organizations? Current community health and long-term care organizations?
5. Does changing to a shared governance model change nurses' roles? If so, how?
6. What is the governance structure of the nursing organization with which you are most familiar?
7. What questions should be asked to determine the level of decentralization in an organization?

CASE STUDY

The purpose of this case study is to consider one example of implementing change in a large academic teaching hospital in Houston, Texas, that has had shared governance in place in the department of nursing since 1987. The case study describes an actual scenario that took place in 2004 as related by D. Thompson, RN, chairman of the Staff Nurse Professional Practice Council at St. Luke's Episcopal Hospital.

Rosemary Luquire, RN, PhD, is the senior vice president of patient care and chief nursing officer of St. Luke's Episcopal Hospital, a 600-bed teaching hospital in a large metropolitan area known as the Texas Medical Center of Houston, Texas. Dr. Luquire is well respected among her peers and subordinates. She is seen to be a no-nonsense, "tells it like it is" leader. She reports to the executive vice president, who directly reports to the president and chief executive officer of the health system. Dr. Luquire has two vice presidents, six directors, and one manager who report directly to her. Dr. Luquire has regularly scheduled meetings with each of her direct reports. She encourages them to meet regularly with personnel who report to them. She has an approachable personality, such that nurses who know her throughout the hospital call her by her first name when they see her in the halls or the cafeteria. In meetings where medical staff are in attendance, she is addressed formally as Dr. Luquire.

1. Based on the information presented thus far, can you determine what type of organizational structure is in place? Centralized or decentralized? Explain.
2. What factors do you look for when determining whether an institution has a centralized or decentralized organizational structure?

The health care system has an online source of information that is accessible to all employees of the system. Newsworthy articles, access to policies of the system, new equipment and innovations, and upcoming education and training events are all announced and broadcast via this method. One special section, known as "Talk to the Executives" gives employees the opportunity to ask questions of the executive level of management of the institution. Questions are submitted and printed in this section of the online newspaper, and the appropriate executive responds to the question online.

A recently submitted question asked, "Can the dress code policy be changed so that clinical staff

may wear brown and/or black shoes? The current policy demands that all clinical staff wear white shoes. White shoes are difficult to keep clean and looking presentable." Since the question referred to staff in the clinical areas, the question was referred to Dr. Luquire to answer. Her first thought was "Oh no, clinical staff have always worn white shoes. How will brown or black shoes look?" However, in her response to the questioner, she agreed to consider the request. She took the issue to the Staff Nurse Professional Practice Council (SNPPC). The group agreed to thoroughly study the issue and come back to her with a recommendation. A small task force of the SNPPC researched the topic of wearing brown or black shoes in clinical settings. They did a literature review, but found no scientific evidence supporting or rejecting the proposed idea. After much discussion the task force took the proposal back to the SNPPC. The members of the SNPPC took the information back to their nursing units, where it was further discussed. The following month a proposal was placed on the agenda for action. The SNPPC voted to amend the dress code to enable staff in clinical areas to wear white, brown, or black shoes. The recommendation was taken back to Dr. Luquire, where it was signed into action. Despite her personal preference, she supported the recommendation of the SNPPC since there was no scientific basis for rejecting the proposal. The decision was then announced through the SNPPC as well as through the online news.

1. Based on the additional information given in the case study, how would you classify Dr. Luquire's organizational style? Centralized or decentralized? Explain.
2. How does an institution with shared governance differ from an institution without shared governance?
3. What key factors in the case study help you to determine whether this is an example of shared governance, participative management, or autocratic rule?
4. Identify some leadership behaviors that develop in professional nurses as a result

CRITICAL THINKING EXERCISE

Esther Brown complains bitterly as she sees the new schedule posted in the nurses' lounge. Once again she finds herself scheduled to work on the days that she requested to be off. As Dorothy Troy reads on the bulletin board that she has been assigned to do unit-based chart reviews for the next 3 months, she also voices her complaints. "The nurse manager didn't even ask me; she just assigned me! I've never even done it before!" Several staff nurses also are disgruntled because of unresolved issues on the nursing unit. Nursing staff are regularly absent from work, necessitating the use of registry nurses to maintain adequate staffing ratios. The continuity of patient care is suffering. Patients complain regularly that staff members do not answer their call lights promptly.

Physicians complain to administration that they can never find a nurse when they need one. And, when they do find a nurse, the nurse can never tell the physicians anything about their patients. The nurse manager is frustrated, exhausted, and discouraged. She laments that she wants to do a good job, but just can't get everything done.

1. What are the areas of concern in this scenario?
2. What should Nurse Brown do?
3. What should Nurse Troy do?
4. What strategies would you offer to the nurse manager to improve the situation on the unit?
5. Does this unit represent an example of centralized or decentralized decision making? Explain.

---

of practicing in a shared governance environment.

5. Describe some ways that registered nurses may be involved in governance of the nursing unit when shared governance is fully functioning.

Reference: St. Luke's Episcopal Hospital. *Shared leadership* (NURSAD-007/IP/500). Houston, TX: St. Luke's Episcopal Hospital.

REFERENCES

Aiken, L.H., Lake, E.T., Sochalski, J., & Sloane, D.M. (1997). Design of an outcomes study of the organization of hospital AIDS care. *Research in the Sociology of Health Care, 14*, 3-26.

Aiken, L.H., Clarke, S.P., Sloane, D.M., Sochalski, J., & Silber, J.H. (2002). Hospital nurse staffing and patient mortality, nurse burnout, and job dissatisfaction. *Journal of the American Medical Association, 288*(16), 1987-1993.

American Hospital Association (AHA) Commission on Workforce for Hospitals and Health Systems. (2002). *In our hands: How leaders can build a thriving workforce.* Chicago: AHA.

Argyris, C. (1994). Good communication that blocks learning. *Harvard Business Review, 72*(4), 77-85.

Beyers, M. (1999). The management of nursing services. In L.F. Wolper (Ed.), *Health care administration: Planning, implementing, and managing organized delivery systems.* (3rd ed.) (pp. 349-370). Gaithersburg, MD: Aspen.

Brooks, B.A. (2004, 31 January). Measuring the impact of shared governance. *Online Journal of Issues in Nursing, 9(1),* Manuscript 1a. Retrieved September 15, 2004, from *www.nursingworld.org/ojin/topic23/tpc23_1a.htm*

David, F.R. (1987). *Concepts of strategic management.* Columbus, OH: Merrill.

DeBaca, V., Jones, K., & Tornabeni, J. (1993). A cost-benefit analysis of shared governance. *Journal of Nursing Administration, 23*(7/8), 50-57.

Drucker, P.F. (1999). *Management challenges for the 21st century.* New York: Harper Collins.

Finkler, S.A., Kovner, C.T., Knickman, J.R., & Hendrickson, G. (1994). Innovation in nursing: A benefit/cost analysis. *Nursing Economic$, 12*(1), 18-27.

Green, A., & Jordan, C. (2004). Common denominators: Shared governance and workplace advocacy—Strategies for nurses to gain control over their practice. *Online Journal of Issues in Nursing. 9*(1), Manuscript 6. Retrieved September 15, 2004, from *www.nursingworld.org/ojin/topic23/tpc23_6.htm*

George, V., Burke, L.J., Rodgers, B., Duthie, N., Hoffmann, M.L., Koceja, V., et al. (2002). Developing staff nurse shared leadership behavior in professional nursing practice. *Nursing Administration Quarterly, 26*(3), 44-59.

Havens, D.S. (1998). An update on nursing involvement in hospital governance: 1990-1996. *Nursing Economic$, 16*(1), 6-11.

Herrick, L.M. (1998). Shared governance in an academic health center. In J.A. Dienemann (Ed.), *Nursing administration: Managing patient care,* (2nd ed.) (pp. 417-424). Stamford, CT: Appleton & Lange.

Herrin, D.M. (2004, 31 January). Shared governance: A nurse executive response. *Online Journal of Issues in Nursing.*

9(1), Manuscript 1b. Retrieved September 15, 2004, from *www.nursingworld.org/ojin/topic23/tpc23_ 1b.htm*

Hess, R., Jr. (1994). Shared governance: Innovation or imitation? *Nursing Economic$, 12*(1), 28-34.

Hess, R.G. (2004, 31 January). From bedside to boardroom—Nursing shared governance. *Online Journal of Issues in Nursing. 9*(1), Manuscript 1. Retrieved September 15, 2004, from *www.nursingworld.org/ojin/topic23/tpc23_1.htm*

Institute of Medicine (IOM). (2004). *Keeping patients safe: Transforming the work environment of nurses.* Washington, DC: The National Academies Press.

Joint Commission on Accreditation of Healthcare Organizations (JCAHO). (2002). *Healthcare at the crossroads: Strategies for addressing the evolving nursing crisis.* Oak Brook, IL: JCAHO.

Johnson, S. (1998). *Who moved my cheese?* New York: G.P. Putnam's Sons.

Jones, C., Stasiowski, S., Simons, B., Boyd, N., & Lucas, M. (1993). Shared governance and the nursing practice environment. *Nursing Economic$, 11*(4), 208-214.

Kouzes, J.M., & Posner B.Z. (1993). *Leadership Practices Inventory (LPI): Participant's workbook and LPI form.* San Francisco: Jossey-Bass.

Ludemann, R.S., & Brown, C. (1989). Staff perceptions of shared governance. *Nursing Administration Quarterly, 13*(4), 49-56.

Maas, M., & Specht, J. (1990). Nursing professionalization and self-governance: A model from long-term care. In G. Mayer, M. Madden, & E. Lawrenz (Eds.), *Patient care delivery models* (pp. 151-168). Rockville, MD: Aspen.

McClure, M.L., & Hinshaw, A.S. (2002). *Magnet hospitals revisited: Attraction and retention of professional nurses.* Washington, DC: American Nurses Publishing.

Miller, G.J. (1992). *Managerial dilemmas: The political economy of hierarchy.* New York: Cambridge University Press.

Minnen, T., Berger, E., Ames, A., Dubree, M., Baker, W., & Spinella, J. (1993). Sustaining work redesign innovations through shared governance. *Journal of Nursing Administration, 23*(7/8), 35-40.

North, D.C. (1990). *Institutions, institutional change and economic performance.* New York: Cambridge University Press.

Orsburn, J.D., Moran, L., Musselwaite, E., & Zenger, J.H. (1990). *Self-directed work teams.* Homewood, IL: Business One Irwin.

Porter-O'Grady, T. (1987). Shared governance and new organizational models. *Nursing Economic$, 5*(6), 281-286.

Porter-O'Grady, T. (2001). Is shared governance still relevant? *Journal of Nursing Administration, 31*(10), 468-473.

Porter-O'Grady, T. (2003a). Of hubris and hope: Transforming nursing for a new age. *Nursing Economic$, 21*(2), 59-64.

Porter-O'Grady, T. (2003b). Researching shared governance: A futility of focus. *Journal of Nursing Administration, 33*(4), 251-252.

Porter-O'Grady, T., Hawkins, M.A., & Parker, M.L. (1997). *Whole-systems shared governance: Architecture for integration.* Gaithersburg, MD: Aspen.

Porter-O'Grady, T., & Malloch, K. (2002). *Quantum leadership: A textbook of new leadership.* Gaithersburg, MD: Aspen.

Prince, S.B. (1997). Shared governance: Sharing power and opportunity. *Journal of Nursing Administration, 27*(3), 28-35.

The Call to the Nursing Profession. (2002). *Nursing's agenda for the future: A call to the nation.* Washington, DC: American Nurses Publishing.

The Robert Wood Johnson Foundation. (2002). *Health care's human crisis: The American nursing shortage.* Princeton, NJ: The Robert Wood Johnson Foundation.

Scott, J.G, Sochalski, J., & Aiken, L. (1999). Review of magnet hospital research: Findings and implications for professional nursing practice. *Journal of Nursing Administration, 29*(1), 9-19.

Straub, J.T. & Attner, R.F. (1994). *Introduction to business* (5th ed.). Belmont, CA: Wadsworth.

Thompson, B., Hateley, P., Molloy, R., Fernandez, S., Madigan, A.L., Thrower, C., et al. (2004). A journey, not an event—Implementation of shared governance in a NHS trust. *Online Journal of Issues in Nursing, 9*(1), Manuscript 3. Retrieved October 31, 2004, from *www.nursingworld.org/ojin/topic23/tpc23_3.htm*

Westrope, R.A., Vaughn, L., Bott, M., & Taunton, R.L. (1995). Shared governance: From vision to reality. *Journal of Nursing Administration, 25*(12), 45-54.

Zelauskas, B., & Howes, D.G. (1992). The effects of implementing a professional practice model. *Journal of Nursing Administration, 22*(7/8), 18-23.

13

Data Management and Informatics

Jacqueline Moss

CHAPTER OBJECTIVES

- Highlight the importance of data management for decision making
- Define and describe computer applications in nursing, nursing informatics, and management information systems
- Analyze information needs in health care
- Classify nursing's data needs
- Appraise the implementation of a computerized patient record
- Explore nursing informatics
- Describe a nursing minimum data set for administrative practice
- Integrate effectiveness research and nursing informatics
- Analyze the need for a standardized and retrievable management data set
- Speculate about future informatics trends
- Exercise critical thinking to conceptualize and analyze possible solutions to a practice exercise

The information age has truly arrived. In the last 30 years, society has seen the widespread adoption of the personal computer, cell phone, personal digital assistant, satellite, and cable television. Information can now be transmitted across the world, immediately, in a variety of formats. Information technology has changed the way people work, play, learn, manage their personal lives, and view the world. Consequently, information has become a commodity to be bought, sold, and managed.

The business of health care information management is growing by leaps and bounds. Management of the health care industry and care delivery relies extensively on the collection and analysis of data. Data can provide information about the patient, provider, outcomes, and processes of care delivery (Mills et al., 1996). These data are collected from many individuals practicing in different specialties and must be integrated, coordinated, and managed. In addition, the increasing demand to use these data for performance measurement and reporting to managed care customers, regulators, and accrediting bodies comes at a time of acquisition and merger within the health care industry (Currie, 1998). Regulatory and governmental agencies require the collection of data to measure performance (e.g., Joint Commission on Accreditation of Healthcare Organizations [JCAHO]), the organization of these data into specific formats (e.g., Medicare/Medicaid), and adequate protections to ensure the confidentiality of these data (e.g., Health Insurance Portability and Accountability Act [HIPPA]). To meet these demands, administrators need data that can be compared across multiple settings, both geographically and clinically.

DEFINITIONS

Computer applications in nursing administration can be understood best as arising from the intersection of three areas: nursing administration, informatics, and effectiveness research or research on client outcomes. The computer is a tool for managing complexity and controlling and coordinating large volumes of data (Mowry & Korpman, 1986). The electronic computer has made knowledge-based systems possible.

As a part of the larger domain of technology, informatics is a combination of computer science with information science. **Nursing informatics** is defined as the management and processing of nursing data, information, and knowledge to support the practice of nursing and the delivery of nursing care (Graves & Corcoran, 1989). It involves the use of information management technologies to facilitate nursing practice, education, administration, and research (Schwirian, 1986). *Effectiveness research* is defined as the study of relationships among health care problems, interventions, outcomes, and costs, generally by analyzing large databases or using epidemiological methods.

A **management information system (MIS)** is defined as an integrated system for collecting, storing, retrieving, and processing a collective set of data. The data are transformed from storage into knowledge that is directly useful and applicable in the process of directing and controlling resources and their application to the achievement of specific management objectives (Ein-Dor & Segev, 1978; Hanson, 1982). An automated MIS is "a combination of hardware, software, and people for the purpose of accomplishing a specific task" (Newbold, 1998, p. 323). An MIS is essentially a system that provides information that managers use in decision-making processes. Applications may process, store, and retrieve information, estimate the outcomes of alternative decisions, or assist in communicating decisions (Peterson & Hannah, 1988). The 10 criteria, or desirable characteristics, for a good MIS are (1) informative, (2) relevant, (3) sensitive, (4) unbiased, (5) comprehensive, (6) timely, (7) action-oriented, (8) uniform, (9) performance-targeted, and (10) cost-effective (Austin, 1979). An example of a component of an MIS is a workload management system (WMS). WMS examples include nursing acuity systems and laboratory workload systems. Staffing and scheduling automated systems also are a part of a WMS, which is a part of an MIS for operational management activities (Davidson & Sanders, 1998).

Automated information systems also are used for the collection of clinical data related to the direct care of clients and managing care processes. Information systems support clinical data gathering in areas such as laboratory test results, medication administration, and vital signs documentation. Narrative reports are less often included. Clinical information systems are used to maintain data on indicators of quality, adverse events, adherence to standards, and identification of potential problems via clinical alerts and on assistance with clinical

▲ LEADING & MANAGING DEFINED

Nursing Informatics

The management and processing of nursing data, information, and knowledge to support the practice of nursing and the delivery of nursing care.

Management Information System (MIS)

An integrated system for collecting, storing, retrieving, and processing a collective set of data; the data are transformed from storage into knowledge that is directly useful and applicable in the process of directing and controlling resources and their application to the achievement of specific management objectives.

decisions via decision support systems such as the selection of appropriate antibiotics (Davidson & Sanders, 1998).

A *clinical data repository* is defined as a physical or logical compilation of client data pertaining to health. This compilation may also be called an *information warehouse* or simply a *data repository*. Data are stored longitudinally over multiple episodes of care. The primary purpose is to facilitate easy retrieval of data (ANA, 1997).

NURSING'S DATA NEEDS

Nursing's data needs fall into four domains. Nurses need data about client care, provider staffing, administration of care and the organization, and knowledge-based research for evidence-based practice. The first three are distinct areas, but research, the fourth domain, interacts with all of the other three. The four areas and the sources for the data are as follows:

1. *Client:* Client care/clinical care and its evaluation, clinical data, and client outcomes. Source: the client's health care record.
2. *Provider:* Professional data, caregiver outcomes, and decision maker variables. Source: personnel records, national data banks, and links to client records.
3. *Administrative:* Management and resource oversight, administrative data, system outcomes, and contextual variables. Source: administrative, fiscal, and regulatory data.
4. *Research:* Knowledge base development. Source: existing and newly gathered data and relational databases.

Table 13.1 displays examples of outcomes and variables to be measured in relation to the three distinct domains of nursing's data needs.

Table 13.1

Outcomes and Variables in Three Domains of Nursing Data Needs		
Domain	Outcomes	Variables
Client	Client satisfaction	Attitudes/beliefs
	Achieved care outcomes	Diagnosis, gender, age
	Costs	Marital status
	Access to care	Support system
		Satisfaction
		Level of dependency
		Severity of illness
		Intensity of nursing care
Provider	Job enrichment	Attitudes/beliefs
	Job/work satisfaction	Education
	Physician satisfaction	Years of experience
	Job stress	Age
	Intent to leave	Work excitement
Administrative	Costs	Agency philosophy
	Productivity	Priorities
	Turnover	Organizational structure
	Income	Fiscal data
		Climate
		Policies and procedures
		Conflict

For example, in the client domain, the cost of care to the client is an important outcome for which data are needed to manage care. Intensity of nursing care is one variable that may be measured to monitor and control costs.

The collection and analysis of data is a critical thrust of current health services research. Data analysis is aimed at cost, quality, and effectiveness outcomes. McCormick (1988) acknowledged the significant contribution that computer technology can make to the documentation of nursing practice. However, this contribution rests on structuring the input logically, providing adequate processing and memory, and assuring valid and reliable output. Clear definition, valid linkage between datasets, and clear coding of input are essential in securing meaningful output that has utility. The aggregation of information over time and how this aggregation affects the quality of information is especially important to uniform datasets. Similarly, the reliable and valid aggregation of nursing management information is important for policy and resource allocation strategies in nursing administration.

NURSING INFORMATICS

Recognized by the American Nurses Association (ANA) as a nursing specialty in 1992, informatics is one of the fastest growing practice areas in health care. As defined by Graves and Corcoran, "nursing informatics is a combination of computer science, information science and nursing science designed to assist in the management and processing of nursing data, information and knowledge to support the practice of nursing and the delivery of nursing care" (1989, p. 227). *Data* are defined as discrete, objective entities, without interpretation; *information* as data that are structured, organized, or interpreted; and *knowledge* as synthesized information with identified relationships.

The focus of nursing informatics practice is the organization, analysis, and dissemination of information, not the computer itself (Abbott & Lee, 2001). Nursing informatics specialists assist practitioners by providing information to enhance decision making and the delivery of safe patient care. Although these specialists may not be directly involved with care delivery, their work is integrally related to clinical and administrative practice. Nursing informatics specialists participate in the analysis, design, and implementation of information and communication systems; effectiveness and informatics research; and the education of nurses in informatics and information technology.

The first master's degree in nursing informatics was offered by the University of Maryland in 1989. In 1992 that same university followed with the first doctoral program in nursing informatics. Now, programs in nursing informatics can be found throughout the United States. These programs offer a variety of educational options, including master's degrees, post-master's certificates, and doctoral degrees. In addition, nurses can obtain certification in nursing informatics from the American Nurses Credentialing Center (ANCC).

ELECTRONIC HEALTH RECORD

In 1965 El Camino Hospital in Mountain View, California, began one of the first attempts to develop an electronic health record (EHR). Along with Technicon Medical Information Systems and Lockheed Missiles and Space Company, an information system was created that communicated physicians' orders, retrieved laboratory results, and supported the documentation of nursing care (Staggers et al., 2001). The development of early information systems designed to support an EHR was confined to large tertiary care centers and federal agencies such as the Veterans Administration and the National Institutes of Health. The high cost of these systems and the fee-for-service reimbursement structure for health care costs provided little incentive for most health care institutions to change the way they were managing health care data.

The shift from a retrospective fee-for-service to a prospective managed care financial structure for the payment of medical services changed the way patient data were perceived and shared

Research Note

Source: Snyder-Halpern, R. (1999). Assessing health care setting readiness for point of care computerized clinical decision support system innovations. *Outcomes Management for Nursing Practice, 3*(3), 118-127.

Purpose

Despite the promise that clinical practice guidelines have as high-quality and cost-effective elements in clinical decision support systems, there has been erratic diffusion and adoption of these evidence-based guidelines. Despite documented success, knowledge-based systems have had limited use in health care settings. The purpose of this article was to describe a clinical information technology innovation model and its use to assess readiness for a clinical decision support system in one hospital.

Discussion

Computerized clinical decision support systems are an advanced clinical information technology useful for bringing evidence-based clinical knowledge to clinicians at the point of care. These systems support the clinician's natural clinical decision making processes by allowing linkage of real-time data to evidence-based clinical knowledge. Recent advances in clinical information system technology have helped the development of integrated clinical information systems. However, despite documented success, knowledge-based advisory systems for clinicians have had limited use in health care settings. In this article, a Clinical Information Technology Innovation Model was displayed and explained. The key concepts are external environmental factors, health care setting characteristics, innovation readiness, innovation customization process, and innovation implementation process. Innovation readiness mediates the interactions among all components. This model was used to guide decision making about an acute pain management knowledge-based system project. The article reports a case illustration of the application of their model to the acute pain management area. The setting, background, purpose, implementation, and innovation readiness assessment outcomes of the project are described. The project was designed to develop and implement a real-time, rule-based knowledge system to assist cardiovascular step down unit RNs with the management of acute pain secondary to CABG surgery in one hospital. The hospital's evidence-based pain management program guidelines were the knowledge source. Project implementation was coordinated by a design team.

Application to Practice

The author describes clinical information technology as a challenging and risky innovation endeavor. It is all-encompassing, complex, and multifaceted, making management and conceptualization of the innovation process difficult. A combination of both high and low readiness factors emerged, but most of the indicators revealed that this hospital was not ready for the innovation. The project was discontinued. However, four recommendations emerged: use an interdisciplinary team approach, maximize knowledge and functional readiness through a comprehensive assessment, improve readiness by developing the basic information processing architecture, and make a strategic commitment to developing structures to support clinicians' information requirements. The model outlines a useful and systematic assessment framework.

(Staggers et al., 2001). Currently, patient data are of interest not only to health care providers but also to managed care organizations and governmental payors, who want to ensure that their money is spent in the most effective way to produce the best patient outcomes. These data are also scrutinized by health care providers to ensure that patient needs are being met in the most efficient and cost-effective manner.

Harvesting these data from traditional paper documentation systems is expensive and inefficient. Those conducting chart reviews to collect data are frequently confronted with incomplete and inconsistent documentation. Using standards for data collection, an EHR could be accessed across health networks, linking clinical and business processes, reducing data replication and increasing the availability and accessibility of information. Well-designed computerized information systems can facilitate the collection of complete and accurate data in a form that is easily accessible to enhance clinical practice, analyze patient outcomes, or manage institutional resources.

The purpose of an EHR is to document patient care in a single repository as a clinical, financial, and legal record. The electronic format makes the record available as a communication device among health care members regardless of their location. Through this method data are archived and can be used for research and quality improvement (Young, 2000). The EHR is a virtual record. It does not originate from one place. It is a compilation of information from a variety of integrated systems.

In 2004 President George W. Bush announced the creation of the position of National Health Information Technology Coordinator at the Department of Health and Human Services (HHS). The coordinator's role is to provide the leadership to develop the standards and infrastructure necessary to harness the use of information technology to improve patient care and reduce health care costs (Phoenix Health Systems, 2004). The central focus of the President's Consolidated Health Informatics Initiative (CHI) is for each American to have an EHR by 2014. The HHS and other federal agencies will adopt 15 standards for the exchange of electronic information across the federal government. To facilitate the development of interoperable EHR systems across the country, the standardized vocabulary, SNOMED CT, has been made available for free download through the National Library of Medicine (USDHHS, 2004).

Much of the recent push for the development of an EHR has been related to the public's awareness regarding the frequency of medical errors in health care. An estimated 23,000 hospital patients die each year as a result of an adverse drug event (Kimmel & Sensmeier, 2002). Most errors (49%) that result in adverse drug events occur when the drug is ordered. Ordering errors identified include the following: wrong dose, wrong choice of drug, known allergy, wrong frequency, and drug-drug interaction (Bates et al., 1995). Handwritten medication orders are often incomplete or contain illegible penmanship. A study of handwritten medication orders in three hospital units found that over a 48-hour period 20% of medication orders and 78% of signatures were either illegible or legible only with effort. In this same study, 24% of medication orders were found to be incomplete (Winslow et al., 1997). Integrating an EHR with pharmacy, laboratory, and clinical information systems allows the implementation of computerized provider order entry (CPOE), decision support systems (DSS), and medication administration systems (MAS) designed to reduce errors in health care systems.

The cost of implementing technological solutions in health care is extremely expensive, and it has been difficult to show a return on investment (ROI) for these expenditures. However, an estimated $12.7 to $36 billion could be saved annually from the national implementation of an EHR through the associated reduction in adverse events, unnecessary clinical procedures, and staff time, along with more rapid record retrieval (Staggers et al., 2001). The growing trend is to regard these expenditures as part of the cost of institutional infrastructure and to tie them to the cost savings gained by improving patient outcomes. The Leapfrog Group, a coalition of major employers, is requiring that health care organizations have CPOE in place if they want to continue to provide care to their employees. Due in part to the documented cost of medication errors, 67% of health care organizations plan to add computerized provider order entry (CPOE) in the next few years (Ball, 2003).

Effectiveness

The first person to analyze patient outcomes associated with nursing care delivery was Florence Nightingale in the nineteenth century. After that time, research into patient outcomes was not emphasized until health care cost and quality became social and policy issues (Maas et al., 1996). Health care systems are struggling to contain costs and determine effectiveness for their survival in a managed care environment. Current measures that focus solely on reduced mortality, length of stay, and hospital costs provide little information about the quality of health care provided. Computer technology and the development of nursing classification systems have made the measurement and evaluation of nursing-sensitive outcomes feasible.

Nurses spend approximately 50% of their time coordinating and documenting patient information (Meadows, 2002). Unfortunately, these data are generally documented in a format that is difficult to access and analyze. Nursing informatics specialists work to organize and aggregate these data for decision making in care delivery management and the analysis of patient outcomes. These activities require data that are organized in nursing outcomes databases. Without clinical outcomes databases that reflect nursing care, data available in current billing systems will be used for generic outcome evaluation. Nursing outcome databases are critical for two reasons: (1) nurses must be able to measure and document how nurses influence patient outcomes, and (2) the study of nursing-sensitive outcomes will allow comparisons between interventional strategies and advance the science of nursing care delivery (Iowa Intervention Project, 1997).

Formulation of the Nursing Minimum Data Set (NMDS) was an effort to standardize the collection of essential nursing information for comparison of nursing data across patient populations. The NMDS identifies the data essential for inclusion in clinical information systems necessary to support decision making in clinical and administrative nursing practice. Three categories of data elements are included in the NMDS: nursing care, demographic, and service. Data elements related to nursing care include nursing diagnosis, intervention, outcome, and intensity of nursing care (Werley & Lang, 1988). Using the NMDS as

a guide helps to ensure that data are collected regarding institutional structure (having the right things), process (doing things right), and outcomes (having the right things happen). Linking structure, process, and outcomes is necessary for the accurate evaluation of efficiency and effectiveness (Donabedian, 1986).

STANDARDIZED CLINICAL TERMINOLOGY

Nurses spend a great deal of their time collecting and documenting information related to patient care delivery. Vast amounts of data are compiled, describing every detail of the patient's encounter with the health care system. Unfortunately, these data are rarely recorded in a way that makes them amenable to analysis. When charting the description of the same surgical incision, five different nurses may chart five different entries. They may describe the size of the wound in centimeters or inches. The wound color could be depicted as pink, slightly reddened, or slightly inflamed. When different terms are used to describe the same observable fact, it is difficult to know that everyone is referring to the same phenomenon.

Norma Lang, a pioneer in nursing informatics, once wrote "If we cannot name it, we cannot control it, practice it, research it, teach it, finance it, or put it into public policy" (Clark & Lang, 1992, p. 109). For nearly 30 years, nurses have been striving to develop classification systems that itemize the diagnoses, interventions, and most recently, outcomes of the professional domain. Often, this process has been fraught with controversy and disagreement, resulting in multiple approaches to classification. Much of the time, these disagreements were viewed as divisive and disruptive to the profession. However, the result has been a richer, more inclusive representation of "what nurses do" in different practice environments. Currently, 13 standardized terminologies are recognized by the American Nurses Association (ANA). These include terminologies for nursing administration, home health care, perioperative nursing, acute care, and also a terminology for describing nursing care internationally. The ANA-recognized terminologies for nursing are as follows: North American Nursing Diagnosis Association, Inc. (NANDA), Nursing Interventions Classification System (NIC), Nursing Outcomes Classification System (NOC), Nursing Management Minimum Data Set (NMMDS), Home Health Care Classifications (HHCC), Omaha System, Patient Care Data Set (PCDS), SNOMED CT, Nursing Minimum Data Set (NMDS), International Classification for Nursing (ICNP), ABCcodes, and Logical Observation Identifier Names & Codes (LOINC) (NIDSEC, 2004).

Terminology structures most commonly used in health care are classification systems. Classification systems are noncombinatorial hierarchical languages designed to categorize objects (Ingenerf, 1995). In health care classification systems, objects classified are generally patient diagnosis and care interventions. Nursing classifications, also referred to as interface terminologies, are generally implemented at the point of care to describe clinical practice (Coenen et al., 2001).

However, most classification terminologies lack the conceptual structure necessary for their direct incorporation in modern object-oriented computer database systems (Button et al., 1998). Concept-oriented or reference terminologies have the potential to provide the necessary structure for documentation in modern computer database systems. On the other hand, concept-oriented terminologies require the user to combine terms, making them awkward for their direct use as a documentation tool (Hardiker & Rector, 2001). Therefore recent efforts have centered on the development of reference terminologies that can serve as intermediaries between standardized nursing documentation and computer database systems. Classification systems can help provide the terms used in documenting practice, and the reference terminology model can provide the structure for their organization in the computer database.

A reference terminology model (RTM) depicts the system of concepts that provide the structure for the organization of documentation terms (Bakken et al., 2001). In recent years, progress has been made in the development of reference terminology models that represent the domain concepts of diagnoses and intervention in nursing. Prominent in these efforts is the work of the European Standardization Committee (CEN TC 251). The CEN combined the efforts of groups working on the International Classification for Nursing Practice (ICNP) and Telenurse ID projects, producing a proposed categorical structure for nursing diagnosis and intervention. This work was continued by the International Standards Organization (ISO) Technical Committee ISO/TC 215 Health Informatics, Working Group 3 Health Concept Representation (ISO/TC 215/WG 3). The efforts of the ISO working group focused specifically on the conceptual structure required by a nursing reference terminology model (ISO, 2002). The resulting conceptual structure for nursing diagnoses and interventions were designed to integrate with evolving multidisciplinary terminology standards. Through the use of these terminology models, diagnosis and intervention terms contained within existing clinical classification systems can be mapped for harmonization across medical and nursing terminologies.

The ISO RTM for Nursing Action is composed of six categories designed to describe nursing interventions in a modern object-oriented computer database. The six categories included in the ISO RTM for Nursing Action are action, target, recipient of care, means, route, and site (ISO, 2002). By using these categories to guide the decomposition and mapping of nursing documentation, the ability of the model to support nursing documentation can be evaluated (Moss et al., 2003), the ability of the documentation to meet regulatory requirements can be evaluated (Moss, 2003), and the structure of formal terminology systems can be enhanced (Hardiker, 2003).

NURSING MANAGEMENT MINIMUM DATA SET

Awareness of the need for standardized, uniformly collected, retrievable, and comparable service-related management data elements, combined with the awareness of their unavailability in practice, was the impetus for the research to develop and test a Nursing Management Minimum Data Set (NMMDS) (Huber et al., 1997; Huber et al., 1992) (Figure 13.1).

Building on the NMDS, the NMMDS specifically identified variables essential to nurse managers for decision making about nursing care effectiveness. For example, the NMMDS can be linked to the nursing care elements of intensity/staff mix to provide an enhanced assessment of the consumption of health care resources to produce specific client care outcomes for a specific age cohort, racial/ethnic group, or geographical region.

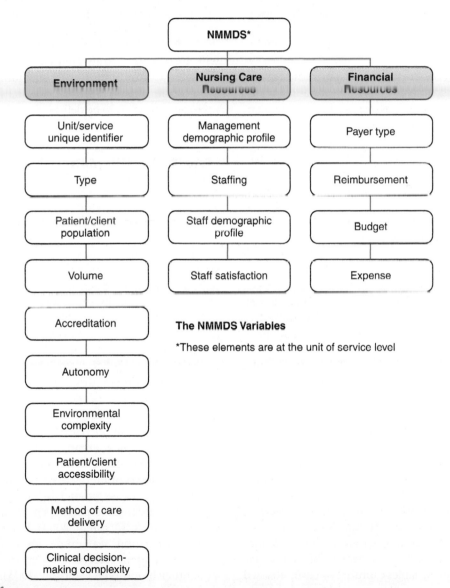

Figure 13.1
The 18 elements of the Nursing Management Minimum Data Set (NMMDS). (Copyright D. Huber & C. Delaney, Iowa City, IA.)

Linkage to the NMDS service elements, specifically the expected payer of the bill, would assist in isolating budgetary elements.

The NMMDS identified 18 elements potentially critical to evaluating the impact of nursing interventions on client outcomes. The NMMDS work has the potential of facilitating the linking and augmenting of the other minimum health data sets by providing information uniquely important to nursing administrative decisions and thus to the evaluation of nursing services for cost and quality outcomes of care delivery.

The NMMDS work helps to clarify and expand the data points that tap contextual variables, which intervene between provider actions and client outcomes. Despite the use of the NMDS in nursing research and practice, the fourth element of intensity is often ignored. The focus of the NMDS is limited to the first three nursing variables of diagnosis, interventions, and outcomes. For example, Blewitt and Jones (1996) reported a pilot study using elements of the NMDS in a sample of clients undergoing parathyroidectomy. After reviewing the four elements of the NMDS, they noted that their study focused on diagnosis, intervention, and outcomes. This strategy ignores the important impact of contextual variables. To fully capture outcomes for quality and effectiveness determinations, multiple domains need to be included (Huber & Oermann, 1999). This is especially important since "the effectiveness of nursing interventions is especially sensitive to the influences of organizational structures and processes" (Maas et al., 1999, p. 4).

Nursing needs a standardized data set that will facilitate decision making and policy development in such areas as job satisfaction, turnover, cost of nursing services, allocation of nursing personnel, and comparison of nursing care delivery models. Such a data set would foster data collection, retrieval, analysis, and comparison of nursing management outcomes across settings, populations, time intervals, and geographical regions. Using a core of variables captured by computerized information systems, data essential to nursing care delivery management can be analyzed and used to meet nursing's goals and objectives. Management information systems join large database development efforts and other information software applications to enhance nursing leadership and management. The future points to further developments and refinements to augment the practice of nursing. The future will hold more computer power, portable computers and hand-held terminals, voice input, videodisk technology, expert systems, artificial intelligence, and more advanced decision support and modeling systems. There will be greater connectedness and outreach linkages. Computing is the medium of communication in the future; information is the message that needs to be delivered (Ball & Douglas, 1988).

LEADERSHIP AND MANAGEMENT IMPLICATIONS

The Institute of Medicine (IOM) landmark report on medical errors in the United States was based, in part, on the landmark study of medical errors conducted by Lucian Leape. Leape found that all seven of the most frequent medical errors cited were due to impaired access to information. These errors were primarily the result of system design faults and accounted for 78% of the total errors uncovered (Leape et al., 1995).

Technological applications have the capability to change system processes to improve communication and information access, and thereby decrease errors and adverse events (Moss et al., 2002). However, inadequate information system design can actually *increase* rather than decrease the risk for medical errors. In January of 2003, Cedars-Sinai Medical Center suspended the use of a $43 million computerized system for physician order entry because physicians complained that the system endangered patient safety and required too much work (Ornstein, 2003). In another case, poor information system design resulted in a transplant patient receiving organs from a donor of another blood type (Stenson, 2003). Although information regarding the donor's blood type was listed in a computerized database, no system was

◬ LEADERSHIP & MANAGEMENT **BEHAVIORS**

Leadership Behaviors

- Envisions a structure to capture data needs
- Projects data needs
- Enables followers to use data and information
- Models knowledge-based practice
- Uses electronic data management resources
- Uses data and information for power and political advantage

Management Behaviors

- Identifies needed data
- Plans for the collection of data

- Organizes data collection
- Uses electronic resources
- Analyzes data
- Uses information strategically

Overlap Areas

- Identifies data and information needs

---

in place for cross-checking this information with that of the recipient's blood type.

Implementation of technology to improve the documentation and delivery of health care will require organizational change in a technical, structural, and behavioral sense (Ball, 2003). Strategically planning for the design and implementation of health care information systems requires the participation and collaboration of all stakeholders within the organizational system. Implementing information systems designed without the involvement and buy-in of representatives from all user groups often results in poorly designed systems that fail to gain acceptance and fail to meet institutional needs.

Increasingly, nurse managers are being asked to participate in the selection, design, and implementation of institutional information systems. It is implicitly acknowledged that collecting, sharing, and analyzing information will positively affect the quality of care delivered. However, too often in the past the documentation of nursing care has not been included in the collection of organizational data. The result of this has been that nursing practice and its contribution to institutional effectiveness have not been visible in the analysis of organizational data. Nursing leaders are in the position of ensuring that information systems are selected that collect nursing data and support the way nurses work. Effective information

system structure requires the determination of the appropriate information system requirements for the specific users' needs (Moss & Xiao, 2004). Successful information systems are those with the ability to accurately measure and analyze the efficiency and effectiveness of care.

CURRENT ISSUES AND TRENDS

Nursing and health care organizations are calling for the redesign of the existing work environment to improve clinician and client satisfaction, client outcomes, and the profitability of all health care organizations. The American Organization of Nurse Executives (AONE) has called for the redesign of work through the use of technology to augment nursing practice during this period of a decreasing and aging workforce (Kennedy, 2003). The purpose of this mandate is twofold: (1) to improve the work environment and attract more individuals to the profession and (2) to use technology to enable aging nurses to remain active in direct-care roles.

Toward this goal, system designers are focusing on how to communicate information for the automation and coordination of health care work. According to Stetson and colleagues (2001) there is no instance in which coordination of care takes place in the absence of communication, and there is no instance in which clinical information

Research Note

Source: Moss, J., & Xiao, Y. (2004). Improving operating room coordination: Communication pattern assessment. *Journal of Nursing Administration, 34*(2), 93-100.

Purpose

Operating room (OR) charge nurses are responsible for balancing the work of nurses, surgeons, anesthesiologists, and technicians to ensure safe and effective patient care. Coordination of this work requires intense communication. In fact, communication, or the lack of it, has been shown to be a major contributor to error in health care. Health care work is highly dynamic. Providers perform multiple tasks simultaneously with frequent interruptions. Even when only 10 seconds separates the intention from the interruption, workers may lose their train of thought and errors can occur. Automating information access and delivery and therefore decreasing communication load may reduce the number of medical errors. The purpose of this study was three-fold: to evaluate a methodology for determining information needs through a data collection tool, to document OR charge nurse communication patterns with the tool, and to characterize the information needs in articulation work.

Discussion

Prior to introducing technology that changes work processes, the information types and communication patterns among health care professionals need to be understood. Inadequately designed information and communication systems can actually increase the risk for error. In this study, the communication of OR charge nurses, in four operating rooms, was recorded on a data collection tool by a trained observer. The tool was designed to answer the following questions:

- What the purposes of the communication?
- Who is involved in communication?
- What media or modes of communication are used?
- What is the duration of communication for each episode?

A total of 2074 communication episodes were observed during the course of approximately 100 hours. The number of communications between charge nurses and other staff ranged from 32 to 74 per hour. Coordinating equipment was the most frequent reason for communication in all surgical suites, averaging 39% of total communication episodes. Communication regarding equipment management was related to the location of equipment and the status of equipment. Equipment status could be characterized as dirty, clean, or sterile. Preparing patients for surgery ranked second in frequency of communication episodes at 26%. Communication most frequently occurred between the charge nurse and OR nurses and was face-to-face. These communications episodes were short. The mean duration of communication related to preparing patients was 31 seconds, and the mean duration of communications regarding equipment management was 40 seconds.

Application to Practice

Determining aspects of health care delivery that can be automated can help reduce errors, control costs, and improve patient outcomes. The short duration and lack of negotiation associated with equipment management and patient preparedness in this study supports the automation of information delivery for these functions in OR management. Examples of possible solutions for the automation of equipment management include the use of bar coding and global positioning equipment to track equipment location and status. Global positioning could also be used to track patients' locations throughout the hospital as they move between departments preparing for surgery. Steps in the patient's preparation for surgery could be posted electronically as they are completed. For example, as laboratory work, anesthesia assessments, and the completion of surgical permits are performed, these milestones could be posted on an electronic whiteboard or hospital intranet to allow access to all team members at varying locations.

exchange occurs in the absence of clinical communication (Stetson et al., 2001). Technological solutions to enable this goal exist to enhance the communication of information through voice, video, imaging, or text. In the past, tasks supported by computers have been classified as information tasks and those supported by telephones as communication tasks (Coiera, 2000). With the use of telephones for information processing and computers for distance conferencing, these distinctions have tended to blur. It is now possible to integrate cell phones, hand-held devices, global positioning systems, bar code scanners, and medication administration systems with traditional information systems through a wireless intranet, for the immediate communication of information to the correct person, at the correct time, in the correct format.

The integration of these systems can also enhance the efficiency of the collection and aggregation of clinical data for use in the management of workload and staffing. Calculating acuity data directly from nursing documentation and treatment plans can more accurately reflect scheduling needs for immediate online retrieval (Kennedy, 2003). This documentation can also be used to determine the quality of care delivered on an institutional, unit, or individual basis. Comparisons can be made between the efficiency and effectiveness of care between units, or the data can be used for an individual nurse's performance evaluation.

Summary

- Critical data and information to support nursing decision making are essential.
- Computerized data make real-time analysis possible and swift.
- Computer applications in nursing administration can be understood best as arising from nursing administration, informatics, and effectiveness research.
- Nursing informatics is the management and processing of nursing data, information, and knowledge to support the practice of nursing and the delivery of nursing care.

- A management information system (MIS) is an integrated system for collecting, storing, retrieving, and processing a collective set of data from storage into knowledge.
- The information collected in health care is used to establish reimbursement, determine access to health care, define services, monitor the quality of care, direct health care policy, and affect the standard of care delivered.
- Information systems that support nursing administrative practice and provide essential decision support are being developed and utilized.
- Nursing's data needs lie in the areas of the client, the provider, administration, and research.
- Nursing's data have been described as being "invisible."
- Computerized nursing management information, standardized language, and the development of and access to uniform nursing management data sets would enhance the collection, retrieval, analysis, and comparison of nursing's "invisible" data.

Study Questions

1. What restraining forces impede the use of nursing data for the analysis of nursing care?
2. What can nursing data be used for?
3. What are advantages that might be seen with the implementation of an EHR?
4. What difference can nurses who manage health care services make to the design and implementation of an EHR?
5. What impact will information/communication technology have on nursing care delivery in the future?

Case Study

Dennis Fowler is the vice-president for nursing at a busy university hospital. The hospital is in the process of determining documentation requirements for a proposed clinical information system. Mr. Fowler has asked each unit manager to identify their nursing documentation needs.

CRITICAL THINKING EXERCISE

No nurse wants to make a mistake. However, the nurses on this busy and short-staffed medical-surgical floor of an acute care tertiary-level hospital know that medication errors frequently happen. The nurse manager meets with the Nurse Manager Council from time to time to discuss this problem of high rates of medication errors. The discussion focuses on the extent and causes of the problem. Crisis management allows little time for systematic problem analysis. Short-staffing leaves nurses exhausted from running from task to task. Now the administration has announced the purchase of a new computer system for the hospital. Nurses will enter all the data, including medication orders handwritten by physicians. The nurse managers are afraid that the nurses will rebel over one more burdensome duty.

1. What problem(s) can you identify in this scenario?
2. What makes this (or these) problematic?
3. What should the nurse manager do?
4. What factors do the nurses and the nurse manager need to assess and analyze?
5. What data needs might the nurses anticipate?
6. What can the nurse manager do to form a persuasive data management plan?

Sandy Jones is the manager of the hospital's nephrology unit. Ms. Jones formed a committee consisting of clinical leaders on her unit and requested that the nursing informatics specialist for their area, Jill Ross, be a member of this committee.

Ms. Ross, the nursing informatics specialist, suggested using the categories of the Nursing Minimum Data Set (NMDS) as a guide to the collection and organization of data requirements for documentation. Using these categories helped guide their evaluation of data for the examination of nursing process, patient demographics, organizational structure, and outcomes of care.

The committee started by reviewing all current documentation tools used by nurses on the unit and reviewing the literature related to computerized nursing documentation. Next, they visited several similar nursing units at other hospitals in the area that had already implemented computerized nursing documentation. Then, they identified the patient outcomes that were important for their unit to track on their particular patient group and what data were needed to analyze these outcomes. Finally, they observed nurses as they provided and documented patient care and questioned them regarding their documentation practices. This work provided them with a list of data point categories they felt were necessary to document and analyze patient care on their unit.

Mr. Fowler has compiled all of the documentation requirements collected from each unit in the hospital. He has asked hospital nursing informatics specialists and nursing leaders to assist in the selection of a nursing documentation system. The documentation system selected must meet the general documentation needs of the hospital but also must be adaptable to different nursing contexts. The committee's first task is to create a document that identifies specific data, nursing language, and organizational requirements for the proposed information system.

REFERENCES

Abbott, P.A., & Lee, S.M. (2001). Informatics: A new dimension in nursing. *Imprint, 48*(3), 51-52.

American Nurses Association (ANA). (1997). *NIDSEC standards and scoring guidelines.* Washington, DC: ANA.

Austin, C. (1979). *Information systems for hospital administration.* Ann Arbor, MI: Health Administration Press.

Bakken, S., Warren, J., Lundberg, C., Casey, A., Correia, C., Konicek, D., et al. (2001, September). *An evaluation of the utility of the CEN categorial structure for nursing diagnoses as a terminology model for integrating nursing diagnosis concepts into SNOMED.* Paper presented at the MEDINFO 2001, Amsterdam.

Ball, M., & Douglas, J. (1988). Integrating nursing and informatics. In M. Ball, K. Hannah, U. Jelger, & H. Peterson (Eds.), *Nursing informatics: Where caring and technology meet* (pp. 11-17). New York: Springer-Verlag.

Ball, M. J. (2003). Hospital information systems: Perspectives on problems and prospects, 1979 and 2002. *International Journal of Medical Informatics, 69*(2003), 83-89.

Bates, D., Cullen, D., Laird, N., Petersen, L., Small, S., Servi, D., et al. (1995). Incidence of adverse drug events and potential adverse drug events: Implications for prevention. *The Journal of the American Medical Association, 274*(1), 29-34.

Blewitt, D.K., & Jones, K.R. (1996). Using elements of the nursing minimum data set for determining outcomes. *Journal of Nursing Administration, 26*(6), 48-56.

Button, P., Androwich, I., Hibben, L., Kern, V., Madden, G., Marek, K., et al. (1998). Challenges and issues related to implementation of nursing vocabularies in computer-based systems. *Journal of the American Medical Informatics Association, 5*(4), 332-334.

Clark, J.L., & Lang, N. (1992). Nursing's next advance: An internal classification for nursing practice. *International Nursing Review, 39*(4), 109-111.

Coenen, A., Marin, H., Park, H., & Bakken, S. (2001). Collaborative efforts for representing nursing concepts in computer-based systems: International perspectives. *Journal of the American Medical Informatics Association, 8*(3), 202-211.

Coicra, E. (2000). When conversation is better than computation. *Journal of the American Informatics Association, 7*(3), 277-286.

Currie, G. (1998). The strategic role of health informatics in integrated delivery systems. *Journal for Healthcare Quality, 20*(5), 4-7.

Davidson, A.M., & Sanders, C.B. (1998). Data management and integrated information systems. In S.A. Price, M.W. Koch, & S. Bassett (Eds.), *Health care resource management: Present and future challenges.* (pp. 155-164). St Louis: Mosby.

Donabedian, A. (1986). Criteria and standards for quality assessment and monitoring. *Quarterly Review Bulletin, 12*(3), 99-100.

Ein-Dor, P., & Segev, E. (1978). *Managing management information systems.* Toronto, Ontario, Canada: Lexington Books.

Graves, J., & Corcoran, S. (1989). The study of nursing informatics. *Image: Journal of Nursing Scholarship, 21*(4), 227-231.

Hanson, R. (1982). Applying management information to staffing. *Journal of Nursing Administration, 12*(10), 5-9.

Hardiker, N. (2003). Determining sources for nursing terminology systems. *Journal of Biomedical Informatics, 35*, 279-286.

Hardiker, N., & Rector, A. (2001). Structural validation of nursing technologies. *Journal of the American Medical Informatics Association, 8*(3), 212-221.

Huber, D., & Oermann, M. (1999). Do outcomes equal quality? *Outcomes Management for Nursing Practice, 3*(1), 1-3.

Huber, D., Schumacher, L., & Delaney, C. (1997). Nursing management minimum data set (NMMDS). *Journal of Nursing Administration, 27*(4), 42-48.

Huber, D.G., Delaney, C., Crossley, J., Mehmert, M., & Ellerbe, S. (1992). A nursing management minimum data set: Significance and development. *Journal of Nursing Administration, 22*(7/8), 35-40.

Ingenerf, J. (1995, July). *Taxonomic vocabularies in medicine: The intention of usage determines different established structures.* Paper presented at the MEDINFO 95, Vancouver, British Columbia.

International Organization for Standardization (ISO). (2002). *Health informatics—Integration of a reference terminology model for nursing* (Committee Document No. ISO/TC 215/N 142). Geneva, Switzerland: ISO.

Iowa Intervention Project (1997). *Nursing outcomes classification (NOC).* St Louis: Mosby.

Kennedy, R. (2003). The nursing shortage and the role of technology. *Nursing Outlook, 51*(Suppl), 33-34.

Kimmel, K., & Sensmeier, J. (2002). *A technological approach to enhancing patient safety.* Chicago: HIMMS.

Leape, L., Bates, D., Cullen, D., Cooper, J., Demonaco, H., Gallivan, T., et al. (1995). Systems analysis of adverse drug events. *Journal of the American Medical Association, 274*(1), 35-43.

Maas, M., Johnson, M., & Moorhead, S. (1996). Classifying nursing-sensitive patient outcomes. *Image: Journal of Nursing Scholarship, 28*(4), 295-301.

Maas, M.I., Delaney, C., & Huber, D. (1999). Contextual variables and assessment of the outcome effects of nursing interventions. *Outcomes Management for Nursing Practice, 3*(1), 4-6.

McCormick, K. (1988). Conceptual considerations, decision criteria, and guidelines for the nursing minimum data set from a research perspective. In H. Werley, & N. Lang (Eds.), *Identification of the nursing minimum data set* (pp. 34-47). New York: Springer.

Meadows, G. (2002). Nursing informatics: An evolving specialty. *Nursing Economic$, 20*(6), 300-301.

Mills, M., Romano, C., & Heller, B. (1996). *Information management in nursing and health care.* Philadelphia: Springhouse.

Moss, J. (2003). A method for evaluating nursing documentation. *Health IT Advisory Report, 4*(8), 14-17.

Moss, J., & Xiao, Y. (2004). Improving operating room coordination: Communication pattern assessment. *Journal of Nursing Administration, 34*(2), 93-100.

Moss, J., Coenen, A., & Mills, M. (2003). Evaluation of the draft international standard for a reference terminology model for nursing actions. *Journal of Biomedical Informatics, 36*(4-5), 271-278.

Moss, J., Xiao, Y., & Zubaidah, S. (2002). The operating room charge nurse: Coordinator and communicator. *Journal of the American Medical Informatics Association, 9*(6 Suppl), 70-74.

Mowry, M., & Korpman, R. (1986). *Managing health care costs, quality, and technology: Product line strategies for nursing.* Rockville, MD: Aspen.

Newbold, S. (1998). Information systems for managing patient care. In J.A. Dienemann (Ed.), *Nursing administration: managing patient care* (2nd ed.) (pp. 323-338). Stamford, CT: Appleton & Lange.

Nursing Information & Data Set Evaluation Center (NIDSEC). (2004). *ANA recognized terminologies that support nursing practice.* Atlanta: American Nurses Publishing. Retrieved May 28, 2004, from *www.nursingworld.org/nidsec*

Ornstein, C. (2003). *Hospital heeds doctors, suspends use of software.* Retrieved December 18, 2003, from *www.latimes.com/news/printedition/california/la-me-cedars22jan22,0,15283.story?*

Peterson, M., & Hannah, K. (1988). Nursing management information systems. In M. Ball, K. Hannah, U. Jelger, & H. Peterson (Eds.), *Nursing informatics: Where caring and technology meet.* (pp. 190-205). New York: Springer-Verlag.

Phoenix Health Systems (2004). *HHS fact sheet: Harnessing information technology to improve healthcare.* Montgomery Village, MD: Phoenix Health Systems. Retrieved May 31, 2004, from *www.hipaadvisory.com/news/NewsArchives/2004/0426bush.htm*

Schwirian, P.M. (1986). The NI pyramid—A model for research in nursing informatics. *Computers in Nursing, 4*(3), 134-136.

Staggers, N., Bagley Thompson, C., & Snyder-Halpern, R. (2001). History and trends in clinical information systems in the United States. *Journal of Nursing Scholarship, 33*(1), 75-81.

Stenson, R. (2003). *Failure to check database, misunderstanding led to teen's death.* Oakland, CA: California HealthCare Foundation. Retrieved December 18, 2003, from *www.ihealthbeat.org/index.cfm?Action=dspItem&itemID=99054*

Stetson, P., McKnight, K., Bakken, S., Curran, C., Kubose, T., Cimino, J. (2001). *Development of an ontology to model medical errors, information needs, and the clinical communication space.* Paper presented at the AMIA Annual Symposium, Washington, DC, November 5.

U.S. Department of Health and Human Services (USDHHS). (2004). *Secretary Thompson, seeking fastest possible results, names first health information technology coordinator.* Washington, DC: HHS. Retrieved May 20, 2004, from *www.dhhs.gov/news/press/2004pres/20040506.html*

Werley, H., & Lang, N. (Eds). (1988). *Identification of the nursing minimum data set.* New York: Springer.

Winslow, E., Nestor, V., Davidoff, S., Thompson, P., & Borum, J. (1997). Legibility and completeness of physicians' handwritten medication orders. *Heart & Lung: The Journal of Acute & Critical Care, 26*(2), 158-164.

Young, K. (2000). *Informatics for healthcare professionals.* Philadelphia: F.A. Davis.

14

Strategic Management

Belinda E. Puetz

CHAPTER OBJECTIVES

- Draw conclusions about the importance of strategic management
- Define and describe strategic management, organizational vision or mission, strategy, tactics, strategic plan, and objectives
- Examine the elements of strategic planning
- Analyze the strategic planning process
- Apply strategic planning to the nursing process
- Exercise critical thinking to conceptualize and analyze possible solutions to a practice exercise

Strategic management is an approach to doing business that involves assessing the environment, knowing the competition, establishing successful performance, achieving targets, and evaluating success. This approach has long been used in business to ensure a competitive advantage over similar enterprises. Because of the changes in health care over the past decades, it has become imperative for health care organizations, as well, to function as businesses. Those that do not do so fail to remain viable for long.

Managed care reimbursement, shortages of health care workers, particularly nurses, and the proliferation of health care ventures have necessitated the use of strategic management to obtain and maintain a competitive advantage. Success of an enterprise depends on its competitive advantage—that is, how well it does something compared with similar efforts and how well it is able to continuously achieve superior performance. Examples abound: Nordstrom is known for its customer service; McDonalds for its fast, friendly service and consistent food; Starbuck's for its custom-made coffee served in a pleasant atmosphere (Collins & Porras, 1994). All of these businesses employ strategic management to set them apart from their competition and to increase their market share and, ultimately, their profit.

Strategic management involves strategic planning and implementation. It provides a "game plan" for operating a business, establishing a competitive position, ensuring customer satisfaction, and reaching strategic objectives or goals. Although most strategic management occurs at the "macro" level (that is, the executive levels of the health care institution), it can benefit the "micro" level as well, such as the nursing division, department, or unit. Strategic management prepares nurses to adapt to the environment in which they practice, an environment that is ever changing and demanding, as they respond to the changes in the external environment in which the health care institution is located. Strategic management helps nurses achieve their goals, whether those goals relate to the workplace or to the profession.

DEFINITIONS

Thinking and behaving strategically are prime methods for nurses to be proactive in a complex, fast-changing, rapid-cycle environment. The overarching concept is strategic management, which

▲ LEADING & MANAGING DEFINED

Strategic Management

Management of an organization based on its vision or mission.

Organizational Vision or Mission

A guiding framework that describes what the organization views as its business and future direction.

Strategy

Competitive move or business approach designed to produce a successful outcome.

Tactics

Choices for action that are made to implement a strategy.

Strategic Plan

Document specifying the action plan for actualizing the organization's mission.

Objectives

The financial or performance-based, short- or long-range targets that an enterprise wishes to achieve.

includes strategic planning and also focuses on strategy implementation. The terms associated with an organization's use of strategy include *strategic management, organizational vision or mission, strategy, strategic plan,* and *objectives*. **Strategic management** is defined as the management of an organization based on its vision or mission. **Organizational vision or mission** is a guiding framework that describes what the organization views as its business and future direction. **Strategy** is a competitive move or business approach designed to produce a successful outcome. **Tactics** are operational choices for action that are made to implement a strategy. A **strategic plan** is a document that specifies an action plan for actualizing the mission. This includes the strategy, goals, and objectives; and it consists of the who, what, by when, where, and in general terms, the costs involved. **Objectives** are defined as the targets an organization wants to achieve. These can be financial or performance-based and short- or long-range targets.

STRATEGIC PLANNING PROCESS

Strategic management generally begins with a strategic planning process, triggered by recognition of the need for an organization to establish its competitive position in the marketplace or to address some other felt need (e.g., seeking Magnet recognition, applying for the Malcolm Baldridge award, or simply to establish future directions). The following are questions to be answered in the strategic planning process:

- Where are we currently?
- Where do we want to go?
- How will we get there?

The components of the nursing process— assessment, planning, implementation, and evaluation—are similar to those employed in strategic management, as follows:

- Developing a strategic mission or vision
- Setting objectives
- Developing strategies to achieve the objectives
- Implementing the strategies
- Evaluating the results

The strategic plan provides a framework for strategic management, taking into consideration both external and internal environmental factors.

Developing a Mission and Vision

The first step of the strategic planning process is to identify the organization's vision or mission. This requires a determination of what the organization is, what business it is in and for whom, and where the business seeks to be in the future. The mission statement reflects the vision of what the organization seeks to do and to become;

it provides a clear view of what the organization is trying to accomplish, and it indicates its intent to carve out a particular position in the industry or field. For instance, Baptist Health Care in Pensacola, Florida, a recent recipient of the Malcolm Baldrige award, has as its mission "To provide superior service based on Christian values to improve the quality of life for people and communities served" (Baptist Health Care, 2004, p. 20). Thus the organization sees providing superior service based on Christian values as what it is trying to accomplish. Baptist Health Care's vision is "to be the best health system in America" (Baptist Health Care, 2004, p. 1). This statement clearly reflects what the organization seeks to become, and it certainly describes Baptist Health Care's intent to stake out a particular position in the health care industry.

In the strategic planning process, questions that assist the planners to arrive at a specific vision and mission include the following:

- What business are we in now?
- What business do we want to be in?
- What do our customers expect of us now?
- What will be the customers' expectations in the future?
- Who are our customers now?
- Who will be our customers in the future?
- Who are our current stakeholders (other than customers)?
- How will those stakeholders change in the future? What about their expectations?
- Who are our primary competitors currently?
- Who will be our competitors in the future?
- What about partners, now and in the future?
- What will be the effect of technology?
- What is happening in the environment now and in the future that may affect us?

Generally, addressing this latter question involves consideration of both external environmental factors (e.g., activities of regulatory bodies) and internal environmental factors (e.g., financial and human resources). The assessment of future environmental impact takes the form of assumptions. These assumptions encompass the sociodemographic, political, economic, and technological aspects of the external environment. Of course,

these assumptions are merely "best guesses," because it is impossible to predict the future with any certainty.

Responses to these questions by the principals involved in an organization (e.g., executive management, supervisory staff, department heads) will shape an organization's strategic plan and, as a result, its strategic management. Involving individuals at all levels of the organization (e.g., staff nurses, clerical workers) in addition to those at the top of the hierarchy will ensure a variety of perspectives and more "buy in" to the final product. In fact, experts in strategic planning recommend that the process occur from the "bottom up and involve everyone in the organization (Peters, 1987).

Crafting a vision with the input of many individuals has the advantage of being a result of many perspectives, and it also engages those individuals in helping to make the vision a reality. When everyone involved in an institution shares the vision, then individuals know where the organization is going and can be instrumental in helping get it there through their daily activities. As the old saying goes, "If you don't know where you're going, then any path will take you there." Conversely, if all of the individuals in the institution know where they are going, they will all take the same path.

Setting Objectives

Once the organization's mission and vision have been established, the next step in strategic planning is to develop the ways and means to get there. Thus strategic goals and objectives are crafted. These objectives generally define the "who," "what," and "where," of the strategies to be implemented. Focusing the objectives allows individuals to recognize where the organization currently is, where it wants to go, and what time it will take to get there. Absence of strategic objectives results in individuals trying to move in too many directions without a coordinated plan or not moving at all because of confusion about the organization's direction.

The strategic objectives provide a way of converting the rather abstract mission of an organization into concrete terms—targets of performance that, taken together, will achieve the mission.

Objectives also offer a way of measuring progress toward achieving the organization's mission. These objectives generally are written to reflect not what *is* but what *should be*—activities that encourage the individuals implementing them to be creative, to stretch beyond their current limits, and challenge themselves to improve their performance. These objectives must be achievable, however, lest individuals lose faith that they can accomplish them. If the strategic objectives are challenging but achievable, they will prevent employees of an institution from becoming complacent or from settling only for the status quo.

Objectives generally are written in terms of financial outcomes that relate to improvements in an organization's fiscal health and those that will result in a stronger position for the institution in the industry. For example, a for-profit hospital may set a financial objective to increase earnings growth by a specific percentage each year. A specific strategic objective might be to achieve lower overall costs than competitors or to attain technological advantage.

Developing an Implementation Strategy

The third step in the strategic planning process is to decide how to achieve the financial and strategic objectives that were established, how to obtain a competitive advantage over rivals in the field or industry, how to respond to changing conditions both externally and internally, how to defend against adverse conditions, and how to grow the business to increase market share. The strategies that are developed must be planned in advance and must also be able to be adapted to outside influences. Thus objectives are the targeted results and outcomes, and the strategy is how to achieve that outcome. The strategy must be deliberate and purposeful (planned and intentional) and also flexible enough to be responsive to events that are unanticipated when the strategy is developed. For example, new opportunities may arise that were unknown at the time a strategic objective was developed; these opportunities could greatly increase an organization's competitive position. Changes in a product line or service provided by

an organization may necessitate a change in a strategic objective.

Basically, an organization's strategy consists of how it treats its customers and stakeholders; how it responds to changes in the industry and marketplace; how it capitalizes on new opportunities; how it manages its operations; how it grows and develops; and how it achieves its financial and strategic objectives. The challenge is to involve key people in the organization in developing this strategy so that these individuals can champion the implementation of the strategy. The desired outcome is to ensure that the strategy is timely, responsive, innovative, creative, and designed to take advantage of opportunities as they arise.

The benefits of strategic management cannot be overemphasized. In today's business climate, particularly in the health care environment, survival is tenuous and success is fraught with difficulty. A good management strategy helps an organization remain strong enough to withstand competition, overcome obstacles, and achieve peak performance. The organization's strategy must be flexible in order to respond appropriately to the following:

- Evolving needs and preferences of customers and stakeholders
- Advances in technology
- Changes in political climate and regulatory requirements
- New opportunities
- Altered market conditions
- Disasters and crises

The organization's strategic plan must include these aspects: where the organization is currently and where it is headed, how it plans to get to its desired future through short- and long-term performance targets (i.e., strategic objectives), and what will be done to achieve these outcomes. The strategic plan encompasses the organization's mission and vision, strategic and financial objectives, and a strategy for achieving the objectives.

Implementing the Strategy

Once the strategy has been explicated, the next step is to implement it. Implementation involves trying out the activities in a way that determines how best to close the gap between how things are done and what it takes to achieve the strategy. For example, given an objective related to improvement of the financial bottom line, the first step is to determine current cost and then compare it with desired cost to decide what needs to be changed to reach the desired, lower cost.

Strategy must be implemented proficiently and efficiently, as well as in a timely manner, if it is to be effective. For this to occur, the organization must attend to its capabilities, the reward structure, available support systems, and the organizational culture. If any of these characteristics are not in place, implementation of the strategy will surely fail. If, for example, employees are not rewarded in ways that are meaningful to them to implement a strategy, it is highly unlikely that they will initiate or maintain efforts to implement the strategy. If the organizational culture does not support innovation or risk taking, or if the prevailing attitude is "if it's not broke, don't fix it," efforts to improve performance or outcomes will be doomed.

Implementing strategy is closely linked to an organization's operations; it involves managing, budgeting, motivating, changing culture, supervising, and leading. Strategic planning and implementation are managerial processes that perform the following functions:

- Demonstrate leadership in implementation of strategy
- Reward those who carry out strategy successfully
- Allocate necessary resources to activities critical to strategy
- Formulate policies and procedures that support identified strategy
- Initiate continuous quality improvement activities
- Develop and reward best practices
- Maintain a culture that supports strategy

Evaluating Effectiveness

The final step in strategic management is to evaluate the outcomes of the strategic planning process and the implementation of strategy. This evaluation component is an ongoing process;

it is not a static endeavor. Because of the nature of health care environments, things change, and it is necessary to constantly evaluate performance and strategy, use the data collected to decide how things are going, and make changes as indicated. Changes that may need to be made range from adjusting the organization's long-term direction, raising or lowering performance expectations, or modifying a strategy, depending on what the situation requires.

It may be—and often is—necessary to make midcourse corrections to the strategic plan, the strategic objectives, or the strategy. The evaluation process should facilitate identification of the areas in which changes need to be made. The need for changes should not be interpreted as failure of the process; rather, elements of the plan may flounder for a variety of reasons, such as diminished focus on the strategic plan, lack of commitment on the part of employees (who may not have initially been part of the process of developing the plan), and the inability to create a balance between staying the course and making corrections in midcourse.

Part of the evaluative process of a strategic plan is an annual review of the plan, the assumptions underlying it, and the feedback received from performance data, activity reports, market indications, and customer surveys. Also, an environmental scan and analysis should be undertaken to ensure that the conditions that affect the organization, its mission, vision, and strategic plan have not changed to a level sufficient to necessitate change in the organization itself.

Environmental analysis incorporates an internal analysis such as a review of the mission statement and value system, as well as an external analysis. The analysis needs to review four areas: strengths, weaknesses, opportunities, and threats (SWOT). The key principle is that the more systematically and carefully environmental factors and key trends are assessed, the greater the likelihood that the impact of change will be accurately gauged (Fidellow & Hogan, 1998). The following four questions can be explored (Martin, 1998):

1. For threats and opportunities, what might we do?
2. For internal competencies, what can we do?

3. For values of key implementers, what do we want to do?
4. For societal responsibilities, what should we do?

The SWOT method is one of the most popular ways to develop strategic plans for an organization. In this approach, strengths and weaknesses internal to the organization are identified. These strengths and weaknesses generally are related to resources, programs, and operations in key areas of the organization, examples of which include the following:

- *Operations:* efficiency, capacity, processes
- *Management:* systems, expertise, resources
- *Products:* quality, features, prices
- *Finances:* resources, performance

Once identified, these components are analyzed for the purpose of drafting a picture of the critical features of the organization, its achievements and failures, and its good and bad points.

The external components are described as opportunities and threats, and they are identified in the same manner as the internal factors. Opportunities and threats may include changes in the following:

- Industry
- Marketplace
- Economy
- Political climate
- Technology
- Competition

Once identified, these strengths, weaknesses, opportunities, and threats must be analyzed for their impact on the organization. Questions from the analysis include the following (Below et al., 1987):

- Have we identified the critical issues facing the organization?
- Do we have sufficient information to select the critical issues?
- Are we using adequate judgment to agree on these critical issues?
- Have we sufficiently discussed the root causes of the critical issues?
- Are we able to arrive at conclusions about the causes of these critical issues?

- Can we defend our conclusions both inside and outside of the organization?

Once satisfied with the responses to these questions, priorities must be established for the critical issues so that strategies are based on the priority issues. For example, a change in the market for the organization's services may be a threat, but a low priority, so that the organization determines it is not essential to target resources (e.g., human, financial) to deal with the threat, when it is a higher priority to take advantage of an opportunity involving technology. The SWOT analysis often leads to future strategies, in which the organization determines to do the following:

- Build on strengths
- Resolve or minimize weaknesses
- Exploit opportunities
- Avoid threats

The strategies identified through the SWOT analysis can be shaped into a strategic plan on which strategic management is based. The more carefully the analysis is done, the more reliable the strategic plan. A plan based on faulty assumptions or careless analysis will not serve the organization well and, indeed, may lead eventually to its demise.

ELEMENTS OF A STRATEGIC PLAN

Most strategic plans result in a written document. This document can be written by the individuals involved in the strategic planning process or, more likely, by the individual who facilitated the strategic planning process (i.e., consultant or employee). Generally, strategic plan documents contain the following sections:

- *Executive summary:* a two- to three-page encapsulation of the essence of the plan, written in language understandable by all potential readers, since many will not venture beyond the first few pages of the document
- *Background:* A description of the institution, its history, and current state, including its accomplishments, as well as the situation that prompted the strategic planning process
- *Mission, vision, and values:* Should describe the philosophy of the organization

- *Goals and strategies:* Should describe the target objectives and the strategies identified to ensure achievement of the objectives
- *Appendices:* Includes all the documentation related to the strategic planning process so that the reader obtains a sense of the background information used by the strategic planners in order to arrive at the strategic plan

Appendix materials can include the following elements:

- Annual reports of the institution
- SWOT analysis results
- Financial information
- Environmental scan results
- Staffing information
- Current and projected programs and services

Other materials can be included as desired. Caution should be exercised, however, not to include confidential data that should not be viewed by "outsiders."

The strategic plan should be disseminated widely throughout the institution. It is not necessary to reproduce the document in its entirety for distribution to everyone in the institution. A decision needs to be made about which parts of the strategic plan are appropriate for the individuals who will receive it. Some will need the entire plan; others only the executive summary; and still others perhaps need only the goals and strategies.

In any case, the strategic plan should be communicated to stakeholders: board members, management, and staff. Copies should be included in orientation programs for new employees. The institution's vision and mission should be displayed in public areas (e.g., waiting rooms, cafeteria) as well as in areas reserved for employees. The strategic plan tenets should be incorporated into all of the institution's policies and procedures.

Copies of the plan can also be provided to trade or professional associations with which the institution is associated. The public relations or community outreach department in the institution can use the strategic plan as the basis for a media campaign to educate the community and other publics about the institution's vision and mission.

Patients can be provided with a condensed summary of the strategic plan on admission, particularly those sections related to their care.

IMPLEMENTATION OF THE STRATEGIC PLAN

It is often at this point that strategic management fails. Strategic plans are developed and then allowed to languish, as the necessary commitment to implementation is not realized for whatever reason. Often the reason is conflicting priorities. Executives and staff in health care organizations have a myriad of tasks facing them, and implementing strategic objectives adds another burden to an already overwhelming workload. To overcome this obstacle, the strategic plan must be integrated into the organization's daily activities. Everyone must be committed to implementing the strategic plan, from the leaders to the staff at all levels and in all departments. Focusing on the strategic plan and its meaning to the viability and future of the institution is imperative.

It also is necessary to develop a business or action plan based on the strategic plan. Those individuals who will be responsible for implementing the strategic objectives need to develop this plan. It should include the following elements:

- A priority order for achieving the strategic objectives or outcomes
- The determination of who (individual or group) will be responsible for achieving these objectives
- An indication of available or necessary financial support
- A timetable outlining when achievement of the objectives can be expected

It may also be advisable to include interim activities and timeframes if the strategic objective is long-term or complex, so that progress can be monitored.

The action plan often breaks the strategic plan into manageable components, particularly for those individuals who were not directly involved in crafting the strategic plan. The action plan, then, must become a living document so that it is

Research Note

Source: Roderer, C.A. (2001). Strategic planning for the recruitment and retention of health care professionals. *Oncology Issues, 16*(5), 31-34.

Purpose

The purpose of this article was to describe strategies hospitals can use to recruit and retain health care professionals, including nurses.

Discussion

The strategies employed were incorporated in categories such as managing and mentoring, recognizing and rewarding employees, compensation and benefit strategies, recruiting strategies, and "growing your own." Managing and mentoring includes managers being sensitive to a culturally diverse staff and managing with respect rather than with authority. The author cautioned that the institution's mission statement must be clear and valued by all employees. Recognition and rewards for employees encompassed equitable and competitive compensation but also flexible scheduling, childcare centers, stress reduction programs, and financial planning for employees. Compensation and benefits described bonuses for referral, weekend work and project completion, and profit sharing, as well as financial incentives for certification or degree completion. Recruitment programs extended beyond the typical classified ads to direct mailing campaigns, billboards, and cinema advertising. "Growing your own" involved tuition reimbursement, internship programs, and scholarship programs for employees' children. The author concluded that employers need to use a strategic plan to ensure that their employment practices were competitive in this era of critical labor shortages.

Application to Practice

This article demonstrated the process of strategic planning to achieve a goal: sufficient individuals to staff hospitals. The author described the strategic objectives and the tactics that can be used to achieve this goal. Not all of the objectives and tactics will be relevant to each institution. Regardless of the applicability of the objectives, it is apparent that strategically planning and managing to avert a shortage of employees will produce a better result than leaving recruitment and retention to chance.

---

constantly referenced, consulted, and discussed. The action plan should be reviewed and updated at intervals. Actions that have been completed or those that do not move the organization toward achievement of its goals should be deleted, and new actions based on existing environmental conditions should be added.

Ensuring that the action plan remains at the forefront of daily activities, whether in an institution as a whole, a department, or a unit, often requires a "champion." This is an individual who is passionate and committed to the process and who can inspire others to be as well. Often, a champion appears as the strategic planning process unfolds; generally, this individual contributes freely, is engaged in the work groups, and expresses interest in the process. Champions can be selected as well, but those who volunteer are usually more enthusiastic about the work than those who are "drafted."

LEADERSHIP AND MANAGEMENT IMPLICATIONS

Strategic management is useful for nursing leaders and managers because it can be used to analyze the environment for opportunities and threats; to set measurable, achievable goals and plans; and to help determine the future of the nursing area, such as a department or unit. Success in strategic

⚠ LEADERSHIP & MANAGEMENT **BEHAVIORS**

Leadership Behaviors

- Involves subordinates in the strategic planning process
- Inspires a vision
- Develops strategic plans and tactics
- Creates new or unique products or services
- Assesses current market position
- Establishes organizational priorities
- Forecasts resource requirements
- Analyzes key vision implications
- Creates the environment to encourage participation in the development of strategic plans

Management Behaviors

- Develops operational and action plans and tactics
- Develops control and evaluation plans

- Monitors implementation of strategy and tactics
- Organizes the strategic planning committee
- Conducts surveys and data collection
- Ensures that strategies are sound operationally

Overlap Areas

- Participates in the strategic planning process
- Ensures strategic plan implementation
- Involves all employees in the strategic planning process

planning and implementing that strategic plan will position nursing well in an institution. The process provides an opportunity for nursing to shine, because the similarities between the nursing process and the strategic planning process allow nurses to shortcut the learning curve and begin to move forward with the implementation phase while others may still be grappling with the planning process. Nursing skills and abilities make it relatively easy to plan strategically, and nurses, as 24-hour workers, can approach implementation as an ongoing, continuous, and seamless process. Nursing's involvement with continuous quality improvement and performance improvement systems provides a basis for involvement in strategic planning that is systematic and thorough.

Implementation of the organization's strategic plan can be useful in unifying staff on a nursing unit or in a department. Collaboration and cooperation among staff generally are required to accomplish strategic objectives. Working together to accomplish a strategic objective keeps staff engaged. Involvement in decisions that ultimately will affect them is essential and often results in positive spin-offs; for example, staff members feel

a sense of ownership in the process and pride in their accomplishments.

Involvement in strategic planning at the institution-wide level provides an opportunity for nurses to be recognized for their contributions and often lessens the feelings of being disenfranchised. Although it is admittedly a lot of work, the benefits of engaging in strategic planning and then implementing that plan far outweigh the disadvantages.

A strategic plan should be realistic and make sense to nurses at all levels. Participation and input help shape the organization's future and that of the nurses employed in that institution.

CURRENT ISSUES AND TRENDS

The focus on the nursing shortage underscores the need to retain nurses in the workplace. Those institutions that successfully retain nurses, particularly those that have obtained Magnet designation from the American Nurses Credentialing Center (ANCC), generally do so because they demonstrate excellence in the delivery of nursing services to patients, promote quality in an environment that supports professional practice, and provide a mechanism for the dissemination of "best practices" in nursing services (ANCC, 2002). Nurses seek out these institutions for their employment, and students look to them for clinical experiences and, after graduation, for employment. Increasingly, schools and colleges of nursing choose Magnet hospitals as sites for clinical affiliations of students.

Aiken and colleagues (2000) reported that nurses in Magnet organizations are more satisfied with their jobs, and patients in Magnet hospitals rate the care they receive more favorably. These authors also reported patient outcomes that ranged from increased satisfaction to shorter length of stay and lower disease-specific mortality rates.

This process of becoming a Magnet health care institution is similar to that of strategic planning. The assessment, goal setting, implementation, and evaluation phases are the basis of the application and site visit processes required for Magnet recognition.

Strategic planning is not reserved for activities such as seeking Magnet recognition, however. Any business venture will benefit from having a strategic plan. The plan provides for assessment of the environment, including current and future opportunities, and identification of specific, measurable, realistic ways of taking advantage of those opportunities. Most important, perhaps, the business plan answers the question, "What business are we in?" In so many instances, nurses have found themselves in businesses other than nursing. Clearly defining a mission and vision will help a nursing unit or department focus its efforts on its core business.

Woods (2001) described how evidence-based methods were used to create a strategic plan for recruitment and retention of staff. Crossan (2003) described the process of strategic management and called for nurses to employ strategic management in their institutions, particularly in the area of policy development. (See the *Suggested Readings* for further inquiry into strategic management.)

Nurses in entrepreneurial roles benefit from a clearly defined business plan, which provides direction and often serves as a vehicle for obtaining outside funding for the venture. Puetz and Shinn (1997) called for nurses who sought to become consultants in their area of expertise to develop a business plan prior to proceeding.

Nurses in all areas of practice and in all employment settings can use strategic planning principles to explore programs, projects, and services. Whether those are new or the strategic planning process is used to determine which programs, projects, and services to discontinue, the process of assessment, setting objectives, implementation, and evaluation guides these activities.

Strategic planning and strategic management are necessary components of business in today's competitive and highly unstable environment. Strategic planning is a process similar to the nursing process, with defined and specific steps to be taken to ensure a comprehensive and thorough process. Strategic management involves implementation of the strategic plan to ensure that the organization is responsive to changes in its environment, as well as to internal events.

Strategic planning and strategic management are not reserved exclusively for organizations. Individuals, such as nurses, can use these techniques to determine their own direction and establish objectives to ensure that they meet the goals they have set for themselves.

Summary

- Competition and competitive advantage are pressures that can be helped with strategic management.
- Strategic management includes both strategic planning and strategy implementation.
- Strategic planning prepares the nurse for readiness to respond.
- A strategy is an integrated plan of action.
- Tactics are choices used to implement strategy.
- Strategic planning is a continuous process of making decisions.
- A strategic plan is a written document.

- Strategic planning is a systematic approach to meeting goals and objectives.
- The strategic management process has five components.
- The strategic planning process results in a written document.
- Strategic planning can be a vehicle for nurse participation and input.

Study Questions

1. What is strategic planning and how does it differ from strategic management?
2. How can nurses use strategic management to improve the care they provide patients?
3. What are some ways to ensure that a strategic plan actually is implemented?
4. What should be included in a strategic plan for nursing?

CASE STUDY

Nurse Kory Danielson is the director of an adolescent substance abuse comprehensive assessment clinic affiliated with a university health care center. This clinic was developed and has been operating for 4 years based on financing from a federal government grant. The grant funding will expire in 1 year. Although a grant resubmission is underway, continued funding from the federal government is uncertain. The other employees are becoming anxious about their job options. A formal program evaluation is underway, but the data will not be analyzed for 9 months.

Nurse Danielson calls a whole clinic staff meeting to begin the strategic planning process. First, a set of questions are posed and discussed: Where are we currently? Where do we want to go? How will we get there? The group has been provided with the clinic's mission, vision, and purpose statements along with current goals and objectives. A number of unanswered questions arise, such as, Do we need to start charging for services and billing insurance carriers?

The meeting is productive, but exhausting. Nurse Danielson knows that closure to this initial planning needs to be facilitated. The question "So what do we do next?" has generated many fruitful ideas. The top three suggestions are (1) to do a formal SWOT analysis, (2) to investigate whether a professor from the College of Business or a representative from the Service Corps of Retired Executives (SCORE) can come and work with the group on a business plan, and (3) to form an outreach team that will present and promote the clinic within the community by means of presentations and personal liaison.

The group divides into three groups to tackle the three suggestions, gather information, and formulate a plan for the group. Nurse Danielson begins to plan for a formal strategic planning session within a month.

CRITICAL THINKING EXERCISE

Nurse Martha Smith serves on the Board of Directors of the local chapter of her specialty nursing organization. One of the chapter's activities is to establish a high school-to-nursing school program to recruit youngsters into nursing. Nurse Smith wishes to use the unit on which she is manager as the location where the high school students can "shadow" nurses. Because of clinical affiliations by local colleges and universities and preceptorship programs for new orientees, nursing staff on the unit are overloaded already. Nurse Smith is convinced of the value of the chapter's program and believes that it is her responsibility as a chapter leader to help implement this program in her setting.

1. Is there a problem here? Why is it a problem?
2. How should Nurse Smith approach the problem?
3. What is the likelihood of success in this situation?
4. What elements of strategic planning and strategic management will be helpful here?

REFERENCES

Aiken, L., Havens, D., & Sloane, D. (2000). The magnet nursing services recognition program: A comparison of two groups of magnet hospitals. *American Journal of Nursing, 100,* 26-35.

American Nurses Credentialing Center (ANCC). (2003). *The magnet recognition program for excellence in nursing service, health care organization, instructions and application process manual.* Washington, DC: ANCC.

Baptist Health Care. (2004). *Baptist Health Care—Mission, values, vision.* Pensacola, FL: BHC. Retrieved May 13, 2004, from *www.ebaptisthealth care.org*

Below, P.J., Morrisey, G.L., & Acomb, B.L. (1987). *The executive guide to strategic planning.* San Francisco: Jossey-Bass.

Collins, J.C., & Porras, J.I. (1994). *Built to last: Successful habits of visionary companies.* New York: HarperBusiness.

Crossan, F. (2003). Strategic management and nurses: Building foundations. *Journal of Nursing Management, 11*(5), 331-335.

Fidellow, J.A., & Hogan, M. (1998). Strategic planning: Implementing a foundation. *Nursing Management, 29*(6), 34, 36.

Martin, M. (1998). Achieving the right balance with strategic planning. *Nursing Management, 29*(5), 30-31.

Peters, T. (1987). *Thriving on chaos.* New York: HarperCollins.

Puetz, B.E., & Shinn, L.J. (1997). *The nurse consultant's handbook.* New York: Springer.

Woods, S.L. (2001). Using evidence-based approaches to strategically respond to the nursing shortage. *Critical Care Nursing Clinics of North America, 13*(4), 511-519.

SUGGESTED READINGS

Benko, C., & McFarlan, F.W. (2003). *Connecting the dots: Aligning projects with objectives in unpredictable times.* Boston: Harvard Business School Press.

Bradford, R.W., & Duncan, J.P. (1999). *Simplified strategic planning.* Worcester, MA: Chandler House Press.

Bryson, J.M. (1995). *Creating and implementing your strategic plan* (rev. ed.). San Francisco: Jossey-Bass.

David, F. (2002). *Strategic management: Concepts and cases* (9th ed.). Upper Saddle River, NJ: Prentice-Hall.

Goodstein, L., Nolan, T., & Pfeiffer, J.W. (1993). *Applied strategic planning.* New York: McGraw-Hill Trade.

Hunger, J.D., & Wheelen, T.L. (2003). *Essentials of strategic management* (3rd ed.). Upper Saddle River, NJ: Prentice-Hall.

Kaplan, R.S., & Norton, D.P. (1996). Using the balanced scorecard as a strategic management system. *Harvard Business Review, 74*(1), 75-85.

Morrisey, G.L. (1995). *A guide to long-range planning: Creating your strategic journey.* San Francisco: Jossey-Bass.

Steiner, G.A. (1997). *Strategic planning.* New York: The Free Press.

Wheelen, T., & Hunger, J.D (2004). *Strategic management and business policy* (9th ed.). Upper Saddle River, NJ: Prentice-Hall.

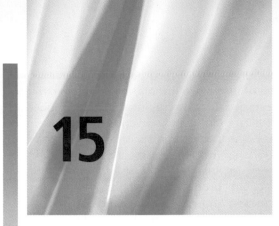

15

Marketing

Dana Woods

Marketing is a business administration concept related to the activities of product development, sales, influence, positioning, persuasion, and image projection. As an offshoot of capitalism, marketing is concerned with paying attention to stimulating and meeting consumer demand. In the most basic terms, marketing is defined as "meeting needs profitably." In a societal context, marketing involves "identifying and meeting human and social needs" (Kotler, 2000, p. 2).

Understanding and satisfying buyer wants and needs is a critical part of successful business marketing. Because nurses are at the center of care delivery—the primary product of health care organizations—they are in a unique position to understand what customers need. This is true regardless of which of its multiple customers (e.g., patients, physicians, payers) a health care organization may serve (Woods, 2002).

Marketing a service such as health care may be dramatically different, from an implementation standpoint, from marketing a consumer product such as a soft drink. However, the underlying concepts are universal. The business goal of a for-profit company is to maximize value so that shareholders will eventually benefit from their financial investment. The business goal of a non-profit organization, which includes many health care organizations, is to fulfill its mission of meeting consumer needs. To achieve its business goal, either organization must be financially viable, because without sustaining infrastructures and investing in new technologies neither a hospital nor a soft drink company will be able to satisfy its customer needs for very long. "No money, no mission" is a maxim for both.

The operation of free market economies provides a perspective on how the principles of marketing apply to nursing and health care. However, marketing health care services has its challenges because the traditional rules of an efficient free market often do not apply. Supply and demand, foundational elements of a free market, are significantly distorted in the health care market for several reasons. First, because of the third-party payer system, the end customer—the patient or potential patient—rarely acts like a typical consumer. In fact, the patient is but one of several customers that a health care service provider must satisfy. Furthermore, the seller of services—for example, a hospital—does not have the same control over the market price of its product that a typical product provider enjoys. Add to this a nearly unlimited demand for services, and health care presents itself as an industry that is neither efficient nor compliant with the rules of free market economy (Alward & Camunas, 1991; Woods, 2002). Is it any wonder that the American health care system is often described as broken and in disarray?

In this turbulent market, it is imperative that a health care organization be deliberate when scanning its environment, setting relevant strategic objectives, and planning effectively to achieve those objectives, no matter which of several possible scenarios plays out in the future. Gone are the days when an organization developed separate organization-wide strategic and marketing plans. Without a marketing orientation that ensures customers' needs are met, the most impressive-looking strategic plans are worthless (Schnaars, 1991).

Although formerly marketing was seen as a for-profit business strategy, it has become more widely used in not-for-profit and health care organizations as well. Highly competitive, resource-constrained environments set up conditions necessitating effective marketing. Marketing theory can be used and applied to enhance client care, nursing, and organizations (Alward & Camunas, 1991). This is because marketing can be thought of as the art of finding, developing, and profiting from opportunities (Kotler, 1999). In times of fiscal crisis or financial uncertainty, marketing is an especially critical survival strategy. For example, in the early 1980s hospitals turned to marketing strategies when diagnosis-related groups (DRGs) became the basis for reimbursement (Alward & Camunas, 1991).

Although nurses experience the impact of a marketing orientation in their daily lives as consumers, they are unlikely to be exposed to it as an essential ingredient of their professional practice. Because of its for-profit roots, the term *marketing* often carries a negative connotation when applied to health care. Critics have described marketing in a variety of negative ways: a waste of scarce health care dollars; intrusive; associated with high-pressure sales, manipulation, and the promotion of low-quality products; stimulating competition; and creating unnecessary demand (Alward & Camunas, 1991). Some nurses may feel that marketing does not have a legitimate place in nursing. However, Kotler's simple but profound definition of marketing, "meeting needs profitably," makes it consistent with, not contrary to, nursing practice (Kotler, 2000, p. 2). Marketing's primary benefits are improved satisfaction of customers, the target market; improved attraction of marketing resources such as nurses, physicians, funding, etc.; and improved efficiency in marketing activities, which contributes to better stewardship of financial and human resources (Kotler & Clarke, 1987).

Whether or not they realize it, nurses, as essential providers of the health care product, are engaged in marketing every day. An exceptional health care organization realizes this and ensures that all caregivers and support staff are informed and thoughtful about what it takes to meet customer needs. In exceptional organizations, marketing is more than a department; it is at the core of the business framework.

DEFINITIONS

Marketing is a process that relates to transactions when goods and services are exchanged in a market. It seeks to achieve an organization's strategic goals through the analysis, planning, implementation and control of systematically developed programs that generate voluntary exchanges of values with target markets (Kotler & Clarke, 1987).

A **market** can be defined broadly or narrowly. Originally, a market was the physical place where buyers and sellers assembled. Economists now see a market as a collection of buyers and sellers who transact (in person, by phone, by mail, or

◭ LEADING & MANAGING **DEFINED**

Market

A set of actual or potential buyers and users of goods, services, and ideas.

Marketing

A social and managerial process in which individuals or groups obtain what they need and want by exchanging products and values with others.

Marketing Mix

An individualized blend of marketing tools and tactics implemented to achieve goals.

Marketing Orientation

The focusing of energy on the identification of the needs and wants of customers and on the delivery of services that create satisfaction.

Market Share

The percentage of the total market for a product or service that is captured by an organization or producer.

Market Research

The systematic process for studying a marketing problem by designing a study, collecting, and analyzing the data, and using information from the findings.

Needs

Basic biological, psychological, and social requirements.

Wants

Desires or preferences satisfied by specific goods and services and influenced by external cues.

Service

Any act or performance that one party can offer to another that is essentially intangible and does not result in the ownership of anything.

Product

Anything that can be offered to a market to satisfy a want or need.

---

electronically) around a specific product group. From a marketer's perspective, the "industry" sells and the "market" buys (Kotler, 2003). Thus **marketing** is a social and managerial process in which individuals or groups obtain what they need and want by creating, offering and exchanging products and services of value with others (Kotler, 2000). Exchange is the act of getting a desired product from someone by offering something in return (Kotler, 2000). It is the defining concept that underlies marketing. By extension, "marketing comprises the set of activities that facilitate transactions in an exchange economy" (Graham, 1993, p. 2).

Marketing mix is an individualized blend of marketing tools or tactics an organization uses to achieve its objectives (Kotler, 2000). A **marketing orientation**, also called a *customer orientation,* is the focusing of energy on the identification of the needs and wants of customers and on the delivery

of services that create satisfaction (Alward & Camunas, 1991). **Market share** is the percentage of the total available market for a product or service that is captured by an organization or producer. **Market research** is the systematic process for studying marketing problems or opportunities by designing a study, collecting and analyzing the data, and using information from the findings to refine strategic and/or operational plans (Alward & Camunas, 1991).

The marketing process is similar to the nursing process—a framework designed to identify, analyze, and solve problems. Skillful marketing is carefully structured. It uses analysis, planning, implementation, and control of programs designed to create voluntary exchanges of values between an organization and target markets in order to achieve objectives. Organizations need to design offerings to match the target market's needs and wants, using communication, price, and distribution to effectively inform, motivate, and deliver services to the market (Kotler & Clarke, 1987).

The marketing process is designed to manage relationships. It is important to determine who the key customers *are* and who they *should be*. The primary markets for most nurses are patients, physicians, and the employing organization. For hospitals and other health care organizations, patients, payers, employees, and physicians are the primary markets. The basis for a marketing orientation is assessment of the needs and wants of customers in one's markets. The needs and wants of every party to the exchange must be considered.

Needs can be basic biological, psychological, and social. For example, a hospital patient may require safety, pain management, compassionate care, sterile conditions, and prevention of complications. These are needs. **Wants** are desires or preferences satisfied by specific goods and **services** and influenced by external cues. A hospital patient's wants may include a quiet and spacious room, good food, and cable television. Wants and needs can be satisfied through goods, services, or ideas that are collectively called **products** (Alward & Camunas, 1991). "A *product* is anything that can be offered to a market to satisfy a want or need" (Kotler, 2000, p. 394).

BACKGROUND

Marketing occurs within the framework of a voluntary exchange, which in health care is often complex. When an employer selects a third-party payer, the result can make it difficult for a patient to connect with a hospital or a physician. In managed care, the exchange is multidimensional, requiring appropriate physician-hospital-payer contracts. Therefore health care organizations must be thoughtful and savvy about each dimension of the exchanges in which they seek to engage. Careful monitoring of the market environment and shrewd contracting is essential if a health care organization seeks to achieve significant market share.

Terms and phrases such as *patient-centered care, staying close to the customer,* and *an obsession*

with service reflect a marketing or customer orientation. Organizational culture, philosophy, and values all need to align for true customer-centeredness. A marketing orientation contains five attributes: a customer-oriented philosophy, an integrated marketing organization, adequate marketing information, strategic orientation, and operational efficiency (Alward & Camunas, 1991; Kotler & Clarke, 1987). A marketing orientation is the foundation for the marketing process. A successful marketing orientation means that energy is devoted to identifying customers' needs and wants and delivering satisfying services.

MARKETING STRATEGY

Strategy and research are the key elements of marketing. Strategy evolves from mission and planning. Research uncovers, analyzes, and monitors the needs and preferences of target markets. Strategic planning sets the overall frame for an organization. Defining the business, determining the mission, and formulating long-term objectives form the basis of an organization's strategic plan. This cannot be effectively done without investing adequate time and resources in evaluating the environment in which an organization is competing for customers. Environmental scanning is a critical step in the strategic planning process. A formal environmental scan includes systematic review of the following:

- Demographic and societal trends relevant to the business
- The organization's position in the market compared with that of its competitors
- Internal business performance indicators—for example, financial results, utilization trends, quality indicators, customer characteristics, etc.
- Market research
- The strength of suppliers and partners

Compilation, review and analysis of the environmental scan must involve every functional area in an organization, including its nurse leaders. Not only must this information be shared, but all key stakeholders must participate in the planning process. What good is accurate market information when only a handful of people have access to it?

Marketing strategy is based on how target markets are defined. Markets are both broad and narrow. Mass marketing offers a product to an entire market. Niche marketing focuses on capturing a small, but important, part of the market. Consider the difference between a full-service community hospital and a children's hospital. The former serves a broad market, the latter targets very specific customers—children and their families. Three critical concepts product differentiation, segmentation, and positioning—are essential to become fluent in the language of marketing. Table 15.1 gives the definitions of these terms, along with an example of each.

Segmentation cannot be achieved without differentiation; yet differentiation does not require segmentation (Schnaars, 1991). A product offering's differentiation is typically what cements its position in the market against competitors.

By analyzing the competitive market, a hospital can determine key strategies to meet the unmet needs in its service area. A small rural community hospital in a market 200 miles from any other hospital will adopt very different strategies for defining and serving its market than will a large suburban hospital in a market with four other hospitals within a 25-mile radius. The rural hospital would likely position itself as a full-service facility capable of meeting the most frequently occurring needs of the mass population. For example, its profile of services is likely to include women's services, emergency care, diagnostic care, and general surgery. On the other hand, the large suburban hospital in a highly competitive market might seek to differentiate itself from competitors by creating a specialty center for heart disease or cancer. However, product lines are not the only way to differentiate. Differentiation based on quality measures and other distinctions such as Joint Commission on Accreditation of Healthcare Organizations (JCAHO) accreditation scores, the Malcolm Baldrige National Quality Award, and the Magnet Recognition Program® are becoming more prevalent.

Table 15.1

Critical Marketing Concepts	
Definition	Example
Product differentiation is "the act of designing a set of meaningful differences to distinguish the company's offering from competitors' offerings" (Kotler, 2000, p. 287).	*Example:* Nordstrom differentiates itself from other department stores by offering highly personalized and excellent customer service.
Segmentation is described as "a merchandising strategy by which products are adjusted to serve a particular group of users" (Schnaars, 1991, p. 101).	*Example:* Nike makes and promotes different shoe products for specific customer groups—runners, hikers, basketball players, etc.
Positioning "is the act of designing the company's offering and image to occupy a distinctive place in the target market's mind" (Kotler, 2000, p. 298).	*Example:* Rolls Royce designs, prices, and promotes cars to achieve a desired position in the small extreme luxury market, compared with Saturn, which strives to appeal to a broader market of economy-minded buyers.

Setting marketing strategy is a shared responsibility within a health care organization. This critical activity must be guided by the strategic plan with input from every key stakeholder group—including nurses—who are engaged in meeting customer needs. Likewise, the organization's marketing team must be engaged from the start when new products and services are planned. With multiple perspectives represented at the planning table, an organization will respond more effectively to the needs and challenges of its market.

THE MARKETING PROCESS: IMPLEMENTING STRATEGY

Effective marketing evolves from a five-step linear process that includes: (1) research, (2) segmentation, (3) mix, (4) implementation, and (5) control. The process is represented visually as follows (Kotler, 1999, pp. 60-61):

$$R \rightarrow STP \rightarrow MM \rightarrow I \rightarrow C$$

where
R = research (i.e., market research)
STP = segmentation, targeting, and positioning
MM = marketing mix
I = implementation
C = control (getting feedback, evaluating results, and revising or improving STP strategy and MM tactics)

The process begins with rigorous marketing research (R) to uncover opportunities and provide strategic planning data. Target segments (STP) are determined, and a positioning of the product or service is strategized. Then the optimal tactical marketing mix (MM) is established. The marketing plan is implemented (I) and controlled (C) for effectiveness (Kotler, 1999).

Determining a marketing mix is one aspect of the marketing process. This is the stage in which specific tactics are custom designed to influence the buyer's decision to purchase the product or service. The tactics chosen for the marketing mix become the basis for operational marketing activities. From the seller's point of view, the marketing mix emerges as a unique combination of the four *P*s of (1) product, (2) price, (3) place, and (4) promotion. From the customer's point of view, the marketing mix emerges from the four *C*s of (1) customer solution, (2) cost, (3) convenience, and (4) communication (Kotler, 2000). Table 15.2 displays the marketing mix applied to health care.

A product is the basis of any business. It is whatever is offered to satisfy a market's need, desire, or preference. Products generally include objects, services, and ideas. They can be at the core, tangible, or augmented levels in relation to the market. A core product is what the client seeks in order to satisfy a basic need. A tangible product has characteristics such as style, quality, packaging, added features, and brand name. Augmented products include added services and benefits (Alward & Camunas, 1991; Kotler, 1999).

A *service* "is any act or performance that one party can offer to another that is essentially intangible and does not result in the ownership of anything. Its production may or may not be tied to a physical product" (Kotler, 2000, p. 428). Services are differentiated from products that are goods by four characteristics: (1) intangibility, (2) inseparability, (3) variability, and (4) perishability. Services are actions. Their performance varies according to circumstances related to both the provider and the recipient. They are sold first and then simultaneously produced and consumed. Services cannot be saved, stored, resold, or returned (Kotler, 2000).

Health, an intangible product, is the ultimate outcome desired from the health care industry. Nursing is a service within the industry. To successfully market itself, nursing must define and clearly articulate the features of its service. Yet articulating the unique contribution of nurses has long been a struggle for individual nurses and for the profession. Quality care is one ideal and intangible product of nursing services. Kramer and Schmalenberg (1988) noted that the product of a hospital is a high-quality, accessible, cost-effective service called client-centered care. Zander (1992) identified nursing as a business with a product of enhanced client outcomes and contained costs.

The eternal question lingers: What is nursing? One way to formulate an answer that best

Table 15.2

The Four *P*s and *C*s of the Marketing Mix Applied to Health Care			
Four *P*s	Four *C*s	General Description	Health Care Applications
Product	Customer solution	Product variety Quality Design Features Packaging Brand name	Product/service lines Patient outcomes Service quality Physical plant design/décor Hospital "name" Health care system "name" and reputation
Price	Customer cost	List price Discounts Allowances Payment period Credit terms	Cash prices Contract price/reimbursement • PPO • HMO • Medical groups

Place	Convenience	Location
		Coverage
		Assortments
		Inventory
		Channels
		Transport
			Health care system location, including
			   clinics or other service branches
			Adjacent medical offices
			Ancillary services on site
			Referral relationship with physicians,
			   medical groups, insurance providers, etc.
			External patient transportation such as
			   vans, taxi vouchers, etc.

Promotion	Communication	Sales promotion Advertising Sales force Public relations Direct marketing	Physician relations Advertising Community events and outreach Media relations Direct mail

From Woods, D. (2002). Realizing your marketing influence. Part 1: Meeting patient needs through collaboration. *Journal of Nursing Administration, 32*(4), 189-195.

communicates a vision of professional nursing is to describe the process and product of nursing as the use of expertise to solve problems for patients and their families. How often do nurses explain the value of what they have done? Are patients and families—for that matter, even hospital administrators or physician colleagues—aware of the contribution of nursing, especially when that contribution may be invisible (except in its absence), such as in the case of preventing an adverse outcome? To convey the importance of the content of nursing, experts advise that nurses describe the complexity of the care they provide and the clinical judgments they use, being deliberate in differentiating their role from other caregivers (Buresh & Gordon, 2000).

Nurses must capitalize on their unique service attributes when planning a health care marketing strategy or mix. Some specific nursing-related service benefits for clients include competence and technical ability in care, compassion and caring, comfort and amenities, convenience, curative ability, and coping augmentation. These attributes need to be balanced by cost considerations in order to promote value positioning. In the case of hospitals, it has long been understood that the primary criterion for hospitalizing a patient is determining what level of nursing care and intervention he or she requires (Woods, 2002).

The marketing process includes deliberate steps taken to design an effective marketing plan for specific products or services that are integrated in an organization-wide strategic plan. Creating total value is one way to differentiate and position a product or service. Translating a product or service into a benefits package and emphasizing purchase value and use value can help to advance marketing objectives (Alward & Camunas, 1991; Kotler, 1999).

Ensuring that nursing is provided with the necessary resources to, in turn, ensure positive patient outcomes is one of the most critical features that the health care product can offer to meet customer needs. For nursing, the core of patient care, marketing strategy should be analyzed and employed so that nursing services and strategic organizational goals are aligned.

LEADERSHIP AND MANAGEMENT IMPLICATIONS

Marketing comprises "the analysis, planning, and control of exchanges in order to develop and hold relationships with priority clients, suppliers, partners, and relevant publics, such as employers, other health care providers, and the media" (Harvey, 1998, p. 189). Thus understanding the motivations and reasons for transactions between organizations and clients is central to the practice of marketing in health care.

Adopting a marketing orientation has both leadership and management implications for nurses. An analysis of the internal and external landscape helps to identify primary markets for nursing services. Patients are the first obvious market. However, other health care providers and even the pool of potential nurse employees can be primary markets for nursing. Nurse leaders are responsible for developing ways to articulate the value of the nursing product to purchasers and strategic partners. Nurse leaders can also develop nursing internally with an eye toward marketing to prospective employees and retaining current ones—a critical consideration with the indefinite nursing shortage that lies ahead.

Profound ethical issues and controversies abound in health care. End-of-life care, organ procurement, reproductive technology and parenting, human gene therapy, and health care costs are but a few examples (Alward & Camunas, 1991). A unique layer of ethical issues may arise around the marketing of health care, one in which marketing ethics is also amplified.

There is an inherent order to things in marketing. If a health care system or provider has not developed a product or service to conform to the standards of its own strategic plan, promoting the product or service can present an ethical challenge. For example, can a hospital, in good conscience, promote the opening of a state-of-the-art cancer facility when it has not invested in recruiting and orienting competent specialized nurses, physicians, and other caregivers? This is an example of where the product is not just the building, the equipment, and the beds. In fact, here it is the caregivers who are the product's primary feature. Attaching an elegant sign to a building and filling the building with the latest equipment does not make it a cancer center (Woods & Cardin, 2002). These issues challenge nurse leaders and managers who may envision effective marketing strategies yet confront ethical dilemmas when seeking to implement them.

In the marketing context, nurse leaders contribute vision for meeting current and future customer needs and creating and supporting the systems that maximize nurses' contributions to excellent patient care. Leaders analyze and translate environmental data to support good decision making at all levels in the organization. Managers contribute further by actively participating in the delivery of services, providing and communicating data that support day-to-day decision making and ensuring that optimal systems and resources are present to meet patient care standards.

Research Note

Source: Needleman, J., Buerhaus, P., Mattke, S., Stewart, M., & Zelevinsky, K. (2002). Nurse-staffing levels and the quality of care in hospitals. *New England Journal of Medicine, 346*(22), 1715-1722.

Purpose

To determine whether lower levels of staffing by nurses in hospitals are associated with an increased risk for complications or death in patients.

Discussion

To test the hypothesis that there is a correlation between the level of nurse staffing and adverse patient outcomes, Needleman and colleagues used administrative data from 799 hospitals in 11 states to explore the relationship between the amount of care provided by nurses and patients' outcomes. They studied 25 total adverse outcomes for medical and surgical patients—11 were common to medical and surgical patients, 3 were specific to surgical patients—that were suspected of being sensitive to nurse staffing levels. Among the adverse "nurse-sensitive" outcomes were urinary tract infection, pneumonia, metabolic derangement, and "failure to rescue." Perhaps the most significant, failure to rescue, is described as the death of a patient with one of five life-threatening complications—pneumonia, shock or cardiac arrest, upper gastrointestinal bleeding, sepsis, or deep venous thrombosis—for which early identification by nurses and medical and nursing interventions can influence the risk for death.

Of the 25 adverse outcomes studied, registered nurse staffing levels were associated with 8. Based on the evidence, Needleman and colleagues (p. 1715) concluded that "a higher proportion of hours of nursing care by registered nurses and a greater number of hours of care by registered nurses per day are associated with better care for hospitalized patients."

Needleman and colleagues also reported that "a higher proportion of total hours of nursing care provided by registered nurses was more frequently associated with lower rates of adverse outcomes than was a greater number of registered nurse hours per day" (p. 1720). Their study looked not only at registered nurse hours but also at licensed practical nurses and aides. However, they found no similar evidence related to staffing with licensed practical/vocational nurses or aides.

Based on the findings, the researchers offered the following recommendation:

"Given the evidence that such staffing levels are associated with adverse outcomes, as well as the current and projected shortages of hospital-based registered nurses, systems should be developed for the routine monitoring, in large numbers of hospitals, of hospital outcomes that are sensitive to the levels of staffing by nurses. Beyond monitoring, hospital administrators, accrediting agencies, insurers, and regulators should take action to ensure that an adequate nursing staff is available to protect patients and to improve the quality of care" (p. 1720).

Application to Practice

The implications of this landmark study are significant for promoting the unique contribution of registered nurses to high-quality patient care, given the evidence for lower adverse events with greater RN staffing. Nurse leaders can incorporate these findings into strategic planning and resource allocation of RN staff. A hospital can develop and promote points of differentiation based on availability of nursing care and its related outcomes. Knowing the importance of adequate registered nurse staffing, a hospital could employ marketing concepts to recruit and retain an optimal number of nurses in the face of a growing global nursing shortage.

▲ LEADERSHIP & MANAGEMENT **BEHAVIORS**

Leadership Behaviors

- Envisions effective market exchanges
- Anticipates customer expectations based on environmental scanning data
- Inspires others to identify and meet customers' needs and wants
- Implements strategic marketing planning
- Role-models effective communication, collaboration, and relationship building
- Finds and develops new opportunities

Management Behaviors

- Analyzes markets and market segments
- Plans marketing mix and tactics

- Monitors performance and market share
- Controls customer relationships

Overlap Areas

- Promotes healthy work environments that sustain marketable nursing services of high quality
- Contributes to the marketing process
- Recognizes and promotes the value of the contribution that nurses make
- Links nursing to the organization's marketing plan and activities

CURRENT ISSUES AND TRENDS

Change is such a pervasive characteristic of the health care industry that achieving or sustaining market leadership over competitors in the turbulence of today's health care industry may seem daunting. However, environmental turbulence and rapid change can also bring forth clarity in the difference between competitors' resources and capabilities. This can lead to greater dispersion of profitability in the health care industry (Grant, 1991). Making good strategic decisions in the face of industry turbulence can set an organization apart from competitors far more rapidly than in a stable market. The key is to be ready with the services or products that consumers need to help them cope with the change. Helpful strategies include analyzing the business in five categories: (1) outputs, (2) personnel, (3) resources, (4) operations, and (5) customers. A series of questions then can be asked, as follows (Zell, 2002):

- Can we adapt to the change?
- How are we going to do this?
- What can we add to meet our customers' needs under the change scenario?
- Who will be responsible for this development?
- How will it integrate into our present products and services?

Gathering and analyzing information will lay the foundation for proactive capitalization on change opportunities. Change may open the door to new products, services, or ventures.

A variety of trends are currently present in the marketing of nursing and health care services—none more concerning than the protracted nursing shortage that is predicted to linger for decades to come. There is growing evidence that insufficient nurse staffing in hospitals is one of the greatest dangers to patient care the hospital industry has ever faced (JCAHO, 2002; Needleman et al., 2002). Hospitals that are able to preserve and optimize this scarce resource will benefit with a distinct advantage over competitors that fail to optimize their nursing resources. As the public becomes further educated about the dangers of the nursing shortage and the related problem of medical errors, hospitals are increasingly promoting the experience and skill of nursing staff as a point of differentiation.

Hospitals increasingly showcase national recognition to differentiate themselves from their competitors—not only in the eyes of patients, but also to attract nurses, physicians, and other employees. National recognition may include the following:

- American Association of Critical-Care Nurses Beacon Award for Critical Care Excellence

- American Nurses Credentialing Center Magnet Recognition Program®
- High JCAHO accreditation score
- Malcolm Baldrige National Quality Award
- *U.S. News & World Report's* list of "America's Best Hospitals"

Outside hospitals, nurses are developing integrated marketing plans for home health agencies to ensure increased market share and profitability (Hughes & Van Vleet, 1999). Service guarantees also have been used as a strategy to market health care systems and services (Levy, 1999). Furthermore, advanced practice nurses are conducting and disseminating growing evidence of their value in the health care provider industry (Kleinpell, 2001).

Summary

- Marketing is a business concept related to the activities of determining and meeting customer wants and needs.
- Marketing is a social and managerial process.
- Marketing capitalizes on opportunities.
- Changes in health care create market opportunities for nurses.
- Nurse leaders and managers need to adopt a marketing orientation. A marketing orientation is a focus on customers.
- Marketing is widely employed in competitive and resource-constrained environments like health care.
- Marketing must be central to and included in organizational strategic planning.
- A marketing mix is a blend of tools and tactics to elicit the desired response from the target markets.
- A marketing mix is based on product, price, place, and promotion or customer solution, cost, convenience, and communication.
- Marketing results in voluntary transactions and exchanges in a market.
- The marketing process uses research, segmentation, mix, implementation, and control.
- The primary elements of marketing are strategy and research. Marketing strategies and tactics

help to position to reach goals. Market research is the systematic study of markets.

Study Questions

1. Do nurses have a marketing orientation? Why? Why not?
2. What is the product of nursing? Of health care?
3. How can nurses identify market opportunities for their services? What are the next steps once those opportunities are identified?
4. How are value and positioning important for nurses?
5. What role do nurses play in designing the marketing mix?
6. How might important target groups view nurses? How can nurses influence this perception?

CASE STUDY

The leadership team of a 220-bed community hospital is struggling with a decision about how best to use its vacant seventh floor. The floor has been empty for 2 years since the institution's leadership decided to close the transitional care unit as a result of the high complexity and low reimbursement associated with new regulations for skilled nursing facilities.

Of the several options the team is considering, one is a cardiac surgical suite and acuity-adaptable intensive care unit. The team has done some preliminary environmental scanning, and based on what has been learned, they believe there is compelling evidence to suggest that the market demand for cardiac surgery will continue to grow dramatically as Baby Boomers reach their senior years.

Although there is consensus that this idea is the strongest option they have considered, a few major concerns still exist The first concern, naturally, is the significant capital investment the hospital will have to make to retrofit the floor to serve as a state-of-the-art surgical suite. It is uncertain how long it will take the hospital to get a return on the investment. The second concern is whether they

CRITICAL THINKING EXERCISE

Luisa Herrera is a nurse in a community hospital maternity center. She is at the end of her rope and considering leaving her job. As one of a handful of nurses in her hospital who speak fluent Spanish, she is frequently asked to interpret for other nurses' patients and their families. Herrera's growing concern is that her own patients and families are not receiving quality care because of her added duties as an interpreter.

The hospital has expended significant financial and human resources promoting itself as the market leader in specialized maternity services for the Latino community. Full-page newspaper advertisements and attractive brochures proclaim in Spanish and English: "With our full complement of bilingual physicians and nurses, we ensure that you and your family will be active participants in every decision affecting your care."

1. What is the problem?
2. What marketing strategy is the hospital trying to adopt?
3. What might have led to the implementation problems Herrera and her colleagues are experiencing?
4. What can Herrera do to become part of a solution?
5. What steps might the hospital take to ensure successful implementation of its strategy?
6. What could prevent this problem from occurring when another new service or feature is launched?

---

will be able to recruit and retain enough qualified nurses to staff the unit in the midst of a severe nursing shortage.

Also a factor is the concern that establishing a robust cardiac surgery service line will exacerbate their already fierce rivalry with a neighboring community hospital located less than a mile away. Many years ago, the two competing hospitals made an informal "gentleman's agreement" that they would not encroach on the other's signature service line. This hospital specializes in maternal-child services and has built a full-service line, including infertility services, a high-risk perinatal center, a state-of-the-art birthing center, and a level III neonatal intensive care unit. The other hospital houses a full-service cardiac center able to accommodate a large volume of patients needing open-heart surgery, stents, angioplasty, cardiac catheterization, and the whole array of cardiac surgical and medical services. For the last decade, both hospitals have tried to refrain from opening competing services in the other's signature specialty areas. To consider a cardiac surgical suite and ICU will require a marketing plan, as well as facility and service planning.

At its regular meeting, the leadership team determined that the prudent next step was for a subcommittee to lead development of a business plan for the proposed cardiac surgical center. The first task of the subcommittee—composed of the director of nursing, critical care nursing and medical directors, marketing director, and chief financial officer—will be to identify who else in the organization should be involved in the business planning. The Director of Marketing was chosen to chair the subcommittee and write the plan.

REFERENCES

Alward, R.R., & Camunas, C. (1991). *The nurse's guide to marketing.* Albany, NY: Delmar Publishers.

Buresh, B., & Gordon, S. (2000). *From silence to voice: What nurses know and must communicate to the public.* Ottawa, Ontario, Canada: Canadian Nurses Association.

Graham, P. (1993). Marketing's domain: A critical review of the development of the marketing concept. *Marketing Bulletin, 4,* 1-11.

Grant, R.M. (1991). *Contemporary strategy analysis* (3rd ed.). Malden, MA: Blackwell Publishers Inc.

Harvey, J.W. (1998). Marketing in the new health care environment. In J.A. Dienemann (Ed.), *Nursing administration: Managing patient care* (2nd ed.) (pp. 185-206). Stamford, CT: Appleton & Lange.

Hughes, M.M., & Van Vleet, J. (1999). Developing a marketing plan for home health care agencies. *Home Health Care Consultant, 6*(4), 33-35.

Joint Commission on Accreditation of Healthcare Organizations (JCAHO). (2002). *Health care at the crossroads: Strategies for addressing the evolving nursing crisis.* Oakbrook Terrace, IL: JCAHO. Retrieved May 31, 2004, from *www.jcaho.org/about+us/public+policy+initiatives/ health+care+at+the+crossroads.pdf*

Kleinpell, R.M. (2001). *Outcome assessment in advanced practice nursing.* New York: Springer.

Kotler, P. (1999). *Kotler on marketing: How to create, win, and dominate markets.* New York: The Free Press.

Kotler, P. (2000). *Marketing management* (Millennium ed.). Upper Saddle River, NJ: Prentice-Hall.

Kotler, P. (2003). *Marketing insights from A to Z.* Hoboken, NJ: John Wiley & Sons, Inc.

Kotler, P., & Clarke, R.N. (1987). *Marketing for health care organizations.* Englewood Cliffs, NJ: Prentice-Hall.

Kramer, M., & Schmalenberg, C. (1988). Magnet hospitals: Institutions of excellence: Part 1. *Journal of Nursing Administration, 18*(1), 13-24.

Levy, J.S. (1999). Marketing service guarantees for health care. *Nursing Economic$, 17*(4), 214-218.

Needleman, J., Buerhaus, P., Mattke, S., Stewart, M., & Zelevinsky, K. (2002). Nurse-staffing levels and the quality of care in hospitals. *New England Journal of Medicine, 346*(22), 1715-1722.

Schnaars, S.P. (1991). *Marketing strategy: Customers and competition* (2nd ed.). New York: The Free Press.

Woods, D. (2002). Realizing your marketing influence. Part 1: Meeting patient needs through collaboration, *Journal of Nursing Administration, 32*(4), 189-195.

Woods, D., & Cardin, S. (2002). Realizing your marketing influence. Part 2: Marketing from the inside out. *Journal of Nursing Administration, 32*(6), 323-330.

Zander, K. (1992). Nursing care delivery methods and quality. *Series on Nursing Administration, 3,* 86-104.

Zell, A.J. (2002). *Change—An opportunity.* Portland, OR: Ambassador of Selling. Retrieved May 31, 2004, from *www.sellingselling.com/articles/opportun.html*

IV

CARE MANAGEMENT

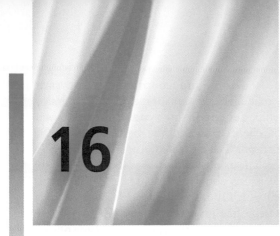

16

Models of Care Delivery

Amy London Deutschendorf

CHAPTER OBJECTIVES

- Associate models of care delivery with organizational structure and process variables
- Define and describe the components of patient care delivery systems
- Classify and define six common nursing care models
- Analyze the advantages and disadvantages of each care delivery system
- Evaluate trends shaping the development and use of care delivery systems in the United States
- Exercise critical thinking to conceptualize and analyze possible solutions to a practice exercise

The goals of successful patient care delivery include high-quality and low-cost care and the achievement of patient outcomes and satisfaction levels. The ability to reach these objectives depends on the organization's approach to the matching of human and material resources with patient characteristics and health care needs. The identification of patient care processes that are necessary to achieve care goals must be done in order to determine health care provider roles most appropriate to the specific process.

The assignment of nursing care staff to clients needing care is a basic activity of health care systems in order to achieve these goals. Assignment is defined as the "downward or lateral transfer of both the responsibility and accountability of an activity from one individual to another" (ANA, 1997, p. 1). The assignment must be within that individual's scope of practice. An element of assignment is delegation, which can be defined as the "transfer of responsibility for the performance of the activity from one individual to another while retaining accountability for the outcome" (p. 1). Both assignment and delegation are methods used by managers to deliver patient care within the structure of the health care system. The determination of the structure and method by which assignments are made is a managerial responsibility. While this is part of a process of developing a model of nursing care delivery, it reflects a unidimensional framework that does not consider the structural and contextual factors that make up a model for professional group practice in a complex health care environment (Anthony et al., 2004).

The determination of a nursing care model or system of care delivery is dependent on organizational structure and processes related to patient care. Examples of structure and process criteria are found in Box 16.1. Trends in the health care environment strongly influence organizational structure. Examples of these trends are found in the "Current Issues and Trends" section of this chapter. Organizational structure and process variables may inhibit or facilitate the work of nurses (Neidlinger & Miller, 1990) and have been closely correlated with quality outcomes (Aiken & Patrician, 2000). Only after careful evaluation of these variables can a model to deliver care be conceived.

Box 16.1

Examples of Structure and Process Criteria

Organizational Structure

Governance
Teaching status
Aggregated units
Technology level
Case/mix
Operating budget
Nursing hours/day
Skill mix
Nurse-to-patient ratio
Use of temporary staff members
Workload
Nursing education/experience
Support for professional development
Continuing education
Expert resources

Organizational Processes

Care delivery model
Care planning
Patient assessment/monitoring
Documentation
Policies/procedures
Support personnel
Supplies
Patient education
Implementation of physician orders
Patient/family communication
Symptom management
Staff communication
Medication administration

Data from The Advisory Board Company. (1999). Understanding the impact of changes in nurse staffing: A review of recent outcomes studies. *Nursing Watch 4*, 1-15. Reprinted from Deutschendorf, A.L. (2003). From past paradigms to future frontiers: Unique care delivery models to facilitate nursing work and quality outcomes. *Journal of Nursing Administration, 33*(1), 52-59.

Nurses deliver and coordinate client care. Nurse managers, in collaboration with nursing leadership, design nursing systems for the provision of client care and the betterment of the organization. The model of care delivery has a direct relationship to the allocation of control over decisions about client care. It is the means through which nurse managers delegate effectively and thereby free up and manage time as a scarce resource. Manthey (1989) said that the type of care delivery system or care model determines whether professional practice exists among the nursing staff on a particular unit because delivery systems define control over nursing decision making. This means that autonomy over practice decisions largely is determined by the care model and the resultant nurse decision-making latitude. The type of care delivery system used has implications for job satisfaction, the character of professional practice, and the amount of authority that is actually transferred to the staff.

DEFINITIONS

A *nursing care model,* or the *system of nursing care delivery,* is often called a care modality. A **care modality** is defined as a method of organizing and delivering nursing care in order to achieve desired patient outcomes. Manthey (1990) identified the basic elements of nursing care delivery systems as clinical decision making, work allocation, communication, and management (Box 16.2). Coordination is a critical component that must be considered in order to manage task interdependencies upon which process and clinical outcomes are reliant. Relational coordination (Gittell et al., 2000) is described as the management of the multiple dimensions of communications and relationships between and among health care providers that are necessary to provide quality and efficient care.

Nursing care delivery models must address both *direct patient care functions* and *indirect patient care functions* (Deutschendorf, 2003) (Box 16.3). The direct patient care functions are facilitated by and dependent on the management (Fox et al., 1999),

⚠ LEADING & MANAGING **DEFINED**

Care Modality

A method of organizing and delivering nursing care in order to achieve desired outcomes.

Private Duty Nursing

One nurse to one client.

Group Nursing

Private duty nurses in group practice.

Total Patient Care

One-shift responsibility for a client.

Functional Nursing

Assignment by functions or tasks.

Team Nursing

Care to a group of clients by a mixed-staff team.

Modular Nursing

Construction of geographic modules to facilitate team nursing.

Primary Nursing

24-hour accountability by a nurse for specific clients from hospital admission through discharge.

Case Management

"A collaborative process of assessment, planning, facilitation and advocacy for options and services to meet an individual's health needs through communication and available resources to promote quality cost-effective outcomes" (CMSA, 2002, p. 5).

Managed Care

The systematic integration and coordination of the financing and delivery of health care.

Critical Path

A written structured care methodology used to standardize care by mapping time and activity sequence for an episode of care.

New and Evolving Types

Mixed models emphasizing outcomes management and integrated professional practice.

---

or indirect, functions. For example, the client care assignment system is an aspect of operations included in indirect patient care functions. It is how the work is distributed. Using human resource decisions such as staffing and skill mix, a framework for the deployment of nursing staff and their assignment to client care can be determined. Although the nurse manager is ultimately accountable for the achievement of direct and indirect patient care functions, the scope of responsibility necessitates appropriate delegation and assignment to competent unit staff. Delegation and assignment of management functions are vital to developing and maintaining professional nursing practice.

Box 16.2

Elements of Nursing Care Delivery

The fundamental elements of any nursing care delivery system are as follows:
- Clinical decision making
- Work allocation
- Communication
- Management
- Coordination

Data from Manthey, M. (1990). Definitions and basic elements of a patient care delivery system with an emphasis on primary nursing. In G. Meyer, M. Madden, & E. Lawrenz (Eds.), *Patient care delivery models* (pp. 201-211). Rockville, MD: Aspen.

Box 16.3

Direct and Indirect Patient Care Functions

Direct Patient Care Functions

Assessment
Monitoring
Prioritizing goals
Care coordination
Therapeutic interventions
Evaluation
Communication
Patient education

Indirect Patient Care Functions

Clinical practice
Education/research
Leadership
Operations
Personnel management
Quality improvement
System coordination
Other

Data from Fox, R.T., Fox, D.H., & Wells, P.J. (1999). Performance of first-line management functions on productivity of hospital unit personnel. *Journal of Nursing Administration, 29*(9), 12-18. Reprinted from Deutschendorf, A.L. (2003). From past paradigms to future frontiers: Unique care delivery models to facilitate nursing work and quality outcomes. *Journal of Nursing Administration, 33*(1), 52-59.

The practice model can be thought of as a link between the problems presented by client populations, the purposes of professional occupations, and the purposes of health care organizations. For any practice model, the degree of integration of the nursing care given to a client, the degree of continuity in assignment of nursing personnel caring for a client, and the type of coordination used to plan and organize the client's care need to be consistent with general client characteristics, available nursing resources, and the organizational support available to nursing (Mark, 1992).

BACKGROUND

Administrators have the responsibility for making decisions about and designing strategies to create a climate and environmental context. Organizational environments exert a strong influence over nursing care delivery, either positive or negative. Nursing care delivery can be seen as the dynamic balance between routine resource management and the structure, process, and content of practice. One outcome is that the system for distribution of nursing personnel must ensure that staff members of the right skill mix and numbers are promptly deployed so that clients are cared for in an appropriate and timely manner. Recent studies have demonstrated the impact of skill mix and nurse staffing on patient outcomes (Aiken et al., 2002; Needleman et al., 2001), further clarifying the need for appropriate role and resource deployment. There are four strategic decisions to make: a philosophy of resource utilization, a choice of delivery system, common and individual practice expectations, and a development of the role of the RN (Manthey, 1991). These four strategic decisions may be made at different levels in any organization. If these decisions are made only by the chief nurse executive, then shared governance and decentralization do not exist.

There are both older and newer systems and models of nursing care delivery in use. The complexity of the health care environment strongly influences organizational decisions regarding patient care. Fiscal responsibility and accountability to the consumer are priorities in an environment of increasing health care costs and health care errors. The development of new models is characterized by changes in the health care climate, including costs, consumer expectations, patient characteristics, and new medical information and technology. Although all models have their advantages and disadvantages, there is no one right way to structure nursing care. The appropriate care delivery model is the one that maximizes existing resources while meeting the objectives of direct and indirect patient care functions (Deutschendorf, 2003). In addition, pieces of

Research Note

Source: Schaffner, J.W., Alleman, S., Ludwig-Beymer, P., Muzynski, J., King, D.J., & Pacura, L.J. (1999). Developing a patient care model for an integrated delivery system. *Journal of Nursing Administration, 29*(9), 43-50.

Purpose

Integrated delivery systems can result from the merger of two or more organizations. The purpose of this article was to describe the process used to define common elements and develop a patient care model for an integrated delivery system that resulted from the merger of two large nonprofit organizations.

Discussion

An integrated health care delivery system needs a consistent patient care delivery model. This is especially difficult when two organizations merge to form an integrated health care delivery system. Advocate Health Care is one such system. After the merger of two separate organizations, there were too many councils and task forces. Variations in care delivery models and the role of the Chief Nurse Executive (CNE) existed. A patient care council was empowered to develop a mechanism for clinical integration by identifying common elements of the CNE role and the patient care delivery model. Retreats were held and facilitators were trained. Then a document was drafted that defined common elements of the patient care model. These elements included the roles of the CNE, first-line managers, staff RNs, and unlicensed assistive personnel. Additional areas of development were the philosophy of nursing and the support functions of staff education and quality measurement using a nursing quality "dashboard" of indicators.

Application to Practice

Because a variety of practice models exist and no one model is superior to others, the approach taken was not to standardize but rather to identify common elements. A common infrastructure relative to roles and responsibilities across the system promoted effectiveness. The care delivery model was developed as a visual guide and orientation to the philosophy of nursing. Indicators and measures of the quality of nursing care and impact on outcomes were developed with reference to the ANA indicators. In the absence of a CNE for the integrated health care delivery system, the patient care council became the mechanism by which a system CNE's functions were fulfilled.

---

older systems often are incorporated into new delivery models as they are developed. Therefore it is important to have an understanding of the variety of models available, both old and new. Pure nursing models (effective in less complex times) have yielded to collaborative practice and interdisciplinary approaches with the proliferation of health care provider roles, expedited care processes, and increased severity of illness.

SIX MAJOR TYPES OF DELIVERY SYSTEMS

Historians mark the emergence of modern nursing from the time of Florence Nightingale's work in the Crimea. She instituted reforms centering on hygiene, cleanliness, and nutrition. She also was the first nurse educator, researcher, and administrator. The Nightingale model was transported to the United States, and nursing practice evolved from there over the course of the twentieth century (Kalisch & Kalisch, 1978).

In the history of American nursing, there have been six major types of nursing care models (Lee, 1993):

1. Private duty
2. Functional
3. Team
4. Primary
5. Case management
6. Current evolving types

Of these six, the four care models of functional, team, primary, and case management are associated with hospital nursing practice. Private duty and case management are associated with public health, home health care, and community health. Private duty, later called *case* or *case management,* was the original way nursing care was delivered; it later became the foundation for public health nursing and community service delivery.

Private Duty Nursing

Private duty nursing, sometimes called *case nursing,* is the oldest care model in the United States. Private duty nursing is defined as one nurse caring for one client. In this model complete and total care is provided by one nurse, but the nurse carries only one client assignment. Originally, when the nurse went into the home, the nurse did the cooking, cleaning, bathing of wounds, and organizing of the household functions, basically functioning as a home manager. In American nursing practice, private duty was the original way that graduate nurses found employment, although some had administrative positions in hospitals and some worked in public health (Reverby, 1987). A form of hospital case nursing evolved between 1900 and the 1930s. When the Great Depression hit, most families were too poor to afford private duty nurses, and so nurses were without jobs. Hospitals then began to employ graduate nurses.

Reverby (1987) noted that during the Depression years a great transformation from private duty to hospital staffing took place in nursing. As the graduate nurses who had been doing private duty moved into the hospital, they wanted to retain the type of care model to which they had become accustomed. Private duty, the idea that one nurse does the total care of one client, was transplanted into hospital settings for as long as nurses were paid by clients. When nurses became employees of hospitals, the kind of client care that private duty allowed was not possible within the organizational structure of hospital staff nursing. The organization of work in hospitals was task-focused, not client-focused (Reverby, 1987).

The advantage of private duty nursing was that the nurse's focus was entirely on one client's needs. This fostered closeness in the nurse-client relationship and increased RN and client satisfaction with care delivery. The disadvantage was that private duty is a costly model because of its low efficiency. Furthermore, job security was tenuous and irregular (Lee, 1993; Reverby, 1987). Other disadvantages were that nurses had little job mobility and were relatively isolated from colleagues.

Two main variations to the basic pattern of private duty nursing developed: group nursing and total patient care. Group nursing was an early alternative model that combined private duty concepts with hospital staff nursing. Total patient care was a hospital care model characterized by 8-hour shift accountability.

Group nursing was a care model proposed in the 1930s by Janet Geister, then the Executive Director of the American Nurses Association (ANA). Defined as nursing group practice, the idea of group nursing in hospitals was similar to divisional private duty in which several clients shared a private nurse. The plan was to reorganize private duty from individual to group practice, both inside and outside the hospital. Thus the registry of private duty nurses would be transformed into a group practice and linked to a community's public health nursing service. Facing political pressure, the plan died. Hospitals also experimented with a group nursing care modality, described as being halfway between a private duty arrangement and graduate nurse hospital staff nursing. Under this plan, clients were grouped together in a special unit in which several clients shared a private nurse. Thus three nurses could do 8-hour shifts for two clients instead of four nurses being needed for 12-hour shifts. The hospital paid the nurses' wages but charged the clients directly as a surcharge on the hospital bill. The advantages included shorter hours for nurses, order and regularity in hospital staffing, steady employment for nurses, slightly cheaper rates for clients, and responsibility for the total care of several clients for the nurse. Nurses obtained the autonomy and care delivery method of private duty without its isolation and uncertainty. Nurses were members of the hospital's staff; yet their time was specifically allocated only to a set number of clients who paid for this service directly. However, economic and political pressures for more efficiency, productivity, and service cut off the adoption of this system in hospitals (Reverby, 1987). It is interesting to note the parallels between group nursing and what eventually came to be the way physicians organized themselves.

Total patient care has been defined as a case method for organizing nursing care in which nurses are responsible for total care of a client but only for the hours in which that specific nurse is present (Glandon et al., 1989; Hegyvary, 1977). The distinguishing feature of total patient care is the shift-only (usually 8-12 hours) accountability for care. Examples initially occurred in intensive care, hospice care, and home health care. The term *total patient care* has come to mean the assignment of each client to a nurse who plans and delivers care during a work shift (McCloskey et al., 1991). Total patient care reemerged in the middle 1990s as a prevalent care delivery system after reengineering and restructuring occurred. The term has become confused with team or primary nursing care delivery systems. Total patient care has been described as a "form of primary nursing" (Reverby, 1987); however, the accountability for patient care coordination throughout the acute episode does not happen. The advantages are the intensity of focus with shift-only responsibility. Significant disadvantages are lack of communication and continuity of care for the client over time. Models of total patient care have contributed to task- and shift-based care that diverts attention from achievement of future patient goals (Bower, 2004).

Functional Nursing

Functional nursing is a care model that uses the division of labor according to specific tasks and technical aspects of the job. It has been defined as work assignment by functions or tasks, such as passing medicine, doing dressing changes, giving baths, or taking vital signs (McCloskey et al., 1991). Under functional nursing, the nurse identifies the tasks to be done for a shift. The work is divided and assigned to personnel, who focus on completing the assigned task. Functional nursing has the advantage of being efficient for taking care of the tasks related to handling a large number of clients.

Functional nursing was the norm in U.S. hospitals from the late 1800s through the end of World War II. Factors such as increases in client acuity, greater complexity of care delivery, and expansion of the number of paying clients increased demand for hospital nursing services. As hospitals searched for ways to improve efficiency and service yet control labor costs, the functional division of tasks was instituted to get the work done. Cyclical shortages of nursing labor, exacerbated during times of war, accelerated staffing shortages and the demands of work. This organization of work, combined with frequent understaffing, forced nurses to be task-oriented rather than client-oriented. It was a major reason why graduate nurses disliked staff nursing as compared with private duty (Reverby, 1987).

In the early 1900s, business and industry concepts of "scientific management" emphasized efficiency. The efficiency was gained by breaking down a work process into its component task steps and then analyzing and timing the steps, establishing standards, and determining the best way to perform each task. Thus managerial control over the planning and execution of work could be established. Assembly lines in factories were one result. Functional nursing was developed as a result of this concern for task analysis and proper division of the nursing workload. Under this model, there might be a "temperature nurse," a "medication nurse," a nurse for the right side of the ward, and a nurse for the left side of the ward (Kalisch & Kalisch, 1978; Reverby, 1987). Functional nursing was less oriented to individualized and holistic client care and more oriented to task accomplishment. One advantage was that there was little confusion about roles and duties. When applied to nursing, this method was efficient and cheap, but nurses and clients hated it. Client satisfaction dropped under this kind of care delivery system. Clients felt that they could not identify who was their nurse caretaker.

Team Nursing

Team nursing is a care model that uses a group of people led by a knowledgeable nurse. It is a delivery approach that provides care to a group of clients by coordinating a team of RNs, licensed practical nurses (LPNs), and aides under the supervision of one nurse, called the team leader (Glandon et al., 1989; Hegyvary, 1977). Team nursing has been defined as the assignment of a group of clients to a small group of workers under the direction of a team leader. Each team member provides most of the care to his or her assigned clients, although some tasks (e.g., medications) may be assigned separately (McCloskey et al., 1991).

Team nursing is designed to make use of each member's capabilities to meet the nursing needs of his or her group of clients. It is a delegation of care to a designated team of staff members. The staff members have various levels of expertise, but they are formed into a team. The nurse leader takes into account the level of expertise, and then divides the assignments accordingly so that the clients who are assigned to a team of caregivers have their needs appropriately met. Team nursing developed in the early 1950s in response to a shortage of RNs and in reaction to the dissatisfaction with functional nursing.

The advantages of team nursing are that each member's particular capabilities can be used to the maximum. This model supports group productivity and the growth of team members. Communication is vital. A sense of contribution via the team can be fostered. Oversight for novice nurses and temporary personnel can be facilitated. However, it takes a skilled RN to be a team leader. Furthermore, an RN team member may not be functioning up to his or her full potential because of being assigned an ancillary role, which creates some underutilization of the RN personnel.

One variation of team nursing is **modular nursing**. Modular nursing is based on the existence of specific facilities and on actual structural and spatial changes to enable hospital nurses to stay near the bedside. Structural modules based on client acuity are clustered in larger districts based on geography. Nurses are stationed near their clients, and a wider range of responsibility is delegated to them. Open design and convenient access architecture provide for decentralization of care delivery based on the spatial arrangement of the unit and enhanced communication (Magargal, 1987). The development of an innovative new care delivery system needs to be in synchrony with the philosophy of care (Guild et al., 1994). Modular nursing is a spatial arrangement resulting in a care delivery system that has philosophy of care implications. The essential features of modular nursing are as follows (Anderson & Hughes, 1993):

- A module consists of a group of nurses and a group of clients.
- Clients are grouped by spatial or floor-plan clustering.
- Nurse/client assignment is standardized.
- Modular care planning rounds occur regularly.
- A unit-based modular committee is established.

In one facility, decentralizing nursing activity to three modular substations for a 50-bed unit allowed for a reduction in RN skill mix from 63% to 46% (Abts et al., 1994).

Functional nursing was a precursor of team nursing. Both models emphasized efficiency and care delivery with limited RNs. However, team nursing corrected some deficiencies in care fragmentation and regimentation that were a problem with functional nursing.

Primary Nursing

Primary nursing began in the 1970s as a way to overcome the discontent with functional and team nursing's emphasis on tasks and discrete functions that directed nurses' attention away from holistic care of the client. This matched a societal trend toward accountability as well as nursing's rising level of professionalism. Primary nursing is an approach in which a nurse has responsibility and accountability for the continuous guidance of specific clients from hospital admission through discharge. Thus the primary nurse provides for the total nursing process for the client during a period of hospitalization (Glandon et al., 1989; Hegyvary, 1977). Primary nursing has been defined as the assignment in a hospital of each client to a primary nurse who plans, delivers, and monitors care under a 24-hour responsibility from admission to discharge (McCloskey et al., 1991). The hallmark of the primary nursing concept is the 24-hour accountability element. Autonomy, authority, and accountability in the primary nurse's role are basic to primary nursing. When the nurse is not actually taking care of clients, an associate delivers the care. However, the primary nurse makes the care and treatment coordination decisions, supervising the entire stay, 24 hours per day, for the length of the hospital stay. This increases continuity of care and consistency in assignments. Primary nursing does not mean that the primary nurse takes care of clients 24 hours a day. Rather, the 24-hour accountability is for the supervision and delegation of client care. Primary nursing has been called the first formal professional model in hospital nursing (Zander, 1992).

The advantages of primary nursing include a focus on the client's needs, greater nurse autonomy, and greater continuity of care. Primary nursing eventually came to be associated with all-RN staffing but has moved away from that position. Problems in the implementation of primary nursing have include the wide variation in its operationalization and implementation. The result has been confusion and lack of a structure to enable primary nurse autonomy. Under cost-containment pressure, an all-RN staff is difficult to justify. Total accountability may create burnout, and a poorly prepared RN may feel threatened by primary nursing.

Research conducted to compare team nursing with primary nursing care models has found higher quality of nursing care, higher levels of nurse satisfaction, increased continuity of care, improved nurse retention, and positive client outcomes with primary nursing. Levels of client satisfaction were equal, and cost comparisons were inconclusive between the two models (Gardner, 1991; Lang & Clinton, 1984; Lee, 1993).

Private duty was a precursor of primary nursing (Poulin, 1985). Both care delivery models emphasized the closeness of the nurse-client relationship, but primary nursing was more cost-effective. Primary nursing was a care model that evolved in reaction to the desire of RNs to return to more direct and active care instead of supervision of ancillary workers as in the team nursing care model. This approach promoted greater RN professional authority, accountability, autonomy, and continuity of care. Initially, an all-RN staff was thought to be needed. Compatible support systems were needed for a primary nursing care model to be effective. Primary nursing is highly sensitive to human resource distribution, skill mix, staff competency levels, and client care needs. However, as budget constraints, shortened lengths of stay, increased client severity, and pressures for cost containment in hospitals grew in the late 1980s and early 1990s, it was difficult to maintain primary nursing care models (Cohen & Cesta, 2005).

Case Management

Case management is the fastest-growing form of a "new" care delivery model. It has been defined as both a process and a care delivery model. Case management has developed as a method to *manage care*. **Managed care** is care coordination that is organized to achieve specific client outcomes, given fiscal and other resource constraints. Managed care has been defined as "the systematic integration and coordination of the financing and delivery of health care" (Grimaldi, 1996, p. 6).

The Case Management Society of America (CMSA) is the professional organization for case managers in practice. It is a multidisciplinary organization. The CMSA definition of case management is "a collaborative process of assessment, planning, facilitation and advocacy for options and services to meet an individual's health needs through communication and available resources to promote quality cost-effective outcomes" (CMSA, 2002, p. 5).

In nursing, the ANA first defined nursing case management as a system of health assessment, planning, service procurement, service delivery, service coordination, and monitoring through which the multiple service needs of clients are met (ANA, 1988; Zander, 1990). Hospital acute care case management today is an attempt to reconfigure the delivery of hospital care away from previous care models. Case management and care coordination have been the care delivery models used for years by public health and community health nurses (Mikulencak, 1993). In these settings, case management has been client-needs centered, rather than shift-, unit-, or system-centered. Case management can occur inside or outside the hospital only, extend across the health care continuum, or be linked to a population focus (Lee, 1993; Lyon, 1993).

Case management in acute care hospital nursing has been defined as a system of client care delivery that focuses on the achievement of client outcomes within effective and appropriate time frames and resources. Case management has components of health services delivery, coordination, and monitoring through which multiple service needs of clients are met. Hospital-based acute care nursing case management is focused on an entire episode of illness, crossing all settings in which the client receives care. Care is directed by a case manager who is not always a nurse and can be unit- or population-focused.

Case management is associated with the use of critical paths. Critical paths are one type of structured care methodology. Structured care methodologies (SCMs) are streamlined interdisciplinary tools used to "identify best practices, facilitate standardization of care, and provide a mechanism for variance tracking, quality enhancement, outcomes measurement, and outcomes research" (Cole & Houston, 1999, p. 53). Other examples of SCMs are evidenced-based algorithms, protocols, standards of care, order sets, and clinical practice guidelines. The use of best evidence is considered the gold standard to reduce practice variation in an environment focused on patient outcomes. Critical paths outline time and the sequence of events for an episode-of-care delivery. Resources appropriate in amount and sequence to a specific case type and individual client are managed for length of stay, critical events and timing, and anticipated outcomes. A **critical path** is a written plan that identifies key, critical, or predictable incidents that must occur at set times to achieve client outcomes within an appropriate length of stay in a hospital setting. The critical path is a tracking system for health outcomes, complications, activity, and teaching/learning (Fuszard, 1988).

In the face of strong economic external forces, acute care hospitals turned to case management. Nursing did not wish to return to team nursing care delivery and the associated issues of care fragmentation and the use of nurse extenders. Instead, nurses advocated the use of professional practice care delivery models. Case management was seen as a way to incorporate and build on the strengths of earlier care models yet provide a professional practice model for nurses. The risk with case management models is that integration into unit care delivery may not occur. Care goals for the patient, as determined by the case manager, may not be communicated to the bedside nurse. The case manager becomes the care coordinator and decision maker for care planning, and the unit nursing staff may become more focused on technical tasks.

'New' Types

Nursing shortages and health care reform have had a strong impact on the creation of **new and evolving types** of patient care delivery models. Staff mix models were retooled in the late 1980s as a result of a severe nursing shortage and in an attempt to complement the work of the professional nurse with the use of nursing extenders (Eastbaugh & Regan-Donavan, 1990; Manthey, 1989; Powers et al., 1990). In an era of managed care, fiscal restraint became a driver for restructuring, reengineering, and redesign. Nurses were perceived as more "costly than cost-effective" as a result of their 24-hour responsibility for patient care and contribution to the overall labor budget (Hall, 1997). As a result many of the newer models for patient care are staff mix models, in which nurses are partnered with a variety of "extenders" or multiskilled workers. Outcome studies have clearly demonstrated the negative impact of "substitution models" in which extenders have not been utilized to complement nurses but rather served as replacements, thereby increasing RN-to-patient ratios (Aiken et al., 2002; Needleman et al., 2001). The determination of the most effective models to fully utilize professional nursing skills in patient care while minimizing tasks that can be safely delegated continues to evolve.

Many new models identified in the literature are mixed models, some form of second-generation primary nursing or professional practice models that emphasize outcomes management, collaboration, the use of a variety of caregivers with variable competency and preparation, and integrated practice (Bard et al., 1994; Jones-Schenk & Hartley, 1993; Lengacher et al., 1993; Parkman & Loveridge, 1994; Wolf et al., 1994; Zander, 1992). Concepts of accountability, cost containment, effectiveness, seamless continuum of care, integration, multidisciplinary collaboration, new roles, alteration in skill mix, and new assignment systems are key components. All seek to reconfigure nursing's work within resource constraints, care needs, and current ideas about professional nursing practice.

Patient-focused or patient-centered care is one model developed to meet the needs of organizations that are reengineered to be more competitive and cost-effective. Patient-centered care is defined as "the redesign of patient care in the acute care setting so that hospital resources and personnel are organized around the patient's health care needs" (Maehling, 1995, p. 62). It is part of a redesign effort to realign the structure and processes involved in delivering care to center around the patient to improve efficiency and resource use. Patients are aggregated according to care requirements or similar service demands (as opposed to similar diagnoses). Protocols or pathways form a central point of focus. Key factors in the implementation of a patient-focused model are the cross-training and multiskilling of

team members for task performance and increased flexibility (Higginbotham, 1999). With a patient-focused approach there is an ongoing process to seek out and determine what is important to the person receiving care. This approach adopts the perspective of the person receiving care and strives to establish mutual goals between patient and provider in order to meet unique needs. To reach this complexity challenge, horizontal structures with an emphasis on relationships and effective working partnership are built (Comack et al., 1999).

More recently, patient-focused care teams have been configured that are made up of RNs, LPNs, respiratory therapists, housekeepers, dietitians and nursing technicians, with the RN as the leader of the team. The advantage of patient-focused care redesigns is that they center systems and services closer to the patient. This strong customer focus may increase patient satisfaction and conserve resources. However, implicit in these redesign efforts is a series of significant work group and culture changes affecting the financial operations and cost structure of hospitals. It also requires a commitment for initial allocation of resources to achieve ultimate financial and clinical outcomes. Multiskilling can be fraught with problems because delegation of nursing tasks must be defined and separated from those requiring nursing assessment. Outcome studies on the implementation of patient focused care vary in terms of provider and patient satisfaction, costs, and clinical outcomes (Barry-Walker, 2000; Seago, 1999). However, measures may not be based on "pure" patient-focused care models.

Because the acute care environment is multifaceted around multiple levels of care, patient types, diseases, and providers, a single organizational model for patient care delivery may be unrealistic. Deutschendorf (2003) proposed the development of unit-based models that incorporate an evaluation of structure and process criteria that influence direct and indirect patient care functions to determine an appropriate model. Nursing units that have a large percentage of novice nurses in an environment of increased activity and severity of

Research Note

Source: Potter, P., & Grant, E. (2004). Understanding RN and unlicensed assistive personnel working relationships in designing care delivery strategies. *Journal of Nursing Administration, 34*(1), 19-25.

Purpose

Unlicensed assistive personnel (UAP) are used to support nursing care in many care delivery models. Although many studies have focused on the perceptions of RNs who have worked with UAPs, few studies have examined the working relationships between the RN and the UAP from the perspective of the UAP. The purpose of this qualitative investigation was to determine characteristics of working relationships between the RN and UAP and the care delivery models that influence those relationships.

Discussion

RNs in the current work environment face many barriers to the delivery of safe care. Contributions to unit stress may include difficult working relationships with other health care providers and nursing extenders. The author of this study conducted separate focus groups for RNs and UAPs in order to determine characteristics that influenced working relationships in a total patient care delivery model. Participants were asked to relate the "good" and "difficult" working relationships and practices on their units. Factors that influenced collaborative working relationships were trust, good communication, and mutual respect. How RNs and UAPs were assigned had a significant bearing on trust and communication. When UAPs were assigned to more than one RN, communication deteriorated. The researchers found that variation in UAP orientation influenced how work roles were perceived and that experienced UAPs exhibited a level of "knowing" not previously evident in the literature.

Application to Practice

With health care workforce shortages, the use of nurse extenders is unlikely to disappear. This study reveals perceptions that have a direct impact on future care delivery designs. The use of extenders can be greatly enhanced by one-to-one assignments of RN and UAP, RN mentoring of UAPs, and collaborative care planning and establishment of priorities. Thus the collective "knowing" that is essential for patient care in an increasingly health care environment can be maximized.

---

illness may benefit from a modified "team" approach to ensure appropriate oversight and continuity of care. The existence of care provider roles that support direct and indirect patient care functions are evaluated and potentially realigned as appropriate. Tables 16.1 and 16.2 display examples of both direct and nondirect patient care function–related roles.

Interdependent practice by health care providers has become paramount to the achievement of patient outcomes as the complexity of acute care has dramatically changed over the last decade. Previous practice models that were either "nursing" or "medical" are single-discipline-focused in an environment where there are many structures of rationality and points of view. The increase of health care errors, brought to our attention with the pivotal Institute of Medicine Report *To Err Is Human: Building a Safer Health System* (Kohn et al., 2000), is a symptom of care delivery process and structures that have become dysfunctional, disorganized, and inappropriate. O'Rourke (2003) proposed a conceptual framework that incorporates individual practice, team practice, and organizational practice in order to determine the patient care model. She is a proponent of an "interdisciplinary professional practice model approach to care delivery" because it is developed

Table 16.1

Roles Associated with Direct Patient Care Functions	
Direct Patient Care Roles	Functions
Registered nurse (RN)	Complex care, critical thinking, leadership, delegation, oversight, teaching, care coordination, independent decision making
Licensed practical nurse (LPN)	Assistance, collaboration, intervention, data collection, some patient education
Unlicensed assistive personnel (UAP)	Defined skills, activities of daily living, limited scope of competency, complementary rather than substitution
Unit secretary	Physician orders, supplies, clerical, phone, laboratory/diagnostic results
Ancillary services (e.g., social worker, respiratory therapist, nutritionist, physical therapist)	Focused care based on intensity and professional scope
Case manager	Clinical care coordination, discharge planning, outcome management

From Deutschendorf, A.L. (2003). From past paradigms to future frontiers: Unique care delivery models to facilitate nursing work and quality outcomes. *Journal of Nursing Administration, 33*(1), 52-59.

Table 16.2

Roles Associated with Indirect or Management Patient Care Functions	
Indirect Patient Care Roles	Functions
Assistant manager	Staffing scheduling, evaluation, clinical resource provision
Charge nurse	Unit care coordination, problem solving, communication
Secretary	Clerical support, record keeping, supplies
Clinical nurse specialist	Practice consultation, education, episodic case management, performance improvement
Educational specialist	Staff development, orientation, adult learning, broad-based program education/implementation, preceptor and charge nurse development
Advanced/leveled nurses/ professional practice teams	Performance improvement application into education and practice at unit level, unit resource, unit development of practice and education standards

From Deutschendorf, A.L. (2003). From past paradigms to future frontiers: Unique care delivery models to facilitate nursing work and quality outcomes. *Journal of Nursing Administration, 33*(1), 52-59.

based on "scope of practice, regulation, and professional association standards." (O'Rourke, 2003, p. 97). Because of the nature of complex knowledge work, models are needed that enhance the professional practice of all disciplines, clarify accountability for outcomes, and focus decision making at the point of service (Comack et al., 1999).

Fundamentally, a nursing care delivery system is the way clients' needs are matched to nursing resources. Through some complex relationships, the nursing care delivery system influences the quality of nursing care provided and its cost. A number of nursing care models have been developed, and there is evidence of evolutionary changes and repeating cycles (Barnum, 1990). Over time, nursing care delivery methods were changed and adapted to better fit external forces and the balance of the needs of clients and the needs of employing organizations. With these changes came variations in assignment systems, skill mix, and the role of the nurse. Nursing care delivery has become more complex, and nurses have evolved professional practice models. Future trends point to greater integration and multidisciplinary team collaboration models for service delivery as health care reform drives changes in the organizations within the health care industry.

LEADERSHIP AND MANAGEMENT IMPLICATIONS

The current health care environment is dynamic and continues to change at a rapid pace. Health care costs continue to rise. Nursing, as a major percentage of the health care labor force, must be able to demonstrate its effectiveness in producing financial and clinical outcomes. Although outcome studies in recent years have clearly linked professional staffing ratios to clinical outcomes, including patient morbidity and mortality, the focus on nursing recruitment and retention to alleviate the most recent nursing shortage has resulted in increased costs. Nursing salaries have increased, as well as monies spent for temporary nurses used to achieve adequate staffing ratios. Nurse retention significantly lowers costs associated with turnover (up to two times a nurse's salary) and is associated with nursing satisfaction (Atencio et al., 2003). Multiple studies have demonstrated the relationship of nursing satisfaction to work environment,

◣ LEADERSHIP & MANAGEMENT BEHAVIORS

Leadership Behaviors

- Envisions an effective and professional care delivery system
- Considers structure and process variables that impede and facilitate care delivery
- Enables professionals to deliver quality and cost-effective care
- Communicates about delivery of care issues
- Mentors and engages staff in change processes
- Influences shared decision making about care models
- Balances tensions from competing stakeholders
- Delegates

Management Behaviors

- Plans a care delivery modality
- Organizes staff for client care assignments

- Communicates clearly
- Delegates assignments
- Monitors resource utilization
- Evaluates the effectiveness of care delivery
- Makes care delivery system adjustments as needed
- Implements care delivery system changes

Overlap Areas

- Develops a care modality
- Communicates
- Delegates

leadership, and perceptions of autonomy, which include the method in which care is delivered.

Nursing leaders and managers have the responsibility to facilitate the design of care delivery models that meet the objectives of cost containment, patient satisfaction, and quality outcomes. It is critical that caregiver costs, roles, and activities be clearly understood. Exploring ways to maximize nursing hours without increasing numbers of nurses should be a priority (Lambrinos et al., 2004). Staff mix models employing both professional nurses and unlicensed personnel must be carefully constructed to ensure communication and coordination of care (Hall & Doran, 2004). Direct patient care functions that may be delegated must be determined and defined as those tasks that may be separated from nursing assessment, provide the most assistance to the nurse, and pose the least risk for the patient. Preserving and developing professional nursing roles is vital in the creation of interdisciplinary models (O'Rourke, 2003). The nurse leader and manager need to be aware of the structures and processes in their clinical domains that support or hinder

Research Note

Source: Hall, L., & Doran, D. (2004). Nurse staffing, care delivery model, and patient care quality. *Journal of Nursing Care Quality. 19*(1), 27-33.

Purpose

Throughout the 1990s restructuring efforts resulted in changes in care delivery models. Many studies have been conducted describing nurses' perceptions of restructuring and redesign. The purpose of this article was to determine how nurses perceive effectiveness and quality of care and the relationships to staffing mix and care delivery models. Whether quality outcomes varied with the type of care delivery model and nurse staffing was explored.

Discussion

A descriptive study was performed, using surveys administered to RN staff and unit managers from 77 adult medical, surgical, and obstetrical units in 19 urban teaching hospitals in Ontario, Canada. Quality outcome data included perceptions of the quality of care, communication, and patient care coordination. Staffing variables were characterized according to staff mix and included combinations of RN/unregulated workers (URW), RN/LPN, RN only, and RN/LPN/URW. Types of care delivery models included team, primary care, and total patient care. Nurses perceived that an all-RN staff had a positive impact on patient care quality, including individualized approaches to communication and coordination. A staff mix that combined RNs with LPNs was perceived to have a negative impact, whereas ironically, a staffing pattern that combined both professional and nonprofessional workers (RNs, LPNs, and URWs) was considered to have a positive impact on quality. Nurses who practiced under a total patient care delivery model perceived a negative impact on patient care quality and care coordination. Team and primary care models were considered to facilitate communication and patient care coordination.

Application to Practice

Collaboration among a myriad of health care providers is essential for effective care coordination in any care delivery model. Much emphasis has been placed on defining roles and responsibilities among RNs and unregulated or unlicensed care providers in a team relationship. There is less distinction in the literature regarding the practice of licensed nurses (RNs and LPNs), especially as it relates to patient care models. Aspects of RN and LPN roles may become muddied in a total patient care delivery model. It is necessary that attention to role definition for all licensed nursing providers be carefully determined to ensure appropriate practice and safe care delivery. In a complex environment, models that emphasize team relationships may demonstrate increased quality outcomes.

patient care. Understanding the "context" in which nurses practice must occur in order to find solutions to nurse staffing and patient care issues. Houser (2003) identified contextual factors that influence the delivery of patient care to be leadership, teamwork, resources, staff stability, expertise, and workload. Support for structure changes needs to occur at the executive nursing leadership level in order to successfully accomplish changes in care delivery method.

Managing the changes associated with redesign and reengineering of care delivery is the responsibility of nursing leaders and managers. Staff nurses undergoing changes in roles and care delivery models may have feelings of uncertainty, distrust, role ambiguity, and powerless (Ingersoll et al., 1999) unless they are fully engaged in the process. Staff nurses who perceived their managers as powerful in the organization were more likely to perceive their own ability to influence change (Ingersoll et al., 1999). Nurses' involvement in decision making enhances their feelings of autonomy. The effective nursing leader must ensure consistent and frequent communication about changes while enlisting input from the bedside caregivers. Mentoring staff to participate in the creation of new care delivery methods is an aspect of effective leadership.

Although there appears to be no one right model of care, nurses will be involved in the planning for care delivery, tinkering with improvements in the current model, exploring new models developed by others, or attempting to develop their own new model of care delivery. The leadership and management challenge is to balance risk taking and adoption of innovations with the pragmatic necessity to be systematic, evaluative, and realistic. Consistency with operating systems and available resources is a key driving component for evaluating a care delivery model (Armstrong & Stetler, 1991). The central components of practice that need to be considered in the construction of a nursing care delivery model are the direct and indirect patient care functions; provider roles, competencies, and experience; fiscal accountability; patient characteristics and case mix severity;

clinical service intensity; practice guidelines; and new medical information and technology (Deutschendorf, 2003). Nurses' autonomy and job satisfaction is affected by the work environment and the structure of the care model used. Leadership is needed to strike a balance between nurses' needs and preferences and those of clients, physicians, and organizations.

CURRENT ISSUES AND TRENDS

Influential Trends

A number of social, technological, environmental, economic, and political trends have shaped and influenced the type of nursing care delivery systems in use in U.S. hospitals. From 1900 to 1950, the following trends were influential (Lee, 1993):

- The status of women and expectations of altruism
- The apprenticeship model of nursing education
- Advances in health care scientific knowledge
- Transfer of equipment-based technologies from physicians to nurses
- Task analysis and division of labor
- Hospital control of nursing education
- Patient location by disease diagnosis
- Cyclic nurse shortages precipitated by epidemics, war, and the peak of the efficiency movement in nursing care delivery
- The Great Depression
- The strike as a negotiation strategy
- Passage of state registration laws
- Upgrading of nursing education standards
- Unsatisfactory working conditions in hospitals and inadequate salaries for nurses

From 1950 until the late 1980s, general health care trends continued to encourage the professionalism of nursing practice. General trends that were influential included the following (Lee, 1993):

- Changes in demographics, social mores, and lifestyle patterns
- Advances in professional self-regulation and nursing knowledge
- Changes in the role of the nurse and in nursing education

- Swings in the organization of hospital nursing care delivery from functional (before the 1950s) to team (early 1950s) to primary nursing (1970s) to case management (late 1980s)
- Participatory management and shared governance
- Cycles of nurse staffing shortages
- Increasing hospital patient acuities
- Political activism, advocacy, legislation, and regulation
- Rise of consumer concern about cost, quality, and access
- Health care reform movement and legislation
- Expansion of hospital and health care service
- Mergers and integration
- Emerging role of advanced practice nurses
- The rise of nursing centers and nurse-run clinics
- Beginning shifts in emphasis to community health care and primary prevention
- Changing professional opportunities for women

The nursing shortage in the late 1980s resulted in increased nursing salaries and an exploration of alternative approaches to patient care delivery, including the expanded use of nurse extenders. At the same time the escalation of health care costs resulted in shifts in the health care industry, including restructured reimbursement and finance mechanisms. The federal prospective payment system and managed care emerged as methods to control spiraling health care costs and limited hospital services to the acutely ill (Gerardi, 2005). Efficiency and effectiveness became paramount in determining care delivery. As the hospital work environment became increasingly stressful and alternative professional opportunities for women increased, a severe nursing shortage developed in the late 1990s. The following trends emerged in the 1990s and have driven the current state of nursing practice (Deutschendorf, 2003):

- Increased severity of illness and complexity of care
- Fewer patient admissions
- Decreased lengths of stay
- Rapid patient turnover
- Objective of acute care as "stabilization and transition"

- Renewed focus on productivity and efficiency
- Changes in the focus of health care delivery from episodic acute care to a continuum of health care services, including prevention, ambulatory care, and chronic illness care
- An aging patient population living with chronic illness
- Focus on patient function rather than cure
- Proliferation of new medical information and technology
- Consumer and regulatory demand for competency and quality outcomes
- Evidenced-based medicine and practice
- Restructuring and reengineering care delivery models
- Rising consumer expectations
- New communication and computing technologies
- An aging nursing population
- Work ethic changes emphasizing personal versus professional role and time over money

Nursing care trends that emerged as a response to the rapid environmental changes include the following (Aiken et al., 2000; Corey-Lisle et al., 1999; Deutschendorf, 2003; Harrison, 1999; Ritter-Teitel, 2002):

- Frequently chaotic and undefined care delivery models, including increasing scopes of care
- An exodus of experienced nurses
- Changes in staffing patterns, including increased staff/patient ratios and changes in skill mix
- Emphasis on task completion
- Underutilization of professional nursing and lack of system supports for nursing
- Loss of expert resources such as advanced practice nurses
- Decreased patient exposure and lack of continuity due to 12-hour shifts and patient turnover
- Application of nursing process (assessment, planning, intervention, and continued evaluation) not geared to rapidly changing patient conditions
- Increased requirements for clinical and multidisciplinary documentation

- Determination of evidenced-based nursing practice
- Interdisciplinary and collaborative practice models
- Increased span of control by managers
- Decreased opportunities for professional development

The challenges for patient care in the future are massive. The work environment of the nurse is dramatically different from any other time. Cost containment and demand for quality outcomes will continue to drive systems of patient care delivery. The "age of information" will test the ability of the system to integrate discovery into safe practice. Even though recent studies (Aiken et al., 2002) have demonstrated the relationship between nurse-to-patient ratios and patient outcomes and have resulted in increased focus on the nurse's work environment and value, dramatic evaluation must occur to create a vision for health care delivery models of the future. Professional nursing has an opportunity and an obligation to participate in shaping future models that address the changes in patient populations as well as clinical and financial trends. The American Organization of Nurse Executives (AONE) is creating a strategy focused on the future development of care delivery models based on the complexities of the current and future health care milieu (Haase-Herrick, 2004). Guiding principles address the following: nursing work as knowledge and caring, patient/client-directed care, "critical synthesis" of knowledge, incorporation of technology, and management of care throughout the continuum (Haase-Herrick, 2004). Operationalization of the guiding principles can only occur after careful examination and creation of supporting organizational structures and processes.

Both recurring themes and new evolutionary issues can be seen in a review of trends affecting care delivery systems. Clearly, forces and pressures outside of professional nursing work to influence nursing care models. Although it is not known which is the best model for each nursing care setting, the evaluation of restructured systems must include specific quality, financial, and patient satisfaction outcomes. Nurses are urged to examine their client populations, come to grips with the business aspects of health care, and remain vigilant in analyzing emerging economic and clinical trends in order to be active participants in the creation of patient care delivery models of the future.

Summary

- Goals of patient care delivery include the provision of high-quality and low-cost care to achieve clinical outcomes and patient satisfaction.
- Assignment and delegation are methods used by organizations to provide patient care within the context of patient care delivery.
- Organizational structure and processes influence the determination of the care delivery model.
- Professional practice is a structural variable that influences the selection of care delivery models.
- A nursing care model is a method of organizing and delivering nursing care.
- The six types of nursing care models are private duty, functional, team, primary, case management, and evolving types.
- Private duty means one RN to one client.
- Total patient care is responsibility for all aspects of patient care for a designated shift
- Functional nursing is assignment to tasks.
- Team nursing is the care of a group of clients by a skill-mixed team.
- Primary nursing is 24-hour accountability by an RN for specific clients over a hospital stay.
- Case management is the coordination and monitoring of services across the continuum of health care.
- Evolving care models focus on effectiveness, resource management, and professional practice.
- Social, technological, environmental, economic, and political trends have shaped and influenced nursing care delivery systems.

Study Questions

1. What is the role of nursing leadership in determining a model for patient care delivery?
2. How do nurses decide which nursing care delivery system to use?

3. What are the structure and process variables that influence nursing practice and patient care delivery?

4. Why are nursing care delivery systems being revised and restructured?

5. What issues arise when the care delivery system is changed?

6. What common themes emerge among the newest care delivery systems being developed? How do they compare with older models?

7. What care delivery system best fits a merger of hospital and community agencies? Or are multiple care models needed?

8. How should the implementation of new care delivery systems be evaluated?

CASE STUDY

Overview

Memorial Medical Center was a 400-bed teaching hospital. The care delivery model for all areas was total patient care, with RNs of differing experiences having shift responsibility for a group of seven to eight patients on medical and surgical floors. The third floor was a general medical unit with 72 beds. Patient diagnoses included cardiovascular (with telemetry monitoring), renal, pulmonary, oncology, and gastrointestinal diagnoses. An interim patient care manager had responsibility for the unit. Charge nurses were responsible for daily operations and frequently had patient assignments. Novice nurses accounted for 30% of the staff. Certified nursing assistants were occasionally assigned to a nurse but were more likely to be assigned tasks. Their responsibilities included basic custodial care and did not include simple technical skills. They were frequently assigned as "sitters," thus removing them from direct patient care.

There were many patient and physician complaints regarding the nursing care provided. Reporting of significant incidents had increased. The nursing director for the area conducted a comprehensive assessment of patient care to determine whether changes in the method of care delivery were needed.

Findings

It was found that patient care delivery at Memorial Medical Center was fragmented, with functions being performed among multiple caregivers with little communication. It was believed that staff did not have the opportunity to develop skills and expertise in specialty areas as a result of the scope of patient problems. Nursing assessments and reassessments were not timely or complete, and evidence of nursing care planning was limited in clinical documentation. Nurses were frequently unaware of the patient's diagnosis and medical plan of care. Nursing tasks were the focus of care, and evidence of critical thinking for decision making was lacking, especially among novice nurses. Care coordination was performed by the case manager but was not communicated to the bedside nurse. Discharge planning was usually not considered at time of admission and frequently delayed discharge. Communication of the plan of care from shift to shift and from caregiver to caregiver was inadequate because of a lack of continuity (with 12-hour shifts), problem identification, and prioritization. Nurses were not comfortable with delegation of tasks to the CNAs and frequently assumed nonnursing functions. There was no mechanism of oversight or support for novice or temporary nursing staff.

Care Delivery Redesign

The nursing director and the nursing vice president agreed that care delivery redesign was necessary to meet the objectives of quality patient care. The nursing director began by forming a team of multidisciplinary care providers and nursing staff who worked on the third floor. The group was surveyed as to their perceptions of patient care processes on the unit. Objectives for the redesign were constructed based on feedback from the staff, as well as a review of the literature. Staff members expressed anxiety regarding changes, but all agreed that transformation was necessary to improve the quality of care and working conditions.

It was determined that the third floor of Memorial Medical Center should be split into two separate units to maximize exposure to, and "knowing" of, specific patient populations. Patients were aggregated based on intensity of service, acuity, and diagnosis (cardiovascular/pulmonary and oncology/renal, with telemetry available on the cardiovascular unit). Staff members were assigned permanently on each unit based on preference, but with an understanding that rotation to the sister unit was available after 6 months.

Because many members of the staff were inexperienced and temporary nurses were used to fill vacancies, it was decided to implement a modular approach to care delivery. A module consisted of 16 to 20 patients with an experienced nurse partnered with novice or agency nurses and 1 to 2 CNAs. Complete intershift report was taken by the module members, facilitating communication and continuity if one staff member was off the unit or not scheduled the following day. Daily discharge planning rounds were established, at minimum for all new admissions, and included participation from module members and the interdisciplinary team.

A new level of CNA was established to increase simple skills that could be performed. This competency was validated in a skills lab. Skills were defined that could provide the most benefit to nurses and the least risk to patients (i.e., performance of ECGs). Nurses and CNAs attended team-building workshops to facilitate understanding of delegation responsibilities and roles. A unit secretary position was approved for all shifts to assume clerical responsibilities for patient care.

The patient care manager remained responsible for both areas; however, a permanent charge nurse position without direct patient care responsibility was established on each unit.

Evaluation

Process, quality, and financial outcome indicators were established prior to redesign. Since clinical outcomes must follow successful implementation of processes, it was decided to measure process indicators for 6 months and then quality indicators at 6 months, 1 year, 18 months, and 2 years. At the end of the first year nursing satisfaction and perceptions of quality care delivery were improved, including facilitation of assessment, monitoring, achievement of care goals, organization of care, delegation, patient teaching, documentation, and continuity. Agency usage was down, and attrition of new graduates was reduced by 20%. Patient satisfaction scores were beginning to demonstrate

---

CRITICAL THINKING EXERCISE

Nurse Manager Lisa Beach has just assumed responsibility for a 32-bed surgical/orthopedic unit that includes trauma patients. She has a vacancy rate of 20%, which is filled with per diem and hospital pool nurses. The activity on the unit is great, with a patient turnover of up to one-third for a 24-hour period. Patient acuity is high, as is service intensity. Most of the patients require some type of posthospital care, including acute rehabilitation, skilled nursing, and home care. Nurse Manager Beach is concerned about recent increases in the average length of stay on the unit and patient/family complaints. Nurses have complained about workload, even though the average nurse-to-patient ratio is 1:6 to 1:7. She has decided that process redesign is in order and has obtained permission from her nursing director to explore care delivery model alternatives for implementation.

1. What should the first step be in planning for a new care delivery model?
2. How can Nurse Manager Beach engage the staff in this change?
3. What care delivery models would be appropriate to meet objectives of direct patient care functions on this unit?
4. What are the direct and indirect patient care functions that are not currently being performed?
5. What roles might be needed to support direct and indirect patient care functions on this unit?
6. How would the nurse manager evaluate implementation of a new model of care delivery?

improvement with regard to pain management, discharge preparation, and meeting of care needs. Although the incidence of pressure ulcers remained constant, patient falls were reduced.

It was demonstrated that careful and deliberate planning with the participation of stakeholders and end-users can result in a successful project. Care delivery models can be established that maximize existing resources, provide oversight and mentoring of staff, and ultimately result in improved patient care.

REFERENCES

Abts, D., Hofer, M., & Leafgreen, P. (1994). Redefining care delivery: A modular system. *Nursing Management, 25*(2), 40-46.

Aiken, L.H., Clarke, S.P., Sloane, D.M., Sochalski, J., & Silber, J.H. (2002). Hospital nurse staffing and patient mortality, nurse burnout, and job dissatisfaction. *Journal of the American Medical Association, 288*(16), 1987-1993.

Aiken, L.H., & Patrician, P.A. (2000). Measuring organizational traits of hospitals: The Revised Nursing Work Index. *Nursing Research, 49*(3), 146-153.

American Nurses Association (ANA). (1988). *Nursing case management.* (Publ. No. NS-32). Kansas City, MO: ANA.

American Nurses Association (ANA). (1997). *Definitions related to ANA 1992 position statements on unlicensed assistive personnel.* Washington, DC: ANA. Retrieved May 25, 2004, from *www.nursingworld.org/readroom/position/uap/uapuse.htm*

Anderson, C., & Hughes, E. (1993). Implementing modular nursing in a long-term care facility. *Journal of Nursing Administration, 23*(6), 29-35.

Anthony, M.K., Brennan, P.F., O'Brien, R., & Suwannaroop, N. (2004). Measurement of nursing practice models using multiattribute utility theory: Relationship to patient and organizational outcomes. *Quality Management in Health Care, 13*(1), 40-52.

Armstrong, D., & Stetler, C. (1991). Strategic considerations in developing a delivery model. *Nursing Economic$, 9*(2), 112-115.

Atencio, B.L., Cohen, J., & Gorenberg, B. (2003). Nurse retention: Is it worth it? *Nursing Economic$, 21*(6), 262-268, 299, 259.

Bard, J., Jimenez, F., & Tornack, R. (1994). An outcome-focused, community-based health support program. *Journal of Nursing Administration, 24*(3), 48-54.

Barnum, B. (1990). Cycles of nursing. *Nursing and Health Care, 11*(8), 395.

Barry-Walker, J. (2000). The impact of systems redesign on staff, patient, and financial outcomes. *Journal of Nursing Administration, 30*(2), 77-89.

Bower, K.A. (2004). Patient care management as a global nursing concern. *Nursing Administration Quarterly, 28*(1), 39-43.

Case Management Society of America (CMSA). (2002). *Standards of practice for case management* (2nd ed.) Little Rock, AR: CMSA.

Cohen, E.L., & Cesta, T.G. (2005). *Nursing case management: From essentials to advanced practice applications* (4th ed.). St Louis: Elsevier Mosby.

Cole, L., & Houston, S. (1999). Structured care methodologies: Evolution and use in patient care delivery. *Outcomes Management for Nursing Practice, 3*(2), 53-59.

Comack, M., Paech, G., & Porter-O'Grady, T. (1999). From structure to culture: A journey of transformation. In S.P. Smith & D.L. Flarey (Eds.), *Process-centered health care organizations* (pp. 45-67). Gaithersburg, MD: Aspen

Corey-Lisle, P., Tarzian, A.J., Cohen, M.Z., & Trinkoff, A.M. (1999). Health care reform: Its effects on nurses. *Journal of Nursing Administration, 29*(3), 30-37.

Deutschendorf, A.L. (2003). From past paradigms to future frontiers: unique care delivery models to facilitate nursing work and quality outcomes. *Journal of Nursing Administration, 33*(1), 52-59.

Eastaugh, S.R., & Regan-Donovan, M. (1990). Nurse extenders offer a way to trim staff expenses. *Healthcare Financial Management, 44*(4), 58-60, 62.

Fox, R.T., Fox, D.H., & Wells, P.J. (1999). Performance of first-line management functions on productivity of hospital unit personnel. *Journal of Nursing Administration, 29*(9), 12-18.

Fuszard, B. (1988). What is case management? *The Facilitator, 4*(1), 3-4.

Gardner, K. (1991). A summary of findings of a five-year comparison study of primary and team nursing. *Nursing Research, 40*(2), 113-117.

Gerardi, T. (2005). The managed care market. In E.L. Cohen & T.G. Cesta (Eds.), *Nursing case management: From essentials to advanced practice applications* (4th ed.) (pp. 210-218). St. Louis: Elsevier Mosby.

Gittell, J.H., Fairfield, K.M., Bierbaum, B., Head, W., Jackson, R., Kelly, M., et al. (2000). Impact of relational coordination on quality of care, postoperative pain and functioning, and length of stay: A nine-hospital study of surgical patients. *Medical Care, 38*(8), 807-819.

Glandon, G., Colbert, K., & Thomasma, M. (1989). Nursing delivery models and RN mix: Cost implications. *Nursing Management, 20*(5), 30-33.

Grimaldi, P.L. (1996, October). A glossary of managed care terms. *Nursing Management, 24*(10, Spec Suppl), 5-7.

Guild, S., Ledwin, R., Sanford, D., & Winter, T. (1994). Development of an innovative nursing care delivery system. *Journal of Nursing Administration, 24*(3), 23-29.

Haase-Herrick, K. (2004). The nurse of the future. Fewer workers, new technologies and older patients place RNs at center stage. *Modern Healthcare, 34*(16), 18.

Hall, L.M. (1997). Staff mix models: Complementary or substitution roles for nurses. *Nursing Administration Quarterly, 21*(2), 31-39.

Hall, L.M., & Doran, D. (2004). Nurse staffing, care delivery model, and patient care quality. *Journal of Nursing Care Quality, 19*(1), 27-33.

Harrison, J.K. (1999). Influence of managed care on professional nursing practice. *Image, Journal of Nursing Scholarship, 31*(2), 161-166.

Hegyvary, S. (1977). Foundations of primary nursing. *Nursing Clinics of North America, 12*(6), 187-196.

Higginbotham, P. (1999). Teams: The essential work unit. In S.P. Smith & D.L. Flarey (Eds.), *Process-centered health care organizations* (pp. 113-117). Gaithersburg, MD: Aspen.

Houser, J. (2003). A model for evaluating the context of nursing care delivery. *Journal of Nursing Administration, 33*(1), 39-47.

Ingersoll, G.L., Cook, J.A., Fogel, S., Applegate, M., & Frank, B. (1999). The effect of patient-focused redesign on midlevel nurse managers' role responsibilities and work environment. *Journal of Nursing Administration, 29*(5), 21-27.

Jones-Schenk, J., & Hartley, P. (1993). Organization for communication and integration. *Journal of Nursing Administration, 23*(10), 30-33.

Kalisch, P., & Kalisch, B. (1978). *The advance of American nursing*. Boston: Little, Brown.

Kohn, L.T., Corrigan, J., & Donaldson, M.S. (2000). *To err is human: Building a safer health system*. Washington, DC: National Academies Press.

Lambrinos, J., LaPosta, M.J., & Cohen, A. (2004). Increasing nursing hours without increasing nurses: A natural experiment at an academic medical center. *Journal of Nursing Administration, 34*(4), 195-199.

Lang, N., & Clinton, J. (1984). Assessment of quality of nursing care. *Annual Review of Nursing Research, 2*, 135-163.

Lee, J. (1993). A history of care models in nursing. *Series on Nursing Administration, 5*, 20-38.

Lengacher, C., Mabe, P., Bowling, C., Heinemann, D., Kent, K., & Cott, M. (1993). Redesigning nursing practice: The partners in patient care model. *Journal of Nursing Administration, 23*(12), 31-37.

Lyon, J. (1993). Models of nursing care delivery and case management: Clarification of terms. *Nursing Economic$, 11*(3), 163-169.

Maehling, J.A.S. (1995). Process reengineering: Strategies for analysis and redesign. In S.S. Blancett & D.L. Flarey (Eds.), *Reengineering nursing and health care: The handbook for organizational transformation* (pp. 61-74). Gaithersburg, MD: Aspen.

Magargal, P. (1987). Modular nursing: Nurses rediscover nursing. *Nursing Management, 18*(11), 98-104.

Manthey, M. (1989). Of bandwagons and partnerships. *Nursing Management, 20*(8), 22-23.

Manthey, M. (1990). Definitions and basic elements of a patient care delivery system with an emphasis on primary nursing. In G. Mayer, M. Madden, & E. Lawrenz (Eds.), *Patient care delivery models* (pp. 201-211). Rockville, MD: Aspen.

Manthey, M. (1991). Delivery systems and practice models: A dynamic balance. *Nursing Management, 22*(1), 28-30.

Mark, B. (1992). Characteristics of nursing practice models. *Journal of Nursing Administration, 22*(11), 57-63.

McCloskey, J., Blegen, M., & Gardner, D. (1991). Who helps you with your work? *American Journal of Nursing, 91*(4), 43-46.

Mikulencak, M. (1993). Public health stands as a proven model for future delivery systems. *The American Nurse, 25*(6), 18.

Needleman, J., Buerhaus, P.I., Mattke, S., Stewart, M., & Zelevinsky, K. (2001). *Nurse staffing and patient outcomes in hospitals* (Contract No. 230-99-0021). U.S. Department of Health and Human Resources, Health Resources and Services Administration.

Neidlinger, S., & Miller, M. (1990). Nursing care delivery systems: A nursing administration practice perspective. *Journal of Nursing Administration, 20*(10), 43-49.

O'Rourke, M.W. (2003). Rebuilding a professional practice model. The return of role-based practice accountability. *Nursing Administration Quarterly, 27*(2), 95-105.

Parkman, C., & Loveridge, C. (1994). From nursing service to professional practice. *Nursing Management, 25*(3), 63-68.

Poulin, M. (1985). Configuration of nursing practice. In American Nurses Association (Ed.), *Issues in professional practice* (pp. 1-14). Kansas City, MO: ANA.

Powers, P.H., Dickey, C.A., & Ford, A. (1990). Evaluating an RN/co-worker model. *Journal of Nursing Administration, 20*(3), 11-15.

Reverby, S. (1987). *Ordered to care: The dilemma of American nursing 1850-1945*. Cambridge, MA: Cambridge University Press.

Ritter-Teitel, J. (2002). The impact of restructuring on professional nursing practice. *Journal of Nursing Administration, 32*(1), 31-41.

Seago, J.A. (1999). Evaluation of a hospital work redesign: Patient-focused care. *Journal of Nursing Administration, 29*(11), 31-38.

Wolf, G., Boland, S., & Aukerman, M. (1994). A transformational model for the practice of professional nursing. Part 2: Implementation of the model. *Journal of Nursing Administration, 24*(5), 38-46.

Zander, K. (1990). Case management: A golden opportunity for whom? In J. McCloskey & H. Grace (Eds.), *Current issues in nursing* (3rd ed.) (pp. 199-204). St Louis: Mosby.

Zander, K. (1992). Nursing care delivery methods and quality. *Series on Nursing Administration, 3*, 86-104.

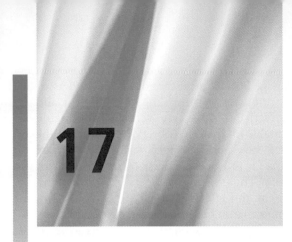

17

Case Management

Diane L. Huber

CHAPTER OBJECTIVES

- Dramatize the importance of case management
- Define and describe managed care and case management
- Differentiate case management from managed care
- Trace the history of case management
- Compare differences in definitions and models of case management
- Analyze the development of case management in nursing
- Outline the main service components in case management models
- Analyze nursing role changes under case management and managed care
- Exercise critical thinking to conceptualize and analyze possible solutions to a practice exercise

ase management is an intervention strategy used by health care providers and systems to advocate for clients, coordinate health care delivery, and facilitate outcomes of both cost and quality. Arising out of pressures for cost containment, and later valued for quality control in the midst of alarming medical errors, case management came to be seen by health plans, and later hospitals, as a major solution to serious problems of mission and margin.

Previously a strategy in social services, rehabilitation, and public health, by the 1990s case management was a popular way to address coordination of care for the ill and the poor and for managing catastrophic injury or illness. Case managers were deployed to decrease fragmentation, reduce expense by streamlining care, and control costs by linking, advocating, coordinating, negotiating, educating, and monitoring. As case management became more popular, case managers' employment settings shifted to hospitals.

Nurses have delivered case management services since the beginning. Nurses have emerged as the majority of case managers, especially in hospitals, in part because of the function of determining medical necessity for health care payment and because of complex medical discharge planning needs (Zander, 2002). Zander called case management "the nursing process applied at a system level" (2002, p. 58). This is because case management services by nurses are designed to produce a balance between the demands of the mission (quality health care) and the operational margin (costs and resources). Case management has grown in conjunction with the experience of risk by payors and providers (Zander, 2002).

Case management has garnered considerable attention in health care. It has been suggested that the processes associated with case management have the potential to save money, improve effectiveness, and maintain or improve the quality of care (Cook, 1998). However, a diversity of case management approaches exists. For example, "case management may describe a patient care delivery system, a professional practice model, a group of activities that a nurse performs within an organizational setting, or a separate service provided by private practitioners" (Goodwin, 1994, p. 29). The term *case management* can be specific to an institution, refer to services rendered to a population or community, or be a separate service provided by independent case managers or health insurance companies (Goodwin, 1994). Case management is an interdisciplinary strategy that crosses settings and sites of care. Models have been implemented in many settings, including acute care, long-term care, and community health care (Huber, 2005; Zander, 2002). Case management is a central component of integrating and coordinating care across the continuum. It is focused on the individual recipient of services.

Case management is an approach to managing care and service delivery that is designed to coordinate care, decrease costs, and promote access to appropriate and needed services. Case management has a heritage more than a century old but has gained wide implementation and popularity as systems of managed health care have emerged. Managed health care, more simply called managed care, has gained momentum as a response to national concern over rising health care costs and expenditures, increasing care fragmentation, and lack of continuity and access under fee-for-service reimbursement. Managed care has evolved as the economic and health services delivery strategy by which costs could be managed while ensuring access to appropriate care levels. By the end of the 1990s, health maintenance organizations (HMOs) had become the most predominant form of health care coverage among U.S. businesses with more than 100 employees (Beilman et al., 1998; Coleman, 1999; Tahan, 1998). Case management is a major strategy used by managed care reimbursement systems.

Internal and external pressures on the health care delivery system have been intensifying. A convergence of cost, quality, and access demands has combined to create a complex and volatile environment. Complexity arises from the simultaneous balancing of needs for quality, productivity, and flexibility. Health care providers are directed to manage both clinical care outcomes and associated resources by providing cost-efficient and cost-effective health care services and being accountable for the value of services relative to the costs of those services. Specifically, the pressure on nurses is to balance quality of care with client advocacy. Thus nurses need to demonstrate and document the effect of nursing care on client outcomes and on the efficiency and price competitiveness of provided services. The benefits achieved need to exceed the costs incurred. Furthermore, nurses need to demonstrate that they can provide services more cost-effectively than other providers (Hicks et al., 1992). The mounting pressures on the health care delivery system since the mid-1980s have provided an impetus for the explosive growth of case management as both an economically important strategy for controlling costs and an opportunity for hope and improvement during economic hard times.

Like health care, case management as a professional practice role is in transition. For example, the Case Management Society of America (CMSA), the organization representing case managers, was founded in 1990. Since then it has grown to an international nonprofit organization dedicated to the support and development of the profession of case management. It has 70 affiliated and pending chapters and more than 8300 individual members. It has promulgated the following:

- Standards of Practice (CMSA, 2002)
- Ethical Statement on Case Management Practice
- Support of a certification program through the Commission for Case Manager Certification (CCMC), which is an independent separate entity

In 1997 CMSA formed an Education Committee and the Council for Case Management Accountability (formerly called Center for Case Management Accountability) to establish evidence-based standards of practice (CMSA, 2004a). Subsequent state of the science papers have been issued on patient adherence and patient involvement and empowerment (CMSA, 2004b).

Because a major role of case managers is to manage risk and coordinate care, case managers are in demand. The case management industry is playing an increasingly important role in this managed care environment. The number of case managers rose from an estimated 5,000 to 10,000 in 1985 to a total in the range of 50,000 to 100,000 in 1995. This is a tenfold increase in 10 years (Chan et al., 1999). The estimate is that more than 100,000 case managers practice in the United States (CCMC, 2004). These case managers come from diverse training backgrounds, disciplines, and practice settings, including nursing, social work, occupational health, and rehabilitation counseling. CCMC has certified more than 27,000 individuals as case managers (CCMC, 2004).

The case manager role was one of the fastest-growing roles in health care in the 1990s, especially in nursing (Haw, 1996). Clients with highly complex or extended-term health care needs are a major focus for cost containment, and case management is the approach of choice for these clients (Conti, 1996).

DEFINITIONS

Managed Care

Managed care is defined as follows:

> ... the systematic integration and coordination of the financing and delivery of health care. These activities are performed by health plans that try to provide their members with prepaid access to high-quality care at relatively low cost and usually are at least partly at risk for the cost of care. The health plans may rely on physician gatekeepers and prior authorization mechanisms to minimize unnecessary or inappropriate utilization. (Grimaldi, 1996, p. 6)

Managed care is one form of a health care reimbursement strategy that also fostered the evolution of organizations and businesses. The generic term *managed care* has been applied to mean a wide variety of organizational structures, prepayment arrangements, negotiated discounts, and agreements for prior authorization and audit of performance, all designed to lower costs and maximize the value of received services and the resources used. The three most commonly associated managed care-related organizational structures are health maintenance organizations (HMOs), preferred provider organizations (PPOs), and privately managed indemnity health insurance plans. Some interpretations of the term *managed care* carry the connotation of financial arrangements that place restrictions on providers and consumers to influence price, site of care delivery, or use of health care services (Hicks et al., 1992). Utilization review and gatekeeper functions are emphasized. What is managed in managed care are the financial aspects.

▲ LEADING & MANAGING **DEFINED**

Managed Care	**Case Management**
The systematic integration and coordination of the financing and delivery of health care; these activities are performed by health plans that try to provide their members with prepaid access to high-quality care at relatively low cost and usually are at least partly at risk for the cost of care; the health plans may rely on physician gatekeepers and prior authorization mechanisms to minimize unnecessary or inappropriate utilization.	A collaborative process of assessment, planning, facilitation, and advocacy for options and services to meet an individual's health needs through communication and available resources to promote high-quality, cost-effective outcomes.

In the nursing literature, the term *managed care* was first used to describe the process of managing and coordinating care delivery in hospitals. It was defined as a clinical system that organizes and sequences the process of caregiving at the client-provider level. The objective is to better achieve cost and quality outcomes (Zander, 1991). Managed care serves to restructure the tools and systems used in client care. It is based on a process of anticipating and describing care requirements in advance and then comparing actual occurrences to the anticipated path. Managed care was seen as project management at the provider-client level and as a unit-based care that is organized to achieve specific client outcomes, given fiscal and other resource constraints. Resources appropriate in amount and sequence to a specific case type and individual client are managed for length of stay, critical events and timing, and anticipated outcomes (Hampton, 1993; Zander, 1992).

Confusion has arisen over the variability in the definitions of the terms associated with managed care and case management. Definitions are fluid because of the evolving and volatile nature of the health care industry. "With health care changing by the nanosecond and managed care entities growing, mixing and mutating even more quickly, the words used to describe, distinguish and categorize various entities and activities are confusing even the most sophisticated professionals" (Grimaldi, 1996, p. 5). However, managed care has now come to refer to a reimbursement strategy of arrangements and organizations, such as HMOs, that incorporate mechanisms aimed at resource allocation and utilization management designed to eliminate waste, fragmentation, and duplication in order to drive down costs.

Managed care refers to a system that provides the structure and focus for managing the use, cost, quality, and effectiveness of health services. Managed care is the umbrella under which case management may be one cost-containment strategy. However, in some instances case management has evolved into meaning a separate hospital professional nursing care delivery model that is unit-based and focused on support for standardized patterns of care and length of hospitalization. Case management differs from managed care in that the focus for delivery of care is based on an entire hospitalization for a targeted DRG group and is not geographically confined to the patient's unit. It implies consistency of coordinator or provider across health care settings. Both managed care and case management employ critical paths, case management care plans, and variance analysis.

A commonly used form of managed care financial reimbursement is called capitated reimbursement, or capitation. *Capitation* is defined as "a fixed dollar amount that a health plan or provider is paid (usually monthly) to furnish specific kinds of medical services that an insured person needs, regardless of the volume of care needed" (Grimaldi, 1996, p. 5). Capitation is a mechanism for paying health care providers that transfers financial risk to the provider and away from the health plan or covered individual. Capitation also refers to the basis on which payment rates are made for providing health services to a defined population over a set period. The typical case is one in which the provider receives an advance amount that is a negotiated payment, usually called a per-member-per-month (pmpm) payment. Capitated reimbursement systems shift risk to providers because payments remain the same, a flat amount per month, despite how much care is needed or how much care costs to deliver.

Case Management

Multiple disciplines lay claim to case management. **Case management** is a term that refers to client-focused strategies designed to coordinate care (Bower, 1992). It concentrates on the coordination and integration of health services for clients with complex or extraordinarily costly health problems (Grimaldi, 1996). Case management has a strong interdisciplinary component. There have been a variety of definitions of case management, often reflecting the perspective of a specific discipline. As the professional organization representing case managers, CMSA's definition comprises the generally accepted description of case management.

This organization defined *case management* as follows:

> Case management is a collaborative process of assessment, planning, facilitation and advocacy for options and services to meet an individual's health needs through communication and available resources to promote quality cost-effective outcomes. (CMSA, 2002, p. 5)

Because definitions and related models of case management are so varied, clarity is needed. The first step is to locate and identify the definition used. The second step is to appreciate multidisciplinary perspectives. For example, both nursing and social work have their own definitions. By comparison to CMSA, the American Nurses Association (ANA) first defined case management in 1988 in a way similar to the New England Medical Center's definition of acute care nursing case management. Case management, as a general concept, has been defined as a system of health assessment, planning, service procurement, service delivery, service coordination, and monitoring through which the multiple service needs of clients are met (ANA, 1988; Zander, 1990). The current definition by ANA in the American Nurses Credentialing Center (ANCC) catalog is as follows:

> Nursing case management is a dynamic and systematic collaborative approach to provide and coordinate health care services to a defined population. The framework for nursing case management includes five components: assessment, planning, implementation, evaluation, and interaction. (ANCC, 2004, p. 10)

From the social work perspective, case management is defined as a specialized practice designed to coordinate the services needed to sustain the most vulnerable populations that are at the greatest risk (Raiff & Shore, 1993). According to the National Association of Social Workers (NASW), social work case management is defined as follows:

> ... a method of providing services whereby a professional social worker assesses the needs of

the client and the client's family, when appropriate, and arranges, coordinates, monitors, evaluates, and advocates for a package of multiple services to meet the specific client's complex needs. (NASW, 1992, p. 5)

Despite the variety of definitions, the general meaning of case management is any method of linking, managing, or organizing services to meet client needs. CCMC noted the following:

> Case management is an advanced practice of health care professionals to coordinate and facilitate access to the treatment and care in a timely, efficient and cost-effective manner. This involves identifying appropriate providers and treatment options that meet an individual's health needs. (2004a, p. 1)

Thus case management entails the coordination and sequencing of care. It helps to tighten the plan of care and link direct caregivers and services across facility and service boundaries.

Acute care hospital nursing case management is a system in which the accountability for the care management of clients in a specific diagnosis-related group (DRG) category, disease group, or other population over an entire hospitalization is assigned to a registered nurse (RN). The nurse case manager coordinates care across the continuum of services. Hospital nursing case management usually is targeted at high-risk populations. Although all clients need to have their care coordinated, case management functions best to coordinate health care services for high-risk populations across community, acute, and long-term care settings (Simpson, 1993). Zander (1991) defined case management as a matrix model at the clinician-provider level in acute care.

Case management in acute care nursing is an attempt to reconfigure the delivery of hospital care into a more integrated system management care modality. Case management and care coordination have been the care delivery modality employed by public health and community health nurses (Mikulencak, 1993). In these settings, case management has been centered on client needs rather than shift- or unit-centered. Case management can occur in the hospital only, extend across the health care continuum, or be linked to a population focus (Lee, 1993).

Case management is described as a system of client care delivery that focuses on the achievement of client outcomes within effective and appropriate time frames and resources. It is a system of health services delivery, coordination, and monitoring through which multiple service needs of clients are met. Case management is an umbrella program in a health care facility for systems management. Case management operates at the intersection of organizational systems and the delivery of clinical care. It is focused on an entire chronic or catastrophic condition or conditions, crossing all settings in which the client receives care. New services across the continuum of health care are incorporated as needed. Care is directed by a case manager, often a nurse, and focuses on a multidisciplinary team effort.

A term related to case management is *disease management*, which is defined as a comprehensive, integrated approach to care and reimbursement based on a disease's natural course. The goal is to address the disease condition with maximum effectiveness and efficiency (Zitter, 1997). Disease management programs contain a series of clinical processes and services across the health care continuum that rely on informatics to identify and manage a medical or chronic condition in a particular at-risk population to improve care, promote wellness, and manage or reduce costs (Ward & Rieve, 1997). Such disease state case management programs are population-based approaches to the identification and management of chronic conditions. Health status is assessed, plans of care are developed, and data are collected to evaluate the effectiveness of the program (Levitt et al., 1998). These programs are focused on the group level of aggregation and may be community-focused or population health-focused.

Critical Pathways

A *critical pathway* is a written plan that identifies key, critical, or predictable incidents that must occur at set times to achieve client outcomes within an appropriate time frame, such as a length of stay in a hospital setting. Critical pathways are tools used to help providers identify, measure, and analyze care processes and desired patient outcomes (Renholm et al., 2002). They detail essential care steps and describe the expected progress. They include time-dependent functions and organize and integrate provider interventions in a multidisciplinary format and across multiple settings or levels of care (Cesta & Tahan, 2003). Providing an overview of the whole process, critical pathways are best practice tools that identify and document the standardized, interdisciplinary processes that need to occur for a patient to move toward a desired outcome in a defined period of time. Elements include all providers' assessments and interventions, laboratory and other diagnostic tests, treatments, consultations, activity level, patient and family education, discharge planning, and desired outcomes (Renholm et al., 2002). Critical pathways have been described as protocols of interdisciplinary treatments, based on professional standards of practice and placed in order on a decision tree (Simpson, 1993).

Critical pathways are called by a variety of names, such as critical path, coordinated care path, clinical pathway, clinical protocol, care track, or care step. They are case management tools that map out the plan of care and guide and document care within a framework that reflects the research, experience, and consensus priorities of a multidisciplinary group of providers actively engaged in providing care to the target population. Critical pathways are cause-and-effect visual grids or paths to direct care toward goals. They show key incidents and expected behaviors. Critical pathway elements include an index of problems, a timeline, a variance record, and the path or grid. Critical pathways are one form of structured care methodologies, or streamlined interdisciplinary tools, that identify best practices and facilitate standardization of care (Cole & Houston, 1999).

A critical pathway is a document that organizes the sequence of events for an episode of care. Both processes and outcomes are incorporated. Some see critical paths as creating a cookbook approach to care delivery. However, critical paths do organize and sequence the usual path of client care and form a standard of care. Variances are noted and analyzed. The process of developing and using critical paths encourages both critical thinking and accountability. Critical paths can be used to educate, prepare, and orient and to negotiate expectations and care roles with clients. Critical paths can and should be individualized to each client. They are major tools of outcomes management and coordination of care delivery.

Benchmarking and evidence-based practice are used in constructing and evaluating critical pathways. Benchmarks form a frame of reference against which an institution can compare itself relative to others. Benchmarking is a useful strategy for helping to understand internal processes and performance levels. Benchmarks help identify performance gaps. Consensus benchmarks can be established by professional societies, health systems, national databases, or texts and manuals (Cesta & Tahan, 2003).

Critical pathways display expected outcomes. A difference between what was expected and what actually occurred is called a variance. A *variance* is a deviation from a standard. Variances can be either positive or negative. Sources of variance include client- and family-related, systems-related, or provider-related factors. A process needs to be in place to document, collect, and analyze variances for trends and opportunities for cost reduction and quality improvement (Cesta & Tahan, 2003). A literature review revealed that the use of critical pathways has a positive impact on patient care outcomes (Renholm et al., 2002).

BACKGROUND

Case Management Models

A variety of case management models has arisen; some are nursing models, others are nonnursing models. The core elements center around a case manager who coordinates and monitors the care given to clients by multiple services in an attempt to decrease service fragmentation and improve

---

Box **17.1**

Service Components of Management Models

1. Client identification and outreach
2. Individual assessment and diagnosis
3. Service planning and resource identification
4. Linking clients to needed services
5. Service implementation and coordination
6. Monitoring service delivery
7. Advocacy
8. Evaluation

Data from Weil, M., & Karls, J.M. (1985). *Case management in human service practice: A systematic approach to mobilizing resources for clients.* San Francisco: Jossey-Bass.

---

the quality of care (Rheaume et al., 1994). Weil and Karls (1985) identified eight main service components common to all case management models (Box 17.1).

Case management exists in many contexts and settings, including insurance-based programs, employer-based programs, workers' compensation programs, social services programs, independent practice, medical practice, nursing practice, public health nursing and Visiting Nurse Association practices, maternal-child settings, and mental health settings. Case management can simultaneously be described as a system, a role, a technology, a process, and a service (Bower, 1992).

As a *system,* case management is assessment and problem identification; planning; procurement, delivery, and coordination of services; and monitoring to ensure that the multiple services needs of the client are met. It is a clinical system that focuses on the achievement of client outcomes within effective and appropriate time frames and resources. It focuses on the entire episode of illness, crossing all settings in which the client receives care. As a *role,* it provides clients with a practitioner who actively coordinates their care. As a *technology,* case management generates tools and techniques to organize care that maximize the timing and sequencing of multiple, often complex, care activities. As a *process,* it expands on the component of the nursing process to view health issues and respond to the needs of clients along the care continuum and across multiple settings. As a *service,* it provides both facilitating and gatekeeping functions for the client. The ultimate goal is to achieve planned care outcomes by brokering services across the health care continuum (Bower, 1992).

"Case management refers to patient-focused strategies to coordinate care" (Bower, 1992, p. 2). It can be thought of as the system or design for moving a recipient through the health care system. A model of case management will be designed for a large, rather generic target group or population (e.g., hospitalized, long-term care, chronic care, rehabilitation) or for a specified "expanse" on the health care continuum (e.g., an episode in one setting, in one organization, or for the whole continuum). A model of case management will specify the standards for care and resource use, relationships, and responsibilities in a more general sense. The nurse may or may not be a direct care provider.

Several organizing frameworks or methods of classification have been considered in grouping case management models. Because of the variability in how case management programs are set up, classification into model types helps to describe and better compare them. The following are common ways of describing case management models:

- Organizational models vs. practice models
- External vs. internal case management models
- Episodic vs. continuity models
- Provider vs. purchaser models
- Hospital-based case management models vs. community-based models
- Case management programs that cross the continuum of care

Using these distinctions, case management models can be understood in terms of perspective (e.g., organization or providers), scope (e.g., services inside an organization), and time (e.g., one episode or across time and settings).

The literature provides many types of case management models and applies many labels to those models. Each author tends to follow a different list of models and definitions. Although each model makes a contribution to the understanding of case management within a discipline, none has received uniform acceptance within a specific field and none are generic enough to be widely adopted across the various human service fields that practice case management (Ridgely & Willenbring, 1992). However, two factors are common across all case management models: the core component is coordination of care, and the core principle is advocacy.

The diversity of case management models in the various disciplines makes it difficult to generalize about the models. In addition to coordination of care, advocacy, brokering of services, and resource management, there are fairly common process elements in case management models regardless of the specific discipline. The models are typically tailored to fit unique target groups, vulnerable populations, settings, or other factors found in the discipline.

Nursing and health care models tend to focus on the management of health/illness or disease or the rehabilitation needs of an individual or population. These models are sometimes called medical models, medical-social models, or disease management models. In the nursing literature, there has been some confusion about whether or not case management is a care delivery model or an intervention that entails a process. In both nursing and social work, there is a differentiation between case management designed to *deliver* services and case management designed to *coordinate* the provision of services (Ridgely & Willenbring, 1992).

Case management programs use principles of client advocacy to precisely target strategies that will manage and coordinate care. Beyond common functions, there is great diversity in the specific manifestation and configuration of each case management model. That is the result of case management taking many different forms. The form that is applied depends on the following:

- Basic client care needs that are to be addressed
- The level of care needs that are to be addressed

- The discipline and professional identity of the case manager
- The environment in which the client is situated
- The organization for which the case manager is working

There are two basic models identified in the nursing literature: the New England model of acute care nursing case management and the community-based model of Carondelet St. Mary's.

The New England Medical Center model is an extension of primary nursing methodology called nursing case management and is focused on the acute care hospital episode (Zander, 1990, 1991, 1992, 1994, 2002). This model exemplifies organization-specific models; it is hospital-based case management, or "modified primary nursing within-the-walls." It is best known for structuring the episode of care. In the mid-1980s this model was introduced at the New England Medical Center, using principles of planning and concurrent management from engineering and other fields to extend primary nursing into outcomes management. The goal was to balance cost, process, and outcomes. The New England model is a client-centered approach instituted during episodes of acute illness. It focuses on outcomes, resource utilization, and nursing accountability (Clark, 1996). Written, standardized documents such as case management plans, timelines, and critical paths were developed and evolved into CareMap® tools that formed the basis for a comprehensive hospital case management system at the New England Medical Center. The complete CareMap® system includes the following:

- Variance analysis
- Use of an outcome-time focus in all multidisciplinary communication
- Case consultation and health care team meetings for clients at more-than-acceptable variance
- Continuous quality improvement

The New England model defines case management as a care delivery model called nursing case management.

Carondelet St. Mary's Community Nursing Network, or the Arizona Model (Forbes, 1999), uses professional nurse case managers (bachelor's and master's level), organized as a nursing HMO, at the hub of a network to broker services. This model type is known as a beyond-the-walls, medical-social, across-the-continuum of care model. It is best known for its innovative work in moving beyond the episode of care and into the continuum. This hospital-to-community model uses case managers to follow the movement of high-risk clients from acute care to community to long-term care settings. Case managers are responsible for clients with chronic health problems, and the relationship is long-term (Clark, 1996).

There are four models in social work: broker, primary therapist, interdisciplinary team, and comprehensive. Social casework emphasizes the development of new resources, linkages to existing service agencies, coordination of care, advocacy, and teaching. Casework typically includes increasing the individual's self-reliance and independence, as well as coordinating and integrating care (Ridgely & Willenbring, 1992). The emphasis is on vulnerable populations.

The broker model emphasizes the case manager's traditional linkage function. Clients are linked to a network of providers and service coverage using assessment, referral, and ensuring the availability of service activities (Raiff & Shore, 1993). The broker approach is sometimes described as a generalist approach. The case manager is a professional responsible for an individual client or a set of clients. The generalist carries out all case management functions and provides the basic direct service, coordination, and advocacy necessary in all case management programs (Weil & Karls, 1985). The primary goal is to increase the likelihood that clients will receive the right services, in proper sequence, and in a timely fashion. To achieve this, the case manager plans a comprehensive service package and negotiates through barriers that prevent clients from accessing needed services. Cost savings may or may not be an explicit goal, but such savings may be expected because the case manager facilitates better access to cost-effective alternatives, achieves better coordination and less duplication of services across agencies, reduces utilization of more expensive and less effective sites of care or services, and diverts clients from admissions (Ridgely & Willenbring, 1992).

In the primary therapist model, the case manager's relationship to the client is primarily therapeutic, and case management functions are undertaken as a part of, or an extension of, therapeutic intervention. The client has one person to relate to about treatment, service access, and case coordination. However, the therapist may feel that case management is a secondary activity to therapeutic work (Weil & Karls, 1985).

The interdisciplinary team model uses a specialized interdisciplinary team in which each member has a specific responsibility for service activities in his or her area of expertise. In combination, the activities of these specialized case managers constitute a complete case management process. The team might divide responsibilities by activity, such as intake, service linkage, and case monitoring (Weil & Karls, 1985). Team structures vary considerably. In some, all case managers on the team are interchangeable and serve the total group of clients. Other programs consist of multidisciplinary teams in which each professional provides specific services to the clients assigned to the team. In other cases, individual case managers carry individual caseloads but provide backup assistance to each other. Despite being called "teams," the specific configuration actually may be critical to the program's success (Ridgely & Willenbring, 1992).

The comprehensive service center model is used in service centers that provide comprehensive services, including social and emotional support, vocational training, and residential facilities. This type of program is often rehabilitative (Weil & Karls, 1985) and is seen in areas such as developmental disabilities and long-term physical disabilities. A personal strengths model may be used to help clients focus on and achieve goals (Huber, 2005).

Other models of case management in health care include independent practice or private case management. Private case management covers those services contracted for by individuals or families or those subcontracted for by other groups. This approach arose because of the concern over rising health care costs and the confusion that accompanies the choices consumers must make. The case manager has three main functions: coordination, advocacy, and counseling (Clark, 1996). Some examples include entrepreneurial or small independent case managers and practice in for-profit, large, national case management companies.

Long-term care, rehabilitation, occupational health, workers' compensation, pharmacy, and medical case management models exist. Many medical models fall within disease management programs.

Insurance models include broker, gatekeeper, catastrophic, HMO types, and governmental models. The broker model within insurance companies includes an emphasis on linkage with no provision of direct services. It is similar to the broker in the social work models except for a strong emphasis on conserving benefits utilization.

Gatekeeper (managed care) models manage access to services and promote the use of cost-effective alternatives to expensive services (Ridgely & Willenbring, 1992). They can produce cost savings by managing care, including substituting less costly, more appropriate services, and sometimes simply by not authorizing higher-cost services. Rather than facilitating access, gatekeepers must restrict access to control utilization and, thereby, costs. The ability of these case managers to create savings depends on the availability of appropriate cost-effective alternatives, case manager authority within the care system, and case manager ability to control financing for the care they deem appropriate (Ridgely & Willenbring, 1992). The case manager functions much like a purchasing agent (Clark, 1996).

Focused on catastrophic diseases or events such as acquired immunodeficiency syndrome (AIDS) or brain injuries, catastrophic case management is often used with workers' compensation cases and life-care planning. It is designed to manage and maximize the benefits, which may be capped at a lifetime maximum. Early warning strategies are adopted to detect the potential for high-cost cases and to deal with both clients and service providers proactively to optimize and economize the health services used (Cline, 1990).

In HMO (managed care) models, prospective or capitated reimbursement systems put providers at financial risk. This creates pressure on providers to control total costs, provide and promote prevention-oriented services, and substitute lower-cost services, preferably without sacrificing quality. One example of managed care models is integrated health care, defined as a network of organizations that provides or arranges to provide a coordinated continuum of services to a defined population and is held accountable for the population's health status (Shortell et al., 1993). Federal, state, and local government agencies also manage and reimburse care via programs such as Medicare, Medicaid, and Workers' Compensation.

Few interdisciplinary models exist. The following two were described in the literature:

1. One model for acute care case management for nurses and social workers has been described (Dzyacky, 1998). It is a program designed to integrate utilization management functions with discharge planning and separate the practice of social work from discharge planning activities. Discharge planning tasks were divided into two categories—simple and complex. Case facilitator nurses became responsible for simple discharge planning cases; social workers handled the complex category.

2. One model for nurse-social worker collaboration in managed care also has been presented (Hawkins et al., 1998). Called the Biopsychosocial Individual and Systems Intervention Model, it is derived from a combination of interdisciplinary collaboration models at the organizational and administrative levels and a case management intervention approach for individuals and small systems levels. Nurses and social workers are assumed to collaborate as equal partners in interdisciplinary team case management using a transdisciplinary model.

History of Case Management

Different disciplines lay claim to case management; thus the history of its development of varies according to the perspective of the specific discipline reporting it. The social work perspective is that the roots of case management descend from social work's historical tradition and the work of Mary Richmond in the era of the early settlement houses and charity organization societies (Raiff & Shore, 1993). This was a social casework concept at the turn of the twentieth century. Since the 1970s there has been a resurgence in case management as a result of shifts in the locus and financing of health care and human services and problems with service fragmentation and inaccessibility.

The insurance companies' perspective is that case management arose in insurance companies because of the need to manage catastrophic and high-cost cases. For example, Liberty Mutual is often credited with having pioneered the concept of in-house case management/rehabilitation programs in insurance companies in 1943 as a cost-containment measure for workers' compensation. This concept was expanded in 1966 by the Insurance Company of North America (now CIGNA) when it started an in-house program incorporating vocational rehabilitation and case management that later became Intracorp. Some view George Welch of CIGNA as the true father of modern case management, as demonstrated in the following perspective:

> Case management as part of the insurance industry or other third-party payer systems seems to have had two somewhat separate origins: the worker's compensation system and the accident and health insurance system. (Siefker et al., 1998, p. 3)

The history of case management in nursing began with private duty nursing, the oldest care modality in U.S. nursing. With the rise of the early settlement houses, there was a concern for coordination of health care services for immigrants and the poor. This was the beginning of public and human services in the United States. Both nurses and social workers were key initiators. The Henry Street Settlement was founded in

1895 by two nurses (identified as social workers), Lillian Wald and Mary Brewster. In 1902 Lillian Wald founded the first school of nursing. By 1900, visiting nurse services were established to provide comprehensive community services and case coordination (Tahan, 1998).

Community service coordination, a forerunner of case management, began at the turn of the twentieth century in public health programs. The Visiting Nurse Service was one of the very first community health programs. Providing service coordination has always been a focus of public health nursing. Service coordination has since evolved into case management, but case management considerably expands on coordination of community services. The concept of a continuum of care was used after World War II to describe the extended community services needed for mental health clients. The term *case management* first appeared in the early 1970s in social welfare literature, followed by a use in the nursing literature. The 1981 Omnibus Budget Reconciliation Act plus Medicare prospective reimbursement encouraged comprehensive, coordinated services. As a result of changing reimbursement structures, insurers have been focused on programs to contain the rising costs of health care. Case management emerged in the fields of psychiatry and social work in the 1920s, was used by visiting nurses in the 1930s, developed and flourished in acute care in the 1980s, and was found in all settings in the 1990s (Cesta & Tahan, 2003).

In nursing, case management historically has been the care delivery model associated with public health and community health nursing. Thus it was operational in settings outside hospitals and operated without the umbrella of managed care. In these settings, case management focused on accountability of process and outcomes of care delivery. Traditional case management principles also were operational in several care models that evolved over time. Case management also was used in social service agencies, community mental health services, rehabilitation settings, and long-term care.

In the 1960s, contemporaneous with government legislation enacting Medicare and Medicaid coverage, the insurance industry began to evolve case management models (Siefker et al., 1998). This preemergence decade set the stage for a series of dramatic evolutionary changes in case management practice each decade since the 1960s.

Many trace the "rise" of case management models to the 1970s. Certainly the last 35 years or so have brought about an amazing pace of change. The effects have been dramatic. In the 1970s, as the federal government began to analyze actuarial data on health care costs, expenditures, and projections, case management became a considered strategy in the rise of health maintenance organizations (HMOs), long-term care demonstration grants, and social work efforts to manage the deinstitutionalization of the chronically mentally ill. The 1970s saw the rise of both solo providers of case management services (independent companies) and of large national case management companies. Models of catastrophic case management and workers' compensation predominated, and the certification as Certified Rehabilitation Counselor (CRC) began.

The 1980s was a decade of rapid spread and wild growth in case management models. With the advent of diagnosis related groups (DRGs) and prospective payment mechanisms, case management came to be seen as one answer to cost stabilization and cost predictability. It spread into models of social health maintenance organizations and other insurance settings. Independent case management companies grew and thrived. The Certified Disability Management Specialist (CDMS) certification was begun, and the New England Medical Center's nursing case management (acute care) model was developed and disseminated into hospital-based case management settings.

The decade of the 1990s was a time of reevaluation. Rapid growth leveled off, and hospitals began downsizing their number of registered nurses. However, interest that had been sparked in the 1980s carried over into the 1990s as health care providers, payors, employers, health plans, and professional organizations struggled to integrate case management practice and identify the knowledge base. Two groups merged to form the professional organization representing case management practice, the Case Management Society of America (CMSA). The Commission for Case Manager Certification (CCMC) was begun and offered the Certified Case Manager (CCM) credential. A proliferation of other certifications, usually within provider disciplines, occurred. CMSA developed and published the standards of practice for case management in 1995 and updated this in 2002. Both CMSA and CCMC adopted the same consensus definition of case management, although CMSA later modified its definition in 2002. The managed care technique of utilization management became more closely aligned with case management. Models of case management also proliferated, usually within hospitals and the acute care sector, but without standardization. Jobs for case managers began to shift into acute care, the insurance industry, and large private companies. Organizational accreditation for case management programs was introduced by the Commission on Accreditation of Rehabilitation Facilities (CARF) and the Utilization Review Accreditation Commission (URAC). Rigorous research results began to emerge to demonstrate the value of case management models. Case management models came under scrutiny for their value and cost-effectiveness. Interest arose in using case management principles and applying them to populations with chronic diseases, which was the preemergence phase of disease management.

The Case Management Process

Sometimes called *care management, outcomes management,* or *clinical resource management,* case management has elements related to access, decision support, and outcomes achievement. Increasingly, the element of organizational compliance has become associated with case management. Other case management functions are access, utilization review and management, discharge planning or transition management, episode tracking and continuous quality improvement, health prevention and disease management, and contracting. These functions may be stand-alone or combined in various ways, especially in hospitals (Zander, 2002).

According to the CMSA's *Standards of Practice for Case Management* (2002), the key functions of a case manager are assessment, planning, facilitation, and advocacy. Collaboration with the client and with those involved in the client's care is essential. Specialized skill and knowledge are needed in positive relationship building; effective communication; negotiation; knowledge of contractual and risk arrangements; ability to affect change, perform evaluation, plan and organize, and promote autonomy; and knowledge about funding sources, health care services, human behavior, health care financing, and clinical standards and outcomes. The process of case management begins with the identification of individuals with high-cost, complex care needs who can benefit from case management services. The case management intervention begins with first contact with the client and/or family and continues as an ongoing relationship until termination.

Assessment

To develop a plan of care, a comprehensive assessment of health needs is done. Tools such as surveys or questionnaires, assessment batteries, telephone assessment strategies, or electronic communication may be used. Interviews of the client and/or family, physician and other providers, and other health care team members are important. Assessment needs to cover health behaviors, cultural influences, and belief and values systems and must include identification of potential barriers, negotiating realistic goals, and searching for alternatives (CMSA, 2002).

Planning

To maximize the client's health status and achieve goals and outcomes, planning is done with the client, family, health care providers, payors, and the community. The plan of care needs to be evidence-based and individualized. The goal of planning is to derive an action plan that is appropriate, fiscally responsible, high-quality, evidence-based, and feasible. Contingency plans need to be in place for variances. Reevaluation should be ongoing (CMSA, 2002).

Facilitation

Facilitation uses strategies of communication and coordination and the involvement of the client and family throughout the case management process. Facilitation also is focused on linking parts of the service delivery system and streamlining care delivery. Coordination and education are key strategies (CMSA, 2002).

Advocacy

Case management advocacy is a function related to client empowerment, autonomy, and self-determination. Advocacy actions are supportive and educative and represent the client's best interests. Representing the client's best interest includes advocating for early referral, necessary funding, appropriate treatment, and timely coordination of services. When conflicts arise, the case manager advocates for the needs of the client (CMSA, 2002).

CASE MANAGEMENT IMPLEMENTATION

"Nursing case management will continue to evolve as a strong method to provide decision support to and procurement and evaluation of resources for patients, families, physicians, and organizations" (Zander, 2002, p. 58). In hospitals, case management has become a popular and effective means to decrease length of stay and secure important outcomes. In managed care arenas, case management has been identified as a major strategy for cost containment that also folds in quality control.

Persuasive arguments exist for implementing case management: "The success of case management in increasing the use of community-based services among a variety of chronically ill and medically fragile populations and in decreasing the frequency and length of stay of hospitalization is well documented" (Erkel, 1993, p. 27). Despite this assertion, one research synthesis of 18 studies of inpatient case management published between 1988 and 1995 revealed inconsistent findings

across studies. The author concluded that there were not enough data to endorse case management programs conclusively (Cook, 1998). However, one randomized, controlled clinical trial in primary care clinics in a group model HMO compared diabetes control in clients receiving nurse case management and clients receiving usual care; significant results for improved glycemic control were found with nurse case management (Aubert et al., 1998). It appears that nurse case management can be significantly more effective in helping certain client groups attain positive outcomes and should be implemented where indicated. Close follow-up, continuous reinforcement, and systematic treatment adjustments helped adult clients with diabetes.

Four basic principles guide nursing case management:

1. Coordination and integration of a continuum of holistic care
2. Promotion and preservation of health through periods of transition and risk
3. Conservation and allocation of scarce resources
4. Provision of follow-up care that tracks and guides service delivery over the long term and across episodes and settings

Thus the nurse case manager remains in a relationship with clients over time and across boundaries. The nursing concept of discharge is replaced by accompaniment as the nurse follows the client, acting to connect and coordinate a broad continuum of sites and services (Hinitz-Satterfield et al., 1993). Nurses "accompany" clients in a cognitive and communication sense. Only in certain models will nurses literally provide care across the continuum.

Coordination and continuity are the keys to managing care over the health care continuum and across organizational boundaries. Thus care must be managed carefully within each area or unit and between health care areas. Case management focuses on provider continuity; managed care focuses on the continuity of the plan. Both must be integrated into the care delivery system using a systems perspective (Falk & Bower, 1994).

Research Note

Source: Aubert, R.E., Herman, W.H., Waters, J., Moore, W., Sutton, D., Peterson, B.L., et al. (1998). Nurse case management to improve glycemic control in diabetic patients in a health maintenance organization. *Annals of Internal Medicine, 129*(8), 605-612.

Purpose

Previous research has demonstrated that keeping patients with type 1 and type 2 diabetes mellitus in near-normal glycemic control reduces the development and progression of microvascular and neuropathic complications by about 50%. The purpose of this study was to compare diabetes control in patients receiving nurse case management and those receiving usual care.

Discussion

The American Diabetes Association has recommended that all persons with diabetes attempt to achieve near-normalization of blood glucose levels. However, this is not routinely followed in practice. Bringing research knowledge into use in practice can be difficult. Furthermore, methods to achieve diabetes control are resource-intensive. Nurse case management has been an integral part of clinical trials therapy and has proven to be effective in care after acute myocardial infarction; it may also be effective for glycemic control. A 12-month randomized clinical trial was conducted to compare a nurse case management model of diabetes care with the usual care in a primary care setting. The diabetes registry of a health maintenance organization (HMO) in Florida was used to obtain the treatment sample of 100 subjects, who provided 12-month follow-up data. The nurse case management diabetes program (intervention) included close follow-up, continuous reinforcement of meal planning and exercise, and systematic treatment adjustments. In clients randomly assigned to the nurse case management intervention, HbA_{1c} values significantly decreased and were consistent across baseline and subsamples. Furthermore, subjects in the intervention group reported better general health status than did those receiving the usual care. An increased loss to follow-up was noted in younger patients in the intervention group.

Application to Practice

This research showed that a nurse case management diabetes program can significantly assist people with diabetes to achieve near-normal control of blood sugar levels and thus reduce morbidity rates. This research is the first prospective, randomized controlled clinical trial of diabetes nurse case management to be published. The research demonstrates the value of nurse case management as a strategy for implementing national health guidelines in clinical practice. The existence of an organized system of health care delivery and a centralized database facilitated the study. Furthermore, in looking at subgroups, it is possible that nurse case management may be less suited to the more mobile and active lifestyle of younger patients. It is important to know both when to use and when *not* to use case management as an intervention.

The unit or area is the most basic locus at which to begin the coordination of care. In nursing, the care delivery system functions to coordinate care at the unit level. Coordination and continuity can be shift-based or unit-based. If the existing care delivery system does not accomplish goals of coordinating care, then a unit-based role with accountability for coordinating care across time will need to be developed (Falk & Bower, 1994).

Despite widespread dissemination of case management as a provider intervention and system strategy, there still remain some problem areas. These include the confusion over definitions and identification of exactly what case management is.

Organizations also have struggled with whether and how to internally combine or separate case management and related functions. With an emphasis on financial viability or "margin," case management programs have been analyzed and challenged to justify the allocation of scarce resources to them.

Controversies exist in the field regarding methods and measurements to assess the value of case management. The two basic outcomes categories to be captured are clinical outcomes and financial outcomes. For clinical outcomes, CMSA (Braden, 2002) identified the following six direct outcomes of case management:

1. Patient knowledge
2. Patient involvement
3. Patient's participation in care
4. Patient empowerment
5. Patient adherence
6. Coordination of care

Thus changes (improvement) in a key indicator such as patient knowledge can be a direct measure of the clinical effectiveness of a case management intervention. When the outcome of improved patient knowledge is linked by research evidence about improved patient knowledge reducing chronic relapse or use of health care resources, then the effectiveness of case management is further strengthened.

Proving financial gain has been somewhat more problematic for case management. In some areas such as diabetes, congestive heart failure, and mental health, case management has acknowledged acceptance. In other areas such as substance abuse treatment, financial benefit has been difficult to demonstrate. This is partly because case management is an intensive one-on-one service delivered by expert providers. In adding on a service cost, case management programs do not result in the same dramatic savings as reducing a day of hospital care or eliminating a procedure or treatment. The Centers for Medicare & Medicaid Services (CMS) have noted this dilemma, as follows:

> In the past, we have conducted several demonstrations of case management for chronic illnesses, including the national channeling demonstration and the Alzheimer's Disease demonstration. The evaluations of these demonstrations found that none of them showed sufficient savings to cover the additional costs of case management.
>
> There are several possible reasons for the lack of positive results. First, the most appropriate individuals were not always targeted and enrolled into the demonstration. In many cases, the sites enrolled patients with less severe, and therefore less costly conditions, making it more difficult to achieve cost savings by avoiding normal utilization patterns of acute or long-term medical care. The disease management demonstration Web site www.cms.hhs.gov/healthplans/research/DMDemo.asp contains additional information about these demonstrations.
>
> We are currently conducting other demonstrations that test either case or disease management. In one demonstration, Lovelace Health Systems in Albuquerque, New Mexico was chosen to operate demonstrations of intensive case management services for high-risk patients with congestive heart failure and diabetes to improve the clinical outcomes, quality of life, and satisfaction with services. The other is a larger scale demonstration involving 15 sites authorized by the Balanced Budget Act (BBA) of 1997 (Pub. L. 105-33, enacted on August 5, 1997) to evaluate methods such as case management and disease management that improve the quality of care for beneficiaries with a chronic illness. The coordinated care demonstration was designed based on the findings of a review of best practices for coordinating care in the private sector. More information about the Coordinated Care Demonstration can be found on our Web site www.cms.hhs.gov/healthplans/research/coorcare.asp (CMS, 2003, pp. 9675-9676)

Fortunately, research is beginning to emerge and be identified to substantiate savings from case management interventions. Peer-reviewed research studies on effectiveness include Allen and colleagues (2002), Fitzgerald and colleagues (1994), Goodwin and colleagues (2003), Laramee and colleagues (2003), Norris and colleagues (2002), Riegel and colleagues (2002), Sesperez and colleagues (2001), and Weiman (1995).

DEVELOPMENT OF CASE MANAGEMENT PROGRAMS

Case management programs are structured around roles and functions of case managers. The case manager's role balances the aspects of provider, care coordinator, and financial manager. The ANCC (1997) identified case manager roles as advocate, facilitator, provider, liaison, coordinator, collaborator, broker, educator, negotiator, evaluator, communicator, risk manager, mentor, consultant, and researcher. Case management functions were identified as care coordination, facilitation and brokerage, education, advocacy, discharge planning, resource management, and outcomes management.

For provider-based case managers, a case management program can be built based on CMSA's Standards of Practice for Case Management (2002). The practice components identified in the standards document can be used as the foundation for establishing a step-by-step process. Following the standards as an outline emphasizes comprehensiveness and professional practice (Birmingham, 1996). Job descriptions also can be revised or composed to reflect the CMSA's Standards of Practice.

Case management programs are developed using a number of situation-specific elements. Two initial assessments are helpful: assessment of the organization and assessment of client populations. The organizational assessment focuses on identification of resources, whereas the client population assessment focuses on how care is experienced by clients and the characteristics of client populations served by the organizations. (Box 17.2 lists related assessment questions.) If case management is used for specific client populations, priority would go to clients who demonstrate the following (Falk & Bower, 1994):

- Have a high rate of recidivism or frequent emergency department encounters
- Have unpredictable needs for care

Box 17.2

Case Management Assessment Questions

Organizational Assessment

- What clinical and support services are needed?
- When in the client experience are services most appropriately provided?
- How should services be provided?
- Where are services best delivered?
- Who are the most appropriate providers?
- Where and by whom are services best managed?

Client Assessment

- What are the major client populations served by the organizations—by volume, diagnosis, cost, payer mix, and high-intensity/resource use outliers?
- What is the service path followed by client populations—by entry point, internal flow, discharge, and recidivism?
- What groups of clients fall into high-risk categories—by volume?
- What clients are at risk for less than desired outcomes—by morbidity, mortality, infection rates, falls, and clinical outcomes?

- Have significant complications, comorbidities, or variances in usual care patterns
- Fall into high-risk profiles
- Are high-cost

The general process for the development of a case management program can be synthesized as follows:

1. Assess the organization and the client population served. This assessment provides a baseline for implementation.
2. Identify high-volume or high-risk case types. This assessment will indicate priority areas for care coordination.
3. Determine the usual client care problems, issues, or difficulties related to the high-volume or high-risk case types. Determine desired goals.

4. Form an interdisciplinary care team of the interrelated care providers who will be involved with the case types.
5. Develop and design a multidisciplinary critical pathway for each selected case type. The path should outline and specify measurable clinical outcomes, key professional care processes, and exact corresponding timelines as based on practice patterns, professional standards of care, and length-of-stay parameters. The input and involvement of the client and each provider group, in relation to achieving client outcomes, should be clearly specified. The pathway would mark the occurrence of routine treatments, tests, consults, client activities, medications, diet, educational interventions, and discharge planning. Variance from the path triggers analysis and intervention.
6. Develop a pilot program or trial site.
7. Evaluate the pilot program and consider system-wide implementation. Review the pilot program's articulation with the existing mode of nursing care delivery.

Research Note

Source: Harrison, J.P., Nolin, J., & Suero, E. (2004). The effect of case management on U.S. hospitals. *Nursing Economic$,* *22*(2), 64-70.

Purpose

Case management (CM) has been shown to be an effective strategy in acute care, long-term care, and outpatient settings with diverse populations and conditions. Well-designed programs are important for effective use of hospital resources and reduction of costs. Demonstrated benefits have been shown for increasing quality of care, patient and family satisfaction, patient adherence, and increased quality of life. The purpose of this research was to evaluate which characteristics distinguish between hospitals with and without case management models. Do they have unique market characteristics, more efficient management, or greater profitability? Hospital CM programs (n = 2725) and hospitals without (n = 1714) as drawn from the American Hospital Association annual survey were analyzed on 11 variables. The Area Resource File and the Centers for Medicare & Medicaid Services' (CMS) Minimum Data Set also were sources of data. Data were analyzed for mean differences, correlations, and by multivariate logistic regression to identify significant relationships.

Discussion

Hospitals with CM programs were more likely to be located in markets with higher incomes and fewer elderly, have higher return on assets and occupancy rates, have lower operating expenses per discharge, be larger, have more clinical services, and have more enrolled capitated lives. Of these, the percentage of elderly, HMO penetration, return on assets, and number of clinical services were related most significantly to hospitals with CM programs. Thus the profile of hospitals with CM programs is as follows: likely to be found in efficient, complex hospitals with a variety of services in a market with high HMO penetration and a smaller Medicare population.

Application to Practice

Case management programs are more prevalent in larger, more complex hospitals, and CM may be critical to coordination of care across services and to improving operational efficiency as a competitive advantage to HMOs. There was a strong positive relationship between CM and an increasing return on assets. Hospitals without CM need to consider using CM as a strategy to improve efficiency and profitability. As size and complexity of a hospital increases, CM becomes more important. Successful coordination of chronic care across the continuum is a key strategy for financial profitability for hospitals.

Tahan (1996) mapped out a 10-step process for developing case management plans: (1) design the format, (2) select the target population, (3) organize the interdisciplinary team, (4) educate the team, (5) examine the current process, (6) review the literature, (7) establish the length of the plan, (8) develop the content, (9) conduct a pilot study, and (10) standardize the plan. These processes emphasize the interdisciplinary team approaches needed and highlight the importance of preparing people and the organization to facilitate success.

Some research is beginning to emerge that evaluates case management programs (see Research Note). Harrison and colleagues (2004) found a link between hospital profitability and the existence of case management programs. Larger hospitals with high clinical complexity and a growing managed care population tended to benefit the most from full case management programs.

LEADERSHIP AND MANAGEMENT IMPLICATIONS

All nursing roles contain a component of management. This may range from basic clinical care management to executive leadership of an organization. McClure (1991) has noted that nurses have two roles: (1) caregiver and (2) care coordinator. Nurses in management positions in an organizational hierarchy are organization managers and coordination specialists who integrate units and systems. Management of client care by nurses makes them clinical managers. The shift to managed care in integrated health systems has highlighted case management as a key strategy for nursing practice management and empowerment of nurses. It also has made multidisciplinary collaboration an imperative.

Future effectiveness is thought to be based on decisions about what types of organizational structures and nursing care delivery systems best enable nurse-managed client care and best support nurses in practice. One related question is, How much management does a nurse require? One assessment is the extent to which a nurse provides client care or manages the care of clients. Case management is one specific approach to redesigning care delivery for client care improvement. This may mean that some traditional management practices and habits will need to be changed or discarded. Case management has come to be a part of care delivery management that emphasizes the expertise of nurses.

Mark (1992) advocated an approach to determining the organization of practice that begins

⚠ LEADERSHIP & MANAGEMENT **BEHAVIORS**

Leadership Behaviors

- Enables nurses to coordinate care
- Creates a vision of high-quality and cost-effective care delivery
- Communicates care management concepts
- Integrates clinical nursing practice
- Evaluates care delivery systems
- Influences policy and organizational systems
- Inspires a multidisciplinary team

Management Behaviors

- Develops critical paths
- Tracks variances

- Integrates clinical nursing practice
- Communicates care management needs
- Organizes nursing care delivery
- Directs others in coordinating care
- Evaluates care coordination
- Influences employees to implement managed care

Overlap Areas

- Integrates clinical nursing practice
- Communicates
- Evaluates care delivery

with clients at the core of care delivery systems. Then the goals, roles, and activities valued by nursing staff, medical staff, critical support services, and other stakeholders can be explored. A new practice model and structure can then be created to be consistent with client characteristics, nursing resources, and available organizational support. Various practice models incorporate dimensions of the following:

- Degree of integration of nursing care given to a client
- Degree of continuity of assignment of nurses to clients
- Type of coordination used to plan and organize care

As nursing care delivery systems evolve, the configuration of these dimensions will need to be addressed and evaluated. Nurse leaders can examine the state of health care management in their organizations and develop strategies to implement coordination of care models to best meet client, organizational, societal, and professional priorities (Kelly, 1992). Given the interdisciplinary nature of case management, model development and success may require a "buy in" by other health care disciplines and other organizational stakeholders. Physicians and hospital administrators are crucial stakeholders for the success of case management programs.

Another leadership and management implication is the human resources deployment of personnel for case management. Who should be a case manager? What roles and functions should case managers be assigned? How much secretarial/clerical support is needed? How will case managers be organized? Given the decision to implement a case management program, leaders and managers will need to make these personnel and systems decisions. In addition, appropriate credentialing for the job is a consideration. Certification typically is an official credential of an individual granted by a nationally recognized agency based on eligibility and passing a national exam. It affirms an advanced degree of competence and is a peer review process (Cesta & Tahan, 2003). Individual certification, as a mark of

professional achievement, is more rigorous than a certificate of attendance or merit and differentiated from accreditation, which is a review of an agency or program. Some accreditation bodies are granting "certification" to programs. This essentially is a certificate of achievement or quality designation.

CURRENT ISSUES AND TRENDS

"Effective and efficient patient management is important in all health care environments because it influences clinical and financial outcomes as well as capacity" (Bower, 2004, p. 39). Case management is a premier strategy to manage patient care within and across settings. This is a major concern in both nursing and health care. Case management operates at the nexus of care coordination of systems and between and among parts of the health care delivery system.

Case management as a process and intervention strategy continues to grow and develop. Trends and issues in case management reflect its complexity and centrality to health care delivery systems.

Crossing the millennium, the first decade of the 2000s is shaping up to be the decade of standardization and precision in case management models. Certification and accreditation are becoming imperatives for case managers and their programs. Multi-interdisciplinary team models are becoming the norm. Automated systems are required for documentation and population health management because they efficiently integrate, identify, risk stratify, capture, and report care trends and alert providers to variance in outcomes. Value and return on investment are imperatives for case management models. Because chronic diseases are on the rise and consume a significant segment of financial resources, disease management programs for populations with chronic diseases also are blossoming and are increasing in sophistication.

Top trends in case management include establishing definitions; shifting case management roles, job functions, and employment settings; and demonstrating outcomes and financial return on investment. Patient safety and other consumer issues have resulted in greater consumer communication and education. Chronic care management is an emerging idea around which the integration of case management and disease management will likely occur. Outcomes research is growing and needs to expand. Nurses are employed by hospitals as case managers; thus the nurse shortage has had an impact on case management. Education for case management needs to be addressed, as well as the confusion around certificates, certification, and continuing education. Multidisciplinary teams are becoming the norm for case management. Relationships with physicians need to be collaborative and collegial. There is a trend toward increasing legislation and rules and regulations in case management practice. Interest in legal and ethical issues in case management practice continues to grow.

Case management is growing as a role and a job for nurses. As organizations struggle with definitions, models, and organizational arrangement choices, nurses will increasingly have opportunities and challenges related to implementing case management roles and functions.

In the shift of nursing care delivery systems toward case management, the balance between nurses' roles may shift. Some of the primary caregiving component may be exchanged for care coordination roles. This is the movement away from service provision and into service coordination as the central component of nurses' practice. The expansion of coordination roles may influence the character and nature of nurse-client relationships (Rheaume et al., 1994). Even case management has undergone radical, rapid change during the past 20 years. Initially, case managers concentrated on catastrophic cases. However, the emphasis now is shifting to focus on population segments, either those specifically at risk or entire populations. Requirements for a broader focus and new technologies for tracking large groups of people have assisted this evolution (Howe, 1999).

Continued pressure for cost-effective health care has pushed payors such as Medicare into managed care arrangements. Managed care organizations use case management as one strategy to control costs.

The nurse case manager is pivotal to overseeing critical paths and facilitating interventions and coordination activities. There is opportunity in the strategic economic importance of the case management process. However, it must be remembered that the common thread weaving through various forms of managed care is the placing of constraints through the use of rewards, penalties, and mandates on both consumers and providers to modify their production/consumption of health care services (Hicks et al., 1992). As systems evolve, new challenges and role changes arise. Many former assumptions about what is appropriate and many former activities and roles will be challenged and rethought. This will take leadership, creativity, innovation, and risk taking.

Another current trend related to case management organizations is the push for accountability and accreditation. For example, the American Accreditation Health Care Commission/Utilization Review Accreditation Commission (URAC) has approved standards for case management organizations. These standards will serve as the basis for accreditation of case management programs. Since a variety of settings and organizational types exist, the standards were designed to accommodate a wide variety of managed care organizations. The standards are divided into nine sections: (1) structure and organization, (2) staff structure and qualifications, (3) staff management and development, (4) information management, (5) quality improvement, (6) oversight of delegated functions, (7) case management process, (8) ethics, and (9) complaints (D'Andrea, 1999).

Summary

- Cost, quality, and access pressures in health care have provided an impetus for case management and managed care.
- Managed care is a clinical system that organizes and sequences caregiving by providers.
- Case management is a system of health assessment and service coordination.
- A critical path is a written plan that identifies key incidents needed to achieve client outcomes.

- *Managed care* is a broader term than *case management.*
- Case management is a nursing care model historically associated with community health nursing but now adapted to acute care hospitals.
- There are a variety of case management models.
- In developing case management programs, both the organization and client populations should be assessed.
- One of nursing's two main roles is care coordinator.
- Organizational structures and nursing care delivery systems need to mesh to support nurses and clients.

Study Questions

1. What are the goals of case management?
2. What are the goals of managed care? How do they compare with those of case management?
3. What are the outcomes anticipated by case management? By managed care?
4. How does case management affect the role of the nurse?
5. Who should be the case manager? Who should lead the multidisciplinary team?
6. Does the public health model apply to hospital settings? Why or why not?
7. Do all clients need case management?

CASE STUDY

The conference room was packed. Tension filled the air. No one wanted to speak up or "tip their hand" by stating a position. The group was gathered to address a serious issue: what to do about the exponential rise in obesity-related health care costs. First, there was the practical matter of illness, disability, and expense associated with the physical and organ-systems damage as a result of nutrition and weight-bearing issues. Then there was the genuine concern for shortened lifespan or decreased quality of life.

However, the pall hanging over the group was an unspoken concern for being labeled as discriminatory toward overweight people. The challenge for the group leader was to initiate a balanced dialogue that moved the group into strategy and action.

The group leader began with a review of the data on incidence and prevalence, local population statistics, the evidence base for health effects, cost figures, and recent media attention on this issue. This generated a lively discussion. Many problems and issues were identified. The next step was to identify a desired action plan. Was it better to implement a case management program for targeted individuals identified as high-risk/high-cost or to implement a disease management program for the entire population?

CRITICAL THINKING EXERCISE

Nurse Christopher Huber works at a community mental health center. The incidence of clients exhibiting problems with dual diagnoses (mental illness plus substance abuse) has been rising. Getting authorization for third-party payment remains a major challenge. Nurse Huber suspects that there is a greater incidence and prevalence of dual diagnosis than appears to be recognized. Little program coordination exists to handle such complex cases. Furthermore, there appears to be a link between dual diagnoses, homelessness, and crime. Nurse Huber has heard that there is some funding available or possible through government payment sources for "case management." He wonders whether case management is effective for clients with dual diagnoses.

1. What is the problem?
2. Whose problem is it?
3. What should Nurse Huber do first?
4. What approach to care coordination should Nurse Huber take?
5. What other resources might Nurse Huber enlist?
6. How can Nurse Huber develop an interdisciplinary approach?

REFERENCES

Allen, J.K., Blumenthal, R.S., Margolis, S., Young, D.R., Miller, E.R. III, & Kelly, K. (2002). Nurse case management of hypercholesterolemia in patients with coronary heart disease: Results of a randomized clinical trial. *American Heart Journal, 144*(4), 678-686.

American Nurses Association (ANA). (1988). *Nursing Case Management* (Publ. No. NS-32). Kansas City, MO: ANA.

American Nurses Credentialing Center (ANCC). (2004). *ANCC certification: Specialty nursing, nursing administration (Basic, Advanced) clinical nurse specialist (Community Health & Home Health).* Washington, DC: ANCC.

Aubert, R.E., Herman, W.H., Waters, J., Moore, W., Sutton, D., Peterson, B.L., et al. (1998). Nurse case management to improve glycemic control in diabetic patients in a health maintenance organization: A randomized, controlled trial. *Annals of Internal Medicine, 129*(8), 605-612.

Beilman, J.P., Sowell, R.L., Knox, M., & Phillips, K.D. (1998). Case management at what expense? A case study of the emotional costs of case management. *Nursing Case Management, 3*(2), 89 95.

Birmingham, J. (1996). How to apply CMSA's standards of practice for case management in a capitated environ ment. *Journal of Care Management, 2*(5), 9-10, 12, 14, 16-18, 20, 22.

Bower, K.A. (1992). *Case management by nurses.* Kansas City, MO: American Nurses Publishing.

Bower, K.A. (2004). Patient care management as a global nursing concern. *Nursing Administration Quarterly, 28*(1), 39-43.

Braden, C.J. (2002). *State of the science paper #2: Involvement/participation, empowerment and knowledge outcome indicators of case management.* Little Rock, AR: Case Management Society of America.

Case Management Society of America (CMSA). (2002). *Standards of practice for case management.* Little Rock, AR: CMSA.

Case Management Society of America (CMSA). (2004a). *CMSA history.* Little Rock, AR: CMSA. Retrieved July 15, 2004, from *www.cmsa.org/Aboutus/History.aspx*

Case Management Society of America (CMSA). (2004b). *CMSA's state of the science papers.* Little Rock, AR: CMSA. Retrieved July 15, 2004, from *www.cmsa.org/Products/StateOfTheSciencePapers.aspx*

Centers for Medicare & Medicaid Services (CMS). (2003). Medicare program; demonstration: Capitated disease management for beneficiaries with chronic illnesses. *Federal Register, 68*(40), 9673-9680.

Cesta, T.G., & Tahan, H.A. (2003). *The case manager's survival guide: Winning strategies for clinical practice* (2nd ed.). St Louis: Mosby.

Chan, F., Leahy, M.J., McMahon, B.Y., Mirch, M., & DeVinney, D. (1999). Foundational knowledge and major practice domains of case management. *Journal of Care Management, 5*(1), 10-30.

Clark, K.A. (1996). Alternate case management models. In D.L. Flarey & S.S. Blancett (Eds.), *Handbook of nursing case management* (pp. 295-304). Gaithersburg, MD: Aspen.

Cline, B.G. (1990). Case management: Organizational models and administrative methods. *Caring, 9*(7), 14-18.

Cole, L., & Houston, S. (1999). Structured care methodologies: Evolution and use in patient care delivery. *Outcomes Management for Nursing Practice, 3*(2), 53-59.

Coleman, J.R. (1999). Integrated case management: The 21st century challenge for HMO case managers, Part 1. *The Case Manager, 10*(5), 28-34.

Commission for Case Manager Certification (CCMC). (2004). *Case manager certification. CCMC backgrounder. About case management.* Rolling Meadows, IL: CCMC. Retrieved July 15, 2004, from *www.ccmcertification.org/pages/12frame_cat123.html*

Conti, R.M. (1996). Nurse case manager roles: Implications for practice and education. *Nursing Administration Quarterly, 21*(1), 67-80.

Cook, T.H. (1998). The effectiveness of inpatient case management: Fact or fiction? *Journal of Nursing Administration, 28*(4), 36-46.

D'Andrea, G. (1999). URAC finalizes accreditation standards for case management organizations. *The Case Manager, 10*(5), 23-25.

Dzyacky, S.C. (1998). An acute care case management model for nurses and social workers. *Nursing Case Management, 3*(5), 208-215.

Erkel, E.E. (1993). The impact of case management in preventive services. *Journal of Nursing Administration, 23*(1), 27-32.

Falk, C., & Bower, K. (1994). Managing care across department, organization, and setting boundaries. *Series on Nursing Administration, 6,* 161-176.

Fitzgerald, J.F., Smith, D.M., Martin, D.K., Freedman, J.A., & Katz, B.P. (1994). A case manager intervention to reduce readmissions. *Archives of Internal Medicine, 154*(15), 1721-1729.

Forbes, M.A. (1999). The practice of professional nurse case management. *Nursing Case Management, 4*(1), 28-33.

Goodwin, D.R. (1994). Nursing case management activities: How they differ between employment settings. *Journal of Nursing Administration, 24*(2), 29-34.

Goodwin, J.S., Satish, S., Anderson, E.T., Nattinger, A.B. & Freeman, J.L. (2003). Effect of nurse case management on the treatment of older women with breast cancer. *Journal of the American Geriatrics Society, 51*(9), 1252-1259.

Grimaldi, P.L. (1996). A glossary of managed care terms. *Nursing Management,* Special Supplement (October), *27*(10), 5-7.

Hampton, D. (1993). Implementing a managed care framework through care maps. *Journal of Nursing Administration, 23*(5), 21-27.

Harrison, J.P., Nolin, J., & Suero, E. (2004). The effect of case management on U.S. hospitals. *Nursing Economic$, 22*(2), 64-70.

Haw, M.A. (1996). Case management education in universities: A national survey. *Journal of Care Management, 2*(6), 10-23.

Hawkins, J.W., Veeder, N.W., & Pearce, C.W. (1998). *Nurse-social worker collaboration in managed care.* New York: Springer.

Hicks, L., Stallmeyer, J., & Coleman, J. (1992). Nursing challenges in managed care. *Nursing Economic$, 10*(4), 265-276.

Hinitz-Satterfield, P., Miller, E., & Hagan, E. (1993). Managed care and new roles for nursing: Utilization and case management in a health maintenance organization. *Series on Nursing Administration, 5,* 83-99.

Howe, R. (1999). Case management in managed care: Past, present, future. *The Case Manager, 10*(5), 37-40.

Huber, D.L. (2005). The diversity of service delivery models. *Disease management: A guide for case managers.* Philadelphia: Saunders.

Kelly, K. (1992). Managing care: A search for role clarity. *Journal of Nursing Administration, 22*(3), 9-10.

Laramee, A.S., Levinsky, S.K., Sargent, J., Ross, R., & Callas, P. (2003). Case management in a heterogeneous congestive heart failure population: A randomized controlled trial. *Archives of Internal Medicine, 163*(7), 809-817.

Lee, J. (1993). A history of care modalities in nursing. *Series on Nursing Administration, 5,* 20-38.

Levitt, D.A., Starz, T.W., & Higgins, R. (1998). Disease state case management in an academic medical center utilizing osteoarthritis-of-the-knee model. *Journal of Care Management, 4*(5), 45, 48, 51-52, 54, 56.

Mark, B. (1992). Characteristics of nursing practice models. *Journal of Nursing Administration, 22*(11), 57-63.

McClure, M. (1991). Introduction. In I.E. Goertzen (Ed.), *Differentiating nursing practice: Into the twenty-first century* (pp. 1-11). Kansas City, MO: American Academy of Nursing.

Mikulencak, M. (1993). Public health stands as a proven model for future delivery systems. *The American Nurse, 25*(6), 18.

National Association of Social Workers (NASW). (1992). *NASW standards for social work case management.* Washington, DC: NASW.

Norris, S.L., Nichols, P.J., Caspersen, C.J., Glasgow, R.E., Engelgau, M.M., Jack, L. Jr., et al. (2002). The effectiveness of disease and case management for people with diabetes: A systematic review. *American Journal of Preventive Medicine, 22*(4 Suppl), 1-25.

Raiff, N.R., & Shore, B.K. (1993). *Advanced case management: New strategies for the nineties.* Newbury Park, CA: Sage.

Renholm, M., Leino-Kilpi, H., & Suominen, T. (2002). Critical pathways: A systematic review. *Journal of Nursing Administration, 32*(4), 196-202.

Rheaume, A., Frisch, S., Smith, A., & Kennedy, C. (1994). Case management and nursing practice. *Journal of Nursing Administration, 24*(3), 30-36.

Ridgely, M.S., & Willenbring, M.C. (1992). Application of case management to drug abuse treatment: Overview of models and research issues. *NIDA Monograph, 127,* 12-33.

Riegel, B., Carlson, B., Kopp, Z., LePetri, B., Glaser, B., & Unger, A. (2002). Effect of a standardized nurse case-management telephone intervention on resource use in patients with chronic heart failure. *Archives of Internal Medicine, 162*(6), 705-712.

Sesperez, J., Wilson, S., Jalaludin, B., Seger, M., & Sugrue, M. (2001). Trauma case management and clinical pathways: Prospective evaluation of their effect on selected patient outcomes in five key trauma conditions. *Journal of Trauma: Injury Infection and Critical Care, 50*(4), 643-649.

Shortell, S.M., Anderson, D.A., Gilles, R.R., Mitchell, J.B., & Morgan, K.L. (1993). The holographic organization. *Healthcare Forum Journal, 36*(2), 20-26.

Siefker, J.M., Garrett, M.B., Van Genderen, A., & Weis, M.J. (1998). *Fundamentals of case management: Guidelines for practicing case managers.* St Louis: Mosby.

Simpson, R. (1993). Case-managed care in tomorrow's information network. *Nursing Management, 24*(7), 14-16.

Tahan, H.A. (1996). A ten-step process to develop case management plans. *Nursing Case Management, 1*(3), 112-121.

Tahan, H.A. (1998). Case management: A heritage more than a century old. *Nursing Case Management, 3*(2), 55-60.

Ward, M.D., & Rieve, J.A. (1997). The role of case management in disease management. In W.E. Todd, & D. Nash (Eds.), *Disease management: A systems approach to improving patient outcomes* (pp. 235-259). Chicago: American Hospital Publishing.

Weil, M., & Karls, J.M. (1985). *Case management in human service practice: A systematic approach to mobilizing resources for clients.* San Francisco: Jossey-Bass.

Weiman, M.G. (1995). Case management. A means to improve quality and control the costs of cure in children with acute myelogenous leukemia. *Journal of Pediatric Hematology and Oncology, 17*(3), 248-253.

Zander, K. (1990). Case management: A golden opportunity for whom? In J. McCloskey & H. Grace (Eds.), *Current issues in nursing* (3rd ed.) (pp. 199-204). St Louis: Mosby.

Zander, K. (1991). Case management in acute care: Making the connections. *The Case Manager, 2*(1), 39-43.

Zander, K. (1992). Nursing care delivery methods and quality. *Series on Nursing Administration, 3,* 86-104.

Zander, K. (1994). Nurses and case management: To control or collaborate? In J. McCloskey & H. Grace (Eds.), *Current issues in nursing* (4th ed.) (pp. 254-260). St Louis: Mosby.

Zander, K. (2002). Nursing case management in the 21st century: Intervening where margin meets mission. *Nursing Administration Quarterly, 26*(5), 58-67.

Zitter, M. (1997). A new paradigm in health care delivery: Disease management. In W.E. Todd & D. Nash (Eds.), *Disease management: A systems approach to improving patient outcomes* (pp. 1-25). Chicago: American Hospital Publishing.

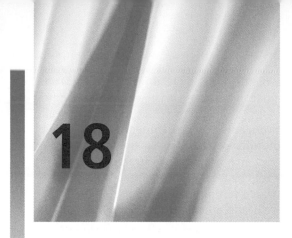

18

Disease Management

Diane L. Huber

CHAPTER OBJECTIVES

- Identify disease and population-based care management forces
- Define and describe disease management and population-based care management
- Discuss distinguishing features of disease management
- Outline the process of population-based program planning
- Illustrate population-based risk assessment
- Integrate chronic conditions care with disease management
- Examine current trends in disease management and population-based care
- Exercise critical thinking to conceptualize and analyze possible solutions to a practice exercise

Disease management (DM) is an important and effective intervention designed to coordinate care and services delivery for better outcomes and lower costs. It is one of three initiatives that are used in the realm of coordination of care: case management, DM, and population health management. First is case management, which basically involves an intensive focus on an individual patient in relation to one or more health conditions. Case management is often triggered by complex, high-cost, or high-volume conditions. The second initiative is DM, which moves up a level of aggregation. DM generally involves an intensive focus on a disease or health condition of a population group, which is subsequently applied to individuals. It often is used to address chronic conditions. The third initiative, which moves up yet another level of aggregation, is population health management (PHM). PHM is a community-based population strategy, such as devising health strategies for all adolescents in a school system or all elders in a community. DM, then, is a population-based strategy for the management of groups needing specialized health care services.

Two major forces have triggered the rise and proliferation of DM programs: (1) the proliferation of managed care systems as a prevailing form of organized health care delivery [the influence of health plans] and (2) the national attention generated by the Institute of Medicine's (IOM, 2004) health care quality initiative, *Crossing the Quality Chasm: The IOM Health Care Quality Initiative.* Health plans led the charge to address the care coordination and service integration needs of clusters of members who had identifiable health conditions, generally chronic in nature. The IOM launched in 1996 an ongoing effort focused on the assessment and improvement of the United States' quality of health care. Now in its third phase, the IOM's 2001 document, *Crossing the Quality Chasm: A New Health System for the 21st Century,* highlighted the need for profound changes in the environment of care, including revamping practices that fragment the care system. The report identified the coordination of care across patient conditions, services, and settings over time as a major organizational challenge yet a key dimension of patient-centered care.

Certain diseases manifest in clinical conditions that need careful, extended management in order to achieve the greatest possible health or quality of life and avoid potentially large costs. In an acute care, episodic-based care and reimbursement system, care coordination is too often ignored by providers.

Disease management programs were developed and implemented largely as managed care health plan initiatives. They have evolved into proven and effective strategies to make groups of individuals healthier while saving scarce health care coverage dollars (Lipold, 2002). The federal government's Centers for Medicare & Medicaid Services (CMS) has taken notice of DM programs, sponsored DM demonstration projects, and encouraged contracting with DM vendors for outsourced medical management programs (Lewis, 2004) because DM has been found to be effective in selected populations.

Disease management efforts usually target people with chronic conditions for which long-term management, patient education, and close monitoring of symptoms can minimize or prevent complications and acute exacerbations. Reducing emergency department visits and hospitalizations saves money and is better for the health of people. Thus DM programs aim to help individuals cope with chronic conditions in a way that reduces detrimental clinical and functional effects and the need for and cost of medical care (Johnson, 2003).

There is widespread recognition that health care delivery can and must be improved. Clearly, the pressures to provide access to care, maintain a high level of quality, and control expenditures are converging on a traditionally fragmented and acute care-focused system. Projections are that sociodemographic and economic tidal waves are set to converge into a "perfect storm" of crisis over health care in the near future. These tidal waves include the aging of the U.S. population, the effect of the maturing of the Baby Boom generation, high pharmaceutical costs, advancing medical technology, dramatic increases in chronic health conditions, and U.S. government budget deficits. The solutions are not easy or obvious. However, DM is one major innovative strategy that is being closely watched, carefully analyzed, and undergoing research testing to determine its potential to improve health outcomes across multiple populations while lowering costs and improving patient satisfaction with care delivery (Huber, 2005).

In addition, the community has become a more viable focus of care than at any other time in the past 60 years (Naylor & Buhler-Wilkerson, 1999). Social and economic pressures demand that health care organizations focus on ways to provide cost-effective population-based care. Hall (1998) stated, "In a capitated, managed-care environment, health care organizations contract to provide the entire continuum of care to a given population at a per capital rate" (p. 40). Thus viability rests on the ability to respond appropriately to the needs of a specific population group. This requires accurate identification of the population's needs along with subsequent development of essential, relevant, and cost-effective programs that provide planned interventions and create aggregate change (Hall, 1998).

DEFINITIONS

Disease Management

To better understand **disease management (DM),** the term needs to be defined and differentiated from similar terms. Although there are various definitions of disease management, the standardized definition is the one developed by the Disease Management Association of America (DMAA; *www.dmaa.org*), the professional trade organization that represents the disease management community. The definition of disease management promulgated by DMAA is as follows:

> Disease management is a system of coordinated health care interventions and communications

⚠ LEADING & MANAGING **DEFINED**

Disease Management	**Population-Based Care Management**
A comprehensive, integrated approach to care and reimbursement based on a disease's natural course.	The integration and coordination of health services to a specified population.
Population	**Community**
A collection of individuals who have in common one or more personal or environmental characteristics.	A locally based entity composed of systems of formal organizations reflecting societal institutions, informal groups, and aggregates.

for populations with conditions in which patient self-care efforts are significant. Disease management:

- Supports the physician or practitioner/ patient relationship and plan of care,
- Emphasizes prevention of exacerbations and complications utilizing evidence-based practice guidelines and patient empowerment strategies, and
- Evaluates clinical, humanistic, and economic outcomes on an going [sic] basis with the goal of improving overall health. (2004, p. 1)

It is seductive to think of disease management as the management of a disease. At least two major characteristics that distinguish disease management programs would be overlooked by viewing this strategy as the medical management of a disease. First, this would imply that disease management fell within the domain of physician practice. DMAA has stressed the multidisciplinary nature of disease management, although medical care is a central component. Clearly, the management effort in disease management programs is aimed at a population or group, and it is targeted at health, not just the cure of diseases. Second, this would imply that only diseases were of concern. This connotation would leave out behavioral health domains and other conditions such as obesity or high-risk pregnancies. Although discrete and specific diseases are a large segment of disease management efforts, it is important to revisit the definitions and note the emphasis on

populations and conditions. Some advocate the use of "population health management" as a substitute for "disease management" because it is more specific to the breadth of disease management efforts. Zitter (1997) noted that population-based care was based on disease management principles. The Chronic Care Model (Improving Chronic Illness Care, 2004; Wagner, 1998) best displays a population health management conceptualization of chronic disease management (Figure 18.1).

The following six components of any disease management program have been identified by DMAA:

1. Population identification processes
2. Evidence-based practice guidelines
3. Collaborative practice models to include physician and support-service providers
4. Patient self-management education (may include primary prevention, behavior modification programs, and compliance/surveillance)
5. Process and outcomes measurement, evaluation, and management
6. Routine reporting/feedback loop (may include communication with patient, physician, health plan and ancillary providers, and practice profiling)

According to DMAA, "Full Service Disease Management Programs must include all 6 components. Programs consisting of fewer components are Disease Management Support Services" (2004, p. 1).

These components have been reformulated into a flow schematic model by Wilson and

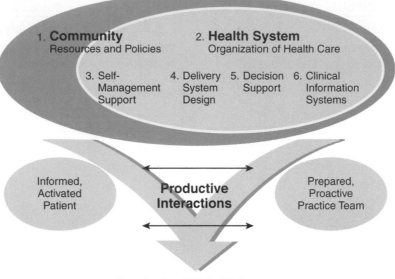

Figure 18.1
The Chronic Care Model. (From Wagner, E.H. [1998]. Chronic disease management: What will it take to improve care for chronic illness? *Effective Clinical Practice, 1,* 2-4. Copyright American College of Physicians, Philadelphia.)

MacDowell (2003), where population selection and evidence-based guidelines flow to providers and patients, which flow to measures and evaluation, which has a feedback loop to providers and patients. The DMAA components have been formulated into an evaluation checklist in Table 18.1.

Related Definitions

To help readers understand the concept of disease management (DM), several related definitions are presented. The first major distinction is between case management and DM.

Case Management Defined

There are two major definitions of case management that emerge from among a variety of definitions in the field. The first is the definition established by the Case Management Society of America (CMSA), the major professional association representing case management practice. This is considered to be the generally accepted

standardized definition. CMSA's definition of case management is as follows:

> Case management is a collaborative process of assessment, planning, facilitation, and advocacy for options and services to meet an individual's health needs through communication and available resources to promote quality cost-effective outcomes. (2002, p. 1)

The definition by the Commission for Case Manager Certification (CCMC) remains the consensus definition adopted by a consortium of case management groups and first issued in 1995. The CCMC definition of case management follows:

> Case management is a collaborative process that assesses, plans, implements, coordinates, monitors, and evaluates options and services required to meet an individual's health needs, using communication and available resources to promote quality, cost-effective outcomes. (2004, p. 2)

Table 18.1

Checklist to Evaluate Disease Management Programs		
Component	Present (yes); Absent (no)	Specific Method or Metric Used
Population identification and selection		
Risk assessment		
Risk stratification		
Use of evidence-based practice guidelines		
Type of practice model		
Collaborative mechanism		
Single-discipline predominates (identify)		
Patient self-management		
Education		
Primary prevention		
Behavior modification		
Lifestyle change motivation		
Telephone contact		
Health advocates		
Compliance/adherence		
Surveillance		
Process, outcomes management		
Process identification and measurement		
Process evaluation		
Outcomes identification and measurement		
Outcomes evaluation		
Process and outcomes management		
Feedback loop		
Communication to:		
Patient		
Physician		
Health plan		
Ancillary providers		
Practice profiling		

From Coggeshall Press. (2004). Coralville: IA.

Other case management definitions exist. Most are discipline-specific and promulgated by professional organizations representing provider disciplines such as nursing, pharmacy, or social work. Of note is an attempt to formulate a "consumer friendly" definition of case management by the Case Management Leadership Coalition (CMLC). This definition is "Case managers work with people to get the health care and other community services they need, when they need them, and for the best value" (CMSA, 2004, p. 37).

Differentiation of Case Management and Disease Management

It is not immediately clear or obvious how case management and DM are the same or different. This has caused some confusion in the field. Ward and Rieve (1997) noted that DM could be defined

Case Management	...two sides of the same coin...	Disease Management
Assessment	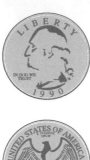	Population identification processes
		Evidence-based practice guidelines
Planning		Collaborative practice models to include physician and support-service providers
		Patient self-management education (may include primary prevention, behavior modification programs, and compliance/surveillance)
Facilitation		Process and outcomes measurement, evaluation, and management
Advocacy		Routine reporting/feedback loop (may include communication with patient, physician, health plan and ancillary providers, and practice profiling).

Figure 18.2

Differentiation of case management and disease management. (From Coggeshall Press. [2004]. Coralville, IA.)

as proactive case management. Case management and DM are distinct and separate strategies, but there is a considerable area of overlap because both are interventions designed to coordinate care for better outcomes and lowered costs. Thus case management and DM might be thought of as looking at two sides of the same coin. Figure 18.2 displays this visually.

Case management generally involves work with an intensive focus on coordinating the care of the individual client in relationship to one or more diseases or health conditions. DM generally involves intensive focus on a disease or health condition in relationship primarily to a population group, with application subsequently to individuals. DM is more population-based than client-centered and more proactive in approach than episodic (Huston, 2001).

Thus case management and DM are two different strategies, employed at two different levels of aggregation. The focus (individual vs. group, episode vs. continuum) varies. However, both are critical interventions for coordination of care and integration of systems.

Other Related Definitions

Concepts of health promotion, the continuum of care, and population health are related to understanding DM. These terms are each defined next.

Health Promotion

The *American Journal of Health Promotion* promulgated the following definition:

> Health promotion is the science and art of helping people change their lifestyle to move toward a state of optimal health. Optimal health is defined as a balance of physical, emotional, social, spiritual, and intellectual health. Lifestyle change can be facilitated through a combination of efforts to enhance awareness, change behavior and create environments that support good health practices. Of the three, supportive environments will probably have the greatest impact in producing lasting change. (1989, pp. 1-2)

This definition clearly outlines health as having the following five distinct domains:

Physical:	Fitness. Nutrition. Medical self-care. Control of substance abuse.
Emotional:	Care for emotional crisis. Stress management.
Social:	Communities. Families. Friends.
Intellectual:	Educational. Achievement. Career development.
Spiritual:	Love. Hope. Charity. (*American Journal of Health Promotion*, 1989, p. 2)

Continuum of Care

A continuum of care is a linkage of health services across health care delivery settings and sites of care. In one view of the continuum of care, Aurora Health Care (2004) listed prevention and early detection, family and community services, primary and specialty care, pharmacies, behavioral health care, emergency care, hospital care, rehabilitation, home care, long-term care, and end-of-life care as components of their continuum of care. From a systems integration perspective, Aikman and colleagues (1998) divided the continuum of care into community care and acute care, with community care on either side of acute care in three overlapping circles. The continuum contained health promotion/illness prevention, public health, primary care, diagnostics/drugs, ambulatory care, acute inpatient, rehabilitative/chronic, long-term care, home services, and palliative care segments.

Both DM and case management programs will vary according to the specific characteristics of the setting of service delivery, the target population, and the scope of the continuum of care. The setting may be acute care, long-term care, community health, or other settings. The target population may be a specific medical disease, chronic condition, age cohort, insurance group members, catchment area, or other group. The continuum of care may be conceived of as within a facility, across the lifespan, across specific transitions, or other defined episode or time span. Clarity in the specification of what the continuum of care encompasses is important for understanding and comparing disease and case management programs.

Population Health Approach

Health Canada noted that using a population health approach signals a shift in thinking to a broader view of health as a capacity or resource, not merely the absence of disease, as follows:

> Population health is an approach to health that aims to improve the health of the entire population and to reduce health inequities among population groups. In order to reach these objectives, it looks at and acts upon the broad range of factors and conditions that have a strong influence on our health. (2004, p. 1)

Income, education, the environment, and biology are examples of broader factors that impact health.

Population-based health care is focused on aggregates and communities. The basic definition of a **population** is a "collection of individuals who have in common one or more personal or environmental characteristics" (Williams, 1996, p. 25). Also called an aggregate, the members of a community who are defined in terms of geography, special interest, disease state, or another common characteristic are a population. The research-related term is *target population*. In community health, population-focused practice is directed toward care for defined populations or subpopulations as opposed to care for individual clients (Williams, 1996). **Population-based care management** is defined as the integration and coordination of health services to a specified population.

A **community** is defined as "a locally-based entity, composed of systems of formal organizations reflecting societal institutions, informal groups, and aggregates. These components are interdependent, and their function is to meet a wide variety of collective needs" (Schuster & Goeppinger, 1996, p. 290). The term *community* can include groups of diverse or similar people living in one geographic location; an interactive link of families, friends and organizations; or systems or groups bound by shared needs and interests (Carroll, 2004). The concept of community includes dimensions of people, place, and function. The community is considered to be the client when the nursing focus is on the collective or common good rather than on the health of an individual. Thus community-oriented nursing practice is directed toward healthy change for the whole community's benefit. The unit of service may be individuals, families, groups, aggregates, institutions, or communities, but the purpose is to affect the entire community (Schuster & Goeppinger, 1996). Thus the term *community* denotes a local entity, whereas the term *population* refers to an aggregate with any common characteristic (not necessarily tied to a place).

The term *community health* involves meeting the collective needs of a group by identifying problems and managing interactions both within the community and between the community and the larger society. Risk factors, health status indicators, functional ability levels, health promotion, health outcomes, and prevention of identified chronic diseases are the focus of data gathering, program planning, and implementation processes and activities. Community participation and partnership are key concepts because active participation in a decision-making process induces a vested interest in the success of any effort to improve the health of a community. Community partnership is a basic tenet of community-oriented approaches. For nurses, the concept of community as client directs the nursing focus to the collective or common good instead of individual health. Population-based care draws on partnership and community as client concepts. These community health concepts also foster culturally competent health care services (Schuster & Goeppinger, 1996).

BACKGROUND

Chronic health conditions pose a formidable challenge to the health care delivery system. The management of chronic conditions is a particular burden for health care payors and employers. Chronic disease creates two particular difficulties for businesses. First, these conditions

---

 Research Note

Source: Boult, C., Kessler, J., Urdangarin, C., Boult, L., & Yedidia, P. (2004). Identifying workers at risk for high health care expenditures: A short questionnaire. *Disease Management, 7*(2), 124-135.

Purpose

Keeping workers healthy and therefore on the job is a prime concern of many employers. Workers' use of health care services can be predicted to some extent by medical conditions and lifestyle habits. Early identification of those at risk allows early intervention. The purpose of this study was to develop and measure the predictive accuracy of a brief questionnaire for risk designed to screen new employees. The 53-item Good Health Survey health risk appraisal instrument was mailed to 15,496 unionized California food processing workers, and researchers obtained records of eligible respondents' (n = 827 of 5656 respondents) health insurance expenditures over the following year. Chi square and multiple linear regression were the statistical methods used.

Discussion

Using multiple linear regression techniques, 8 of the 53 items were identified as predicting future expenditures most accurately. They are the following: age 50+ years, male sex, arthritis causing pain most days, high cholesterol, diabetes, cancer, regular use of medication, and 3+ clinic/MD visits in the previous year. A regression formula for predicting total insurance expenditures was derived. The formula was tested on transportation workers (n = 7445) and their dependents (n = 5562), where respondents classified as high risk had health insurance expenditures 2.4 and 1.8 times greater, respectively, than those identified by the formula as low risk.

Application to Practice

Because response rates partially depend on the length of a questionnaire, condensing to an 8-item form is an important data collection advantage. This 8-item questionnaire and its scoring formula can identify high-risk groups of workers predicted to have high health care expenditures. Organizations can use this tool to identify workers for case management and disease management interventions.

in the workforce lead to diminished productivity. Second, these conditions result in a greater portion of the business's revenue being diverted into health care expenditures (Javors et al., 2003). Further effects are seen on the health care delivery system, society, and individuals' functioning and activities. Of particular concern is the increasing trend of chronic illness in relatively younger people (Javors et al., 2003).

Population and health trends are tracked by governmental agencies such as the U.S. Census Bureau, Centers for Disease Control and Prevention, Bureau of Labor Statistics, and Health Resources and Services Administration, as well as private foundations and organizations. Table 18.2 provides information about these agencies. Clearly, health and health care delivery systems data are continually in flux. However, the available statistics are impressive.

Approximately $1 trillion is spent per year on health care, and about 75% of direct health care expenditures goes to treat chronic diseases and their complications, many of which are preventable (Javors et al., 2003). Almost 50% of all Americans report having one or more chronic diseases. The estimates are that in 2005, 112 million people will have a chronic health condition, costing $539 billion. By 2010 the estimates are for 120 million people and $582 billion in costs (Nobel & Norman, 2003). As Baby Boomers, a group including 28% of the total U.S. population

in 2000 (U.S. Census Bureau, 2001), age in the next decade, chronic disease numbers are projected to rapidly rise. Costs are a considerable pressure, since on average individuals with chronic conditions cost 3.5 times as much to serve as others, and they account for a large proportion of services (80% of all bed days and 69% of hospital admissions) (Nobel & Norman, 2003). The chronic conditions that pose a particular economic burden but can be helped by disease management are characterized by high prevalence, high expense, relatively standardized treatment guidelines, and a significant role played by the member's behavior on the progression of the condition (Cousins & Liu, 2003).

Other forces of change sweeping in DM programs include the following (Ho, 2003):

- Highest health care cost trends in a decade
- Weak economy and softer labor market
- Increase in consumerism
- Heightened demand for increased quality and patient safety
- Up to 300% variance in provider costs and quality

Thus DM has arisen as a major strategy to address these concerns. Attractive features include effective population management, coordination of care for chronic conditions, consistency of care for at-risk populations, customization of care support, encouragement of adherence to treatment, and proactive interventions.

Disease Management Programs

DM programs offered by health plans can be developed in-house or purchased either from a vendor or another organization such as a hospital. In a stratified random sample of 65 health plans, all of which were members of the American Association of Health Plans (AAHP), 64% of the diabetes DM programs were developed in-house, 27% were purchased from a vendor, and 9% were purchased from other sources (Welch et al., 2002). A recent development in the field is employers contracting directly with DM providers. It has been estimated that there are about 200 DM-related service programs available from health

Table 18.2

U.S. Agencies Tracking Population and Health Trends	
Agency	Website Address
U.S. Census Bureau	*www.census.gov*
Centers for Disease Control and Prevention (CDC)	*www.cdc.gov*
Bureau of Labor Statistics	*www.bls.gov*
Health Resources and Services Administration	*www.hrsa.gov*

plans, hospitals, pharmacy benefit management and pharmaceutical companies, and companies specializing in DM (Lipold, 2002).

Proactive outreach is a major strategy of DM programs. Nursing outreach programs are the core element. Personal communications (usually via telephone) between an expert nurse and the health plan participant build a personal relationship, help identify knowledge deficits and counseling needs, facilitate close monitoring and progress toward goals, enhance treatment adherence, and promote clinical and cost stabilization.

The personal nurse, functioning as a personal health advisor, establishes a single point of contact and coordination of care and service for patients having health problems and promotes a trusting relationship. Whether employed by health plan or a contracted outside vendor, the DM provided by nurses functioning as personal health advisors and advocates is central to effective outcomes.

The core of the DM concept is to comprehensively integrate care and reimbursement based on a disease or health condition's natural course. Both clinical and nonclinical interventions are timed to occur where and when they are most likely to have the greatest impact. This sequencing and targeting ideally prevents occurrences or exacerbations, decreases the use of expensive resources, and creates positive health outcomes through the use of prevention and proactive case management strategies. Chronic conditions are the focus, and systematic ways of delivering health care interventions to patients with similar characteristics are the methods used (Zitter, 1997). DM models focus on the identification, conformity, and coordination of a continuum of care across populations with the same or similar disease process (Ward & Rieve, 1997).

Disease Management Models

DMAA has not offered a conceptual model of DM beyond its definition. However, there are two useful models, one for case management and one for DM, that visually illustrate concepts related to population health management across the continuum of care. The case management model (Coggeshall Press, 2004) (Figure 18.3) depicts case management following traditional public health concepts and incorporating concepts of the Pareto Law (2004). The pyramid shows a base of strategies applied to all members, with gradual narrowing and focusing of interventions for greater precision and conservation of resources. Applied to DM, the pyramid visual can be drawn simply as wellness, DM, and case management (Figure 18.4). A model integrating both DM and case management is depicted in Figure 18.5. The entire population (base of the triangle) would be targeted for prevention and assessed for risk identification and stratification. Care coordination and DM would be used for those individuals identified as at-risk. Then case management would be applied as an intervention for the 10% to 20% of the population projected to need intensive intervention, surveillance, and follow-up for complex care needs.

The second model was reported in the literature (Ho, 2003) as PacifiCare Health System's approach to DM. Using the same pyramid visual, segments started at the base with preventive health management (e.g., screening and education), followed by acute episode management, DM, special population care, and catastrophic care management of

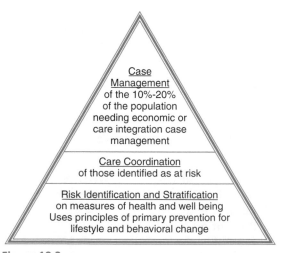

Figure 18.3
Case management model. (From Coggeshall Press. [1999]. Coralville, IA.)

Research Note

Source: Patel, P.H., Welsh, C., & Foggs, M.B. (2004). Improved asthma outcomes using a coordinated care approach in a large medical group. *Disease Management, 7*(2), 102-111.

Purpose

Asthma affects more than 14 million people with costs at $11.3 billion per year. The purpose of this study was to discuss the development of a multidisciplinary asthma disease management (DM) program in one large medical group practice in an urban area and evaluate its outcomes as of 2001. Population data were analyzed from an administrative claims database (n = 3486) at baseline of 1 year (1998-1999) and compared with the follow-up time frame (1999-2000). A medical record audit was conducted to examine recorded adherence with asthma guidelines and documentation. The DM intervention was the development of the patient registry, systematic assessment of asthma control using the Asthma Therapy Assessment Questionnaire, nurse case management, and physician education.

Discussion

At baseline, disease control problems were frequent, and 34% of adult respondents reported missing work because of asthma. Documentation needs for written treatment plans were uncovered. Beneficial results from the program included improved medical record documentation and patient education. Emergency Department visits and hospitalization as related to asthma showed statistically significant decreases. The authors suggested that the greatest determinant of the overall success of the program was a realization that improving patient outcomes is a shared goal of the entire system. This led to the redesign of care processes to improve coordination and continuity of care.

Application to Practice

This DM program was comprehensive and involved an important clinical process redesign using patient and provider education and case management. The program was successful and sustainable based on significant improvement in several essential processes of care and in ED and hospitalization events. These results support the replication of similar programs in other organizations.

complex cases. Such conceptual models assist with understanding and communicating the array of programs and the level at which each is targeted. The coverage of the continuum of care is evident.

A related model that emphasizes aspects of chronic care is called the Chronic Care Model (see Figure 18.1). This model identifies the essential elements of a health care system and community that encourage high-quality chronic disease care. The six basic elements are (1) the community, (2) the health system, (3) self-management support, (4) delivery system design, (5) decision support, and (6) clinical information systems. Developed by the staff of the MacColl Institute for Healthcare Innovation and supported by the Robert Wood Johnson Foundation, the model can be applied to a variety of chronic illnesses, health care

settings, and target populations. The model is being tested by the Improving Chronic Illness Care program. Themes of care coordination and case management fall under the basic elements (Improving Chronic Illness Care, 2004; Wagner, 1998).

History

The genesis of the rise of DM occurred in the late 1980s and into the decade of the 1990s in the U.S. health care delivery system. Nested within the general evolution of case management practice, managed care organizations and health plans began to look closely at DM after initial case management programs had been launched. Further refinements in program quality and cost savings were desired. With some experience in case management to draw upon, the unique challenges of

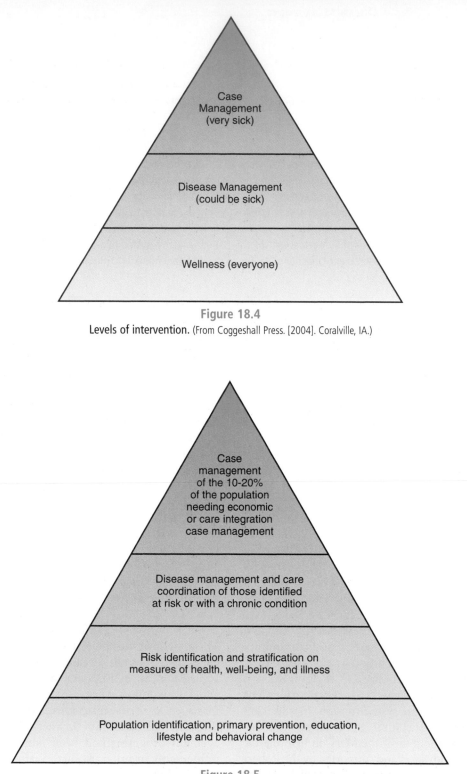

Figure 18.4
Levels of intervention. (From Coggeshall Press. [2004]. Coralville, IA.)

Figure 18.5
Integrated model. (From Coggeshall Press. [2004]. Coralville, IA.)

chronic conditions occurring on a large scale needed to be addressed. In pharmaceutical companies, DM emerged as a way to encourage medication adherence.

DM programs became evident in the 1990s with selected visible exemplars. Programs grew and spread rapidly. Todd and Nash's book *Disease Management: A Systems Approach to Improving Patient Outcomes* was published in 1997. In 1999 DMAA was organized. The years since then have seen the growth and increased sophistication of these broader DM programs for populations with chronic conditions. In a stratified random sample survey of 65 health plans in 2000, Welch and colleagues (2002) found that the prevalence of DM programs in health plans increased considerably between 1996 and 2000. Prevalence rates increased from 45% to 83% for diabetes, from 50% to 77% for asthma, and from 14% to 57% for congestive heart failure. These were thought to be conservative estimates. Other estimates are that revenues in the DM industry grew from $77 million in 1997 to $350 million in 1999, and that in 1999, 56% of employers, 67% of HMOs, and 64% of point of service (POS) plans offered DM to their beneficiaries (Berger et al., 2001). In 2000, health plans spent about $360 million on DM, and the figures for 2002 were expected to be about $510 million (Nobel & Norman, 2003). Projections for 2003 were for $725 million in revenue (Cousins & Liu, 2003).

Todd and Nash (1997) described four generations in the history of DM. This view identifies DM as an evolving phenomenon which is progressing in sophistication. The first generation was distinguished by enhanced services. One or more services outside the usual medical care were added to help address illness care. These developments often were prompted by quality report card or accreditation requirements.

The second generation saw the targeting of the sickest patients because they are the highest risk for generating costs. Outreach, education, and proactive, ongoing follow-up to reduce costly acute care episodes are featured.

The third generation saw the true integration of care and a true population-based focus. Risk identification and stratification occur. All important elements of care are addressed for the population using evidence-based protocols. Treatment is centrally coordinated, and health outcomes and costs are tracked.

The fourth generation will contain a true health management model that focuses on optimizing health through wellness and prevention. Lifelong health education and strong incentives for healthy lifestyle behaviors will be featured. Resources will be allocated based on who is most likely to respond and benefit. DM programs are moving into the third generation and are looking to the future fourth generation.

POPULATION-BASED PROGRAM PLANNING

Both DM and PHM tend to occur within organized programs. Nurses need to have skills and knowledge in health care program planning to best showcase their unique contribution to DM.

Health care program planning emerged in the early 1980s. It began as a key aspect of health education and health promotion endeavors. Early models contained operational planning, program development, and strategic planning. In the late 1980s, business plans became more common as tools for both new ventures and health care program development. Now, program planning also needs to address the evidence base for practice and outcomes evaluation criteria. Programs also must be evaluated for their potential and relative worth in terms of cost, quality, and value (Hall, 1998).

A comprehensive program plan enables an assessment of the potential for success prior to allocating resources, provides a plan to streamline and facilitate implementation, identifies all needed resources, and outlines a way to obtain reliable and valid evaluation data. An integrated population-based program planning model contains the following four components (Hall, 1998):

1. Contextual analysis
2. Implementation plan
3. Budget
4. Evaluation plan

A program outline would discuss the problem, state the need, identify assumptions, and present objectives and standards (Hall, 1998).

Community-focused or population-based care delivery planning follows the nursing process. The six basic steps are as follows (Schuster & Goeppinger, 1996):

1. Establishing the contract partnership
2. Assessing
3. Determining the nursing diagnosis of the problem
4. Planning
5. Implementing interventions
6. Evaluating interventions and outcomes

Assessment involves gathering data, developing a composite database, and interpreting the data. Data gathering usually involves obtaining existing data about the demography of a community. Data such as population characteristic distributions of age, gender, socioeconomic status, and race; vital statistics such as morbidity and mortality; disease incidence and prevalence; community institutions and resources distribution; and health care provider characteristics and distribution are gathered (Schuster & Goeppinger, 1996). Because of the influence of managed care reimbursement, the top few employers in the community might also be determined, since the health care needs and policies of the largest groups of insured individuals will have an influence on community health needs and resources.

Population and community health status may be profiled by vital statistics such as births and deaths, the incidence and prevalence of the leading causes of mortality and morbidity, health risk profiles of selected aggregates, and functional ability levels. The structure of community health may be profiled by the number and location of health facilities such as hospitals and nursing homes, the health-related planning groups, health manpower types and numbers, and health resources utilization patterns. Data may be gathered by existing databases, surveys, interviews of key informants, or published reports. The five key methods of collecting data are (1) informant interviews, (2) participant observation, (3) windshield surveys

(the drive-by equivalent of simple observation), (4) secondary analysis of existing data, and (5) surveys (Schuster & Goeppinger, 1996).

After data gathering and assessment, a nursing diagnosis of the problem is generated. A modification of the nursing diagnosis format can be used. The three parts are "risk of," "among," and "related to." Each part is filled in to identify the problem clearly. The planning phase is then begun. It consists of problem analysis, problem prioritization, goals and objectives determination, and intervention activity development. Problem analysis may use a matrix or spreadsheet to map and identify direct and indirect precursors and consequences; relationships among problems, precursors, and consequences; and supportive data. Origins and impacts of the problem, points for intervention actions, and parties with an interest in the problem and solution need to be identified (Schuster & Goeppinger, 1996).

The problems identified as part of the assessment need to be ranked to determine relative importance. Priorities are established by using predetermined criteria. The following six criteria are recommended (Schuster & Goeppinger, 1996):

1. Community awareness of the problem
2. Community motivation to resolve it
3. The nurse's ability to influence problem solution
4. Availability of relevant expertise
5. Severity of consequences
6. Speed with which resolution can be achieved

The establishment of goals and objectives for high-priority problems needs to be done in precise, clear, behaviorally stated, incremental, and measurable terms. A search for the evidence base for any recommended interventions needs to be done. If standardized evidence-based protocols exist, these should be used. Intervention activities also can be mapped on a spreadsheet, along with a probability rating of the likelihood that the activity will foster achievement of the objective and be implemented. Interventions are then implemented and evaluated. Evaluation criteria include successful intervention implementation, meeting of partnership objectives, problem resolution, participant satisfaction, and development of community strengths. Evaluation of both costs and effectiveness is important. The process includes a feedback loop to renegotiate the partnership if needed (Schuster & Goeppinger, 1996).

POPULATION-BASED RISK ASSESSMENT

The aggregate health care costs of chronic conditions increase yearly as individuals grow older. Older individuals tend to have chronic conditions that require complex care. It is estimated that one-third to one-half of all health care spending is consumed by the elderly. With the shift in demographic trends toward increasing numbers of elderly, there is a shift in the need for preventive care and chronic illness management services (Coleman, 1999). To meet this challenge, managed care organizations have created infrastructures of population-based risk assessment, demand management (self-management and decision support systems such as call centers), DM, and case management.

Illustrating the continuum of care as spanning the well and worried well (self-directed care and primary care), the acutely ill (secondary and tertiary care), and the chronically ill (tertiary care and long-term care), Coleman (1999) identified the corresponding infrastructure. Demand management spans the entire continuum. Case management and DM cover primary care through long-term care and focus on acute and chronic conditions. Case management is identified as valuable for high-volume, high-risk conditions and those who have catastrophic illnesses.

To be effective at individual and population-based care management, both case and DM programs need to identify, assess, and define the populations to be served early in the program planning effort. After the population has been defined, individuals within the population need to be selected and assessed for the appropriateness of case or disease management as an intervention. Profile characteristics may be age, number of chronic illnesses, or number of medications. Sometimes a survey such as a health assessment

questionnaire is used to screen for high-risk indicators (Aliotta, 1996).

Population-based risk identification is an innovation that helps to determine the best use of staff and clinical resources while also identifying the long-term health needs of groups and populations. Risk identification can be comprehensive when it spans health promotion, wellness, chronic disease, illness, and disability. It can be specific when identifying persons at risk for high-cost, high-intensity, or long-term health care needs. Levels of risk are primary (prevention), secondary (early detection), and tertiary (management of an episode of care) (Burgess, 1999).

A more detailed model of population care management contains these six levels: population needs assessment, identification of health services, targeted health planning, wellness and prevention, care management, and case management (Qudah & Brannon, 1996). Population-based risk identification leads to referring individuals into case management and DM programs. "Disease management is largely an ambulatory care program" (Goldstein, 1998, p. 102). Extended case management often is targeted at persons with complex conditions, multiple diagnoses, or extended-term care requirements. Cost effectively managing populations requires careful risk identification and then the application of population-based principles and care strategies.

Zitter (1997) outlined the following six key success factors for the development and implementation of any DM program:

1. Understanding the course of the disease
2. Targeting patients likely to benefit from the intervention
3. Focusing on prevention and resolution
4. Increasing patient adherence through education
5. Providing full care continuity
6. Establishing integrated data management systems

The selection of a specific DM program for initiation and implementation can be guided by an analysis of the environment and potential target populations. Nobel and Norman (2003) identified the following four modules used by effective DM programs:

1. Candidate identification and stratification
2. Enrollee recruitment
3. The intervention itself
4. Evaluation

Each module contributes an important link in the process, and the four combine to form a process loop. Timely access to critical information is needed in each of the four modules.

Gillespie (2002) outlined the following seven criteria useful in the selection of a condition as a candidate for implementing a DM program:

1. Availability of treatment guidelines with consensus about the appropriateness and effectiveness of care
2. Generally recognized problems in therapy that are well documented in the medical literature
3. Large practice variation and a variety of drug treatment modalities
4. Large number of patients with the disease whose therapy could be improved
5. Preventable acute events that are often associated with the chronic disease (e.g., an emergency department or urgent care visit)
6. Outcomes that can be defined and measured in standardized and objective ways and that can be modified by application of appropriate

therapy (e.g., decreased number of emergency department visits or hospitalizations)
7. The potential for cost savings within a short period (less than 2 years) (p. 226)

In a stratified random sample survey of 65 health plans in 2000, Welch and colleagues (2002) found that virtually all DM programs exhibited the following characteristics:

- Used evidence-based guidelines
- Identified the population with a disease
- Stratified the population by risk
- Matched the intervention with the need
- Educated patients in self management
- Evaluated the program's process and outcomes

LEADERSHIP AND MANAGEMENT IMPLICATIONS

Managing the Continuum of Care

Nurses need to turn the focus of their attention on managing the continuum of care as a basis of nursing practice. Collaboration and communication are essential elements of coordination and integration across a "seamless" continuum of care: "Continuity of patient care involves a series of coordinating linkages across time, settings, providers, and consumers of health care.

◢ LEADERSHIP & MANAGEMENT BEHAVIORS

Leadership Behaviors

- Envisions improved health services for populations
- Encourages interdisciplinary and interorganizational coordination
- Inspires nurses to develop population-based health care plans
- Creates linkages across care settings
- Enables providers to work together to coordinate care delivery

Management Behaviors

- Plans for coordination of population health care
- Organizes interdisciplinary teams

- Directs critical pathways and other population-based care plans
- Manages interorganizational linkages across the continuum of care
- Controls provider actions for coordinated outcomes

Overlap Areas

- Leads population-based care planning
- Motivates providers to coordinate care for populations and communities

Communication is a core task in coordinating patient care" (Anderson & Helms, 1998, p. 255). Continuity of care, as a care management strategy, often requires that clients be tracked through multiple organizations or settings of care. The communication of client data and care needs is fundamental to continuity of care. Therefore coordination of care involves communication across boundaries. This need is increased with the multiple and complex elements of chronic illness management and decreased hospital inpatient stays (Anderson & Helms, 1998). Individual nurses may not see immediate opportunities in their jobs for true continuity of care. However, as the emphasis on DM and PHM accelerates, nurses have a leadership role and opportunity to use their skills creatively with DM and PHM perspectives.

One critical application of managing the continuum of care is the facilitation and management of interdisciplinary, interorganizational communication for continuity of care. This is an imperative because information transfer is necessary for planning, and planning is necessary for continuity of care. Information exchange problems and gaps were found in a study of case management and interorganizational referral communication between a hospital and a home health agency within one health care system (Anderson & Helms, 1998; Anderson & Tredway, 1999). The need for barrier reduction in interorganizational communication is an urgent continuity-of-care need. Resources need to be redirected toward reducing obstacles and facilitating data and information transfer in order to improve the health of individuals and to manage population health care better.

Three major strategies of DM programs are (1) the use of an interdisciplinary team, (2) outcomes evaluation to measure results, and (3) the application of information management technologies. These three core techniques are used with a population health focus in order to improve overall health.

Included in the DMAA definition of DM components is that collaborative practice models include physicians and all support service providers. Provider disciplines have become areas

characterized as "silos" that prevent integrated care. The interdisciplinary team needs to form and collaborate on the total plan of care, with each discipline integrating its expertise. For medical conditions, physicians, nurses, pharmacists, dietitians, social workers, and any other allied health professional with specific expertise need to be incorporated into the team. Communication among and between team members is the key to a successful program.

CURRENT ISSUES AND TRENDS

DM is a current health care trend. The viability of health care organizations may depend on how an organization responds to the needs of specific population bases (Hall, 1998). A current trend is for the development of integrated population-based programs. For example, a children's home-based asthma management and prevention service was developed for a military clinic in the southeastern United States (Hall, 1998). The University of Virginia School of Nursing developed a nurse-managed primary care clinic to serve low-income elderly and disabled housing authority residents (Glick et al., 1996). The Visiting Nurse Service of New York has a Community Nursing Organization Medicare demonstration project to deliver community-focused nursing case management services to elderly clients (Storfjell et al., 1997). Nurses' roles include integrating, coordinating, and advocating for individuals, families, and groups in order to improve continuity and enhance appropriate service use. The disease manager's role is to screen for risks, monitor risk factors over time, and initiate both preventive and treatment measures.

Research results are being reported about population health-related care delivery. For example, Bryan and colleagues (1997) investigated the learning needs of hospital-based nurses preparing to change from acute care to community-based care. A national Delphi study was done to determine competencies for nursing leadership in public health. The results showed four areas of needed competency: (1) political competency, (2) business acumen, (3) program leadership, and (4) management capability (Misener et al., 1997). Outcomes for community health practice have been studied (Alexander & Kroposki, 1999), and a useful measure of population health status has been analyzed (Kindig, 1999). The effects of case management on the context of nursing practice have also been studied (Lynn & Kelly, 1997). Evidence-based guidelines for public health nursing practice have been explored and developed (Strohschein et al., 1999). These research projects are beginning to lay a foundation for evidence-based practice in DM and PHM by showing that DM and PHM are viable programs to address cost and quality issues.

Another current trend is the identification of patient adherence as a driver of disease cost and the need for intervention with clients to foster adherence (Aliotta, 1996, 1999). *Adherence* is the extent to which the client continues a negotiated treatment. *Maintenance* is the extent to which a client continues health behavior without supervision. This compliance/adherence engagement is critical because the ultimate benefit of a treatment plan depends on the extent to which the client implements it. Adherence may directly improve outcomes. For example, poor adherence has been implicated in drug-resistant strains of tuberculosis. Aliotta (1999) stated, "Current best evidence suggests a strong potential for establishing linkages between adherence and better outcomes in the area of chronic illness" (p. 82). Nurses have the skills to deliver adherence interventions.

Information management technologies are critical at every stage of a DM program. Nobel and Norman (2003) divided the information management arena into information gathering, information integration and analysis, and information deployment. Effective programs need timely access to clinical, administrative, financial, and logistical information flows. Once acquired, these large databases need to be analyzed to identify opportunities for effective interventions to enhance the management of care and services. Deployment of information is reflected in strategies of notification, alerts, reports, and assessment of trends and the impact of interventions. There are a variety of emerging information management technologies, such as biometric and handheld devices, that can manage the collection and distribution of information (Nobel & Norman, 2003).

Technological innovations in informatics have made possible the rapid analysis of large databases. In turn, statistical analyses have become more sophisticated. Currently, claims databases are primarily used for data mining and profiling for DM. In the future, related databases such as pharmacy and nursing care are likely to be linked or merged with claims databases for a more robust disease profiling. Two important applications of information management technologies in DM are predictive modeling and calculation of return on investment (ROI). Predictive modeling is the use of statistics to calculate expected costs based on variables such as demographics, diagnoses, pharmacy claims, and survey data (Kramer, 2004). Predictive models have been used in other industries, such as credit card companies and retailers, for years. Applied to DM, predictive models would be able to analyze data to answer questions such as: how much of a cost trend is being driven by age and how much by illness? Which complications and co-morbidities drive costs (Kramer, 2004)?

Calculation of ROI is being attempted in case management (Smith et al., 2003) and DM. ROI is one method used to describe the impact of case or disease management. It is a dollar calculation of the value of cost savings produced by the case or disease manager in exchange for what is spent on the program. It is a desirable benchmark given cost pressures. Although no standardized formula yet exists, there is beginning convergence on the inclusion of hard and soft savings criteria (Smith et al., 2003).

Summary

- Disease management is an innovative strategy for managing chronic conditions.
- Progress needs to be made in health care coordination of chronic conditions and in population health.

- Managed care and the Institute of Medicine are two forces that have emphasized DM and care coordination.
- DM programs have six components for comprehensive care.
- Population-based health care focuses on aggregates and communities.
- A population is a collection of individuals who have a characteristic in common.
- Population-based care management is the integration and coordination of health services to a population.
- DM programs offer coordination, consistency, and customization.
- Community participation and partnership are key elements.
- There are four components of population-based program planning.
- The six steps of population-based care planning follow the nursing process.
- Population-based risk assessment is a part of chronic illness management and resource management.
- Care for a population is depicted as a triangle.
- DM programs use evidence-based guidelines and risk stratification.
- Nurses need to manage the continuum of care and have the skills to address advocacy and adherence.
- Collaboration and communication are essential to care coordination.

Study Questions

1. Which should come first, case management or DM?
2. Should all nurses be doing population-based care management? Why or why not?
3. How can nurses motivate others to facilitate coordination across organizations?
4. What is the role of informatics in disease and population-based care management?
5. How are community health and population-based care management applied in nursing?
6. Why don't all clients need disease management?
7. Who should do disease management?

CASE STUDY

The disease manager (DM) for Big Insurance Company (BIC) is reviewing today's printout from the predictive modeling analysis of pharmacy claims for attention deficit/hyperactivity disorder (ADHD) drugs. Several trends pop out. Of concern is the alarming jump (83% increase) in the number of prescriptions filled for ADHD drugs from 1999 to 2003 and suggestions that ADHD is overdiagnosed. Along with this are concerns of cost (average cost of a 30-day prescription for the popular nonstimulant medication was $108) and therapy adherence. The ADHD drugs are expensive, have side effects, and often are not accompanied by the recommended adjunctive behavioral therapy or dose-to-side-effects adjustment.

The DM then reviews individual claims profiles and selects those with erratic prescription refills. She begins to call individual families for interviews to determine the scope of factors related to adherence. She reaches the mother of Linda, a 15-year-old girl diagnosed with ADHD by a clinical counselor. She was placed on one of the common ADHD drugs, which she does not like to take. Her father is an elementary school teacher, and her mother is a factory worker. The mother relates that Linda is taking her medications "pretty much" and that she needs to take them. She reports no problems except her occasional forgetting to take the drugs. When asked about behavioral therapy, the mother states that Linda's participation in extracurricular events takes up her time so they don't have her doing any therapy sessions. The DM obtains the mother's permission to talk to Linda and arranges a time when Linda can talk to her privately.

The DM calls Linda at the appointed time. She asks Linda to describe her experience of ADHD, the diagnosis, and how things have been going. Linda tells her that she hates taking the medicine and dislikes its side effects. She says that her father complains about the cost and that when she did not want to take her medicine her father told her to take it once a week so her mother would still

CRITICAL THINKING EXERCISE

Nurse Gloria Davis just got her dream job as a case manager for diabetes care in a large integrated delivery system. Nurse Davis is deeply committed to high-quality client care. She has structured an excellent teaching program that is administered through the ambulatory clinics. She has instituted population data collection using the SF-36 and Diabetes Quality of Life tools. Nurse Davis has begun to collect trend data on HbA_{1c} values and frequency of blood glucose instability or complications. The next outcome to measure is client satisfaction. Nurse Davis assumes that client satisfaction is related to compliance with treatment. The first step is a small focus group. In the focus group meeting, Nurse Davis discovers that client interactions with a health care provider are becoming more impersonal. The clients have fewer choices about to whom and where they can go for services, must get complicated authorizations, need to fill out more forms, have to listen to more recorded messages, and are waiting longer for appointments. On clinic days they wait a long time to see their provider only briefly. The process of coming in for care actually makes many of these clients feel worse.

1. What is the problem?
2. Why is it a problem?
3. What are the key issues?
4. What should Nurse Davis do first?
5. How should Nurse Davis handle this situation?
6. What problem-solving style should Nurse Davis use?
7. What leadership and management strategies might be useful?

think she was taking it. The DM begins a list of pro and con adherence factors in her database. An evidence-based treatment plan will be needed.

REFERENCES

Aikman, P., Andress, I., Goodfellow, C., LaBelle, N., & Porter-O'Grady, T. (1998). System integration: A necessity. *Journal of Nursing Administration, 28*(2), 28-34.

Alexander, J., & Kroposki, M. (1999). Outcomes for community health nursing practice. *Journal of Nursing Administration, 29*(5), 49-56.

Aliotta, S.L. (1996). Components of a successful case management program. *Managed Care Quarterly, 4*(2), 38-45.

Aliotta, S. (1999). Patient adherence outcome indicators and measurement in case management and health care. *The Journal of Care Management, 5*(4), 24, 26, 29-31, 81-82.

American Journal of Health Promotion. (1989). *Definition of health promotion.* West Bloomfield, MI. Retrieved January 19, 2004, from *www.healthpromotionjournal.com/*

Anderson, M.A., & Helms, L.B. (1998). Comparison of continuing care communication. *Image, 30*(3), 255-260.

Anderson, M.A., & Tredway, C.A. (1999). Communication: An outcome of case management. *Nursing Case Management, 4*(3), 104-111.

Aurora Health Care. (2004). *Aurora's continuum of care.* Milwaukee, WI: Aurora Health Care. Retrieved February 15, 2004, from *www.aurorahealthcare.org/aboutus/continuum/index.asp*

Berger, J., Slezak, J., Stine, N., McStay, P., O'Leary, B., & Addiego, J. (2001). Economic impact of a diabetes disease management program in a self-insured health plan: Early results. *Disease Management, 4*(2), 65-73.

Bryan, Y.E., Bayley, E.W., Grendel, C., Kingston, M.B., Tuck, M.B., & Wood, L.J. (1997). Preparing to change from acute to community-based care: Learning needs of hospital-based nurses. *Journal of Nursing Administration, 27*(5), 35-44.

Burgess, C.S. (1999). Managed care: The driving force for case management. In E.L. Cohen & V. DeBack (Eds.), *The outcomes mandate: Case management in health care today* (pp. 13-19). St Louis: Mosby.

Carroll, P.L. (2004). *Community health nursing: A practical guide.* Clifton Park, NY: Thomson Delmar Learning.

Case Management Society of America (CMSA). (2002). *Definition of case management.* Little Rock, AR: CMSA. Retrieved January 30, 2004, from *www.cmsa.org/AboutUs/CMDefinition.aspx*

Case Management Society of America (CMSA). (2004). The case report. *The Case Manager, 15*(3), 37.

Centers for Medicare & Medicaid Services (CMS). (2004). *National health care expenditures: Historical overview.* Baltimore: CMS. Retrieved July 12, 2004, from *www.cms.hhs.gov/publications/overview-medicare-medicaid/default2.asp*

Coggeshall Press. (2004). *Care for the total population.* Coralville, IA: Coggeshall Press.

Coleman, J.R. (1999). Integrated case management: The twenty-first century challenge for HMO case managers, part I. *The Case Manager, 10*(5), 28-34.

Commission for Case Manager Certification (CCMC). (2004). *Code of professional conduct for case managers with standards, rules, procedures, and penalties.* Rolling Meadows, IL: CCMC.

Cousins, M.S., & Liu, Y. (2003). Cost savings for a preferred provider organization population with multi-condition disease management: Evaluating program impact using predictive modeling with a control group. *Disease Management,* 6(4), 207-217.

Disease Management Association of America (DMAA). (2004). *Definition of disease management.* Washington, DC: DMAA. Retrieved February 7, 2004, from *www.dmaa.org/definition.html*

Gillespie, J.L. (2002). The value of disease management—Part 3: Balancing cost and quality in the treatment of asthma. *Disease Management,* 5(1), 225-232.

Glick, D.F., Hale, P.J., Kulbok, P.A., & Shettig, J. (1996). Community development theory: Planning a community nursing center. *Journal of Nursing Administration,* 26(7/8), 44-50.

Goldstein, R. (1998). The disease management approach to cost containment. *Nursing Case Management,* 3(3), 99-103.

Hall, P.J. (1998). Planning an integrated population-based program. *Journal of Nursing Administration,* 28(10), 40-47.

Health Canada. (2004). *What is population health?* Ottawa, Ontario, Canada: Health Canada. Retrieved February 15, 2004, from *www.hc-sc.gc.ca/hppb/phdd/approach/index.html*

Ho, S. (2003). The emerging role for health plans: Info-Mediary. *Disease Management,* 6(1 Suppl), 4-10.

Huber, D.L. (2005). Overview of disease management. In D.L. Huber (Ed.), *Disease management: A guide for case managers.* Philadelphia: Saunders.

Huston, C.J. (2001). The role of the case manager in a disease management program. *Lippincott's Case Management,* 6(5), 222-227.

Improving Chronic Illness Care. (2004). *Model elements.* Seattle: MacColl Institute for Healthcare Innovation. Retrieved October 2, 2004, from *www.improvingchroniccare.org/change/model/components.html*

Institute of Medicine (IOM). (2001). *Crossing the quality chasm: A new health system for the 21st century.* Washington, DC: National Academies Press.

Institute of Medicine (IOM). (2004). *Crossing the quality chasm: The IOM health care quality initiative.* Washington, DC: National Academies Press. Retrieved October 2, 2004, from *www.iom.edu/focuson.asp?id=8089*

Javors, J.R., Laws, D., & Bramble, J.E. (2003). Uncontrolled chronic disease: Patient non-compliance or clinical mismanagement? *Disease Management,* 6(3), 169-178.

Johnson, A. (2003). Why we can't wait to implement disease management. *Business and Health Archive, October 15,* 21.

Kindig, D.A. (1999). Purchasing population health: Aligning financial incentives to improve health outcomes. *Nursing Outlook,* 47(1), 15-22.

Kramer, M.S. (2004). Predictive models make smart purchasers. *Business & Health, January 10,* 1-4.

Lewis, A. (2004). Savings opportunities through Medicaid disease management. *Disease Management,* 7(1), 35-46.

Lipold, A.G. (2002). Disease management comes of age, not a moment too soon. *Business and Health Archive, June 19,* 7.

Lynn, M.R., & Kelly, B. (1997). Effects of case management on the nursing context—Perceived quality of care, work satisfaction, and control over practice. *Image,* 29(3), 237-241.

Misener, T.R., Alexander, J., Blaha, A.J., Clarke, P.N., Cover, C.M., Felton, G.M., et al. (1997). National Delphi study to determine competencies for nursing leadership in public health. *Image,* 29(1), 47-51.

Naylor, M.D., & Buhler-Wilkerson, K. (1999). Creating community-based care for the new millennium. *Nursing Outlook,* 47(3), 120-127.

Nobel, J.J., & Norman, G.K. (2003). Emerging information management technologies and the future of disease management. *Disease Management,* 6(4), 219-231.

Pareto Law. (2004). *Pareto principle: "The 80-20 rule."* London: Pareto Law. Retrieved February 7, 2004, from *www.paretolaw.co.uk/paretoprinciple.asp*

Qudah, F.J., & Brannon, M. (1996). Population-based case management. *Quality Management in Health Care,* 5(1), 29-41.

Schuster, G.F., & Goeppinger, J. (1996). Community as client: Using the nursing process to promote health. In M. Stanhope & J. Lancaster (Eds.), *Community health nursing: Promoting health of aggregates, families, and individuals* (4th ed.) (pp. 289-314). St Louis: Mosby.

Smith, D.S., Auerbach, L.P., & Hamill, C.T. (2003). Case management return on investment. *Care Management,* 9(6), 24-48, 42.

Storfjell, J.L., Mitchell, R., & Daly, G.M. (1997). Nurse-managed health care: New York's community nursing organization. *Journal of Nursing Administration,* 27(10), 21-27.

Strohschein, S., Shaffer, M.A., & Lia-Hoagberg, B. (1999). Evidence-based guidelines for public health nursing practice. *Nursing Outlook,* 47(2), 84-89.

Todd, W.E., & Nash, D. (Eds.). (1997). *Disease management: A systems approach to improving patient outcomes.* Chicago: American Hospital Publishing.

U.S. Census Bureau. (2001). *Age: 2000. Census 2000 brief.* Washington, DC: U.S. Census Bureau.

Wagner, E.H. (1998). Chronic disease management: What will it take to improve care for chronic illness? *Effective Clinical Practice,* 1, 2-4.

Ward, M.D., & Rieve, J.A. (1997). The role of case management in disease management. In W.E. Todd & D. Nash (Eds.), *Disease management: A systems approach to improving patient outcomes* (pp. 235-259). Chicago: American Hospital Publishing.

Welch, W. P., Bergsten, C., Cutler, C., Bocchino, C., & Smith, R.I. (2002). Disease management practices of health plans. *The American Journal of Managed Care* 8(4), 353-361.

Williams, C.A. (1996). Community-based population-focused practice: The foundation of specialization in public health nursing. In M. Stanhope & J. Lancaster (Eds.), *Community health nursing: Promoting health of aggregates, families, and individuals* (4th ed.) (pp. 21-33). St Louis: Mosby.

Wilson, T., & MacDowell, M. (2003). Framework for assessing causality in disease management programs: Principles. *Disease Management, 6*(3), 143-158.

Zitter, M. (1997). A new paradigm in health care delivery: Disease management. In W.E. Todd & D. Nash (Eds.), *Disease management: A systems approach to improving patient outcomes* (pp. 1-25). Chicago: American Hospital Publishing.

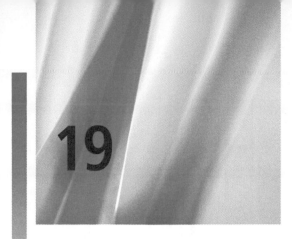

19

Patient and Family Cultural Values

Diane L. Huber

CHAPTER OBJECTIVES

- Develop an awareness of cultural diversity
- Define cultural diversity, cultural competence, and transcultural nursing
- Analyze cultural influences on health care
- Recommend strategies for cultural competence
- Evaluate the impact of cultural competence on nursing practice
- Using critical thinking, conceptualize and analyze possible solutions to a practice exercise

"Throughout the 21st century, efforts to improve health will be shaped by important changes in the U.S. population. As Americans meet this challenge, it will be in the context of a Nation that is growing older, and becoming more racially and ethnically diverse" (Centers for Disease Control and Prevention [CDC], 2003, p. 23).

The need for U.S. health care to meet the challenge of increasing racial and ethnic diversity in the United States has been highlighted by data from the U.S. Census Bureau (Hobbs & Stoops, 2002) (Figure 19.1) and the CDC, which identified the aging character of that population (Figure 19.2). Patient and family cultural values are critical to the provision of quality health care to all Americans because health beliefs and practices and communication styles can affect clinical outcomes. According to McCarty and colleagues (2002), "Despite recent advances in improving the health of the general U.S. population members of minority and ethnic groups are experiencing a widening gap in disease and mortality" (p. 54). For example, language differences are a major barrier in health care delivery. The situation becomes more pressing as the U.S. experiences rapidly increasing minority populations.

GOVERNMENT STANDARDS

The U.S. Department of Health and Human Services (USDHHS) acted at the end of 2000 to make cultural competence a priority in health care, adopting National Standards for Culturally and Linguistically Appropriate Services (CLAS) in Health Care. Fourteen standards were issued by publication in the Federal Register (FR Doc. 00-32685, filed 12-21-00). These standards deal with culturally competent care, language access services, and organizational supports for cultural competence (Box 19.1). Of the 14 standards, 4 (No. 4-7) are mandates required of all recipients of federal funds. One of the 14 standards (No. 14) is suggested for voluntary adoption by health care organizations. The remaining 9 standards (No. 1-3 and 8-13) are recommended for adoption as mandates by federal, state, and national accrediting agencies. Agencies and their staff providing care

(Percent)

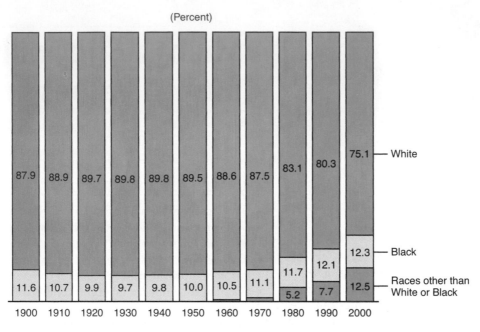

87.9 88.9 89.7 89.8 89.8 89.5 88.6 87.5 83.1 80.3 75.1 — White

12.3 — Black

80.3 12.1

11.7

83.1 5.2 7.7

11.6 10.7 9.9 9.7 9.8 10.0 10.5 11.1 12.5 — Races other than White or Black

1900 1910 1920 1930 1940 1950 1960 1970 1980 1990 2000

Note: In 2000, the percent distribution is based on the reporting of race alone
for Whites and Blacks. Source: U.S. Census Bureau, decennial census of population,
1900 to 2000.

Figure 19.1
Distribution of total population by race: 1900-2000. (Data from Hobbs, F., & Stoops, N. [2002]. *Demographic trends in the 20th century* [U.S. Census Bureau, Census 2000 Special Reports, Series Censr-4]. Washington, DC: U.S. Census Bureau, U.S. Department of Commerce. Retrieved October 8, 2004, from *www.census.gov/prod/2002pubs/censr-4.pdf*)

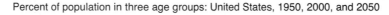

Percent of population in three age groups: United States, 1950, 2000, and 2050

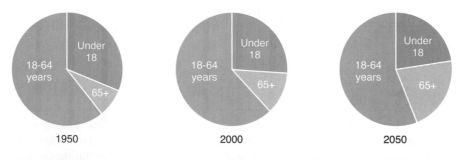

1950 2000 2050

NOTE: See Data Table for data points graphed
and additional notes.

SOURCES: U.S. Census Bureau, 1950 and 2000
decennial censuses and 2050 middle series population
projections.

Figure 19.2
Percentage of the population in three age groups in the United States in 1950, 2000, and 2050. (Data from Centers for Disease Control and Prevention [CDC] [2003]. *Health, United States, 2003 with chartbook on trends in the health of Americans*. Hyattsville, MD: CDC. Retrieved May 4, 2004, from *www.cdc.gov/nchs/data/hus/hus03.pdf*)

Box **19.1**

National Standards for Culturally and Linguistically Appropriate Services (CLAS) in Health Care*

Culturally Competent Care

1. Health care organizations should ensure that patients/consumers receive from all staff members effective, understandable, and respectful care that is provided in a manner compatible with their cultural health beliefs and practices and preferred language.
2. Health care organizations should implement strategies to recruit, retain, and promote at all levels of the organization a diverse staff and leadership that are representative of the demographic characteristics of the service area.
3. Health care organizations should ensure that staff at all levels and across all disciplines receive ongoing education and training in culturally and linguistically appropriate service delivery.

Language Access Services

4. Health care organizations must offer and provide language assistance services, including bilingual staff and interpreter services, at no cost to each patient/consumer with limited English proficiency at all points of contact, in a timely manner during all hours of operation.
5. Health care organizations must provide to patients/consumers in their preferred language both verbal offers and written notices informing them of their right to receive language assistance services.
6. Health care organizations must assure the competence of language assistance provided to limited English proficient patients/consumers by interpreters and bilingual staff. Family and friends should not be used to provide interpretation services (except on request by the patient/consumer).
7. Health care organizations must make available easily understood patient-related materials and post signage in the languages of the commonly encountered groups and/or groups represented in the service area.

Organizational Supports for Cultural Competence

8. Health care organizations should develop, implement, and promote a written strategic plan that outlines clear goals, policies, operational plans, and management accountability/oversight mechanisms to provide culturally and linguistically appropriate services.
9. Health care organizations should conduct initial and ongoing organizational self-assessments of class-related activities and are encouraged to integrate cultural and linguistic competence-related measures into their internal audits, performance improvement programs, patient satisfaction assessments, and outcomes-based evaluations.
10. Health care organizations should ensure that data on the individual patient's/consumer's race, ethnicity, and spoken and written language are collected in health records, integrated into the organization's management information systems, and periodically updated.
11. Health care organizations should maintain a current demographic, cultural, and epidemiological profile of the community as well as a needs assessment to accurately plan for and implement services that respond to the cultural and linguistic characteristics of the service area.

Data from U.S. Department of Health and Human Services (USDHHS). (2000). Washington, DC.
*Issued by the Office of Minority Health (OMH), USDHHS.
Note: CLAS mandates are current federal requirements for all recipients of federal funds (Standards 4, 5, 6, and 7). CLAS guidelines are activities recommended by OMH for adoption as mandates by federal, state, and national accrediting agencies (Standards 1, 2, 3, 8, 9, 10, 11, 12, and 13). CLAS recommendations are suggested by OMH for voluntary adoption by health care organizations (Standard 14).

Continued

Box **19.1**

National Standards for Culturally and Linguistically Appropriate Services (CLAS) in Health Care*—cont'd

Organizational Supports for Cultural Competence—cont'd

12. Health care organizations should develop participatory, collaborative partnerships with communities and utilize a variety of formal and informal mechanisms to facilitate community and patient/consumer involvement in designing and implementing class-related activities.
13. Health care organizations should ensure that conflict and grievance resolution processes are culturally and linguistically sensitive and capable of identifying, preventing, and resolving cross-cultural conflicts or complaints by patients/consumers.
14. Health care organizations are encouraged to regularly make available to the public information about their progress and successful innovations in implementing the class standards and to provide public notice in their communities about the availability of this information.

to clients whose cultures or languages are different from the staff need to be aware of these federal standards and incorporate them into practice. They were developed from current regulations, research, policies, and input from stakeholders (Narayan, 2002).

Cultural Competence in Nursing

Many factors, including the increasing use of advanced technology, electronic communication, and rapid transportation, have brought about an increased awareness of a global community. This growing appreciation for the global community not only has raised the awareness of individuals in one culture to the values of those in other cultures, but also has heightened an awareness of differing values in subcultures within any local community. Nurses need to develop ways of working effectively in cross-cultural circumstances and exhibit respect for cultural differences. Many culturally sensitive areas arise in nursing practice, such as gender roles, religious influences, dietary practices, rites and rituals of birth and death, and language interpretation and comprehension.

The nurse has two significant areas in which cultural diversity must be addressed for successful delivery of health care. First, there must be recognition by nurses of the values of other cultures or subcultures as they relate to health and health care behaviors. This is necessary not only to provide the services needed in a way that respects the values of others but also to facilitate meaningful communication between the nurse and the client, as well as the client's family, to engage positive health practices. To understand and treat human responses to health and illness, the nurse must recognize the multifaceted ways in which cultures define health and illness, develop systems of care, handle developmental stages, and prescribe roles for patients and healers (Dreher, 1996).

Second, the nurse must take positive steps to encourage increased participation in the nursing profession by persons from other cultures and subcultures. The nursing profession is projected to be one of the largest job growth areas among professions in the United States. New nursing job opportunities, along with replacement needs as projected retirements occur, provide a significant opportunity in nursing for increasing the presence of persons who can bring with them an understanding of the values of other cultures and an increase in the diversity and perspectives of those providing nursing care to the population.

DEFINITIONS

Cultural diversity refers to variations with respect to the "thoughts, communications, actions, customs, beliefs, values, and institutions of racial, ethnic, religious, or social groups" (U.S. Department of Health and Human Services [USDHHS], 2000, p. 80873). Cultural diversity means not only that persons are unique but also that there are societal groups, based on religion, gender, ethnicity, sexual orientation, age, birth place, and many other characteristics, who hold strongly ingrained beliefs and values and have a significant influence on feelings and behaviors.

Providing care effectively to persons from the multiplicity of cultures is called cultural and linguistic competence. There are many definitions for cultural and linguistic competence, but transcending those definitions is a sense of something that is a dynamic, cross-cultural interaction. Cultural and linguistic competence is defined as "the ability of health care providers and health care organizations to understand and respond effectively to the cultural and linguistic needs brought by the patient to the health care encounter"

(Agency for Healthcare Research and Quality [AHRQ], 2003, p. 1). Linguistic competence is defined as "providing readily available, culturally appropriate oral and written language services to limited English proficiency (LEP) members through such means as bilingual/bicultural staff, trained medical interpreters, and qualified translators" (AHRQ, 2003, p. 1). Cultural competence is defined as "a set of congruent behaviors, attitudes, and policies that come together in a system or agency or among professionals that enables effective interactions in a cross-cultural framework" (AHRQ, 2003, p. 1). AHRQ (2003) has noted that cultural competence requires that organizations and their people value diversity, assess themselves, manage the dynamics of difference, acquire and institutionalize cultural knowledge, and adapt to diversity and the cultural contexts of the individuals and communities they serve.

Cultural competence, to be properly understood, should be viewed as a process or a journey rather than a destination. The Office of Minority Health ([OMH], 2000) in the U.S. Department of Health and Human Services has developed and

---

⚠ LEADING & MANAGING **DEFINED**

Cultural Competence

The ability to recognize and respond to health-related beliefs and cultural values, disease incidence and prevalence, and treatment efficacy.

Acculturation

Process of incorporating values, beliefs, and behaviors from the host culture into an immigrant's world view.

Cultural Blind Spot

Areas in one language that cannot be expressed well when translated into another language.

Ethnocentrism

Interpretation of the beliefs and behavior of others in terms of one's own cultural values and traditions; belief that one's own culture is superior.

Mutuality

Back-and-forth sharing of power in a relationship.

Proxemics

Nonverbal communication through the use of interpersonal space.

Racism

Belief that some populations are inherently superior or inferior to others.

Stereotype

Making an assumption about another person based on group membership.

promulgated what may be a helpful definition of cultural competence. Cultural competence involves an ongoing expansion and updating of an individual's understanding of different cultures. However, it is equally important to remember that a person's identification with a culture does not necessarily mean that that person agrees with all the dominant beliefs in that culture. In fact, cultural diversity involves differences not only between cultures but also within cultures. A nurse must look at each client individually to make a cultural assessment.

Cultural competence is a crucial link to practicing empathy, understanding, communication, valuing, and caring in health care and nursing care (Box 19.2). Cultural competence also involves recognizing the importance of integrating persons with other values in the process of organizational operations. Cross-cultural comparative perspectives influence health care practices. From this awareness has emerged transcultural nursing.

Transcultural nursing is defined as "a formal area of study and practice focused on comparative holistic cultural care, health, and illness patterns of people with respect to differences and similarities in their cultural values, beliefs, and lifeways with the goal to provide culturally congruent, competent, and compassionate care" (Leininger, 1997, p. 342). Other related terms used in cultural and linguistic competence include **acculturation**, **cultural blind spot**, **ethnocentrism**, **mutuality**, **proxemics**, **racism**, and **stereotype**.

BACKGROUND

The demographic makeup of the U.S. population is changing radically in both the areas of ethnicity and age. According to the U.S. Census Bureau (2004), as follows, the nation's Hispanic and Asian populations continue to grow at much faster rates than the population as a whole:

> The population of Hispanics reached 39.9 million on July 1, 2003, accounting for about one-half of the 9.4 million residents added to the nation's population since Census 2000. Its growth rate of 13.0 percent over the 39-month period was almost four times that of the total population (3.3 percent). The number of people who reported being Asian grew 12.5 percent to 13.5 million.
>
> The U.S. median age continued to rise, from 35.3 years on April 1, 2000, to 35.9 years on July 1, 2003. (p. 1)

The President's Cancer Panel has pointed to these changes and their implications and projected impact on health care:

> The distribution of the four major U.S. population groups (white, black, Hispanic, and Asian American/Pacific Islander) is changing radically, both overall and within each group. Between 1990 and 1995, the Asian/Pacific Islander population grew by just over 20 percent; but between 1990 and the year 2010, this population is expected to increase by about 90 percent. The Hispanic population is expected to increase by about

---

Box 19.2

Examples of Culturally Competent Care

- Striving to overcome cultural, language, and communication barriers
- Providing an environment in which patients/consumers from diverse cultural backgrounds feel comfortable discussing their cultural health beliefs and practices in the context of negotiating treatment options
- Using community workers as a check on the effectiveness of communication and care
- Encouraging patients/consumers to express their spiritual beliefs and cultural practices
- Being familiar with and respectful of various traditional healing systems and beliefs and, where appropriate, integrating these approaches into treatment plans

Data from Office of Minority Health [OMH]. [2000]. Assuring cultural competence in health care: Recommendations for national standards and an outcomes-focused research agenda. *Federal Register, 65*(247), 80865-80879.

80 percent overall over the same period. These enormous increases are not distributed evenly across the country. To illustrate, by the year 2015, the white population in California will become a minority. (President's Cancer Panel, 1997, p. 11)

The U.S. Census Bureau (2000) estimated that Hispanics/Latinos will constitute the largest minority group in the United States by the year 2005. The health status of this medically underserved population makes its projected increase important to health care policy makers and leaders at all levels. An understanding of Hispanic social, cultural, economic, and physical environments is needed if appropriate health care is to be provided. According to the President's Cancer Panel (1997):

It is clear that individuals from racial/ethnic minorities, the poor, and/or the medically under served have not shared equally in the progress that is being made against cancer. ...While poverty does have a great impact on cancer, it is by no means the only significant issue. ... Geographic differences, dietary habits, immigration status, and many other factors must be taken into account. For example, Hispanic Americans in Illinois have the highest breast cancer incidence in the nation, yet nationally, Hispanic women have among the lowest breast cancer rates. Similarly, in Texas, more than 30 percent of breast cancer deaths among Hispanics and blacks were in women under age 50, twice the percentage for white women in the State. (p. 37)

The literature is replete with examples of the failure to obtain parity in positive health care outcomes for members of minority groups: "Despite notable improvement in the overall health of the American people, there are continuing disparities in the burden of illness and death experienced by African Americans, Hispanics, Native Americans, Asian Americans, and other racial/ethnic minorities, compared to the U.S. population as a whole. Over the next decade these groups currently experiencing poorer health status are expected to grow

as a proportion of the total U.S. population" (USDHHS, 1999, p. 1). Clearly, despite being disadvantaged for health care, improving the health status of ethnic minorities benefits the health of the entire nation and must be vigorously addressed. This is an issue of improving the quality of care and effectively managing health care resources for vulnerable populations and the larger community.

The Agency for Healthcare Research and Quality reported that race and ethnicity influence a patient's chance of receiving many specific procedures and treatments, as follows:

Of nine hospital procedures investigated in one study, five were significantly less common among African American patients than among white patients; three of those five were also less common among Hispanics, and two were less common among Asian Americans. Other AHRQ-supported studies have revealed additional disparities in patient care for various conditions and care settings including:

- **Heart disease.** African Americans are 13 percent less likely to undergo coronary angioplasty and one-third less likely to undergo bypass surgery than are whites.
- **Asthma.** Among preschool children hospitalized for asthma, only 7 percent of black and 2 percent of Hispanic children, compared with 21 percent of white children, are prescribed routine medications to prevent future asthma-related hospitalizations.
- **Breast cancer.** The length of time between an abnormal screening mammogram and the followup diagnostic test to determine whether a woman has breast cancer is more than twice as long in Asian American, black, and Hispanic women as in white women.
- **Human immunodeficiency virus (HIV) infection.** African Americans with HIV infection are less likely to be on antiretroviral therapy, less likely to receive prophylaxis for Pneumocystis pneumonia, and less likely to be receiving protease inhibitors than other persons with HIV. An HIV infection data coordinating

center, now under development, will allow researchers to compare contemporary data on HIV care to examine whether disparities in care among groups are being addressed and to identify any new patterns in treatment that arise.

- **Nursing home care.** Asian American, Hispanic, and African American residents of nursing homes are all far less likely than white residents to have sensory and communication aids, such as glasses and hearing aids. A new study of nursing home care is developing measures of disparities in this care setting and their relationship to quality of care.

Identifying that disparities in care exist is important, but it is not enough. Now, researchers are also beginning to focus on why these disparities exist, which disparities actually indicate poor-quality care, and how to develop strategies to address them. (AHRQ, 2000, p. 1)

Disparities in health care among groups often are ascribed to differences in income and access to insurance. Research has shown that both of these factors are important, but they are not the only factors. Physician decisions about referring patients for additional care (e.g., for cardiac catheterization) also are a factor. Research is being done to see how interpersonal processes of the way in which patients and clinicians interact also affect access to health care services and outcomes of care (AHRQ, 2000).

CULTURAL AWARENESS

The population of the United States has been described as a melting pot. As a result of waves of immigration, there has always been cultural diversity. U.S. society has been characterized by its pluralism. Nurses recognize that cultural diversity and awareness is necessary for excellent nursing care (Pasco et al., 2004). There can be a direct impact on how problems, assessments, diagnoses, and intervention strategies are determined. As global trends in mobility, migration, cultural identity importance, and changing roles increase,

there is a greater need for transcultural awareness (Leininger, 1997). Shifts in the site of care to the community, a rise in moral/ethical issues in health care, and a desire by many, but not all, consumers to control and regulate their own health care have created a necessity to know and respect diverse cultural perspectives. This is important for effective and acceptable health care delivery; examples are provided in Box 19.3.

Box **19.3**

Religious/Cultural Prohibitions

Example 1

A female college student from another country sought health care for menstrual pain after arriving in the United States. She went to a physician to obtain a prescription for medication to ease the pain. The physician decided that the woman should have a Pap smear. Being unmarried, the woman could not agree to this for religious prohibition reasons. She tried to explain the situation to both the doctor and the nurse, but neither realized the cultural/religious issue nor seemed to understand the patient's inability to comply. The nurse told the woman, "Whatever your reasons are, you should have the Pap smear first as a diagnostic procedure." The woman refused, left the clinic, and did not return.

Example 2

Ramadan is the holy month of fasting and prayer in the Muslim religious tradition. During Ramadan, Muslims refrain from food and drink from early morning until early evening. Pregnant women, children under the age of 14, and those who are ill are exempt from the fast. However, many Muslims will not take medications during the hours when they are fasting. These patients and others, such as those with diabetes, can benefit from guidance that would help them alter their medication schedules in keeping with their fast.

Without a sense of cultural competence, U.S. health care providers tend to impress on people of other cultures provider-held values of patient autonomy, truth telling, and informed consent in spite of personal or family values regarding health care. When a nurse or other provider "tells" a client that he or she must have some therapy or intervention that does not fit the client's cultural perspective, a real potential for negative feelings and adverse behaviors occurs. If nursing is concerned with client advocacy and engaging with the client on a health care journey, then cultural competence is critical to effectiveness. Valuing the client's perspective and right to choose was once explained thus: If we do not value the client's right to choose, then we should refuse to care for all smokers, drug addicts, or others who persist in nonapproved lifestyle behaviors. To not enable harmful behavior, nurses need to teach, counsel, and use motivational behavioral change strategies.

In seeking cultural competence, nurses also need to recognize their own cultural values. The expectations, attitudes, and behaviors of nurses are affected by their cultures just as surely as the expectations, attitudes, and behaviors of clients are influenced by theirs. This can be a barrier to cultural competence if the nurse does not exhibit self-awareness and sensitivity to others.

There can be direct impacts on client care from culturally mediated practices. For example, national characteristics, culture, and philosophy affect the client's compliance with medication directives (Levy & Hawks, 1995). American, Japanese, and European medical practices reflect differences in the approach to medications. In Japan, where a more conservative approach is practiced, clients generally use lower dosage levels and have less tolerance for side effects. In the United States there is a much greater tolerance of side effects with a greater emphasis on the effectiveness of the medication. The European medical practice reflects patterns between those of the United States and Japan and recognizes diagnoses in some countries that are not used in others. Cultural differences also appear in the length of time that clients are willing to take medications.

Many Southeast Asian cultures prefer short-term medication prescription accompanied by an expectation of quick symptom relief.

CULTURAL ASSESSMENT

Learning to assess cultural backgrounds is a cultural skill-building strategy. It helps the nurse to develop cultural awareness, sensitivity, and competence, and it supplements the nurse's comprehensive assessment as a part of the nursing process. Because addressing cultural issues augments efforts at compliance, the six areas of communication, interpersonal space, social organization, sense of time, environmental control, and biological variations have been suggested for making a comprehensive cultural assessment (Davidhizar et al., 1998).

Cultural assessment tools exist both within and outside of nursing. In nursing, for example, Rosenbaum (1995), using Leininger's theory, displayed a cultural assessment tool to assist with holistic data collection. The elements of this assessment are as follows:

- Cultural affiliation
- Health and care beliefs and practices
- Illness beliefs and customs
- Interpersonal relations
- Spiritual practices
- World view and other social structure features

In health care, Goode (2002) displayed a self-assessment checklist for personnel providing primary health care services. Divided into sections—physical environment, materials, and resources; communication styles; and values and attitudes—this 30-item instrument includes assessment questions such as the frequency of ensuring that printed materials reflect the different cultures of individuals served by the agency, attempting to learn and use key words in other languages, and avoiding imposing values that may conflict or be inconsistent with other cultural groups. This tool provides a useful self-check for providers so that they can heighten awareness and sensitivity.

Mason (1995) presented a questionnaire designed to assess cultural competence training needs of human services organizations and staff. It is divided into sections of knowledge of communities, personal involvement, resources and linkages, staffing, and organizational policies and procedures. Questions include perceptions about how well you are able to describe the communities of color in your service area, whether you interact socially with people of color, whether staff use cultural consultants, if there are people of color on the staff, and whether the agency has culture-specific treatment approaches. Other cultural assessment and differences tools can be found on the Internet (e.g., *www.med.umich.edu/ multicultural/ccp/tools.htm*).

LEADERSHIP AND MANAGEMENT IMPLICATIONS

The Bureau of Health Professions (BHP) of the USDHHS reported that African Americans and Hispanics are underrepresented in the registered nurse workforce relative to their proportion in the overall population, as follows (BHP, 2004):

Estimates from the 2000 Sample Survey of Registered Nurses (HRSA, 2001) indicate that approximately 86.6 percent of RNs are non-Hispanic white, 4.9 percent are non-Hispanic African American, 3.5 percent are Asian; 2 percent are Hispanic; 0.5 percent are American Indian or

Table 19.1

Population Distribution by Ethnicity

Year	Non-Hispanic White (%)	African American (%)	All Others (%)
2000	69.1	12.3	18.6
2005	67.1	12.5	20.4
2010	64.8	12.7	22.5
2015	62.8	12.9	24.3
2020	60.8	13.1	26.1

Modified from Bureau of Health Professions (BHP). (2004). *Middle series projections.* Rockville, MD: National Center for Health Workforce Analysis, BHP, U.S. Department of Health and Human Services.

Alaskan Native, 0.2 percent are Native Hawaiian or Pacific Islander, and 1.2 percent are of two or more racial backgrounds. (Section 3.3.2)

This compares with the BHP report of census projections of population distribution by ethnicity (BHP, 2004), as shown in Table 19.1. This disparity points to the need for nursing to push forward strong cultural competence initiatives. The focus needs to be both on culturally competent client care practices and on a culturally competent workplace environment. Lack of understanding of cultural practices may result in longer hospital stays, noncompliance issues, and loss of meaningful

⚠ LEADERSHIP & MANAGEMENT BEHAVIORS

Leadership Behaviors

- Envisions holistic care, including cultural competence
- Influences others to be culturally sensitive
- Inspires trust and confidence among culturally diverse people
- Leads others toward cultural competence

Management Behaviors

- Coordinates care to include cultural assessment and planning
- Integrates cultural diversity into the workplace

- Plans cultural sensitivity training
- Organizes teams that include culturally diverse workers

Overlap Areas

- Plans for cultural diversity issues
- Motivates others toward culturally competent communication

nurse-client communication. Underrepresentation of racial/ethnic groups in the workforce may inhibit recruitment into the profession because of a lack of role models. The key is being sensitive to differences (Trossman, 1998).

CARING FOR CULTURALLY DIVERSE CLIENTS

Being sensitive to differences incorporates the twin strategies of cognitive awareness of potential issues and building a repertoire of strategies to enhance cultural and linguistic competence. Common sources of cultural differences or approaches can be seen as sources of problems or potential conflicts. Some examples include language and interpretation of communication, eye-contact norms, gender issues, touching and physical contact, food practices, and caregiver acceptability issues (Galanti, 1999).

On the journey toward cultural competence there are road signs and strategies that can help smooth the way. Some are basic common sense, such as stopping to think about others, whereas others require specific knowledge of the client and the client's culture. For instance, it is helpful to remember that what is viewed as polite, caring, quality health care in one culture may be considered rude, uncaring, or even poor health care in another culture. A first step is to try to learn how the client wants to be treated. If the nurse does not know, he or she can start by simply asking. The respect shown for the client's cultural values will be appreciated.

U.S. culture is more informal than most cultures. For instance, people who grew up in a different culture, within the United States or elsewhere, may consider it a lack of respect to address others by their first names, especially when there is a significant difference in age between the caregiver and the client. The caregiver can ask the client how he or she would like to be addressed or address the client by his or her family name. However, in many Asian cultures the family name precedes the given name. Should Chen Lee be called Mr. Chen or Mr. Lee? It is best to ask.

Another road sign to cultural competence involves questioning. When a client is asked if he or she understands, a nod of the head or a yes may not mean that the client cognitively understood the question. This is true for limited English-speaking clients. It is also true for clients who speak English well but cannot hear well. It is not unusual for someone who is hearing-impaired to reply in the affirmative when he or she does not clearly hear the question. For some, a nod is meant to encourage more information so that the listener can piece together the meaning of the communication from further contextual cues. One strategy is to ask open-ended questions that call for specific information and then listen closely to the answer for clues to the client's understanding and hearing of the questions.

Still another road sign to cultural competence involves personal space. Every culture has its own set of rules regarding touching and distance. Nonverbal communication includes the use of space, called *proxemics*. Americans generally perceive four space zones: public (12 feet to limits of sight), social (4-12 feet away), personal (2-4 feet away), and intimate (0-2 feet away) (Figure 19.3). An initial greeting or introduction would occur in social space. A physical examination would occur in intimate space. If people are not sensitive to proxemics, tension or uneasiness can arise when a perceived violation of the meaning of the space zone occurs. This distracts from positive communication (Bremer, 2004). Many Americans feel uncomfortable if someone stands closer than 3 feet away from them for a conversation. On the other hand, many people from the Middle East need to stand close to the person with whom they are conversing. Hispanic clients usually expect the health care provider to shake hands with them at the beginning of a conversation, whereas most Japanese clients may feel very uncomfortable with shaking hands. Touching and closeness may be perceived as either friendly or threatening.

Because U.S. health care may be overwhelming and confusing to many culturally diverse clients, adherence to the following few general guidelines

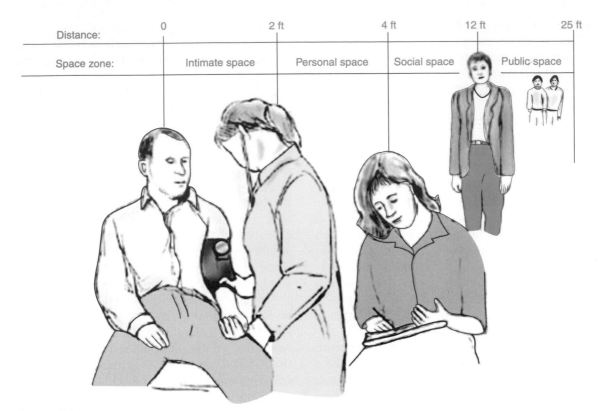

Figure 19.3
Social, personal, and intimate spaces of the patient requiring health care. (Modified from Wilkins, R.L., Krider, S.J., & Sheldon, R.L. [2000]. *Clinical assessment in respiratory care* [4th ed.]. St Louis: Mosby.)

can be helpful for a more culturally competent practice:

- Consider that the nurse's behavior may be interpreted as abrupt, rude, or frightening when it is very different from the client's cultural expectations.
- Be aware that attitudes toward suffering and the etiology of illness may vary.
- Understand that resistance to invasive procedures may be founded in religious beliefs.
- Evaluate the fit of the treatment plan with the client's lifestyle, eating habits, and preferred form of medication to increase the potential for compliance.
- Anticipate that informed consent forms may be frightening if the concept is strange to the client.

- Recognize that clients may be unfamiliar with the role of the nurse as professional staff and may expect care directly from a physician.
- Realize that Americans tend to think in linear terms and emphasize the clock; people from other cultures may not.

STRATEGIES FOR CULTURAL COMPETENCE

Cultural differences in ways of doing things and in beliefs about health and illness are learned and transmitted via cultural environments. Because cultural differences are learned, cultural sensitivity and competence in nursing practice also can be learned.

A culturally competent model of care was developed by Campinha-Bacote (1994). The four

🗎 Research Note

Source: Bartol, G.M., & Richardson, L. (1998). Using literature to create cultural competence. *Image, 30*(1), 75-79.

Purpose

The purpose of this article is to describe how selected literature and reading can be used as a tool to promote cultural competence. Cultural competence is an important skill for nurses in managing a diverse societal environment.

Discussion

The authors stated that cultural competence is a dynamic process of thinking and behaving. Assumptions, knowledge, and meanings from another culture are identified and framed. The culture in which we are raised is a powerful influence on our beliefs and behaviors. Cultural competence begins with knowing one's own culture and then being open and inquiring about others. It is a way of becoming self-aware and understanding how others assign meaning. The authors explore and demonstrate examples from the use of popular literature to show how nurses can learn insight, perspective, and meaning about different points of view.

Application to Practice

Knowledge, sensitivity, and mutual understanding are needed for cultural competence in a diverse society. Culture is learned, and differences among cultural groups exist. Since there is not one single culture, nurses need to learn about important themes in other cultures. Since both health care team members and clients come from diverse cultures, good dialogue, understanding, care delivery strategies, and team relationships will be improved by cultural competence, mutual sensitivity, and better awareness of differences and perspectives that drive health care behaviors.

identified components are (1) cultural awareness, including sensitivity and biases; (2) cultural knowledge, including world views and frameworks; (3) cultural skill, including assessment tools; and (4) cultural encounters, including exposure and practice. Using this model, Campinha-Bacote and colleagues (1996) defined each term and gave examples of how cultural competence concepts can be applied in nursing:

- *Cultural awareness* is a deliberate and cognitive process of becoming aware of and sensitive to the client's culture by becoming aware of the influence of one's own cultural values and learning to avoid imposing them on others. Experiential exercises, field trips, and critical incidents can be used to create an awareness focus.
- *Cultural knowledge* is a process of seeking and obtaining an educational background about the different world views of various cultures. The knowledge base of fields such as transcultural nursing, sociology, psychology, and anthropology can be examined for cultural knowledge.

- *Cultural skill* is the process of learning how to do a cultural assessment, allowing the nurse to identify an individual client's perceptions, beliefs, and practices. Various cultural assessment tools are available in nursing, such as Rosenbaum's (1995), which can be given to nurses as a guide for practicing cultural assessment.
- *Cultural encounter* is a process of directly engaging in cross-cultural interactions. This is a face-to-face experiential encounter. The nurse can structure or be exposed to specific clinical practice experiences that engage the nurse in multiple interactions with a specific cultural group or across cultural groups.

Other strategies for cultural competence include creating systems that train and support nurses and other health personnel in how to assess, problem-solve, and intervene with cultural sensitivity. Available tools can be used to assess the community, the institution, and the individual provider. These heighten awareness of basic differences and compare cultural norms and values.

Patients' health beliefs also can be assessed. Standardized assessment guides lead the practitioner through the areas to assess and can be used for practice simulations and personal improvement feedback.

Systems also can be assessed to determine whether they meet the USDHHS' (2000) CLAS standards. Quick reference "fact sheets" may be developed and posted in a handy place to refresh providers' memories about cultural differences. For example, Table 19.2 summarizes key historical influences, cultural values, and influences on health care use by racial/ethnic minority groups (Glanz, 2003).

Other strategies include incorporating diversity into mission statements, career development and management programs for minority groups (often using mentoring, examining recruitment and retention practices, community involvement

Table 19.2

Major Influences of Racial/Ethnic Minority Groups*			
	Key Historical Influence(s)	Core Cultural Values	Influences on Health Care Use
Mexican American	Mexicans were early migrants to the Americas; over thousands of years and several civilizations they have adapted and acculturated. Eventual settling in Mexico and border areas, then annexation to the United States created adverse social conditions.	Women were held in high regard in Aztec culture but later excluded during the colonial period. Traditional family values survive; loyalty, solidarity, community, and extended family are important, as are cooperation, respect, and the Catholic religion.	Use of *curanderismo*, herbal treatments, and prayer provides healing on emotional, spiritual, and physical levels. Traditional healing complements modern medicine. Revival of positive cultural attributes holds hope for disease-preventing lifestyles.
Puerto Rican	There are two distinct groups: in Puerto Rico and in the U.S. mainland. Island economy has transformed from a rural to an urban, service-based economy. Many in the mainland live in Northeast urban centers (e.g., New York, Philadelphia)	Strong family ties, female-headed and single-parent households are common. Lifestyles differ between U.S. mainland and Puerto Rican groups, but core values and religion cut across regions.	Cost, language, and discrimination are often barriers to care in the U.S. mainland. View that physicians are insensitive is often a barrier.
Cuban American	There have been several waves of immigration to the United States, in 1950s-1960s and later in	Cuban society is highly patriarchal, with men expected to provide for their	A sense of "specialness" and take-charge attitude may promote self-care. Early surveys found high

Table 19.2

Major Influences of Racial/Ethnic Minority Groups*—cont'd		
	Key Historical Influence(s)	Core Cultural Values	Influences on Health Care Use
	the 1980s. Most immigrants have been political exiles fleeing an oppressive government regime.	families; this seems to have led to greater strain on males. Loyalty to family is an important value.	fear and fatalism about cancer. Culturally and linguistically targeted health and cancer care programs seem to have been effective.
African American	First brought to the United States as slaves, African Americans are historically in a disadvantaged position. Racial integration and equal legal rights are relatively recent occurrences.	African-American women are traditionally in a subordinate position. Family and kinship networks are strong, with churches often central to a sense of belonging. Women have a key role in stability and caring for the family and children.	African Americans are more likely to use preventive care if it uses culturally appropriate methods, such as lay peer educators, family and community networks, and community outreach.
Asian American	Wide variations in history exist; there are more than 25 ethnic groups, ranging from fifth generation to recent immigrants and refugees. Experiences in immigration and acculturation in the United States are also widely divergent.	An internal balance or equilibrium is believed to support health; keeping balance between "cold" (yin) and "hot" (yang) elements leads to good health; "chi" is energy circulating through the body.	Access to and use of health care are related to cultural, linguistic, and other social barriers. Traditional healers and herbal medicines are common; Asian Americans may feel no need for Westernized preventive care.
Native Hawaiian	Europeans introduced disease and brought cultural and social disruption to the indigenous Polynesian population. Hawaii, its monarchy overthrown by	Efforts to preserve and enhance cultural heritage and overcome historical displacement have recently	Provision of culturally acceptable services is a continuing problem. Women respond to personal interaction and communication as well as problem solving.

Continued

Table 19.2

Major Influences of Racial/Ethnic Minority Groups*—cont'd

	Key Historical Influence(s)	Core Cultural Values	Influences on Health Care Use
Native Hawaiian—cont'd	Americans, was annexed to the United States in 1898. Intermarriage has reduced the number of ethnically pure Hawaiians.	intensified. Emphasis is on social harmony (lokahi), family ('ohana), inter-dependence/oneness (mana), and ties to the land (malama 'aina). Women are seen as powerful actors.	Traditional healers and remedies are often used. A limited number of Native Hawaiian health professionals is a further barrier.
American Samoan	Residing in the Samoan archipelago of U.S. mainland, American Samoans have a Polynesian heritage and village leadership systems. The United States has influence, and migration patterns are family related.	Communities are tightly unit, with close ties to churches and families. Some adjustment difficulty occurs among migrants, more in Hawaii than in California locales.	Culturally based beliefs about diseases are common, and many prefer traditional healers and herbalists. Belief in supernatural causes of disease may lead to delay in seeking Western health care.
American Indian	Land base and resources were lost with European migration; displacement, relocation to reservations, epidemics, and poverty ensued.	Male-oriented traditions dominated for many years. View of health is holistic, emphasizing harmony/balance in body, mind, spirit, and emotions.	Illness can have natural/supernatural causes; it is taboo to talk about cancer owing to the "power of language." Many are reluctant to "look for illness" (screening).
Alaska Native	Indigenous people were disrupted by European/Western culture and commerce.	Alaska Natives have strong family/communal ties, spirituality, and traditional subsistence lifestyle.	Women may neglect their health in favor of their families; traditional healing practices are common, although communication styles may differ.

From Glanz, K. (2003). *Cancer in women of color monograph.* Bethesda, MD: National Cancer Institute, National Institutes of Health, USDHHS. Retrieved October 8, 2004, from *http://dccps.nci.nih.gov/womenofcolor/pdfs/overview-table3.pdf*
*As with any summary of key dimensions of culture, this table cannot fully convey the depth and variation of influences within these racial/ethnic minority groups. The information included here is respectfully considered a reasonable effort to highlight these factors.

and outreach, diversity dialogue groups, and targeted education and training programs). Building competence in problem solving and intervention techniques can be augmented by practice exercises. Exercises such as analysis of body language can help in understanding cultural differences, as follows:

Silence: You may view silence as awkward; however, other cultures are quite comfortable with periods of silence.

Distance: The most comfortable physical distance between you and another person varies from culture to culture. The typical American generally prefers to be about an arm's length distance away from another person. Hispanics usually prefer closer proximity than most Americans. Allow the other person to establish the proper distance for the interaction.

Eye Contact: The amount of eye contact that is comfortable varies with each culture. Many Americans are brought up to look people straight in the eye. However, some cultures have been taught not to make eye contact. Staring is considered impolite in some groups. However, if you avoid eye contact, or break eye contact too frequently it may be misinterpreted by the participant as disinterest. Sitting next to someone, rather than directly across from them, will reduce eye contact.

Facial Expression: Expression of emotion between people of different cultures varies from very expressive, as with Hispanics, to total non-expressiveness, as with Asians. Many Americans have a tendency to regard people who are more expressive as immature and those with less expression as unfeeling.

Body Language: The position, gestures, and motion of the body can be interpreted differently depending on the culture. The use of hands is a common vehicle for nonverbal expression. A firm handshake may be a positive gesture of goodwill in the Anglo-American culture, but some other cultures prefer only a light touch. Many cultures use handshakes more frequently than do most

Americans, some even as a greeting between husband and wife. Standing with hands on hips may imply anger to some participants. Pointing or beckoning with a finger may appear disrespectful to some cultures. Conservative use of body language is wise when you are uncertain as to what is appropriate within a cultural group. Observing actions and interactions may give you direction. Being open with participants and asking general questions about body language can also help. (ISCOPES, 2003, section on Nonverbal Communication)

Cultural competence practice exercises often use vignettes or case studies. Some examples are presented in the Case Study in this chapter.

CURRENT ISSUES AND TRENDS

Nurses will encounter cultural and linguistic issues in their clinical practice. Some issues that nurses should be alert for include female circumcision, gender and transgender roles, use of alternative and complementary medicine, and religious influences. Professional principles of informed consent and advocacy for the patient may intersect with cultural influences. Nurses need to assess carefully and intervene with cultural sensitivity.

Attracting a Culturally Diverse Workforce

Reaching for cultural competence in the health care workplace requires not only that institutions strive for a greater understanding of the values represented by divergent clients but also that efforts be increased to diversify the makeup of nursing and other health care professions. The Pew Health Professions Commission report (1998) spoke directly to this need:

Not only would renewed commitment to diversity be the fairest way to accommodate all potential medical practitioners, it would be in the best interest of those parts of the population that bear the greatest burdens of poor health. Students that come from medically underserved communities have demonstrated a much greater willingness to return to them to practice. By knowing the language and cultural mores of the population they serve, they offer a more complete and effective kind of care. (p. iv)

Workplace diversity is an issue of both the workforce and the clients. The institutions that take the initiative to strive for cultural competence can engender respect for the similarities and differences that both employees and clients bring to the health care endeavor. Success with cultural competence concerning employees will provide improved understanding for culturally diverse clients. In turn, success with culturally diverse clients will help an institution to recruit and maintain a culturally diverse workforce. The inevitable conflict that can occur when persons with diverse value sets work together will be decreased as success is achieved in cultural competence in interpersonal relationships.

There are both advantages and challenges to cultural diversity in the workplace. The synergy of diverse viewpoints can improve nursing's knowledge base and care strategies. Yet the differences among people can give rise to communication gaps and conflict. The same issues of communication, interpersonal space, social proscriptions, time sense, and other variations in beliefs and behaviors that are so important when interacting with clients need to be balanced and smoothed in work groups and teams. The nurse care manager can employ cultural competence principles in leading and managing work groups. Strategies of respect for differences, exploring beyond the comfort zone, withholding judgment of others, emphasizing the positive, and practicing good communication techniques are strategies for success (Grossman & Taylor, 1995).

Efforts to pursue cultural competence must incorporate the broad base of diversity. The American Association of Colleges of Nursing (AACN) has reiterated the importance of intensifying efforts to increase diversity in programs that prepare nurses (AACN, 2004).

Diversity initiatives in the nursing profession will have a marked opportunity in the coming years since there is a bright outlook for growth in nursing jobs. The U.S. Bureau of Labor Statistics (BLS) (Hecker, 2004) projected that nursing, the largest health care occupation, will grow faster than the average for all other occupations. In fact, in 2004, registered nurses topped the list (ranked No. 1) of the 10 occupations with the largest projected job growth in the years 2002 to 2012. This top-10 list is used in career guidance and may have an impact on nursing school enrollments.

Language Diversity

The BHP (2004) reported that "language and cultural differences also are cited as factors affecting health care utilization. With the growing population of Hispanics in the U.S. and immigration from non-English speaking countries, language is playing an increasingly important role in the provision of health care services" (section 3.2).

The Modern Language Association ([MLA], 2004, p. 1) reported that the 2000 census identified 47.0 million respondents who reported that they spoke other languages than English (18% of the entire population over five years old). Of those respondents, "55% said that they also spoke English 'very well,' 22% that they also spoke English 'well,' 16% that they also spoke English but 'not well,' and 7% that they did not speak English at all." The 2000 census (U.S. Census Bureau, 2003) reported that in addition to English there are seven languages spoken by more than a million persons each in the U.S. (Table 19.3).

Because translation services are expensive, yet CLAS standards need to be met, nurses and other health care providers must be aware of major languages in the community. Creative strategies, interpreter services, and informatics applications can be used to reach linguistic availability.

The Aging Population

A related cultural diversity issue concerns age group-specific factors. Among the characteristics of the elderly population is a low literacy concerning health. Gazmararian and colleagues (1999) reported results of a survey that indicated that more than one-third of U.S. Medicare recipients, aged 65 or older, had inadequate or marginal

Table 19.3

Languages Spoken in the United States	
Language	Number Who Speak Language
English	215,423,557
Spanish or Spanish Creole	28,101,052
Chinese	2,022,143
French (including Patois and Cajun)	1,643,838
German	1,383,442
Tagalog	1,224,241
Vietnamese	1,009,627
Italian	1,008,370

Data from U.S. Census Bureau, U.S. Department of Commerce. (2003). Washington, DC.

health literacy. Health illiteracy appeared to increase with age. Personal interviews assessed health literacy by determining each respondent's ability to understand simple prescription instructions, blood glucose self-monitoring guidelines, instructions preparatory to an upper gastrointestinal (GI) tract x-ray procedure, and a Medicaid "Rights and Responsibilities" document. This research tested 3,260 Medicare recipients in a large managed care organization, revealing that overall, 33.9% of English-speaking and 53.9% of Spanish-speaking respondents either did not have or had only marginal health literacy skills. Since inadequate health literacy may adversely affect costs and care delivery, providers need to assess health literacy skills, especially among elderly clients. Such an assessment can lead to designing more effective educational and communication interventions and materials.

Summary

- Moving to a global community means a greater awareness of cultural diversity.
- Cultural and linguistic competence is needed to improve health care services to clients and to enhance the nursing profession.

- Cultural diversity refers to variety and differences among people and groups.
- Cultural competence means learning and respecting the values of others.
- Transcultural nursing provides a theoretical base for nursing regarding cultural competence.
- Population demographic projections in the United States show a change in ethnicity and age groups.
- Cultural competence is needed to improve client care and avoid adverse outcomes.
- Cultural awareness, knowledge, skill, and encounters help enhance cultural competence.
- Nursing needs to implement strategies to reflect the cultural mix of society within the workforce more closely.

Study Questions

1. Why is cultural competence important for nursing?
2. What are the components of cultural awareness?
3. How do you perform a cultural assessment?
4. How does the nurse apply cultural competence in the workplace?

CASE STUDY

Case 1

Maria, a Hispanic woman with three children, presented with a tumor requiring a hysterectomy. Maria did not speak English, and the health care staff had asked her bilingual son to serve as an interpreter in explaining that Maria needed to sign an informed consent form for the surgery. The son explained the procedure to the mother. Staff noted that he appeared to be translating their explanation to the mother and pointed to his mother's abdomen as he translated. Maria willingly signed the consent form. When Maria learned the next day that she would no longer be able to bear children because her uterus had been removed, she became very agitated. Eventually she threatened to sue the hospital. When the health care staff discussed Maria's agitation with her family, they were told that, because it is not appropriate for a Hispanic male to discuss his mother's private parts with her, Maria's son had explained to her that a tumor would be removed from her abdomen and pointed to the general area. Maria's anger about not being able to bear more children was the result of her role in the Hispanic culture where a Hispanic woman's status is derived in large part from the number of children she produces.

Case 2

A nurse entered the hospital room of an Iranian patient who was scheduled for surgery the next day. Upon entering the room the nurse found the patient huddling on the floor. The patient did not speak English, and the nurse was unable to understand what the patient was mumbling. Assuming that the patient had fallen out of bed, the nurse tried to help the patient climb back into the bed. However, the patient responded by becoming visibly upset. When the patient's English-speaking family arrived, the nurse asked them to talk with the patient about what had happened. The nurse learned that the patient, a Muslim, had not fallen out of bed but rather was practicing her religion in the traditional manner of praying to Mecca.

CRITICAL THINKING EXERCISE

APPLICATIONS OF CULTURAL DIVERSITY TO END-OF-LIFE DECISIONS

Advance care planning for death and the client's right to withdraw, limit, or refuse unwanted therapy is a concept that evolved in Western traditions and is based on specific cultural orientations and views of life. Centering on principles of individual autonomy, the Western view of bioethical decision making at the end of life presumes an ideal client.

Koenig (1997) has identified seven characteristics that this type of client would have: (1) a shared understanding of illness, prognosis, and treatment options with members of the health care team; (2) orientation to the future and desire to maintain "control"; (3) the perception of freedom of choice; (4) openness to discussion of death and dying; (5) a balance between fatalism and belief in human agency that favors the latter; (6) a religious orientation that minimizes the likelihood of divine intervention; and (7) an assumption that the individual is the appropriate decision maker, not the family or extended social group. Clearly, this profile would not fit all persons or cultural orientations. There is growing evidence that clients from diverse cultures have different responses to the notion of advance directives. Koenig (1997) provided three examples that illustrate comparative cultural influences and manifested behaviors in dealing with a terminal prognosis.

Example 1

George is a 59-year-old European American man whose pancreatic cancer was discovered when he collapsed on the street and was taken to the emergency department of the local public hospital. George was quite open in discussing both the cancer diagnosis and the eventual outcome. He used the word *cancer* in discussing his illness, avoiding euphemisms. George's family also was open in talking about the illness. Following his initial surgery, the health care team suggested a treatment regimen of radiation therapy and chemotherapy. George began the treatment course but stopped all treatment soon thereafter because of the unpleasant side effects. He made specific plans for his funeral and began choosing a nursing home/hospice where he could receive end-of-life care, reflecting his desire not to "die at home," which he felt would burden his family.

Example 2

Mr. Lin was diagnosed with cancer in China before he immigrated to the United States with his wife and their two sons. The older son attends junior college and

CRITICAL THINKING EXERCISE—CONT'D

speaks English well, always accompanying his non-English-speaking father to the clinic. Since his arrival in the United States, Mr. Lin received treatment for locally invasive nasopharyngeal cancer, which progressed to the point of being immediately life-threatening because of the high likelihood of hemorrhage from major blood vessels in his neck. He has been treated with both radiation therapy and chemotherapy and is taking traditional Chinese medicine.

The professionals caring for Mr. Lin began with the assumption that he must be fully informed. However, relying on Mr. Lin's son to translate opens up the possibility of conflicting notions of what constitutes appropriate disclosure. This is because many Chinese are not used to telling their ill family member everything. Ill family members are not used to this either. It is believed that the client cannot tolerate this information and will become more ill if told the worst. In this case Mr. Lin and his son chose to maintain ambiguity and thus hope.

Example 3

Elena Alvarez is a 48-year-old woman who has lived in the United States for many years. Originally from El Salvador, she speaks only limited English. Before her diagnosis with ovarian cancer, Ms. Alvarez worked as a child care provider. Her disease has progressed despite surgery and chemotherapy. Elena Alvarez speaks openly about her cancer diagnosis with members of the clinic staff but maintains a complex silence within her family. From the point of view of her health care providers, Ms. Alvarez faces many decision points. She does not experience any personal sense of choice, however, and does not experience health care as including decisions. In the case of Elena Alvarez there is a tension between her belief that no choices exist and the health care team's demands that she make decisions. She feels that in other countries providers tell the family, and the family has influence by deciding what to do. Here the patient is pressed to decide.

These three examples highlight the diverse ways in which individuals respond to health and illness and filter their experiences through cultural values. Notice the number of Koenig's (1997) seven characteristics that were manifested in each of the three client stories. Although U.S. society may mandate asking about advance directives, nurses are advised to practice cultural competence with individual clients and families.

1. What is the problem in each case?
2. Whose problem is it?
3. What should the nurse do in each case?
4. How many of Koenig's seven characteristics are present in each case?
5. How can the nurse be culturally competent in each case?

REFERENCES

Agency for Healthcare Research and Quality (AHRQ). (2000). *Fact sheet: Addressing racial and ethnic disparities in health care* (AHRQ Publ. No. 00-PO41). Rockville, MD: AHRQ. Retrieved June 6, 2004, from *www.ahrq.gov/research/disparit.htm*

Agency for Healthcare Research and Quality (AHRQ). (2003). *What is cultural and linguistic competence?* Rockville, MD: AHRQ. Retrieved September 27, 2004, from *www.ahrq.gov/about/cods/cultcompdef.htm*

American Association of Colleges of Nursing (AACN). (1997). *AACN endorses the Sullivan Commission's report on increasing diversity in the health professions.* Washington, DC: AACN. Retrieved October 8, 2004, from *www.aacn.nche.edu/Media/NewsReleases/SullivanComm04.htm*

Bremer, J. (2004). *Proxemics—How we use space.* Oak Park, IL: Bremer Communications. Retrieved October 8, 2004, from *www.bremercommunications.com/Proxemics_How_We_Use_Space.htm*

Bureau of Health Professions [BHP]. (2004). *Changing demographics and the implications for physicians, nurses, and other health workers.* Rockville, MD: National Center for Health Workforce Analysis, BHP, USDHHS. Retrieved June 24, 2004, from *www.bhpr.hrsa.gov/healthworkforce/reports/changedemo/composition.htm#3.3.2*

Campinha-Bacote, J. (1994). Cultural competence in psychiatric nursing: A conceptual model. *Nursing Clinics of North America, 29*(1), 1-8.

Campinha-Bacote, J., Yahle, T., & Langenkamp, M. (1996). The challenge of cultural diversity for nurse educators. *The Journal of Continuing Education in Nursing, 27*(2), 59-64.

Centers for Disease Control and Prevention (CDC). (2003). *Health, United States, 2003, with chartbook on trends in the health of Americans.* Hyattsville, MD: CDC. Retrieved May 4, 2004, from *www.cdc.gov/nchs/data/hus/hus03.pdf*

Davidhizar, R., Bechtel, G., & Giger, J. (1998). Model helps CMs deliver multicultural care. *Case Management Advisor, 9*(6), 97-100.

Dreher, M.C. (1996). Nursing: A cultural phenomenon. *Reflections, 22*(4), 4.

Galanti, G. (1999). Caring for culturally diverse patients at home. *Home Health Care Consultant, 6*(1), 33-34.

Gazmararian, J.A., Baker, D.W., Williams, M.V., Parker, R.M., Scott, T.L., Green, D.C., et al. (1999). Health literacy among Medicare enrollees in a managed care organization. *Journal of the American Medical Association, 281*(6), 545-551.

Glanz, K. (2003). *Cancer in women of color monograph.* Bethesda, MD: National Cancer Institute, National Institutes of Health, USDHHS. Retrieved October 8, 2004, from *www.dccps.nci.nih.gov/womenofcolor/pdfs/overview-table3.pdf*

Goode, T.D. (2002). *Promoting cultural and linguistic competency.* Washington, DC: National Center for Cultural Competence, Georgetown University Center for Child and Human Development. Retrieved October 10, 2004, from *www.gucchd.georgetown.edu/nccc/nccc11.html*

Grossman, D., & Taylor R. (1995). Cultural diversity on the unit. *American Journal of Nursing, 95*(2), 64-67.

Hecker, D.E. (2004). Occupational employment projections to 2012. *Monthly Labor Review Online, 127*(2). Retrieved October 8, 2004, from *www.bls.gov/opub/mlr/2004/02/art5abs.htm*

Hobbs, F., & Stoops, N. (2002). *Demographic trends in the 20th century* (U.S. Census Bureau, Census 2000 Special Reports, Series Censr-4). Washington, DC: U.S. Census Bureau, U.S. Department of Commerce. Retrieved October 8, 2004, from *www.census.gov/prod/2002pubs/censr-4.pdf*

ISCOPES. (2003). *Cultural competence.* ISCOPES. Washington, DC: The George Washington University. Retrieved October 8, 2004, from *www.gwu.edu/~iscopes/LearningMods_Culture.htm#8*

Koenig, B.A. (1997). Cultural diversity in decision making about care at the end of life. In M.J. Field & C.K. Cassel (Eds.), *Approaching death: Improving care at the end of life* (Appendix E). Washington, DC: National Academies Press.

Leininger, M. (1997). Transcultural nursing research to transform nursing education and practice: 40 years. *Image, 29*(4), 341-347.

Levy, R.A., & Hawks, J.W. (1995). Multicultural medicine and pharmacy management. II. Compliance with medications. *Drug Benefit Trends, 7*(4), 13-14, 24.

Mason, J.L. (1995). *Cultural competence self-assessment questionnaire. A manual for users.* Portland, OR: Research and Training Center on Family Support and Children's Mental Health.

McCarty, L.J., Enslein, J.C., Kelly, L.S., Choi, E., & Tripp-Reimer, T. (2002). Cross-cultural health education: Materials on the World Wide Web. *Journal of Transcultural Nursing, 13*(1), 54-60.

Modern Language Association (2004). *MLA language map FAQ.* New York: MLA. Retrieved June 24, 2004, from *www.www.mla.org/census_about*

Narayan, M.C. (2002). The national standards for culturally and linguistically appropriate services in health care. *Care Management Journals, 3*(2), 77-83.

Office of Minority Health (OMH). (2000). Assuring cultural competence in health care: Recommendations for national standards and an outcomes-focused research agenda. *Federal Register, 65*(247), 80865-80879.

Pasco, C.Y., Morse, J.M., & Olson, J.K. (2004). Cross-cultural relationships between nurses and Filipino Canadian patients. *Journal of Nursing Scholarship, 36*(3), 239-246.

Pew Health Professions Commission. (1998). *Recreating health professional practice for a new century.* San Francisco, CA: The Center for the Health Professions, University of California. Retrieved October 8, 2004, from *www.futurehealth.ucsf.edu/pdf_files/rept4.pdf*

President's Cancer Panel. (1997). *President's cancer panel meeting: Meeting minutes. The real impact in the reduction of cancer morality research.* Bethesda, MD: National Cancer Institute, National Institutes of Health. Retrieved October 8, 2004, from: *www.deainfo.nci.nih.gov/advisory/pcp/archive/pcp0997/minutes.htm#5*

Rosenbaum, J.N. (1995). Teaching cultural sensitivity. *Journal of Nursing Education, 34*(4), 188-189.

Trossman, S. (1998). Diversity: A continuing challenge. *American Nurse, 30*(1), 1, 24-25.

U.S. Census Bureau. (2000). *Census Bureau projects doubling of nation's population by 2100.* Washington, DC: U.S. Census Bureau, U.S. Department of Commerce. Retrieved October 8, 2004, from *www.census.gov/Press-Release/www/2000/cb00-05.html*

U.S. Census Bureau. (2003). *Language use and English-speaking ability: 2000. Census 2000 brief.* Washington, DC: U.S. Census Bureau, U.S. Department of Commerce. Retrieved October 8, 2004, from *www.census.gov/prod/cen2000/doc/sf3.pdf*

U.S. Census Bureau. (2004). *Hispanic and Asian Americans increasing faster than overall population.* Washington, DC: U.S. Census Bureau, U.S. Department of Commerce. Retrieved June 16, 2004, from *www.census.gov/Press-Release/www/releases/archives/race/001839.html*

U.S. Department of Health and Human Services (USDHHS). (1999). *Racial/ethnic disparities in health* (Parklawn Health Library Bulletin No. 471). Rockville, MD: USDHHS.

U.S. Department of Health and Human Services (USDHHS). (2000, 22 December). Office of Minority Health. National standards on culturally and linguistically appropriate services (CLAS) in health care. *Federal Register, 65*(247), 80865-80879. Retrieved May 5, 2004, from *www.frwebgate.access.gpo.gov/cgi-bin/getdoc.cgi?dbname=2000_register&docid=00-32685-filed*

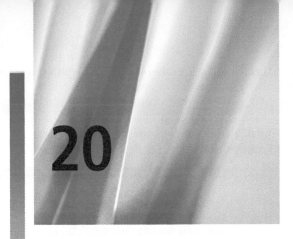

20

Communication, Persuasion, and Negotiation

JoEllen Koerner   Diane L. Huber

CHAPTER OBJECTIVES

eadership is an attempt to influence. The three basic competencies of influencing are diagnosing, adapting, and communicating. For leadership purposes, the skill of communicating means being able to put a message into a form that can be easily understood and accepted by others. Leaders influence others from both personal power and position power bases. One aspect of personal power is the ability to establish rapport by communicating so that the people who will be influenced feel comfortable and have trust and confidence in the leader (Hersey et al., 2001). Basic nursing practice emphasizes therapeutic communication for effectiveness in the nurse-client relationship, and communication in leadership and care management builds on this skill to address the scope of work-related communication issues.

Communication is the lubricant of organizations. It is a vital aspect of both leadership and management. Communication is the basis for interpersonal relationships necessary for professional practice. Humans communicate naturally and frequently. In nursing practice, communication is focused on both client care management and organizational outcomes. As nurses work within organizations to deliver nursing care, they need to be able to work together to reach common goals. Communication can facilitate positive working relationships, or it can contribute to stress, lack of recognition, and feelings of alienation. Organizations face the challenge of creating communication pathways that lead to professional, productive, and comfortable work environments.

DEFINITIONS

Words are, of course, the most powerful drug used by mankind.

Rudyard Kipling

Communication is the art of being able to structure and transmit a message in a way that another can easily understand and accept. **Organizational communication** is defined as the degree to which information is transmitted among the members and parts of an organization. Information can be transmitted through a variety of verbal, written, electronic, and oral communication modes. Some examples are fliers, memos, letters, faxes, e-mail, formal discussions, committees, informal networking, newsletters, videos, bulletin boards, and telephone calls. The basis of communication is information exchange, and accuracy and openness are necessary for building trust.

Communication occurs as both verbal and nonverbal information transmission. **Verbal communication** is both written and spoken (oral). **Nonverbal communication** is unspoken and is composed of affective or expressive behaviors. The effectiveness of verbal communication depends on vocabulary, language, phrases, sentence structure, sentence clarity, rate of speech, diction, tone, rhythm, and volume. Nonverbal behavior includes gestures, facial expression, eye contact, body language, and positioning (Hersey et al., 2001). Art, music, and body language are forms of nonverbal expression.

Communication can be characterized by four distinctions: (1) formal and informal, (2) vertical and horizontal, (3) personal and impersonal, and (4) instrumental and expressive. These distinctions are defined as follows (Price & Mueller, 1986):

- *Formal:* officially transmitted information, supported by organizational sanctions
- *Informal:* unofficial information exchange
- *Vertical:* transmission of information in superior-subordinate relationships
- *Horizontal:* transmission of information among peers
- *Personal:* information transmitted in situations where mutual influence may occur
- *Impersonal:* information exchange without mutual influence
- *Instrumental:* transmittal of information necessary to do the job
- *Expressive:* the residual category of nonjob information transmittal

▲ LEADING & MANAGING DEFINED

Organizational Communication

The degree to which information is transmitted among the members and parts of an organization.

Verbal Communication

Communication through the use of words, either spoken or written.

Nonverbal Communication

Communication that does not use words but rather affective or expressive behaviors.

Persuasion

Human communication designed to influence another to change attitudes or alter behaviors.

Negotiation

A process of give-and-take exchange among persons aimed at resolving problems, conflicts, or disputes.

Bargaining

The exchange of favors or trading activity.

Thus in the complex situations of organizational environments, information of various types is communicated in many different ways. Nurses need to analyze all aspects of communication at work.

Persuasion is defined as a human communication activity designed to influence another to change attitudes or alter behaviors by the use of techniques such as argument, reasoning, or pleading. Persuasion uses knowledge about human psychology and power, status, and communicative ability to influence others to the persuader's point of view. Unless a change is accomplished by using a purely directive strategy, nurses will use persuasion as a major technique for accomplishing goals. Persuasion is a basic, dynamic process of politics. It is the art of getting people to share a similar perception of the truth so that they can work together (Curtin, 1991). The persuader seeks to get another to make a change, initiate some action, or alter activities through the use of language to convince others that one option is more desirable than another. In the ideal situation, the persuader leaves the person with a perception of having choices. People often respond negatively to the concept of persuasion because it sounds manipulative and therefore negative. Persuasion is neither bad nor good. It can be neutral, or it can be used for positive or negative purposes.

Negotiation is defined as a process of give-and-take exchange among persons that is aimed at resolving problems, conflicts, or disputes. **Bargaining**, a closely related term, is the exchanging of favors or trading activity. Negotiation uses a communication process and attempts to settle a problem or a conflict or gain more resources. Both bargaining and negotiating are strategies used to divide the areas of contention so that each party gains something. To reach a level of agreement, a back-and-forth process occurs in which the parties have sequential rounds of offering their position on terms and conditions for settlement. This process is called *negotiation.*

Negotiation has been described as getting what you want. It is a part of everyday life. Every desire and need is a potential occasion for negotiation. Exchanging ideas with the intention of changing relationships and conferring for agreement are negotiations. Negotiation is the process that occurs when individuals engage in resolution to reach an agreement with stated conditions and expectations (Booth, 1993). Negotiation is used when both parties have strong feelings or conflicting views and when there is a need for agreement, resolution, or compromise.

Negotiation can be applied specifically to labor-management disputes and unionization. Nurses may work in settings in which the registered nurses (RNs) and ancillary workers are unionized. In unionized settings, the term *negotiation* takes on a specific collective bargaining connotation. Collective bargaining is a prescribed realm of negotiation in which there are specific laws and rules that govern the negotiating activity. In collective bargaining the concept of negotiation becomes more narrowly defined as a process in which the terms and conditions of work are resolved between the employer and the organized representatives of the employees. Formal unionization limits employers' ability to take unilateral action in selected areas of work life, and it may slow innovation or create some restrictions for nurses.

BACKGROUND

Communication is a process. The classic communication model is a linear model that describes a circular process of a sender who encodes a message, a message channel, a receiver who decodes the message, a set of barriers that may occur between sender and receiver, and feedback between receiver and sender (Anderson & Tredway, 1999). The interpretation of this model in leadership theory describes the elements as the leader; the leader's perceptions; the message in the form of words, nonverbal elements, and paralanguage; the follower; the follower's perceptions; and feedback. The perceptions become filters to the communication process. Active listening, pacing, and rapport are key skills in the leadership communication process (Hersey et al., 2001). All forms of

Research Note

Source: Anderson, M.A., & Tredway, C.A. (1999). Communication: An outcome of case management. *Nursing Case Management, 4*(3), 104-111.

Purpose

Case management is a multidisciplinary system emphasizing collaboration, coordination, and communication to assess, plan, monitor, evaluate, and coordinate options and services among multiple providers and across a variety of settings and sites of health care. Communication is an outcome of case management activities. The purpose of this study was to investigate case management communication outcomes and the influence of selected organizational and medical condition factors on communication.

Discussion

Effective communication in the form of information exchange is needed for the collaborative relationship between case managers and other care providers. Case managers work to ensure continuity of care by overcoming traditional barriers to provider communication by coordinating all services. *Communication* is defined here as the amount and type of referral information transferred from a hospital-based case manager to a home health agency (HHA) using an established case management model for coordinating continuous client care. Information exchange takes the form of a home health referral during the discharge planning phase in the acute care hospital. Despite the importance of appropriate and timely communication, the process is problematic in regard to breakdowns and gaps. Information may be late, unusable, or absent.

The classic communication model of sender, message channel, receiver, barriers, and feedback was used to frame the study. A nonexperimental, retrospective, descriptive design using a closed medical record review of 200 home care medical records at one Midwestern HHA was the structure for this study. Data were collected by using the Referral Data Inventory Tool to identify continuity of care. Results suggested that referrals mainly contained background and medical data, with little psychosocial or nursing data. All referral data were insufficient in amount. Significantly greater amounts and types of referral data were transferred when a phone call followed by the standard transfer form occurred. Results indicated that case managers were absent from the transfer of client information from the hospital to HHA despite a job description containing referral communication responsibilities. A number of barriers to effective communication existed.

Application to Practice

A breakdown in communication between the hospital and HHA was identified and analyzed in relation to communication theory. Models of case management, and the hospital job description in this case, define coordination as a responsibility of the case manager. However, case managers were absent from this role. Delegation of interorganizational referral to others created too many individuals involved in creating and exchanging the message, and a lack of coordination of duties created too many filters. Distortion of message and breakdown in communication resulted. Recommendations included increasing the case managers' involvement and establishing an interdisciplinary team to refine the referral procedure. The HHA also needs to respond with feedback to the acute care hospital as message sender.

the communication process are designed to enhance interpersonal relationships.

Communication and relating are linked to each other in that effective communication enhances interpersonal relations, and positive interpersonal relations promote effective communication. Communication models described in the literature include the sender-receiver, human needs, and transactional analysis models (Grant, 1994).

The sender-receiver model describes communication as messages or signals passed between the sender and the receiver. A single communication can be broken down into the following five steps of information exchange (Grant, 1994):

1. *Message formation:* The message develops in the sender's mind.
2. *Message encoding:* The decision is made by the sender as to verbal and nonverbal components.
3. *Message transmission:* The spoken, written, and/or nonverbal information is expressed.
4. *Message reception:* The receiver receives the information.
5. *Message decoding:* The receiver interprets the message.

Communication can be viewed as a pathway between two people. It occurs in a variety of interactive patterns (Cornell, 1993) (Figure 20.1). What this means is that the equality of exchange may be balanced or skewed. Sometimes people only desire to express themselves or impart information. Therefore they do not engage in listening to the other or in reciprocity of information. When people

take turns, the conversation can be productive and show fewer signs of faulty communication. Listening is a basic and powerful way to understand and connect to another human being.

Perception and interpretation form filters for messages and create a potential for communication breakdown. Both sender and receiver have separate perceptual filters. On both ends, then, what was meant and what was understood may vary.

Problems can occur at any point and result in miscommunication. Successful communication is promoted by using simplicity, clarity, appropriate timing, relevance, adaptation to circumstances, and credibility. On the other hand, successful communication is hindered by actions that distract, cut off communication, insert unhelpful advice, remove the other person's decision-making power, or negate the importance of the other person or of his or her message. Specific behaviors of offering inappropriate reassurance, rejecting the other, agreeing uncritically, stereotyping, belittling, or being egocentric tend to harm or hinder communication (Grant, 1994).

Communication also has been conceptualized within the framework of interpersonal skills or transactional analysis models. These models emphasize therapeutic communication techniques of active listening, attending, questioning, paraphrasing, reflecting feelings, assertion, challenging, confrontation, and interviewing skills (Thies & Williams-Burgess, 1992).

Communication in Groups

Group communication is complex because of the exponential way interactions duplicate as the number of active participants increases. This makes effective communication a greater challenge. To better comprehend what makes group communication effective, social psychologists and communication researchers have conducted communication net studies. In these experiments a few subjects are put into networks with selectively restricted channels of communication, given simple games or tasks, and then observed for patterns of interaction. The researchers observed how members passed messages through others.

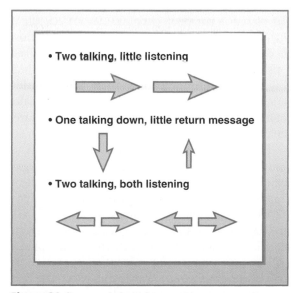

Figure 20.1
Interactive communication patterns. (Data from Cornell D. [1993]. Say the words: Communication techniques. *Nursing Management, 24*[3], 42-44.)

The five communication networks are the wheel, the Y, the chain, the circle, and all-channel. The wheel, Y, and chain formations restrict communication the most and tend to be centralizing and hierarchical. The wheel network, also called a *star pattern,* passes all communication through one person.

Examples occur in autocratic and hierarchical structures of groups or organizations. For instance, the chain style resembles the chain of command in a military organization. In the wheel structure, employees send all information to the boss, and the boss sends selected information to employees. There is little lateral communication. The all-channel form has no communication restrictions. This is an example of an open communication network, in which information and messages are passed everywhere. The circle and the all-channel networks tend to be more democratic configurations. The circle is the least efficient network (Mintzberg, 1993). In a hierarchical network, all members have to pass messages through one person. Sometimes a circle is formed and communication only allowed to either side. In a democratic network, all members can communicate freely. Hierarchical networks organize more quickly, make fewer errors, and have less satisfied members at the periphery. Democratic networks often develop hierarchies by themselves (Mintzberg, 1993). Clearly, there is an association between communication patterns and organizational structure.

In organizations, a parallel finding is that centralized organizations are more efficient in certain circumstances. Horizontally decentralized organizations seem better for morale but tend to become unstable and revert to a more centralized structure to complete tasks. This is especially true for organizations that do simple, repetitive, and unskilled tasks. Complex and knowledge-based work by professional workers tends to pull the organization toward decentralization (Mintzberg, 1993). There seems to be a pattern of relationships among group communication networks, effective communication, and the structure of an organization.

Personal Communication Effectiveness

Communication is a basic aspect of human relationships. Interpersonal competence in communicating is needed for establishing a human-to-human relationship. Nurse-client communication processes form the basis of therapeutic relationships in nursing. Such processes are based on the nurse's interpersonal competence. Interpersonal competence is composed of understanding complex cognitive, behavioral, and cultural factors that influence communication efforts. Social cognitive competency refers to the ability to interpret message content from each participant's point of view. Message competency refers to the ability to use language and nonverbal behaviors in a strategic way to achieve goals (Boggs, 1999). Personal communication effectiveness is derived from knowledge of communication elements and styles and practice in the use of communication channels and styles that are effectively matched to the situation.

Structuring a message for effectiveness is an important concept to consider. The sender has a choice of channels, whether it is by dress, nonverbal behavior, or written or oral communication. To plan for personal effectiveness, a decision is made about what message is desired and how it can be structured so that it will be received positively and will elicit the response preferred. Effectively communicating takes into consideration decisions about how to communicate, including aspects such as message structure, delivery style, and mode of communication.

Effectiveness in communication is related to timing and the choice of channel. In general, people respond positively to personal contact or appeal. For example, it is much more difficult to say no to someone who comes personally to ask for participation than it is to decline a request by email. It is more difficult to say no on the phone to someone who is a colleague than it is to ignore or discard a written note or memo.

Consider the choice of words used in structuring a message. When oral communication is used, the words can be selected with care to structure the presentation for maximum impact. There are certain red flags, or emotionally charged words, to which people respond. Most of the emotion-laden words are superlatives, but there are certain words that are emotionally charged triggers. An example is racist or sexist language. Even though the sender may think he or she is using normal conversation, any hint of discrimination or exclusion may raise sensitivities. Orators and preachers deliberately include inflammatory words as a motivation and persuasion technique. Because people often respond to the inflammatory words and do not listen critically to the message, it may be necessary to deliberately delete certain words. If a person has an emotional response to the choice of words, then the message may be obscured or completely lost.

It is so easy to overlook the basic necessity of checking whether a message was understood. This is especially true in nursing, a field prone to jargon. Whether nurses are teaching clients or delegating work, it is tempting to assume that the instructions given are clear and thus understood. This is not always the case, as one group of nurses discovered. They constructed 34 acontextual sentences using common nursing jargon, such as *vitals, NPO, ambulate, void, stool, flatus,* and *analgesic.* They asked 101 adult clients to define the general meaning of each term. Correct responses ranged from 16% for *flatus* to 98% for *OR, stethoscope,* and *bloodwork.* If communication is key to understanding, then care must be taken to avoid misperceptions in translation (Cochrane et al., 1992). In a complex care environment, the transmission and constancy of information needs to be built into communication systems to decrease medical errors and risks to patient safety (Anthony & Preuss, 2002).

Feedback and Criticism

Feedback is a basic and essential communication principle. It is tied into the concept of delegation: after choosing what to delegate (the right task), matching the task to the delegate's competence (the right person), and making an effective assignment (the right communication), then sharing the evaluation (the right feedback) closes the loop by providing closure and future motivation.

Giving effective feedback provides a sense of recognition for task accomplishment. What is said and how the message is communicated affect the results of an interaction and the working relationships. Clear, timely, tactful communication with shared input and perceptions promotes effectiveness (Hansten & Washburn, 1992).

Part of feedback is learning how to give constructive criticism. Criticism is not inherently negative. It takes time and exposure to giving and receiving positive criticism to be able to take the ideas and use them to improve. Nurses may be targets for criticism for the following reasons (Deering, 1993):

- Being on the front lines
- Being the focus for displaced criticism when others are upset with the system
- Working with people who have health problems
- Working in high-stress environments requiring frequent critical decisions

The most natural human response is to become defensive. Defensive reactions may in turn prompt defensive counterreactions. In such cases, a heated argument, not a civil discussion, ensues. The opportunity to see a problem more clearly evaporates. The three communication techniques recommended to respond effectively to criticism are the following: ask for more information, agree with the critic, and use listening skills to guide the critic toward the real problem source (Deering, 1993).

There are group situations in which feedback, brainstorming, or open discussion is asked for. One of the essential characteristics of followership is to be able to dissent. However, when that dissent is formed as a personal attack or as the defamation of a person, it is not appropriate. Personal attacks merely tear down another person. Constructive criticism is not focused on blame or on a person's characteristics; it is focused on an analysis of the problem. Problem solving is a way of practicing positive communication. When there is a problem with the system or the process, the appropriate communication approach is to use critiquing: balancing the positives and negatives and pointing out problems and solution options.

Giving criticism may be avoided because it tends to provoke defensiveness and arguments. However, conflict may erupt if the skills of positive criticism are not employed to defuse frustrations. The first consideration is when and whether to criticize. The key is to take charge of the situation without losing control of emotions and alienating others. After choosing an appropriate time and place to deliver criticism, communication techniques such as phrasing the criticism in terms of outcomes desired and avoiding blanket statements are helpful. Criticism may have its basis in perception, not reality (Deering, 1993).

Because delivering bad news and critiquing weak performance is a job nobody likes, Manzoni (2002) suggested taking an open approach and being more conscious and careful when framing decisions. Research shows that feedback is more willingly accepted when people feel that (1) the feedback giver is felt to be reliable and has good intentions, (2) the feedback process is fair, consistent, and considerate of facts and opinions, and (3) the feedback communication process is fair, respectful, and supportive.

Appearance and Behavior

Communication behavior includes both the content of the communication and the expression or communication style. Research has shown that 55% of audience interpretations for speaker messages are determined by the speaker's nonverbal communication, such as facial expression and body language; 38% by the speaker's vocal quality, including tone, pitch, volume and variation; and 7% by the literal words. Overall, audiences remember concepts and emotional expression more than the content (Yepsen, 1988). Furthermore, there appear to be gender-based differences in communication behavior. For example, the communication of women may fulfill a socioemotional or expressive function; the communication of men may fulfill a task or instrumental function (Kennedy et al., 1990).

Psychologists have analyzed job interviews and found that they consist of two parts. The first part is what is called the 30-second hurdle because

research has shown that most employers make up their minds about job applicants in the first 30 seconds. This 30-second decision is based on the halo effect. In the context in which psychologists use the term *halo*, it means the effects of the person's first impression. The halo effect radiates out in all directions and can be positive or negative. Unfortunately, first impressions are not always good impressions. It is this initial effect or impression that is extremely difficult, if not impossible, to overcome. Very little content can be expressed in 30 seconds to make a critical difference. Therefore it is not the content of the message that forms the initial impression; it is the packaging. Facial expression, clothing, body posture, and hair form a total image. Appearance and behavior create a dramatic communication. The total picture, both verbal and nonverbal, can and does effectively communicate a message. If this first impression part is received negatively, then the chances of getting the job are slim no matter how brilliantly the second part, the actual interview, is handled (Brothers, 1986). It may be tempting to ignore the impact of appearance and behavior. However, it appears to be a natural human response and one that nurses need to recognize and use effectively.

Professional Communication Effectiveness

> Communication is always influenced by the environment in which it takes place. It does not occur in a vacuum but is shaped by the situation in which the interaction occurs. (Boggs, 1999, pp. 206-207)

For therapeutic nurse-client communication, effectiveness is related to interpersonal sensitivity, interpersonal competence, and the use of communication styles, such as the validation of individual worth, which increase responsiveness and involvement. The style of communication used by a health care provider is known to influence client behavior, especially compliance with treatment (Boggs, 1999).

However, in leadership and care management situations, different issues arise and different styles may be needed. In care management situations in which nurses may be communicating with peers or superiors, effectiveness is still related to interpersonal skill. However, the communication of all aspects of professionalism and collaboration also are needed. For example, the importance of positive messages may be neglected in communication in nursing. These include compliments and positive feedback given to others. Are nurses able to express their needs? Does verbal abuse exist, creating a climate of intimidation in which nurses feel they should not ask questions at all? In what kind of environment is nursing practiced? What kind of person is each nurse in that environment?

Image and Uniforms

Communication includes both verbal and nonverbal modalities, put together so that a message is communicated in a package. One application in nursing relates to image. The problem of image in nursing includes the portrayal of nurses in the media and dissention about uniforms and dress codes.

Nurses have identified their portrayal in the media as a concern related to stereotyping, lack of professionalism, and low esteem (Aber & Hawkins, 1992). Occupational prestige, both internal and external, was an issue during the nurse shortage of the late 1980s (Bream et al., 1992). Clearly, it is easier to recruit into an occupation that has a high prestige in society or pays high salaries. The societal view of nursing is called external prestige. Nurses also need to examine internal prestige, which is how nursing itself values nursing and nurses.

In the past, one media strategy evolved into a national advertising campaign. In 1990 the National Advertising Council, along with nursing's Tri-Council, published a series of ads as a way of helping to alleviate the prevailing nursing shortage of the time. This campaign was called the "National Nursing Image Campaign," and its theme was, "If Caring Were Enough, Anyone Could Be a Nurse." One ad said, "At 10:26 AM Sandy Hardwick brought her 57-year-old cardiac patient back to life. What did you accomplish this morning?" Another ad said, "After 4 years of college,

you look for a job. After nursing school, a job's looking for you." The idea was to convey a different image of nursing: that it is an important and essential service with a strong job market. At the same time, the Nurses of America published Media Watch, a communicative strategy to monitor the media for sexism and negative images of nurses. Their major impact was on the TV program "The Nightingales," which eventually was cancelled. More recently, the Johnson & Johnson Company has sponsored media attention on recruitment into nursing as a career. Called the *Campaign for Nursing's Future,* the Johnson & Johnson Company (2004) targeted their resources to address the nurse shortage. They developed a website (*www.discovernursing.com*) and ran commercials. Brochures, posters, and videos were made available to assist recruitment into nursing. Scholarship grants also were made available.

Another image issue involves attire. Who determines what is appropriate nursing attire? An interesting small-group activity is to ask participants to come up with their ideal professional uniform. Policy committees may have lively discussions about nursing dress codes. This is because clothing is a form of nonverbal communication that stimulates judgmental responses from others (Kalisch & Kalsich, 1985).

Research in the 1980s and 1990s showed that consumers preferred white uniforms with skirts and a cap as a nurse's uniform, possibly because of the persistence of traditional views and images of nursing (Franzoi, 1988; Kucera & Nieswiadomy, 1991). In one research study a series of photos of a woman in three styles of nursing attire were given to students and consumers to rate (Franzoi, 1988). One pose was the traditional white dress, white hose, white shoes, and white cap. The second was a modern style consisting of white slacks and shoes with a multicolored, vertically striped blouse and no cap. The third style was scrubs. The study found that most of the people thought that the person in scrubs was a physician. The people identified the woman in the traditional outfit as a nurse 90% of the time. Overall, 60% of the people preferred the traditional uniform, 35% favored the modern uniform, and only 5% preferred the picture of the person in the scrubs. Although nurses think scrubs are practical and comfortable, the public would prefer to see them in the traditional nurse attire. Although this research is not recent, the relevance of the issue of nursing attire and image remains a practice concern.

The nurse's uniform is both a source of pride and of controversy. The uniform is an identifier. It has been designed to project soberness and respectability as a means of enhancing the image and work of nursing (Houweling, 2004). Practicality prevailed with the popularity of scrubs, but the result has been the inability to clearly distinguish RNs from others. The recognizable, respected symbol is gone, but identity is still important. A suggested solution is the artist-designed RN patch, available for sewing on uniforms, scrubs, or lab coats (Mason & Buhler-Wilkerson, 2004).

Research continues to show that nurses' role identification and competency are a part of indicators of professionalism conveyed by nurses' attire (Lehna et al., 1999). This also appears to be an international issue (Campbell et al., 2000; DeKeyser et al., 2003; Pearson et al., 2001). The choice of style of a uniform and the image it needs to present must be a balance of presenting a professional authority figure, providing security for patients and families, and suggesting an approachable figure (Campbell et al., 2000). The factors related to uniforms include professionalism, status and power, infection control, identity, modesty, symbolism, and occupational health and safety (Pearson et al., 2001). Related issues include what to do about tattoos and body piercings in the OR.

The issue of attire is important for creating a positive perception and communicating an attitude of competence and professionalism. The way nurses dress symbolizes role identity, function, authority, professional image, and confidence in ability and judgment, as well as how nurses feel about themselves (Mangum et al., 1991). It is even possible to find designer uniforms that attempt to blend professional tailoring with the uniform style (Barnum, 1990).

Institutions try to balance the public's perception of a nurse as a female in a white uniform and cap with the practical reality of nursing practice. Caps are not functional for nurses, and they are silly for male nurses. On the other hand, in some health care facilities it is not uncommon to see nursing staff who are dressed in overly casual, soiled, unattractive, tight-fitting, disheveled, revealing, or seductive clothing. In these facilities, the leaders or managers might be concerned about the image that the nurses portray and decide that a certain uniform or dress code is required as a part of enhancing the nurses' image.

Furthermore, organizations may feel the need to be responsive to consumer preferences, choosing to use image and professional polish as a competitive edge (Mangum et al., 1991). Marketing and imaging have become a communication imperative as competition increases in the field of health care. The choice of clothing in itself is an important statement about nurses' professionalism because it affects the degree of trust, confidence, and respect from the consumer.

Organizational Communication

Exchanging ideas and information becomes a basic and pervasive activity in organizations. Communication makes organizations function. Nurses feel the impact of this when communication technology fails, such as when telecommunication lines are disrupted during natural disasters. The inherent need for human communication is magnified when organizations such as health care systems are run by professionals such as nurses, who function as knowledge workers.

Organizations have unique communication systems. They communicate externally with their environment and internally through specific systems, processes, and cultures. When communicating externally, organizations create an image and leave an impression on others. Marketing campaigns are one example. Such communications may fail or succeed, based to some extent on persuasion and perceptual filters.

Five basic internal types of organizational communication systems are (1) downward, (2) upward,

(3) horizontal, (4) grapevine, and (5) network communications. Formal channels are downward, upward, and horizontal modes; informal channels are the grapevine and the network. Networks are similar to the grapevine, but they refer to various groups of people who come together, such as small groups who socialize together or work together on a team (Hersey et al., 2001). With work teams becoming more interdisciplinary or interdepartmental, the concepts of horizontal communication between coworkers and network communication blend and blur. In this case, both formal and informal communication are facilitated in organizations.

Nurse-physician and other interdisciplinary collaborations are important for providing quality care in a cost-effective way. The use of collaborative practice is being promoted in a variety of settings. One application is in the development of critical pathways or other collaborative practice protocols. Collaborative standardization improves physician-nurse communication (Lassen et al., 1997). Another application is interorganizational communication between a hospital and home health agency in regard to discharge referrals (Anderson & Tredway, 1999). Collaboration has been defined as the act of working together. Both interpersonal behaviors and organizational structures are facilitators of or barriers to collaboration. A recognition of differences in perspective and orientation is a necessary step in collaborating with others (Coeling & Cukr, 1998).

Effective organizational communication rests on the choice of styles. Collaboration requires that all parties feel free to speak their mind. The style an individual uses in interacting with others affects communication, trust, and rapport. The communication styles that facilitate collaboration include nonaggressive, affirming, listening, confident, and indirect approaches (Coeling & Cukr, 1998). For business communication, common effectiveness aspects include (Katz & Green, 1997) the following:

- All communication must be receiver-centered.
- Communication should be brief.
- Communication needs to be simple and straightforward rather than complex.

The structure of a communication system in an organization is especially important, both as a barrier to or facilitator of information flow and as a way of promoting collaboration among members. For example, the network of committees, task forces, and work groups provides cross-communication and organizational linkages to facilitate work flow and problem solving. This structure can be a key element in effective communication in an organization. Leaders and managers play a key role in the design or redesign of the committee structure. As organizations work to become flatter, leaner, and more customer-oriented, the committee structure provides a route for communication and collaborative work. This structure can be analyzed and reconfigured to improve organizational communication flows (Ball et al., 1998).

The influence of power and politics pervades all aspects of organizations and organizational communication. For example, leadership and other interpersonal styles affect follower or coworker responses. Since there is a difference in role responsibilities and scope, a gap occurs between the personal and professional interests of nurses as care provider professionals and as nurse managers and system administrators. The approach of being supportive versus being defensive can set the tone for smooth or rough relationships. All parties need to focus on styles, modes, channels, and skills of openness, trust, rapport, and facilitation to decrease the barriers to effective communication in organizations.

Within nursing, power struggles also have occurred between nurses and physicians. Patient care and hospital services rely on the collaborative contributions of both professions. However, physicians have been accorded more power and prestige within health care systems. Nurses may be viewed as subordinates to be delegated to. Communication, negotiation, and persuasion are all wrapped up in the doctor-nurse relationship. At the worst, nurses report verbal abuse from physicians. At the best, both physicians and nurses work within systems where respect is an explicit value expected of all providers and where nurses and doctors practice a style of communication that is factual, collegial, problem-solving, centered on patient care, and designed to build trust and positive relationships. Power and conflict are further discussed in Chapter 24.

Communication in organizations is not a simple sender/receiver/channel concept. Group dynamics and the interaction of multiple people provide complexity and challenges to the communicative process and the influence of perception in organizations. Political and interpersonal subtleties and complexities also need to be taken into account. Consider an example from an employee's perspective about how an organization might communicate when a hospital is laying off nurses. In nursing, there have been periods when downsizing or reductions in force (RIFs) were common, as well as times of nursing shortage. Each institution must make choices when it decides to lay people off. The types of controversies include how to choose who will be laid off, how to tell them, what kind of outplacement help is extended to them, the extent of unionization, and other personnel requirements. Conversely, the messages that organizations send when they are actively recruiting nurses may reflect an attitude of valuing professionalism or of offering short-term inducements.

In life and in the work setting, there are options for increasing one's personal and professional effectiveness. Job satisfaction in nursing can be augmented as nurses perceive themselves to be more effective and more in control of their practice environment and professional work life.

Persuasion

Both persuasion and negotiation are power and conflict interventions. Fundamentally, there are two ways individuals can get what they want: coercion or persuasion. If a person lacks the power to coerce (or is unwilling to exercise coercion because of ethical or practical concerns), persuasion is used as an influence strategy. Bargaining and negotiation are twin influence techniques used to persuade others to resolve conflicts or share resources. These concepts are common in everyday experiences of satisfying needs and wants. They also are an inherent part of human interactions at work. Thus nurses will find that persuasion and negotiation are useful techniques for implementing decisions and gaining resources for quality client care and care management.

Persuasion, rather than force, is the appropriate action to use when the course of events needs to be controlled for any length of time. Persuasion is indicated in at least two circumstances. First, whenever those involved have equivalent or complementary resources in terms of knowledge, skill, or authority, persuasion is to be used. In other words, persuasion may need to be used when dealing with a peer. Second, whenever those involved in the interaction have common or conflicting interests in the outcome of an activity, persuasion is used (Baker, 1986). As nurses work in collaborative, interdisciplinary teams, persuasion becomes an important skill for gaining objectives.

A persuader is any person who tries to get what they want by convincing others to take some action such as working on a committee, reducing the budget, donating money, or funding a project. Persuaders must stimulate and motivate action even if the target is reluctant. They assess the various motives of their targeted audiences. The most common appeals are for self-preservation, money, romance, and recognition (Baker, 1986). Advertising and marketing are excellent examples of common persuasive appeals; an example is trying to get someone to buy a car. Nurses can apply persuasive appeals to their work environment. For example, they can use persuasion when working in interdisciplinary teams or proposing new programs. Nurses may be the targets of persuaders, for example, when vendors try to sell medical equipment or supplies.

Effective persuaders use a variety of techniques designed to garner attention, engage with and hold a focus on their message, motivate others to action, and arouse feelings about issues and needs. They include every listener through voice modulation, eye contact, gestures, and movements. They try to identify themselves with their audience, and they compliment and enlist their audience's attention

(Baker, 1986). First, a persuader has to penetrate the listener's defenses. This is done by identifying with the listener and trying to get the listener to identify with the persuader. This identification process creates feelings of trust and openness to the persuader's message. Then the persuader clarifies the issue at hand as concretely as possible because only then can the persuader maneuver into a position to negotiate. Technique and timing are vital, and credibility and trust essential. Persuaders time their technique to lower the listener's defenses, compliment and enlist the listener's intelligence, clarify the issue at hand, and deliver a message (Baker, 1986).

Nurses can use techniques of persuasion as they manage and lead in health care organizations. For example, a nurse who plans and develops a proposal to implement a new program to provide better access to health care for clients generally will need to obtain funding approval. Either a grant proposal document or an oral presentation may be used for persuasive communication.

A number of social science disciplines have been interested in aspects of persuasion. Speech communication views persuasion as rhetorical skills that process messages. Psychology's interest in persuasion centers on its relationship to motivation. Sociology examines persuasion and the social or cultural environment. Public relations and politics emphasize creating favorable public images. Marketers apply methods to arouse or trigger buying or consumption. Health care applies persuasion to client care and health services (Rappsilber, 1982). For example, nurses try to persuade clients to adopt wellness behaviors. Nurse managers try to persuade nurses to work collaboratively with one another and with other care providers.

Research about the ways people at work influence their colleagues has indicated the following five basic categories of reasons to exert influence (Kipnis & Schmidt, 1980):

1. To obtain assistance with one's own job
2. To get others to do their job
3. To obtain personal benefits
4. To initiate a change in work
5. To improve the individual's job performance

Eight categories of influence tactics have been identified: (1) assertiveness, (2) ingratiation, (3) rationality, (4) sanctions, (5) exchange, (6) upward appeal, (7) blocking, and (8) coalitions. The status of the person that the persuader is trying to influence tends to be the most decisive factor in determining which tactic is chosen (Levenstein, 1982).

Techniques of persuasion can be aimed at changing existing attitudes and behaviors. In some persuasion techniques, the persuader seeks to increase the other person's identification with himself or herself and reduce interpersonal distance. Threats and fear are avoided; rational explanations are used to help change attitudes into actions. The two major persuasion tactics employed are intensification of certain points and the downplaying of other points (Figure 20.2). Intensification uses repetition to imprint a way of responding on the receiver's mind, association or

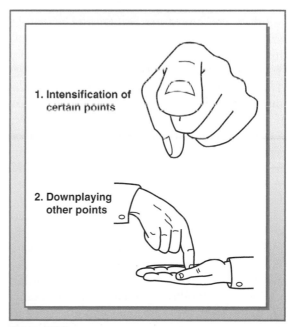

Figure 20.2
Two major persuasion tactics. (Data from Rappsilber, C. [1982]. Persuasion as a mechanism for change. In J. Lancaster & W. Lancaster [Eds.], *The nurse as a change agent: Concepts for advanced nursing practice* [pp. 132-145]. St Louis: Mosby.)

linking of one idea with something held in esteem, and contrasting of one idea to a less desirable one. Downplaying of other points uses tactics of omission, diversion, and confusion. Key information can be withheld or concealed. Jargon and technical language can be used to create miscommunication or an environment that makes people reluctant to ask questions. Effective change strategies and practical persuasive success are linked to choice of technique, audience attributes, effort, ethics, and evaluation (Rappsilber, 1982).

Why are some individuals such effective persuaders? How is it that some people can seem to sell anything yet others are never successful at sales? Effective communicators establish intense rapport. They do so through structuring breathing patterns, body position, and language to mirror those of the other person. Neurolinguistic programming is a communication model dealing with ways to establish rapport. It is based on the study of effective communicators. Individuals have different ways of patterning their thought processes and their concepts of the world. People represent knowledge in different sensory modalities, and this is reflected in their language. For example, "I see what you mean" reflects visual patterning. "I hear you" reflects auditory patterning. "It touches me" reflects kinesthetic patterning. Part of understanding persons targeted for persuasion is to understand their patterning. A basic rule of persuasion is that speaking to another person in his or her language will increase the comfort and trust the person feels, so the persuader is more likely to be successful (Knowles, 1983).

Persuasion can be used to obtain personal benefit, to get others to cooperate, or to satisfy organizational goals (Levenstein, 1982). It enters into interactions with roommates, spouses, or parents and is involved in most situations in which a need must be fulfilled through others. For example, in job interviews, the applicants are trying to persuade an organization to hire them. Applicants will talk positively about themselves. However, it takes an estimated 30 seconds to form an initial opinion and lasting impression or decision about a person during the first meeting. Therefore what

the applicant says is often less persuasive than body language, dress, and overall image.

Persuasion is one of the tools available for nurses to use to accomplish client care goals. Being effective involves having an expanded repertoire of strategies and tactics to use as solutions when problems arise. Theories and techniques of persuasion can be applied to problems of client education, adherence to medical regimens, and functioning of health services (Rappsilber, 1982).

NEGOTIATION

Negotiation is a tool, strategy, or technique useful for avoiding head-on competition or a win-lose conflict outcome. Negotiation employs communication, interpersonal skills, persuasion, the ability to articulate a point of view, and the acknowledgment of the other person's position. Learning to negotiate is a way to acknowledge each party's needs and to reach a win-win conflict solution.

To contrast the strategies of influence, it is important to recognize the difference between win-win and win-lose conflict outcomes. Negotiation for conflict resolution can be one of two basic types: competitive (only one party wins) or cooperative (all parties win). The objective in both cases is to achieve agreement (Smeltzer, 1991). Competitive negotiation brings about a win-lose or lose-lose result and is more associated with persuasion and compromise. However, negotiation as a strategy is more closely associated with cooperative negotiation. Cooperative negotiation is a strategy of pursuing common goals, acknowledging the other party's needs and goals, and incorporating them in resolutions. Satisfaction is the medium of exchange during a negotiation. Win-lose means solely attaining one party's goals, without regard to the other parties or their needs. In a problem-solving modality, participants negotiate to equalize power. In a win-lose modality, one side emphasizes its own power and independence by trying to force its position on the other side. The win-lose strategy incorporates an all-or-nothing posture. Negotiation uses trust as opposed to exploitation of the other party. Thus successful negotiation provides satisfaction to both parties (Laser, 1981).

Successful negotiation involves identifying the needs of the other party. Identifying these needs puts an adversary in a better position to exchange and negotiate by acknowledging the other party's need and incorporating it into a solution. Recognizing personal ambitions and interests and then establishing a constructive dialogue about how to satisfy those needs is a beginning to negotiation. This requires a basic understanding of human interaction and reaction and the possible strategies for negotiation.

Process

Nurses will encounter various situations in which negotiation takes place. For example, nurses negotiate with physicians about client care management needs. They negotiate with one another for distribution of the workload or administration of the work group. Sometimes nurses negotiate over vacation time or coverage of the unit. Negotiations follow a process. First, three criteria need to be met for true negotiation to occur (Smeltzer, 1991): (1) the issue must be negotiable, (2) the negotiators must be interested in both giving and taking, and (3) the parties must trust each other and the negotiating process. Thus nurses can evaluate each negotiation circumstance for the presence of these three criteria. Any negotiation has the following four elements (Laser, 1981):

1. *Goals* that are both conflicting and nonconflicting
2. *Values* that vary as to urgency and priority as information is exchanged
3. *Mutual victory* when both sides realize satisfaction and feel something has been won
4. *Incomplete information* since parties never reveal all information and thereby shift the negotiating power

Negotiation is a back-and-forth process triggered by one party's attempting to alter the current relationship with another party. Despite the issues, it is desirable to maintain the relationship, hence negotiation. However, the climate surrounding a negotiating incident may vary from the parties being defensive to the parties being supportive. In a defensive milieu, there are feelings of superiority and strategies of controlling. In a supportive environment, feelings are focused on the problem issue, and strategies are sincere and problem-focused. Poor listening, inaccurate communication, strong reactions to stress, or failure to disclose information or feelings may contribute to a defensive environment (Smeltzer, 1991).

The process of negotiation may proceed through a series of steps. The following 10 steps are involved in most negotiation processes (Smeltzer, 1991):

1. Preparing for negotiation
2. Communicating a general overview of what is to be accomplished
3. Reviewing why negotiation is required
4. Redefining the issue or issues
5. Selecting when issues will be addressed
6. Encouraging discussion throughout the process
7. Addressing the fall-back or compromise position for both parties on each issue
8. Agreeing in principle during the settlement stage
9. Recapping and summarizing the agreement
10. Monitoring compliance with the agreement after settlement

Nurses should expect negotiations to follow steps similar to the ones presented here. However, the more formal the negotiation process, the more closely the steps will be used in a systematic manner. Nurses preparing to initiate a negotiation will find a review of these steps helpful.

Formal negotiations also use a specific language. A review of terms will clarify the meaning of the language of negotiation. Some terms used in the process of negotiation are *issues, deadlock, impasse, concession,* and *power* (Box 20.1) (Laser, 1981).

There are numerous strategies available for use by nurses in the process of negotiation. The most effective use of a technique occurs when it is deliberately planned or consciously used. Laser (1981) identified four significant strategies for negotiation (Box 20.2). Awareness of strategies enhances a nurse's ability to choose alternative approaches and enhance effectiveness. Successful negotiation is based on deliberate strategy. Suggestions for negotiation tips are displayed in Box 20.3 (Kippenbrock, 1992). Tips for successful negotiation include separating the people from the problem; focusing on interests, not positions; inventing options for mutual gain; and insisting on using objective criteria (Fisher & Ury, 1991).

The strategies of negotiation that are chosen in any situation may depend on whether the climate for negotiation is supportive or defensive. Defensive environments can lead to negotiation mistakes such as poor listening and mismanagement of issues. Progress should be monitored throughout the negotiation to avoid communication blocks and to overcome deadlocks. Needs, power, and timing are the essential components of negotiating (Smeltzer, 1991). Information becomes a critical resource in any negotiation process. Information about a party's needs and awareness can be a strategic power resource and becomes an input to decision making. Both verbal and nonverbal cues are important in negotiating. Information may be altered, filtered, given selectively, or withheld as an advantage-gaining power strategy (Smeltzer, 1991).

Experts also suggest that any negotiator always maintain room to maneuver. It is essential that opening positions contain enough latitude so that both parties can win, yet concessions not drop below minimum requirements (Laser, 1981). Nurses may need to be encouraged to build an experiential base in negotiation. Confidence and skill are built through practice in negotiation in low-risk areas. It is important to remember the influence of information power in negotiation. Assuming that all the facts are known is foolish

---

Box 20.3

Successful Negotiation Tips

- Open the parameters to negotiate as a way of controlling the framing of the issues and areas.
- Prepare thoroughly and completely.
- Dress carefully and be aware of body language and nonverbal aspects.
- Use talking and listening skills for good communication.
- Maintain a positive tone.
- Take calculated risks.
- Work toward a solution that everyone can support.

---

negotiations succeed or fail based on three dimensions of deal making: (1) tactics, (2) deal design, and (3) set-up (Lax & Sebenius, 2003). Tactics are the people and processes such as interpersonal issues, poor communications, and "hardball" attitudes. Deal design relates to value and substance, or how to craft feasible, desirable, value-creating agreements. Set-up is the scope and sequence, or actions taken "away from the table" to approach the right parties in the right order to deal with the right issues. This is done to set up the most promising situation possible for a viable process and valuable agreement.

because it overlooks the secret agenda (or unspoken and purposely concealed position) that is presumed to exist in any negotiation. Thus nurses may need to build careful assessment and healthy skepticism into their negotiations.

Negotiators need to be good listeners, persuaders, and tacticians. Research has shown that

LEADERSHIP AND MANAGEMENT IMPLICATIONS

Communication is a process in which information, perception, and understanding are transmitted from person to person. As an integral part of any relationship, communication is important to nurses. Nurse leaders and managers can view communication as a tool to accomplish work and meet goals. The significance of communication

▲ LEADERSHIP & MANAGEMENT BEHAVIORS

Leadership Behaviors

- Communicates a vision
- Structures messages to inspire
- Motivates by communication strategies
- Projects a professional image
- Models positive communication
- Influences frequent communication
- Coaches followers
- Structures symbols and shared meanings
- Persuades followers to accomplish goals
- Convinces followers to work together
- Invites agreement and commitment
- Negotiates common understandings

Management Behaviors

- Communicates with superiors and subordinates
- Structures messages for clarity

- Directs the performance of others by communication strategies
- Manages organizational goal accomplishment by communicating
- Persuades subordinates to accomplish organizational goals
- Bargains for scarce resources
- Exchanges ideas and plans
- Negotiates agreements and contracts

Overlap Areas

- Communicates with others
- Promotes effective communication
- Persuades others
- Negotiates with others

revolves around its effectiveness and the climate in which communication occurs. Effective communication is enhanced by clear, direct, straightforward, and frequent message transmission. Trust, respect, and empathy are the three ingredients needed to create and foster effective communication.

For leaders, communication is a key element of the role. Leaders are in charge of vision, and the vision needs to be communicated as a compelling image. Such a compelling image is thought to induce enthusiasm and commitment in others. Thus a major part of the leader's role is to communicate a vision. Leaders shape values and norms in a way that binds and bonds individuals and groups. Communication is key to this effort. Visions are communicated by means of managing meaning and creating understanding, commitment, and ownership of a vision. Leaders use communication as a tool for building trust. Trust is the glue that holds leaders and followers together.

Communication is a basic and essential skill for leaders and managers. Communicating, along with diagnosing and adapting, is one of the three basic competencies of influencing and leadership (Hersey et al., 2001). It is a critical and important tool for effectiveness, in engaging and motivating people and in getting work done through others. Structuring messages so that people understand them clearly and avoiding emotion-laden triggers enhances the communication effectiveness of a manager. For example, the communication of accurate (correct, truthful, precise), adequate (sufficient, consistent, repetitious), and applied (useful and appropriate to the nurse's individual needs) information was necessary for directing managed care changes (Apker & Fox, 2002). These communication techniques can foster stronger organizational affiliation while maintaining nurses' strong identification with nursing.

Health care organizations are complex and exist in uncertain environments. Nurse leaders and managers play a crucial role in the management of information and communication for the purpose of effective care coordination and the avoidance of unsafe and error-prone care situations.

Medical errors and patient safety in hospitals have been a focus of the Institute of Medicine. Clearly, providers need high-quality information and effective communication. Nurse administrators are responsible for developing care delivery systems with adequate structure and an effective communication system that enhances care coordination. These systems of communications need to enable patient rescue and safety by coordinating care, preventing information loss, and improving methods of surveillance (Anthony & Preuss, 2002). Interventions have been initiated to augment nurse and physician collaboration in intensive care units (Boyle & Kochinda, 2004) and to capture communication patterns in OR nurses to facilitate automation to reduce adverse events (Moss & Xiao, 2004).

A related concern for the management of information and communication is how to prevent breaches of patient confidentiality. The Health Insurance Portability and Accountability Act (HIPAA) provisions have heightened awareness about and strategies to protect patients' privacy and data security in health care transactions. For example, fax transmissions need to be secure, and security measures need to be taken to protect computerized databases and electronic transmissions. In a series of interviews with 51 patients, Brann and Mattson (2004) identified both internal and external confidentiality breaches, which were categorized into a typology table. Health care providers' actions that disseminate confidential information can create harm to patients. Systems, processes, and structures can be altered to prevent many of these situations.

Acquiring interpersonal relationship skills, including the ability to communicate, is as essential to a leader's personal set of leadership skills as psychomotor skills are for a clinical nurse. Leadership and management ability is predicated on a facility for communication. In nursing leadership and management, skillful communication is essential for effective implementation of the change process. It is an intervention that leaders and managers in nursing use to accomplish their goals. Communication is a key component of case management practice.

Research Note

Source: Boyle, D.K., & Kochinda, C. (2004). Enhancing collaborative communication of nurse and physician leadership in two intensive care units. *Journal of Nursing Administration, 34*(2), 60-70.

Purpose

Poor nurse-physician collaborative communication is one of the factors in increased risk-adjusted mortality and length of stay in ICUs. The purpose of this study was to test an intervention designed to enhance collaborative communication among nurse and physician leaders in two different ICUs. The Analytic Model for Studying ICU Performance was the framework for the study. In this model nurse-physician collaborative communication is one of four predictor variables of ICU outcomes. The study used a pretest-posttest, repeated measures design with follow-ups at baseline, intervention, and 6 months after. ICUs in two hospitals participated. The Collaborative Communication Intervention was targeted to the five dimensions of nurse-physician collaborative communication: leadership, communication, coordination, problem solving/conflict management, and team-oriented culture. The intervention consisted of 23.5 hours of training using six standardized curriculum models: leadership, core skills for communication, guiding conflict resolution, helping others adapt to change, teams, and trust. Evaluation data were gathered pre- and posttest, using a vignette test and a self-perception and staff perceptions questionnaire.

Discussion

The intervention proved feasible and useful. After the intervention, nurse and physician leaders' communication skills significantly increased. Six months after intervention, scores on unit outcome measures showed improvement, including a decrease in personal stress. This was a pilot study and small in scope, but it was intervention-focused and attempted an experimental design.

Application to Practice

ICU nurse and physician leaders have the responsibility to create an environment of collaborative communication as a way to effect a positive work environment and affect outcomes. In this study, collaborative communication improved after a training intervention. Individual skills increased. Other ICUs and potentially other units could benefit from similar skills training interventions.

Language is used by leaders to give meaning to work. Farley (1989) identified six areas of organizational communication that can be assessed for communication problems (Box 20.4). Communication problems may be a source of dissatisfaction. Research has indicated that a positive communication atmosphere, positive communication between staff nurses and immediate superiors, and personal feedback on job performance are related to nurse job satisfaction (Pincus, 1986).

Communication effectiveness becomes crucial in times of disaster. In fact, often one of the key outcomes of disaster drills is to identify breaks in

Box **20.4**

Communication Assessment

- Accessibility of information
- Communication channels
- Clarity of messages
- Span of control
- Flow control/communication load
- The individual communicators

Data from Farley, M. (1989). Assessing communication in organizations. *Journal of Nursing Administration, 19*(12), 27-31.

the communication system so they can be fixed before a real-time event occurs. Argenti (2002) found that in times of extreme crisis the internal communication to employees took precedence. It was most important for the leader to effectively rebuild the morale of employees so that they could then serve customers. The five strategies he recommended are as follows:

1. Get on the scene to lead, decide, and show compassion.
2. Choose your channels carefully because normal flows often are disrupted due to destroyed phone and power lines.
3. Stay focused on the business.
4. Have a contingency and disaster plan in place.
5. Improvise, but from a strong foundation of values, preparation, and training.

A couple of examples from nursing leadership and management are worth considering. In hospital nursing, situations occur in which nurses are sent (*pulling, floating,* or *farming* are the terms used) from the unit where they normally work to another unit. The person who has to deliver the often unpleasant news determines whether to call the unit and leave a little note on the assignment sheet or go to the nurse to talk directly about the change. Some might offer to take the nurse to the other unit, introduce the person to the charge nurse, and smooth out the transition. There are different ways to structure and deliver the message to be effective in difficult situations.

One leadership situation occurs when a nurse presents a proposal to a committee that must be convinced to release the money for a project that is vitally important to the care of clients. Strategic planning and a written business plan are used to determine how to maximize the message delivery. This may include knowing how to structure the communication, nonverbally as well as verbally, so that a positive impression is created to set the stage for a full and impartial hearing.

Leaders and managers always communicate in basic ways, whether they want to or not: they always communicate their attitude and their goals and expectations. Trust or distrust is communicated. Leaders communicate a vision, subtly or directly, and a sense of where they are going and what they expect from their followers.

One technique used for interpersonal effectiveness in groups, collaborative teams, and interdisciplinary work situations is persuasion. The tactics of persuasion are useful when an authoritarian leadership style is not appropriate and the nurse has to convince colleagues to work together.

Harvey (1990) suggested that skillful, positive questioning can persuade people to accept change. People are more willing to commit themselves when they see personal benefits. Positive questioning capitalizes on this fact to establish hopeful, affirmative attitudes. Inviting agreement, commitment, and realization of benefits facilitates necessary changes. Setting a positive and cooperative tone within a work group is each member's responsibility. Nurses frequently may find themselves in situations in which they need to persuade others to cooperate. Therefore, they will need to use strategies of persuasion and negotiation.

The work of successful nurses and managers depends on the ability to negotiate. Nurses need to be able to articulate needs, positions, and justification for resources. The different techniques of conflict resolution and influencing in nursing include bargaining and negotiation as one method of gaining power and persuading others to grant autonomy by using individual and collective action. The use of collective action at both the work group and the larger profession levels can make a difference in terms of autonomy in professional practice, job satisfaction, and a general positive feeling about the profession of nursing.

Human interaction issues are the general arena in which leaders and managers spend most of their time. Power and conflict become important focal points of human interaction in organizations that may need management or resolution through persuasion or negotiations. Both conflict resolution and negotiation techniques can and should be used to manage change. As nurses are confronted with the impact of mergers, downsizing, restructuring and reengineering, and alterations in skill mix, negotiation skills are needed. These skills can help improve relationships and aid managers to function in their designated roles. Negotiation is used to educate clients and other professionals about nurses' roles and contributions, to get a fairer exchange in decision-making autonomy, to interact with vendors, to deal with client complaints, to interact with integrated health systems and group health care purchasers, to deal with unionized employees, to respond to the media, and to negotiate with medical staff and managed care groups to consolidate contracts (Sherer, 1994).

CURRENT ISSUES AND TRENDS

The traditional view of communication follows a linear model of sender, receiver, perceptions and feedback. Although this is useful, nurses need to be equipped with strong communication skills as a foundation for leadership and practice in an interdisciplinary collaborative environment filled with complexity and chaos. Examining an alternative view of communication will help expand nurses' skills at communication.

We are known by the stories we tell.

Anonymous

We are living in the information age. Trillions of documents move through offices each day. Internet traffic doubles every hundred days. Multiple papers, messages, phone calls, and e-mails flood us daily, accompanied by the media in its multiple forms. There is so much stimulation calling for our attention that silence is a scarce resource, and it is in the silence that all is heard.

Why are so many people trying to communicate with one another? What is driving their need to capture another's attention? The answer to that question sets the stage for a very simple, but not easy, process: the process of healthy and effective communication.

Good communication is the glue holding society together (Mulgan, 1997). It is the beacon that guides our life journey. It is the mirror that gives us a quick glimpse of who we are in the eyes of others. It is the vehicle we use to achieve outcomes and results needed to leverage our impact on our

relational world of family, friends, coworkers, communities, and nation-states. Without communication there is no connection. Humans strive for relationship. Thus communication is the thread that weaves our lives into a rich tapestry of meaning and community. It is the essence of being human.

What Do You Want to Say?

To be really great in little things, to be truly noble and heroic in communicating the insipid details of everyday life, is a virtue so rare as to be worthy of canonization.

Harriet Beecher Stowe

Although conversations occur daily, the *gentle art* of communication requires the purposeful development of skills and capacities that become second nature to us, much as many of the clinical skills that nurses rely on in a crisis situation. Reflect on the myriad of conversations that are engaged in each day. Each exchange offers us a chance to learn something new or to verify, amplify, or clarify something already known. A conversation that matters is one that comes from the soul of one to touch the heart of another in a way that heals or transforms. A thoughtless one can leave a wound that never heals.

Typical courses in communication deal with proficiency in obvious and fundamental tasks to be accomplished. However, the gentle ART of communication relies heavily on the subtle and intuitive nuances that give meaning to the exchange. These subtle skills, at the level of intention and intuition, move a good communicator to a person of mastery and wisdom. Six communication techniques help move an individual toward mastery: (1) clarity, (2) intention, (3) engagement, (4) medium, (5) language, and (6) alignment.

Clarity: Know Your Position on the Issue at Hand

Calling a friend for lunch or setting up a meeting agenda or a classroom schedule is asking people for their time and attention. Each encounter benefits from concerted efforts to clarify the purpose. Meaningful communication helps acquire clarity when individuals make decisions for an action today whose outcomes will be experienced at a future time. Following are some questions to ask yourself to improve clarity:

- What is the situation you are encountering or intending to create?
- How did you come to identify this issue as one of importance?
- Who needs to share in your dialogue and information exchange?
- How do you integrate subsequent thoughts on the topic?

A strategic conversation broadens the long view. The exploration of multiple perspectives and differing possible scenarios helps to begin to order perceptions. Clarity around possibilities leads to the selection of a strategy that would work in multiple plausible futures (Schwartz, 1991). It gives friends, colleagues or managers a common vocabulary for talking about shared things.

Conversations of this nature help elicit each person's unspoken assumptions, leading the whole group into a continuous learning cycle. By mixing existing practices, ideas and relationships with an exploration of ideal future states, a flexible and robust blueprint for an evolving world can be created.

Intention: Unlock the Secrets of Your Subconscious Mind

Human beings articulate intentions and dreams. Old patterns, thoughts, and behaviors often are repeated. Although the outcomes are not always great, the path is well worn and well known. There is a comfort to saying and doing things one way, much like wearing a pair of sneakers that have come to "fit" the specific landscape of the foot. Mindless communication repeats specific patterns with variations on a theme. This is the hallmark of an individual's personality—the way people come to know and expect the person to be.

A mindful person, however, begins with an honest exploration of motive before setting something into motion. Questions to ask yourself to elicit intention include the following:

- Why is this gathering or conversation important?
- What issue are you really trying to address?
- What is your personal contribution to this issue?
- Why did you select the "others" to communicate with?
- Have you been here before, how often, and what happened?
- What has and has not worked in the past?
- What outcome are you trying to achieve?

Creating a consistently clear lens for accurate communication occurs when subconscious blocks are dissolved and their hidden messages are integrated into conscious awareness and the activities that flow from that knowing (Csikszentmihalyi, 1993). Couching information in the appropriate social context shapes the understanding of all involved, moving the group toward shared meaning. This forms the foundation for exceptional and effective communication.

Search, find out, remove and reject every assumption till you reach the living waters and the rock of truth. ... Resist your old habits of feeling and thinking: keep on telling yourself: "No, not so, it cannot be so: I am not like this, I do not need it, I do not want it," and one day will surely come when the entire structure of error and confusion will collapse and the ground will be free for a new life.

Sri Nisargadatta

Engagement: How Do You Engage Others?

Attention involves understanding how to focus and work despite an overabundance of "information competition."

John C. Beck

Mini-Exercise

Remember times when you have engaged in an unforgettable conversation? Who was it with? Under what circumstances? What was it that made the event such a treasured memory? Why did the dialogue and exchange leave such deep insight and lasting impression? Can you use this insight in future interactions?

Invitation: Engage the Attention and Commitment of Others

There are several reasons why someone would commit the time and energy to engage in communication. The call to participate is a powerful one when the invitation is sincere. When people truly believe that the communicator respects who they are and what they can bring to the table, they often participate because they know they have something to offer. A commitment from the inside-out transcends one based on reward, mandate or monetary gain. The following questions address engagement:

- Why are you inviting others to your table, or why did you join theirs?
- What is it they bring that you need?
- What do you have that would enrich them?
- What is in it for them, for you, for the patient/organization?

We are moving from being a "watching society" to an active "experience society" in an inherently personal way (Pine & Gilmore, 1999). It is the value of the experience that determines its worth to those engaged. Although there may be misunderstandings, individuals do not have misexperiences. It is experience that is, in the end, a most reliable teacher.

Medium: Select the Right Venue for the Message

The agenda and the audience invited affect communication. A similar message given in oral or written form carries a different impact on the intended audience. The information age offers multiple exciting ways to communicate (Barabasi, 2002). Visual and auditory strategies can be further enhanced using multimedia tools and web-based technologies.

Not all messages are created equal. Using a taxonomy that matches level of depth and complexity of the message with the appropriate medium for delivery supports efficiency both time and resources. Mapping out the basic concepts to be considered and delivering them in a way that allows the participants to achieve the desired outcome is an act of respect. This fosters

trust and authentic participation within the group, key elements to achieving a positive outcome. The following questions help in the decision of which medium to use:

- What are the core elements on the agenda?
- What is the expectation of the participants in relation to each item: acquire information, give advice, make a decision?
- How much time is allowed for the discussion and the decision?
- What form of information delivery will best help achieve the role in timely fashion: verbal report, text, slides, video, CD-ROM, simulation?

Inviting people to a conversation or meeting is only half the task. Engaging and maintaining their attention is the other half. The most important function is not taking information in, but rather screening it out. Individuals pay closest attention to things useful to survival or relevant to their life situation. Once these basic needs are satisfied, their attention moves to less pressing matters. A gathering held in a context of respect, with an agenda that holds "meaning" to the participants, is the one that remains as a top priority today, and a rich memory tomorrow (Davenport & Beck, 2001).

Attention can work for or against us—and misguided attention often is more detrimental.

Thomas H. Davenport and John C. Beck

What Do Others Hear?

Any perception can connect us to reality properly and fully. What we see or hear doesn't have to be pretty, particularly; we can appreciate anything that exists. There is some principle of magic in everything, some living quality. Something living, something real, is taking place in everything.

Chogyam Trungpa

Words are more than they seem. While there are obvious language barriers between cultures, there is another language breech that occurs within a culture. Language is encoded, and spoken words carry different vibrations than written ones.

The intonation of speech has its own signature because subtle variations with emphasis on different sounds are used. Only by listening to others with the whole body and being do individuals come to perceive and understand the "whole" of the message being delivered.

Language: Understand the Spoken and Recognize the Unknown

There are two levels of language recognized in society today. The ordinary language of everyday life is first-level expression. It is oriented to left-brained, linear, logical, and rational thought. When people communicate, they rely heavily on the words of their culture. Much time and energy is spent on selecting the right words to express what is meant. Creation of common definitions helps form a shared understanding within a group. Those shared words emit a vibrational energy that resonates with the energy of the listeners.

Second-level language has a right-brain orientation. It includes the world of intuition, feeling, and spirit. In an effort to convey the meaning of words or scope of vision, individuals resort to metaphors and symbols that are encoded with attributes that go beyond the word itself. These words have a higher energetic sound, and the vibrations affect the physical body differently. Some questions to ask about language are as follows:

- What is the common language that the whole group can understand?
- How do you create a shared definition of key concepts?
- What new thought or unsettling concept can move the group to a greater understanding or conscious awareness?

When a new idea catches a person's attention to its reality, the resulting energy starts to lift the person and guide them to a different place. When individuals are lifted to a higher level, dramatic things can happened. This may also be happening to others in the group or community without them necessarily being conscious of the process. They may be uplifted for a different reason, because not all individuals are working on the same level at the same time. This higher vibrational shift is what creates a new form (Rael, 1993).

Alignment: Maintain Consistency and Congruence

The integrity of the message needs to be vigilantly monitored. Unspoken thoughts and feelings are broadcast energetically in a way that transcends the spoken word. If the same thing is not said at every level of communication, then listeners may misinterpret, distrust, or not even hear the intended message.

Mini-Exercise

Think of your thoughts, feelings, and actions in various settings. There are some people who make us feel comfortable, inviting us to be authentic, playful, funny, strong. Others will bring out our negative behaviors, subservience, self-consciousness, or feelings of inferiority. Watch for personal sabotage.

A key to avoiding becoming congruent with another's negative beliefs is to become aware of bias in others while creating congruence within oneself. From a centered position, an individual will notice a congruence or lack thereof in others and maintain a sense of balance (Peirce, 1997). The following questions can help determine alignment:

- Do you align yourself with the person or group you are engaged with by being clear that your intention is to clarify, educate, entertain, heal, protect, support, or bless?
- Do you carry any hidden agendas or negative emotions that arise from fear, greed, or insecurity?
- How often do you ask to be confirmed?
- When appropriate, do you articulate the subtle or hidden dynamics of the situation out loud, putting confusion on the table and bringing clarity and focus back into the conversation?

When the individual is engaged in meaningful exchange, coming from a spirit of authentic presence and unconditional regard, a sense of trust and openness exists. This happens when a sense of poise is shown: the ability to control emotions while expressing feelings. This is the skill of being detached—able to observe without the need for a specific outcome. From this open space the individual remains fully discerning and can identify the natural next best step. Goodwill is the intention behind all activity. In that potentiating space, truth and transformation can emerge (Price, 1990).

> *Detachment does not mean that I will not get involved; it means to not let outer circumstances throw off my inner balance.*
>
> Harold Klemp

Negotiation: How Do You See the "Whole" Within the 'Hole?'

> *What do we live for if not to make life less difficult for each other?*
>
> George Eliot

One of the most rich and beautiful facts of human existence is the abundance of diversity. It also is one of the most challenging and growth-producing facts of our existence. Diversity sparks multiple ways of knowing and being—and conflict is its natural partner. Best of all, *conflict is the key to intellectual capital.*

Conflict arises when there are differing points of view. Various perspectives see differing parts of the whole. When people come to a neutral table and are free to express opinions while carefully listening to an alternative view, the scope of all parties can be enlarged. A higher order of knowing transcends old perspectives in a way that one person alone cannot acquire.

Information: Gather Appropriate Facts for Engagement and Persuasion

People constantly gather and translate data into frames and mental models so that they can explain reality in certain ways. The scientific research patterns that underpin professional practice have created a specific way of addressing the issue at hand. This is the world view of a scientist. Ironically, over time, knowledge about a phenomenon becomes so dense that less and less can be explained. The paradox of information is that less is more; pure data have limits. Questions to ask about information gathering are as follows:

- What types of data and information support your cause?
- What types of information refute it?
- What information format and sequencing is most effective for the message being delivered?
- What contextual facts or stories must accompany the data so that the proper meaning is derived from them?

It is important to understand the strengths and limitations of various forms of information so that precious focus and scarce resources are not misused. Because nursing is a profession that serves the health needs of society, nurses need to become aware of the physical and social periphery as well as nursing's unique information needs so that tunnel vision is avoided.

> *Attending too closely to information overlooks the social context that helps people understand what that information might mean and why it matters.*
>
> John S. Brown and Paul Duguid (2000)

Well-developed resources for living tend to fall out of sight when people are in an information tunnel. New technologies draw much attention, diverting awareness from the power of the social periphery: the colleagues, communities, and organizations that frame human activities. These vital components, often missing from the data and communications put together in this evolving information age, must be woven into each person's world view and conversation if clarity and focus are to be maintained.

Integration: Care For and About the Whole

The "Law of Opposites" is the third law of the physical universe (Klemp, 2002). This law of physics states that every phenomenon, physical and mental, is the result of a combined meeting of two opposite and yet related factors, along with a third passive middle. This middle is not passive as in negation, but rather an active balancing point for the two factors. For example, a person may strongly voice an opinion at the extreme end of an issue (e.g., euthanasia). In the debate with others who hold a strong view on the opposite side, the "middle ground," or balance point, may emerge. When a person is no longer attracted to one side of an issue to the total exclusion of the other, true freedom exists. This is an internal integration of the whole.

Life is a paradox. Polar opposites exist to hold the world together, for each end is an opposing manifestation of the same phenomenon. The key to living a whole and balanced life is the ability to stand centered in the middle and move toward each pole with grace and ease, not preferring one over the other because true home is at center. Nurses recognize that there is great diversity among people, both in their approaches to health care issues and in their opinions as expressed in communication. Nurses do not seek for "one right answer" or a guaranteed way to communicate to all clients. Rather, standard approaches (the middle ground) are used, and then care—as well as the communications around care—is customized around an acceptance of the person in his or her environment.

Liberation occurs with freedom from false certainty (Block, 2002). A felt need for certainty creates the sense of doubt, and a belief that we are not enough then exists. This leads to an assumption that knowing more or better would lead to knowing what to do. Accepting the fact that some issues are beyond solution helps to make room for the mystery that is life in all its vagary. This opens space for wonder and gratitude, compassion and surrender, forgiveness and grief in both personal and organizational lives. The following are questions to ask about internal integration:

- What are your deepest stereotypes and expectations about the issue and the players involved in the conflict?
- How can you identify the duality in each experience and then locate the middle space pulsing with potential for either pole?
- What skills are needed to hold multiple perspectives without judgment?
- What role do your ambitions play in this debate?

Being open to the possibility of an imperfect and paradoxical world of polarities creates an opening for a more intimate connection with the world. The relationships between seemingly unrelated parts are revealed. This brings depth and joy to life and a delight in living the question rather than in the search for one narrow answer.

All experiences and events in life reflect the Law of Balance. Sooner or later the pendulum swings back. That moment, when both positive and negative forces are in equal proportions, we have the chance to go beyond the normal cause and effect of daily experience.

Harold Klemp

What Are You Trying to Achieve?

Always be a first rate version of yourself rather than a second rate version of someone else.

Judy Garland

We continuously find our way through the multiple relationships, experiences, and resulting perceptions that create insights to continue to grow and evolve. The journey is enriched by a fluid imagination that fosters creativity. It is hampered by a need for control, certainty, a quick fix, or ambition. Fear is the roadblock to realizing potential. What is focused on is what results.

Intuition: Stay With the Natural Flow of Your Life

In order to move into the future with grace, each person must be present in the "now" without distortion. The future is viewed through eyes clouded by old belief systems, including the limitation, victimization, and suffering themes of the age. Individuals start to purposely become more courageous in the choices they make and the messages they give when they are not motivated by fear and limitation. Energy is freed for more direct involvement with life. Relationships and communication are transformed through an innovative dance with possibility (Peirce, 1997).

Trusting intuition, rather than the laws of the tribe, opens the door to experiences that can change a person forever. Through self-observation, more presence will come automatically into each life (Tolle, 1999). The wonder of the moment is experienced as predictable ways of knowing the world are released. The following questions can help enhance intuition:

- How often is your mind focused on the past and the future?
- What is going on inside of you in this moment?
- How fully do you use all of your senses?
- Do you honor your hunches, or do you relinquish them to "reasonable thought"?
- How can you put joy, ease, and a sense of peace into what you are doing?

The choices made demonstrate the degree of conscious awareness. True choice begins the moment the individual releases conditioned patterns and moves into the present moment. This gives people access to their true power and intuition and is a true guide to the destiny they were born to live.

Community: Become a Social Entrepreneur

Nursing is not just moving into the twenty first century but into a reality entwined with the global nursing community and the universal community at large. As the Internet and global communication systems bring everyone closer together, a new generation of social leaders is rising up. Just as business advances new ideas and models to attack problems through an entrepreneur's single-minded vision and fierce determination, a new generation of social leaders is dedicating creativity and passion to create a better world. As "social entrepreneurs" they are creating new ways to approach old problems by using their unique talents to create a meaningful existence for themselves and others (Bornstein, 2004).

Nursing is a universal phenomenon. The nursing profession has a history replete with nurses who became social entrepreneurs long before it was the fashionable thing to do. Within the very fabric of nursing practice rest the stories and memories of nurses who utilized the fabric of human intimacy and mutual responsibility to affect the health and well-being of society. This rich heritage is calling nurses to move beyond the notion of communication and negotiation to a strong commitment to social action. This will require mutual learning about the issues that face humankind, mutual understanding about roles in issues that matter, and a mutual agenda for action to enhance the balance of the earth and all things upon it. Asking the following questions can augment social entrepreneurship:

- What are the universal core health issues facing humanity today?
- What must nursing's role be in addressing these issues?
- How can nurses unite globally around a shared agenda?
- When will nursing begin to advocate for groups and communities in the same way they have been individual patient advocates across time?
- What will happen if we do not take our social responsibility seriously and create an outcome that can change the world?
- When will you begin? How? What is the first step?

Nursing stands at a crossroad. One hundred years ago Florence Nightingale observed that nurses had always had a social calling. She challenged nurses to enlarge that calling with a social consciousness and a social creativity that would transform the health of society. She gave that challenge to all nurses, and the time to accept it and act on it is now. Let us begin.

I believe that there are those who will see their fundamental work not as making decisions, but as making mutual understanding.

Peter Schwartz

Summary

- Communication is the art of being able to structure and transmit a message in a way that another can easily understand and/or accept.
- Communication is defined as the degree to which information is transmitted among the members and parts of an organization.

- Verbal communication is both written and spoken (oral).
- Nonverbal communication is unspoken but affective or expressive behaviors.
- Communication can be characterized by four distinctions: formal/informal, vertical/horizontal, personal/impersonal, and instrumental/expressive.
- Communication models described in the literature include the sender-receiver, human needs, and transactional analysis models.
- Interpersonal relationships include an element of communication.
- A single communication can be broken down into five steps of information exchange.
- Communication occurs in a variety of interactive patterns.
- Perception and interpretation form filters for messages and create a potential for breakdown.
- Effectiveness in communication is related to timing and the choice of channel.
- Feedback is a basic communication principle associated with the concept of delegation.
- Constructive criticism is focused on an analysis of the problem.
- Appearance and behavior add to the total communication to convey a message effectively.
- One issue in nursing is how to project and communicate an attitude of competence and professionalism.
- Group dynamics and the interaction of multiple people provide complexity and challenges to the communicative process and the influence of perception in organizations.
- Communicating, along with diagnosing and adapting, is one of the three basic competencies of influencing and leadership.
- There are six areas of organizational communication that can be assessed for communication problems: (1) accessibility of information, (2) communication channels, (3) clarity of messages, (4) span of control, (5) flow control/communication load, and (6) the individual communicators.
- In nursing, communication techniques can be applied to work-related issues—for example,

verbal abuse, physical violence, and the use of work teams.
- Persuasion and negotiation are influence techniques.
- Persuasion is human communication designed to influence another to modify attitudes or alter behaviors by using argument, reasoning, or entreaty.
- Persuasion is used to generate action or activity.
- Persuasion is used to control the course of events.
- Persuaders use appeals and engage their audience's emotions.
- Successful persuasive communication uses commitment, imagination, and trust.
- There are five categories of reasons to exert influence.
- There are eight types of influence tactics.
- Intensification and downplaying are two common persuasion tactics.
- Persuasion is used both to obtain personal benefit and to satisfy organizational goals.
- Communication is the core of leadership; influencing is achieved through persuasion.
- Negotiation is a give-and-take exchange to resolve conflicts.
- Negotiation often is applied to collective bargaining.
- Negotiation is used to avoid a win-lose outcome.
- Three criteria set the framework for true negotiation.
- There are four elements to the negotiation process.
- There are 10 steps to the negotiation process.
- Four negotiating strategies are the flinch, the deadline, the nibble, and the concession.
- The work of a manager depends on the ability to negotiate.

Study Questions

1. What are the essential components of the communication process?
2. What are the barriers to effective communication in organizations?

3. What problems of communication occur frequently in nursing?

4. Are employer-employee communication problems more common than peer-to-peer difficulties?

5. What solutions tend to help communication effectiveness?

6. What is the relationship of communication skill to leadership effectiveness?

7. What is the leader's role in helping others improve written and oral communication?

8. How important is written communication skill in influencing an individual's image?

9. How do you personally communicate, both verbally and nonverbally?

10. How might you choose some other message or some other channel to increase your personal effectiveness?

11. Do nurses, from the staff nurse to the chief nurse executive, present an image of nursing that you agree or disagree with?

12. What does the ideal nursing uniform look like? Analyze your response.

13. Why do nurses need to look professional?

14. What persuades an individual to become a nurse?

15. What feelings are associated with an interview for a nursing position?

16. What was the last issue you negotiated?

17. What behaviors contribute to cooperative and productive negotiation?

18. What words or actions indicate competitive negotiation?

19. What approaches or strategies of negotiation are most effective for nursing?

20. What factors are facilitators or barriers to collaboration among professionals?

21. Does collective bargaining increase professionalism in nursing?

22. What organizational factors are associated with unionization?

23. Is positional power eroding in nursing? With what forms of negotiation can nurses replace positional power?

CASE STUDY

Caring is a fundamental aspect of nursing practice. Nurses also adhere to ethical principles; for instance, maintaining patient confidentiality. Hospitals identify a list of patient rights, such as the right to privacy and confidentiality in medical care and records. Although nurses perceive that they maintain patient privacy and confidentiality, the patient's experience is quite different. This is a serious ethical problem with possible liability attached.

The chief nurse executive, George Everson, was concerned about breaches of patient confidentiality, especially since there had been several recent patient complaints. He had just finished reading Brann and Mattson's (2004) research after seeing a brief article about it in the local newspaper. Nurse Everson assumed that local media coverage might accelerate other patients' complaints. He decided to do a "walk-about" to get a sense of the situation himself. Nurse Everson discovered by simply walking and loitering in patient care areas that there were frequent occurrences of informal conversations about patients' health status among care providers: in hallways, elevators, and outside patients' rooms. Sometimes dialogues between health care providers and patients could easily be overheard, especially in two-bed patient rooms. Because of open nursing stations, information about patients could be overheard or was directly given to nonpatients. In ambulatory areas or waiting rooms, confidential information about patients was shared with family members or the other people waiting and was overheard in conversations with other providers, referral sources, or insurance companies.

Nurse Everson had heard enough to begin to plan for needed changes. Further assessment of the situation was formally conducted, and an ad hoc committee was formed to analyze and recommend strategies. A variety of action plans were formed: renovation of open spaces and less-private areas, new procedures for registration, conducting telephone calls in private, and more thorough training for all health care providers.

CRITICAL THINKING EXERCISE

Nurse Aminta Parra is in charge of an interdisciplinary team at Sunrise Hospital. The nurses at Sunrise have identified a need to develop a critical pathway for ventilator-dependent patients who are about to be discharged to home with home health care. Nurse Parra knows that these patients have multiple complex care needs. It is urgent that information flow be specific and detailed to make "seamless" the care transfer between the hospital and home care, wherever this may be. First, Nurse Parra had to manage a few physicians who flatly stated that they would not follow a "cookbook" concocted by nurses. Then the dietary representative presented the team with Dietary's protocols and suggested that nurses integrate these since nurses were in charge of the pathway

maintenance. Next, Nurse Parra discovered why the local home health care representative was not returning phone calls and was not able come to team meetings for quite a while: the group was planning a move in 1 month and was just notified of a JCAHO visit in 3 months.

1. What is the problem?
2. Whose problem is it?
3. What should Nurse Parra do?
4. What mode of communication should Nurse Parra use?
5. How can Nurse Parra structure a clear message?
6. To whom should Nurse Parra communicate first? Who else needs to be involved in the communication flow?
7. What leadership and management strategies should Nurse Parra use?

REFERENCES

Aber, C., & Hawkins, J. (1992). Portrayal of nurses in advertisements in medical and nursing journals. *Image, 24*(4), 289-293.

Anderson, M.A., & Tredway, C.A. (1999). Communication: An outcome of case management. *Nursing Case Management, 4*(3), 104-111.

Anthony, M.K., & Preuss, G. (2002). Models of care: The influence of nurse communication on patient safety. *Nursing Economic$, 20*(6), 209-215, 248.

Apker, J., & Fox, D.H. (2002). Communication: Improving RNs' organizational and professional identification in managed care hospitals. *Journal of Nursing Administration, 32*(2), 106-114.

Argenti, P. (2002). Crisis communication: Lessons from 9/11. *Harvard Business Review, 80*(12), 103-109.

Baker, D. (1986). Persuasion: The power is in the art. *Nursing Management, 17*(11), 59.

Ball, J.R., Counts, D., Jones, M.L.H., Vinci, C., & Winn, C. (1998). An organization-wide approach for an effective communication system, Part 1. *Journal of Nursing Administration, 28*(3), 28-34.

Barabasi, A. L. (2002). *Linked: The new science of networks: How everything is connected to everything else and what it means for science, business and everyday life.* Cambridge, MA: Perseus Press.

Barnum, B. (1990). Wear your designer clothes on duty: The Diane Von Furstenberg collection. *Nursing and Healthcare, 11*(9), 484-485.

Block, P. (2002). *The answer to how is yes: Acting on what matters.* San Francisco: Berrett-Koehler Publishers Inc.

Boggs, K.U. (1999). Communication styles. In E. Arnold & K.U. Boggs (Eds.), *Interpersonal relationships: Professional communication skills for nurses* (3rd ed.) (pp. 195-208). Philadelphia: W.B. Saunders.

Booth, R. (1993). Dynamics of conflict and conflict management. In D. Mason, S. Talbott, & J. Leavitt (Eds.), *Policy and politics for nurses: Action and change in the workplace, government, organizations, and community* (2nd ed.) (pp. 149-165). Philadelphia: W.B. Saunders.

Bornstein, D. (2004). Real people building a better world. *Ode, 14.* Retrieved September 17, 2004, from *www.odemagazine.com/article.php?aID=3891*

Boyle, D.K., & Kochinda, C. (2004). Enhancing collaborative communication of nurse and physician leadership in two intensive care units. *Journal of Nursing Administration, 34*(2), 60-70.

Brann, M., & Mattson, M. (2004). Toward a typology of confidentiality breaches in health care communication: An ethic of care analysis of provider practices and patient perceptions. *Health Communication, 16*(2), 229-251.

Bream, T., Bram, K., Bantle, A., & Krenz, K. (1992). Beyond the ordinary image of nursing. *Nursing Management, 23*(12), 44-47.

Brothers, J. (1986, November 16). How to get the job you want. *Parade,* pp. 4-6.

Brown, J.S., & Duguid, P. (2000). *The social life of information.* Boston: Harvard Business School Press.

Campbell, S., O'Malley, C., Watson, D., Charlwood, J., & Lowson, S.M. (2000). The image of children's nurse: A study of the qualities required by families of children's nurses' uniform. *Journal of Clinical Nursing, 9*(1), 71-82.

Cochrane, D., Oberle, K., Nielson, S., Sloan-Roseneck, J., Anderson, K., & Finlay C. (1992). Do they really understand us? *American Journal of Nursing, 92*(7), 19-20.

Coeling, H.V.E., & Cukr, P.L. (1998). Collaboration in practice. In S.A. Price, M.W. Koch, & S. Bassett (Eds.), *Healthcare resource management: Present and future challenges* (pp. 185-202). St Louis: Mosby.

Cornell, D. (1993). Say the words: Communication techniques. *Nursing Management, 24*(3), 42-44.

Csikszentmihalyi, M. (1993). *The evolving self: A psychology for the third millennium.* New York: Harper Collins.

Curtin, L. (1991). Leaders: The organization's pacemakers. *Nursing Management, 22*(3), 6-8.

Davenport, T. H., & Beck, J. C. (2001). *The attention economy: Understanding the new currency of business.* Boston: Harvard Business School Press.

Deering, C. (1993). Giving and taking criticism. *American Journal of Nursing, 93*(12), 56-61.

DeKeyser, F.G., Wruble, A.W., & Margalith, I. (2003). Patients voice issues of dress and address. *Holistic Nursing Practice, 17*(6), 290-294.

Farley, M. (1989). Assessing communication in organizations. *Journal of Nursing Administration, 19*(12), 27-31.

Fisher, R., & Ury, W. (1991). *Getting to yes: Negotiating agreement without giving in.* New York: Penguin Books.

Franzoi, S. (1988). A picture of competence. *American Journal of Nursing, 88*(8), 1109-1112.

Grant, A. (1994). *The professional nurse: Issues and actions.* Springhouse, PA: Springhouse.

Hansten, R., & Washburn, M. (1992). What's your feedback style? *American Journal of Nursing, 92*(12), 56-61.

Harvey, K. (1990). The power of positive questioning. *Nursing Management, 21*(5), 94-96.

Hersey, P., Blanchard, K.H., & Johnson, D.E. (2001). *Management of organizational behavior: Leading human resources* (8th ed.). Upper Saddle River, NJ: Prentice-Hall.

Houweling, L. (2004). Image, function and style: A history of the nursing uniform. *American Journal of Nursing, 104*(4), 40-48.

Johnson & Johnson Company. (2004). *Campaign for nursing's future.* New Brunswick, NJ: Johnson & Johnson. Retrieved July 19, 2004, from *www.jnj.com/our_company/advertising/discover_nursing/*

Kalisch, B., & Kalisch, P. (1985). Dressing for success. *American Journal of Nursing, 85*(8), 887-893.

Katz, J.M., & Green, E. (1997). *Managing quality: A guide to system-wide performance management in healthcare* (2nd ed.). St Louis: Mosby.

Kennedy, C., Camden, C., & Timmerman, G. (1990). Relationships among perceived supervisor communication, nurse morale, and sociocultural variables. *Nursing Administration Quarterly, 14*(4), 38-46.

Kipnis, D., & Schmidt, S. (1980). Intraorganizational influence tactics: Explorations in getting one's way. *Journal of Applied Psychology, 65*(4), 440-452.

Kippenbrock, T. (1992). Power at meetings: Strategies to move people. *Nursing Economic$, 10*(4), 282-286.

Klemp, H. (2002). *The spiritual laws of life.* Minneapolis: Eckankar.

Knowles, R. (1983). Building rapport through neuro-linguistic programming. *American Journal of Nursing, 83*(7), 1010-1014.

Kucera, K., & Nieswiadomy, R. (1991). Nursing attire: The public's preference. *Nursing Management, 22*(10), 68-70.

Laser, R. (1981). I win—you win negotiating. *Journal of Nursing Administration, 11*(11/12), 24-29.

Lassen, A.A., Fosbinder, D.M., Minton, S., & Robins, M.M. (1997). Nurse/physician collaborative practice: Improving healthcare quality while decreasing cost. *Nursing Economic$, 15*(2), 87-91, 104.

Lax, D.A., & Sebenius, J.K. (2003). 3-D negotiation: Playing the whole game. *Harvard Business Review, 81*(11), 64-74.

Lehna, C., Pfoutz, S., Peterson, T.G., Degner, K., Grubaugh, K., Lorenz, L., et al. (1999). Nursing attire: Indicators of professionalism? *Journal of Professional Nursing 15*(3), 192-199.

Levenstein, A. (1982). Tactics of persuasion. *Nursing Management, 13*(11), 40-41.

Mangum, S., Garrison, C., Lind, C., Thackeray, R., & Wyatt, M. (1991). Perceptions of nurses' uniforms. *Image, 23*(2), 127-130.

Manzoni, J. (2002). A better way to deliver bad news. *Harvard Business Review, 80*(9), 114-119.

Mason, D.J., & Buhler-Wilkerson, K. (2004). Who's the RN? *American Journal of Nursing, 104*(4), 11.

Mintzberg, H. (1993). *Structure in fives: Designing effective organizations.* Englewood Cliffs, NJ: Prentice-Hall.

Moss, J., & Xiao, Y. (2004). Improving operating room coordination: Communication pattern assessment. *Journal of Nursing Administration, 34*(2), 93-100.

Mulgan, G. (1997). *Connexity: How to live in a connected world.* Boston: Harvard Business School Press.

Pearson, A., Baker, H., Walsh, K., & Fitzgerald, M. (2001). Contemporary nurses' uniforms—History and traditions. *Journal of Nursing Management, 9*(3), 147-152.

Peirce, P. (1997). *The intuitive way: A guide to living from inner wisdom.* New York: MJF Books.

Pincus, J. (1986). Communication: Key contributor to effectiveness—The research. *Journal of Nursing Administration, 16*(9), 19-25.

Pine, B. J., & Gilmore, J. H. (1999). *The experience economy: Work is theater and every business a stage.* Boston: Harvard Business School Press.

Price, J., & Mueller, C. (1986). *Handbook of organizational measurement.* Marshfield, MA: Pitman.

Price, J.R. (1990). *A spiritual philosophy for the new world.* Carlsbad, CA: Hay House, Inc.

Rael, J. (1993). *Being and vibration.* Tulsa, OK: Council One Books.

Rappsilber, C. (1982). Persuasion as a mechanism for change. In J. Lancaster & W. Lancaster (Eds.), *The nurse as a change agent: Concepts for advanced nursing practice* (pp. 132-145). St Louis: Mosby.

Schwartz, P. (1991). *The art of the long view: Planning for the future in an uncertain world.* New York: Doubleday Press.

Sherer, J. (1994). Resolving conflict (the right way). *Hospitals and Health Networks, 68*(8), 52-55.

Smeltzer, C. (1991). The art of negotiation: An everyday experience. *Journal of Nursing Administration, 21*(7/8), 26-30.

Thies, K., & Williams-Burgess, C. (1992). Communication as a progressive curriculum concept. *Nurse Educator, 17*(2), 39-41.

Tolle, E. (1999). *Practicing the power of now.* Novato, CA: New World Library.

Yepsen, D. (1988, October 5). Molding a candidate for the media. *The Des Moines Register,* p. 7A.

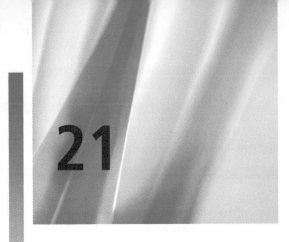

21

All-Hazards Disaster Preparedness

Gene S. Rigotti Karen N. Drenkard

CHAPTER OBJECTIVES

- Overview of all-hazards preparedness
- Define and discuss multiple facets of all-hazards preparedness
- Analyze planning for a comprehensive all-hazards preparedness strategy for health care
- Discuss strategies to resolve implementation issues
- Critique nursing leadership and management implications
- Identify all-hazards preparedness resources
- Exercise critical thinking to conceptualize and analyze possible solutions to a practice exercise

TRANSITIONING THEORY INTO PRACTICE FOR ALL-HAZARDS PREPAREDNESS

September 11, 2001, was a tragic day that touched everyone's lives and changed Americans' perception of a "safe" world forever. Since that time people of all backgrounds have been scrambling to prepare significant others and themselves, their homes, and their workplaces for what might happen. A list of terrorism possibilities is endless: biological mishaps, chemical spills, radiological exposures, nuclear blasts, conventional bombings, agricultural contamination, cyber viruses and other unforeseen cataclysmic events. Thus disaster and bioterrorism preparedness is most appropriately termed **all-hazards disaster preparedness**.

Since September 11, people in every community have been gathering information from a variety of resources, reevaluating personal perspectives about preparing for an inevitable disaster, and planning what they would do in the event of a disaster (Ashcroft, 2001; Myers, 2001; Richter, 2004; Vecchio, 2000). But how does one go about preparing for an event in the workplace, and more specifically, the hospital environment? Traditionally the community hospital is a place of refuge for the sick and wounded. How does all that change in the event of a disaster?

Health care executives across the country are struggling to find their place with regard to participating effectively in all-hazards preparedness. The Health Insurance Portability and Accountability Act (HIPAA), along with the Joint Commission on Accreditation of Healthcare Organizations (JCAHO) require all health care facilities to have detailed all-hazard preparedness plans. Nursing leaders are an integral part of this planning because no one knows better than they do that the measure of success equals the degree of effective planning. Nurse leaders possess the

The authors would like to thank their colleagues: Fran Vasaly, RN, Infection Control Practitioner, Inova Health System; Dan Hanfling, MD, FACEP, Director of Emergency Management and Disaster Medicine, Inova Health System/Inova Fairfax Hospital; Allan Morrison, MD, FACP, FIDSA, Medical Chief of Infection Control, Inova Health System/Inova Fairfax Hospital; Greg Brison, Director of Safety and Security, Inova Alexandria Hospital.

necessary skills, competencies and experience that serve them well in taking on a primary role in disaster preparedness (Lindholm & Uden, 2001).

Effective planning for all-hazards preparedness is an important process, and skill in planning is an essential management competency for nurse leaders. This chapter describes how to orchestrate a multilevel plan for a health care facility. A comprehensive all-hazards preparedness plan will assist in establishing the following: (1) an organized hospital-based plan for both internal and external disasters at the department/unit level, (2) an interhospital plan for effectively collaborating with other hospitals within a health care system and within the local vicinity, (3) a community plan that will integrate the hospital plan with other external community plans, and (4) a national plan that will guide nurse leaders in accessing financial assistance from federal and state all-hazards preparedness resources.

DEFINITIONS

From a health care perspective, a **disaster** is an unforeseen and often sudden event that causes great damage, destruction, and human suffering. Though often caused by nature, disasters can have human origins. Wars and civil disturbances that destroy homelands and displace people are included among the causes of disasters. Other causes can be a building collapse, blizzard, drought, epidemic, earthquake, explosion, fire, flood, hazardous material or transportation incident (such as a chemical spill), hurricane, nuclear incident, tornado, or volcano (Disaster Relief Library, 2004).

There is a wide variety of types and causes of disasters. Disasters can be internal (a catastrophic event that occurs within a facility and is usually handled within the facility, depending on the size of the event) or external (a catastrophic event that affects the community, which may or may not affect the facility). Causes of natural disasters include such things as earthquakes, forest fires, floods, or hurricanes, just to name a few. Disasters also can be caused by human acts; these can include biological, chemical, radiological, nuclear, cyber, or conventional terrorist events.

Other disaster-related definitions are as follows:

All-hazards: A general term that is descriptive of all types of natural and/or human terrorist events.

All-hazards disaster preparedness: Multifaceted internal and external disaster preparedness that establishes action plans for every type of disaster or combination of disaster events

Biological disaster: An incident involving a natural or deliberate outbreak of a pathogen affecting large numbers of adults and children (Inova Health System, 2001a).

Chemical disaster: Exposure to hazardous chemically toxic materials that may produce a wide range of adverse health effects (Inova Health System, 2001b).

Conventional disaster: A catastrophic event caused by the use of weapons such as guns, bombs, missiles, grenades, etc.

Cyber disaster: A catastrophic event affecting large numbers of people and lasting more than a few hours that impacts the ability to use information technology.

Radiological/nuclear disaster: A radiological or nuclear emergency that may result from accidents occurring within a facility (such as the Departments of Nuclear Medicine and Radiation Oncology) or from external sources involving vehicles transporting radioactive

---

◢ LEADING & MANAGING **DEFINED**

All-Hazards Disaster Preparedness	**Disaster**
Action plans for every type of disaster or combination of disaster events.	An unforeseen and often sudden event that causes great damage, destruction, and human suffering.

materials (RAM) or caused by terrorism events involving nuclear weapons or radiologically contaminated conventional weapons (Inova Health System, 2001c).

GETTING STARTED: FIRST STEPS

Starting any project can be confusing and difficult. Beginning the work of establishing a comprehensive all-hazards preparedness plan is no exception. Historically, most hospitals have had some sort of disaster plan in place. Being the leader in the evaluation of the hospital's current disaster plan, in light of the nation's current focus on maintaining a state of constant readiness, can be a complex process. One of the first steps to gaining participation from appropriate stakeholders and moving the evaluation process forward is the creation of an oversight committee, or all-hazards preparedness task force (AHPTF). The nursing executive, often called a chief nurse officer (CNO), will play a pivotal role in facilitating the initial task force.

Creating an All-Hazards Preparedness Task Force

As nurses know, effective projects that create lasting change start with the basic nursing process: assessment, planning, implementation, evaluation, and modification. The all-hazards preparedness task force will similarly follow this process. It is essential to get administrative support regarding the need for an all-hazards preparedness plan. This is best accomplished by establishing a high-level administrative task force whose purpose will be oversight of the multilevel all-hazards preparedness plan development. Whether the hospital is part of a larger health care system or is a free-standing, independent hospital, the AHPTF will function similarly.

Health care systems with multiple facilities are very familiar with the complexity and intricacies of trying to establish a standardized system-wide approach to care needs. In organizations such as these, system-wide executive administrators need to be part of the AHPTF. Having a senior executive administrator of the health care system serve as the chairperson of the task force will provide the leadership needed to communicate the importance of all-hazards preparedness as a system priority. A representative CNO and emergency care physician, serving as co-chairs with the senior executive administrator, will create a dynamic team that is uniquely prepared to tackle any issues that arise. A project facilitator is also helpful in getting the task force started and operational.

Establishing the AHPTF requires that all departments be committed to the tasks at hand and cognizant of the need for consensus building and standardization of processes. Bi-directional communication is imperative. Coordination of the work of the task force members also needs to be addressed. Fortunately, most of the work will be broken down into step-by-step pieces that allow each member to play a vital role and have control over his or her department's contribution to the plan as a whole. The standing membership should be composed of stakeholders representing all areas of the organization. Since not all departments can logistically be on the task force, the members will have large areas of oversight and communication. The AHPTF membership might typically look like that outlined in Table 21.1.

As the team evolves in its work, ad hoc members can be added as needed. Internal ad hoc members might include medical radiology, facility engineering, telecommunications, volunteer support, chaplain services, physician chairs, social work, case management, dietary, respiratory, and laboratory services. External ad hoc members might include public health administrators, government liaison support, police force liaison, public school system liaison, community church representatives, community physicians, and even vendor representatives, who can be contracted to provide such things as oxygen, ice, food, cots, and linens in the event of a disaster.

For the first year, the system-wide AHPTF will most likely need to meet every other week. During this period the task force will perform a gap analysis based on the JCAHO standards and other regulations and start a working action plan to correct

Table 21.1

All-Hazards Preparedness Task Force Membership Responsibilities		
Responsibility Area(s)	Position Title	Detail of Areas Covered
Executive owner (Chair)	Executive administrator	Leads the All-Hazards Preparedness task force as chair. If the hospital is part of a health care system, this person will be a system-wide senior administrator. If the hospital is a freestanding, independent facility, this person will be the hospital's chief operating officer.
Clinical operations (Co-chair)	Chief nurse officer	Represents all nursing and clinical departments. Co-chairs the task force.
Chemical/radiological/ conventional threats (Co-chair)	Emergency department/air care medical director	Represents all aspects of emergency medicine and physician needs related to All-Hazards Preparedness. This person also will co-chair the task force.
Physician liaison(s)	Department chiefs	Serve as spokesperson for physician needs with regard to disaster preparedness. Facilitate communication of timely of information should an event occur. Have oversight for physician credentialing in times of a disaster. Assist in approval of medical standards established for various types of disasters.
COOs from health care system facilities	Chief operating officer(s)	Represent the needs of their facility in establishing an effective All-Hazards Preparedness plan. Facilitate system-wide collaboration in standardizing practices and communicate essential information to employees.
Security	Safety and security director	Serves as liaison for system-wide Safety & Security Departments in the system. Coordinates and synchronizes efforts of all departments as related to All-Hazards Preparedness. Responsible for rapid "lock down" of all entrances and flow of people in the event of a disaster.
Communications	Chief information technology officer	Oversees successful operation of the integrated information system, including telephones, radios, computers and satellite technology, during times of instability. Creates and maintains redundant systems to assure an ability to communicate within facilities, outside to other hospitals, and partners with community.
Messages/media	Marketing director	Plays an active role in communicating the "All-Hazards Preparedness" message to all employees, patients, and community. Acts on behalf of the health care system or hospital in

Table 21.1

All-Hazards Preparedness Task Force Membership Responsibilities—cont'd		
Responsibility Area(s)	Position Title	Detail of Areas Covered
		speaking with press about impending or actual disaster situations.
Human resources	Human resources director	Serves as the staff's voice in meeting the needs of employees during a disaster. Creates manuals to guide staff in preparing for and responding to a disaster.
Financial reimbursement	Chief financial officer	Leads efforts in monitoring financial expenses related to establishing an effective All-Hazards Preparedness plan. Seeks out state/federal reimbursement opportunities for planning.
Government funding	Government affairs director	Serves as a vital link to local, state, and federal boards representing the system financial and operational needs in regards to All-Hazards Preparedness. Advocates for funding related to all-hazards preparedness.
Biological threats	Infectious disease medical director	Serves as the liaison for all infection control (IC) departments in the system.
	Infection control nurse	Coordinates and synchronizes efforts of all IC departments as related to all-hazards preparedness. Responsible for development, dissemination, and understanding of procedures called related to biological events.
Legal	Executive attorney	Advises All-Hazards Preparedness task force in legal matters related to establishing an effective All-Hazards Preparedness plan.
Education planning	Education director	Has oversight for planning and implementing educational efforts for staff and patients. As needed, coordinates "just in time" training for any arising incident. Is an integral partner in planning and implementing internal and external disaster drills.
Logistics	Pharmacy director	Serves as the liaison for all system pharmacies. Has oversight for stockpiling of medications for use in a disaster. Establishes par levels of drugs for use in "patient surge" situations. Establishes contracts with pharmaceutical vendors to ensure adequate supply of medications in the event of a disaster. Has oversight for any medical supply trucks ready for deployment in times of a disaster (e.g., stocking par level of drugs used in a chemical disaster).

Continued

Table 21.1

All-Hazards Preparedness Task Force Membership Responsibilities—cont'd		
Responsibility Area(s)	Position Title	Detail of Areas Covered
Logistics—cont'd	Materials management director	Serves as an active participant on the task force. This liaison is the system representative for all materials management departments. Is very involved in setting par levels for supplies and equipment on the units at the time of a disaster. Establishes contracts with materials management vendors to ensure adequate supply of medications in the event of a disaster (e.g., stocking a supplemental supply truck for use in a disaster).
	Engineering	Directs any operational building redesign needed to prepare hospital for handling a disaster (e.g., decontamination showers).

Courtesy Inova Health System, Falls Church, VA.
NOTE: This assessment tool was developed by Inova Health System based on a bioterrorism preparedness survey created by a committee consisting of representatives from Baylor University's Graduate Program in Healthcare Administration, the U.S. Army Center for Healthcare Education and Studies, and the University of Texas Health Science Center at San Antonio. (For more information, see Drenkard et al., 2002).

any deficiencies. Nursing leaders will play key roles in creating aggressive timelines, often 1 to 2 weeks, for resolving issues on the action plan. The goal should be to have resolutions that are correct but not necessarily perfect. Most resolutions will be modified and enhanced over time as the task force gains more knowledge about all-hazards planning.

From the gap analysis assessment, the task force will establish high-level, multifaceted standards of practice and system-wide goals for all-hazards preparedness. These standards and goals will be implemented at the facility level and department level as directed by the COO, CNO, and emergency department medical director. At this point there is latitude for departments to design and implement the standards and goals based on the unique needs of each area.

Performing an Effective Gap Analysis

There are many ways to perform an all-hazards preparedness gap analysis so that leaders do not have to start from nothing. There are a multitude of online reference websites, including, but not limited to, the following examples: Office of National Preparedness, Health and Human Services, Health and Medical Services Support Plan, the American Hospital Association (AHA), the Centers for Disease Control and Prevention (CDC), and the Hospital Emergency Incident Command System (HEICS) (Pletz et al., 1998) (Box 21.1).

The guiding principle for creating a hospital-specific all-hazards gap analysis is to "keep it simple!" One example of a simple way to assess the current state is to create an emergency preparedness survey that is easy to read and requires the department directors to answer in simple checklists one of two ways: (1) "Yes, we have it" or (2) "No, we don't have it." Survey questions need to be concise and clear. The goal is to begin by identifying the areas where there are gaps in the facility's preparedness plans. Questions should be addressed to appropriate departments, who then assess the items and make a determination of the

Box 21.1

All-Hazards Preparedness Resources

Websites Relevant to All-Hazards Preparedness

Association for Professionals in Infection Control and Epidemiology
www.apic.org
Emergency Preparedness and Response, Centers for Disease Control and Prevention
www.bt.cdc.gov/
Anthrax (Centers for Disease Control and Prevention)
www.bt.cdc.gov/agent/anthrax/index.asp
Botulism (Centers for Disease Control and Prevention)
www.cdc.gov/ncidod/dbmd/diseaseinfo/botulism_g.htm
"What Every Person Needs to Know about the Anthrax Vaccine" (Medical NBC Online Information Server,
    U.S. Army's Office of the Surgeon General)
www.nbc-med.org/SiteContent/HomePage/WhatsNew/anthraxinfo/Anthraxinfo3.htm
Anthrax Vaccine Immunization Program, U.S. Department of Defense
www.anthrax.osd.mil/
Center for Biosecurity, University of Pittsburgh Medical Center
www.upmc-biosecurity.org/
"Guidelines for the Surveillance and Control of Anthrax in Humans and Animals" (World Health Organization)
www.who.int/emc-documents/zoonoses/docs/whoemczdi986.html
Federal Emergency Management Agency
www.fema.gov/
American Red Cross
www.redcross.org
Centers for Disease Control and Prevention
www.cdc.gov/
U.S. Department of Homeland Security
www.dhs.gov/dhspublic/
Press Room, U.S. Department of Homeland Security
www.dhs.gov/dhspublic/interapp/press_release/press_release_0363.xml
Occupational Safety and Health Organization
www.osha.gov/
Homeland Security Presidential Directive-3 (The White House, President George W. Bush)
www.whitehouse.gov/news/releases/2002/03/20020312-5.html
"Members from Three Incident Management Teams Travel to Florida" (American-Firefighter.com)
www.american-firefighter.com/articles/article_2004_09_28_3000.html

Other Sources of Information

U.S. Army Medical Research Institute of Infectious Diseases: 301/619-2833 BIOPORT (producers of anthrax
    vaccine): 517/327-1500
American Red Cross: 202/303-4498
Salvation Army: 888/321-3433
U.S. Public Health Service: 800/872-6367
Domestic Preparedness Information Line: DOMESTIC 800/368-6498
National Response Center: 800/424-8802

current state. A review of the literature and online web searches will assist the team in identifying the areas of assessment (English et al., 1999; Macintyre et al., 2000; McLaughlin, 2001; Wetter et al., 2001). Examples of questions to ask in the survey might include those listed in Box 21.2 (Drenkard et al., 2002).

Once the survey is created, it should be distributed to all stakeholders. Directors should be challenged to complete and return it in 5 working days so that work can be initiated to address outstanding issues. The AHPTF should review the survey results and start an issues list to address deficiencies.

Box **21.2**

Hospital Gap Analysis Survey

Sample Questions

General

- Does your hospital have an internal disaster plan addressing what to do if an emergency occurs only in your facility?
- Does your hospital have an external disaster plan addressing what to do if an emergency occurs in the community and you need to be prepared to respond?
- Do the directors know where to find facility internal and external disaster plans?
- Do the directors know who is in charge of the command center in a disaster?
- Does your department staff know the chain of command in an emergency?
- Does your department know their role in a disaster?
- Does your hospital know their role in the community in an emergency situation?
- Are those in charge identified by a vest or have some sort of distinction?
- Are there specific plans for biological, chemical, nuclear, and conventional emergencies? Do all staff in your department know their role in each emergency?
- Is there a bed and staffing plan for surge capacity for 50 patients? 100 patients? 250 patients? Do you have portable cots contracted for use in a surge situation?
- Does your facility have an operational command center to coordinate the hospitals response in the event of a disaster?
- Is there a central command center phone number to use in the event of a disaster?

Human Resources

- Does your department staff know how to prepare themselves, their significant others, and pets in the event of a disaster?
- Is there a credentialing plan for health care professionals who come to the nearest facility in a disaster to volunteer their services?

Safety and Security

- Does your facility:
  —Have a lockdown plan in case of an emergency?
  —Have a plan for allowing staff to get to work and be allowed entry to hospital during an emergency?
  —Have a plan for facility traffic flow during an emergency?
  —Have multilanguage signage to direct people as to where to go during an emergency?

Box **21.2**

Hospital Gap Analysis Survey—cont'd

Communication

- Does your hospital have emergency-powered phones in case of a disaster?
- Does your facility have a backup radio system and volunteer staff to run it?
- Does your facility have a tiered paging system that can reach multiple staff simultaneously?
- Does your department know the central command center number (if there is one)?
- Is there an on-call procedure for notifying the administrator on-call and opening the command center in the event of a disaster?
- Are there established linkages to the external community (e.q. other hospitals in the reqion, fire department, police, emergency medical system, public schools, public health)?
- Do the telephone operators know how to link patients and families both in your facility and in the community should a disaster occur?
- Is there an on-call list for administrative coverage of the command center? If so, do the telephone operators know how to contact the administrator on-call for the command center?
- Is there a plan for contacting essential employees and administrators in a disaster?

Logistics

- Does your facility have:
  —Backup emergency supplies, pharmaceuticals, and equipment?
  —The ability to release and send pharmaceuticals, medical supplies, and equipment such as respirators to the areas in need in the event of a chemical or biological emergency?
  —Prearranged plans with physicians, ambulances, nearby churches, and nursing homes to clear beds in an emerqency? (What sites can take patients?)
  —Contracts with vendors to bring in food, ice, oxygen, etc.?
- Is there an established written psychosocial role for social work, chaplains, psychiatry, employee health, and case management in the event of a disaster?
- Are there contingency plans for 3 to 5 days for no power, no water, no computers and/or no food?
- Are there contingency plans for staff to report to nearest facility to work?
- Are there contingency plans for childcare during an emergency so that parents can work?
- Is there common nomenclature used during an emergency so that everyone understands what is happening and who has what responsibility?

Clinical Operations

- Does your facility have:
  —Procedures established to maximize staff safety in the event of a disaster?
  —Procedures for fit testing of respiratory masks for staff?
  —Procedures and training for using protective equipment?
  —The ability to track patients until discharge, admission, or death using HIPAA guidelines?
  —Clear established policies and procedures to respond to biological, chemical, nuclear, and conventional emergencies?
  —A decontamination area and detailed step-by-step procedures on how to work in this area?
  —A backup staff to assist with people/patients arriving to the hospital?

Continued

Box **21.2**

Hospital Gap Analysis Survey—cont'd

Clinical Operations—cont'd

- Does your facility have procedures for how to:
  —Open and operate the command center?
  —Track available beds?
  —Track staff working and direct them to a designated area?
  —Track volunteer staff and direct them to a designated area?
  —Track arriving patients and direct them to a designated area?
  —Operate every department of the hospital during an emergency?
  —Track discharged patients and direct them to a designated area?
  —Handle surge capacity situations?
  —Handle OR cases in the event of an emergency?
  —Track biological, chemical, or nuclear events and report them to authorities?

Financial

- Is there an established plan to tracking costs during an emergency?
- Is there a established plan for submitting for disaster reimbursement?

Messages/Media

- Is there an established communication plan in case of an emergency?
- Is there an established communication script in the event of an emergency?
- Is there an alternative communication plan if power, telephones, and radios are not working?

Courtesy Inova Health System. From Drenkard, K., & Rigotti, G. (2002). *Inova Health System survey 2001.* Falls Church, VA: Inova Health System.

Keeping the Momentum Going

Once the gap analysis is completed and the issues are identified, a critical time in development of the comprehensive plan occurs. The work can appear daunting, and it is hard to know where to start. It is at this point that nursing leadership has the opportunity to take a lead. Nurses are experts at creating workable action plans for seemingly impossible obstacles and help others to see the steps to take, because they do this every day in caring for patients. So even though the gap analysis may show multitudes of areas for improvement, issues are solvable one step at a time. The CNO and nurse leaders can help focus the AHPTF and department directors. Focused effort on creating a streamlined, comprehensive internal all-hazards preparedness plan will set the foundation for later steps when

the hospital begins to work externally with the community.

Working the Issues List

Over the next phase, the development of an issues list will become the working action plan used to prioritize and organize work to be done. Subgroups made up of members from the AHPTF can be assigned to lead efforts to resolve issues. Issues need to be constantly added and resolved so that the work will be ongoing as the facility refines plans. Reports from subgroup progress should be relayed to the task force every 2 weeks or monthly, depending on the meeting schedule of the task force. The task force should have oversight for the subgroups and should strive to "clear the road" for subgroup progress as needed. Some common

Research Note

Source: Ghilarducci, D.P., Pirallo, R.G., & Hegmann, K.T. (2000). Hazardous materials readiness of United States level I trauma centers. *The Journal of Occupational Medicine, 42*(7), 683-692.

Purpose

One disaster that could likely confront hospitals and emergency departments is injuries to patients caused by hazardous materials (hazmat) accidents. In such a case, emergency departments will need decontamination capabilities as part of their readiness strategy. The purpose of this study was to assess the level of hazmat readiness of U.S. level I trauma centers and the ability of the centers to safely decontaminate patients. The study asked 10 questions that examined 52 variables. Data were collected about the number of decontamination patients treated annually, the presence or absence of plans, physical resources and equipment available for decontamination, training levels of staff, drills completed, and incidence of staff injury. A 60.9% response rate was obtained from 256 level I trauma centers across the United States. Descriptive statistical data were presented, including percentages, mean, median and ranges in each response category. Data also were sorted by region.

Discussion

Results indicated that only 6% of the national level I trauma centers had all of the necessary equipment required for safe decontamination of patients. Although 83% had some level of hazmat plans, only 30% reported that their plans were complete. Only 30% of staff were adequately trained in decontamination procedures. Only 58% of respondents reported that they had participated in a drill in the last year. Training results indicated 36% of staff had received training. Only 3.2% of facilities reported meeting all 10 of the readiness criteria.

Although hazmat accidents occur frequently, the level of preparation of level I trauma centers appeared inadequate in 2000, a pre-9/11 era. This study can serve as an excellent baseline for a national look at the level of improvement in the area of preparation for a potential chemical terrorist event.

Application to Practice

The reality of the nation's level of preparation for decontamination is evident in this study. This study offers criteria for emergency departments that can serve as a guide for care of decontamination patients. The 10 readiness criteria are as follows:

1. An isolation area capable of segregating contaminated patients from treatment areas prior to decontamination
2. Disposable chemical protective clothing
3. Respiratory protection
4. Showers
5. A treatment area with an isolated ventilation system
6. Hazardous chemical/toxicological desk references
7. A hazmat response plan
8. 10 or more operations-level-trained personnel
9. At least 1 hour of refresher training annually
10. The performance of a hazmat drill within a 1-year period

For nursing directors and chief nursing officers of level I trauma centers, reviewing this list and evaluating their programs is essential in a post-9/11 world. A follow-up research study to mark the improvement in national planning would be a worthwhile contribution.

issues that hospitals may need to address are discussed in the following paragraphs.

Establishing a Common Nomenclature, Structure, and Role Definition for Writing All-Hazards Preparedness Plans

Often the disaster plan on file at the hospital relates specifically to safety and security preparedness. The primary responsibility of the Safety and Security Department, in conjunction with nursing leadership, will be to develop or refine the hospital's internal disaster plan for incidents occurring at the facility. In addition, the external all-hazards preparedness plan, for incidents involving two or more facilities or disaster events occurring in the community, should be addressed as well. The Safety and Security Department should have assigned oversight for facility security, quick lockdown, and management of people flowing in and out of the hospital. Nursing leadership should lead efforts to make sure all facility departments have a plan for what they will do in a disaster situation. Nursing leaders are the coordinators in synchronizing department plans so that everything fits together to meet the staff's, patient's, and hospital's essential needs. Once the disaster plans are complete, every department should have an identified written role.

Helping Staff Overcome Fear Associated with Disaster and All-Hazards Preparedness

It is important to know that the first rule of disaster preparedness is to keep staff safe. In a disaster, the paradigm of keeping the patient safe first needs to change its focus so that the staff members (and their families) feel as safe as possible. This may be a shift in thinking, but the reality is that if staff members do not feel comfortable coming in to work, then the patients' needs cannot be met at all.

Nursing leadership, in partnership with the Human Resources and Education Department leadership, will be needed to develop educational tools to assist staff in creating personal disaster preparedness plans for themselves, significant others, their families, and even their pets. There are many websites available to assist in developing educational tools, such as the Federal Emergency Management Agency (FEMA) or the America Red Cross websites. Tools such as personal disaster preparedness plans should be effectively communicated so that employees know that the facility will "keep staff safe" as their first priority in a disaster. Then when a disaster occurs, the staff will feel as comfortable as possible coming in to work. Arrangements will need to be made for 24-hour child care somewhere close to the hospital or on-site. Employee assistance programs need to be available on an ongoing basis for coping with fear related to a disaster. Having personal protective gear for staff available on site is also critical.

Creating Procedural Addendums to All-Hazards Preparedness Plan

In addition to the overall all-hazards preparedness plans, the hospital will need to define procedures regarding what will be done in any biological, chemical, nuclear/radiological, or conventional disaster, and the surge capacity needs to be related to any of the events. Surge capacity refers to a health care system's ability to rapidly expand or flex up beyond normal capacity to meet an increased demand for qualified peronnel, beds, and medical care services in the event of a large sclae emergency or disaster (Agency for Healthcare Research and Quality, 2005). The AHPTF can assign the creation of each of these procedures to a subgroup. The time frame for completing the initial plans should be about 3 weeks. These teams are often lead by nursing leadership and the emergency medicine director with appropriate ad hoc participation. For example, the Infectious Disease Department, in partnership with Public Health, can co-lead the biological and chemical planning efforts; the Radiology Department can co-lead the nuclear/radiological efforts, partnering closely with local authorities; and nursing and emergency medicine can co-lead the conventional and surge capacity efforts, partnering closely with police, fire, and rescue. The goal with these procedural addendums is to create easy, step-by-step action plans, fact sheets, and algorithms for identifying, intervening, and notifying the appropriate authorities. As with most all-hazards preparedness literature, the most current references will be online. Some essential websites to assist in writing specific hospital procedures include the Centers for Disease Control and Prevention (CDC), the Department of Homeland Security (DHS), and the U.S. Department of Labor's Occupational Safety and Health Administration (OSHA).

In establishing procedural addendums and the overall all-hazards disaster preparedness plan, the general thought in the literature is to plan to be "on your own without external help" for 72 hours should an external disaster occur that impacts the region (Kaji, 2004). Hospital leadership needs to make sure every operating unit and department is prepared. In general, hospitals need to have a conservative stockpile of essential antibiotics for biological threats; antidotes for chemical exposures; basic food and bottled water surpluses for environmental contamination events; pre-planned contracts with local supply companies and businesses for ice, oxygen and gases, and emergency power; alternate communication methods and plans both internally and externally in case of power outage; staff and volunteer credentialing and identification procedures; established entrances for staff during lockdowns; patient identification systems for families in search of loved ones; downtime procedures for cyber threats (these need to be able to extend up to 5 days); and staff ability to bring in their children for care while they are working, just to name a few.

Creating an All-Hazards Planning Subgroup

Even with comprehensive all-hazards preparedness plans and procedural addendums, there will be times when the unexpected happens, as in recent threats and incidents involving anthrax, severe acute respiratory syndrome (SARS), monkey pox, and smallpox. At first no one will know whether these are true terrorist threats or just isolated spontaneous incidents. At all times, the hospital will need to be ready to respond. An ongoing all-hazards planning subgroup should be formed that is chaired by a nurse leader who sits on the

AHPTF, along with key stakeholder membership (including emergency department, infection control, and employee health staff). Based on the changing needs of the events, this planning subgroup will enable the facility to respond quickly to the "just in time" educational needs of the staff, allow for rapid procedural planning to occur related to community needs, and ensure appropriate authority notification in the event of a disaster. For example, the staff will be expected to recognize the symptoms and presentation of smallpox and respond by critical thinking, as follows:

- Triaging and isolating the patient on admission to the emergency department (ED) and placing the patient in the hospital or facility negative pressure room if available
- Obtaining and wearing appropriate personal protective equipment for the staff
- Locking down the department and determining whether the entire hospital should be on lockdown
- Identifying all patient contacts (name, address, telephone number), transport services (EMS), staff, and patients in the waiting room
- Notifying the infection control practitioner, hospital/ facility infectious disease physician or epidemiologist, public health officials, and police.

Developing a Command Center

Should a disaster occur, the hospital will need a dedicated centralized command center where all department directors can report for direction. The four essential elements of a command center, explained in more detail below, are as follows:

1. Setting up the room
2. Developing processes in the command center
3. Establishing the hospital's role in the community
4. Testing the all-hazards preparedness plans and command center

Setting up the room

This center is often located near the Safety and Security Department and is commanded by the administrator on-call along with the CNO, the emergency department medical director, and safety and security director. The room is composed of multiple telephones/telephone lines with speed dial for frequently called numbers, computer access (with both Intranet and Internet capabilities) and printing capability, batch Fax and copying capabilities, alternative phone options (e.g., 800 mz radio technology and/or voice-over Internet protocol technology, a phone system that operates over Internet lines with functioning antenna and people trained to use them), tiered paging capability, television access, and all office-related supplies such as paper, pens, easels, dry erase boards, work table, and phone books.

The command center should be available at a moment's notice and fully functional within minutes. The usual scenario will be that the call comes into the ED. Nursing leadership staff in the ED, along with medical staff, will determine the gravity of the situation and decide whether the incident can be handled in the ED or whether the hospital administrator needs to be contacted. If it is deemed appropriate to contact the hospital administrator, there will be dialogue between nursing leadership, medical leadership, and the administrator to decide whether the command center should be opened. If the command center is to be opened, the hospital administrator will start the process to open the command center and notify any on-call additional staff to come in and assist in the operations of the command center. In the event that the disaster involves the area where the command center is located, hospitals may want to establish a back-up command center in another location. In the case of a multifacility system, the alternate command center could be another hospital.

Developing processes in the command center

Because there may be several rotating on-call administrators who may need to open the command center, the creation of an easy step-by-step short (1- to 2-page) document of how to open, operate, and close down the command center is important. A more extensive manual can also be created, but in times of a disaster the short "How to Open the Command Center" document

is crucial: "EMS transported casualties will start arriving at the nearest hospitals within 30 minutes of the event and the numbers will peak over the next 60 to 90 minutes. Additionally hospitals will experience waves of self-transporting victims and the worried well arriving at facilities" (Kaji, 2004).

If the facility does not have an on-call administrator list, one needs to be established, and staff must know how to reach the on-call person(s). A clear decision matrix should be in place, outlining when to open the command center and who needs to be notified. It may be helpful to create a communication tree identifying the process for notifying administrative team and AHPTF members quickly. Techniques such as using vests to identify people in charge during a disaster with generic nomenclature for roles and a 1-page role and responsibility sheet in each vest pocket are essential in a crisis situation. Color-coded vests may also be useful in identifying roles. All hospital and department all-hazards preparedness plans must be on hand and clearly labeled in the command center, along with in-house phone and pager directories.

Establishing the hospital's role in the community

Once the hospital's internal all-hazards preparedness plans are in place, members of the AHPTF can take a step back and begin to assess their role. More than likely, the hospital will play an important role in the community in the case of a disaster. Knowing how the hospital fits into the disaster response plan from the perspective of such entities as the police and fire departments, the local school system, area physician practices, public health department, and emergency medical systems will be important in coordinating efforts. When working with the community, recognizable nomenclature becomes especially important for communication in crisis situations. More and more hospitals have adopted the Hospital Emergency Incident Command System (HEICS) (Pletz et al., 1998) for their all-hazards preparedness plans, because it allows logical standardization with common nomenclature that is understood both within the hospital environment and in the community setting.

The AHPTF will be instrumental in defining the hospital's role locally in the community, as well as nationally in regard to federal government expectations. On a local level, the chairperson of the task force will partner with public health, local police and fire departments, local school systems, community physicians, regional alliances with other health care facilities, and local emergency management agencies/councils. It will be important to define the hospital's role and the community's role in the emergency situation. Testing of plans using local disaster drills, on a biannual basis, are essential to continually improve processes. The hospital may wish to test its internal all-hazards preparedness plans, along with any planned community drills, to get a full picture of its ability to respond in a disaster.

Nationally, each hospital will play an important role in the political arena by helping local and federal government personnel understand that hospitals, like police and fire departments, are first responders in a disaster. The materials, equipment, and training required for hospitals to prepare adequately for their role in responding to disasters are very expensive. Capital expenditures will be required to create decontamination facilities; purchase personal protective equipment; train and educate staff on effective all-hazards preparedness; stockpile emergency equipment, supplies, and pharmaceuticals; ensure adequate isolation rooms; and outfit a hospital command center. Hospitals need financial assistance to do this well, and the AHPTF members can all be advocates for federal and state funding. It is helpful to establish a financial subgroup whose mission will be to establish a set plan for capturing costs related to the event as the disaster unfolds. This will enable the hospital to submit immediately for any reimbursement funding that becomes available after the event.

Testing the all-hazards preparedness plans and command center

Having comprehensive all-hazards preparedness plans requires frequent (at least biannual) drills to work through problems and allow for a streamlined preparedness plan. There are many types of drills, including the following:

- Internal drills to test specific department and/or hospital responses (e.g., setting up and operating the command center; recognizing a biological event both in the emergency department and on the units; lockdown of the hospital entrances; simulating decontamination processes; operating using downtime procedures during a communications or cyber disaster event; handling various surge capacity situations)
- External drills in collaboration with community agencies and departments (police, fire, and rescue, public health); table-top drills simulating an unknown biological, nuclear/radiological, or chemical scenario and prioritizing the response by departments

All of these drills offer great insight into the merit of the all-hazards preparedness plan and allow facilities the opportunity to modify plans to improve processes.

LEADERSHIP AND MANAGEMENT IMPLICATIONS

Moving Into the Future with Confidence

Within 6 to 12 months nursing leaders can affect change and can ensure that an effective all-hazards preparedness plan is developed for the hospital. The journey towards preparedness is ongoing and constant. Nursing leadership and competencies in disaster planning and crisis management will prove invaluable as health care organizations face a changing future that requires skills of collaboration, outreach, and negotiation (Ehrat, 2001). Clearly, nurse executives are in a position to take a greater role in the planning process for their organizations. Nurse leaders are called upon to take charge, make decisions, implement successfully, then evaluate and modify their action plans. Emotional competencies include good interpersonal skills, excellent and clear communication skills, and calm, controlled delegation

▲ LEADERSHIP & MANAGEMENT **BEHAVIORS**

Leadership Behaviors

- Demonstrates calm
- Commands the environment
- Keeps open communication channels
- Develops strategic long-term plans to protect staff and patients
- Influences policy makers about financial requirements to ensure readiness
- Demonstrates decision making skills
- Serves as a role model for directors in times of crisis
- Seeks creative alternatives when problem solving
- Demonstrates emotional intelligence by being emotionally self-aware and self-managed
- Builds partnerships through networking
- Allocates resources in times of crisis

Management Behaviors

- Stays calm
- Demonstrates controlled delegation
- Communicates clearly
- Leads drills to ensure preparation
- Implements the plans
- Works well on the team
- Thinks critically
- Takes appropriate risks
- Ensures plans are up to date
- Shares critical information with upper levels of leadership to aid in good decision making

Overlap Areas

- Remains calm
- Ensures communication

(Fahlgren & Drenkard, 2002). In addition, being willing to take risks is an important attribute of the nursing leader. Nurse leaders are in a unique position to forge new pathways in the arena of disaster preparedness because of their combination of clinical skills, strong organizational ability, networking expertise, and training in clinical crises. With strong nursing leadership at the managerial and executive level, the management of disasters can be proactively addressed. With proactive planning, a constant state of readiness can be obtained and maintained.

CURRENT ISSUES AND TRENDS

As we move into the "new world order," where all-hazards preparedness is a way of life and knowledge about the level of alertness—low = green; guarded = blue; elevated = yellow; high = orange; severe = red (The White House, 2002)—is an everyday expectation, hospital staff and leadership have begun to settle in at a heightened state of preparedness. If the all-hazards preparedness task force is not diligent in its efforts to keep everyone

focused on preparedness, there may even be a sense of complacency around refining all-hazard preparedness plans on an ongoing basis.

Current nursing and medical literature is focused on specific departments and how they are establishing their unique roles and responsibilities in a disaster. Nursing leaders can use these benchmark articles to springboard units and departments forward in fully assessing and defining their roles in all-hazards preparedness. As the CNO explores the breadth of disaster nursing within his or her facility, care can be enhanced in many ways during a disaster. For instance, closing clinics, emergency care centers, and community health programs during a disaster can free up clinical staff to assist in the hospital's surge capacity planning in a disaster, provide staff for vaccination teams in a biological event, or serve as decontamination help in a chemical exposure event.

One area of all-hazards preparedness that has not been fully developed in many areas, but has great potential, is the role of long-term care (LTC) facilities in disaster planning. The nursing leader can lead the way in establishing a partnership between the hospital and the LTC facility. If the CNO can work with the LTC facility in establishing plans for moving patients out of LTC to receive stable patients from the hospital, then surge capacity stress could be dramatically reduced as more inpatient beds would be made available for the influx of victims during a disaster event.

To effectively manage large-scale events, networking beyond the hospital will be critical to create partnerships with other facilities, hospitals, community agencies, and local, state, and federal departments. There is a trend underway, evidenced by a growing alliance between regional hospitals and the community at large throughout the United States, to strategically plan for allocation and sharing of federal and state resources in the event of a disaster.

As an example, in Virginia, a Regional Hospital Command Center (RHCC) has been established, in which 14 northern Virginia hospitals have been networked to more effectively respond in a disaster. This is accomplished via radio communication and a shared web-based bed availability tracking system, displaying each hospital's ability to take varying levels of patient acuities. These hospitals can directly link with Washington, D.C. hospitals to coordinate efforts during an event and communicate effectively with fire, police, EMS, schools, public health, the emergency operating center (a local command center for overseeing the event), and the field incident commander in coordinating the disaster response and effectively assisting victims. Cohorts of hospitals, fire fighters, EMS, law enforcement, schools, public health, and businesses, similar to the Virginia RHCC noted above, are joining together to form regional alliances and collaborations to leverage their capability to respond in a coordinated manner.

On a national level, the U.S. Department of Homeland Security Secretary Tom Ridge created a National Incident Management System (NIMS), that will further standardize and integrate response practices nationally:

NIMS incorporates incident management best practices developed and proven by thousands of responders and authorities across America. These practices, coupled with consistency and national standardization, will now be carried forward throughout all incident management processes: exercises, qualification and certification, communications interoperability, doctrinal changes, training, and publications, public affairs, equipping, evaluating, and incident management. All of these measures unify the response community as never before (U.S. Department of Homeland Security, 2004, p. 1).

Under the direction of NIMS, Incident Management Assistance Teams (IMAT) are being created to send supplemental assistance to the region impacted by a disaster. These teams consist of "trained personnel from different departments, organizations, agencies, and jurisdictions within a state or DHS Urban Area Security Initiative region, activated to support incident management at major or complex emergency incidents or special events that extend beyond one operational period" (American-Firefighter.com, 2004, p.1). It is likely that hospital leadership, with nursing in the forefront, will take lessons from this benchmark program and partner with other area hospitals and departments to create IMATs, teams ready to assist one another at the site most impacted by a disaster.

Summary

- All-hazards disaster preparedness is essential in strategic planning for hospitals.
- Nursing leaders play a significant role in the successful implementation of a hospital's all-hazards disaster plan.
- Keeping the staff safe is the most important element in the implementation of an effective all-hazards disaster plan.
- Using the nursing process of assessing, planning, implementing, evaluating, and modifying will result in the creation a comprehensive all-hazards disaster preparedness plan.
- It is important to use accepted, standardized terminology when writing the all-hazards disaster plan.

- Having a multidisciplinary hospital-wide team lead by a nurse leader, hospital administrator, and medical leader is essential in creating an effective and workable all-hazards disaster plan.
- Comprehensive all-hazards disaster planning includes internal and external disaster plans, a surge capacity plan, and addendums for biological, chemical, nuclear/radiological, and conventional disasters.
- Collaboration with community resources in a partnership is a requirement of effective all-hazards disaster preparedness.
- All-hazards disaster preparedness is never complete; the plan keeps evolving and expanding to link all facets of effective coordination of care internally, externally, locally, statewide, and nationwide during a disaster event.

Study Questions

1. How does an all-hazards disaster plan differ from a typical disaster plan?
2. What is the difference between an internal disaster plan and an external disaster plan?
3. What is the role of nursing leadership and the chief nurse officer (CNO) in creating an effective all-hazards disaster preparedness plan?
4. Why is it important for each department/unit to define its role and responsibility in a disaster?
5. What types of addendums are needed in addition to the basic all-hazards disaster plan? Why are they important?
6. Why is it important to partner with external resources such as local hospitals, fire, police, and public health in creating and implementing your all-hazards disaster plan?

CASE STUDY

Patients had arrived first at hospitals in Oklahoma, Pennsylvania, and Georgia, states that are far removed from your hospital in Virginia. These patients had presented complaining of aches and fevers and exhibiting unusual rashes. Each patient had visited one of three shopping centers, and

lab tests confirmed that they did not have flu or measles. They had all contracted variola (smallpox).

The federal government began to deploy what was left of the nation's smallpox vaccine stockpile to the states that were first affected. A television news station reported that an epidemiologist projected 3 million cases and a million deaths within 90 days unless everyone was inoculated. Hysteria spread. Then Reuters reported that a variola case was confirmed in Maryland, a state in close proximity to your hospital.

Because the stock of vaccine was nearly depleted, the remaining vaccine would be rationed, and health care providers would be inoculated first, according to the CDC. Vaccine delivery was scheduled to arrive on Monday, 2 days from now.

The press had leaked news of the vaccine distribution, and by Monday morning people began arriving at your hospitals and emergency care centers, first requesting, then demanding the vaccine. The decision was made to restrict entry to the hospital until the crisis passed. Total hospital lockdown of entrances and exits began at 11:00 AM.

What Happens Next

The Safety and Security Department issues the lockdown notice to your hospital after consulting with the ED charge nurse, the ED medical director, the hospital administrator, and chief nurse officer. Entrance to the hospital for patients is restricted to the main ED entrance with a double-door alcove entrance area for triage. Signs in multiple languages are posted on windows and locked doors to direct patients on campus. Security staff wearing protective masks are stationed strategically outside to direct patients already on the campus. Local police are called in to work at the hospital road entrances and to reroute traffic away from the hospital. Only local ambulances and staff with hospital identification are allowed entrance onto the hospital campus. People in the hospital desiring to leave the facility are escorted out after giving their name and contact information to the ED. This information is gathered as a precautionary measure in the event that smallpox is identified in the facility. Staff reporting to work are directed to a separate hospital entrance away from the ED, where they report from and to work in a designated general personnel pool area, which will be operational for as long as the lockdown remains in effect. There, staff receive instruction about any personal protective equipment needed at that time, assignment of staffing for shift, and general updates on the situation. ED staff also receive a 1-page fact sheet on smallpox signs, symptoms, and treatment, along with instructions as to isolation procedures for any high-risk patients arriving either by ambulance or by walk-in.

The general personnel pool is a function of the all-hazards disaster preparedness plan and is set up as needed by the command center. Designated departments should know in advance whether or not they have responsibility for manning this function. In this case, the nursing education staff has the responsibility for set-up of the general personnel pool, and in operating this area, they assess staffing needs and allocate resources. Constant contact is maintained between the general personnel pool area and the command center regarding any staffing needs.

As soon as the lockdown is initiated, the command center is activated. A mandatory 30-minute management meeting is held outlining the internal and external lockdown plan, as well as the communication plan for staff, patients, and the media. Handouts are given with frequently asked questions and answers for managers. Managers are instructed about where to obtain additional N95 masks. Ongoing management briefings are established at set intervals throughout the event to keep everyone informed. The clinical management staff are given a 1-page fact sheet on smallpox and are asked to assess patients in their departments/units who might be at risk and to immediately report findings back to the medical director in the command center. They are asked to assess bed availability in case this is needed. Clinical and support departments such as pharmacy, respiratory therapy, materials management, and nutrition are asked to inventory their supplies

and equipment and report back to the command center with this information.

The psychosocial needs of everyone (staff, patients, visitors) need to be supported. Social workers, clergy, and clinical nurse specialists are reassigned in designated roles to assist with the support needs throughout the hospital. Visitors to the hospital are moved to a designated area of the hospital where they can be counseled and receive information about the situation and their loved ones. It is important to keep visitors away from the patients to reduce exposure to high-risk patients.

Externally the command center staff is working with public health, the local police department, the media, and the external operating center for the county to coordinate next steps. The goal is to lift the lockdown as soon as reasonably possible. Information is disseminated on an ongoing basis as the event unfolds.

Once the lockdown is terminated and the situation has deescalated to the point of closing the command center, it is important to have the key stakeholders involved in a debriefing. The following questions could be used in the debriefing:

- Overall how effective was the lockdown, the operations of the command center, and the communication flow? What could have gone more smoothly, and how could this have been accomplished?
- Was there a clear chain-of-command? Did communications flow logically? Were they helpful?
- What parts of the all-hazards disaster plan helped staff handle this situation? What parts were not helpful and why?
- How were staff and visitors notified about the lockdown (PA announcement, e-mail, media, signs, etc)? Was it effective or not? Why?
- How were the police notified? What was their role? Did their participation work well?
- What entrances were locked, and who was stationed at each entrance? What were the pros and cons of this effort?
- How were persons who arrived at locked entrances informed? Did this work effectively? What could have been done better?

CRITICAL THINKING EXERCISE

The AHPTF has completed standards and goals for all-hazards preparedness. The comprehensive plan calls for ongoing readiness drills. To keep up staff readiness, the following drill is done:

Type of drill: Suspected biological agent

Purpose: To test the emergency department's recognition and management of a patient with a suspected biological agent.

Scenario: At 11 AM, a patient with a highly suspicious rash and history presents at the emergency department.

Patient gives the following history: High fever for 24 hours, malaise, headache, backache with abdominal pain. Patient has a maculopapular rash on the mucosa of the mouth and pharynx. There is some suspicion that a rash has also begun on the face and forearms. Patient arrived at the ED via ambulance and was transported into the ED.

1. What should the nurse do first, based on the history, when the patient arrives?

2. Based on patient's history, is the patient at risk for having a contagious disease?
3. Which addendum in the all-hazards disaster preparedness plan should the nurse refer to in this scenario?
4. What help would the general all-hazards disaster preparedness plan lend in this scenario?
5. What are the subsequent administrative and clinical steps that the nurse should take if the patient is suspected of having a contagious illness?
6. What is the chain of command in notification of a contagious disease event both internally and externally?
7. What is the role of the charge nurse and the nursing director (head nurse) of the Emergency Department?
8. What is the role of the chief nursing officer at the hospital? What departments should be notified to be on alert concerning this event?
9. What should be done to secure the area, keep staff safe and keep patients safe?

- How did the general personnel pool area work for staff reporting and leaving work? Any suggestions for improvements with this process?
- What precautions should be adopted right now to make sure there are no patients admitted with smallpox in the hospital without detection?
- *Internal notifications:* What security measures, if any, should have be taken prior to a lockdown?
- *External notifications:* Were local and state agencies involved appropriately? Who was called? Who was missed? What worked and did not work?
- How should the all-hazards disaster preparedness plan and addendums be enhanced to better meet the needs in a disaster like this one?
- What staff safety procedures should be implemented based on this disaster?
- How can the planning for vaccinations in an event like this one be better organized so that this scenario does not happen again?

- If hospital workers were quarantined until they received the vaccine, how did this go? What worked and did not work well in this situation?
- How well were "external" agencies integrated? Was communication effective or not? What would make that more effective?
- How did communications with the media go? What were the learning opportunities with this?
- Was surge capacity an issue with this scenario? If so, what worked well and what needed improvement?
- What if more ventilators, linens, protective masks had been needed? Could they have been obtained?
- Were staff members all fitted for a protective mask prior to the event? What were the learning opportunities here?
- Was the ED able to treat ill patients with conditions unrelated to the current emergency? What worked well, and what needs to be improved with this process?

- Were resources sufficient to meet the hospital needs?
- If there was a suspect case being transported by EMS, where did they go? Were alternate locations identified?
- How were inpatients being triaged to make room for admissions? Were they discharged home? Were alternate locations identified?
- *Morgue:* Was there enough capacity and capability to house contaminated patients?
- What were the plans if staff did not—or could not—report for duty?
- What processes were in place to address the emotional and supportive needs of the staff?

REFERENCES

Agency for Healthcare Research and Quality. (2005). *Surge capacity and health system preparedness.* Washington, D.C. Retrieved April 12, 2005, from *http://www.hsrnet.net/ahrq/surgecapacity/*

American-Firefighter.com. (2004). *Members from three incident management teams travel to Florida.* Retrieved November 13, 2004, From www.american-firefighter.com/articles/article_2004_09_28_3000.html

Ashcroft, T. (2001). Braced for disaster. *Nursing Management, 32*(5), 49-52.

Disaster Relief Library (2004). Disaster dictionary. Atlanta: American Red Cross, CNN Interactive, and IBM. Retrieved November 13, 2004, from *www.disasterrelief.org/Library/Dictionary/*

Drenkard, K., Rigotti, G., Hanfling, D., Fahlgren, T., & LaFrancois, G. (2002). Health care system disaster preparedness, part 1: Readiness planning. *Journal of Nursing Administration, 32*(9), 461-469.

Ehrat, K. (2001). Executive nurse career progression: Skills, wisdom and realities. *Nursing Administration Quarterly, 25*(4), 36-42.

English, J.F., Cundiff, M.Y., Malone, J.D., Pfeiffer, J.A., Bell, M., Steele, L., et al. (1999). *Bioterrorism readiness plan: A template for healthcare facilities.* Washington, DC: The Advisory Board Company. Retrieved November 5, 2004, from *www.advisory.com*

Fahlgren, T., & Drenkard, K. (2002). Health care system disaster preparedness, Part 2: Nursing executive role in leadership. *Journal of Nursing Administration, 32*(10), 531-537.

Inova Health System. (2001a). *All-hazards disaster preparedness plan. Annex B.* Falls Church, VA: Inova Health System.

Inova Health System. (2001b). *All-hazards disaster preparedness plan. Annex C.* Falls Church, VA: Inova Health System.

Inova Health System. (2001c). *All-hazards disaster preparedness plan. Annex R.* Falls Church, VA: Inova Health System.

Kaji, A.H. (2004). *Hospital disaster preparedness in Los Angeles County.* Los Angeles: University of California Los Angeles. Retrieved November 13, 2004, from *www.ph.ucla.edu/epi/layne/Epidemiology%20226/EPI226.lect.04.ppt* or *www.ph.ucla.edu/epi/layne/EPI226.html*

Lindholm, M., & Uden, G. (2001). Nurse managers' management, direction, and role over time. *Nursing Administration Quarterly, 25*(4), 14-29.

Macintyre, A.G., Christoper, G.W., & Eitzen, E. (2000). Weapons of mass destruction events with contaminated casualties: Effective planning for health care facilities. *Journal of the American Medication Association, 283*(2), 242-249.

McLaughlin, S.B. (2001). *Hazard vulnerability analysis tool.* Chicago: American Society for Healthcare Engineering. Retrieved May 16, 2002, from *www.ashe.org/ashe/membersonly/pdfs/Feb2001TechDoc.pdf*

Myers III, F.E. (2001). Bioterrorism: Responding to militant microbes. *Nursing2001, Hospital Nursing, 31*(9), 32hn1-32hn4.

Pletz, B., Cheu, D., Russell, P., & Nave, E. (1998). *Hospital emergency incident command system update project: About the HEICS III project* (3rd ed.) (Volume I) (Grant Contract #EMS-6040). San Mateo, CA: San Mateo Health Services Agency, Emergency Medical Services. Retrieved June 9, 2004, from *www.emsa.ca.gov/DMS2/HISTORY.HTM*

Richter, P. (2004). *Hospital disaster preparedness: Meeting a requirement or preparing for the worst?* Chicago: American Society for Healthcare Engineering of the American Hospital Association.

The White House. (2002). *Homeland security presidential directive-3.* Washington, DC: The White House, President George W. Bush. Retrieved November 13, 2004, from *www.whitehouse.gov/news/releases/2002/03/20020312-5.html*

U.S. Department of Homeland Security. (2004). *Fact sheet: National incident management system NIMS.* Washington, DC: U.S. Department of Homeland Security. Retrieved November 13, 2004, from *www.dhs.gov/dhspublic/interapp/press_release/press_release_0363.xml*

Vecchio, A. (2000). *Plan for the worst before disaster strikes.* Health Management Technology, *21*(6), 28-30.

Wetter, D.C., Daniel, W.E., & Treser, C.D. (2001). Hospital preparedness for victims of chemical or biological terrorism. *American Journal of Public Health, 91*(5), 710-716.

22

Evidence-Based Practice: Strategies for Nursing Leaders

Laura Cullen

CHAPTER OBJECTIVES

- Define evidence-based practice
- Illustrate use of the Diffusion of Innovations Model when implementing evidence-based practice changes
- Describe effective strategies to use when implementing an evidence-based practice change
- Outline strategies for building an evidence-based practice culture in an organization
- Discuss the role of nurse leaders in promoting evidence-based practice
- Understand the benefits of evidence-based practice
- Describe current trends in evidence-based practice
- Exercise critical thinking to conceptualize and analyze possible solutions to a practice exercise

Nursing has a long history of using research to improve practice, beginning with Florence Nightingale's work, reemphasized with research utilization efforts, and progressing to the current trend in using best evidence in guiding patient care. Using the evidence-based practice (EBP) process to answer clinical questions can be challenging. Multiple strategies are required when implementing practice changes. Implementing EBP projects can be facilitated when considering topic selection and by communicating the practice change with clinician-users in a way that fits within the organizational context. Each of these concepts is outlined with practical implementation strategies in this chapter. Implementing evidence-based practice as an organizational initiative requires additional strategies for success. A building block approach is outlined. The use of EBP has grown, yet the science of translation research on which EBP works is based is still developing. Current issues and trends in translation science are described. The application of evidence-based practice is the responsibility of every nursing leader. This chapter outlines strategies for success.

DEFINITIONS

An understanding of EBP and related concepts such as implementing practice change requires requisite knowledge of a variety of terms. **Evidence-based practice** involves the integration of research and other best evidence with clinical expertise and patient values in health care decision making (Sackett et al., 2000). Evidence-based practice involves a process similar to that of research utilization.

A process of using research findings as a basis for practice is known as **research utilization**. Research utilization encompasses critique of research studies, synthesis of findings, determining applicability of findings, review for application with implementation of scientific findings in practice, evaluating the practice change and dissemination of scientific knowledge.

⚠ LEADING & MANAGING DEFINED

Evidence-Based Practice

The integration of research and other best evidence with clinical expertise and patient values in health care decision making.

Research Utilization

The use of research findings as a basis for practice encompassing critique, synthesis, evaluation, and dissemination of scientific knowledge.

Translational Research

The scientific investigation of methods and variables that influence use of evidence-based practices to improve decision-making in the delivery of health care services.

Audit and Feedback

Ongoing monitoring of critical indicators of practice and periodic reporting of the data/information back to the clinicians responsible for patient care.

Best Practice

Clarity in definition of best practice remains elusive; the goal of best practice is to provide currency, relevancy, and usefulness for interventions in clinical practice.

Change Champion

Practitioner who continually promotes use of evidence-based practices through education, demonstration, and encouragement of colleagues.

Opinion Leaders

Informal leaders who influence their peer groups to evaluate innovations for use in their settings.

Organizational Context

The health system environment in which the proposed evidence-based practice is to be implemented.

Outreach or Academic Detailing

One-on-one discussions with practitioners in their setting to provide information, feedback, and rewards regarding evidence-based practice.

Performance Gap Assessment

A data-driven strategy/intervention that demonstrates an opportunity for practice changes and improvement related to specific indicators.

Practice Guideline

A systematically developed standard, designed to assist both provider and patient in making decisions about appropriate health care for specific clinical circumstances.

Systematic Review

The structured and systematic combination of findings from research into powerful and clinically useful reports to guide practice.

Reinfusion

The planned and systematic process used to promote integration of the evidence-based practice into daily practice following initial pilot evaluation.

Translational research is the scientific investigation of methods and variables that influence rate and extent of adoption of evidence-based practices by individuals and organizations to improve clinical and operational decision making in the delivery of health care services. This includes testing the effect of strategies/interventions for promoting the adoption of evidence-based practices with the outcomes being the rate and extent of health care providers' use of these practices (Titler & Everett, 2001).

Audit and feedback involves ongoing monitoring of critical indicators of practice and providing periodic reporting of the data/information back to the clinicians responsible for patient care (Davis et al., 1995; Oxman et al., 1995; Schoenbaum et al., 1995). Feedback can be aggregated at different levels such as the individual provider, patient care unit, service line, organization, or health system. It is helpful to provide data that compares indicators over time to demonstrate improvements (or lack thereof) in the evidence-based practices.

The use of the term **best practice** is currently very popular. Clarity in definition and use remains elusive: "Although 'best practice' and 'evidence-based practice' are sometimes used interchangeably, the two are different in some important respects" (John A. Hartford Center for Geriatric Nursing Excellence, 2004, p. 1). To promote understanding, it is recommended that the extent of evidence use in "best practices" initiatives be outlined when the term is used. The goal of best practice is to apply "the most recent, relevant and helpful nursing interventions in clinical practice" (John A. Hartford Center for Geriatric Nursing Excellence, 2004, p. 1).

Practitioners from the local peer group who continually promote evidence-based practice are known as **change champions**. They educate colleagues about the evidence-based practice, encourage peers to align their practice with the evidence, demonstrate skills and knowledge necessary to carry out the evidence-based practice, and teach new and existing personnel about the evidence-based practice (Titler & Everett, 2001).

Opinion leaders are informal leaders from the local health care setting who are viewed as important and respected sources of influence among their peer group (e.g., nurses, physicians). Opinion leaders are trusted to evaluate innovations for use in their setting and thus set practice standards and model appropriate behavior (Titler & Everett, 2001).

Organizational context refers to the health system environment in which the proposed evidence-based practice is to be implemented. The core elements that help describe the organizational context include the prevailing culture of the system (e.g., patient-centered), the nature of human relationships in the system, including the leadership styles that are operational (e.g., team work; clear role delineation), and the organization's approach to routine monitoring of performance of systems and services within the organization (Kitson et al., 1998).

Outreach or academic detailing is the use of a marketing strategy in which a trained individual meets one-on-one with practitioners in their setting to provide information about the EBP. Discussions may revolve around provider performance improvement/data or specific issues in using the EBP (Davis et al., 1995; Jiang et al., 1997; Pippalla et al., 1995).

Performance gap assessment is a strategy of demonstrating an opportunity for improvement at baseline outlining current practice related to specific indicators (Oxman et al., 1995; Schoenbaum et al., 1995). This data-driven strategy/intervention is used early in the implementation to garner commitment for practice changes.

A **practice guideline** is a statement designed to assist provider and patient in making decisions about appropriate health care for specific clinical circumstances (Sackett et al., 2000). Guidelines are systematically developed, link the evidence with health outcomes (benefits and harms), and continue to require subjective judgments when making decisions for use (Woolf & Atkins, 2001).

A rigorous scientific process used to combine findings from research (usually randomized controlled trials) into a powerful and clinically useful report to guide practice is known as a **systematic review**. Components of a systematic review include the following: question being reviewed, search strategies, selection criteria/inclusion or exclusion criteria, review/appraisal methods, study descriptions, synthesis method (e.g., meta-analysis), results, and implications (Titler, 2002b).

MODELS

The best process to use when addressing clinical issues depends on the question at hand and the extent of research or other evidence available on the topic. Several processes may be used to improve care, from quality/performance improvement to EBP to the conduct of research. For questions that can be addressed through quality improvement, improvements can be brought to the patient care level quickly and efficiently (see Chapter 39 for a more detailed description of quality improvement). Clinical questions with little or no research, which include patient risk, may be good questions to answer by conducting research. The shift from research utilization to evidence-based practice reflects the realization that not all clinical questions have been answered through research; thus other forms of evidence (e.g., lower rigor research, case studies, or expert opinion) may be required to find the answer. An emphasis on use of EBP includes the application of the best available evidence and also represents a desire to improve patient outcomes with a consideration for patient values and preferences when making patient care decisions. Thus EBP is a broader, scientific process for improving health care, building on what has been learned from quality improvement, research utilization, and the conduct of research.

Evidence-based practice work in nursing has led to the development of several models to guide nursing practice (Goode & Piedalue, 1999; Rosswurm & Larrabee, 1999; Rycroft-Malone et al., 2002; Stetler, 2001; Titler et al., 2001, and others). The challenge for clinicians is to successfully implement practice changes using a model as a guide during implementation. It has been said that "invention is hard, but implementation is much more difficult" (Berwick, 2003, p. 1970). The Diffusion of Innovations Model (Rogers, 2003) has been adapted to support the hard work of implementing practice change in health care (Titler & Everett, 2001). Rogers (2003) defined diffusion of an innovation as a process by which (1) an *innovation* (2) is *communicated* through certain *channels* (3) over *time* (4) among the members of a *social* system. In other words, multifaceted, interactive strategies or interventions (i.e., communicating through certain channels) are required to support clinicians' adoption of a practice change (i.e., innovation) that is adapted to work within their

organization (i.e., social system). As such, the Diffusion of Innovations Model is widely used to guide implementation of practice changes. Components to consider when planning for adoption of evidence-based practice include consideration of the topic and strategies for communicating the practice change with clinician-users within the context of their organization (Titler & Everett, 2001). Each variable will be considered in turn.

TOPIC SELECTION

Topic selection is an important first step in the EBP process. When choosing a topic, it is essential to consider clinical interest or issues, the amount of organizational commitment, and adoptability of the practice change(s). Clinical issues valued by the organization are more likely to be allocated resources and successfully adopted. Organizations often articulate important values as broad concepts (e.g., improving patient satisfaction, managing pain, or risk reduction), requiring nurse leaders to adapt these values into a clinically relevant practice issue to address (e.g., improving patient satisfaction with discharge education, appropriate pain assessment, and management for patients following surgery or assessment of fall risk). Adoption of evidence-based practices will be promoted when topics are clinically relevant and are priorities for clinicians and the organization. The work of a project team will be facilitated when the topic is narrow and specific, providing a clear goal (e.g., every 4-hour pain assessment following abdominal surgery; daily assessment of fall risk for psychiatric patients).

Topic selection is one variable that will affect how readily a practice change is adopted. Topics most easily integrated into clinical practice through the evidence-based practice process incorporate the following considerations (Nutley et al., 2002; Rogers, 2003):

- *Staff involvement in topic selection:* Greater staff involvement in topic selection improves buy-in and adoption.
- *Complexity of the intervention:* Simplified interventions help promote adoption.

- *Interest and commitment to topic:* Buy-in by staff (e.g., through involvement in topic selection) promotes adoption.
- *Observability of impact of practice change:* Practices that directly show an impact will promote adoption (e.g., changes in tissue when using an antidote for IV infiltration were reported by Montgomery and Budreau [1996] and Montgomery et al., [1999].)
- *Centrality to the day-to-day work:* Addressing high-volume patient care issues or procedures improves the opportunity for reinforcement of the "correct" practice when integrating the practice change, thus promoting adoption.
- *Technical/clinical versus administrative focus:* Use of a bottom-up or "pull" approach will promote adoption.
- *Pervasiveness/extent of change required:* Small incremental changes are more readily adopted.
- *Radicalness or extent the practice differs from the "norm":* Traditional practices are harder to change and radical innovations are more difficult to implement.
- *Uncertainty about outcomes:* Certain/clear expected outcomes facilitate demonstrating the need for the change and adoption of the change.
- *Appeal to local power holders:* Selecting topics that appeal to local power holders promotes buy-in and adoption.
- *Additional resources needed:* Simple interventions requiring few resources are more readily adopted.

Practice questions generated by clinicians in a bottom-up approach will promote adoption by addressing real issues faced in day-to-day practice and promoting commitment to the process. Interventions with the least amount of complexity are more likely to be carried out as intended. Researchers should look for a simple solution to a problem first. Procedures done frequently or clinical issues found often in day-to-day practice are also good topics to address and promote adoption because they provide frequent opportunities to reinforce the new practice. For example, when the process used for endotracheal suction in the MICU was revised, many factors promoted adoption. The fact that suction is done multiple times each day, by every nurse and respiratory therapist, was one facilitator for the practice change. Thus, centrality of the new practice in the day-to-day work of the clinicians promotes adoption. Small practice changes will also be adopted more readily. The more "radical" the proposed practice change—or the more "sacred cows" to address in implementation—the slower uptake will occur. Often nurses find it difficult to eliminate traditions, even when they are ineffective (see chapter Case Study). In fact, traditional practices provide wonderful topics to address through the evidence-based practice process. An additional consideration when selecting an EBP topic is that of clinician buy-in and level of evidence available. Use of a bottom-up approach (what is important to nurses at the bedside) for topic selection can be facilitated to improve adoption. Clinicians will "pull" the practice change into their care instead of having the change "pushed" down from above or outside the organization (Kirchhoff, 2004). When multiple potential topics must be prioritized, the use of established selection criteria is helpful when setting priorities (Titler, 2002a, 2002b).

Topic selection must fit within the local organizational context. Interventions to support adoption of practice changes include localizing the practice guideline and the development of practice prompts (Titler & Everett, 2001). Guidelines that are available and have been developed to address practice questions (Box 22.1) may need to be adapted for each patient population. Localization refers to the process of modifying a practice guideline to fit the needs of the patient population and organization in the local setting. Reinvention may even be necessary if significant revisions are needed to successfully implement an EBP in a local setting (Berwick, 2003). Both localization and reinvention can be effective in adapting an evidence-based practice to the needs of the population based on cultural values or availability of resources or equipment, and they are effective strategies to promote staff buy-in. The development of practice prompts can also trigger practitioners

Box 22.1

Examples of Organizations Publishing Practice Guidelines

American Association of Critical Care Nurses:
www.aacn.org

Association of Women's Health. Obstetric, and Neonatal Nurses: *www.awhonn.org*

Centers for Disease Control and Prevention:
www.cdc.gov

Gerontology Nursing Intervention Research Center:
www.nursing.uiowa.edu/centers/gnirc/

National Guideline Clearinghouse:
www.guideline.gov

Oncology Nursing Society: *www.ons.org*

Registered Nurses Association of Ontario:
www.rnao.org

The Joanna Briggs Institute: *www.joannabriggs.edu.au*

U.S. Preventive Services Task Force:
www.ahrq.gov/clinic/uspstfix.htm

Critiquing the evidence requires skill development and practice. Critique of the evidence is important for knowledge building, team building, and development of a guide for practice within the local setting. Synthesis of the evidence is essential in building a practice guide or guideline, which often takes the form of an organizational policy or procedure. The work of many international and national professional organizations in the EBP movement has been on critique, synthesis, and dissemination of the evidence. Evidence summaries disseminated by specialty organizations provide a good starting point for both topic selection and review of the best available evidence. Beginning with a national guideline can help teams avoid duplication of effort and accelerate the synthesis process. Critiquing the evidence is an essential step, but it should not be a barrier to progress. It is important to avoid the pitfall of getting stuck in the literature and instead move forward with implementation.

COMMUNICATING THE PRACTICE CHANGE

Implementation of change can be complex. Because of this, understanding and using effective implementation strategies are important. Communicating the practice change or guideline to clinicians requires a systematic process to support adoption. Interventions to improve adoption include interactive education, use of opinion leaders (informal leaders in the setting) and change champions (peer group leaders), core group strategies, outreach or academic detailing, and use of action plans. Education is essential to develop an understanding of why and how the EBP is done, but education alone will not result in use of the practice guideline. Communicating the practice change through mass education is just the beginning. To achieve "take off" in adoption of the practice, interactive and repetitive strategies are required (Gladwell, 2000; Rogers, 2003).

to use an evidence-based practice. Practice prompts are designed to provide "just-in-time" clinically relevant information to guide practice by providing reminders to busy clinicians. Practice prompts may include computer generated clinical reminders or decision support, algorithms, quick reference guides, or pocket cards.

Once a topic is selected, the team gathers, critiques, and synthesizes the best available evidence. The credibility of the evidence is evaluated through the critique process. The credibility of this evidence or the practice guideline may affect adoption. The process for critiquing different kinds of evidence has been outlined elsewhere, as follows:

- Quantitative research (Heermann & Craft, 2002)
- Qualitative research (Speziale, 2002)
- Systematic reviews (Titler, 2002b)
- Guidelines (Burgers et al., 2003; *www.agreecollaboration.org*)
- Websites (Morris et al., 2001)

In addition to education, multifaceted interventions are needed to communicate the practice change to clinicians. Using an opinion leader within each discipline to promote the practice change (e.g., nurse or physician opinion leader) can be very effective (Berner et al., 2003; Locock et al., 2001; Soumerai et al., 1998; Thomson O'Brien et al., 2003a). Opinion leaders are often the early adopters of innovative practices. The best opinion leaders are respected clinical experts who are influential among their peers, set the practice standard, and role-model practice. Opinion leaders are responsible for modeling practice, influencing their peers, altering the norms or expected behaviors of the group and affecting the organizational structures to support the practice (e.g., revising documentation to trigger the appropriate practice).

Change champions can partner with opinion leaders to "sell" the practice change to their colleagues, educating and demonstrating use of the new practice in day-to-day care. Change champions can network with colleagues to troubleshoot implementation of the new practice and bring issues back to the multidisciplinary team responsible for the evidence-based practice project. A core group approach to implementation involves development of a small group of experts responsible for bringing the practice change to a designated subgroup of practitioners by dividing up the work of personally connecting with each clinician. For example, a nurse from the core group may have responsibility for the implementation of a new hand scrub procedure on the evening shift and may collaborate with four to five people who routinely work the evening shift. The core group member is responsible for tracking the education and providing outreach for each of the people to whom they are assigned. A tree approach is used, but roles are not distinctly delineated and will overlap.

Use of outreach or academic detailing is an effective strategy to promote adoption of the practice guideline. Use of outreach with opinion leaders can be quite potent (Thomson O'Brien et al., 2003b). The process involves providing individualized education and feedback to clinicians. Through outreach an expert meets individually with clinicians, provides a synthesis of the evidence, answers their questions, gives feedback

on their use of the practice guideline and encouragement to integrate the practice, and provides recognition and rewards for use of the practice. Recognition can take many forms, from large formal awards to small informal approaches (e.g., distributing memo pad containing the project logo or creating a "star board" of successful adopters). All these discussions can occur in a brief amount of time in the office or clinical area and can be very persuasive.

Development of an action plan as a strategy for communicating the practice change can guide the team's work and communicate needs and successes to power brokers and organizational leaders. Through the action plan, each step in the EBP process is outlined, with strategies to promote adoption, including a clear statement of accountability with a timeline (Titler, 2002b). While developing the action plan, a reinfusion plan should also be included. **Reinfusion** or reinforcement of the practice change will be needed on an ongoing basis until the evaluation demonstrates that the practice has been integrated into daily care (see *Leading & Management Defined*). This is because integration of practice changes takes time and commitment to follow through and see an improvement. Thus a plan for reinfusion or reinforcement needs to be made (Stenger et al., 2001). In the action plan, periodic updates for organizational leaders should be included throughout the project. Brief memos are effective in providing updates on progress, challenges, resources (used or needed), and evaluation results. Sharing project successes with organizational leaders is essential to maintain their support and access to organizational resources. Using multiple interactive strategies to effectively communicate the need for the practice change will support adoption by clinician-users.

USERS OF THE PRACTICE GUIDELINE

Influencing clinicians as users of the new practice and organizational leaders as supporters of the evidence-based practice process can best be accomplished with data. Reporting results to clinicians

Research Note

Source: Thomson O'Brien, M.A., Oxman, A.D., Haynes, R.B., Davis, D.A., Freemantle, N., & Harvey, E.L. (2004). *Local opinion leaders: Effects on professional practice and health care outcomes (Cochrane Review)* (The Cochrane Library, Issue 3). Oxford, England: The Cochrane Collaboration.

Purpose

The purpose was to develop a systematic review describing the impact of opinion leaders on clinician practices and on health care outcomes when implementing practice changes. Two reviewers critiqued potential studies for inclusion using the Cochrane Effective Practice and Organization of Care group checklist and extracted data independently. Main study results were tabulated, and differences attributable to the intervention were summarized. Eight randomized control studies were included in the analysis, six reporting on professional practice behaviors and at least one health care outcome. General management of a variety of clinical conditions was studied (i.e., acute myocardial infarction, cancer pain, osteoarthritis, rheumatoid arthritis, chronic lung disease, vaginal birth after caesarean section, labor and delivery, and urinary catheter care). The theoretical framework uses the Diffusion of Innovations Model and the social influences model of behavior change theories; both indicate local opinion leaders set practice standards and role-model behavior that can promote adoption of evidence-based practice changes.

Discussion

A handful of randomized control trials have tested use of opinion leaders as an intervention to promote adoption of evidence-based practice changes and evaluated the impact on patient outcomes. Most studies included in this analysis found at least some practice improvements with use of opinion leaders. Opinion leaders significantly improved practice in experimental groups in only two of the eight studies included in the analysis. The exact impact of this intervention was difficult to assess given the difficulty identifying and defining the opinion leader role. Seven of the eight studies used the same method for identifying the opinion leader, providing some consistency, yet a limited description of the process. The implementation window and timing of the evaluation varied across studies, adding to the difficulty of comparing the impact of opinion leaders. Despite the methodological inconsistencies and analytical limitations, opinion leaders appear to improve health care practices and may thus improve patient outcomes. Use of opinion leaders is more effective than other interventions alone and more effective when used in combination with additional interventions.

Application to Practice

A number of interventions to promote adoption of evidence-based practices have been tested. There are a limited number of randomized control studies evaluating use of the opinion leader intervention. Use of opinion leaders is an effective method for creating and supporting practice changes. It is not yet possible to identify when use of opinion leaders is likely to be most effective, how to best identify opinion leaders, or the most important components of the opinion leader's role. The most potent interventions supporting adoption of evidence-based practice involves use of opinion leaders in combination with other interventions. For example, clinical outreach by the opinion leader is a powerful strategy to employ when creating practice change. Opinion leaders are effective at establishing existing and revising practice standards and modeling practice changes necessary for adoption of evidence-based practice. There is a growing body of research identifying strategies that promote adoption of evidence-based practice changes. Use of multiple, interactive, and repetitive strategies is necessary to promote adoption of evidence-based practices to improve patient care and outcomes. Interventions for implementing evidence-based practice can be effective by communicating the practice change with clinicians-users in a way that fits within the organizational context.

supports clinical decision making, and several strategies are effective. Use of performance gap assessment demonstrates a difference between the organization's, unit's, or practitioner's baseline data and the achievable outcomes based on the evidence. Thus the "gap" between current performance and desired performance is demonstrated. Sharing performance gap assessment results with experts is influential in establishing the need for change and promoting commitment to the practice guideline. Evaluation findings may also be shared throughout the implementation process by concurrent monitoring using audit-feedback. The use of audit-feedback involves ongoing monitoring of critical indicators to illustrate progress as well as opportunities for improvement. Results can be trended over time to demonstrate change. Issues to be addressed in data collection and reporting include the following: reasonable sample sizes to use, key indicators to monitor, data source(s), frequency of data collection, appropriate denominators to use, and time frames for reporting (e.g., monthly, quarterly). Comparison of pre-and post-group results may be evaluated using descriptive and/or inferential statistical analyses, and statistical process controls may be used for the interpretation of trended data. Feedback of audit results with discussion and decisions for focusing improvements will facilitate adoption (Foy et al., 2002; Jamtvedt et al., 2004; Thomson O'Brien et al., 2003a). This is a common process improvement technique used to facilitate change.

Two additional strategies of trying the change and using focus groups can also be effective in promoting implementation. Clinicians given the opportunity to try the change through a pilot and then give feedback may be more likely to use the new practice and be more actively involved in implementation. Understanding that the practice change will be evaluated and that their feedback will be incorporated in testing the new practice will ease clinicians' concerns about premature adoption of practices with uncertain outcomes. Focus groups provide the opportunity for practitioners to give feedback and suggest improvements

in a facilitated group discussion (Krueger & Casey, 2000). An objective facilitator, without previous involvement with the project or program, should leading focus group discussions. Focus group suggestions can then be incorporated with other evaluation results in planning revisions of the practice guideline following the pilot.

Focus group discussions require participant consent, explicit discussion of group rules (e.g., equal participation and open discussions to remain confidential), audio taping of discussion, transcription, and analysis. Focus groups can provide a depth of discussion and insight not available in a quantitative evaluation. Feedback of evaluation results is essential to encourage clinician participation. Clinicians tend to buy into the need for the practice change when they understand the evidence and see data as informative, thus demonstrating an opportunity for practice improvement within their organization.

Organizational Context

Organizational systems designed to support clinical practice must be revised to incorporate evidence-based practices if adoption is to occur. A "fix the system" approach is now commonly used in quality improvement as well. Practice change will be facilitated when documentation, policies and procedures, and education include the essential components from the practice guideline. Regardless of whether paper or automated systems are used, documentation systems are designed to support clinical practice and must capture the essential elements of the guideline that practitioners are expected to perform. The documentation system can serve as a "trigger" to assess important risk factors (e.g., risk for falling or risk for pressure ulcer development), patient conditions (e.g., pain intensity, duration, or location), and outcomes of care (e.g., development of pressure ulcers). Automated documentation systems may also provide the opportunity for decision support to assist clinicians in the implementation of evidence-based practice guidelines.

The need for education regarding a practice change is fundamental. The organization can support use of evidence-based practices by incorporating education about the practice guideline into orientation for new hires, competency review for current employees, and education for senior leadership. Education is a necessary first step but is insufficient alone to create a practice change. An additional strategy is to incorporate the practice change into organizational policies and procedures. The clinical practice committee responsible for policies and procedures includes experts in the process of development, approval, and use of policies. The policy and procedure committee includes clinical experts representing varied clinical services; these experts can provide an excellent critique of a new policy or procedure and make recommendations supporting the adaptation of guidelines for use within their organization.

The quality improvement committee also can support EBP. The quality improvement process supports reporting of evaluation findings within the organization. The quality improvement committee has report forms, a reporting system, and an established process for use of the results to continuously improve practice, until the practice reaches the established goal and becomes integrated. Using the quality improvement system for reporting evidence-based practice changes provides efficient communication within the existing organizational infrastructure. The quality improvement process also supports ongoing planning, monitoring, and reinfusion of the expected care delivery, supporting successful adoption and integration of evidence-based practices.

Successes need to be celebrated along the implementation path. Celebrations help build a culture that supports and expects the use of evidence in practice. The celebration should include formal recognition from high-level organizational leaders, visibility for the project champions, accessibility to practitioners within the organization, and a clear articulation of the benefits of the evidence-based practice project. Celebrations provide the opportunity to put practitioners in the spotlight for doing great work. Recognition can clearly articulate the benefits to and commitment of the organization. Celebrating successes

will promote buy-in and commitment to the EBP process and will strengthen the foundation for future projects. Multifaceted, interactive strategies are essential when implementing EBPs; making them fun will help too.

Organizational Infrastructure

Strategies for implementing evidence-based practices occur at both the project/clinical level and the organizational level. Titler and colleagues (2002) stated that integrating EBP at the organization or social system level can be accomplished through a building block approach, and that providing leadership for EBP can focus on the following:

> … four major building blocks: (1) Incorporating evidence-based practice terminology into the mission, vision, strategic plan, and performance appraisals of staff; (2) Integrating the work of EBP into the governance structure of nursing departments and the health care system; (3) Demonstrating the value of evidence-based practice through administrative behaviors of the chief nurse executive; and (4) Establishing explicit expectations about EBP for nursing leaders (e.g., nurse managers and advanced practice nurses) who create a culture that values clinical inquiry. (p. 26)

Development of a mission and vision statement inclusive of EBP provides a foundation for the work of EBP at all levels of the organization and begins the process of building a culture in which evidence-based health care practices are the expected norm. The vision statement can stretch the current bounds of EBP and promote work that leads staff to "reach" for a higher standard. An example of a vision statement might be that the organization will develop a center of excellence for EBP and be seen as a leader in use of evidence-based practices in care delivery. To support the vision, an infrastructure for EBP is needed as another building block. The infrastructure should take advantage of the expertise currently available and not be added work in an already busy work place. A committee with expertise in the research and quality improvement processes will have the requisite skills. In many organizations, the clinical practice committee may have the right membership to develop expertise in the EBP processes. Critical skills include critique and synthesis of the evidence, development of an evaluation plan, statistical analysis, and reporting of results. The right committee or council will differ in each organization but should reflect the expertise and functions needed to promote evidence-based practices.

The value of EBP must be "lived" through the behaviors of nursing leadership. Action steps for building a culture that values EBP can be included in the departmental strategic plan. Discussion during committee meetings can stimulate interest in and use of EBP; include an EBP item on each agenda. Accountability is outlined in committee functions. An organizational culture that promotes use of evidence values nurses questioning their practice, provides education about EBP, adopts an EBP model, and recognizes and rewards the work. Recruiting and hiring nurses with interest in EBP will also help build the desired culture. Orientation can contain EBP concepts and protocols, with new staff learning from colleagues who can share experiences from EBP project teams. This provides recognition for the work done, sets the expectation that EBP is important in clinical care, and demonstrates that nurses have authority over their practice. EBP must be alive in daily practice, not just "pulled off the shelf" when organizational leaders appear in the clinical area. Another building block involves the use of EBP components in performance appraisals for all roles. Leadership is needed across all organizational levels and roles when implementing EBP changes.

LEADERSHIP ROLES IN PROMOTING PRACTICE

Many roles are essential and complementary in the work of EBP. From the chief nurse executive through nurse managers, advanced practice nurses, and staff nurses, everyone has a role in EBP work. Nurse executives are responsible for creating a culture in which clinicians expect EBP, creating the capacity to accomplish EBP, and developing and sustaining a vision inclusive of EBP, an important building block for EBP. The strategies discussed in building an organizational infrastructure for EBP will be effective in developing the culture, building the capacity, and sustaining the vision. The nurse manager is responsible for developing the unit culture, parallel to that of the nurse executive. The nurse manager sets the expectations for the unit, discusses the importance of the work of EBP with the unit nurses and other disciplines, supports the team with time to work on the project, is a project cheerleader, tracks progress, facilitates moving the project through appropriate committees, and allocates resources as needed. The nurse manager's commitment is critical to project success and can make a significant impact on project outcomes.

The advanced practice nurse partners with the project team leaders and plays an important role in project development. Advanced practice nurses can function as opinion leaders and mentors. They have the ability to take on the most challenging steps in the process, lead a team, identify potential roadblocks, facilitate problem solving throughout implementation and evaluation, and provide expertise in the EBP process. As EBP experts, advanced practice nurses are in the ideal position to tackle the most challenging steps in the process. Critique and synthesis of the evidence, development of an evaluation plan, and analysis of results are steps that utilize the expertise of the advanced practice nurse. These nurses may also act as cheerleaders and mentors for the team. The path to improving care can be bumpy, and teams will need encouragement to address the barriers and sustain the commitment and momentum.

Staff nurses are ideally positioned for working on EBP projects. As bedside clinicians, they are the key to quality and use of evidence-based practices. Staff nurses can function as change champions and core group members within their current functions. The staff nurse also can function as an opinion leader or even project director (Cullen & Titler, 2004). Integration of practice changes through the EBP process can be complex. Education is necessary but alone is insufficient to change practice (Camiletti & Huffman, 1998). As Stonestreet and Lamb-Harvard (1994) stated, "Facilitating the actual change in practice is perhaps the most difficult challenge facing nursing individuals and organizations" (p. 144). Programs are needed to help staff nurses integrate evidence-based practice change into care delivery (Hinds et al., 2000; Lacey, 1995; Newman et al., 2000; Tranmer et al., 1995). When staff nurses receive sufficient support, they are effective at integrating evidence-based practice changes into care delivery and find the experience to be empowering (Cullen & Titler, 2004). Staff nurses are expert clinicians who have the skills to collaborate and problem-solve by finding many creative solutions. They are a critical component in providing quality care through implementation of EBPs.

One important role that will keep the project moving forward is that of the project director. The project director is responsible for establishing meeting schedules and timelines with the group, running the meetings, delegating work assignments, and overseeing the process and progress. The focus of the project direct must always be on moving the project forward, despite challenges,

as a key strategy for success. The project director may orchestrate discussions for identifying potential barriers, addressing those barriers that cannot be avoided but continuing to move forward despite distractions. Staff nurses can function as project directors if they are given sufficient support and mentorship (Cullen & Titler, 2004). Staff nurses and nursing leaders work together with complementary skills and expertise to address challenges and issues inherent in EBP.

LEADERSHIP AND MANAGEMENT IMPLICATIONS

Regardless of job title, all nurses have a role in making EBP changes successful. A multifaceted approach is needed when integrating EBP at the project or organizational level. Change is difficult. Combining strategies to build on existing strengths should be considered. For example, educational offerings may already exist in familiar formats (e.g., posters or inservices); adding new approaches can stimulate interest (executive summaries, resource manuals, or selected research references). Identifying those nurses and physicians who are innovative and influential among their peers to function as opinion leaders is important.

◮ LEADERSHIP & MANAGEMENT BEHAVIORS

Leadership Behaviors

- Inspires evidence-based practice focus and challenges all practice interventions regarding evidence base
- Enables the identification and use of evidence-based knowledge to drive practice and improve outcomes
- Describes a vision for both client and systems outcomes based on evidence
- Enables evidence-based practice using organizational systems to support care delivery based on evidence (e.g., computerized documentation)
- Removes barriers to use of evidence in practice
- Articulates the value of evidence-based practice

Management Behaviors

- Identifies outcomes of care and service based on evidence
- Evaluates the consistency, quantity, and quality of evidence base for practice
- Manages the process of practice based on evidence
- Analyzes variances
- Takes corrective action when variances occur

Overlap Areas

- Determines evidence base for management and practice
- Leads and manages implementation of innovations

Outreach, along with audit and feedback, should be included throughout implementation. Simple solutions should be sought first; creativity becomes important when addressing barriers. Staff nurses can often bring fresh approaches to use when addressing challenges.

A building block approach should be considered when developing the organizational culture and capacity for EBP. EBP should be incorporated into strategic documents, including the mission statement, vision, strategic plan, job descriptions, performance appraisals, and committee functions. Leadership that demonstrates and expects EBP will promote its use in clinical and operational decision making. Dialogue must be conducted during important meetings about use of EBP for decision making. Prioritizing and holding leaders accountable for the work are essential. The use of multiple, interactive strategies will promote adoption of EBP at all levels in the organization.

CURRENT ISSUES AND TRENDS

EBP is a priority. Sigma Theta Tau International recently held international "think tanks" to identify priorities in nursing. Development of evidence-based nursing was identified as an international priority (Sigma Theta Tau International, 2003). To support nurses in development and implementation of evidence in practice, Sigma Theta Tau International is developing *Nursing Knowledge International*, an initiative to provide the latest resources on research, education, and practice. Its website (*www.nursingknowledge.org*) will post new developments.

A number of groups and organizations are working to support EBP; yet many issues remain. Current issues in EBP include its use in operational decision making, development of the field of translation research, testing of implementation strategies, and development of educational programs. Use of the EBP process for clinical decision making has lead to expecting use of the same process for operational decision making. Research is available on managerial topics such as nursing retention, collaboration, scheduling, use

of information systems in health care, and quality improvement. A national guideline is available on nurse retention (Tang, 2002), and a review of interventions to promote collaboration can be accessed through the Cochrane Collaboration (Zwarenstein & Bryant, 2004). Expansion of the use of evidence-based decision making from clinical topics to operational issues is a natural progression resulting from successful implementation of practice changes based on research and other best evidence.

Research is still needed to address a number of issues that would promote adoption of evidence-based health care practices. Translation research involves the conduct of research that evaluates factors influencing the rate and extent of adoption of evidence-based practices, whether by individuals or organizations, which improve clinical and operational decision making in the delivery of health care services (Titler & Everett, 2001). The science of translation research is young and warrants further development (U.S. Invitational Conference, 2004). Because translation research is a relatively young field of study, many fundamental issues have not been fully addressed (e.g., gaining consensus on definitions of terms). Translation research models also need to be further developed and tested. Measurement of the rate and extent of adoption of EBP is difficult, and methodologies have not yet been fully developed (Dawson, 2004; Titler, 2004; Tripp-Reimer & Doebbeling, 2004). This chapter has outlined a number of implementation strategies that are effective in promoting adoption of EBP, but the impact of these strategies individually and in combination has not been adequately measured, and additional research is needed in this area. It is clear that the organizational culture or context affects adoption of evidence-based practices (Kirchhoff, 2004; McCormack et al., 2002; Rycroft-Malone et al., 2002). Assessing organizational readiness and developing organizational interventions to improve use of evidence-based practices has not been done. Participants at the U.S. Invitational Conference: Advancing Quality Care Through Translation Research, held

October 13-14, 2003, identified priority areas for translation research. Proceedings from the conference are available in *Worldview on Evidence-Based Nursing,* a new evidence-based practice journal developed by Sigma Theta Tau International (U.S. Invitational Conference, 2004), or on CD-ROM (*www.uihealthcare.com/depts/nursing/rqom/ evidencebasedpractice/index.html*). A larger pool of experts is needed to promote research and use of evidence in practice. How will we prepare researchers, educators, and clinicians in translation research and EBP (Williams, 2004)?

CONCLUSION

So why is research not used in practice? In studying the barriers to research utilization, several challenges in uptake/adoption of research findings have been identified. Indeed, it takes 10 20 years for most innovations to find their way into practice (medical or nursing practice) for the following five reasons:

1. The research findings are not disseminated in a way that clinicians can readily apply/use the results.
2. Clinicians are not well versed in critique and synthesis of research findings.
3. The usual continuing education methods are ineffective in creating practice changes.
4. Clinicians do not have ready access to the research synthesis findings (although finding guidelines based on research has become much easier as a result of the Internet).
5. Time limitations—Clinicians have very little time to consider and apply new innovations in practice, and evaluation of the impact of the innovations/guidelines is even more difficult.

It is clear in the literature (research and non-research) that programs actively promoting adoption of evidence-based practices are effective (e.g., the Evidence-Based Practice Staff Nurse Internship). Interventions to promote adoption of practice changes must be multifaceted, interactive, and repetitive and include a great deal of positive reinforcement. It is easy to underestimate the extent to which intervention is required to create a practice change.

Another reason research findings are not always directly applied in practice is that they do not always work in practice the same way they did in research (i.e., heterogeneous population, multiple providers, or difference in setting). The application of research results in practice requires pilot testing with an evaluation to see whether the findings actually work as intended; sometimes interesting and unexpected results are obtained through piloting of the research-based protocols (Rakel, 2003; Rakel et al., 1994; Redus et al., 2002). Additionally, the lack of infrastructure to support this work creates problems for clinicians. Use of the EBP process is an ideal way for clinicians to positively improve patient outcomes and demonstrate the impact of nursing care, and nurses find using evidence-based nursing practice very empowering as well. To promote use of research findings or EBP, an organizational infrastructure must integrate this work into the daily practices of the organization and avoid the problem of creating additional work. The work of the EBP process must be built into existing work and organizational structures (e.g., committee work, unit QI work, and educational activities). Another important dimension to creating a work environment supportive of EBP is building an effective infrastructure (e.g., job expectations and performance criteria at all levels, mission statement, or strategic initiatives). Effective implementation strategies are needed at the project and organizational levels. Given what is known about effective implementation of EBP, how will nurses face the challenge of making nursing care evidence-based?

Summary

- Nurses use the evidence-based practice process to answer clinical questions.
- Not all clinical questions have been answered by research.
- EBP involves integration of best evidence with clinical expertise and patient values in decision making.

- EBP emphasizes use of the best available evidence.
- Rogers' Diffusion of Innovations Model is often used as a framework for EBP practice changes.
- An innovation is communicated to clinician-users through channels over time within a social system.
- Important components are the topic and strategies for communicating the practice change to clinician-users within the context of the organization.
- Nurses have leadership roles in EBP at all levels.
- EBP is a priority in nursing.
- Current issues include how to best translate research evidence and operationalize EBP.
- Time limitations continue to be a challenge in adoption of EBP innovations.

Study Questions

1. What process is used to identify topics for development of an evidence-based practice project?
2. What implementation strategies are effective in supporting adoption of a practice change?
3. What are the four building blocks used to develop the organizational structures supporting an evidence-based practice environment? How can nurses put these in place?
4. What is the role of the nurse manager in developing an evidence-based practice culture?
5. What current nursing issues can be addressed through translation research?
6. How is EBP used in a multidisplinary team?

CASE STUDY

A member of your general surgery unit staff approaches you with a practice question. This senior nurse wants to know whether bowel sounds are a good indicator for return of gastrointestinal (GI) motility for her patients after surgery. As a nurse manager, you recognize this as an opportunity to build an evidence-based practice project for your unit. The following benefits are anticipated:

- Improving care
- Empowering staff nurses
- Developing a new unit culture that uses evidence in daily practice

What Are Your Next Steps?

You recognize that you will need a strong team, a review of the evidence, an implementation plan, and an evaluation method. Partnering with experts in the organization will best match the skills and expertise needed. The staff nurse raising the question is the unit quality improvement coordinator. She is already an opinion leader and is ideally suited to lead a team; you are committed to helping her. The team develops an action plan and divides responsibility for the project. Team members tackle each of the following: literature review, development of a survey of current nursing practice within the hospital, notifying physicians of the practice review, development of a physician practice survey, development of an educational poster based on the literature review, and developing strategies for implementing a potential practice change.

An early obstacle occurs when you cannot find any research on auscultation of bowel sounds. This is a good time to add a team member who can tackle the search, critique, and synthesis of the evidence. The nursing survey is revised and sent to a national group of experts to determine current practice trends. Certified wound, ostomy, and continence nurse practitioners are identified as appropriate experts to provide the team with the necessary guidance. Simultaneously, the physician's practice survey is sent to general surgeons within the organization. A secondary analysis of basic science research, a small body of other literature, and the surveys indicate that bowel sound assessment is not the best indicator of return of GI motility following abdominal surgery. A change in practice is needed.

A traditional practice, such as bowel sound assessment, can be difficult to change. Multiple interventions are needed. The team decides to use

CRITICAL THINKING EXERCISE

Nurse Maria Garcia works for a managed care type of Health Maintenance Organization (HMO). The nurses at the HMO have noticed a problem with women's health care—little assessment or counseling regarding menopause is being done. Nurse Garcia sees menopause counseling as a prime opportunity for nurses to deliver needed preventive and wellness care to adult women and their families. Furthermore, the National Committee for Quality Assurance (NCQA) that accredits managed care organizations is projected to include menopause counseling in its HEDIS data set. It already has developed a national database of standardized performance and accreditation information for benchmarking. Nurse Garcia wants to take the lead in developing a

menopause counseling program. However, the following questions have arisen:
- What is the evidence base for implementing this program?
- What should be included in the program?
- What patients should be targeted?
- What change steps need to be taken?
  1. What is the problem?
  2. Why is it a problem?
  3. What are the key issues?
  4. What should Nurse Garcia do first?
  5. How should Nurse Garcia handle this situation?
  6. What evidence is needed?
  7. What outcomes should be used for this new program?

multiple strategies for implementation: opinion leaders, change champions, audit-feedback, educational posters, a resource manual, practice prompts, and documentation changes. Processes and outcomes are reviewed through the evaluation process. The team reviews nursing knowledge, compliance with documentation of return of GI motility, nurses' perception of facilitators of the practice change, and rates of bowel obstruction and paralytic ileus. The data suggest that nursing documentation of return of flatus improves (60% pre-group; 69% post-group) and documentation of first bowel movement also improves (60% pre-group; 88% post-group) and could be better, so a task force works with the nursing informatics group to revise the documentation process. Bowel obstruction rates are lower in the post-group (0%) than in the pre-group (4%), and paralytic ileus rates decrease from 12.5% in the pre-group to 0% in the post-group, creating some confidence that eliminating bowel assessment is not causing any patient harm.

This project was successful in many ways; yet like so many EBP projects, additional work is needed. The unit quality improvement coordinator will now complete reinfusion and integration through the unit's quality improvement efforts.

A fundamental practice question has been answered, and patient care improvements continue through the EBP process (Madsen et al., in press).

REFERENCES

Berner, E., Baker, C., Funkhouser, E., Heudebert, G., Allison, J., Fargason, C., et al. (2003). Do local opinion leaders augment hospital quality improvement efforts? A randomized trial to promote adherence to unstable angina guidelines. *Medical Care, 41*(3), 420-431.

Berwick, D. (2003). Disseminating innovations in health care. *Journal of the American Medical Association, 289*(15), 1969-1975.

Burgers, J.S., Cluzeau, F.A., Hanna, S.E., Hunt, C., Grol, R., & the AGREE Collaboration. (2003). Characteristics of high quality guidelines: Evaluation of 86 clinical guidelines developed in ten European countries and Canada. *International Journal for Technology Assessment in Health Care, 19*(1), 148-157.

Camiletti, Y.A., & Huffman, M.C. (1998). Research utilization: Evaluation of initiatives in a public health nursing division. *Canadian Journal of Nursing Administration, 11*(2), 59-77.

Cullen, L., & Titler, M.G. (2004). Promoting evidence-based practice: An internship for staff nurses. *Worldviews on Evidence-Based Nursing, 1*(4), 215-223.

Davis, D.A., Thomson, M.A., Oxman, A.D., & Haynes, R.B. (1995). Changing physician performance: A systematic review of the effect of continuing medical education strategies. *Journal of the American Medical Association, 274*(9), 700-705.

Dawson, J. (2004). Quantitative analytical methods in translation research. *Worldviews on Evidence-Based Nursing, 1*(Suppl 1), S60-S64.

Foy, R., MacLennan, G., Grimshaw, J., Penney, G., Campbell, M., & Grol, R. (2002). Attributes of clinical recommendations that influence change in practice following audit and feedback. *Journal of Clinical Epidemiology, 55,* 717-722.

Gladwell, M. (2000). *The tipping point: How little things can make a big difference.* Boston: Little Brown.

Goode, C.J., & Piedalue, F. (1999). Evidence-based clinical practice. *Journal of Nursing Administration, 29*(6), 15-21.

Heermann, J., & Craft, B. (2002). Evaluating quantitative research. In G. LoBiondo-Wood & J. Haber (Eds), *Nursing research* (5th ed., pp. 165-102). St Louis: Mosby.

Hinds, P., Gattuso, J., & Morrell, A. (2000). Creating a hospital-based nursing research fellowship program for staff nurses. *Journal of Nursing Administration, 30*(6), 317-324.

Jamtvedt, G., Young, J.M., Kristoffersen, D.T., Thomson O'Brien, M.A., & Oxman, A.D. (2004). Audit and feedback: Effects on professional practice and health care outcomes (Cochrane Review). *The Cochrane Library, Issue 1.* Chichester, UK: John Wiley & Sons, Ltd.

Jiang, H.J., Fieselmann, J.F., Hendryx, M.S., & Bock, M.J. (1997). Assessing the impact of patient characteristics and process performance on rural intensive care unit hospital mortality rates. *Critical Care Medicine, 25*(5), 773-778.

John A Hartford Center for Geriatric Nursing Excellence. (2004). *Best Practices.* Iowa City, IA: The University of Iowa College of Nursing. Retrieved March 2, 2004, from *www.nursing.uiowa.edu/hartford/nurse/bestpractice/best_practice.htm*

Kirchhoff, K. (2004). State-of-the-science of translation research: from demonstration projects to intervention testing. *Worldviews on Evidence-Based Nursing, 1*(Suppl 1), S6-S12.

Kitson, A., Harvey, G., & McCormack, B. (1998). Enabling the implementation of evidence based practice: A conceptual framework. *Quality in Health Care, 7*(3), 149-158.

Krueger, R., & Casey, M. (2000). *Focus groups: a practical guide for applied research* (3rd ed.). Thousand Oaks, CA: Sage Publications, Inc.

Lacey, E. (1995). Facilitating research-based practice by educational interventions. *Nurse Education Today, 16,* 296-301.

Locock, L., Dopson, S., Chambers, D., & Gabbay, J. (2001). Understanding the role of opinion leaders in improving clinical effectiveness. *Social Science & Medicine, 53,* 745-757.

Madsen, D., Seabolt, T., Cullen, L., Folkedahl, B., Mueller, T., & Richardson, C. (in press). Why listen to bowel sounds? *American Journal of Nursing.*

McCormack, B., Kitson, A., Harvey, G., Rycroft-Malone, J., Titchen, A., & Seers, K. (2002). Getting evidence into practice: The meaning of 'context.' *Journal of Advanced Nursing, 38*(1), 94-104.

Montgomery, L., & Budreau, G. (1996). Implementing a clinical practice guideline to improve pediatric intravenous infiltration outcomes. *AACN Clinical Issues, 7*(3), 411-424.

Montgomery, L., Hanrahan, K., Kottman, K., Otto, A., Barrett, T., & Hermiston, B. (1999). Guideline for IV infiltrations in pediatric patients. *Pediatric Nursing, 25*(2), 167-169, 173-180.

Morris, M., Scott-Findlay, S., & Estabrooks, C. (2001). Evidence-based nursing web sites: Finding the best resources. *AACN Clinical Issues, 12*(4), 578-587.

Newman, K., Pyne, T., Leigh, S., Rounce, K., & Cowling, A. (2000). Personal and organizational competencies requisite for the adoption and implementation of evidence-based health care. *Health Services Management Research, 13,* 97-110.

Nutley, S., Davies, H., & Walter, W. (2002). *Conceptual synthesis 1: Learning from the diffusion of innovation.* St. Andrews, England: University of London.

Oxman, A.D., Thomson, M.A., Davis, D.A., & Haynes, R.B. (1995). No magic bullets: A systematic review of 102 trials of interventions to improve professional practice. *Canadian Medical Association Journal, 153*(10), 1423-1431.

Pippalla, R.S., Riley, D.A., & Chinburapa, V. (1995). Influencing the prescribing behavior of physicians: A metaevaluation. *Journal of Clinical Pharmacy and Therapeutics, 20,* 189-198.

Rakel, B.A. (2003). *Piloting the practice change.* Iowa City, IA: Department of Nursing Services and Patient Care, The University of Iowa Hospitals and Clinics.

Rakel, B.A., Titler, M.G., Goode, C.J., Barry-Walker, J., Budreau, G., & Buckwalter, K.C. (1994). Nasogastric and nasointestinal feeding tube placement: An integrative review of research. *AACN Clinical Issues in Critical Care Nursing, 5*(2), 194-206, 218-199, 223.

Redus, K., Cullen, L., Matthews, G., Wagner, M., Pottinger, J., Swartzendruber, S., et al. (2002). *Safety in the real world: Fall risk assessment.* Paper presented at the 9th National Evidence-Based Practice Conference, Iowa City, IA.

Rogers, E. (2003). *Diffusion of Innovations* (5th ed.). New York: Free Press.

Rosswurm, M., & Larrabee, J. (1999). Clinical scholarship. A model for change to evidence-based practice. *Image: The Journal of Nursing Scholarship, 31*(4), 317-322.

Rycroft-Malone, J., Harvey, G., Kitson, A., McCormack, B., & Titchen, A. (2002). Getting evidence into practice: Ingredients for change. *Nursing Standard, 16*(37), 38-43.

Sackett, D.L., Straus, S.E., Richardson, W.S., Rosenberg, W., & Haynes, R.B. (2000). *Evidence-based medicine: How to practice and teach EBM.* London: Churchill Livingstone.

Schoenbaum, S.C., Sundwall, D.N., Bergman, D., Buckle, J.M., Chernov, A., George, J.H.C., et al. (1995). *Using clinical practice guidelines to evaluate quality of care, Volume 2: Methods.* Rockville, MD: U.S. Department of Health and Human Services, Public Health Service, Agency for Health care Research and Quality.

Sigma Theta Tau International. (2003). *Arista3 report executive summary. Nurses and health: A global future.* Indianapolis, IN: Sigma Theta Tau International, Honor Society for Nursing.

Soumerai, S.B., McLaughlin, T.J., Gurwitz, J.H., Guadagnoli, E., Hauptman, P.J., Borbas, C., et al. (1998). Effect of local medical opinion leaders on quality of care for acute myocardial infarction: A randomized controlled trial. *Journal of the American Medication Society, 279*(17), 1358-1363.

Speziale, H. (2002). Evaluating qualitative research. In G. LoBiondo-Wood & J. Haber (Eds), *Nursing research* (5th ed.) (pp. 165-182). St Louis: Mosby.

Stenger, K., Schooley, K., & Moss, L. (2001). Moving to evidence-based practice for pain management in the critical care setting. *Critical Care Nursing Clinics of North America, 13*(2), 319-327.

Stetler, C. (2001). Updating the Stetler Model of Research Utilization to facilitate evidence-based practice. *Nursing Outlook, 49*(6), 272-279.

Stonestreet, J.S., & Lamb-Havard, J. (1994). Organizational strategies to promote research-based practice. *AACN Clinical Issues, 5*(2), 133-146.

Tang, J.H.C. (2002). *Evidence-based practice protocol: Nurse retention.* Iowa City, IA: The University of Iowa College of Nursing, Gerontological Nursing Interventions Research Center Research Dissemination Core.

Thomson O'Brien, M.A., Oxman, A.D., Davis, D.A., Haynes, R.B., Freemantle, N., & Harvey, E.L. (2003a). *Audit and feedback versus alternative strategies: Effects on professional practice and health care outcomes* (The Cochrane Library, Issue 2). Oxford, England: The Cochrane Collaboration.

Thomson O'Brien, M.A., Oxman, A.D., Davis, D.A., Haynes, R.B., Freemantle, N., & Harvey, E.L. (2003b). *Educational outreach visits: Effects on professional practice and health care outcomes* (The Cochrane Library, Issue 2). Oxford, England: The Cochrane Collaboration.

Titler, M.G. (2002a). Use of research in practice. In G. LoBiondo-Wood, & J. Haber (Eds.), *Nursing research* (5th ed.). St Louis: Mosby.

Titler, M.G. (2002b). *Toolkit for promoting evidence-based practice.* Iowa City, IA: Research, Quality and Outcomes Management, Department of Nursing Services and Patient Care, The University of Iowa Hospitals and Clinics.

Titler, M.G. (2004). Methods in translation science. *Worldviews on Evidence-Based Nursing, 1*, 38-48.

Titler, M. G., Cullen, L., & Ardery, G. (2002). Evidence-based practice: an administrative perspective. *Reflections on Nursing Leadership, 28*(2), 26-27, 46.

Titler, M.G., & Everett, L.Q. (2001). Translating research into practice: Considerations for critical care investigators. *Critical Care Nursing Clinics of North American, 13*(4), 587-604.

Titler, M.G., Kleiber, C., Steelman, V., Rakel, B.A., Budreau, G., Everett, L.Q., et al. (2001). The Iowa Model of Evidence-Based Practice to Promote Quality Care. *Critical Care Nursing Clinics of North American, 13*(4), 497-509.

Tranmer, J.E., Kisilevsky, B.S., & Muir, D.W. (1995). A nursing research utilization strategy for staff nurses in the acute care setting. *Journal of Nursing Administration, 25*(4), 21-29.

Tripp-Reimer, T., & Doebbeling, B. (2004). Qualitative perspectives in translational research. *Worldviews on Evidence-Based Nursing, 1*(Suppl 1), S65-S72.

U.S. Invitational Conference. (2004). *Advancing quality care through translation research.* (Set of 2 CD-Roms). Conference Proceedings. Iowa City, IA: University of Iowa Hospitals and Clinics.

Williams, C.A. (2004). Preparing the next generation of scientists in translation research. *Worldviews on Evidence-Based Nursing, 1*(S1), S73-S77.

Woolf, S.H., & Atkins, D. (2001). The evolving role of prevention in health care. Contributions of the U.S. Preventive Services Task Force. *American Journal of Preventive Medicine, 20*(3, Suppl 1), 13-20.

Zwarenstein, M., & Bryant, W. (2004). *Interventions to promote collaboration between nurses and doctors (Cochrane Review)* (The Cochrane Library, Issue 1). Oxford, England: The Cochrane Collaboration.

HUMAN RESOURCES MANAGEMENT

V

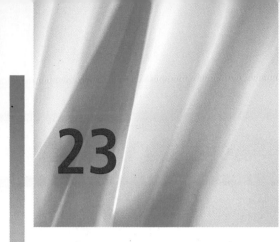

23

Motivation

Richard W. Redman

CHAPTER OBJECTIVES

- Define and describe motivation
- Examine the content and process motivation theories
- Differentiate between internal and external motivation
- Critique classic theories of motivation
- Analyze motivation in organizations
- Evaluate motivation in nursing
- Analyze the link between motivation and leadership and management
- Exercise critical thinking to conceptualize and analyze possible solutions to a practice exercise

The concept of motivation seems to pervade daily life. It may manifest in a negative way, as when someone is *not motivated* to do something, or more positively, as when someone is particularly "pumped" (i.e., excited and motivated) to get something done. A central characteristic of motivation is some type of energy, drive, or will to behave in a certain way or to get something accomplished.

Motivation has been described as the ability to get individuals to do what one wants them to do—when and how one wants it done. Motivated people have a sense of forward drive as an identifying characteristic, as well as a sense of energy, enthusiasm, and goal-directedness.

Motivation is central to a number of issues important to nurses and nursing practice. It is a factor in how nurses feel about professional issues and about the workplace or practice setting. It has implications for leadership as nurses struggle with the challenge of how to get members of a team or workgroup to do something they may not want to do. Also, motivation theory can provide insights into the process of trying to understand how patients' behaviors are related to health and illness activities and the challenge this relationship presents to nurses as they help patients take on more responsibility for their health.

First, this chapter examines the large body of motivation theory and reviews some of the different approaches to explaining motivation and behavior. Next, some applications of these theories are considered from the perspective of nursing and health services research. Finally, key principles from motivation theories are presented and applied to professional nursing practice.

DEFINITIONS

The term **motivation** comes from the Latin word *movere*, meaning "to move." Although it has multiple definitions, three common components are embodied in the term *motivation*. Motivation describes factors that are believed to energize human behavior in some way. It also refers to the

▲ LEADING & MANAGING DEFINED

Motivation The degree to which an individual is moved or aroused to achieve a goal or purpose.	**Motives or Needs** Wants, drives, or impulses.
Activity A basic unit of human behavior.	**Motivation to Work** The degree to which members of an organization are willing to work.

mechanisms of how and where that behavior will be directed. Finally, it encompasses insights on how that behavior is sustained over time. Essentially, motivation means the degree to which an individual is moved or aroused to expend effort to achieve some goal or purpose (Rainey, 2001).

Motivation also is used to describe the process of activating human behavior. It implies a sense of movement, excitement, and expectancy. Motivation is a catalyst to move individuals toward goals.

The basic unit of human behavior is an **activity** or a discrete action. People vary in both their ability and their willingness to do any activity. Motivation is the willingness aspect. **Motives or needs** are the wants, drives, or impulses within an individual. They are the drives to action and the reasons for behavior. Motives are directed toward goals and are the energizing forces that become an incentive to strive for the desired rewards outside the individual. Activity is generally focused on the need(s) with the greatest strength at any given point in time.

Motivation to work is the degree to which members of an organization are willing to fulfill their role or to do their job. There are energizing forces within individuals that drive them to behave and environmental forces that trigger these drives. The idea of goal orientation means that human behavior is directed *toward* something. To analyze motivation from a systems orientation means to look at the forces within individuals, as well as those in the environment that feed back to either reinforce the intensity of a drive or to discourage a course of action and redirect efforts. For example, motivation can be sparked as a result of persuasive

communication that occurs between a leader and a follower.

The most powerful source of motivation is thought to be internal, intrinsic drives. To effectively motivate, leaders need to discover in their followers some internal or external need or trigger that arouses a desire, energizes the will, and serves as a basis for action or thought.

MOTIVATION THEORY

A large body of literature that includes several theories of motivation has developed over the years. Although these theories initially focused on behavior in general, the primary focus eventually shifted to motivation as it relates to work; thus most motivation theories are focused on motivation and behavior in the workplace and are found in the business and organizational sciences literature. Motivation theory permeates nearly all aspects of management sciences today, including elements of leadership, teams, job performance, change management, and decision making. It is seen by managers as an essential component in the job performance equation on all levels. Researchers see theories of motivation as fundamental to developing evidence-based policies and guidelines for effective management practices that can be applied in all types of work environments (Steers et al., 2004).

Rainey (2001) described motivation theories as the foundation for thousands of research studies on the topic. However, the volume of theories and research projects has not resulted in one single theory that everyone agrees on. Rainey (2001) noted that motivation is best viewed as an umbrella construct that embraces a set of concepts and issues rather than a single variable or theory with a precise operational definition.

Motivation theories often reflect an interaction between processes or factors internal to the individual and stimuli or forces in the external environment. Each of these components is emphasized and valued to varying degrees in a given theory. As the social, behavioral, and biological sciences have matured over time, motivation theories have reflected these developments. Some theories focus primarily on personality and genetic characteristics, explaining motivation as primarily originating in innate characteristics of the individual. Eventually, theories became more social in their orientation, recognizing the importance of work groups or cultural factors as influencing variables in shaping motivation within an individual (D'Aunno et al., 2000). Today, theories generally contain elements that are found within individuals as well as in the social or professional environment where individuals work.

Given the large number of motivation theories that are available, schemas for grouping them have been developed. Box 23.1 presents two ways to categorize the large number of motivation theories that exist. The more common method is to group them as either content or process theories. Content theories describe behavior based on factors that exist primarily within the individual. Most of these factors focus on needs, drives, or forces within an individual that result in the person directing behavior in some particular way. Process theories examine behavior as a function of human decision-making processes and often include components in the environment that motivate people to behave in various ways (Porter et al., 2003).

Development in this area of theory progressed gradually over the last century. Initially, theories focused on instincts as a driving force and included concepts such as fear, curiosity, or sociability. The theories were referred to as content theories and eventually evolved into a variety of need theories. Eventually, the theories became more oriented

---

Box 23.1

Approaches to Categorizing Motivation Theories

I. Schema developed by Porter, Bigley, & Steers (2003).
   A. Content theories (factors primarily within the individual)
      1. Maslow's hierarchy of needs
      2. McClelland's needs for achievement, power, and affiliation
      3. Herzberg's two-factor theory
   B. Process theories (focus on the psychological or behavioral processes)
      1. Operant conditioning
      2. Vroom's expectancy theory
      3. Goal-setting theory
II. Schema developed by Mitchell & Daniels (2003)
   A. Internal motivation theories
      1. Thoughtful (based on cognitive approaches)
         a. Expectancy theory
         b. Goal-setting theory
      2. Not rational (non-cognitive; based on individual differences)
         a. Personality theory
         b. Genetic theory
   B. External motivation theories
      1. Job design or characteristics model
      2. Social theories: groups and culture

---

toward drives and reinforcement through interaction with the environment, thus becoming more behaviorally oriented. These theories view individuals in a learning relationship between their actions and consequences for those actions. This behavioralist view of individuals is still a central theme in many motivation theories today. As theories developed more of a focus on process, they became more cognitive in their underpinnings, attempting to explain and understand the thought processes involved in determining how people will behave, especially in the workplace.

This work culminated in a focus on goal-setting theory, which is the dominant perspective today (Steers et al., 2004).

Regardless of the particular theoretical perspective on work motivation, most researchers would agree that the best way to view work performance is as an interaction effect between abilities and motivation (O'Reilly & Chatman, 1999). It might be seen in terms of the following simple formula:

$$Performance = Ability \times Motivation$$

An individual can have strong abilities to perform a task or set of responsibilities, but if the individual is not motivated to perform or to do them well, he or she will not do so. The reverse can also be envisioned, where someone is highly motivated to do his or her best, but the person simply does not have the abilities or skill to successfully perform a task or carry out a set of responsibilities. In this sense, motivation might best be viewed as a moderator of ability.

There are too many motivation theories available to examine all of them here. Instead, a few examples from the content and process categories have been selected with the intent to depict how they are used to explain and predict behavior.

Content Theories

The content theories are based on factors that exist primarily within the individual. These often describe instincts, needs, or drives within the individual that result in an individual behaving in some particular manner. The classic theory in this category was called the *need satisfaction model.*

Need Satisfaction Model

To motivate is not an easy task. Knowledge about how individuals pursue the satisfaction of needs helps nurses understand motivation. A special process is involved with motivation. First, a need is felt. For example, a felt need is something like needing to get a job or earn money. Next, there is some sort of activity or behavioral response to the felt need. Then the goal either is attained or blocked. If the goal desired to reduce the feeling of need is blocked, frustration results. At this point

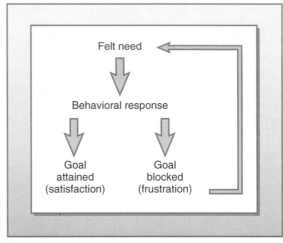

Figure 23.1
Need Satisfaction Model. (Data from Schweiger, J. [1980]. *The nurse as manager.* New York: John Wiley & Sons.)

another round of the process is initiated in an attempt to reduce the frustration. This process forms the core of the need satisfaction model (Schweiger, 1980) (Figure 23.1). For example, a nurse assesses that a client is in pain and determines that comfort measures are not sufficient to alleviate the pain or the client-felt need. The nurse, in a behavioral response, contacts the physician for a pain medication order. This results in either attaining the goal if successful or in frustration if unsuccessful. If unsuccessful, new behaviors are called for because frustration has become the new felt need.

In general, motivational theories are based on the relationship of attitudes, needs, and behaviors. Motivation can be either internal or external, called *intrinsic* or *extrinsic. Internal motivation* is that which arises from within an individual and is aimed at a sense of personal accomplishment. *External motivation* is motivation that arises from outside an individual, where something or somebody becomes an incentive. External motivation is related to the application of rewards or punishments. For example, a grade given for performance on an examination is an external motivator. Weight loss, smoking cessation, and chemical dependency rehabilitation programs all deal with internal versus external motivation and the challenge of finding the right combination to overcome strong urges and behavioral or lifestyle choices.

A person's attitudes and values create the internal versus external orientation. Some circumstances involve a combination of both internal and external motivators. For example, nurses may work at a rapid pace because they enjoy feeling a sense of achievement, an internal motivator, but also because they are given an external motivator in the form of a heavy assignment. Personal philosophy, values, beliefs, and assumptions are the foundations for motivation. To understand an individual's internal motivation, one must understanding the person's beliefs, values, and assumptions (Figure 23.2).

The need satisfaction model provides insight into understanding human behavior. This model has been the basis for many theories of motivation, including Maslow's (1954) hierarchy of needs theory, Alderfer's (1969) ERG theory, Herzberg's (Herzberg et al., 1959) motivation-hygiene theory, and McClelland's (1961, 1976) need for achievement theory. Some theorists have focused on specific human drives deemed to be important. Some examples are the achievement motive, the affiliation motive, the need for equity, the need for activity and exploration, the need for competence, and the self-actualization motive (Lawler, 1973).

Going beyond a description of needs, one group of motivation theories uses a cognitive premise as its base. The cognitive theories assume that individuals reason, think, and consider the consequences of their behavior. Thus the focus is on the thought and evaluative processes individuals use in participating and performing in the workplace. These theories examine the attractiveness of outcomes to individuals and are categorized as expectancy theories. Expectancy, equity, and goal-setting theories are included, although goal-setting has been viewed primarily as a technique rather than a theory. Vroom's (1964) expectancy theory is a major example of the cognitive theories (Lawler, 1973; Steers & Porter, 1987). As applied to working in organizations, theories of motivation are discussed in connection with job satisfaction. Herzberg's theory is an example. Job satisfaction is an internal subjective state related to an affective reaction to motivated job behavior. It is related to organizational outcomes such as absenteeism and turnover, which are costly to organizations and influence their effectiveness (Lawler, 1973; Price & Mueller, 1986). Motivation as applied to

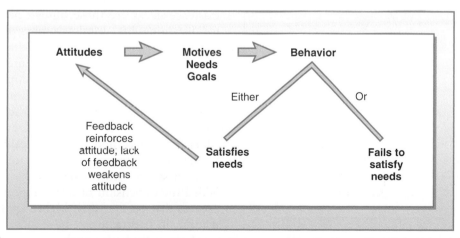

Figure 23.2
Relationship of attitudes, motives, and behavior. (Data from Schweiger, J. [1980]. *The nurse as manager*. New York: John Wiley & Sons; and Steers, R., & Porter, L. [1987]. *Motivation and work behavior* [4th ed.]. New York: McGraw-Hill.)

the work environment also is the focus of Hackman and Oldham's (1979) job characteristics theory. Finally, McGregor's (1960) Theory X and Theory Y are related to motivation. Not truly a theory of human motivation, McGregor's X-Y theory describes managerial attitudes toward employees and is more specific to assumptions about what motivates people to work. Three examples of content theories that will be described in more detail here are Maslow's, Herzberg's, and McClelland's theories.

Maslow's Hierarchy of Needs Theory

Maslow (1954) arrayed human needs along a hierarchy from most basic to most sophisticated. This progression can be thought of as stair steps or as a pyramid (Figure 23.3). At the bottom, or base, are the most basic needs, the *physiological* drives for food, sleep, clothing, and shelter. These needs are usually associated with the survival needs for which humans seek to acquire money. The majority of an individual's activity will be at this level until the needs are fulfilled sufficiently to sustain the body. When physiological needs are fulfilled, other levels of needs emerge and dominate.

The second level in the Maslow's hierarchy is *safety and security* needs. These are needs to be free of the fear of physical harm and deprivation of basic physiological needs. Employee benefit plans are aimed at security needs. The third level is *belonging* needs that relate to the drive for affiliation and love. These are social needs. In nursing, work group social support and cohesion meet some belonging needs. The next level is *esteem and ego* needs. These are needs to achieve independence, respect, and recognition from others. Satisfaction of esteem needs results in prestige, self-confidence, power, and a feeling of usefulness. Recognition is an important esteem motivator in nursing. The highest level of the hierarchy of needs, at the apex, is *self-actualization* needs. These relate to the need to maximize one's potential and achieve a sense of personal fulfillment, competence, and accomplishment. This need is individual and internal. In Maslow's theoretical framework, needs at the lower levels must be fulfilled before those at a higher level can emerge and have energy devoted to them (Maslow, 1954). Maslow's theory applies to people in general and is not specific to work or organizational behavior.

Alderfer (1969) modified Maslow's (1954) work by collapsing the five hierarchical levels into three sets of needs: existence needs, relatedness needs, and growth needs. According to Alderfer's model, existence needs are those human needs specific to sustaining life. Maslow's physiological and safety/security needs would be included in existence needs. Relatedness needs are needs for meaningful interpersonal relationships, similar to Maslow's belonging needs. Growth needs are the needs for self-esteem and self-actualization, similar to Maslow's self-actualization needs. Alderfer's (1969) model has been called the ERG theory, the acronym standing for *existence*, *relatedness*, and *growth* needs. The ERG theory added the dimension of a frustration-regression process that occurs when higher level needs are continually frustrated.

Maslow's theory is one that is familiar to nurses because it is often used to explain patient or client behavior. However, it is one of the early theories

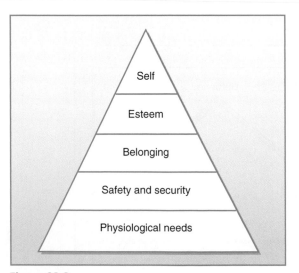

Figure 23.3

Maslow's hierarchy of human needs. (Data from Maslow, A. [1954]. *Motivation and personality*. New York: Harper & Row.)

that, over time, has diminished in value. Although Maslow's theory is quoted extensively, it has not held up well when research has been conducted to test it. The five-step hierarchy has never been confirmed through research, although studies have provided some support for a two-step hierarchy with lower level needs that deal with material and security needs and higher level needs that deal with an emphasis on achievement and challenge. The theory remains attractive, in spite of its lack of empirical verification. The idea of individuals having growth needs and motives and that some needs are more important than others continues to hold intuitive appeal. Although Maslow's theory is not used in management sciences today, as one of the early motivation theories, it has had a significant influence on the development of many other content theories (Rainey, 2001).

Herzberg's Motivation-Hygiene Theory

Herzberg (Herzberg et al., 1959) applied Maslow's general theory of motivation specifically to work motivation. Herzberg's motivation-hygiene, or two-factor, theory proposed that there are two different categories of needs, which are independent and affect behavior in different ways: hygienes and motivators (Figure 23.4). The hygiene or maintenance factors are security, status, money, working conditions, interpersonal relations, supervision, and policies and administration. The hygienes are related to the environment and conditions of the job. They are not growth-producing motivators for employees; they only prevent lost productivity due to job dissatisfaction. On the other hand, the motivators seem to be effective in motivating toward superior performance and positively affecting job satisfaction. They are related to the job itself. The motivators are growth and development, advancement, increased responsibility for work, challenging work, recognition, and achievement.

In Herzberg's theory, work motivation is seen as composed of job satisfaction and dissatisfaction. Satisfaction is not a continuum, with of satisfaction on one end and dissatisfaction on the other. Rather, satisfaction and dissatisfaction were seen as two independent continuua: (1) no satisfaction to high satisfaction and (2) no dissatisfaction to high dissatisfaction. The hygiene factors are essentially equivalent to Maslow's lower-level

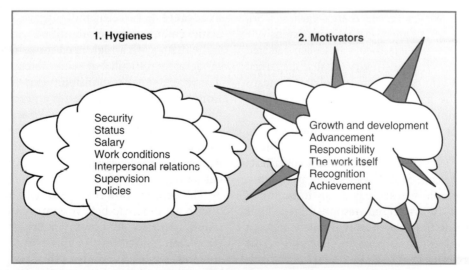

Figure 23.4
Herzberg's factors. (Data from Herzberg, F., Mausner, B., & Snyderman, B. [1959]. *The motivation to work*. New York: John Wiley & Sons.)

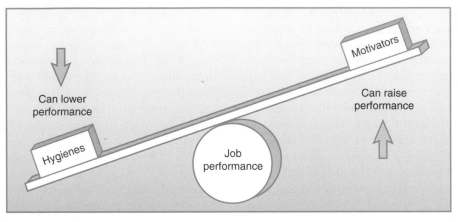

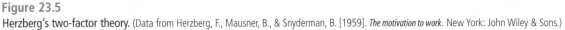

Figure 23.5
Herzberg's two-factor theory. (Data from Herzberg, F., Mausner, B., & Snyderman, B. [1959]. *The motivation to work*. New York: John Wiley & Sons.)

factors, whereas the motivators are higher-level factors (Figure 23.5). In other words, there must be enough of the hygiene factors so that the employee is not dissatisfied. Enough of the motivators need to be present to be personally rewarding.

Herzberg's two-factor theory was one of the first motivation theories to be developed that focused specifically on work motivation and the identification of ways that jobs might be enriched to address motivational needs that employees bring to the workplace. Herzberg's earliest work appeared in 1959 and was refined extensively through the 1970s. The theory has been referred to as a "job enrichment" theory because it sparked a number of strategies to enrich jobs as a means to address the motivator factors and, hopefully, job satisfaction (Herzberg, 2003; Miner, 2002).

This theory resulted in much controversy in the workplace. Part of the controversy was due to viewing pay as a factor that does not contribute to job satisfaction. Most surveys rank pay highly, and many employees see pay as an indicator of achievement or increased responsibility. Thus some critics do not see conceptual clarity between intrinsic and extrinsic rewards. Regardless, the theory has contributed to an increased understanding of the importance of restructuring work so that it is interesting and stimulating and provides

opportunities to satisfy motivation for growth and fulfillment. (Rainey, 2001).

McClelland's Theory

McClelland (1961, 1976) identified three basic needs that people possess in varying degrees: the need for achievement, the need for power, and the need for affiliation. Each person tends to have one predominant need. The **need for achievement** is the strong desire to overcome challenges, to excel, to advance or succeed, and to grow. The need for achievement can be identified and assessed. Individuals with a high need for achievement set moderately difficult but achievable goals and like to take personal responsibility for finding solutions to problems. Included is a need for competence, or a strong desire to make a contribution or to produce some visible outcome and to do quality work. Those who exhibit high need for achievement are eager for responsibility, take calculated risks, and desire concrete feedback.

The **need for power** is the urge to be in control and to get others to behave contrary to what they would naturally do. Power is a drive to influence people and situations. People with a pure need for power need to control other people and the environment around them. They desire to make an impact, be influential, be in charge, and gain

⚠ LEADING & MANAGING **DEFINED**

Need for Achievement	Need for Affiliation
The strong desire to overcome challenges, to excel, to advance or succeed, and to grow.	The desire to work in a pleasant environment and the desire for friendly, close relationships.

Need for Power

The need to be in control and to get others to behave contrary to what they would naturally do.

personal influence and prestige more than they desire productivity.

The **need for affiliation** is the desire to work in a pleasant environment and the need for friendly, close relationships. Affiliation is a drive to relate to people. People who have a high need for affiliation seek out meaningful friendships, want to be respected and liked, avoid decisions that oppose the group, and are more interested in high morale than productivity.

McClelland and Boyatzis (1982) studied individuals with long tenure in management positions and found a "leadership motive pattern" that enabled effectiveness at higher levels of an organization. The features of a leadership motive pattern are moderately high levels of the need for power and low needs for affiliation, with high levels of self-control. Absent is the need for achievement motive, which was associated with managerial success at lower management levels in nontechnical areas (Henderson, 1993). Thus theories of needs motivation have been related to leadership and management by investigating which characteristics or combinations of characteristics can be used to predict job "fit" or success.

Henderson (1993) found that nurse managers' and nurse executives' profiles did not fit the profile of successful managers described by McClelland and Boyatzis (1982). Specifically, about one-third of respondents showed no power motive preference. There may be a variety of explanations for this, such as differences in industry versus service sector, female role socialization, the position of nurse executives in the hierarchy,

individual characteristics of age or education, or the type, complexity, or culture of the setting. It is possible that profiles change over time. Measurement tools may not be precise or setting-specific enough to detect relationships. Thus theories and measures need to be evaluated as data are gathered for decision making and prediction.

McClelland's (1961, 1976) framework can be used for self-assessment and to assess and influence others. Self-assessment is an analysis of which of these types most represents an individual. Once self-assessment has been completed, others in the environment can be evaluated for their highest need motivation. Communication is enhanced, and conflicts are diminished as effective strategies are employed to meet individuals' needs. People are motivated by different needs, and understanding the basic types helps nurses learn to work with a diversity of personalities in actual work situations. The idea is to match the individual's need structure to the assignment in the organization. To plant individuals in a place where they will grow is a key to productivity and success.

Process Theories

Process theories of motivation concentrate on behavioral and psychological processes in motivation as opposed to needs and drives that may influence motivation. Three classic process theories are highlighted in this chapter: (1) operant conditioning, (2) expectancy theory, and (3) goal-setting theory.

Operant Conditioning

A classic approach to motivation that focuses primarily on processes in the external environment is operant conditioning. Nurses are familiar with behavior modification, which also derives directly from operant conditioning theory. In this theory, behavior and motivation are shaped primarily as the result of responses to stimuli in the environment. People respond to stimuli that they view as rewarding, and they avoid stimuli that they view as undesirable or punishing. Generally, this theoretical perspective does not focus to any degree on the internal processes operating within the individual and emphasizes the process of shaping behavior through environmental stimuli such as rewards. In the current business literature, a series of books on the "one minute manager," based on operant conditioning, have been published over the past two decades (e.g., Blanchard et al., 1999).

Expectancy Theory

Expectancy theory is built on the basic premise that individuals seek to do what they think will produce desirable results and minimize undesired results. This theory poses that individuals in the work setting will engage in behaviors that they expect will lead to valued outcomes. Different work-related activities are viewed as having positive or negative valences (similar to the electron valences in chemistry). Outcomes of behavior are viewed as having positive or negative assessments, and an employee will be motivated to perform those behaviors with the highest valences, or the highest probability of leading to very good results (Pinder, 1998).

Lewin (1935) described behavior as a function of characteristics in both the person and the environment. Thus motivation can be influenced by the nature of the individual and by the policies and practices of the organization. Lewin (1935) introduced the concept of valence, defined as the attractiveness of an outcome. Later theories introduced the concept of expectancy, defined as the likelihood that an action will lead to a certain outcome. The general expectancy theory framework views behavior as determined by the multiplication of valence with expectancy.

Vroom's (1964) VIE theory is the most well-known expectancy theory and is the one applied to work settings (VIE stands for *valence-instrumentality-expectancy*). Instrumentality is a belief about the probability that behavior will lead to other second-level outcomes. All three VIE variables are beliefs held by individuals related to what they expect will happen. Vroom (1964) postulated that behavior results from conscious choices among alternatives. The choice behaviors are related to perception and the formation of attitudes and beliefs. Humans naturally choose to maximize pleasure and minimize pain. The combinations of VIE, which Vroom represented symbolically by mathematical equations, interact to create a motivational force for action. In the context of work, individuals will pursue the level of performance that they believe will maximize their overall best interest (Steers & Porter, 1987).

Vroom's (1964) VIE theory was refined by Porter and Lawler (1968), who found that employee effort was determined jointly by two factors: (1) the individual's assessment of the value of certain outcomes and (2) the degree to which there is a belief that the person's effort will lead to the attainment of valued rewards. Both beliefs must be in place for further effort to be elicited. However, there is a distinction between actions and outcomes that indicates effort may not result in job performance. Furthermore, performance and satisfaction may or may not be related, depending on a variety of factors (Lawler, 1973; Steers & Porter, 1987).

Nurses attempting to use VIE theory try to structure rewards on an individualized basis. However, it is difficult to assess the actual needs of employees, so their values and attitudes are assessed as a proxy for actual needs. Managers work to assign personnel to jobs for which they are capable of performing. For example, nurses would operationalize this theory when delegating to unlicensed assistive personnel by structuring assignments to meet needs and preferences. Nurses' latitude of freedom may be constrained in organizations by policies and procedures, precedents, or union contracts (Steers & Porter, 1987).

Expectancy theory is a prominent and well-regarded theory of work motivation, even though it has not held up well in research, which is most likely due to the complexities of trying to identify and measure, in terms of valences, what is important to the individual. The theory also proposes that individuals compute complex equations in their mind before they act, which is also difficult to measure (Rainey, 2001). Nonetheless, expectancy theory is viewed as an important conceptual framework that has made valuable contributions and insights regarding motivation in the workplace. The fact that perceptions about reward expectancies exist is an important contribution.

Goal-Setting Theory

Goal-setting theory is the most prominent and valued motivation theory at the present time. Its basic premise is simple: goals serve as targets for human behavior. In turn, difficult, specific goals lead to higher performance than vague or nonexistent goals. Difficult goals direct attention and effort toward the task, serve to mobilize action, and motivate the individual to search for strategies that will lead to effective performance. A component of this theory is self-efficacy, a concept that is quite familiar to nurses and used to describe health behaviors in patients. Self-efficacy relates to a person's confidence and sense of capability in accomplishing goals. Self-efficacy is enhanced by the goals that are set before an individual. This approach to motivation relies heavily on cognitive processes. Because behavior is intentional, it arises from the deliberate actions and conscious choices to accomplish specific goals. In essence, people act in ways that are consistent with the intentions and goals (Pinder, 1998).

This theory fits nicely into many work settings, where goals are used to help individuals define their performance and to grow over time. Many management principles are based on a collaborative goal-setting between employee and manager as a way to guide work behavior and to set a framework for evaluation of performance (Rainey, 2001).

The use of periodic feedback is an important tool to help individuals attain their desired goals and to encourage or motivate them to continue to strive for successful accomplishment of targeted goals.

Job Characteristics Model

The job characteristics model describes how the characteristics of a job and the individual differences among workers interact to affect motivation, job satisfaction, and productivity at work (Hackman & Oldham, 1979). The model is often used as a framework to analyze the design of jobs and how that affects motivation and job satisfaction in workers. Frequently, the redesign of work in health care organizations is based in the diagnostic methods that are part of the job characteristics model (Redman & Ketefian, 1995).

The job characteristics model depicts core dimensions of any job (skill variety, task identity, task significance, autonomy, and feedback), psychological state of the worker (the meaningfulness of work to the employee, the degree of responsibility an employee has for the outcomes of his or her work), and personal or work outcomes (level of performance, job satisfaction). These factors interact in ways that influence both how employees feel about their work and their motivation to perform at certain levels of productivity (Hackman & Oldham, 1979). When using this approach to redesign work, attempts are made to increase the motivation potential of a job. This might be done, for example, by increasing the employee's autonomy or the significance of his or her work. The job characteristics model is viewed as an important framework for enriching jobs in a way that will affect employee motivation, satisfaction, and productivity.

Related Theories of Work Motivation

Organizations that employ nurses seek to manage scarce human resources in a way that best coordinates and motivates nurses as employees. However, the best way to do this is not immediately obvious. Traditional bureaucratic organizations use close supervision and tight control of employees. Human relations or human resources models utilize limited participation or decentralization to enhance employee morale and cooperation. Because motivation is a complex yet critical element, it has been extensively investigated. Two related theories of work motivation are McGregor's Theory X and Theory Y and the famous Hawthorne studies.

McGregor's Theory X and Theory Y

A manager's philosophy about people, attitudes, and assumptions plays a role in his or her choice of motivational strategies. The assumptions about the nature of people that Theory X managers bring to the workplace are based on a belief that people who work for an employer are lazy. These managers assume that employees dislike responsibility, prefer to be directed, resist change, and want safety. At the same time, however, Theory X managers assume that employees are rational in that they can be motivated. The accompanying belief is that people are motivated by money and the threat of punishment. Thus, if the workers are lazy, management must be active. Managers need to impose structure and control and closely supervise employees, since external control is necessary to deal with unreliable, irresponsible, and immature workers. This view of human nature and motivation is called Theory X (McGregor, 1960).

Challenging the conventional Theory X view of the day, McGregor (1960) proposed Theory Y (Box 23.2). In a democratic society, the Theory X view of human nature and the managerial practices based on it may not be correct and appropriate. Thus management approaches based on Theory X may fail to motivate individuals toward organizational goals. Theory Y assumes that people are not lazy and unreliable by nature, but rather that people can be self-directed and creative if they are properly motivated.

Theory Y acknowledges that the behavior of people is complex. Under certain conditions people will accept responsibility; they are not necessarily passive; and creativity exists in all levels of the organization. Theory Y managers truly believe that motivation can be unlocked by creating and

---

Box 23.2

Managerial Assumptions

Theory X

People:
- Dislike work
- Need control and force to make them work
- Like to be directed
- Lack ambition

Theory Y

People:
- Like to work
- Can be self-disciplined for objectives to which they are committed
- Will accept responsibility

---

fostering an environment that is motivating. They view this as their job as a manager. These managers think people do like to work, can be self-directed, and will accept responsibility given an environment in which to grow, accomplish, and feel a sense of self-esteem and autonomy. It is the manager's job to create a motivating environment within the system of work. McGregor's (1960) Theory X and Theory Y is not so much a motivation theory as it is a theory about managers' beliefs, which then translates into the ways they choose to motivate their employees.

Hawthorne Studies

Industrial efficiency experts have been interested in determining what mix of physical conditions, work hours, and work methods are ideal to stimulate maximum productive output by workers. Unlocking the secrets of the motivation to work and the relationship between motivation and productivity has been a universal management concern.

In 1924 a famous experiment that came to be known as the *Hawthorne studies* was conducted at the Hawthorne plant of Western Electric, outside Chicago. A team of researchers went into the plant to find out what motivated people. The purpose of the study was to test the effect of working conditions, including such diverse variables as lighting and pay, on productivity.

The researchers had reliable data on the production line, and they knew exactly how long it took a worker to wire a telephone. The regular production line was used as a control. For the experiments, the researchers pulled five workers off the assembly line and put them in a room, creating a mock production line so that the researchers could control and manipulate variables. The first variable was lighting. When more lights were added, production went up. Other variables included scheduled rest periods, company lunches, and shorter work weeks. After introduction of each variable, production went up. To test the strength of association of working conditions and productivity, all the innovations were suddenly withdrawn. Surprisingly, production went up to a new all-time high. All the researchers were able to conclude was that changes in physical working conditions alone had nothing to do with productivity. It must have been something else: specifically, productivity must be tied to the human aspects, such as the attention lavished on the workers. At this point, the research was refocused, and employee interviews were conducted to explore the human relations aspects.

The Hawthorne studies resulted in a new awareness about the need to study and understand human interpersonal relationships at work. The most significant factor affecting organizational productivity was job-related interpersonal relationships, not just pay or working conditions. When informal groups identified with management and the workers felt competent, productivity increased. Furthermore, the findings pointed to involving workers in the planning, organizing, and controlling of their own work as a way to secure workers' positive cooperation. Out of the Hawthorne studies came the phrases "the Hawthorne effect," to refer to attention paid to employees, and "the informal organization," to denote the web of interpersonal relationships beyond management control. Insights gained

from the Hawthorne experiments began the human relations era of management theory with its emphasis on human motivation at work.

Clearly, the behavior of people is complex. Therefore motivation is not a simplistic matter. The motivation of human beings is not reducible to a formula as simple as "people are motivated by money." The differences in motivation stem from the differences in people. However, in creating circumstances in which people are more likely to become self-motivated, managers can consider the following list of needs that employees expect of their employers (McConnell, 1998):

- Capable, respected leadership
- Decent and safe surroundings
- Acceptance as a member of a group
- Recognition and other feedback
- Fair treatment
- A reasonable sense of job security
- Knowledge of the results of individual effort
- Knowledge of the organization's policies, rules, and regulations
- Recognition for special effort
- Respect for individual beliefs
- Assurance that others are doing their fair share of the work
- Fair monetary compensation

Although motivating aspects can be identified and prioritized by nurses, no simple protocol automatically produces motivation in nurses. This is because motivation is internal to the individual and driven by unique combinations of complex factors.

RESEARCH FINDINGS ON MOTIVATION IN NURSING

A number of examples of research addressing work motivation in nursing practice can be found in the literature. Typically, the focus of work motivation research looks at how motivation of employees is associated with various dependent variables such as job satisfaction, desire to continue in one's job, or commitment to the organization. Often the focus is on conditions of the work environment that may have a positive or negative impact on nurses in terms of how they feel about their work, their positions, and the organization where they are employed. A few studies are high-lighted here to illustrate the diversity of studies and the different motivation theories that frame the investigations.

Rantz and colleagues (1996) conducted a series of interviews with nurses in different types of roles to find out what types of factors in their jobs were most closely related to their motivation. Interpersonal relations with colleagues at work ranked as the most important factor. Recognition at work, the amount of responsibility, and the nature of the work itself were also identified as critical motivating factors. These factors were deemed as areas that could be addressed in the work setting to enhance the motivation and job satisfaction of nurses (Rantz et al., 1996). This study used Herzberg's two-factor theory as its framework.

A study of home health care nurses was conducted to examine the impact of increasing workloads on the motivation of the nurses. These increased workloads had created a variety of addi-tional demands and stress for the public health nurses. These changes had a direct effect on the motivation of the nurses—motivation decreased when the responsibilities and the workload was felt to be overwhelming by the nurses. In this study, information about work goals was a strong predictor of positive work motivation (Laamanen et al., 1999). These findings fit nicely with goal-setting theory.

Tzeng (2002) studied staff nurses in acute care hospitals to identify what factors would predict the nurses' intent to stay in their positions at the hospital. The most significant predictor was the work motivation of the nurses and how they felt their jobs provided opportunities for them to meet their motivational needs. The quality of the work environment moderated their levels of work motivation. Those nurses who felt rewarded had positions in which they were involved in decision making and felt valued by the hospital; they also had increased levels of motivation and were less likely to leave their position. This study contains

elements of Herzberg's two-factor theory, expectancy theory, and goal-setting theory.

A similar study found that various aspects of the work environment have a greater impact than personality variables on how individuals feel about their work (Laschinger et al., 2001). In general, work experiences are a strong predictor of affective feelings about work and, based on various theories of motivation, can have an impact on employee motivation and job performance.

The issue of quality of the work environment and its relationship to how nurses feel about their jobs and the organizations they work for is a con-sistent finding in the research literature. This is a major theme in the magnet hospital movement, based on the idea that hospitals which create positive working environments supporting profes-sional nursing practice will have more committed employees, a better employee retention rate, and provide better patient care as well (McClure & Hinshaw, 2002). These research findings relate to the various motivation theories on how work and the work environment interact with motivational needs and desires of the employee. The result is improved work performance and better quality work for the organization.

LEADERSHIP AND MANAGEMENT IMPLICATIONS

Motivation is a key concept of leadership and management in nursing. The art of leading and managing groups of professionals requires cre-ative, interesting, and continuous ways to make people feel good about what they are doing. In a service industry with professional employees, human relations variables are important for pro-ductivity, since the work is dependent on the knowledge, skill, and work effort of human beings. Motivation is important for understand-ing why people work and why some people are highly productive and others are not, as well as for comprehending complex relationships related to teamwork and productivity in organizations. Organizations have a vital interest in productivity. The trend in work life is to emphasize working

Research Note

Source: Laschinger, H.K., Finegan, J., & Shamian, J. (2001). The impact of workplace empowerment, organizational trust on staff nurses' work satisfaction and organizational commitment. *Health Care Management Review, 26*(3), 7-23.

Purpose

The purpose of this study was to assess the impact of current hospital restructuring and job reengineering on nurses who are directly affected by these initiatives. Specifically, the investigation tested a model that links staff nurses' workplace empowerment, organizational trust, job satisfaction, and commitment to the organization. All of these factors are related directly or indirectly to work motivation in nurses. Five research instruments were distributed to 600 staff nurses in urban tertiary care hospitals in Ontario, Canada. A response rate of 73% (412 nurses) was obtained.

Discussion

The analyses indicated that the nurses perceived their work settings to be only moderately empowering, and they did not perceive their jobs to offer a high degree of formal power over decision making and clinical judgment. They reported higher confidence and trust in their peers than in their managers. In addition, they were not very satisfied with their jobs. The testing of the proposed model revealed that the degree of workplace empowerment, or ability to make decisions that affect their work, perceived by the nurses was strongly related to their trust of management, job satisfaction, and a willingness to exert effort in the workplace as well as continue to work at the same organization. The results suggest that fostering work environments that increase nurses' perceptions of empowerment will have positive effects on the organizational members and increase organizational effectiveness as well.

Application to Practice

The factors addressed in this study continue to demonstrate the important relationship between creating motivating work environments and how nurses feel about their jobs. The creation of work environments that encourage professional nursing practice by giving nurses control over their decision making will improve job satisfaction and the motivational attitudes that affect job performance, ultimately leading to improved quality of patient care. The implication for managers is to focus less on control and more on facilitation of nurses' work. Both nurses and managers must be willing to work together to create work environments that foster motivation, work satisfaction, and commitment to organizational goals to provide high-quality nursing care.

LEADERSHIP & MANAGEMENT BEHAVIORS

Leadership Behaviors

- Enables others through high expectations
- Recognizes contributions
- Celebrates accomplishments
- Creates social support networks
- Fosters collaboration
- Communicates an inspiring vision
- Motivates followers
- Sets an example of high motivation
- Provides opportunities for growth and development

Management Behaviors

- Plans motivating rewards
- Links rewards to performance

- Directs others to achieve organizational goals
- Evaluates effectiveness of motivation strategies
- Motivates subordinates
- Provides opportunities for subordinates to achieve
- Provides valued rewards

Overlap Areas

- Motivates others
- Provides opportunities for need satisfaction

harder and being more effective. This requires some internal or external force to move human beings to continuous high levels of productivity. Motivation, along with the structures set up in organizations to motivate human beings, has an effect on outcomes such as performance, turnover, and absenteeism.

Clearly, there is no single theory or model that fits all situations or predicts with accuracy what motivates individuals or how they will behave in a given situation. There are a variety of theories, each one providing some insight. Over time, the earlier theories have influenced and helped to refine the theories developed at later points in time. Given the complexities of human behavior and the rapid pace of change in contemporary work environments, it is unlikely that a definitive theory on motivation will be developed in the near future. That notwithstanding, it is possible to derive some general principles from the various motivation theories that exist to serve as guides for both work behavior and nursing practice. Generalizations from motivation theory follow:

- *The complexities of human behavior will likely never be explained by one simple theory.* However, motivation theories help nurses to identify that individuals, in general, will seek outcomes that are positive for them and try to avoid outcomes that are negative. Knowing this, motivation theory suggests how important it is for nurses to understand what it is that they value as positive and negative outcomes for themselves (Amabile, 1997). The same applies to work with patients. Motivation theory is likely to provide important insights in terms of how and why nurses behave as they do. Although it may not explain the *why*, it likely will predict the *what*. Nurse leaders and managers can use this theory to create positively motivating work environments.
- *Nurses are aware of individual differences as they work with patients.* This same variation in behavior is evident in motivation and work behavior as well. Although it seems simplistic, more often than not nurses expect all employees to work in the same way or perform at the same level. However, individuals vary on almost

every dimension because of fundamental factors such as values, needs, personality, and culture. Individuals have unique genetic and personal backgrounds that shape who they are—including wants, reactions, and motives (Mitchell & Daniels, 2003). Given this variation, it is very important that time be spent getting to know oneself, colleagues, and patients and reflecting on how the unique components of every individual can come together to influence his or her motives and behavior. Recognizing the variation and uniqueness in those with whom we work will help nurses and leaders and managers to understand their motivations and why they behave as they do.

- *Goals are important, regardless of the task at hand.* Whether focusing on team members or patients, it is always important to have established goals that are understand by all in order to see successful behavior (Nicholson, 2003). There is no guarantee that people will perform accordingly because of the phenomenon of individual variation. However, it is quite likely that if shared goals do not exist, not everyone will behave in a predictable manner. Goals are a major motivating factor, and specific goals are generally preferred to ambiguity. Setting goals and contracts with individual employees is a powerful way to motivate individuals (Rousseau, 2004). Once goals have been set, preferably in collaboration with those who will be affected by them, there is a higher probability that individuals will be motivated to perform accordingly.
- *Incentives and rewards are always important.* Regardless of the motivation theory that seems to work best for a given situation, nurse leaders and managers need to remember the importance of giving feedback to individuals so that they receive cues on how they are doing and what else they might need to do. Nurses value recognition for doing a task well, and rewards work well in recognition programs (Kane & Montgomery, 1998). These do not have to be monetary rewards; being recognized and praised is often as important as money (Morse, 2003). This is especially important in the

current health care environment, which is continually challenged by diminishing resources.

- *Equity is important.* Nurses are social beings, and all people tend to compare themselves with those around them. This is equally true in the workplace. If variations in performance are noted yet rewards and recognition are given to all, even individuals who may be performing at a substandard level, nurses will likely have a negative reaction. Nurses want to be treated fairly and want to see consistency from leaders and managers when they compare themselves with others. Motives can vary, but nurses anticipate that, as individuals, they will be treated fairly and equitably.

CURRENT ISSUES AND TRENDS

Although the work on theory development about motivation seemed to slow down by the 1990s, there is a growing need for further work in this area (Ambrose & Kulik, 1999; Locke & Latham, 2004). In an assessment of the state of motivation theory development, Steers and colleagues (2004) pointed out that not all of the insights to be made about motivation have been accomplished. One reason is the dramatic changes that have occurred in the workplace over the last decade. Companies, including the health care industry, have downsized and restructured with regularity. The workforce is increasingly diverse, information technology has dramatically changed how much of our work is transacted, and the distribution of power and the role of teams keep evolving. All of these forces have an impact on the motivation of employees, regardless of the theory that seems to fit best in a given situation.

Another major challenge for motivation theory is the rapid diversification in society. Cultural differences can have a profound impact on motivation and job attitudes, although is it not always clear why or how culture influences motivational processes. Often differences are seen in behavior across national boundaries, but the underlying dynamics are not obvious. Nearly all motivational theories have been developed in the United States

and, as a result, have integrated American cultural values extensively (Lachman, 1997). When these theories are applied in other countries or with workers of different cultures, they often do not work well to explain or predict motivation or behavior in the way we would expect. Cultural differences are important variables that influence both individual behavior and environmental characteristics. There is a growing body of evidence suggesting that cultural differences influence work values, motivation, and job attitudes. This evidence suggests that existing theories need to be reexamined and that new theories of motivation no doubt need to be developed (Hofstede, 1993; Sanchez-Runde & Steers, 2001). As society becomes increasingly diverse, this need will become more critical.

Summary

- Motivation is important in a service industry such as nursing.
- Motivation and human relations variables are important for productivity.
- Motivation is a state of mind in which a person views goals.
- Motivation is a process of activating human behavior.
- Motivation to work is the willingness to work.
- Motivation is a process of felt need, behavior, goal attainment/blockage, frustration, and cycle repetition.
- Motivation can be either internal or external.
- There are many theories of motivation.
- Maslow described a hierarchy of five levels of needs.
- Alderfer collapsed Maslow's theory into three levels.
- Herzberg applied Maslow's theory to work motivation.
- Herzberg identified hygiene and motivator factors related to satisfaction and dissatisfaction.
- McClelland identified three basic needs.
- Vroom represents the cognitive motivational theories.
- McGregor differentiated managers' attitudes into Theory X and Theory Y.

- The Hawthorne studies highlighted the importance of human interaction factors in work motivation.
- Personal and economic rewards are powerful motivators in nursing.
- The core of what motivates nurses is the work itself.
- Motivation is complex.
- The manager's job is to create an environment that fosters motivated behavior.

Study Questions

1. How do you stay motivated to love nursing for the rest of your life?
2. Does loving nursing guarantee quality care?
3. What is the motivation to enter nursing as a career? Is this changing?
4. How does real-world nursing practice compare with what motivation theories say?
5. What positive incentives are most important to nurses? To you personally?
6. What are the elements of a motivating environment?
7. Is it manipulative or Machiavellian to deliberately plan and implement rewards and incentives to get other people to perform? Do you ever do this?
8. Under cost-containment pressures, what is the effect on nurses of relying on recognition as the organizational motivation strategy?

CASE STUDY

John Smith is in his third year as a staff nurse in the surgical ICU at a large teaching hospital. The acuity level of the patients continues to increase as the number of staff nurses available in the ICU continues to decrease. The nursing shortage has affected the staffing ratios in the hospital and in Nurse Smith's unit. Increasingly, he is working mandatory overtime, has fewer days off, and is exhausted. Nurse Smith notices that the ICU is relying increasingly on external agency nurses. The agency nurses make more money, have better control over their schedules, and do not have to work mandatory overtime. He feels as though the hospital and nursing administration do not recognize the depth of the staffing problem and are doing little to address the working conditions. Morale on the unit continues to decline, staff nurses are quitting, and no new hires are found to take their place. Nurse Smith, too, is ready to quit and go to work for an agency where he'll make more money and have better control over his schedule.

1. What are the key factors in the ICU work environment, and how are they affecting the staff nurses?
2. How might motivation theories be used to analyze the situation?
3. What next steps would you take if you were the nurse manager in this ICU?

CRITICAL THINKING EXERCISE

Staff nurses in a coronary step-down unit feel as though they are spending most of their time "performing tasks" and moving patients quickly to discharge. They have little opportunity to be involved in patient education activities. The nurses want to be involved in designing programs that will educate patients about risk factors and lifestyle changes that will promote better health in the future. However, the nurse manager and the physicians do not see this as important. The job satisfaction of the nurses continues to decline on the unit.

1. How would you characterize the work environment on this unit?
2. What insights might be obtained from motivation theories?
3. What kinds of change might be implemented that would improve job satisfaction and increase the motivation of the staff?

REFERENCES

Alderfer, C. (1969). A new theory of human needs. *Organizational Behavior and Human Performance, 4*, 142-175.

Amabile, T.M. (1997). Motivating creativity in organizations: On doing what you love and loving what you do. *California Management Review, 40*(1), 39-58.

Ambrose, M.L., & Kulik, C.T. (1999). Old friends, new faces: Motivation research in the 1990s. *Journal of Management, 25*(3), 231-292.

Blanchard, K., Edington, D.W., & Blanchard, M. (1999). *The one minute manager balances work and life.* New York: W. Morrow.

D'Aunno, T.A., Fottler, M.D., & O'Connor, S.J. (2000). Motivating people. In S.M. Shortell & A.D. Kaluzny. *Health care management: Organization design and behavior.* Albany, NY: Delmar.

Hackman, J., & Oldham, G. (1979). *Work redesign.* Reading, MA: Addison-Wesley.

Henderson, M. (1993). Measuring managerial motivation: the power management inventory. *Journal of Nursing Measurement, 1*(1), 67-80.

Herzberg, F., Mausner, B., & Snyderman, B. (1959). *The motivation to work.* New York: John Wiley & Sons.

Herzberg, F. (2003). One more time: How do you motivate employees? *Harvard Business Review, 81*(1), 87-96.

Hofstede, G. (1993). Cultural constraints in management theories. *Academy of Management Executive, 7*(1), 81-94.

Kane, K., & Montgomery, K. (1998). A framework for understanding disempowerment in organizations. *Human Resource Management, 37*(3-4), 263-275.

Laamanen, R., Broms, U., Happola, A., & Brommels, M. (1999). Changes in the work and motivation of staff delivering home care services in Finland. *Public Health Nursing, 16*(1), 60-71.

Lachman, R. (1997). Taking another look at the elephant: Are we still (half) blind? Comments on the cross-cultural analysis of achievement motivation. *Journal of Organizational Behavior, 18*(7), 317-321.

Laschinger, H.K., Finegan, J., & Shamian, HJ. (2001). The impact of workplace empowerment, organizational trust on staff nurses' work satisfaction and organizational commitment. *Health Care Management Review, 26*(3), 7-23.

Lawler, III, E. (1973). *Motivation in work organizations.* Monterey, CA: Brooks/Cole Publishing.

Lewin, K. (1935). *A dynamic theory of personality.* New York: McGraw-Hill.

Locke, E., & Latham, G.P. (2004). What should we do about motivation theory? Six recommendations for the 21st century. *Academy of Management Review, 29*(3), 388-403.

Maslow, A. (1954). *Motivation and personality.* New York: Harper & Row.

McClelland, D. (1961). *The achieving society.* Princeton, NJ: Van Nostrand.

McClelland, D. (1976). Power is the great motivation. *Harvard Business Review, 54*(2), 100-110.

McClelland, D., & Boyatzis, R. (1982). Leadership motive patterns and long-term success in management. *Journal of Applied Psychology, 67*, 737-743.

McClure, M.L., & Hinshaw, A.S. (2002). *Magnet hospitals revisited: Attraction and retention of professional nurses.* Washington, DC: American Nurses Publishing.

McConnell, C.R. (1998). Employee involvement: motivation or manipulation? *Health Care Supervisor, 16*(3), 69-85.

McGregor, D. (1960). *The human side of enterprise.* New York: McGraw Hill.

Miner, J.B. (2002). *Organizational behavior: Foundations, theories and analyses.* New York: Oxford University Press.

Mitchell, T., & Daniels, D. (2003). Observations and commentary on recent research in work motivation. In L.W. Porter, G.A. Bigley, & R.M. Steers (Eds.), *Motivation and work behavior* (7th ed.) (pp. 26-44). Boston: McGraw-Hill/Irwin.

Morse, G. (2003). Why we misread motives: We think other people are more mercenary than they really are. *Harvard Business Review, 81*(1), 18-19.

Nicholson, N. (2003). How to motivate your problem people. *Harvard Business Review, 81*(1), 57-65.

O'Reilly, C.A., & Chatman, J.A. (1999). Working smarter and harder: A longitudinal study of managerial success. In L.W. Porter, G.A. Bigley, & R.M. Steers (Eds.), *Motivation and work behavior* (7th ed.) (pp. 603-627). Boston: McGraw-Hill/Irwin.

Pinder, C.C. (1998). *Work motivation in organizational behavior.* Upper Saddle River, NJ: Prentice-Hall.

Porter, L., Bigley, G.A., & Steers, R.M. (Ed.). (2003). *Motivation and work behavior.* (7th ed.). Boston: McGraw-Hill/Irwin.

Porter, L., & Lawler, E. (1968). *Managerial attitudes and performance.* Homewood, IL: Dorsey Press.

Price, J., & Mueller, C. (1986). *Handbook of organizational measurement.* Marshfield, MA: Pitman.

Rainey, H.G. (2001). Work motivation. In R.T. Golembiewski (Ed.), *Handbook of organizational behavior* (2nd ed.) (pp. 19-42). New York: Marcel Dekker, Inc.

Rantz, M.J., Scott, J., & Porter, R. (1996). Employee motivation: New perspectives of the age-old challenge of work motivation. *Nursing Forum, 31*(3), 29-36.

Redman, R.W., & Ketefian, S. (1995). Conceptual and methodological issues in work redesign. In K. Kelly & M. Maas (Ed.) *Series on nursing administration: Health care work redesign.* (Vol. VII). Thousand Oaks, CA: Sage Publications.

Rousseau, D.M. (2004). Psychological contracts in the workplace: Understanding the ties that motivate. *Academy of Management Executive, 18*(1), 120-127.

Sanchez-Runde, C.J., & Steers, R.M. (2001). Cultural influences on work motivation and performance. In L.W. Porter, G.A. Bigley, & R.M. Steers (Eds.). *Motivation and work behavior* (7th ed.) (pp. 357-374). Boston: McGraw-Hill/Irwin.

Schweiger, J. (1980). *The nurse as manager.* New York: John Wiley & Sons.

Steers, R., & Porter, L. (1987). *Motivation and work behavior* (4th ed.). New York: McGraw-Hill.

Steers, R.M., Mowday, R.T., & Shapiro, D.L. (2004). The future of work motivation theory. *Academy of Management Review, 29*(3), 379-387.

Tzeng, H.M. (2002). The influence of nurses' working motivation and job satisfaction on intention to quit: An empirical investigation in Taiwan. *International Journal of Nursing Studies, 39*(8), 867-878.

Vroom, V. (1964). *Work and motivation.* New York: John Wiley & Sons.

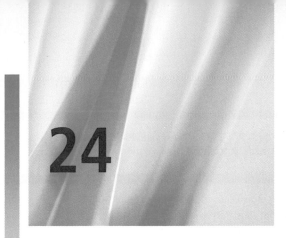

24

Power and Conflict

Kathleen B. Cox

// POWER

For many nurses, power has had a negative connotation. With major issues and challenges facing the health care delivery system in the United States and the nature of work in today's complex health care organizations, it is imperative that nurses accept the reality and legitimacy of power. Although the United States has one of the most sophisticated health care systems in the world, there are major issues related to costs, access, and quality. The United States spends more on health care than any other industrialized country. Health care spending rose to $1.6 trillion in 2002, up from $1.4 trillion in 2001 and $1.3 trillion in 2000. The health care share of GDP increased to 14.1% in 2001 and 14.9% in 2002 (Centers for Medicare & Medicaid Services [CMS], 2004). In addition, an estimated 15.2% of the population, or 43.6 million people, were without health insurance during 2003, up from 14.6% in 2001 (Mills & Bhandari, 2003). Minority Americans face serious disparities in disease incidence, morbidity, and mortality, as well as in the health care they receive (Modlin, 2003). Finally, the Institute of Medicine's (IOM) landmark report in 2000 estimated that 44,000 to 98,000 people die each year as a result of medical errors (Kohn et al., 2000). The chaos and uncertainty in the health care environment provide unlimited opportunities for the profession of nursing. As the largest health care profession, nursing must use power and influence as a legitimate tool to facilitate change in health care organizations and the health care system.

DEFINITIONS

Although power connotes strength and ability, the term *power* has different meanings. It can mean the ability to compel obedience, control, or dominate; or it can be a delegated right or privilege as

⚠ LEADING & MANAGING **DEFINED**

Power

The capability of acting or producing some sort of effect, the potential capacity to exert influence.

Relational Aspect of Power

Power is a property of a social relationship.

Dependency Aspect of Power

Power resides in the other's dependency on the powerful one.

Sanctioning Aspect of Power

Power is an active, direct manipulation of another's outcomes.

Empowerment

Giving individuals the authority, responsibility and freedom to act on what they know and instilling the confidence to do so.

---

occurs in the power to enact the staff nurse role. **Power** can be defined as the capability of acting or producing some sort of an effect, usually associated with the ability to influence the allocation of scarce resources. Other definitions identify power as the potential capacity to exert influence, characteristically backed by a means to coerce compliance. A key element to power is its aspect of being potential as well as actual.

There are three formal dimensions of power, as follows (Bacharach & Lawler, 1980):

1. The relational aspect
2. The dependence aspect
3. The sanctioning aspect

The **relational aspect of power** suggests that power is a property of a social relationship. Many definitions (Bierstedt, 1950; Blau, 1964; Kaplan, 1964; Mechanic, 1962) indicate that power has to do with relationships between two or more actors in which the behavior of one is affected by the other. Weber (1947) defined power as "the probability that one actor within a social relationship will be in a position to carry out his own will, despite resistance, and regardless of the basis on which this probability rests" (p. 52). Dahl (1957) also defined power as an interactive process and stated that "A has power over B to the extent that he can get B to do something B would not otherwise do" (pp. 202-203).

The second formal aspect, the **dependency aspect of power**, was addressed by Emerson (1957),

who suggested that power resides implicitly in the other's dependency:

> Social relations commonly entail ties of mutual dependence between the parties. A depends on B if he aspires to goals or gratifications whose achievement is facilitated by appropriate actions on B's part. By virtue of mutual dependency, it is more or less imperative to each party that he be able to control or influence the other's conduct. At the same time, these ties of mutual dependence imply that each party is in a position, to some degree, to grant or deny, facilitate or hinder, the other's gratification. Thus, it would appear that the power to control or influence the other resides in control over the things he values, which may range all the way from oil resources to ego-support, depending on the relation in question. (p. 32)

Dependency is particularly evident in organizations that require interdependence of personnel and subunits. Daft (2003) defined *interdependence* as the extent to which departments depend on each other for resources or materials to accomplish their task. The highest level of interdependence is reciprocal interdependence. Reciprocal interdependence exists when the output of operation A is the input to operation B, and the output of operation B is the input back again to operation A. Daft noted that hospitals are excellent examples of reciprocal interdependence because they provide coordinated services to patients.

The third formal aspect, the **sanctioning aspect of power**, is the active component of the power relationship, referring to the direct manipulations of the other's outcomes. Sanctions can consist of manipulations of rewards, punishments, or both. Sanctions are a significant part of the process through which parties actually affect one another. In summary, power is a property of a social relationship between two or more actors, in which one is dependent on the other. Sanctions are applied in the form of rewards, punishments, or both.

Empowerment

Empowerment is a corollary concept to power in groups and organizations. **Empowerment** is defined as giving individuals the authority, responsibility, and freedom to act on what they know and instilling in them belief and confidence in their own ability to achieve and succeed (Kramer & Schmalenberg, 1990). Thus empowerment has two meanings: the transfer of actual power and the inspiring of self-confidence. Both aspects enable others to act. Empowerment is a key leadership component.

Employee empowerment became a popular topic in the 1990s, especially in the business literature. With an emphasis on customer service and improving the bottom line through capitalizing on the creative and innovative energy of employees, businesses sought a strategic advantage. Empowerment programs were developed to improve productivity, lower costs, or raise customer satisfaction. However, growing evidence suggests that these empowerment programs fail to meet either managers' or employees' expectations, possibly because while empowerment programs promise employees power, they may not deliver on the promise (Hardy & Leiba-O'Sullivan, 1998).

Empowerment initiatives take two forms. First is the relational approach. The aim here is to improve performance by decentralizing power by delegating power, authority, and decision making. In theory, this reduces organizational barriers to getting the job done. Self-managing teams are one example (Hardy & Leiba-O'Sullivan, 1998).

The second empowerment strategy is the motivational approach. With this approach, there is less delegation of power and more emphasis on open communication and inspirational goal setting. The affective domain is emphasized, with feelings of ownership, responsibility, capability, commitment, and involvement. The goal is to improve employees' self-efficacy, ability to cope with adversity, and willingness to act independently and responsibly. Increasing self-efficacy and decreasing feelings of powerlessness have been linked to effective performance. Examples are training programs for group dynamics and group problem solving.

AUTHORITY AND INFLUENCE

Authority and influence are two major content dimensions of power (Bacharach & Lawler, 1980). There have been three conceptualizations of authority and influence. Some authors equate these terms; others tend to equate power with influence and assert that authority is a special case of power. Still others view authority and influence as distinctly different dimensions of power. Several points of contrast are summarized in Table 24.1.

Influence Tactics

Kipnis and colleagues (1980) were among the first to investigate the influence behavior of managers. Content analysis lead to the identification of 370 different forms of influence behavior, which were condensed into 14 categories. Subsequently, factor analysis brought about the following eight forms of influence behavior:

1. *Assertiveness* means expressing one's own position to another without inhibiting the rights of others.
2. *Ingratiation* means trying to make the other person feel important: giving praise or sympathizing. Ingratiation is attempting to advance oneself by trying to make another person feel important.

Table 24.1

Authority and Influence Contrasted

Authority	Influence
Authority is a static, structural aspect of power in organizations.	Influence is the dynamic, tactical element.
Authority is the formal aspect of power.	Influence is the informal aspect.
Authority refers to the formally sanctioned right to make decisions.	Influence is not sanctioned by the organization and is, therefore, not a matter of organizational rights.
Authority implies involuntary submission by subordinates.	Influence implies voluntary submission and does not necessarily entail a superior-subordinate relationship.
Authority flows downward, and it is unidirectional.	Influence is multidirectional and can flow upward, downward, or horizontally.
The source of authority is solely structural.	The source of influence may be personal characteristics, expertise, or opportunity.
Authority is circumscribed.	The domain, scope, and legitimacy of influence are typically ambiguous.

3. *Rationality* means using logical and rational arguments, providing pertinent information, presenting reasons, and laying an idea out in a logical, structured way.

4. *Sanctions* are threats. Positive sanctions, or rewards, are addressed within motivation mechanisms.

5. *Exchange* means that to persuade, an exchange is offered; this is sometimes called "scratching each other's back."

6. *Upward appeal* means going to a higher authority: the childhood threat of "if you don't play by my rules, I am going to go tell mom." Upward appeal simply means taking the appeal to a higher authority to arbitrate.

7. *Blocking* means deliberately keeping others from getting their way, threatening to stop working with them, ignoring them, not being friendly, or simply attempting to make sure others cannot accomplish their aims.

8. *Coalitions* are the result of a group of people getting together to speak or negotiate as one voice.

In their three-nation study of managerial influence styles, Kipnis and colleagues (1984) identified the most-to-least–popular strategies (Table 24.2).

Yukl and Falbe (1991) continued the work of Kipnis and colleagues (1980). They developed an instrument, the Influence Behavior Questionnaire (IBQ), to measure the influence behavior of managers. In later studies, the IBQ was developed further and psychometric tests were performed (Yukl et al., 1992; Yukl et al., 1993). The nine tactics cover a wide range of influence behavior relevant for managerial effectiveness or, in a broader sense, for getting things done in an organization. Influence tactics are identified in Table 24.3.

SOURCES OF POWER

Individual Sources of Power

Although multiple mechanisms of power have been identified, the most widely accepted power base classification is French and Raven's (1959) five sources of power. Their original conceptualization identified the following five power sources (Box 24.1):

1. Reward
2. Coercive

Table 24.2

Most-to-Least–Popular Managerial Influence Strategies Used in All Countries		
Strategy's Popularity	Managers Influencing Superiors	Managers Influencing Subordinates
Most popular ↑ ↓ Least popular	Reason Coalition Friendliness Bargaining Assertiveness Higher authority	Reason Assertiveness Friendliness Evaluation Bargaining Higher authority Sanction

Modified from Kipnis, D., Schmidt, S.M., Swaffin-Smith, C. & Wilkinson, I. (1984). Patterns of managerial influence: Shotgun managers, tacticians, and bystanders. *Organizational Dynamics, 12*(3), 58-67.

Table 24.3

Definitions of Influence Tactics	
Tactic	Definition
Rational persuasion	The agent uses logical arguments and factual evidence to persuade the target that a proposal or request is viable and likely to result in the attainment of task objectives.
Inspiration appeals	The agent makes a request or proposal that arouses target enthusiasm by appealing to his or her values, ideals, and aspirations or by increasing target self-confidence.
Consultation	The agent seeks target participation in planning a strategy, activity, or change for which target support and assistance are desired, or the agent is willing to modify a proposal to deal with target concerns and suggestions.
Ingratiation	The agent uses praise, flattery, friendly behavior, or helpful behavior to get the target in a "good mood" or to think favorably of the agent before asking for something.
Personal appeals	The agent appeals to target feelings of loyalty and friendship toward him or her before asking for something.
Exchange	The agent offers an exchange of favors, indicates willingness to reciprocate at a later time, or promises a share of the benefits if the target helps to accomplish a task.
Coalition tactics	The agent seeks the aid of others to persuade the target to do something or uses the support of others as a reason for the target to agree as well.
Legitimating tactics	The agent seeks to establish the legitimacy of a request by claiming the authority or right to make it or by verifying that it is consistent with organizational policies, rules, practices, or traditions.
Pressure	The agent uses demands, threats, frequent checking, or persistent reminders to influence the target to do what the agent wants.

From Yukl, G., Falbe, C., & Joo, Y.Y. (1993). Patterns of influence behavior for managers. *Group and Organization Management, 18*(1), 5-28.

Box **24.1**

French and Raven's Five Sources of Power

1. *Reward power* is giving something of value. For example, in nursing, rewards may be a pay raise, praise, a promotion, or a job on the day shift. Reward power is based on the ability to deliver desired rewards.
2. *Coercive power* is force against the will. For example, in nursing coercive power can be the threat of firing, of disciplinary action, or other negative consequences. Coercive power is the power derived from an ability to threaten punishment and deliver penalties. It is a source of power used to apply pressure so that others will meet what is demanded.
3. *Expert power* means the use of expertise. It is knowledge, competence, communication, and personal power all combined in a reservoir of knowledge and experience. Expert power is a source of power held by those with some special knowledge, skill, or competence in a particular area. For example, the nurse with the greatest expertise in wound dressings will be sought out by other people in the work environment for this expertise. Expertise is an artful combination of skill and knowledge. It may be founded on depth of knowledge and/or psychomotor skill. In the use of knowledge and skill is power: because people need you or can benefit from your expertise, power exists. Therefore the use of expertise can be structured to accomplish or influence movement or action toward certain goals.
4. *Referent power* is a little more difficult to understand because it is subtle. It is the use of charisma to influence others. The followers of someone with referent power respond positively to the interpersonal communication and image of the charismatic person. In organizations, this translates into an informal leadership based on liking, charisma, or personal power. Referent power comes from the affinity other people have for someone. They admire the personal qualities, problem-solving ability, style, or the dedication the person brings to the work. Referent power can be viewed as an inspirational power, because people's admiration for someone allows that person to influence without having to offer rewards or threaten punishments. For example, in the political arena, occasionally there are charismatic political figures or orators. Their influence comes from their followers' liking or identification with them. An example in nursing is Florence Nightingale, who became a symbol of professional nursing. There is an emotional upsweep felt by associating with a charismatic person. Referent power is a personal liking and identification experienced by others. Followers attribute referent power to a leader on the basis of the leader's personal characteristics and interpersonal appeal. Physical attractiveness may contribute to referent power.
5. *Legitimate power* means position power. It is the right to command within the organizational structure, based on the hierarchical position held. The President of the United States has power because of holding the position. Legitimate power is the most common source of power. It is what most often is called *authority*. The authority of position gives the person the right to act, order, and direct others. However, leadership and influence need not be confined to those with authority. Every person possesses the ability to tap different sources of power to use in a variety of situations.

Data from French, J., & Raven, B. (1959). The bases of social power. In D. Cartwright (Ed.), *Studies in social power* (pp. 150-167). Ann Arbor, MI: University of Michigan, Institute for Social Research.

---

3. Expert
4. Referent
5. Legitimate

When reward power is used, people comply because doing so produces positive benefits.

Coercive power depends on fear. An individual reacts to the fear of the negative consequences that might occur for failure to comply. Referent power is based on admiration for a person who has desirable resources or personal traits.

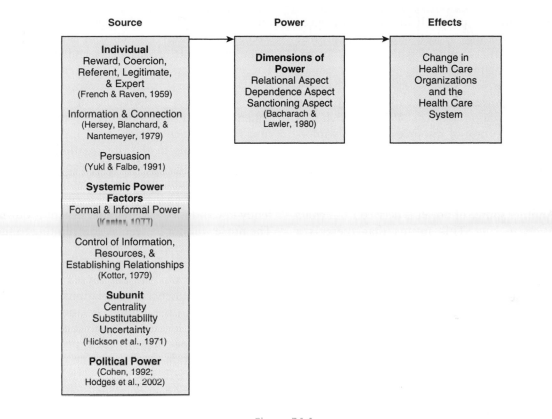

Figure 24 1
Conceptual framework for power.

Legitimate power represents the power a person receives as a result of his or her position in the formal organizational hierarchy. Expert power results from expertise, special skill, or knowledge. The problem with the French and Raven typology is that the list is not exhaustive and it ignores organizational sources of power. Figure 24.1 shows a combined conceptual framework for power that blends elements of multiple theories of power.

Other Sources of Power

Raven and Kruglanski (1975) and Hersey and colleagues (1979) identified two additional sources of power: (1) connection power and (2) information power. A third type of power also has been identified: (3) group decision-making power (Liberatore et al., 1989). These three other sources of power are related to groups and organizations specifically, as opposed to French and Raven's (1959) original five sources of power that relate more to an individual.

Within organizations, the power of connections comes from networking or knowing people and from being able to go across lines laterally to gather information. For example, this occurs when a nurse knows a colleague in another facility with whom to exchange information. For a nurse to know what effective nursing interventions are being used by other institutions helps the institution to be competitive and current. *Connection power* is one strategy to get information accurately and reliably. It also may be manifested as power based on having connections with powerful others. Connection power is based on another's perception that the influencer has access to powerful persons or groups.

Information is power. If information is given away, its power may be lost. This is especially true in situations that require negotiation. If information is used strategically, its possession can be a strong source of power. *Information power* is a source of power that can stem from any person in the organization. Kanter's (1977) research suggested that control of resources, especially information, is a major organizational power source. Information power is based on another's perception that the influencer either possesses or has access to information valuable to another.

Another source of power is derived from *group decision making*. This means that there is a creative synergy and force created when a group comes together, makes decisions, and acts as a united front. For example, some professional groups have formed strong lobbies to influence state and national legislation. With more than 2.5 million licensed registered nurses in the United States, group decision making with resultant unity of action could be a powerful strategy for nurses to use to advance nursing's goals or policy agenda.

Persuasive power is an additional source of power identified by later researchers investigating French and Ravens' (1959) taxonomy. Persuasive power refers to skill in making rational appeals (Yukl & Falbe, 1991). Yukl and Falbe (1991) differentiated between position power and personal power. According to these authors, position power consists of legitimate, reward coercive, and information power. Personal power consists of expert, referent, persuasive power.

In her structural theory of organizational behavior, Kanter (1977) asserted that "those with sufficient power are able to accomplish the tasks required to achieve organizational goals" (p. 166). Conditions in the work environment influence how much productive power is available to employees. According to Kanter, formal and informal systemic structures are the sources of workplace empowerment. Job discretion, recognition, and relevance to organizational goals are important dimensions of formal power. High levels of job discretion ensure that work is non-routinized

and permit flexibility, adaptation, and creativity. Recognition reflects visibility of an employee's accomplishments among peers and supervisors. For example, an innovative staff development director or nurse manager whose techniques are reported in a respected nursing journal will enhance his or her influence in the hospital. Finally, relevance of job responsibilities and accomplishments to the organization's strategic plan or current problems is also important. A nurse who publishes will probably not accrue much power when the hospital's census is consistently low and Medicare reimbursement is down. The nurse will not be seen as contributing to the solution of pressing organizational problems. Another key systemic structure is informal power, which comes from the employee's network of interpersonal alliances or relationships within and outside an organization. Relationships with people at higher hierarchical levels confer approval, prestige, and backing, whereas peer networks provide reputation and "grapevine" information (Kanter, 1977).

In Kanter's model, individuals with high levels of formal and informal power have access to structures of productive power within an organization. These structures include lines of information, lines of support and lines of resources/supply. The lines of information involve formal information that is necessary to carry out a job, as well as informal information that concerns the current state of affairs within an organization. Lines of support include positive feedback from superiors and important others, as well as support for job autonomy. Lines of resources address the ability to obtain the materials, money, and rewards necessary for achieving job demands. Access to opportunity for professional growth and movement in the organization completes the necessary tools for success at work. Kanter claimed that working in these conditions has a positive impact on employees, that is, increased feelings of self-efficacy and job satisfaction, higher motivation, and less burnout. These empowering conditions create more productive work environments because employees are highly effective and more satisfied with their jobs, more committed to organizational goals, more likely to try out innovative approaches to work, and less likely to be stressed at work or to change jobs.

Kanter's theory has been tested extensively in nursing populations. These populations have been found to be only moderately empowered, with varying levels of access to information, support, opportunity, and resources (Laschinger & Havens, 1997; Laschinger et al., 2001b). Higher levels of structural empowerment have been associated with higher levels of organizational commitment (Laschinger et al., 2000), greater participation in organizational decision-making (Laschinger et al., 1997), higher levels of job autonomy (Sabiston & Laschinger 1995), higher levels of job satisfaction (Laschinger & Havens 1997; Laschinger et al., 2001a), and greater organizational trust (Laschinger et al., 2000). All these findings lend support to Kanter's theory.

Kotter (1979) maintained that the basic methods for acquiring and maintaining power are gaining control over tangible resources, obtaining information and control of information channels, and establishing favorable relationships. Basically, acquiring and maintaining power is an exercise in developing credibility by getting people to feel obligated in some way, building a good professional reputation through visible achievement, encouraging identification by trying to look and behave in ways that others respect, and finally, creating perceived dependence either for help or security. The keys to success at gaining power are as follows:

- Be sensitive to where power exists in the organization
- Take calculated risks
- Recognize that all actions can affect power and avoid actions that will decrease it
- Try to move up in the organizational hierarchy and toward positions that control a strategic contingency for the organization

In summary, control of information and resources and development of support systems are common elements in both Kanter's and Kotter's theories.

THE POWER OF THE SUBUNIT

Subunit or horizontal power pertains to relationships across departments. Daft (2003) noted that while each department makes a unique contribution to organizational success, some contributions are greater than others. Pfeffer (1981) identified the following structural determinants of power within organizations:

- *Power is derived from dependence.* Simply stated, power comes from having something that someone else wants or needs and being in control of the performance or resource so that there are few, if any, alternative sources for obtaining what is desired.
- *Power is derived from providing resources.* Organizations require a continuing provision of resources such as personnel, money, customers, and technology in order to continue to function. Those subunits or individuals within the organization that can provide the most critical and difficult-to-obtain resources come to have power in organizations. Their power is derived from their ability to furnish those resources upon which the organization most depends.
- *Power is derived from coping with uncertainty.* Coping with uncertainty is a critical resource in the organization since it ensures organizational survival and adaptation to external constraints.
- *Power is derived from being irreplaceable.* Members must not only provide a critical resource for the organization but also prevent themselves from being readily replaced in that function. The degree of substitutability is not a fixed thing, however, so one might expect that various strategies will be employed by individuals and subunits who are interested in enhancing their power within the organization. Some of these might involve the availability of documentation, use of specialized language, centralization of knowledge, and maintenance of externally-based sources of expertise.
- *Power is derived from the ability to affect the decision process.* Because decisions are made in a sequential process, it is possible for an individual

to acquire power because of his or her ability to affect the premises of basic values or objectives used in making any decision. A person can gain power by influencing the information about the alternatives being considered in the decision process.

- *Power is derived if there is a shared consensus within the organizational subunit.* If individuals within a subunit share a common perspective, set of values or definition of the situation, they are likely to act and speak in a consistent manner and present to the larger organization an easily articulated and understood position and perspective. Such a consensus can serve to enhance the power of the subunit among other organizational members.

The strategic contingencies theory of intra-organization power proposed by Hickson and colleagues (1971) specified the conditions for the differentiation of power among organizational subunits. The strategic contingencies theory of power relates the power of a subunit to its coping with uncertainty, substitutability, and centrality, through the control of strategic contingencies. *First,* according to strategic contingencies theory, a unit will become powerful if it is able to control scarce resources that are important to the organization as a whole. *Second,* a unit will become powerful if it is able to control uncertainty. Organizations fear the unknown, because unanticipated events create havoc with financial commitments, long-range plans, and tomorrow's operations. Sources of uncertainty include a change in governmental policies, changes in supply and demand, and an unexpected downturn in the economy. *Third,* a unit will become powerful it its activities are central to the workflow of the organization. Subunits may influence the work of most other subunits. Centrality also exists when a subunit has an especially crucial impact on the quantity or quality of the organizations key product or service. A subunit's activities are more central when their impact is more immediate. Several studies in the management literature have provided support for this theory (Crozier, 1964; Hinings et al., 1974; Salancik & Pfeffer, 1974). Dennis (1983) suggested

that the nursing profession would do well to listen to and study the advice of Hinings and colleagues (1974): "For dominant power, take advantage of immediacy, reduce your substitutability, and then make a bid for a decisive area of uncertainty … but don't get involved in a network of interaction links before you can dominate it" (p. 56). In other words, find ways to help the organization decrease uncertainty, position yourself to be central rather than peripheral, and make your function indispensable or nonsubstitutable.

The Theory of Group Power within Organizations was developed from a synthesis and reformulation of King's (1981) interacting systems framework and the Strategic Contingencies Theory of Power (Hickson et al., 1971). Variables within the Strategic Contingencies Theory of Power and their relationships were reformulated within King's framework. These variables are controlling the effects of environmental forces, position, resources, and role. Sieloff (2003) noted that although nursing groups are proposed to have a power capacity resulting from controlling the effects of environment forces, position, resources, and role, not all nursing groups have acted powerfully. Therefore four additional concepts were added to the theory as variables that intervened between a nursing group's power capacity and its ability to actualize that power capacity. These concepts are communication competency, goal/outcome competency, nurse leader's power competency, and power perspective. Every nursing group has a power capacity. The group has the potential to achieve their goals and become a more visible contributor to the progress of the organization. The value of the theory is that it provides nurse leaders at all levels with strategies that could be implemented to improve a nursing group's actualized power (Sieloff, 2003).

LEADERSHIP AND MANAGEMENT IMPLICATIONS

Robbins and Langton (1999) differentiated between power and leadership and indicated that the two concepts are closely intertwined. Leaders use power

Research Note

Source: Sieloff, C.L. (2003). Measuring nursing power within organizations. *Journal of Nursing Scholarship, 35*(2), 183-187.

Purpose

The Sieloff-King Assessment of Departmental Power (SKADP) was originally designed to measure the power of nursing departments within the hospital. The instrument has been revised and renamed. The purpose of the study was to describe psychometric evaluation of the 36-item Sieloff-King Assessment of Group Power within Organizations (SKAGPO) instrument. A survey of 357 chief nurse executives in the United States was conducted to evaluate the psychometric properties of the SKAGPO. Psychometric evaluation of the SKAGPO included the following: (1) internal consistency reliability using Cronbach's alpha coefficient, split-half with the equal-length Spearman Brown Correction Formula, and item analysis; (2) concurrent criterion-related validity; and (3) factor analysis.

Discussion

Cronbach's alpha coefficient for the SKAGPO was 0.92. Subscales' alpha ranged from 0.63 to 0.88. Item-total correlations ranged from 0.24 to 0.68 with an average item-total correlation of 0.48 (n = 334). Concurrent criterion-related validity was supported with a correlation of 0.63 between the SKAGPO and the criterion. An exploratory factor analysis with varimax rotation resulted in eight factors that explained 61.1% of variance. The factors were controlling the effects of environmental forces, position, power perspective, resources, role, chief nurse executive's power competency, communication competency, and goal and outcome competency. Results of the analysis provided support for the reliability and validity of the revised instrument.

Application to Practice

It is critical for nurses to understand that power is a legitimate tool and can be used to facilitate change and achieve goals. As an abstract concept, power is very difficult to measure. The research is relevant because it is one of the first studies to identify the reliability and validity of an instrument designed to estimate the level of nursing power within the organization. The new measure may possibly be used not only to measure power of nursing in organizations, but also to explore the relationships between power and other variables of interest to nursing administrators. As such, the new measure has the potential to increase our understanding of power in organizations.

as a means of attaining group goals. Leaders achieve goals, and power is a means of facilitating goal achievement. One of the main differences between the two concepts relates to goal compatibility. Power requires dependence, but it does not require goal compatibility. On the other hand, leadership requires congruence between the goals of the leader and those being led. In addition, power focuses on intimidation, whereas leadership focuses on downward influence. Power maximizes the importance of lateral and upward influence, but leadership minimizes the importance of lateral and upward influence. Finally, power focuses on tactics for gaining compliance, whereas

leadership research focuses on answers (Robbins & Langton, 1999).

POWER AND LEADERSHIP

Power and leadership are closely connected and highly intertwined concepts. This is because power is one of the vehicles by which a leader influences followers to take action. Nurses may be inclined to avoid an acknowledgement or analysis of power. However, to lead and manage, nurses need to acquire, possess, and use power.

Hersey and colleagues (2001) described the relationships among concepts of style of leadership, readiness level of followers, and power base use. They indicated that the readiness of the followers dictates which leadership style is likely to be successful and which power base would most successfully influence followers' behavior. Combining these concepts maximizes the leader's probability of success. Thus nurses should be able to use Situational Leadership Theory to assess and predict style choice and power source use based on the situation and readiness of followers.

Readiness is the ability and willingness of individuals or groups to take responsibility for directing their own behavior in a situation. There appears to be a direct relationship between the level of readiness in individuals and groups and the power base type that has a high probability of effectiveness for use with them (Figure 24.2). Readiness is a task-specific concept. At the lowest level of readiness, coercive power is most appropriate. As people move to higher readiness levels, connection power, then reward, then legitimate, then referent, then information, and finally, expert power impact the behavior of people. At the highest level the followers have competence and confidence, and they are most responsive to expert power (Hersey et al., 2001).

If power is the basic energy needed to initiate and sustain action, then power is a quality without which a leader cannot lead. Power is fundamental to leadership, in that leadership may be the wise use of power. This is especially true for transformative leadership (Bennis & Nanus, 1985). Power need is highly desirable in leaders and managers. This is because power is necessary in influencing others. Assertiveness and self-confidence are associated with power and leadership. Leadership may be characterized as power in the service of others (Kouzes & Posner, 1987). For nurses, this may mean that they need to view power as an integral part of their professional roles in care management and client advocacy. Nursing leadership requires a willingness and ability to take on a power role and to expand the use of power bases.

All of these theories provide insight into the nature of power. Although the strategic contingencies theory specified the conditions for the differentiation of power among organizational subunits, certainly the principles of uncertainty, centrality, and substitutability can be applied to increase the power of the nursing profession within organizations and also within the health care system. In addition, Sieloff's (2003) notion of

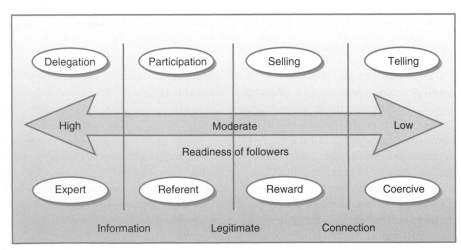

Figure 24.2
Power related to leadership. (Data from Hersey, P., Blanchard, K.H., & Johnson, D.E. [1996]. *Management of organizational behavior: Utilizing human resources* [7th ed.]. Upper Saddle River, NJ: Prentice-Hall.)

leadership behaviors that foster nursing group power is also relevant.

Uncertainty

Nurses must demonstrate that they can cope with uncertainty. Examples of uncertainties include, but are not limited to, patient safety, the aging population, chronic and other diseases, bioterrorism, and technology, as well as access, costs, and quality of health care.

Quality of Care and Patient Safety

In November 1999, the Institute of Medicine (IOM) issued a comprehensive report on medical errors, *To Err Is Human: Building a Safer Health System* (Kohn et al., 2000). Speaking to the seriousness of the problem and issuing a call for action on the part of nurses and others, the report indicated that it is not acceptable for patients to be harmed by the health care system. Obviously, nurses who are directly involved with patients must play a key role in the assessment of organizational safety, creation of safer systems, and implementation and evaluation of those systems.

Aging Population

The population's increasing longevity is a source of uncertainty and a driving force for the development of improved services for the elderly. The number of elderly, defined as the population "age 65 and over," will grow by more than 50% between 2000 and 2020 and by an estimated 127% by 2050. Furthermore, the relative size of the elderly population is projected to increase from 12.6% of the population in 2000 to an estimated 16.5% in 2020. Between 2030 and 2050, one in five Americans will be elderly (U.S. Department of Health and Human Services, Bureau of Health Professions [USDHHS, BHP], 2003). Nurses can increase power by demonstrating that they can maintain the health of the elderly and provide skilled nursing care in home and community settings.

Technology

The rapid growth in information technology has already had an impact on health care delivery, and nurses need to be skilled in the use of computer technology. Developing expertise in new technology for diagnosis and treatment as well as telemedicine will enable nursing to become invaluable and indispensable.

Use of health care websites by consumers tripled in 2002 as individuals spent more time exploring their options before making health care decisions (Stokowski, 2004). However, many consumers will need assistance in understanding their options and making the decisions that are best for them. In a recent Harris poll, 92% of consumers indicated they trusted the information nurses gave to them (Ulrich, 2001); therefore nurses are well positioned to assume a central role as advisors and teachers.

The quality of consumer health information on the Internet is an important issue for nursing. The large volume of health information resources available on the Internet has great potential to improve health, but it is increasingly difficult to determine which resources are accurate or appropriate for users. Because of the potential for harm from misleading and inaccurate health information, the profession has a responsibility to ensure the availability and accuracy of information obtained through the Internet. Developing expertise in the use of computer technology is another way of becoming invaluable and indispensable and of demonstrating the ability to cope with uncertainty.

Chronic Disease

For millions of Americans, living with chronic disease is a way of life. Research is needed to determine best practices for care and management of chronic disease. In order to turn the tide on chronic disease, nurses need to be at the forefront of efforts to provide education for young and old clients on healthy lifestyles including diet, exercise, and stress management (Stokowski, 2004). By demonstrating the ability to handle this uncertainty, nursing can assume a central role in improving the care of the chronically ill.

Other Diseases

Recent years have seen the appearance of antibiotic-resistant infections, lethal strains of influenza,

West Nile virus, SARS, mad-cow disease, and drug-resistant tuberculosis. In addition, the AIDS virus continues to mutate and spread, and the threat of bioterrorism carries the risk for infecting millions with smallpox or anthrax. Nurses must demonstrate that they can contain and prevent the spread of these infectious diseases. They must increase their awareness of the threat of communicable diseases and their role in preventing and managing the public health crises they represent (Stokowski, 2004).

Cost and Access

In addition to coping with organizational uncertainties, the profession must be prepared to cope with uncertainties in the health care system. As noted earlier, access, cost, and quality are major uncertainties in the health care system. With health care costs and the number of uninsured increasing, nurse-managed health centers (NMHCs) could help meet the need for cost-effective quality care and for improving access. These health centers have been in existence for about 25 to 30 years. There are approximately 200 NMHCs located in rural communities, homeless shelters, senior centers, public housing, churches, urban storefronts, elementary schools, and on Native-American reservations. The centers serve vulnerable populations such as the poor, the elderly, the uninsured, and those with cultural or language barriers that hinder access to health care (Report of the National Nursing Summit Addressing Nurse-Managed Health Centers, 2002). Although financial sustainability is the top issue facing these health centers, they offer another way of demonstrating nursing's ability to cope with uncertainty.

Centrality and Substitutability

Professional nurses have a high degree of centrality within health care organizations. They are critical to the operation of most health care organizations, and without nurses, many health care facilities would not be able to offer services. Nursing must maintain that power by becoming irreplaceable. Strong chief nurse executives with strong formal power are needed to create conditions within the organization and the health care system that make nurses difficult to replace. Nagle (1999) cautioned that unless we profile the value of registered nurses, other care providers will be substituted. In other words, the profession must demonstrate its economic value. During the early 1990s, restructuring and redesigning care delivery was initiated in order to contain costs. Decisions were made to replace registered nurses with less skilled unlicensed personnel because nurses were seen as too costly. Also, new models of patient-centered care delivered by cross-trained unlicensed personnel were implemented. Because there was little or no evidence of nursing services in hospital billing systems, nursing was not able to veto those cost-driven decisions. Consequently, authority in decision making—such as arguing to direct cost-cutting to more appropriate targets than direct-care nursing staff—has been nearly impossible (Kany, 2004).

Also, there has been a dearth of research establishing and quantifying the relationship between nursing staffing and patient outcomes (Kany, 2004). Fortunately, this situation is changing. For example, Unruh (2003) has demonstrated that a 10% increase in nurse staffing was associated with fewer adverse patient events. Aiken and colleagues' (2002) study demonstrated that in hospitals with high patient-to-nurse ratios, surgical patients experience higher risk-adjusted 30-day mortality and failure-to-rescue rates, and nurses are more likely to experience burnout and job dissatisfaction. Without documentation of the value of this profession, nursing will be excluded from decision making on a range of issues, at all levels within health care facilities.

CONFLICT

The same turbulent health care environment that demands the use of power also creates the conditions that breed conflict. Health care in the United States has gone through dramatic changes in recent decades. Change increases conflict in organizations (Gardner, 1992; Johnson, 1994), may be counterproductive to patients (Forte, 1997), and has a negative impact on teamwork (Cox, 2001) and work satisfaction (Cox, 2001; Gardner, 1992).

Managers spend about 20% of their time dealing with conflict, and they rate conflict management skills as equally important or slightly more important than planning, communication, motivation, and decision making (McElhaney, 1996). Caudron (2000) reported that line managers list managing conflict as seventh on the top 10 list of priorities. Given the effect that conflict has on patients, teamwork, work satisfaction, and the time that managers spend on conflict, it is imperative that nurses at all levels understand the nature of conflict and the approaches to managing conflict.

Most people know when conflict exists because it is a part of everyday experience. Conflict is a part of life that arises because of the complexity of human relationships. Conflict has its origin in the fact that each person is unique and possesses a value system, philosophy, personality structure, preferences, and styles. Understanding how to maneuver around and manage conflict situations increases the ability to be more effective both in personal and professional roles.

DEFINITIONS

There are many definitions and uses of the term *conflict* (Albanese, 1981). As a noun, *conflict* is defined as "a state of open, often prolonged fighting; a battle or war" (*American Heritage College Dictionary*, 1997, p. 292). Another use of the noun form is "a state of disharmony between incompatible or antithetical person, ideas, or interests, i.e., a clash" (*American Heritage College Dictionary*, 1997, p. 292). From a psychological perspective, conflict is "a psychic struggle resulting from the opposition or simultaneous functioning of mutually exclusive impulses, desires, or tendencies" (*American Heritage College Dictionary*, 1997, p. 292). In a work of drama or fiction, conflict is "the opposition between characters or forces in a work of drama or fiction." As a verb, *conflict* means "to be in or come into opposition" (*American Heritage College Dictionary*, 1997, p. 292).

Conflict is defined here as a clash or struggle that occurs when a real or perceived threat or difference exists in the desires, thoughts, attitudes, feelings, or behaviors of two or more parties (Deutsch, 1973). It exists as a tension or struggle arising from mutually exclusive or opposing actions, thoughts, opinions, or feelings. Conflict can be internal or external to an individual or group. It can be positive as well as negative.

⚠ LEADING & MANAGING **DEFINED**

Conflict

A clash or struggle that occurs when a real or perceived threat or difference exists in the desires, thoughts, attitudes, feelings, or behaviors of two or more parties.

Organizational Conflict

The struggle for scarce organizational resources.

Job Conflict

A perceived opposition or antagonistic process at the individual-organization level.

Competitive Conflict

Rules-based conflict with the goal to win or beat an opponent.

Disruptive Conflict

Activity designed to attack, defeat, or eliminate an opponent through disruption.

Organizational conflict is defined as the struggle for scarce organizational resources (Coser, 1956). Values, goals, roles, or structural elements may be the specific locus of the struggle for scarce organizational resources. For example, two parties may be in opposition because of perceived differences in goals, a struggle over scarce resources, or interference in goal attainment. This opposition prevents cooperation (Deutsch, 1973). **Job conflict** is defined as a perceived opposition or antagonistic process at the individual-organization interface (Gardner, 1992). Conflict levels have an effect on productivity, morale, and teamwork in organizations (Gardner, 1992). Conflict serves to bind a group together, preserve a group by serving as a safety valve for hostility, integrate and stabilize a group, and promote growth through innovation, creativity, and change (Coser, 1956).

A review of the literature revealed several definitions of conflict. Social conflict is a struggle between opponents over values and claims to scarce status, power, and resources (Coser, 1956). According to Deutsch (1973), a conflict exists whenever incompatible activities occur. Conflict occurs when one party is interfering, disrupting, obstructing, or in some other way making another party's actions less effective. Wall (1985) defined conflict as a process in which two or more parties attempt to frustrate the other's goal attainment. The factors underlying conflict are threefold: (1) interdependence, (2) differences in goals, and (3) differences in perceptions. Conrad (1990) indicated that conflicts are communicative interactions among people who are interdependent and who perceive that their interests are incompatible, inconsistent, or in tension. Conflict is thus the interaction of interdependent people who perceive incompatible goals and interference from each other in achieving those goals (Folger et al., 1997). Wall and Callister (1995) defined conflict as a process in which one party perceives that its interests are being opposed or negatively affected by another party. Walton (1966) defined conflict as opposition processes in any of several forms such as hostility, decreased communication, distrust, sabotage, verbal abuse, and coercive tactics.

Interpersonal conflict is a dynamic process that occurs between interdependent parties as they experience negative emotional reactions to perceived disagreements and interference with the attainment of their goals (Barki & Hartwick, 2001).

VIEWS OF CONFLICT

Robbins (2003) described transitions in conflict thought. The traditional view of conflict argued that conflict must be avoided; it indicated a malfunctioning with the group. This early approach assumed that all conflict was bad. By definition, it was harmful and was to be avoided. This view was consistent with the prevailing attitudes about group behavior in the 1930s and 1940s. Conflict was seen as a dysfunctional outcome resulting from poor communication, a lack of openness and trust between people, and the failure of managers to be responsive to their employees.

The human relations view argues that conflict is a natural and inevitable outcome in any group and that it need not be evil. Rather, it has the potential to be a positive force in determining group performance. Conflict was viewed as a natural occurrence in all groups and organizations. Since it was natural and inevitable, conflict should be accepted. Conflict cannot be eliminated and may even contribute to group performance. The human relations view dominated conflict theory from the late 1940s through the mid-1970s.

The interactionist approach proposes that conflict can be a positive force in a group and explicitly argues that some conflict is absolutely necessary for a group to perform effectively. This approach encourages conflict on the grounds that a harmonious, peaceful, tranquil, and cooperative group is prone to becoming static and nonresponsive to needs for change and innovation. Group leaders maintain enough conflict to keep the group viable, self-critical, and creative. Whether a conflict is good or bad depends on the type of conflict.

Conflict can be competitive or disruptive. **Competitive conflict** is similar to games and sports, where rules are followed and the goal is to

---

Box 24.2

Effects of Conflict

Constructive Effects

- Improves decision quality
- Stimulates creativity
- Encourages interest
- Provides a forum to release tension
- Fosters change

Destructive Effects

- Constricts communication
- Decreases cohesiveness
- Explodes in fighting
- Hinders performance

---

winning but rather on disrupting the opponent. The feelings and actions generated by competitive conflict focus on the positive; for disruptive conflict, feelings, and actions focus on the negative (Filley, 1975).

Conflict is functional or constructive when it improves the quality of decisions, stimulates creativity and innovation, encourages interest and curiosity, provides a medium through which problems can be aired and tensions released, and fosters an environment of self-evaluation and change (Box 24.2). On the other hand, dysfunctional or destructive outcomes include a retarding of communication, reduction in group cohesiveness, and subordination of group goals to the primacy of infighting between members (Robbins, 2003). Extremely high or low levels of conflict hinder performance. An optimal level is high enough to prevent stagnation and stimulates creativity, releases tension, and initiates change. However, it is not so high as to be disruptive or counterproductive (Brown, 1983) (Figure 24.3).

win or beat an opponent. A **disruptive conflict** is some activity designed to attack, defeat, or eliminate an opponent. It is not based in rules jointly agreed to, and its objective is not focused on

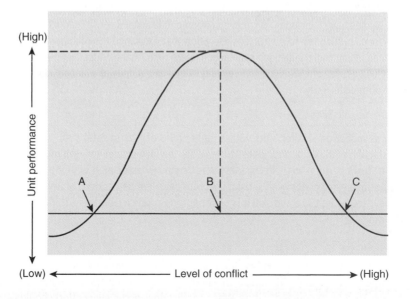

Figure 24.3
Conflict and unit performance. (From Brown, L.D. [1983]. *Managing conflict at organizational interfaces*. Reading, MA: Addison-Wesley/Pearson Education.)

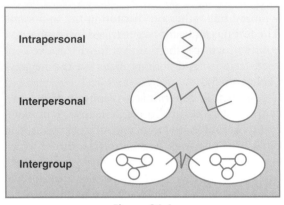

Figure 24.4
Types of conflict.

LEVELS OF CONFLICT

Thomas (1992) noted two broad types of conflict. The first refers to incompatible response tendencies within an individual, which Rahim and Bonoma (1979) referred to as *intrapersonal conflict* (Figure 24.4). *Intrapersonal conflict* means discord, tension, or stress inside, or internal to, an individual that results from unmet needs, expectations, or goals. Intrapersonal conflict is conflict that generates from within an individual (Rahim, 1983a, 1983b, 1983c). It often is manifested as a conflict over two competing roles. For example, a parent with a sick child who has to go to work faces a conflict: the need to take care of the sick child against the need to make a living. A nursing example occurs when the nurse determines that a client needs teaching or counseling,

Research Note

Source: Cox, K.B. (2000). The effect of unit morale and interpersonal relations on conflict in the nursing unit. *Journal of Advanced Nursing, 35*(1), 17-25.

Purpose

Health care organizations face major changes, and these changes are likely to increase conflict in organizations. Although numerous studies have focused on conflict management, few have considered causes and effects of conflict in nursing units. This investigation tested a structural equation that examined the relationships among individual and contextual variables and intragroup conflict, job satisfaction, team performance effectiveness, and anticipated turnover. The nonrandom sample consisted of 141 nurses employed on 13 inpatient units at a state-supported, 597-bed academic medical center in a Southeastern city.

Discussion

Intragroup conflict was higher on smaller units with a higher ratio of RNs to total staff. Intragroup conflict was not associated with satisfaction with pay or anticipated turnover. In the final model, the unit morale and the interpersonal relations dimension of team performance effectiveness was negatively associated with intragroup conflict and anticipated turnover and positively associated with satisfaction with pay. High perceptions of unit morale and interpersonal relations buffered the effect of unit size and skill mix on intragroup conflict. Goodness of fit statistics indicated a good fit of the model to data.

Application to Practice

Findings of this study indicated that there is less intragroup conflict on units where there are high perceptions of unit morale and interpersonal relations. In view of this finding, nurse administrators should strive to create a work environment that supports a team-oriented culture. When conflict does occur, every effort should be made to manage conflict in order to create a win-win situation.

but the organization's assignment system is set up in a way that does not provide an adequate amount of time. When other priorities compete, then an internal or intrapersonal conflict of roles exists.

The second use refers to conflicts that occur between different individuals, groups, organizations, or other social units. Rahim and Bonoma (1979) identified these as interpersonal conflict, a category that includes intragroup conflict, intergroup conflict, and interorganizational conflict. *Interpersonal* means conflict emerging between two or more people, such as between two nurses, a doctor and a nurse, or a nurse manager and a staff nurse (Rahim & Bonoma, 1979). If the conflict originates between two or more individuals, it is called *interpersonal* (Rahim & Bonoma, 1979). In this case, two people have a disagreement, conflict, or clash. Either their values or styles do not match, or there is a misunderstanding or miscommunication between them. Interpersonal conflict can be viewed as happening between two individuals or among individuals within a group. When it specifically involves multiple individuals within a group, interpersonal conflict is called *intragroup conflict*, which refers to disagreements or differences among the members of a group or its subgroups with regard to goals, functions, or activities of the group.

Intergroup conflict refers to disagreements or differences between the members of two or more groups or their representatives over authority, territory, and resources. Interorganizational conflict occurs across organizations (Rahim & Bonoma, 1979). Intergroup conflict occurs between two or more groups (Rahim, 1983b). It is conflict occurring between two distinct groups of people. For example, physicians and nurses may disagree about policies on third-party reimbursement for services, or lay midwives may seek to perform home deliveries without being prepared as licensed nurse midwives. Sometimes the conflict arises between departments or units as groups. For example, hospital nurses might find themselves in conflict with central purchasing if supplies are provided that do not meet nursing's needs or are defective.

TYPES OF CONFLICT

Three broad types of conflicts have been identified: relationship, task, and process. *Relationship conflict,* an awareness of interpersonal incompatibilities, includes affective components such as feeling tension and friction (Rahim & Bonoma, 1979). Relationship conflict involves personal issues such as dislike among group members and feelings such as annoyance, frustration, and irritation. This definition is consistent with past categorizations of conflict that distinguish between affective and cognitive conflict (Amason, 1996; Pinkley, 1990). Results of a meta-analysis revealed strong negative correlations between relationship conflict and team performance and also strong negative correlations between relationship conflict and team member satisfaction (DeDreu & Weingart, 2003).

Task conflict is an awareness of differences in viewpoints and opinions about a group task. Similar to cognitive conflict, it pertains to conflict about ideas and differences of opinion about the task (Amason & Sapienza, 1997). Task conflicts may coincide with animated discussions and personal excitement but, by definition, are void of the intense interpersonal negative emotions that are more commonly associated with relationship conflict.

Recent studies have identified a third unique type of conflict, labeled *process conflict* (Jehn, 1995, 1997; Jehn et al., 1999). It is defined as an awareness of controversies about aspects of how task accomplishment will proceed. More specifically, process conflict pertains to issues of duty and resource delegation, such as who should do what and how much responsibility different people should get. For example, when group members disagree about whose responsibility it is to complete a specific duty, they are experiencing process conflict.

STAGE MODELS OF CONFLICT

Pondy (1967), Filley (1975), Thomas (1976), and Robbins (2003) described conflict dynamics across a temporal sequence of stages or phases.

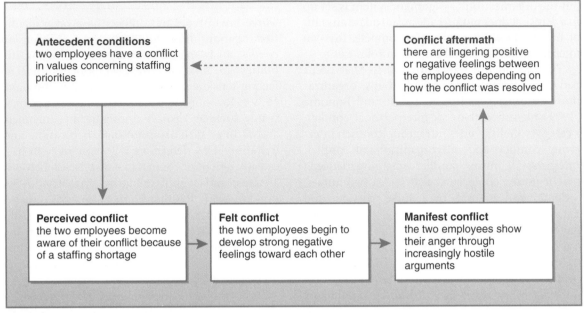

Figure 24.5

Pondy's stages of conflict. (Data from Pondy, L.R. [1967]. Organizational conflict: Concepts and models. *Administrative Science Quarterly*, 12, 296-320.)

These models provide significant insight into understanding the nature of conflict phenomena. Pondy's model consisted of the following four stages (Figure 24.5):

1. Latent (antecedent conditions)
2. Perception and feeling
3. Behavior manifestation (manifest)
4. Aftermath

The process begins with antecedent conditions such as unclear roles, competition for scarce resources, the quest for autonomy, or subunits with divergent goals. The process, depending on how it is handled, may be cyclical with the conflict aftermath becoming the antecedent conditions for a future conflict episode. The antecedent conditions form a background. This background leads to perceived conflict and then to felt conflict, which arises at an emotional level. One party senses that there is a problem and feels an emotional reaction beginning. These stages of perceived and felt conflict initiate manifest behavior. The conflict tension causes action. In this stage the individual may verbalize negativity, attack another person, or try to change the situation or the environment as a way of reducing the tension.

At the stage of manifest behavior, visible evidence of conflict occurs. Subsequently, either the conflict is resolved or suppressed. For example, ventilating strong emotions by verbal expression may not resolve the problem, but it calms an individual and suppresses the problem for a period of time. In the aftermath of this process, there will be new attitudes or feelings between the parties. These may be positive feelings because coping occurred and the individual felt positive and constructive in the resolution of the conflict. However, negative feelings may arise because of an inability to do anything to resolve the conflict or because the other person had more power. The negative feelings may fester. The memory of the conflict and feelings about how it was processed may linger and provide antecedent conditions for another cycle of conflict. Thus there is an aftermath to the conflict even if it is temporarily resolved. This is a residual effect from having had conflict or tension with which the individual invested psychological energy and emotion.

Filley's (1975) model is composed of the following six stages:

1. Antecedent conditions
2. Perceived conflict
3. Felt conflict
4. Manifest behavior
5. Resolution or suppression
6. Conflict aftermath

An emotional cycle of conflict was proposed as a process model of conflict by Thomas (1976). In this model the conflict process begins as frustration, an affective-emotional trigger. Thomas's model (1976) bears a strong resemblance to Pondy's (1967). Frustration is one antecedent condition to conflict. Conceptualization is a form of cognition or perception of conflict. Frustration is an affective response, a form of felt conflict. Behavior and interaction both compare to Pondy's manifest conflict stage. Both models conclude with an outcome or aftermath conditions.

The Thomas process model depicted the following five major concepts (Figure 24.6):

1. Frustration
2. Conceptualization
3. Behavior
4. Others' reactions (interaction)
5. Outcome

The five stages of the Robbins (2003) model are as follows:

1. Potential opposition
2. Cognition and personalization
3. Intentions
4. Behavior
5. Functional or dysfunctional outcomes

Commonalities in the Stage Models

The models of Pondy (1967), Filley (1975), Thomas (1976), and Robbins (1994, 2003) are similar in that all indicate that conflict follows

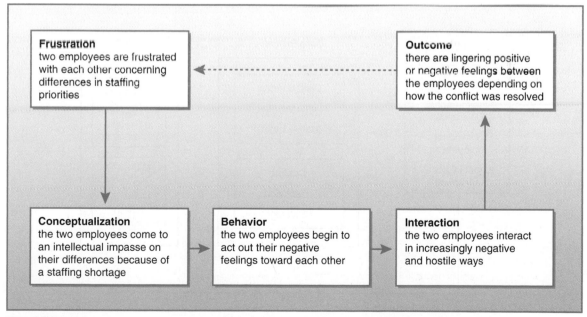

Figure 24.6
Thomas's conflict process events. (Data from Thomas, K.W. [1976]. Conflict and conflict management. In M.D. Dunnette [Ed.], *The handbook of industrial and organizational psychology* [pp. 889-935]. Chicago: Rand McNally.)

a predictable course, though they differ in the number of identifiable stages or elements in a particular pattern. The following elements exist in all the models:

- Causes identified as conditions that occur prior to the conflict
- Core processes, including the perception that conflict exists, followed by some kind of affective state or emotional response
- Conflict behaviors, including a variety of behaviors from very subtle to violent
- Effect that includes outcomes such as resolution or aftermath consequences

Cause, Core Process, Effect

Wall and Callister (1995) described a generic model of conflict that is presented in Figure 24.7. As with any social process, there are causes and a core process that have effects. These effects in turn have an impact on the original cause. This conflict cycle takes place within a context (environment), and the cycle flows through numerous iterations. Wall and Callister indicated that the model is a

general one that displays how the major pieces in the conflict puzzle fit together. The value of this model is that concepts from all other models may be subsumed under the major concepts of this generic model. In addition, the simplicity of the model facilitates the discussion of conflict according to cause, core process, and effect.

Causes of Conflict

According to Wall and Callister (1995), conditions that occur prior to conflict are identified as causes. Pondy (1967) identified the underlying sources of organizational conflict. These are competition for scarce resources, drives for autonomy, and divergence of subunit goals. In Filley's (1975) model, antecedent conditions include the following: ambiguous jurisdictions, conflict of interest, communication barriers, dependence of one party, differentiation in organization, association of the parties, need for consensus, behavior regulations, and unresolved prior conflicts. According to Rahim and Bonoma (1979), sources of intragroup conflict include leadership style, task structure,

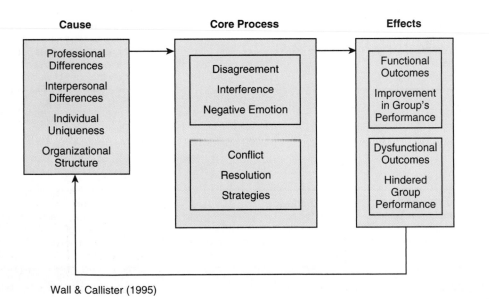

Wall & Callister (1995)

Figure 24.7

Conceptual framework for conflict. (Data from Wall, J.A., & Callister, R.R. [1995]. Conflict and its management. *Journal of Management, 21,* 515-558.)

group composition and size, cohesiveness and groupthink, and external threats and their outcomes. Intergroup conflict is generated from system differentiation, task interdependence, scarce resources, jurisdictional ambiguity, and separation of knowledge from authority.

Potential sources of conflict in nursing include unclear roles and duties, conflict of interest, communication barriers, dependence on one another, relationship differences, response to regulation, unresolved prior conflict, and finally, unique health care conflicts such as those that occur between nurses and physicians and between nurses and unlicensed assistive personnel (Hansten & Washburn, 1998).

The Core Process of Conflict

Although conflict has been defined in many different ways, three general dimensions are thought to underlie these definitions: disagreement, interference, and negative emotion (Barki & Hartwick, 2001). These three dimensions can be viewed as reflecting cognitive, behavioral, and affective manifestations of interpersonal conflict. Disagreement is the most commonly discussed and assessed cognition in the literature. Although a number of different behaviors have been associated with and may be typical of conflict, they do not always indicate the existence of conflict. Conflict exists when the behavior of one party interferes with or opposes another party's attainment of its own interests, objectives, or goals. Finally, a number of affective states have been associated with conflict. However, it is the negative emotions such as fear, anger, anxiety, and frustration that have been used to characterize conflict. Barki and Harwick (2001) proposed that interpersonal conflict exists only when disagreement, interference, and negative emotion are present in the situation.

Effects of Conflict

Robbins (2003) described functional and dysfunctional outcomes of conflict for groups in organizations. Functional outcomes result in an improvement in the group's performance. Conflict is constructive when it improves the quality of decisions, stimulates creativity and innovation, encourages interest and curiosity, provides the medium through which problems can be aired and tensions released, and fosters an environment of self-evaluation and change. On the other hand, if the group's performance is hindered, the outcome would be described as dysfunctional. Among the more undesirable consequences are a retarding of communication, reductions in group cohesiveness, and subordination of group goals to the primacy of infighting. At the extreme, conflict can bring group functioning to a halt and potentially threaten a group's survival. Excessive levels of conflict can hinder group effectiveness, resulting in reduced productivity (Robbins, 2003).

Positive outcomes in nursing include better patient care and patient satisfaction, improved relationships, improved communications, personal and professional growth, efficient use of resources, increased staff satisfaction, and improved collaboration. On the other hand, negative outcomes include hostility, gossip, burnout, lack of professional growth, increased turnover, lack of professional collaboration, and less efficient use of resources. In addition, patient care could suffer and destructive behaviors could prevail (Hansten & Washburn, 1998).

Conflict Scales

There are two conflict inventories available to measure conflict. The Rahim Organizational Conflict Inventory-I (Rahim, 1983b, 1983c) is designed to measure three dimensions of conflict: intrapersonal, intragroup, and intergroup. The Perceived Conflict Scale (Gardner, 1992) contains four subscales of conflict: intrapersonal, interpersonal, intergroup/other departments, and intergroup/support services. This scale is designed to measure conflict in nursing. The scales can be used not only for objective measurement to determine how much conflict exists, but also to determine the causes and effects of conflict and the relationship of conflict to other variables of interest to nursing administrators. Barki and Hardwick's (2001) proposed dimensions of disagreement, interference, and negative emotion have implications for the development of another instrument containing items that reflect the three dimensions. If the psychometric properties of the new scale are strong, it could contribute to our understanding of conflict.

CONFLICT MANAGEMENT

There are many views about conflict management. Clearly conflict is managed via the style and the strategy chosen by the conflict manager. Several conflict styles and strategies exist, meaning that individuals have choices. The ability to select among styles and strategies if something is not working provides flexibility for the person dealing with conflict.

Managing conflict relates to determining whether the level is too high or too low. Assessment of levels and sources is the first step in conflict assessment. The goal of conflict management is to stimulate growth and coping behavior but avoid reaching the point where conflict seems overwhelming. Conflict is an inherent element of change and is manifested in resistance to change. This indicates that nurses need to be alert to the predictability of resistance and conflict in any change process.

Personal styles and the interaction of styles contribute to conflict moments. The reality is that most people are more comfortable around people who are similar to them. If people are very different in terms of personality and styles, then how the styles interact contributes to conflict potential. Awareness of one's own style and the recognition of other people's styles contribute to effective management of conflict.

Multiple factors must be considered in conflict management. The important factors can form the basis for conflict management behaviors needed by nurses. These behaviors have been listed in a conflict management checklist (Box 24.3). The checklist can be used as a review or assessment for critically analyzing conflict situations.

A companion tool is a series of systematic steps that have been recommended for nurses to use in handling conflict situations (Mallory, 1981)

Box 24.3

Conflict-Management Checklist

✓ Identify the boundaries of the conflict, the areas of agreement and disagreement, and the extent of each person's aims.

✓ Understand the factors that limit the possibilities of managing the conflict constructively.

✓ Be aware of whether more than one issue is involved.

✓ Be open to the ideas, feelings, and attitudes expressed by the people involved.

✓ Be willing to accept outside help to mediate the conflict.

(Figure 24.8). The advantage of following a systematic approach to handling conflict is that the nurse becomes a better problem solver. This is especially important in conflict situations, which have a significant component of strong human emotions. The emotions may need to be defused before the content issues can be tackled.

Conflict-Management Strategies

It is important to take action as soon as a conflict surfaces so that bad feelings will not linger and grow. Conflict in groups adds the complexity of multiple parties to the conflict situation. Usually the best place for a work group to clear the air is in a group meeting. During such meetings issues can be defined and strategies worked out for managing the points of disagreement. Three overall frameworks or postures for conflict management are the defensive, compromise, and creative problem-solving modes.

The *defensive mode* produces feelings of winning in some and loss in others. There are several conflict resolution strategies that adopt a defensive mode. Sometimes if creative problem solving and compromise fail, this may be the only way to decrease some of the destructive effects of conflict. Or a defensive mode may be used initially to gain time to calm down or to think about how to

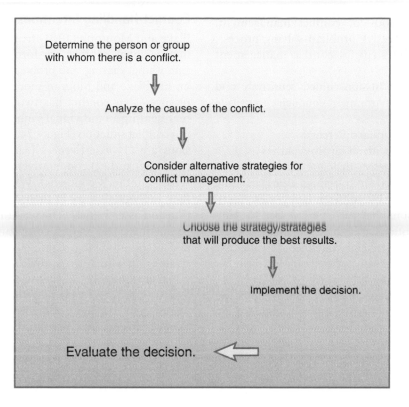

Figure 24.8
Handling conflict situations. (Data from Mallory, G. [1981]. Believe it or not, conflict can be healthy once you understand it and learn to manage it. *Nursing, 11*[6], 97-101.)

proceed. Following are ways to defensively solve a conflict:

- *Separate the contending parties.* For example, people may be assigned to different shifts or teams or different days off and on.
- *Suppress the conflict.* For example, people may decide not to talk about their differences.
- *Restrict or isolate the conflict.* For example, the parties can agree to disagree about a conflict and move on to items that they do agree about.
- *Smooth it over or finesse it through an organizational change.* For example, sometimes it is possible to solve conflicts by restructuring around the issue.
- *Avoid the conflict to diminish the destructive effects.* For example, people can change the

subject whenever the conflict arises or avoid the party or parties involved.

The second mode of conflict management is compromise. With a *compromise* each party wins something and loses something. In the settlement, each side gives up a part of its demands. Thus each side may "go halfway" or "split the difference." A compromise comes about when both sides want harmony or an end to the conflict and are willing to give up something to settle the difference.

The third mode of conflict management is creative problem solving. Use of a *creative problem-solving* mode produces feelings of gain and no feelings of loss for all conflict participants. All parties work together collaboratively to arrive at a solution that satisfies everyone, and all parties feel that they win. Creative problem solving is the most effective mode of conflict management. As part of the creative problem-solving process, the following five steps for conflict management can be identified:

1. Initiate a discussion, timed sensitively and held in an environment conducive to private discussion.
2. Respect individual differences.
3. Be empathic with all involved parties.
4. Have an assertive dialogue that consists of separating facts from feelings, clearly defining the central issue, differentiating viewpoints, making sure that each person clearly states their intentions, framing the main issue based on common principles, and being an attentive listener consciously focused on what the other person is saying.
5. Agree on a solution that balances the power and satisfies all parties, so that a consensus on a win-win solution is reached.

Conflict-Handling Intentions

Blake and Mouton's (1964) five styles of handling interpersonal conflict are forcing, withdrawing, smoothing, sharing, and problem solving. Building on the Blake and Mouton model, Thomas (1976) reported that conflict has two dimensions, each representing an individual's intention with respect to a conflict situation (Figure 24.9). The two dimensions are (1) assertiveness (satisfying one's own concerns) and (2) cooperativeness (attempting to satisfy another's concerns). When handling conflict, individuals vary in their degree of cooperation and assertiveness. The resulting behaviors are competing, collaborating, compromising, avoiding, and accommodating. Competing is an assertive strategy in which an individual's concerns are satisfied at the other's expense. Collaborating is an assertive, cooperative strategy in which individuals work together to find a mutually satisfying solution. Compromising incorporates both assertiveness

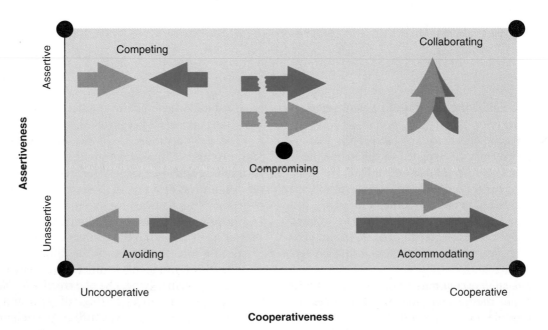

Figure 24.9
Dimensions of conflict-handling intentions. (From Thomas, K. [1992]. Conflict and negotiation processes in organizations. In M.D. Dunnette & L.M. Hough [Eds.], *Handbook of industrial and organizational psychology* [2nd ed., Vol. 3] [p. 668]. Palo Alto, CA: Consulting Psychologists Press.)

and cooperating. In compromising, each individual involved in the conflict must give something up in order to resolve the situation. Avoiding is an unassertive, uncooperative strategy used when an individual postpones or sidesteps an issue. Accommodating is an unassertive, cooperative strategy used when an individual focuses on the concerns of the other while neglecting his own.

Conflict-Resolution Strategies

Conflicts can be a source of chronic frustration, or they can lead to increased effectiveness in organizations and groups. It takes leadership and management to solve them creatively so that people exist more cooperatively with others. Leadership and management of conflict resolution has implications for work group morale and productivity. A fair proportion of a leader's or manager's time is spent on handling conflict.

Conflict management techniques stress the importance of communication, assertive dialogue, and coming from a point of empathy. Thus during conflict situations, the more that individuals look at the total situation and use positive communication techniques, the closer they will come to a path toward successful resolution. Conflict resolution techniques have been identified, described, and categorized in a variety of ways by a variety of authors. Some terms have been used interchangeably, and some terms have similar but slightly different meanings. The following is an overall list for methods or strategies for conflict resolution (Figure 24.10):

- *Avoiding:* This is the strategy of avoiding conflict at all costs. Some people never acknowledge that a conflict exists. The individual's posture is, "If I do not acknowledge there is a problem, then there is no problem." It is sometimes reflected in the phrase, "leave well enough alone."
- *Withholding or withdrawing:* In this avoidance strategy, one party opts out of participation. They remove themselves from the situation. This does not resolve the conflict. However, this strategy does give individuals a chance to calm down or to avoid a confrontation.
- *Smoothing over or reassuring:* This is the strategy of saying "Everything will be OK." By maintaining surface harmony, parties do not withdraw but simply attempt to make everyone feel good. It is similar to "smoothing ruffled feathers." Smoothing over or reassuring strategies use verbal communication to defuse strong emotions.
- *Accommodating:* This strategy is used when there is a large power differential. The more powerful party is accommodated to preserve harmony or build up social credits. What this means is that the party of lesser power gives up his or her position in deference to the more powerful party. Accommodation may be used when one party has a vested interest that is relatively unimportant to the other party. "Kill the enemy with kindness" is the related phrase.
- *Forcing:* This technique is a dominance move and an arbitrary way to manage conflict. An issue may be forced on the table by issuing orders or by putting it to a majority-rules vote. The hallmark phrase is "Let's vote on it." Forcing is an all-out power strategy to win while the other party loses.
- *Competing:* This is an assertive strategy where one party's needs are satisfied at the other's expense. Competing is an all-out effort to win at any cost. It is sometimes reflected in the phrase "Might makes right." Competing strategies tend to follow rules and be similar to games and athletic contests. Applying for a job is a form of competition.
- *Compromising:* This strategy is called "splitting the difference." It is useful when goals or values are markedly different. It is a staple of conflict management.
- *Confronting:* This technique is called *assertive problem solving* and is focused on the issues. Individuals speak for themselves, but in a way that decreases defensiveness and allows another person to hear the message. It is a staple of conflict management but requires courage. "I" messages are used; "you" messages are avoided.

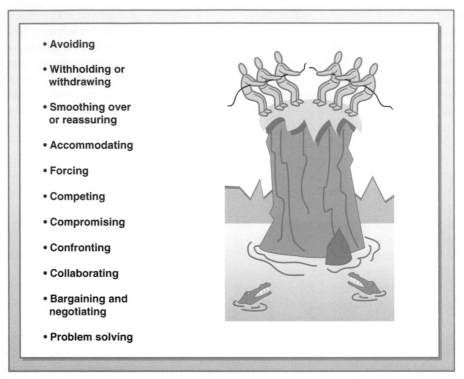

- Avoiding
- Withholding or withdrawing
- Smoothing over or reassuring
- Accommodating
- Forcing
- Competing
- Compromising
- Confronting
- Collaborating
- Bargaining and negotiating
- Problem solving

Figure 24.10
Strategies for conflict resolution. (Data from *American Journal of Nursing* [AJN]. [1987]. *Conflict management* [videotape]. New York: American Journal of Nursing Company; Barton, A. [1991]. Conflict resolution by nurse managers. *Nursing Management, 22*[5], 83-86; Mallory, G. [1981]. Believe it or not conflict can be healthy once you understand it and learn to manage it. *Nursing, 11*[6], 97-101; and Thomas, K. [1976]. Conflict and conflict management. In M. Dunnette (Ed.), *The handbook of industrial and organizational psychology* [pp. 889-935]. Chicago: Rand McNally.)

- *Collaborating:* This is an assertive and cooperative strategy in which the parties work together to find a mutually satisfying solution. It is invoked with the phrase "Two heads are better than one."
- *Bargaining and negotiating:* These strategies are attempts to divide the rewards, power, or benefits so that everyone gets something. They involve both parties in a back-and-forth effort at some level of agreement. The process may be formal or informal.
- *Problem solving:* This strategy's goal is to try to find an acceptable, workable solution for all parties. It is designed to generate feelings of gain by all parties. The problem-solving process

is employed to reach a mutually agreeable solution to the conflict.

Face Negotiation Theory

Face negotiation is the focus of a theory developed by Ting-Toomey to describe and explain differences in responses to conflict on the basis of cultural backgrounds (Ting-Toomey, 1988; Ting-Toomey & Kurogi, 1998). This theory draws on the idea that *face* is a metaphor for our public identity, or self-image, and is an important element of social situations throughout the world. Specifically, face is "a projected image of one's self in a relational situation" (Ting-Toomey, 1988, p. 215). In the theory, *facework* refers to specific verbal and nonverbal messages that help to maintain and restore face loss and to uphold and honor face gain. All individuals want others to see them in a certain way, even though they may not be consciously aware of this desire.

Ting-Toomey (1988) originally considered face negotiation theory as a way to explain differences in conflict communication styles stemming from cultural preferences for individualism versus collectivism. She proposed that those in cultures best described as collectivistic would be more likely to seek to uphold "other-face," whereas those in individualistic cultures would more like seek to uphold "self-face."

Face negotiation theory builds on the five-style dual-concern framework developed by Rahim (1983a) and is based on the degree to which a person is concerned with self-interest, as well as with the interests of others. The five styles are problem solving (also called *integrating, collaborating,* or *cooperating*), forcing (also called *competing* or *dominating*), avoiding (also called *suppressing* or *withdrawing*), yielding (also called *obliging, accommodating,* or *smoothing*), and compromising (Putnam & Poole, 1987; Rahim, 2001). The theory posits that collectivistic cultures favor the avoiding, yielding, and compromising styles; in contrast, individualistic cultures reputedly favor forcing and problem-solving styles (Ting-Toomey, 1988).

In 1998, the face negotiation theory was revised; and the dimension of self-construal (self-image) was discussed in terms of the independent and interdependent self, or the degree to which people conceive of themselves as relatively autonomous from, or connected to, others (Ting-Toomey & Kurogi, 1998). The revised theory posits that the degree to which people see themselves as autonomous (independent; self-face) or connected to others (interdependent; other-face) is a better predictor of conflict interaction than their cultural or ethnic background. Ting-Toomey and Kurogi (1998) also added the concept of power to the theory to explain communicative differences based on the cultural dimension of power distance. In low-power distance cultures, differences in treatment based on status are less accepted. On the other hand, in high-power distance culture, differences in treatment based on status are more accepted. The authors proposed that individuals of different status levels in low-power distance cultures are more likely to use the forcing style to resolve conflict, whereas in high-power distance cultures those in lower-status roles may use styles such as yielding.

Recent cross-cultural empirical tests of the revised face negotiation theory supported much of the theory (Oetzel & Ting-Toomey, 2003; Oetzel et al., 2001). The 2001 study involved a cross-cultural comparison of four national cultures (Oetzel et al., 2001). The purpose of the study was to investigate face and facework during conflicts across four national cultures: China, Germany, Japan, and the United States. A questionnaire was administered to 768 participants in the four national cultures, in their respective languages, to measure 3 face concerns and 11 facework behaviors. The major findings of the study were as follows:

- Self-construals had the strongest effects on face concerns and facework, with independence positively associated with self-face and dominating facework and interdependence positively associated with other- and mutual-face and integrating and avoiding facework.
- Power distance had small, positive effects on all three face concerns and avoiding and dominating facework.
- Individualistic, small-power distance cultures had less other-face concern and avoiding facework and more dominating facework than collectivistic, large-power distance cultures.
- Germans had more self- and mutual-face concerns and used defending more than Americans.
- Chinese had more self-face concern and involved a third party more than Japanese.
- Relational closeness and status only had small effects on face concerns and facework behavior.

In the 2003 study of face-negotiation theory, Oetzel and Ting-Toomey tested the underlying assumption that face mediates the relationship between cultural or individual level variables and conflict styles. The sample included 768 participants and was drawn from the Oetzel and colleagues (2001) study. That previous study involved a cross-cultural comparison of the four national cultures, whereas the 2003 study tested the face-negotiation theory across all cultures.

The major findings of the 2003 study were as follows:

- Cultural individualism-collectivism had direct effects on conflict styles, as well as mediated effects through self-construal and face concerns.
- Independent self-construal was associated positively with self-face concern and interdependent self-construal was associated positively with other-face concern.
- Self-face concern was associated positively with dominating conflict styles and other-face concern was associated positively with avoiding and integrating conflict styles.
- Face concerns accounted for all of the total variance explained (100% of 19% total explained) in dominating, most of the total variance explained in integrating (70% of 20% total explained), and some of the total variance explained in avoiding (38% of 21% total explained) when considering face concerns, cultural individualism-collectivism, and self-construals.

Oetzel and Ting-Toomey (2003) noted that the findings empirically validated the face-negotiation theory (Ting-Toomey, 1988; Ting-Toomey & Kurogi, 1998). They concluded that this study provides a further step in understanding the complex nature of face and conflict behavior. The findings provide supportive evidence of the face-negotiation theory, especially that face concerns provide a mediating link between cultural values and conflict behavior. The authors also suggested that these findings are particularly significant given the relatively large sample size across four national cultures. Oetzel and Ting-Toomey (2003) pointed out that face-negotiation theory is a popular theoretical framework for research and practice, and their research further substantiates the usefulness of the theory. However, the authors noted that

despite this support, future research is needed to better understand how face is negotiated in cross-cultural and intercultural conflicts to create more harmonious multicultural relationships. The theory has relevance for nursing, and future research efforts should be directed toward testing the theory with samples of nursing personnel.

Results of the studies indicated that nursing administrators need to be more attuned to face issues in the conflict dialogue process. The findings of the Oetzel and Ting-Toomey 2003 study demonstrated that display of other-face concern, which is maintaining the poise or pride of the other person and being sensitive to the other person's self-worth, can lead to a collaborative, win-win integrative approach or an avoiding approach. In contrast, individuals who are more concerned with maintaining self-pride or self-image during a conflict episode would devote effort to defending their conflict position to the neglect of other-face validation issue. The theory clearly has implications for nursing research and nursing administration.

Conflict-Resolution Outcomes

Whatever the conflict resolution style used, the individual must be aware of the outcome that results from the strategy selected. The outcomes of conflict are what actually happens as a result of the conflict management process. There are three ways in which conflicts resolve: (1) win-lose, (2) lose-lose, and (3) win-win (Filley, 1975) (Box 24.4).

A *win-lose* situation is one in which one party's views, ideas, or opinions predominate and the other side's are ignored. Putting something to a majority vote creates a win-lose situation in which the majority wins and the minority loses. A *lose-lose* situation is one in which the conflict deteriorates to the point where both parties end up losing. Strategies of averaging, using bribes, using a third-party to arbitrate, or trading may result in a lose-lose outcome. The *win-win* outcome is an attempt to make sure that each party gains something and that there is a solution acceptable to all parties. Problem solving, consensus building, and integrative decision making are techniques aimed toward a win-win outcome.

Box **24.4**

Conflict-Resolution Outcomes

Win-Lose

One party exerts dominance.

Lose-Lose

Neither side wins.

Win-Win

An attempt is made to meet the needs of both parties simultaneously.

Data from Filley, A. (1975). *Interpersonal conflict resolution.* Glenview, IL: Scott, Foresman, and Filley, A., House, R., & Kerr, S. (1976). *Managerial process and organizational behavior.* Glenview, IL: Scott, Foresman.

Managing clients or other nursing personnel places the nurse in many conflict resolution situations. The leader's role is to use positive communication techniques and alternatives to come to a resolution of conflicts. Many institutions have no officially sanctioned way to handle hostility among their members. Effective conflict management techniques establish a common etiquette to lessen conflict tension, increase mutual respect, engender confidence, and increase power through willing collaboration in the endeavors of the organization.

Filley (1975) described the win-win resolution as the optimum conflict management. Win-lose and lose-lose resolutions also occur, but effective managers should seek win-win resolutions. Win-win strategies focus on problem solving.

Negotiation is a fundamental form of conflict resolution. Negotiation includes bargaining power, distributive bargaining, integrative bargaining, and mediation. Bargaining power refers to another person's inducement to agree to terms. Distributive bargaining is what either side gains at the expense of the other. In integrative bargaining, the focus shifts to problem solving, and negotiators reach a solution that enhances both parties and produces high joint benefits. Mediation is a process in which a third party encourages the two parties in conflict to acknowledge that they have injured the other but are also dependent on each other (Hampton et al., 1987).

Integrative bargaining tends to be more cooperative, and distributive bargaining tends to be more competitive. In general, integrative bargaining is superior to distributive bargaining. Fisher and colleagues (1992) proposed an alternative called *principled negotiation.* This approach calls for negotiators to use the following five fundamental principles to negotiate effectively with each other instead of against each other:

1. Separate the people from the problem.
2. Negotiate about interests, not positions.
3. Invent options for mutual gain.
4. Insist on objective decision criteria.
5. Know your BATNA (best alternative to a negotiated agreement).

Although there is no one best method of conflict resolution, competence in managing conflict is essential.

Conflict-Resolution Inventories

Two instruments have been developed to measure conflict handling styles. In the Organizational Conflict Inventory-II, Rahim (1983b, 1983c) divided the handling of interpersonal conflict into the two dimensions of concern for self and concern for others, both in high and low degrees, to form a grid. Rahim then adapted Blake and Mouton's (1964) five types of handling interpersonal conflict (forcing, withdrawing, smoothing, compromising, and problem solving) into five styles of handling interpersonal conflict: (1) avoiding, (2) obliging, (3) compromising, (4) integrating, and (5) dominating. The inventory measures the five identified styles.

Thomas and Kilmann (1974) also developed a style assessment and diagnosis inventory, called the Thomas-Kilmann Conflict Mode Instrument (TKI). Their grid uses dimensions of assertiveness and cooperativeness on high to low degrees. The five styles are avoiding, accommodating, compromising, competing, and collaborating. This model blends a description of an individual's behavior on assertiveness and cooperativeness dimensions in situations where the concerns of two people appear to be incompatible. The behaviors of individuals are thought to be a function of both personal predispositions and situational contingencies. Avoiding is low on both assertiveness and cooperativeness; collaborating is high on both aspects. Competing is high on assertiveness and low on cooperativeness; accommodating is low on assertiveness and high on cooperativeness. Compromising is in the middle. All modes have some use in specific situations (Barton, 1991).

Studies of Conflict Management in Nursing

Several studies used the TKI (Thomas & Kilmann, 1974) to measure staff nurses' and nurse administrators' ways of managing conflict. Hightower's (1986) investigation of hierarchical conflicts by 160 predominantly female (98%) nurse managers revealed that avoidance was the most frequently used conflict handling style, followed by compromise, collaboration, competition, and accommodation. Findings of Woodtli's (1987) study of 167 deans of baccalaureate nursing programs indicated that compromising was used most frequently. This was followed by collaborating, avoiding, accommodating, and competing. Cavanagh (1991) studied 145 staff nurses and 82 nurse managers in eight West Coast hospitals. Findings indicated that both staff nurses and nurse managers used avoidance as their major method of handling conflict. However, nurse managers used compromise almost as frequently as avoidance. Barton (1991) studied 69 nurse managers in a large private, nonprofit teaching hospital in the Midwest. Findings of Barton's studying indicated that compromising was the most frequently used conflict handling style followed by collaborating, avoiding, accommodating, and competing. In summary, avoiding and compromising were the most frequently used conflict handling intentions in nursing. It is interesting to note that none of the nurses used collaboration as their major conflict handling intention, and only the deans in Woodtli's study and nurse managers

in Barton's study used collaboration with any frequency. Results of these studies have implications for including content on conflict resolution skills in all nursing curricula.

LEADERSHIP AND MANAGEMENT IMPLICATIONS

Organizational Conflict

Thomas (1976) further identified a structural model of conflict concerned with underlying conditions that influence the process of conflict and its resolution in organizations. This macro model, or "big picture," of conflict examines four factors that seem to influence the way conflict is handled in organizations: behavioral predispositions of individuals, social pressure in the environment, the organization's incentive structure, and rules and procedures. The different levels of power exist as a result of the bureaucratic hierarchy and the resultant position power.

Organizational conflict is a form of interpersonal conflict that is generated from aspects of the institution, such as the style of management, rules, procedures, and communication channels. Conflicts that arise when an individual's needs and goals cannot be met within the system are generally organizational. Conflict may be necessary to groups and organizations. Conflict serves to unify and bind together a group by setting boundaries and strengthening a group's identity. Conflict may help stabilize a group by serving as a test of opposing interests within the group. Conflict may help integrate a group by distributing power. Conflict may be necessary for the growth of a group and its members. Conflict serves to stimulate creativity, innovation, and change (Coser, 1956).

Organizational leadership sets a tone for conflict and conflict management (Barton, 1991). This occurs because leaders and managers model behaviors of positive or negative conflict management and choose when and how to intervene in conflict situations. Choice of intervention style and timing of conflict management are a function

⚠ LEADERSHIP & MANAGEMENT **BEHAVIORS**

Leadership Behaviors

- Empowers followers
- Encourages the acquisition and use of power to accomplish group goals
- Models the constructive use of power
- Mentors and supports others
- Builds connections
- Enables group decision making
- Is visible and relates to others
- Demonstrates expertise
- Enables followers to use power to manage conflicts
- Models constructive conflict resolution
- Encourages growth-producing conflict
- Mentors and supports followers in conflict management
- Builds conflict interventions
- Is visible in conflict situations
- Collaborates with others

Management Behaviors

- Uses power to obtain resources
- Manages power and conflict moments
- Negotiates from a power base
- Uses information strategically
- Gives rewards and punishments
- Exercises legitimate authority to accomplish work
- Plans for conflict management
- Organizes the environment to decrease frustration
- Directs subordinates in resolving conflicts
- Negotiates conflict resolutions
- Competes and bargains for scarce resources

Overlap Areas

- Uses power to achieve goals
- Uses power sources
- Manages conflicts
- Resolves conflicts

of the individuals' behavioral predispositions and environmental pressure coupled with the organization's reward structure and coordination and control methods.

Specifically related to organizational conflict and the focus on groups in organizations, Pondy (1967) identified three strategies to use when attempting to resolve organizational conflicts. The strategies are bargaining; using rules, procedures, and administrative control; and using a systems integrator. Bargaining might be useful when there is a conflict over scarce monetary resources. The administrative control approach might be helpful when there is a need to clarify role boundaries. The systems integrator approach might be appropriate in a matrix structure or where there is a need to coordinate personnel in vertical and horizontal structures (Booth, 1993).

Sources of Conflict in Organizations

The sources of conflict frequently encountered in organizations are power, communication, goals, values, resources, roles, and personalities. Conflict arises from a variety of sources. Power clashes lead to conflict. This happens if one person has more power than another. For example, in organizations there are relationships between and among individuals with unequal power such as that between physicians and nurses.

Another source of conflict is the misunderstanding or breakdown of communication. Conflicts can be the result of clashes between deep-seated, sincere, but diametrically opposed views. Communication may be used to clarify opposing views. Since values are internalized, they are not easily changed but may be clarified by communication or become a barrier as a result of miscommunication. Conflict situations often arise suddenly with the awareness of conflict existing on an emotional level. Emotional intensity may be the first element communicated. The emotional reaction may include responses such as frustration or wanting to lash out with a strong verbal communication.

The roots or causes of conflict are many and varied. Other general sources of conflict that occur frequently in organizations are different goals, different ways to reach a goal, different values, overlapping or unclear designation of responsibility, lack of information, and personality conflicts. Unresolvable conflicts will need to be carefully managed within any work group in order to balance conflict levels. For example, nurses may thrive when the conflict level is sufficient to stimulate a clash of ideas that leads to creativity and innovation or growth. However, nurses may expend energy in nonproductive activity if the conflict level is too high or becomes destructive.

Conflict appears to be an inherent part of the work of nursing. Nurses are prime candidates for conflict because of the need to work collaboratively with people of varying social, ethnic, and educational backgrounds. Collaboration implies a distribution of power, yet nurses may be employed in a hierarchical system. Nurses find that working in groups creates a situation in which there are a number of different colleagues and a variety of client types and personalities with which to work. These are complex interrelationships. Added to the complexity is the fact that there are multiple providers requiring coordination and communication to manage the care for any client. For example, those involved may include physicians, nurses, nurse managers, ancillary personnel, the client, and the client's family.

Within health care, there is interdependence among members. This situation also provides conditions ripe for conflict to arise. Multiple care providers rely on one another to carry out portions of the work. For example, physicians are dependent on nurses in order to achieve certain client outcomes, nurses are dependent on physicians in order to achieve certain client outcomes, and both nurses and physicians are dependent on a variety of assistive or allied care workers to deliver the therapies or promote client outcomes. Nurses and physicians also have a dependence on each other's expertise. For example, nurses need the physician to write an order for pain medication if medication would be the appropriate

intervention for pain. When physicians write an order for certain therapies, they rely on nurses to assess and evaluate the client, coordinate the care, get the laboratory results ordered and processed, and ensure that therapy is delivered. The complexity of the interrelationships and the nature of interdependent work create conflict moments for nurses. This coincides with Kotter's (1979) ideas about dependency, power, and conflict in organizations. He viewed power as a mechanism to resolve conflict.

The source of a conflict can be interpersonal or organizational in nature. Furthermore, these categories often overlap. In some cases the conflict situation grows to involve multiple groups or pairs of groups.

Personal and organizational goals and values may clash over general policies. *General policy* refers to the course of action taken by an institution, department, or unit. Policies are the guidelines developed to handle specific issues. They are designed to give guidance about standardized ways to make decisions in recurring circumstances. However, professionals and care providers may approach situations with diverse viewpoints about the "best" way to handle a specific problem. Disputes between nurses, physicians, and assistive personnel arise over methods and procedures involving specific diagnostic, therapeutic, clerical, or managerial routines. Clashes may result when a nurse's professional judgment as an autonomous professional intersects with standardized policies developed by the institution and designed to produce uniform behavior.

Resource allocation is an issue associated with the definition of organizational conflict. Cost containment strategies have created conflict over scarce resources in organizations. Nurses often are placed in the center of this conflict. The scarcer the resources, the greater the potential for conflict.

Power divisions occur across organizational and interpersonal lines to produce role conflicts. Role conflicts often manifest themselves in role overload and role ambiguity. Role overload is a common source of nursing conflict. It occurs when nurses are expected to perform the work of other employees or disciplines in addition to providing nursing care. The result of overload often is burnout. Another facet of role conflict, role ambiguity, occurs when the nurse's responsibility expands faster than is officially recognized. When roles are unclear, conflict can surface.

Another stress point for conflict in nursing occurs at the point at which the individual's needs intersect with the organization's needs and goals. Role stress and strain are a reality in the work existence of nurses. For example, other decision makers in the environment may hold one view about what the nurse's role should be, whereas nurses may have an entirely different view, and the two views may conflict. For example, nurses consider a part of their role to be client advocacy. When an unfavorable outcome occurs, the nurse's client advocacy role may be placed in opposition to the institution's image or legal liability needs. Furthermore, nurses as individuals may have a need for job security, practice autonomy, or pay equity. These needs may be in conflict with the organization's needs to hold down labor costs or control the practice decisions of its largest category of workers.

Sometimes conflict stems from individuals' attitudes, personalities, and personal behavior. Personal behavior refers to style, mannerisms, or work habits. Chronic lateness is an example of a personal behavior that frequently causes conflict. In all cases it is important for leaders and managers to separate issues related to persons and personalities from issues arising from the actual problem or problems.

Whatever the cause, when a conflict occurs, an individual can expect that more information will be needed to process the conflict constructively. Similar to problem solving, conflict situations require information gathering and clear problem definition. However, the conflict may be difficult to define, especially if more than one causative factor contributes to the tension. Furthermore, the conflict may involve a covert, less obvious issue than what is presented on the surface. Conflicts often appear larger and more difficult to manage

than what actually can be done about them. For example, intense or high levels of emotion are a part of conflict. Both the emotional and issues content of the conflict will need to be managed. By identifying both the areas of agreement and disagreement and then defining the extent of each party's aims, a nurse leader or manager can begin the process of constructively reducing a seemingly overwhelming conflict to a manageable and functional one.

Clearly, if not handled productively, conflicts can be a disruptive rather than a creative force. Conflict involves energy. Within an organization it usually is not effective to consistently avoid or suppress conflict because conflict can be the first process that occurs in an attempt to create changes or to innovate. If managed appropriately, conflict can motivate people to look at situations and others in new ways. It can lead to increased productivity and harmony. Modes of behavior such as aggressive, hurtful competition maximize the destructive effects of conflict. For nurses, the techniques of problem solving form a useful basis for handling conflict. However, nurses need to cultivate an understanding of conflict and an attitude of self-confidence in constructive conflict management.

A related issue for nurse leaders and managers is the need to address cross-cultural conflicts, especially between high- and low-context cultures. Chapter 28 provides further information on the differences between high- and low-context cultures. Intergenerational and other cultural issues are further discussed in Chapters 19 and 28.

When conflict does occur, there are several strategies to manage the conflict. *First,* the negative emotion associated with the conflict situation needs to be reversed. Strategies such as visualization, breathing techniques, exercise, and expressing thoughts in writing can help to put the situation in the proper perspective and dissipate negative emotions. The situation can be viewed as a chance to learn, grow, and transform negative emotions (Adlersberg & Ottem, 2004).

Second, an appropriate approach to manage the situation needs to be carefully chosen. The choice of the most appropriate approach depends on a considered balancing of variables such as the situation itself, the time urgency needed to make the decision, the power and status of the players, importance of the issue, and the maturity of the individuals involved in the conflict. Although most of us prefer certain approaches to others, the consistent use of one style may limit an individual's ability to manage conflict. With learning and experience, other approaches that are appropriate for the situation can be chosen.

Third, the key to resolving most conflict situations is good communication skills. Techniques such as active listening, open questions, paraphrasing, and clarifying inconsistencies should be used. The use of assertive statements that begin with "I" allows the expression of thoughts, feelings, and needs without attacking or blaming the other person (Adlersberg & Ottem, 2004).

Finally, the goal of conflict resolution is to create a win-win situation for all. Although it is not realistic to think that every conflict can be resolved in such an ideal fashion, win-win solutions are a worthy goal requiring hard work, creativity, and sound strategy.

CURRENT ISSUES AND TRENDS

Political Power

As the nation's largest health care profession, nursing has the potential to be a mighty force in the health policy arena (Hodges et al., 2002). It is crucial that nursing become involved in the political process at the local, state, and national levels. Government bodies control many issues that affect nurses such as nurse practice acts, funding for nursing education and research, reimbursement issues, resource allocation, and health care reform. Development of coalitions and supporters within organizations and communities and building networks and relationships with other health care professionals, government leaders, and policymakers will increase power in the political arena. To participate effectively and communicate effectively with congressional delegates, nurses must

have thorough knowledge of the issue, an awareness of data to support a position, and knowledge of the legislation under consideration (Hodges et al., 2002).

Although today is an extremely turbulent time in health care, it is also a time of tremendous opportunity for the nursing profession. Nursing must accept the legitimacy of power and take advantage of the opportunity. There is a need for consideration of status and power issues at all levels of nursing education (Cohen, 1992). Including the concept of power in nursing curricula will better prepare nurses to participate in social and political decisions affecting health care. By creating dependency through becoming irreplaceable, demonstrating the ability to cope with uncertainty, and participating in the political process, the nursing profession will be able to establish its power base and use that power to facilitate change in health care organizations and the health care system.

As has always been the case, nurses derive their core power from being the health care providers whom the public most trusts. Caring generates power in relationships, and nurses can nurture this as a power source. Benner (1984) identified six types of power exercised by nurses (Box 24.5). Benner's (1984) six types of nursing practice-derived power can be compared to French and Raven's (1959) five sources of power for individuals. For instance, transformational and participative/affirmative nursing practice power types would be similar to referent power. Integrative, advocacy, healing, and problem-solving types of power would be similar to expert power. French and Raven's (1959) legitimate, reward, and coercive power sources are more frequently applied to nurses as care managers than to nurses as care providers.

Individually, nurses can use power concepts to establish a power base and gain power in their work setting. For example, nurses can use information and expertise to construct powerful, persuasive arguments. Nurses can collect and analyze data that can be strategically used or controlled. They can be visible and persistent in goal pursuit. They can be creative and challenge the

---

Box 24.5

Power Exhibited by Nurses in Client Care

- *Transformational power:* the ability to assist clients to transform their self-image
- *Integrative power:* the ability to help clients return to normal lives
- *Advocacy power:* the ability to remove obstacles
- *Healing power:* the ability to create a healing climate and nurse-client relationship
- *Participative/affirmative power:* the ability to draw strength from a caring interaction with a client
- *Problem-solving power:* the ability, through caring, to be sensitive to cues and search for solutions to problems

---

system to innovate. Nurses can use group power strategies such as networking, connecting, and collaborating to achieve professional goals.

Summary

- Power is a basic element in human relations and organizational behavior.
- Power is the capability to produce effects and allocate scarce resources.
- Power is the ability to exert influence over others by persuasion or coercion.
- Attitudes and values affect the use of power.
- Power is both personal and professional.
- French and Raven identified five sources of power.
- Three other power sources are connection, information, and group decision making.
- Perceptions and prestige are intertwined with power.
- Nurses derive power from nursing practice.
- Nurses can use a variety of sources of power and political strategies.
- Empowerment means developing a structure and environment where people are motivated to excel.

- Conflict is a part of life and everyday experience.
- Conflict is a clash when threat or difference exists among people.
- Organizational conflict is a struggle for scarce resources.
- There are both positive and negative aspects to conflict.
- Types of conflict include intrapersonal, interpersonal, and intergroup.
- Conflict can be competitive or disruptive.
- There are stages to the conflict process.
- There are many sources of conflict, but power clashes are at the root of conflict.
- Conflict is an occupational hazard for nurses.
- There is power in managing conflict.
- Nurses can follow a series of steps in handling conflict situations.
- There are three general strategies for conflict management.
- There are ten different conflict resolution techniques.
- Conflict outcomes are win-lose, lose-lose, or win-win.

Study Questions

Power

1. Think of a manager who has had the most influence over you. Why was that individual influential?
2. What types of power are you most comfortable with? Which types would you consider difficult to cope with?
3. Think about yourself as acting with strength and power and feeling the most satisfied about it. What kinds of things would you be doing?
4. How do you react in situations in which you feel powerless? Why do you respond in this way?
5. Does a lack of power affect the way that you feel about situations?
6. When you are trying to control a situation, what makes you feel comfortable or uncomfortable?

7. How can power principles be structured to advance nursing professional goals?

8. What are your sources of power? What other sources of power can you develop?

Conflict

1. What types of conflict are most common among nursing staff?

2. What sources of conflict are most common in nursing practice?

3. Does the way your immediate superior handles conflict help or hinder you?

4. Is there one best way to handle the conflicts most common to nursing practice? Why or why not?

5. What is the difference between functional and dysfunctional conflict? What determines functionality?

6. What are the components of the conflict process model? From your own experience, give an example of how a conflict episode proceeded through the stages.

7. What are the largest obstacles to effective conflict resolution?

8. Identify a couple of specific situations you are currently facing that involve conflict. Apply the steps in the chapter to the conflict you identify.

CASE STUDY

Sabrina Faoro has worked for a 300-bed nonprofit community hospital since graduating from nursing school 15 years ago. She has worked her way up from a staff nurse and is now the Director for Women's Services in this hospital. She reports to the Chief Nursing Officer who is the Vice President (VP) of Patient Services and has been very happy with her position.

However, 6 months ago, Nurse Faoro's boss of many years retired, and a new Chief Nursing Officer was hired. During this time span, the new VP has become more aggressive and powerful. In meetings, she wants to do all the talking, disagrees with any input, and targets anyone who makes comments outside her suggestions. It appears as though she wants followers to do what she wants rather than brainstorm ideas, as had been the custom. In addition, the new VP is a micromanager, and Nurse Faoro and the new VP have had many disagreements about unit policies. Nurse Faoro believes that the VP has made every effort to block her efforts, and she feels that she no longer has the decision making authority that she once had.

Nurse Faoro makes an appointment with the new VP to discuss her concerns. During the meeting, the VP becomes extremely angry and suggests that Nurse Faoro has been resistant ever since the VP's arrival 6 months ago. The VP also states to Nurse Faoro, "Your evaluation may reflect this resistance." Nurse Faoro knows that the President of the Hospital has great confidence in the new VP. She is extremely upset, dreads going to work each day, and fears that she might have to leave her position.

Nurse Faoro takes a personal "time out" for reflection and analysis. When she calms down, she realizes that leadership styles and power and control approaches in the hospital have changed. She reviews her power sources and reasons that her expert power and connection power are an advantage. She realizes that her current approach to the VP is resulting in conflict. Nurse Faoro determines that she needs to convert this approach to a problem-solving mode.

At the next administrative meeting the VP outlines a new agenda for change. Rather than pointing out barriers, Nurse Faoro notes with respect and empathy that nursing services need to be positioned for innovation and improvement through internal program changes. She offers the benefit of her expertise from a recent department overhaul she has undertaken on Women's Services. Because the other nursing directors respect Nurse Faoro as a peer, they too move into a problem-solving dialogue. This opens the discussion and reframes it. The VP relaxes some and also engages in creative problem solving with the group.

CRITICAL THINKING EXERCISE

Scenario 1

Julie Paulsen recently moved to the area because of her husband's transfer and was pleased to accept the nurse manager position on the orthopedic unit of a community hospital. She has had considerable experience in management and is anxious to begin her new position. Unfortunately, three of the staff nurses on the day shift have banded together against their new manager. They feel that one of them should have gotten the job. The three have done everything to sabotage the Nurse Paulsen's leadership and have managed to influence some of the other staff against her. They continually complain among themselves about policies, new ideas, and the new manager. In meetings when Nurse Paulsen announces changes that are going to be implemented, they roll their eyes, cross their arms, sigh, and say "I don't see why we have to change." When Nurse Paulsen asks for input, they are silent. Many of the things these nurses do are so subtle and underhanded that it is difficult to call attention to them.

Scenario 2

Mia Cardona recently graduated from the university college of nursing and was delighted when she was assigned to the evening shift on the telemetry unit. She is hard-working, highly motivated, and eager to learn. The evening charge nurse, Charlie Waychoff, has been working at the hospital for more than 20 years and on the telemetry unit for the past 15 years. Nurse Waychoff is an excellent clinician and is an integral part of keeping many functions of the unit running on the evening shift.

In some cases, he is the only one who knows how some of the equipment on the unit works.

Nurse Waychoff is assigned as Nurse Cardona's preceptor during her orientation. From the beginning, he makes it clear that he does not like to precept new graduates. In fact, Nurse Waychoff states that he has such a heavy workload that he can't find the time to orient new graduates. He has frequently assigned Nurse Cardona to complex patients with very little supervision. When she asks questions, Nurse Waychoff does not give complete information. On one occasion he criticizes Nurse Cardona in front of a patient for not recognizing a second-degree heart block on the patient's monitor. Today he criticized her for her technique during a dressing change. Nurse Cardona is beginning to lose confidence, and she has begun to experience fear, anxiety, sadness, frustration, mistrust, and nervousness. She is reluctant to discuss the situation with Nurse Waychoff for fear of retaliation, and she is reluctant discuss the situation with the nurse manager on the day shift. She fears the nurse manager will think that she is "thin skinned" or can't get along with her coworkers.

1. What are the dimensions of power and conflict evident in these case studies?
2. How is it possible to turn the situations around?
3. How can win-win situations be created?
4. What power and conflict resolution strategies might be helpful?
5. Which communication techniques would be most constructive?

REFERENCES

Adlersberg, M., & Ottem, P. (2004). *Managing conflict.* Vancouver, British Columbia: Registered Nurses Association of British Columbia. Retrieved June 3, 2004, from *www.rnabc.bc.ca/registrants/nursing_practice/articles/conflpg1.htm*

Aiken, L.H., Clarke, S.P., Sloane, D.M., Sochalski, J., & Silber, J.H. (2002). Hospital nurse staffing and patient mortality, nurse burnout, and job dissatisfaction. *Journal of the American Medical Association, 288,* 1987-1993.

Albanese, R. (1981). *Managing: Toward accountability for performance* (3rd ed.). Homewood, IL: Richard D. Irwin, Inc.

Amason, A. (1996). Distinguishing effects of functional and dysfunctional conflict on strategic decision making: Resolving a paradox for top management teams. *Academy of Management Journal, 39,* 123-148.

Amason, A., & Sapienza, H. (1997). The effects of top management team size and interaction norms on cognitive and affective conflict. *Journal of Management, 23,* 496-516.

American Heritage College Dictionary (3rd ed.). (1997). Boston: Houghton Mifflin.

Bacharach, S.B., & Lawler, E.J. (1980). *Power and politics in organizations.* San Francisco: Jossey-Bass.

Barki, H., & Hartwick, J. (2001). Interpersonal conflict and its management in information system development. *MIS Quarterly, 25,* 195-228.

Barton, A. (1991). Conflict resolution by nurse managers. *Nursing Management, 22*(5), 83-86.

Benner, P. (1984). *From novice to expert: Excellence and power in clinical nursing practice.* Menlo Park, CA: Addison-Wesley.

Bennis, W., & Nanus, B. (1985). *Leaders: The strategies for taking charge.* New York: Harper & Row.

Bierstedt, R. (1950). An analysis of power. *American Sociological Review, 15,* 730-738.

Blake, R., & Mouton, J.S. (1964). *The managerial grid.* Houston: Gulf Publishing.

Blau, P.M. (1964). *Exchange and power in social life.* New York: Wiley.

Booth, R. (1993). Dynamics of conflict and conflict management. In D. Mason, S. Talbott, & J. Leavitt (Eds.), *Policy and politics for nurses: Action and change in the workplace, government, organizations, and community* (2nd ed.) (pp. 149-165). Philadelphia: Saunders.

Brown, L.D. (1983). *Managing conflict at organizational interfaces.* Reading, MA: Addison-Wesley Publishing Co.

Caudron, S. (2000). Keeping team conflict alive. *Public Management, 82*(2), 5-9.

Cavanagh, S. (1991). The conflict management style of staff nurses and nurse managers. *Journal of Advanced Nursing, 16,* 1254-1260.

Centers for Medicare & Medicaid Services (CMS). (2004, January 8). *Health care spending reaches 1.6 trillion in 2002.* Baltimore: CMS, U.S. Department of Health and Human Services. Retrieved May 15, 2004, from *www.cms. hhs.gov/media/press/release.asp?Counter=935*

Cohen, L.B. (1992). Power and change in health care: Challenge for nursing. *Journal of Nursing Education, 31,* 113 116.

Conrad, C. (1990). *Strategic organizational communication: An integrated perspective* (2nd ed.). Fort Worth, TX: Holt, Rinehart, and Winston.

Coser, L.A. (1956). *The functions of social conflict.* Glencoe, IL: Free Press.

Cox, K.B. (2001). The mediating effects of unit morale and interpersonal relations on conflict in the nursing unit. *Journal of Advanced Nursing, 35*(1), 17-25.

Crozier, M. (1964). *The bureaucratic phenomenon.* Chicago: University of Chicago Press.

Daft, R.L. (2003). *Organization theory and design* (8th ed.). Cincinnati, OH: South Western Educational Publishing.

Dahl, R.A. (1957). The concept of power. *Behavioral Science, 2,* 210-218.

DeDreu, C.K.W., & Weingart, L.R. (2003). Task versus relationship conflict, team performance, and team member satisfaction: A meta-analysis. *Journal of Applied Psychology, 88*(4), 741-750.

Dennis K.E. (1983). Nursing's power in the organization: What research has shown. *Nursing Administration Quarterly, 8,* 47-57.

Deutsch, M. (1973). *The resolution of conflict: Constructive and destructive processes.* New Haven, CT: Yale University Press.

Emerson, R.M. (1957). Power-dependence relations. *American Sociological Review, 27*(1), 31-40.

Filley, A.C. (1975). *Interpersonal conflict resolution.* Glenview, IL: Scott, Foresman and Company.

Fisher, R., Ury, W., & Patton, B. (1992). *Getting to yes: Negotiating agreement without giving in* (2nd ed.). New York: Penguin Books.

Folger, J.P., Poole, M.S., & Stutman, R.K. (1997). *Working through conflict: Strategies for relationships, groups, and organizations.* New York: Longman.

Forte, P.S. (1997). The high cost of conflict. *Nursing Economics, 15,* 119-123.

French, J., & Raven, B. (1959). The bases of social power. In D. Cartwright (Ed.), *Studies in social power* (pp. 150-167). Ann Arbor, MI: University of Michigan, Institute for Social Research.

Gardner, D.L. (1992). Conflict and retention of new graduate nurses. *Western Journal of Nursing Research, 14,* 76-85.

Hampton, D.R., Summer, C.E., & Webber, R.A. (1987). *Organization behavior and the practice of management.* Glenview, IL: Scott, Foresman.

Hansten, R., & Washburn, M. (1998). *Clinical delegation skills: A handbook for professional practice* (2nd ed.). Gaithersburg, MD: Aspen Publishers.

Hardy, C., & Leiba-O'Sullivan, S. (1998). The power behind empowerment: implications for research and practice. *Human Relations, 51*(4), 451-483.

Hersey, P., Blanchard, K.H., & Johnson, D.E. (2001). *Management of organizational behavior: Leading human resources* (8th ed.). Upper Saddle River, NJ: Prentice-Hall.

Hersey, P., Blanchard, K.H., & Natemeyer, W.E. (1979). Situational leadership, perception, and the impact of power. *Group and Organization Studies, 4,* 418-428.

Hickson, D.J., Hinings, C.R., Lee, C.A., Schneck, R.E., & Pennings, J.M. (1971). A strategic contingencies theory of intraorganizational power. *Administrative Science Quarterly, 16,* 216-229.

Hightower, T. (1986). Subordinate choice of conflict handling modes. *Nursing Administration Quarterly, 11*(1), 29-34.

Hinings, C.R., Hickson, D.J., Pennings, J.M., & Schneck, R.E. (1974). Structural conditions of intraorganizational power. *Administrative Science Quarterly, 19,* 22-42.

Hodges, L.C., Williams, B.G., & Carman, D.D. (2002). Taking political responsibility for nursing's future. *MEDSURG Nursing, 11*(1), 15-24.

Jehn, K.A. (1995). A multimethod examination of the benefits and detriments of intragroup conflict. *Administrative Science Quarterly, 40,* 256-282.

Jehn, K.A. (1997). A qualitative analysis of conflict types and dimensions in organizational groups. *Administrative Science Quarterly, 42,* 530-557.

Jehn, K.A., Northcraft, G., & Neale, M. (1999). Why differences make a difference: A field study of diversity, conflict, and performance in workgroups. *Administrative Science Quarterly, 44,* 741-763.

Johnson, M. (1994). Conflict and nursing professionalization. In J.M. McCloskey & H.K. Grace (Eds.), *Current issues in nursing* (4th ed.) (pp. 643-649). St Louis: Mosby.

Kany, K. (2004, May 31). Nursing in the next decade: Implications for health care and for patient safety. *Online Journal of Issues in Nursing, 9*(2), 3. Retrieved June 15, 2004, from *www.nursingworld.org/ojin/topic24/tpc24_3.htm*

Kanter, R.M. (1977). *Men and women of the corporation.* New York: Basic Books.

Kaplan, A. (1964). Power in perspective. In R.L. Kahn & E. Boulding (Eds.), *Power and conflict in organizations* (pp. 11-32). London: Tavistock.

King, I.M. (1981). *A theory for nursing: Systems, concepts, process.* New York: Wiley & Sons.

Kipnis, D., Schmidt, S.M., Swaffin-Smith, C., & Wilkinson, I. (1984). Patterns of managerial influence: Shotgun managers, tacticians, and bystanders. *Organizational Dynamics, 12*(3), 58-67.

Kipnis, D., Schmidt, S.M., & Wilkinson, I. (1980). Intraorganizational influence tactics: Explorations in getting one's way. *Journal of Applied Psychology, 65*(4), 440-452.

Kohn, L.T., Corrigan, J.M., & Donaldson, M.S. (Eds.). (2000). Committee on quality of healthcare in America. Institute of Medicine of the National Academies. *To err is human: Building a safer health system.* Washington, DC: National Academies Press.

Kotter J.P. (1979). *Power in management-How to understand, acquire, and use it.* New York: AMACOM.

Kouzes, J., & Posner, B. (1987). *The leadership challenge: How to get extraordinary things done in organizations.* San Francisco: Jossey-Bass.

Kramer, M., & Schmalenberg, C. (1990). Fundamental lessons in leadership. In E. Simendinger, T. Moore, & M. Kramer (Eds.), *The successful nurse executive: A guide for every nurse manager* (pp. 5-21). Ann Arbor, MI: Health Administration Press.

Laschinger, H.K., Finegan, J., & Shamian, J. (2001a). The impact of workplace empowerment, organizational trust on staff nurses' work satisfaction and organizational commitment. *Health Care Management Review, 26*(3), 7-23.

Laschinger, H.K., Finegan, J., Shamian, J., & Wilk, P. (2001b). Impact of structural and psychological empowerment on job strain in nursing work settings: Expanding Kanter's model. *Journal of Nursing Administration, 31*(5), 260-272.

Laschinger, H.K., Finegan, J., Shamian, J., & Casier, S. (2000). Organizational trust and empowerment in restructured healthcare settings: Effects on staff nurse commitment. *Journal of Nursing Administration, 30*(9), 413-425.

Laschinger, H.K., & Havens, D.S. (1997). The effect of workplace empowerment on staff nurses' occupational mental health and work effectiveness. *Journal of Nursing Administration, 27*(6), 4-50.

Laschinger, H.K., Sabiston, J.A., & Kutszcher, L. (1997). Empowerment and staff nurse decision involvement in nursing work environments: Testing Kanter's theory of structural power in organizations. *Research in Nursing and Health, 20,* 341-352.

Liberatore, P., Brown-Williams, R., Brucker, J., Dukes, N., Kimmcy, L., McCarthy, K., et al. (1989). A group approach to problem-solving. *Nursing Management, 20*(9), 68-72.

Mallory, G. (1981). Believe it or not conflict can be healthy once you understand it and learn to manage it. *Nursing, 11*(6), 97-101.

McElhaney, R. (1996). Conflict management in nursing administration. *Nursing Management, 24*(5), 65-66.

Mechanic, D. (1962). Sources of power in lower participants in complex organizations. *Administrative Science Quarterly, 7,* 349-364.

Mills, R.J., & Bhandari, S. (2003). *Health insurance coverage in the United States: 2002.* Washington, DC: U.S. Census Bureua, U.S. Department of Commerce. Retrieved May 30, 2004, from *www.census.gov/prod/2003pubs/p60-223.pdf*

Modlin, C.S. (2003). Culture, race, and disparities in health care. *Cleveland Clinic Journal of Medicine, 70,* 283-288.

Nagle, L. (1999). A matter of extinction or distinction. *Western Journal of Nursing Research, 21*(1), 71-82.

Oetzel, J.G., & Ting-Toomey, S. (2003). Face concerns in interpersonal conflict: A cross-cultural empirical test of the face negotiation theory. *Communication Research, 30*(6), 599-624.

Oetzel, J.G., Ting-Toomey, S., Masumoto, T., Yokochi, Y., Pan, X., Takai, J., et al. (2001). Face and facework in conflict: A cross-cultural comparison of China, Germany, Japan, and the United States. *Communication Monographs, 68,* 235-258.

Pfeffer, J. (1981). *Power in organizations.* Boston: Pitman Books Ltd.

Pinckley, R. (1990). Dimensions of the conflict frame: Disputant interpretations of conflict. *Journal of Applied Psychology, 75,* 117-128.

Pondy, L.R. (1967). Organizational conflict: Concepts and models. *Administrative Science Quarterly, 12,* 296-320.

Putnam, L.L., & Poole, M.S. (1987). Conflict and negotiation. In F. M. Jablin, L.L. Putnam, K. Roberts, & L.W. Porter (Eds.), *Handbook of organizational communication* (pp. 549-599). Newbury Park, CA: Sage.

Rahim, M.A. (1983a). A measure of styles of handling interpersonal conflict. *Academy of Management Journal, 26,* 368-376.

Rahim, M. A. (1983b). Measurement of organizational conflict. *The Journal of General Psychology, 109,* 189-199.

Rahim, M. (1983c). *Rahim organizational conflict inventories: Experimental edition: Professional manual.* Palo Alto, CA: Consulting Psychologists Press.

Rahim, M.A. (2001). *Managing conflict in organizations* (3rd ed.). Westport, CT: Quorum.

Rahim, M.A., & Bonoma, T.V. (1979). Managing organizational conflict: A model for diagnosis and intervention. *Psychological Reports, 44,* 1323-1344.

Raven, B., & Kruglanski, W. (1975). Conflict and power. In P. Swingle (Ed.), *The structure of conflict* (pp. 177-219). New York: Academic Press.

Report of the National Nursing Summit Addressing Nurse-Managed Health Centers. (2002, December 3-4). Dearborn, MI: Michigan Academic Consortium. Retrieved June 15, 2004, from *www.nursing.umich.edu/ocp/nursing_summit_12-02.pdf*

Robbins, S.P. (1994). *Essentials of organizational behavior* (4th ed.). Englewood Cliffs, NJ: Prentice-Hall.

Robbins, S.P. (2003). *Organizational behavior* (10th ed.). Engelwood Cliffs, NJ: Prentice-Hall.

Robbins, S.P., & Langton, N. (1999). *Organizational behavior, concepts, controversies, applications* (Canadian ed.). Scarborough, Ontario: Prentice-Hall Canada.

Sabiston, J.A., & Laschinger, H.K. (1995). Staff nurse empowerment and perceived autonomy. Testing Kanter's theory of structural power in organizations. *Journal of Nursing Administration, 25*(9), 42-50.

Salancik, G.R., & Pfeffer, J. (1974). Organizational decision making as a political process: The case of a university budget. *Administrative Science Quarterly, 19*(1), 453-473.

Sieloff, C.L. (2003). Measuring nursing power within organizations. *Journal of Nursing Scholarship, 32,* 183-187.

Stokowski, L. (2004). Trends in nursing: 2004 and beyond. *Topics in Advanced Practice Nursing eJournal, 4*(1). Retrieved June 15, 2004, from *www.medscape.com/viewarticle/466711* (online access granted after free registration)

Thomas, K. (1992). Conflict and negotiation processes in organizations. In M.D. Dunnette & L.M. Hough (Eds.), *The handbook of industrial and organizational psychology* (2nd ed., Vol. 3) (pp. 651-717). Palo Alto, CA: Consulting Psychologist Press.

Thomas, K.W. (1976). Conflict and conflict management. In M.D. Dunnette (Ed.), *The handbook of industrial and organizational psychology* (pp. 889-935). Chicago: Rand McNally.

Thomas, K.W., & Kilmann, R.H. (1974). *Thomas Kilmann Conflict Mode Instrument.* Tuxedo, NY: Xicom, Inc.

Ting-Toomey, S. (1988). Intercultural conflict styles: A face-negotiation theory. In Y.Y. Kim & W. Gudykunst (Eds.), *Theories in intercultural communication* (pp. 213-235). Newbury Park, CA: Sage.

Ting-Toomey, S., & Kurogi, A. (1998). Facework competence in intercultural conflict: An updated face-negotiation theory. *International Journal of Intercultural Relations, 22,* 187-225.

Ulrich, B. (2001). A matter of trust. *NurseWeek,* p. 1. Retrieved 6/15/04 from *www.nurseweek.com/ednote/01/121701a_print.html*

Unruh, L. (2003). Licensed nurse staffing and adverse events in hospitals. *Medical Care, 41,* 142-152.

U.S. Department of Health and Human Services, Health Resources and Services Administration, Bureau of Health Professions (USDHHS, HRSA, BHPR). (2003). *Changing demographics: Implications for physicians, nurses, and other health workers.* Washington, DC: USDHHS. Retrieved June 15, 2004, from *www.bhpr.hrsa.gov/healthworkforce/reports/changedemo/Content.htm*

Wall, J.A. (1985). *Negotiation, theory and practice.* Glenview, IL : Scott, Foresman.

Wall, J.A., & Callister, R.R. (1995). Conflict and its management. *Journal of Management, 21,* 515-558.

Walton, R.E. (1966). Theory of conflict in lateral organizational relationships. In J.R. Lawrence, (Ed.), *Operational research and the social sciences* (pp. 409-426). London: Tavistock Publications.

Weber, M. (1947). *The theory of social and economic organization* (A.M. Henderson & T. Parsons, Trans.). New York: Oxford University Press. (Original work published 1923).

Woodtli, A.O. (1987). Deans of nursing: Perceived sources of conflict and conflict handling modes. *Journal of Nursing Education, 26,* 272-277.

Yukl, G., & Falbe, C.M. (1991). Importance of different power sources in downward and lateral relations. *Journal of Applied Psychology, 76*(3), 416-423.

Yukl, G., Falbe, C., & Joo, Y.Y. (1993). Patterns off influence behavior for managers. *Group and Organization Management, 18*(1), 5-28.

Yukl, G., Lepsinger, R., & Lucia, T. (1992). Preliminary report on development and validation of the Influence Behavior Questionnaire. In K.E. Clark, M.B. Clar, & D.P. Campbell (Eds.), *The impact of leadership* (pp. 417-427). Greensboro, NC: Center for Creative Leadership.

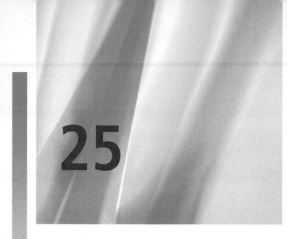

25

Delegation

Maureen T. Marthaler   Diane L. Huber

CHAPTER OBJECTIVES

- Define and describe delegation, delegator, delegatee, and supervision
- Analyze the relationships among delegation, responsibility, and accountability
- Outline the seven elements of delegation
- Examine the five steps in the process of delegating
- Evaluate delegation pitfalls
- Analyze the legal and regulatory aspects of delegation and supervision
- Analyze the use of and delegation to registered nurses, licensed practical nurses, and unlicensed assistive personnel
- Exercise critical thinking to conceptualize and analyze possible solutions to a practice exercise

Delegation is a fundamental aspect of every nurse's job. The effective assignment of work to others is essential in every type of health care setting and organization. Furthermore, effective delegation skills are important for managers whose function is to get work done through the labor of others (Poteet, 1989). For most nursing jobs the zone of responsibility exceeds one person's ability to complete all the tasks (Figure 25.1). This is especially true for the care coordination aspects of nursing care management. Thus nurses need to delegate parts of nursing care delivery to others because, at some point, it becomes impossible to do it all by oneself.

Throughout the history of nursing, nurses have delegated to personnel in the health care environment, whether to a fellow nurse, student, licensed practical nurse/licensed vocational nurse (LPN/LVN), orderlies or technicians, corpsman, nursing assistant, or some other form of nurse extender. In the 1800s, delegation was identified by Florence Nightingale (1859) as a critical skill: "But then again to look at all these things yourself does not mean to do them yourself. ... But can you not insure that it is done when not done by yourself?" (p. 17).

Clearly, the cycles of the nurse shortage in the 1980s and 2000s have created a pressing need for more nurses or substitutes for nurses. Meeting the public's increasing demand for quality health care that is both accessible and affordable has created a demand for health care providers and maximized the stress on every health care worker. As a result, the identification of which tasks are appropriate to nursing, which of these tasks can be delegated, and to whom they can be delegated is imperative. Delegation issues have become connected to issues of work overload, safety and quality of care, mix of staff, job security and turf, and nurses' job satisfaction. Delegation of non-nursing tasks also helps reduce health care costs by making more efficient use of nursing time and the facility's resources (Fisher, 2000).

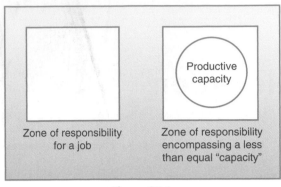

Figure 25.1
Zones of responsibility.

DEFINITIONS

Delegation in nursing is defined as transferring to a competent individual the authority to perform a selected nursing task in a selected situation (National Council of State Boards of Nursing [NCSBN], 1995). The American Nurses Association (ANA) also defined *delegation* as the transfer of responsibility for the performance of a task from one individual to another. Delegation essentially is getting things done through other people (ANA, 1996). The goal of delegation is workload distribution. It relies on trust. The **delegator** is the person making the delegation. The **delegatee** is the person receiving the delegation. **Supervision** in nursing is defined as the provision of guidance or direction, evaluation, and follow-up by the licensed nurse for

accomplishment of a nursing task delegated to unlicensed assistive personnel (UAP) (NCSBN, 1995). Supervision is the active process of directing, guiding, and influencing the outcome of an individual's performance of an activity or task. Within the clinical setting supervision can be categorized as on-site or off-site in nature (ANA, 1996).

The ANA (1996) defined unlicensed assistive personnel (UAP) as individuals who are trained to function in an assistive role to the registered professional nurse in the provision of patient/client care activities as delegated by and under the supervision of the registered professional nurse. In the past a nurse extender meant a nursing assistant or a corpsman. A nurse extender was an ancillary person trained to perform some basic client care tasks who may have been given a client assignment. Today, there are many names for and types of nurse extenders, and they can be classified according to clinical and nonclinical job duties (Gardner, 1991; Hall, 1997). The basic distinction is whether the nurse extender performs direct client care. Nurse extenders range from LPNs and LVNs to UAP, who have no formal health care education or training. Alterations in the skill-mix percentage of RNs to UAP have been moving toward an increase in UAP and a decrease in RNs. Nurses argue that inadequate staffing ratios can create a potentially dangerous circumstance for client care and safety. In California, nurses have minimum nurse-client ratios in acute care hospitals that were passed in legislation.

◭ LEADING & MANAGING DEFINED

Delegation

The transfer of responsibility for the performance of a task from one person to a competent other.

Delegator

The person making the delegation.

Delegatee

The person receiving the delegation.

Supervision

The provision of guidance or direction, evaluation, and follow-up by the licensed nurse for accomplishment of a nursing task or activity delegated to unlicensed assistive personnel, with initial direction and periodic inspection of the actual accomplishment of the task or activity.

Client care activities include all tasks and activities, mental and physical, necessary to care for clients and produce nursing and health outcomes. Nursing activities involve tasks and direct client contact, as well as the full scope of the nursing process. Delegating certain activities, performed by nurses but not limited to them, does not mean nursing itself is delegated. Core activities of the nursing process require specialized knowledge and judgment that only the nurse has. Nonnursing tasks are those necessary to support the patient environment. They can be categorized as cleaning, running errands, clerical, stocking, and maintenance not involving patient contact (American Association of Critical-Care Nurses [AACN], 1995).

BACKGROUND

Delegation of care originated from physician responsibilities being delegated to nurses. Nurses began to assume more and more tasks deemed as nursing care to the point that they could not be completed by the nurse in the limited time frame. Thus phlebotomists, respiratory therapists, physical therapists, and UAP emerged to help provide more comprehensive care. The establishment of the health care team formed around these specialists needing to coordinate work. With this work structure the need to delegate work arose.

The NCSBN issued conceptual and historical papers in 1990 on delegation as a dynamic decision-making process and formulated practical guidelines for delegation. An updated document was published in 1995 to provide resources for boards of nursing, health policy makers, and health care providers on delegation and the roles of licensed and unlicensed health care workers (NCSBN, 1995). This work remains an important standardized framework for nursing delegation.

The NCSBN (1995) further identified the delegating nurse as being responsible for an individualized assessment of the client and situational circumstances. This involves an assessment of each person's competency prior to delegating any task.

Box 25.1

Delegation Checklist

✓ How is the task to be done?
✓ When is the task to be done?
✓ Where is the task to be done?
✓ By whom is the task to be done?
✓ What is the responsibility and authority for decision making (approves, is responsible, is consulted, is informed)?

Questions that the delegating nurse should ask before delegating include the following:

- What is the task to be delegated?
- Is the task complex or simple?
- How much intensive decision making is needed to complete the task?

Additional factors to be considered besides the task include the staff available, the client's needs, the potential delegate's competency, and the level of supervision available. Box 25.1 displays a series of questions that can form a delegation checklist.

A key element is to assess the competency of the staff available for delegation. Assignments must fall within the person's scope of practice. The delegatee must understand the assignment and be competent. The nurse's delegation responsibilities also include assessing the competency of the person and assessing how much supervision time is needed. The nurse's two main legal responsibilities when making work assignments are (1) to appropriately delegate duties and (2) to adequately supervise afterward (Barter & Furmidge, 1994). Both factors may vary depending on the situation and the delegatee's job maturity or readiness. The amount of time needed to supervise after delegation and the needed proximity of the supervisor affect the nurse's workload. Clearly, there is a difference between delegating tasks to a fellow RN and delegating to LPN/LVNs or UAP. To ease the time and effort it takes for each nurse to assess every other care provider's competency level, organizations develop standardized job descriptions and some related job scope policies for the system.

However, individual skill sets vary, despite standardized competency assessments. For example, applying a splint to a wrist would naturally occur more frequently in an emergency department than on a maternity floor. Thus the nurse needs to determine individual competency for each instance of delegation.

In a visual model format, the NCSBN (1998a) illustrated the plotting of RN, LPN, and UAP roles. This framework contains the two axes of client competency and self-care deficit. This selection of role-appropriate assignment to personnel is placed in the context of the client's needs. Consultation and coordination are identified as key RN roles. Companion documents include *The Continuum of Care Framework* (NCSBN, 1998b), which is a one-page table outlining and differentiating RN versus assistive roles, and a resource paper for regulatory agencies (NCSBN, 1998c).

The NCSBN (1997a) developed an algorithm tool based on the delegation decision tree from the Ohio Board of Nursing. It gives specific assessment questions and indicates the path to follow in delegation decision making. This decision tree can be accessed at the NCSBN website (*www.ncsbn.org/pdfs/delegationtree.pdf*) for easy review by students and nurses in practice. This caution should be noted: the tool must be altered to make it consistent with each state's nurse practice act and scope of practice. The NCSBN (1997b) developed a companion instrument, the Delegation Decision-Making Grid, which provides a scoring mechanism for the following seven critical elements to be considered when making delegation decisions:

1. Level of client
2. Level of UAP competence
3. Level of licensed nurse competence
4. Potential for harm
5. Frequency
6. Level of decision making
7. Ability for self-care

As a group, the NCSBN documents provide easy-to-use guidelines to address common issues and assist with structural assessment needs for making delegation decisions.

PROCESS OF DELEGATION

Delegation is a decision-making process that requires expert nurse judgment. The decision to delegate should incorporate critical thinking and sound clinical decision making. The process is to give a directive, set a time frame, and have periodic reviewing from the beginning of the task through its end. In most cases it is recommended for the delegator and the delegatee to agree on the task, circumstances, and time frame and then to arrange for feedback in which the delegatee reports or the delegator evaluates progress towards completion of the task. One way to make certain that both delegator and delegatee understand what the task is and how to complete it effectively is to follow up a verbal directive with written instructions so that each person can refer to them later. Figure 25.2 displays a sample delegation tracking form. This form can be used by the delegator when initially assigning a task as a vehicle for clear communication with the delegatee and verification of expectations and consensus. The task should specify a time frame in which the entire task is to be completed.

Decisions to delegate need to be carefully and thoroughly evaluated. General guidelines have been suggested. A reasonable first decision rule is to be able to delegate the care of clients whose care requirements are routine and standard. Once it is assessed that the person to be delegated to has the minimal competencies required for safe care, and if the outcomes of care are relatively predictable, delegation is considered safe. If the client's reaction to illness and hospitalization is not threatening to his or her mental health or sense of self, it also is relatively safe to assume that that this care can be delegated to a UAP. For example, a client experiencing an acute episode of hypertension would be assigned to the RN as opposed to the UAP. As for the LPN/LVN's assignment, the nurse will delegate the care of clients who are not experiencing life-threatening situations.

In making a decision to delegate nursing tasks, the following five factors can be assessed (AACN, 1995):

1. Potential for harm
2. Complexity of task

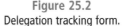

Date _____

Task outcome _____

Task steps _____

Task location _____

Delegator _____

Delegatee _____

Time frame _____

Decision responsibility/authority _____

Next communication _____

Other _____

Figure 25.2
Delegation tracking form.

3. Problem solving and innovation required
4. Unpredictability of the outcome
5. Level of patient interaction

The NCSBN (1995) presented a format for the delegation decision-making process. The decision to delegate needs to be consistent with the nursing process. Thus the nurse needs to ensure appropriate assessment, planning, implementation, and evaluation in a continuous process.

First the nurse determines the legal scope of delegation as set forth in the state's Nurse Practice Act. Then the qualifications of both the delegator and the delegatee are determined. When this baseline is in place, the licensed nurse enters the continuous process of delegation decision-making. The situation is assessed, and a plan for specific task delegation is established, taking into consideration patient needs, available resources, and patient safety. The nurse needs to ensure accountability for the acts and process of delegation. This includes supervision of the performance of the entire task, any necessary intervention, and evaluation of the task performance and the delegation itself.

The process of delegation can be further facilitated by utilizing The Five Rights of Delegation outlined by the NCSBN (1995) as follows:

1. Right Task
2. Right Circumstance
3. Right Person
4. Right Direction/Communication
5. Right Supervision

When determining the *right task* to delegate, the nurse will determine whether the task falls within the guidelines of established agency policies and procedures, the ANA Code of Ethics, and legal regulations for practice. The nurse then must consider whether the task can be delegated to any other staff members.

The *right circumstance* to perform the task indicates the delegatee has the available resources, equipment, safe environment, and supervision to complete the task correctly. The *right person* will have the education and competency to perform the task. The right person delegated to will therefore be legally acceptable to complete the task.

The *right direction/communication* of delegated tasks will be a clear, concise description of the task, including its objective, limits, and expectations. The nurse will allow for clarification without the fear of repercussions.

The *right supervision* of a task will include appropriate monitoring, intervention, evaluation, and feedback as deemed necessary. A process for staff reporting both the task completion and the client's response back to the RN should be in place.

The five "rights" can quickly help to analyze whether a delegation decision will most likely result in a safe outcome. To facilitate the delegation process in a way that will ensure the client's personal health needs are addressed and the nurse's professional goals are achieved, effective communication techniques must be used (Marthaler, 2003). Box 25.2 outlines a personal checklist for the delegator to use for self-evaluation.

True delegation is real to the delegatee. The delegator lets the delegatee go on their own, but only after instilling in them the highest standards of performance and adherence to a shared vision. The delegatee then functions within the standards set by the delegator, who has given authority to do the job, make independent decisions, and be responsible for seeing that the job is done well. True delegation trust is earned over time. For the new nurse who basically has to prove his or her ability to complete tasks, this sometimes can take

up to 2 years to occur. Effective delegation requires that the delegatee have the authority to accompany the responsibility. The delegator monitors task completion and is alert for variances or other problems.

No matter what method the nurse uses for delegation, the essence of the task being delegated is often overlooked. Recognition of the potential vulnerability of the client, and thus the presence of an inherently moral element to health care practice, has raised concerns in relation to proper moral regard and respect for clients (Niven & Scott, 2003). This means that nursing judgment about which tasks are to be delegated requires consideration of the client's needs at that particular time. For example, obtaining the vital signs on a client who is dying may be a reasonable delegation to a UAP. However, because a nurse has spent a lot of time explaining the process of the "do-not-resuscitate" status to the family, a trusting relationship has been established. The client or family members' preferences for treatment/ care need to be considered in delegating care activities.

An issue that arises in practice is whether delegation can safely occur when the responsible delegator is not physically present to supervise. According to the Association of Operating Room Nurses (AORN, 2004) off-site (indirect) delegation is defined as follows: direction provided through various means of written and verbal communications. For example, the nurse manager will make a list of tasks to be completed—i.e., check code cart, clean kitchen, clean break room, and restock IV bags. The tasks will be assigned to RNs, UAP, LPN /LVN, or the unit secretary. The delegated tasks are assigned to reflect the ability, experience, and education of the individual.

The ultimate responsibility and accountability rests with the delegator because, in the end, the delegator is accountable to his or her own superiors for fulfilling the responsibility to get the job done right and on time. Thus true delegation or off-site delegation means giving up some of the authority and holding onto the ultimate responsibility and accountability.

Box **25.2**

Delegator's Checklist

✓ Develop a good attitude
✓ Decide what to delegate
✓ Select the right person
✓ Communicate responsibilities
✓ Grant authority
✓ Provide support
✓ Monitor the delegation
✓ Evaluate

Data from Nelson, R. (1994). *Empowering employees through delegation.* Burr Ridge, IL: Richard D. Irwin.

DELEGATION PITFALLS AND SOLUTIONS

Although it is in everyone's best interest to delegate, the process may be undermined from within the health care setting. Delegation suggests that work is being moved from one member of the primary health care team to another in a downward direction (Richards et al., 2000). As a result, the nurse most commonly delegates to UAP. Both RNs and those to whom they delegate have psychological responses to the act of delegation. The UAP sometimes resents the nurse delegating tasks that could be completed by the nurse. On the other hand, the nurse may find it difficult to let go of control. When tasks are delegated, strong feelings and reactions occur, including the nurse's desire to keep control. At times, the nurse reclaims some of the delegated responsibility. Nothing is more demoralizing for delegatees than to discover that the delegator has undercut their responsibility. Nurses who are novice, insecure, or need to feel indispensable are most likely to resist delegation or to "renege" on it later. Their motto is, "If you want a job done right, you have to do it yourself." Box 25.3 displays reasons for reluctance to delegate.

When called on to delegate something important, nurses may suddenly discover that, for some reason, they do not trust their coworkers quite as much as they thought they did. How can work be delegated to people if they are not trusted? On the other hand, how can health care providers earn the trust of the nurse who does not delegate to them? This is a real dilemma, facing both delegator and delegatee. The absence of trust by the delegator is based on one of the most powerful of all feelings: fear. This fear is very real for the nurse, especially when it involves a loss of control.

There is an emotional reality that surrounds delegation. Delegation inevitably involves risk. Ignorance of the capabilities or the scope of practice of health care team members can cause detrimental outcomes. Likewise, overdelegating tasks can be dangerous (e.g., allowing a nursing assistant in nursing school to start an intravenous line or asking an LPN/LVN to give discharge instructions because you are good friends and a favor is owed). Delegating a task that is completed incorrectly translates into potentially harming a patient and possibly incurring a lawsuit.

Conversely, successful delegation of a task may be threatening to a nurse's self-esteem or seen as a nurse's failure to personally accomplish work. This is a natural emotion (i.e., the fear that a delegatee might surpass the nurse in ability or prestige), especially for individuals in a new role or job such as a new nurse manager or graduate nurse. The ability to delegate appropriately should be viewed as an achievement and be rewarded, not seen as a weakness or laziness.

In nursing, conventional wisdom and anecdotal experiences indicate how difficult it can be for nurses to delegate effectively. In fact, some nurses may find themselves unable to delegate. Historically, the RN was responsible for providing most of the direct client care. Therefore nurses became used to providing care themselves and may not have learned how to delegate. Similarly, graduate nurses typically have had limited experience delegating in nursing school, and they have been delivering direct client care the vast majority of their time in the clinical arena.

Underdelegation can also be the result of a lack of motivation to delegate. Some nurses may find that they need to delegate, direct, and supervise others; yet they have no power over the rewards and disciplinary action that motivates cooperation. This issue is especially acute in

---

Box 25.3

Delegation Reluctance

- The "I can do it better myself" fallacy trap
- Lack of ability to direct
- Lack of confidence in subordinates
- Lack of confidence in self
- Aversion to taking a risk
- Need to feel indispensable and difficulty letting go
- Fear of losing authority or personal satisfaction

Data from *Delegating* [videotape]. (1981). Del Mar, CA: McGraw-Hill; and Poteet, G. (1989). Nursing administrators and delegation. *Nursing Administration Quarterly, 13*(3), 23-32.

unionized environments. The new graduate nurse may have a tendency to underdelegate to seek recognition from coworkers that all of his or her tasks were completed by his or her own personal effort. Unfortunately, the new graduate may then be reprimanded for high overtime. Nurses who do not delegate well may feel inadequate about not being able to complete all of the tasks associated with care. Delegators are reluctant to delegate because they feel that they need to do it themselves, lack the ability to direct, lack confidence in subordinates and self, have an aversion to taking a risk, have a fear of letting go, and have a fear of losing authority or personal job satisfaction (Poteet, 1989).

At times delegatees attempt to avoid delegation by fostering a myth that the delegators are so indispensable that they need to do the work themselves. The illusion of the delegator's indispensability can be actively fostered by the delegatees. Sometimes this belief is genuine, but it may instead be a way for delegatees to avoid being delegated to and, therefore, to avoid or feel reluctant to accept more responsibility. Delegatees may fear criticism regarding mistakes because they lack confidence in their own abilities. The most common complaint delegates make is that they already have more work that than can handle, when in fact, the delegated tasks are not extra work but a part of their job description. Additionally, they may not have confidence in their own abilities. This can be a matter of reminding delegatees that they do have the necessary skills and abilities, especially if they would push themselves a little bit. The delegator may feel that the delegatees do have the job maturity, knowledge, and ability to handle the task, but the delegatees may feel that positive incentives are not present. From the delgatees' perspective, why take on something extra or put in more effort if the perception is that they are not going to be rewarded? Box 25.4 outlines reasons why delegatees avoid delegation responsibilities.

Delegators sometimes reestablish their claim on authority by hovering after a task has been delegated. Hovering, or "breathing down somebody's

---

> **Box 25.4**
>
> ### Why Delegatees Avoid Responsibilities
>
> - Fear of criticism for mistakes
> - Lack necessary information and resources to do a good job
> - Overwhelming workload
> - Lack of self-confidence regarding ability to successfully delegate
> - Positive incentives may not be sufficient motivators
> - Delegator's personality and preferences may interfere with the delegation process
> - Ease of seeking answers from the delegator than deciding on their own how to deal with problems

---

neck," usually conveys a feeling of distrust. This behavior may lead to the delegatee feeling that he or she really *does* lack ability. Delegation is not meant to intimidate or isolate the delegator or delegatee. The goal of delegating is to provide client-centered care in the most efficient way. Delegating appropriate tasks to the right person, who can complete the task in an established time frame and who understands that the completed task, will allow care to be completed in a timely manner. Equally important, delegation can stimulate interest in a nursing career, maintain competencies, spark new interests, and prevent monotony.

Solutions to pitfalls of delegation are straightforward. Licensed nurses and UAP experience positive events when a routine observation occurs following delegation (Anthony et al., 2000). Recognizing the importance of the process of supervision and its implications for educational opportunities that focus on delegation competencies is essential for RNs. Peer staff or nurse managers can be consulted regarding delegating nursing activities to UAP or LPN/LVN to ensure accuracy. Detailed and specific activities need to be communicated to the delegatee. Knowledge of the delegatee's performance will enhance trust and confidence in their abilities by the RN.

LEGAL ASPECTS OF DELEGATION AND SUPERVISION

Nurses are accountable for following their state nurse practice act, standards of professional practice, policies of the health care organization, and ethical-legal models of behavior (Marthaler, 2003). Each state's legislature has set up a board of nursing whose function is to interpret and enforce the law. When this body interprets the law, the formal interpretations become administrative rules that have the force of law. State nurse practice acts and their official interpretations constitute a body of rules, codified within the legal regulatory system, that govern nursing practice and provide direction about delegation and supervision. The American Nurses Association (ANA) and each state's nurses association are the bodies that speak for the profession of nursing to define and guide the professional practice of nursing through definitions, standards of practice, and statements about delegation and supervision.

Standards of care are used to determine whether the minimum level of care has been delivered. The term *malpractice* refers to an improper performance of professional duties; a failure to meet the standards of care that result in harm to another person (Zerwekh & Claborn, 2003). When a nurse deviates from the internal standards of care of an organization, the nurse can be liable for malpractice or negligence. This includes acts of delegation and supervision.

The Iowa Board of Nursing (2003) website defines *accountability* as being obligated to answer for one's acts, including the act of supervision. The RN is expected to recognize and understand the legal implications of accountability by knowing what accountability is and what it means in terms of nursing practice. Accountability includes acts of supervision, among other things. In a legal sense, *supervision* means personally observing a function or activity, providing leadership in the process of nursing care, delegating functions or activities while retaining the accountability, and evaluating or determining that nursing care being provided is adequate and delivered appropriately. Although this document is dated, the definitions and principles of the law related to supervision have not changed.

Delegation is considered to be part of the nurse's role. Nurses delegate, and they are delegated to. The nurse delegator is accountable to assess the situation and accountable for the decision to delegate. When a nurse delegates, the task must be performed in accordance with established standards of practice, policies, and procedures (NCSBN, 1995). The nurse is ultimately accountable for the appropriateness and supervision of the delegated tasks. Thus the nurse delegator may incur liability if found negligent in the process of delegating and supervising. The person delegated to is accountable for accepting the delegation and for the actions in carrying out the delegated tasks (Box 25.5). Therefore accountability is shared by both the delegator and delegatee. The nurse is accountable for supervision, follow-up, intervention, and corrective action in the event of an error. Assessment, evaluation, and nursing judgment should not be delegated; tasks and procedures may be delegated. Although others may suggest which acts to delegate, the individual nurse ultimately decides the appropriateness of delegation in a specific situation (NCSBN, 1995).

Box **25.5**

Who Has Accountability?

Delegator
- Own acts
- Acts of delegation
- Acts of supervision
- Assessment of the situation
- Follow-up
- Intervention
- Corrective active

Delegatee
- Own acts
- Accepting the delegation
- Appropriate notification and reporting
- Accomplishing the task

Delegating also requires skillful written and verbal communication to avoid liability. If it is not documented, it is considered that it was not done. Clear documentation of assignments and additional clarification of the delegated tasks for each health care team member is required when delegating. Courts view written communication as an important reminder of "tasks" and attention to clients (Kraus & Cameron, 2004). It is the nurse's responsibility to keep current with updates in the literature and guideline changes in the standards of care of delegation. The institution is responsible for informing nurses of all changes in policy through e-mail, memos, inservices, or staff meetings.

The legal issues associated with delegation include the following:

- The RN remains legally responsible for activities delegated.
- The RN is accountable for appropriateness of delegated task and its accurate completion.
- The organization for which the RN, UAP, and LPN/LVN work for is liable for their negligence or malpractice.
- Unlicensed assistive personnel cannot supervise other UAP.
- UAP cannot redelegate to another UAP or nursing student.
- UAP cannot complete a pain assessment.
- LPN/LVN cannot complete discharge teaching.

The state administrative code also identifies nursing behavior that constitutes illegal conduct. This includes delegating nursing functions to others contrary to statute or state rules. Such nursing behavior is subject to licensure discipline. The state regulatory body can use any measure of discipline across the continuum, including revoking a license. In a legal sense, negligence or malpractice consists of failure of a professional person to act in accordance with the prevalent professional standards or failure to foresee possibilities and consequences that a professional person, having the necessary skill and training to act professionally, should foresee. The nurse must perform at a level that exceeds or equals that of a reasonably prudent professional RN. Generally, practice

issues are tested in courts of law. In this process, expert witnesses are used to interpret the standard of a reasonably prudent professional RN.

The nurse has an obligation or duty to act in the event of a breakdown in client care wherever in the chain that breakdown occurs. This means that the nurse is never permitted under law to passively observe substandard care. Delegation and supervision are key areas in which such issues may arise. The most common situation is of a fellow nurse or other health care provider demonstrably or clearly failing to provide the appropriate care to clients. Substandard care also may come about when a health care agency fails to exercise its corporate duty in providing sufficient numbers of RNs with appropriate delegation and supervision skills to ensure quality care. Under both of these circumstances, the nurse must act and cannot hide behind the fact that "the doctor knows best" or that "the administration does not listen to nurses."

In the event the health care agency is compromising care, the nurse will initiate an assessment of how much client safety is being compromised. If there is clear actual or potential harm, the nurse must act directly. If the situation is ambiguous, such as an ethical issue, then the nurse must take some action appropriate to the circumstance. For example, this may be reported to the immediate superior, or there may be a refusal to participate if that is appropriate.

Some situations are less complex and clearer as to the appropriate actions to take. For example, when an intensive care unit (ICU) nurse walks away from the bedside of a client who is comatose with an intracranial pressure screw in place and leaves the side rails down, client safety is clearly compromised and action must be taken (i.e., raising the side rails). As another example, if an inappropriate dose of a chemotherapy drug is ordered, action must be taken regarding seeking clarification of the order with the health care provider who wrote it. However, many situations are not this clear and instead fall into a "gray area." For example, providers use a variety of practice patterns. Situations are complex and multidimensional. Ethical values may be at odds. One provider might not have complete information about an observed situation. For example, behaviors manifested because of physical or psychological organic illness may be interpreted as the result of substance abuse. Thus the nurse's assessment and judgment are critical components of delegation and supervision.

Legal and ethical issues surround the tensions and trade-offs between quality and cost. For example, what constitutes an "unsafe" level of nurse staffing is not clear. Nurses face uncomfortable situations when deciding between labor budget pressures and staffing for clients' care needs. At what point does the nurse take action to report "unsafe" staffing levels? What action strategies are effective? How does the nurse who calls the fire department to report serious overcrowding of clients into hallways reconcile the duty to protect client safety with accusations of insubordination and potential job termination? It is not uncommon for the nurse to find conflicts between an employer's expectations and the nursing standards of care, resulting in problems such as having insufficient time or staffing to adhere to the standards taught in nursing school or receiving poor evaluations for taking too long to render care (Martin & Cain, 2003).

Clearly, client safety and the obligation to do no harm is a fundamental starting point. The nurse can analyze the situation and decide on a strategy. A framework for ethical analysis can be chosen to help clarify values and ethical choices. A legal analysis can be done to assess whether the elements of a malpractice claim appear to be in evidence: duty, breach of duty, proximate cause,

Research Note

Source: McGlung, T.M. (2000). Assessing the reported financial benefits of unlicensed assistive personnel in nursing. *Journal of Nursing Administration 30*(11), 530-534.

Purpose

To review highlights of several studies reported in the past decade that describe the use of UAP in nursing care models and assess their justification.

Discussion

The use of UAP in the late 1980s and early 1990s was solely based on reducing cost. Today, it can be argued the use of UAP is due to the diminishing supply of RNs. In 1990 nursing aide positions were increased by 100% for every RN position vacancy. Cost containment was implemented, but the quality of care suffered. This resulted in the development of job descriptions of UAP by nurse executives, states, and agencies; but they were still inconsistent across settings and sites. In 1991 a new care model using a multiskilled technician type of UAP teamed with an RN changed the patient-to-staff ratio from 5:1 to 7:1 patient-to-RN/UAP team without any budget changes or quality of care changes. In two studies involving critical care units using UAP paired with an RN, a savings of $52,000 was reported, and this decreased the expense per patient-day. Measuring start-up costs, exploring UAP models, and relying on a random mix of subjective and quantifiable measures are suggestions for further research in this area.

Application to Practice

The use of UAP and other unlicensed personnel to provide client care at a reduced cost continues to happen. The lack of nurses, an increase in jobs for nurses, or the events of the nurse shortage have increased the need for additional client care providers. Nursing shortages are positive for nurses but detrimental to client care. Positive outcomes for nurses include consideration of staffing ratios, salary and benefit increases, and recognizing that nurses do not have to complete all of the care. Some care needs to be delegated.

and damages. Other assessments can be done by consulting organizational policies and standards, the state's nurse practice act and administrative rulings from the board of nursing, Code of Ethics for nurses (ANA, 2001) and standards of practice, and standards and guidelines of specialty organizations. A clear legal duty to act is more urgent than is a question of ethics. Through reasoned investigation and analysis of the situation, the nurse then decides whether to act immediately, investigate further, document, report, or analyze the situation for future decision making. The standards of "reasonable," "prudent," and "good faith" form the foundations for legal and ethical decision-making strategies.

Nurses at all levels should be clear regarding their legal accountability when delegating. Questions regarding situations that may occur include these: What is my responsibility if a student creates an error or is negligent in caring for my client? What are the legal parameters of delegating to a UAP who has had only 2 weeks of training? What can I delegate and to whom?

LEADERSHIP AND MANAGEMENT IMPLICATIONS

Managers and administrators know that the quality of care delivered to clients can be affected by the type of working relationships that exist between RNs and UAP (Potter & Grant, 2004). Delegation is a critical yet very difficult leadership and management skill. All nurses need to build a delegation competency. Delegation means giving up some of the authority and holding onto the ultimate responsibility and accountability. Delegation benefits both nurses and organizations by gaining freedom, time, and greater efficiency from its effective implementation. Unfortunately, the amount of delegation by nurses varies (Richards et al., 2000). Delegation is directly related to leadership effectiveness and the use of leadership styles. It appears that leaders and managers may adopt one of two problem-solving styles: adaptation or innovation. Adaptors generate ideas to solve problems. Innovators detach the problem, critically think about it, and search for a solution. Individuals tend to remain in an organizational

⚠ LEADERSHIP & MANAGEMENT **BEHAVIORS**

Leadership Behaviors

- Enables followers to learn delegation and supervision skills
- Creates a positive work climate and teamwork
- Matches leadership style to readiness of followers and situation
- Is visible and available
- Communicates clearly
- Uses interpersonal relationship facilitation to aid group functioning
- Delegates
- Facilitates delegation and acceptance of responsibility

Management Behaviors

- Coaches subordinates to improve task maturity
- Performs careful assessments of abilities

- Makes assignments to match skills and abilities
- Monitors performance through supervision
- Documents
- Evaluates task accomplishment
- Disciplines employees
- Communicates clearly
- Delegates

Overlap Areas

- Facilitates delegation and acceptance of responsibility
- Communicates clearly
- Delegates

environment that has a problem-solving style that matches their personal inclination (Adams, 1993). The same may be true for styles of delegation. Individuals may adopt unique styles, and these styles may be a "fit" or a mismatch.

Leader behaviors for delegation and supervision include being around, being available, and helping the delegatee through the task actions and decisions. Coaching actions of delegation are also employed. Providing guidance and leadership in the development of the nurse's ability to delegate is an important aspect of RN skill building. Delegation is a managerial technique that helps people build skills and confidence. It is hard work and may not come naturally. However, mentored guidance and leadership in building the skills related to delegation enhance individuals and build high-performing teams.

Nursing practice in community health or home health care settings may include supervision and delegation of tasks off-site. The importance of the skills involved in assessing the competencies of UAP cannot be overestimated (McIntosh, 2003). Careful assessment, regular visits, and complete documentation are used when delegating in these settings (Barter & Furmidge, 1994).

Certain aspects of managerial work should never be delegated. These are discipline, praise, recognition, and morale issues. Sending others to do the manager's corrective directing is a counterproductive approach to a problem requiring attention. When a problem needs to be addressed in a direct, calm, unemotional and fact-finding/clarifying approach, the manager is the best person to handle the situation. Additionally, the manager should handle the discipline of employees. The direct managerial intervention of discipline maintains a climate within the work group, communicates a message, and shows discharge of duty. For example, if there is an area in which client care is not bringing about quality results or if there is some problem with regard to the delivery of client care, the manager needs to be directly active in the resolution of the problem. At the same time, praise and recognition are powerful motivators if given by managers and supervisors. The last area

not to be delegated by the manager relates to morale issues. Morale, and its associated aspects of motivation and job satisfaction, should be addressed directly as a function of leadership and organizational management. Leadership style and the interpersonal and communication skills of the leader have a strong influence on employees' morale.

CURRENT ISSUES AND TRENDS

Changes in the delivery of health care have increased the complexity of the RN's role, created greater pressure for, and enhanced the importance of delegation and supervision. Tangible changes have occurred in practice that have made the job of a nurse better in some ways and more difficult in others. The environment is becoming safer; in many facilities a computer is readily available on every unit to provide accurate and up-to-date information; delegation of care continues to evolve within health care teams and from the nurse to UAP. All jobs in the health care team have been expanded. Is this the result of delegation? Or was delegation the result of expanded roles?

According to the ANA, "Staffing should be based on achieving quality of patient care indices, meeting organizational outcomes, and ensuring that the quality of the nurse's work life is appropriate" (1999, p. 3). Outsourcing of qualified foreign registered nurses is a natural choice to many nurse executives because historically the United States has welcomed immigrants with diverse skills and qualifications to be part of the American economy (Dikaya & Appelet II, 2004) In 2002, there were 12,762 first-time NCLEX-RN® examination candidates listing education codes from other countries. Outsourcing with foreign nurses into permanent positions is used to keep health care costs down in some cases. Another form of outsourcing is the use of staffing agency or "traveler" nurses, which has become a significant budgetary outlay. Delegation and supervision issues related to outsourced or traveler staff take on a different character and urgency because these RNs are not part of the regular unit employees of the organization. Foreign nurses hold a nursing degree equivalent to a U.S. nursing degree and have had training to successfully complete the national licensure exam, thus indicating their capabilities to care for clients. Their unit orientation, familiarity with policies and procedures, and ability to know and reassess the competency of UAP and other team members may need to be customized and managed differently from that of regular unit employees. To that end, agency nurses will be assigned those clients on the unit who are not the sickest. As the organization becomes more familiar with the agency or traveler nurse and credibility has been established, delegation of tasks will become more extensive.

The highly competitive marketplace of health care triggered widespread restructuring and redesign initiatives in the mid-1990s. Altering the makeup of the care delivery team and cross-training to provide multiskilled personnel were components of many redesign efforts. Nursing has criticized the lack of published evaluations of these initiatives. Advocates of redesign argue that delivery systems become more client centered. However, the fear remains that such redesign opens a potential for undesirable trade-offs between costs and quality of care. Reports from the nursing community allege unsafe redesign-related alterations in the numbers and mixes of nursing personnel available to provide care (Havens & Aiken, 1999). Tremendous shifts in staff mix have occurred in hospitals as the use of UAP as a part of the care delivery team has increased. These shifts have resulted in a significant change in the skill level of the care providers assigned to client care and sometimes have been an issue related to patient safety. The most prevalent influence on staff mix has been financial forces (Hall, 1997).

The National Center for Health Workforce Analysis (2002) of the Health Resources and Services Administration (HRSA), Bureau of Health Professions, developed supply and demand projections for registered nurses. In 2000, the supply of full-time equivalent (FTE) registered nurses was estimated at 1.89 million, while the demand was estimated at 2 million. This is a shortage of

110,000 or 6%. Based on what is known about trends, the shortage is expected to grow until 2010 and reach 12%.

Interestingly, although cost containment produces downsizing and a dramatic increase in the use of UAP, a nursing shortage cycle also tends to create a pressure for the substitution of less prepared personnel. The ANA's *Joint Statement on Maintaining Professional and Legal Standards During a Shortage of Nursing Personnel* (ANA, 1992) noted that during a time of RN shortage there is a predictable trend to deregulate, remove, or reduce barriers to entry into the marketplace and substitute less prepared persons for expediency. Such shifts create serious allied issues related to delegation and supervision for RNs as they attempt to work in environments of fewer RNs and more non-RN personnel.

The end of the 1990s saw economic forces and health care costs come to an intersection. Changes in the health care system led to changes in the numbers and types of personnel who deliver direct care to clients (Potter & Grant, 2004). A decrease in the number of licensed caregivers and an increase in the number of UAP occurred. Hospitals had restructured, redesigned, and downsized RNs without paying attention to evidence-based practice changes or known effects on delegation, supervision, and client safety. The ANA (1997) also issued a position statement on restructuring and work redesign. The association noted that there was no evidence that nursing has contributed to escalating health care costs and that nursing averages 23% of hospital labor costs. Despite hospital executives' rating of nursing care as the most important contributor to hospital quality, hospitals targeted RNs for layoffs. The work responsibilities of RNs were increased, and simultaneously workers with less skill were substituted for them. Such profit-driven health care strategies created fears that the quality of client care had eroded and client safety had been compromised (ANA, 1997).

This "de-skilling" became visible in the 1996 settlement of a lawsuit in Ohio over the 1994 death of a client who underwent a hysterectomy and died because her caregivers were client care technicians, not RNs. The technicians missed the signs and symptoms of infection and shock (*AJN*, 1996a). Such reports sparked a round of legislative hearings and debate about regulating UAP by boards of nursing. The issues became contentious as nurses reported low morale, high workload stress, and a shifting of blame for unsafe care onto nurses who were labeled inflexible and not aware of how to delegate. Nurses insisted that mandated nurse-to-patient staffing ratios be enacted in laws. Hospital officials contended that these reports were exaggerated; nursing administrators opposed mandated staffing ratios (*AJN*, 1996b). These issues of the recent past set a precedent for future rounds of organizational cost-containment initiatives.

Problems related to delegation arise whenever new staff-mix models are introduced. Recent models of nursing care delivery include a form of primary nursing and client-focused care in which RNs independently manage and direct the care of a group of clients. Managing a group of clients is different from managing and directing care provided by other providers, such as was common with team nursing. Thus previous models did not use the RN's supervisory and delegation skills in the same fashion as contemporary models require. It is possible that excluding RNs from the in-depth development of UAP roles contributed to problems with delegation (Hall, 1997). On a positive note, as health care becomes more complex, the knowledge and skill base of UAP is growing with the expansion of training opportunities, greater experiential learning, and opportunities to make more money (McIntosh et al., 2000). Delegation and supervision always will be intertwined with issues surrounding the use of nurse extenders and UAP.

The Tri-Council for Nursing (1990) has stated that it is extremely important that UAP be used in a way that ensures appropriate delegation and assignment of nursing functions and adequate supervision of those to whom nursing activities are delegated. The Joint Commission on Accreditation of Healthcare Organizations (JCAHO, 2004) stated that effective staffing has been linked to positive client outcomes and improved quality and safety of care. Concerns about declining quality of care and nurse staffing shortages led to legislation mandating minimum nurse-to-patient ratios in the state of California (Hodge et al., 2004). Suggested minimum ratios ranged from a low of 3:1 to as many as 10:1 clients per nurse for medical-surgical units. However, hospitals say that they must trim costs, that ratios have little to do with clients' needs, and that this is a turf issue about RN job security (Anders, 1994; Sherer, 1993).

Decisions about the use of UAP focus on what tasks they are to do and which ones belong only to the RN. Some guidelines include routine care needs, predictable outcomes, and nonthreatening illness states (Box 25.6). The nursing profession is challenged to find ways to balance the tension between professional judgment about care needs and the fiscal pressures of the organization.

Hiring UAP increases an organization's responsibility for screening, orientation, and training. The direct care RNs assumes a major responsibility for supplementing minimally trained UAP and for supervising their delegated tasks (Barter & Furmidge, 1994). The ANA's position statement (1992) and the NCSBN's position paper (1995) recommended that nursing's bottom line remain "what is best for the client." The Institute of Medicine (IOM, 2003) released a report titled *Patient Safety: Achieving a New Standard for Care*, which noted that "to achieve an acceptable standard of patient safety ... all health care settings [should] establish comprehensive patient safety

---

Box **25.6**

Delegation to UAP

Clients whose ...

... care requirements are routine and standardized
... outcomes are predictable
... reaction to illness and hospitalization is not threatening to their mental health

programs operated by trained personnel within a culture of safety" (pp. 169-170). Thus staffing patterns and methods of care delivery should be scrutinized in terms of client outcomes and basic safety.

Delegation as a part of the RN's role occurs within the context of a care delivery system. The skill mix and care modality structure that best fit care delivery needs vary over time and in specific settings and sites. Developing skills for managing role conflict, such as negotiation and delegation, is a useful strategy (Kleinman, 2004). Learning when and how to delegate is a key skill for developing effective nurse leaders and managers and for maintaining quality of care under conditions of rising client acuity, fiscal pressures, and shorter lengths of hospital stays (Hansten, 1991). Furthermore, the nurse ultimately decides and is accountable for appropriate and safe delegation, even when faced with employer pressure and staffing problems (NCSBN, 1990).

Summary

- Delegation is essential for every nurse in all health care delivery organizations.
- Delegation is the transferring to a competent individual the authority to perform a selected nursing task in a selected nursing situation.
- Supervision is the provision of guidance or direction, evaluation, and follow up by the licensed nurse for accomplishment of a delegated nursing task.
- Delegation involves an assessment of competency.
- The delegation process involves selecting a capable person, explaining the task and outcomes, giving authority and means to do the task, and keeping in contact.
- When strong feelings and reactions occur, managers may be reluctant to delegate or subordinates may resist delegation.
- Delegation and supervision are part of the nurse's role.
- Laws and regulations influence delegation and supervision in nursing.

- The nurse ultimately must decide about appropriate and safe delegation.
- Delegation is related to leadership effectiveness.
- Delegation and supervision are issues surrounding the use of UAP.
- Client satisfaction and outcomes of care should be the same when delegation is used.

Study Questions

1. What does your state's nurse practice act say about delegation and supervision?
2. Should a nursing student delegate nursing activities?
3. How often is delegating to unlicensed personnel (UAP) performed in your work setting?
4. How comfortable do you feel with delegation?
5. How can the nurse delegate to assist others to develop further?
6. What criteria can be used to assess co-workers' competency?
7. How do competency criteria differ for RNs, LPN/LVNs, UAP, and nursing students?
8. What routine tasks can RNs delegate to others?
9. When you delegate your work, what type of work do you then perform ?
10. What is a safe or minimum nurse-to-client ratio? Does this differ across care settings?
11. When and what is a nurse responsible for during client care and delivery coordination?
12. What type of relationships have you observed among RNs, LPN/LVNs, and UAP? Were they positive? If not, what changes could be implemented to help the relationships?

CASE STUDY

The shift began very busy. The nurse finished admitting a patient who was scheduled for surgery within the hour. The consent had not been signed, and the surgeon's cell phone was breaking up when he was phoned, so no orders had been received. Another patient going for surgery needed Ancef (cefazolin) 1 g, administered IV piggyback, 30 minutes before surgery as a pre-op medication.

CRITICAL THINKING EXERCISE

The staff on the oncology unit for the day shift (7 AM to 3 PM) for nine patients includes Sherry Trader, the charge nurse; James, Fair, a staff nurse; and Julie Coggeshall, a UAP.

A 54-year-old woman admitted with the diagnosis of breast cancer is scheduled for a radical mastectomy at 10:30 AM. The patient is nonverbal to Nurse Fair, the nurse assigned to the patient. Nurse Fair reports to the charge nurse that he has never prepared a patient who was undergoing a mastectomy. The charge nurse indicates to Nurse Fair that the forms are no different from those for any other surgery.

1. What are the key issues to consider when delegating care to this patient?
2. What is the problem presented in this case?
3. Why is this a problem?
4. What are the possible solutions?
5. Who and what should be delegated for this patient?

The surgery department had called to say "pre-op the patient."

The nurse asked a UAP to hang the piggyback as a big favor. The UAP completed the task. A few minutes later the patient went into respiratory arrest. The medication was not the patient's, and the patient was allergic to the medication that was hung. Was the task delegated to the UAP appropriate? What should the nurse do?

REFERENCES

Adams, C. (1993). The impact of problem-solving styles of nurse executives and executive officers on tenure. *Journal of Nursing Administration, 23*(12), 38-43.

American Association of Critical-Care Nurses (AACN). (1995). *Delegation: A tool for success in the changing workplace.* Aliso Viejo, CA: AACN.

American Journal of Nursing (AJN). (1996a). $3 million suit exposes "de-skilling." *American Journal of Nursing, 96*(11), 70.

American Journal of Nursing (AJN). (1996b). Pennsylvania lawmakers probe RN cuts, grill hospitals on UAP use. *American Journal of Nursing, 96*(11), 71-72.

American Nurses Association (ANA). (1992). *Joint statement on maintaining professional and legal standards during a shortage of nursing personnel.* Washington, DC: ANA.

American Nurses Association (ANA). (1996). *Registered professional nurses & unlicensed assistive personnel.* Washington, DC: ANA.

American Nurses Association (ANA). (1997). *Restructuring, work redesign, and the job and career security of registered nurses.* Washington, DC: ANA.

American Nurses Association (ANA). (1999). *Principles for nurse staffing.* Washington, DC: ANA.

American Nurses Association (ANA). (2001). *Code of ethics for nurses with interpretive statements.* Washington, DC: ANA.

Anders, G. (1994, January 20). Nurses decry cost-cutting plan that uses aides to do more jobs. *The Wall Street Journal,* p. B1.

Anthony, M.K., Standing, T. & Hertz, J.E. (2000). Factors influencing outcomes after delegation to unlicensed assistive personnel. *Journal of Nursing Administration 30*(10), 474-480.

Association of Operating Room Nurses (AORN). (2004) *Official statement on unlicensed assistive personnel.* Denver: AORN.

Barter, M., & Furmidge, M. (1994). Unlicensed assistive personnel: Issues relating to delegation and supervision. *Journal of Nursing Administration, 24*(4), 36-40.

Dikaya, Z.A., & Applet II, H.F. (2004). Foreign registered nurses. *Journal of Nursing Administration, 34*(7/8), 379-383.

Fisher, M. (2000). Do you have delegation savvy? *Nursing 2000, 30*(12), 58-59.

Gardner, D. (1991). Issues related to the use of nurse extenders. *Journal of Nursing Administration, 21*(10), 40-45.

Hall, L.M. (1997). Staff mix models: Complementary or substitution roles for nurses. *Nursing Administration Quarterly, 21*(2), 31-39.

Hansten, R. (1991). Delegation: Learning when and how to let go. *Nursing91, 21*(2), 126-133.

Havens, D.S., & Aiken, L.H. (1999). Shaping systems to promote desired outcomes: the magnet hospital model. *Journal of Nursing Administration, 29*(2), 14-20.

Hodge, M.B., Romano, P.S., Harvey, D., & Samuels, S.J. (2004). Licensed caregiver characteristics and staffing in California acute care hospital units. *Journal of Nursing Administration, 34*(3), 125-133.

Institute of Medicine (IOM). (2003). *Patient safety: Achieving a new standard for care.* Washington, DC: National Academies Press.

Iowa Board of Nursing (2003). *Nursing practice for registered nurses/licensed practical nurses.* Des Moines, Iowa: The State of Iowa. Retrieved September 23, 2004, from *www.state.ia.us/nursing/nursing_practice.html*

Joint Commisssion on Accreditation of Healthcare Organizations (JCAHO). (2004). *Staffing effectiveness standard.* Oakbrook Terrace, IL: JCAHO. Retrieved October 11, 2004 from *www.jcaho.org/accredited+ organizations/hospitals/standards/draft+standards/ staffingeffectivenessstandard0804.pdf*

Kleinman, C.S. (2004). Leadership strategies in reducing staff nurse role conflict. *Journal of Nursing Administration 34*(7/8), 322-424.

Kraus, K., & Cameron, M.E. (2004). Legal and ethical issues: Communication and malpractice lawsuits. *Journal of Nursing Administration, 34*(1), 3.

Marthaler, M. (2003). Delegation of nursing care. In P. Kelly-Heidenthal (Ed.), *Nursing leadership and management* (pp. 266-279). Clifton Park, NY: Delmar.

Martin J., & Cain S.K. (2003). Legal aspects of patient care. In P. Kelly-Heidenthal (Ed.), *Nursing leadership and management* (pp. 266-279). Clifton Park, NY: Delmar.

McIntosh, J. (2003). Questions we should ask about community nursing practice. *Primary Health Care Research and Development, 4,* 137-145.

McIntosh, J., Moriarty, D., Lugton, J., & Carney, O. (2000). Evolutionary change in the use of skills within the district nursing team: A study in two Health Board areas in Scotland. *Journal of Advanced Nursing 32,* 783-790.

National Center for Health Workforce Analysis. (2002). *Projected supply, demand, and shortages of registered nurses: 2000-2020.* Washington, DC: Bureau of Health Professions, Health Resources and Services Administration, USDHHS.

National Council of State Boards of Nursing (NCSBN). (1990). *Concept paper on delegation.* Chicago: NCSBN.

National Council of State Boards of Nursing (NCSBN). (1995). *Delegation: Concepts and decision-making process.* Chicago: NCSBN. Retrieved September 17, 2004, from *www.ncsbn.org/regulation/uap_delegation_documents_ delegation.asp*

National Council of State Boards of Nursing (NCSBN). (1997a). *Delegation decision-making tree.* Chicago: NCSBN.

National Council of State Boards of Nursing (NCSBN). (1997b). *Delegation decision-making grid.* Chicago: NCSBN.

National Council of State Boards of Nursing (NCSBN). (1998a). *Diagram to illustrate roles of nurse and AP.* Chicago: NCSBN.

National Council of State Boards of Nursing (NCSBN). (1998b). *The continuum of care framework.* Chicago: NCSBN.

National Council of State Boards of Nursing (NCSBN). (1998c). *The continuum of care: A regulatory perspective.* Chicago: NCSBN.

Niven, C., & Scott, P. (2003). The need for accurate perception and informed judgment in determining the appropriate use of the nursing resource: Hear the patient's voice. *Nursing Philosophy, 4,* 201-210.

Nightingale, F. (1859). *Notes on nursing: What it is and what it is not.* London: Harrison & Sons.

Poteet, G. (1989). Nursing administrators and delegation. *Nursing Administration Quarterly, 13*(3), 23-32.

Potter, P., & Grant, E. (2004). Understanding RN and unlicensed assistive personnel working relationships in designing care delivery strategies. *Journal of Nursing Administration, 34*(1), 19-25.

Richards, A., Carley, J., Jenkins-Clarke, S., & Richards, D. (2000). Skill mix between nurses and doctors working in primary care-delegation or allocation: A review of the literature. *International Journal of Nursing Studies, 37,* 185-197.

Sherer, J. (1993). Nurses call for regulations on hospital staffing ratios. *Hospitals & Health Networks, 67*(14), 56.

Tri-Council for Nursing. (1990). *Statement on assistive personnel to the registered nurse.* Washington, DC: American Association of Colleges of Nursing.

Zerwekh, J., & Claborn, J.C. (2003). *Nursing today: Transition and trends* (4th ed.). Philadelphia: Saunders.

26

Team Building and Working with Effective Groups

Jo Manion   Diane L. Huber

CHAPTER OBJECTIVES

- Highlight the emergence of teamwork as a knowledge work strategy
- Define a group, committee, team, and team building
- Outline the elements of group interactions
- Evaluate the reasons why people join groups
- Compare the advantages and disadvantages of using groups in organizations
- Identify the points on the continuum of group decision-making power
- Explain committee structure and function
- Differentiate among work groups, pseudoteams, and true teams
- Examine the dynamics of work groups and interdisciplinary teams
- Relate the leader's function in committee work and effective meetings
- Discuss constructive group member roles
- Identify the types of disruptive group members
- Exercise critical thinking to conceptualize and analyze possible solutions to a practice exercise

Nurse leaders in today's health care organizations must be skilled group facilitators with an exquisite ability to manage and lead the collective work of people. A significant percentage of work completed in organizations today is done through collective efforts, either in work groups, committees, or teams. Understanding the characteristics of each of these entities as well as basic principles for attaining successful outcomes increases the leader's effectiveness.

In the 1990s, many health care organizations attempted to convert their traditional hierarchical, bureaucratic structures to a team-based structure, with varying degrees of success. Many of these efforts were less than successful at the broad organizational level; yet the factors driving these changes still exist. "The appreciation of 'teamwork,' intensified during these years and has developed as a major management concept" (Spitzer, 1998, p. 169). There are various reasons why teamwork is the new imperative. Changing reimbursement, managed care organizations, increasing complexity, technology advances, rapid information dissemination at the worker level, and the shift to a knowledge worker-based service society are some of the social and economic forces operative in health care. These forces converged to create great change in health care delivery.

A major trend in the late 1990s, creating successful teams was thought to provide the strength and structure to deal with work complexities and changes (Brown, 1998). When the redesign, integration, merger, and partnering strategies settle, a decentralized and organic structure called the *knowledge organization* emerges with a growing emphasis on the role of teams. Although interdisciplinary teams have always played an important role in home care, hospice, and other community settings, hospitals and large health care organizations are placing more emphasis on teams as a part of their core structure.

"Knowledge has become so complex and specialized that virtually no single individual can be effective alone" (Sorrells-Jones & Weaver, 1999, p. 15). Because knowledge workers are specialists, the only way for them to be adequately productive is to work in groups or teams. Thus as the focus shifts to building knowledge work teams, a tandem concern is raised about how to help these teams be more effective and productive (Drucker, 1993; Sorrells-Jones & Weaver, 1999).

Developing effective teams of professionals from different disciplines has proven to be difficult. However, effective knowledge work teams can create a form of synergism in which the outcome is greater than the sum of individual efforts. Such synergism confers a competitive edge and boosts productivity under conditions of constrained resources. Developing a team-based structure is one way to enlist employee participation. Such teams capitalize on possibilities for improved productivity, better decisions, and process innovation. Thus the development of flexibility and responsiveness in well-designed teams holds the potential for positive solutions to health care delivery problems (Manion et al., 1996). Team building is a strategy for designing, implementing, developing, and nurturing work teams in organizations. These work teams are a specialized subset of the many types of groups that form or are formed in organizations. Group work is a major managerial strategy for accomplishing work through others.

Nurses do not do their work in isolation. In many nursing care delivery settings, nurses function in a work group environment or as a part of a team. Although many times these teams are composed of all nursing personnel, nurses are increasingly becoming involved in interdisciplinary work teams. There are some occupations in which people work in relative isolation from others, but that is not the reality of the work of nursing. As health care restructures and becomes more complex, a greater value is being placed on high-performing and cohesive work groups. This is because complexity and cost-control factors in the environment have encouraged the use of interdisciplinary work teams. Therefore nurses need to learn how to function constructively in group situations.

In nursing, group process theory relates to both how to be therapeutic with clients and how to work as an employee within an organization that is often large and complex. Nursing has at its core both a caring and a coordinative function. The nurse's coordinative role is at the hub of all client care information. For example, nurses collect, process, and integrate the initial assessment and laboratory data, handle the tracking of all therapeutic interventions for the client, and often are at the bedside for surveillance of minute-by-minute changes. Furthermore, if pain medications are given in a hospital, nurses track whether or not that intervention has worked, whether or not alternative pain strategies might be needed, and what psychological reaction the client might have. Clients and families note that a physician may visit a hospital unit once a day and may not recognize the fine distinctions of change in a client's condition. Nurses predominate in actual client care in home health, long-term care, and hospice settings. The nurse is involved more intimately and more proximately than any of the other health care givers in managing the total health care of the client. Therefore understanding and developing skill in group process and group dynamics is essential within the context of leadership and management in nursing because of the group functioning and coordinative aspects of nursing practice.

Nurses have to work collaboratively, not only with other nurses and their nurse manager, but also with people who do not share the same professional background, such as those in the administrative structure of the organization, other providers, the supply department, or the legal staff. These interpersonal and collaborative activities shape the essence of nursing practice. In addition, there are generational differences and issues of cultural diversity (see Chapters 19 and 28) that contribute to how people frame issues differently and thus affect how people work in groups. Therefore, as the environment of health care becomes more collaborative, nurses need strong group process and interaction skills to communicate clearly and collaborate effectively with a variety of health care workers.

DEFINITIONS

A **group** is defined as any collection of interconnected individuals working together for some purpose. Groups are important in organizations not only because of informal network dynamics but also because of the formation and functioning of formal committees and teams.

A **committee** is a relatively stable and formally composed group. Committees are a subset of groups; they are a specific type of group in that they are stable, meet periodically, and have an identified purpose that is part of the organizational structure. There is a mechanism for maintaining and selecting members. Typically, committees have official status and sanction within an organization. For example, there is

a policy and procedure committee or a quality assurance/improvement committee.

Team building is defined as the process of deliberately creating and unifying a group into a functioning work unit so that specific goals are accomplished (Farley & Stoner, 1989). A **team** was defined by Katzenbach and Smith (1993) as "a small number of people with complementary skills who are committed to a common purpose, performance goals, and approach for which they hold themselves mutually accountable" (p. 45). Manion and colleagues (1996) modified this definition slightly for health care by noting that the members need to be consistent. This was in reaction to confusion in terminology for many people in health care with a past history of team nursing, where whoever was present on a given shift was on the team. In this type of team nursing model, members could vary from shift to shift and from day to day, reducing the overall performance outcomes of the team. Team nursing was an assignment pattern and work allocation methodology rather than a true team model.

The distinction between a work group and a true team is crucial. The mistake made by many

▲ LEADING & MANAGING **DEFINED**

Group

Any collection of interconnected individuals working together for some purpose.

Committee

A relatively stable and formally composed group; a subset of a group.

Team Building

The process of deliberately creating and unifying a group into a functioning work unit so that specific goals are accomplished.

Team

A small number of consistent people with complementary skills, a shared purpose that entails collective work, specific performance goals, common approaches to the work, and who hold themselves mutually accountable for outcomes.

Work Group

Collection of individuals who are led by a strong and focused leader.

Pseudoteam

A group of people who think they are a team but are not; characterized by confusion over purpose or a highly politicized purpose, dysfunctional and unhealthy interpersonal relationships and communication patterns, lack of clarity about goals, and no evaluation criteria.

health care leaders in the 1990s was assuming that simply calling a group a *team* actually made them a team. As Katzenbach and Smith (1993) noted repeatedly, the group only becomes a true team by doing its collective work. The team goes through a developmental process that takes time and the investment of energy in order to materialize. There are many collective entities in today's organizations that are called a team, yet clearly function more as a work group than a true team.

A **work group** is a collection of individuals who are led by a strong, clearly focused leader. They come together to share information and ideas, and they may even mutually make some decisions. However, the members of the work group have individual work products for which they are responsible. For example, in a patient care unit, the unit secretary has certain responsibilities as does the charge nurse, the patient care nurse, and the manager. The boundaries remain pretty clearly separated when the collective entity is a work group. Each person may feel individual accountability, but there is little to no collective accountability.

This is in contrast with a true team, which is a collective entity in which the leadership rotates and is shared by various members of the team, depending on appropriateness and fit of skills and abilities. In a true team, there are collective work products—for example, the provision of quality patient care to all of the patients housed in the department. There is group as well as individual accountability. If one member of the team is having a problem, it is not just that person's problem, but the problem of and for the whole team to resolve. An example of team thinking is "No one sits down until we can all sit down" or "No one goes home until we all go home." If quality outcomes are difficult for one team member, all team members are affected by this and become engaged in helping the affected team member to meet expectations.

Another collective entity apparent in many organizations is a **pseudoteam**. This is a group of people who believe they are already a team, although clearly they fall short of the definition.

Characteristics of a pseudoteam include confusion over their purpose, unhealthy or toxic interpersonal issues and communication patterns, members who put individual needs and ambition above the needs of the team, the presence of hierarchical rituals that preclude full participation of all members, unclear goals, and a lack of evaluation criteria. The true danger of pseudoteams is that these people think they are already a team and thus see no need for improvement. As a result, they do not grow and develop, but rather they just become more and more dysfunctional as time goes by.

BACKGROUND

Group interactions are a pervasive element of the health care environment in which nurses work. A basic understanding of groups helps nurses function more effectively. These principles apply to any group, whether an actual team, a committee, or an informal group effort. Group interactions are composed of the following elements (Book & Galvin, 1975) (Figure 26.1):

- The *process* that the group undergoes to reach outcomes: This relates to the unique way the group interrelates and begins to work together. The leader can assess group process through observation. What is the process that this group goes through in accomplishing its task?
- The *standards* that regulate the group's behavior: This relates to the specific values and norms that are chosen for group processing. Which ones are chosen; which are discarded?
- The process of *problem solving* or *decision making* that the group adopts: Does the group solve problems? How are decisions made? Are they group decisions made by consensus, or are they individual decisions made with group input (as occurs when the group participates but the decision is made by a leader or manager)?
- The *communication* that occurs among group members: What are the internal patterns and styles of communication among group members? To whom does the group communicate?

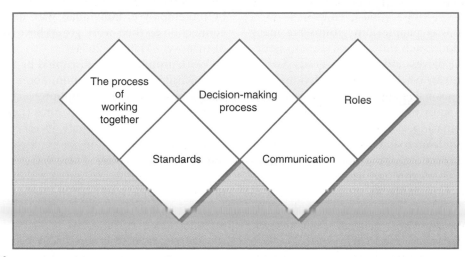

Figure 26.1
Group process elements. (Data from Book, C., & Galvin, K. [1975]. *Instruction in and about small group discussion*. Falls Church, VA: Speech Communication Association.)

Do they report as a subcommittee to a full committee? If a team, does the team have frequent communication with external team leaders? What are the internal and external modes of communication for group input and output?

- The *roles* played by each member: There are a variety of group roles. Members may take on different roles in different situations. For self-awareness, knowing what part one played in his or her family helps an individual recognize roles that he or she might gravitate toward in groups. It is important to remember when assessing group interactions that roles in the group are not always clearly established by the leader or the group. In this situation each group member moves in and out of group roles that best suit him or her. Clarity in the more formal roles, such as team leader, facilitator, recorder, and time-keeper is important to avoid confusion and unnecessary conflict.

Groups tend to go through a series of stages in their work and development. Farley and Stoner (1989) identified these as (1) orientation, (2) adaptation, (3) emergence, and (4) working. The *first stage*, orientation, occurs when the group first forms and the members begin to relate to one another and the task. The group needs to develop trust and define boundaries in order to establish involvement and identification. The *second stage* of adaptation occurs as the group begins to develop a collective identity and differentiate roles. The group needs a facilitative structure and climate to maximize its processing and to develop roles, rules, norms, and a common language. The *third stage* of emergence occurs as control issues arise. Disputes, disagreements, confrontations, alliances, and power struggles mark this stage of determining control over the group in order to emerge with a more consolidated identity. The *final stage* of working occurs when conflict and dissension dissipate and the group achieves greater cohesion through negotiation. The group is now primarily focused on decision making and productivity. The stages may overlap and are not necessarily sequential. The group leader pays attention to the stage of the group as a way of monitoring the group's development and progress. For example, the leader may need to be more alert to the need to intervene personally in the orientation stage than in the working stage when the group has achieved a higher level of maturity.

WHY PEOPLE JOIN GROUPS

The reasons why people join groups are many and may include such things as a desire to satisfy psychological drives and primary needs. Group participation can be desirable to individuals for a variety of reasons. For example, interaction with people and a sense of self-achievement may result from participating. Psychological satisfaction can be derived from making a contribution, being with people, accomplishing goals, and demonstrating outcomes through group participation. Groups provide an outlet for affiliation needs—to make friends or meet and mix with people. There are a number of ways in which groups at all levels fulfill socialization and friendship needs.

In nursing, the formation of groups occurs primarily for one of two reasons: (1) to provide a personal or professional socialization and exchange forum or (2) to provide a mechanism for work accomplishment. Groups can be social, professional, or organizational in purpose. The following are some reasons why groups would be established in organizations:

- Group activities can create a sense of status and esteem.
- Groups allow an individual to test and establish reality.
- Groups function as a mechanism for getting a job done.
- The work to be accomplished requires the complexity of knowledge and skill only possible in a group.

"The ebb and flow of work done by groups is a major part of the working environment of hospital nurses" (Leppa, 1996, p. 23). The work group provides an institutional and professional identity for an individual nurse. Cooperative teamwork and trust form the basis of a nurse's work. Work groups become a focus for interpersonal relationships, support, and social integration. Interpersonal relationship elements such as work group cohesion, communication, and social integration remain consistent moderate-level predictors of nursing job satisfaction (Blegen, 1993). Additionally, being part of a healthy group or team is also related to the level of organizational commitment by the employee. Individuals with an emotional connection to their work group have lower levels of turnover (Manion, 2004).

Work groups can be disrupted by factors such as downsizing, reorganization, absenteeism, and turnover. Work group disruption has been shown to be linked to negative outcomes (Leppa, 1996). In a study of four hospitals, interpersonal relations were found to be an important part of nurses' job satisfaction. There was a relationship between work group disruption and interpersonal relations (Leppa, 1996). Things get done because of relationships among people; nurses need to build successful collaborative relationships among multiple levels of colleagues, key people, organizations, and clients (Laramee, 1999).

A breakdown in working relationships can lead to a strike vote in a collective bargaining environment (Ponte et al., 1998). Furthermore, informal work group norms exert a strong influence on nurses' behavior and can contribute to forms of nursing deviance. Work group relationships can reinforce behaviors and reinforce rationalization, thus leading to deviant behaviors becoming passively or actively accepted. Such strong work group norms can be seen in the extreme. For example, in one study of nurses in practice, nurses used work group norms to neutralize opposition to and reinforce behaviors of drug theft and use (Dabney, 1995). Clearly, there is a strong relationship between work groups, interpersonal relationships, and outcomes such as nurses' behaviors and perceptions. Work group relationships are a powerful mechanism influencing both good and bad outcomes in nursing practice.

ADVANTAGES OF GROUPS

There are advantages to group work. For example, groups are one vehicle for solving problems. Veninga (1982) identified the following five major advantages of group problem solving over individual problem solving:

1. *Greater knowledge and information:* Obtaining a broader and wider range of knowledge and experiences creates a higher-quality input into

group problem solving. The insights of one member can stimulate the thinking of others (Beachy & Biester, 1986). With the increased specialization of health care workers today, this is especially true.

2. *Increased acceptance of solutions:* If there is a decision to be made in an organization, people can get together in a group to talk about it so that the people themselves are more committed to the decision. When individuals who are going to be affected by a decision are part of the decision-making process, they are more likely to be committed to implementing the decision.

3. *More approaches to a problem:* Complex problems typically are more manageable when a number of perspectives are mixed together to address the problem. The advantages include blending and complementing individual learning and problem-solving styles to capitalize on strength through diversity.

4. *Individual expression:* Groups allow for individual expression, and in organizations specifically, there may be few mechanisms for expression of individual perspectives. Sharing information and getting input is done best in groups (Veninga, 1982). Sometimes groups allow people to express themselves, for example, if they are anxious about a change or if morale is low.

5. *Lower costs:* If the group is functioning in a positive and constructive manner, the use of a group can be less expensive than the use of individual effort to accomplish a task. Group decision making is cost-effective if it saves time. For example, when a group meets for one session as opposed to the leader meeting multiple times with multiple individuals, time is saved by the leader and possibly by the group members. Furthermore, cost-effectiveness may result through the division of labor (Beachy & Biester, 1986).

It is imperative that the purpose of the group be established and assessed when the group is part of a larger organization. This means that all members need to have a clear definition of the work of

Table 26.1

Committee Cost Analysis			
Members	Salary/ Hour ($)	Benefits/ Hour ($)	Cost ($)
Nurse 1	25	7	32
Nurse 2	25	7	32
Pharmacist	37	9	46
Nurse manager	30	8	38
Physician	120	N/A	120
		TOTAL:	268

the group. Either the leader needs to disseminate this information or the followers need to ask for clarification. Then evaluation of the stated purpose should occur periodically. Is it a functioning group? Is it accomplishing the task to which it was assigned? If not, should the group be disbanded? Sometimes when the work output of a group of nurses is analyzed, meetings appear to be very costly endeavors. For example, when the number of hours spent by all committee members is multiplied by their individual hourly salary and fringe benefit cost and added together to compute a committee total, the sum of costs for the group may be astounding (Table 26.1). This is another reason for paying attention to how well the group is functioning.

A well-tuned and functioning group is positive for an organization. Often such a group is less expensive and time-consuming in terms of solving problems. Participation and involvement in a group decision typically results in individuals being more committed to a decision, even if there is disagreement.

DISADVANTAGES OF GROUPS

Group decision making can be derailed at a number of points in the process. The three disadvantages commonly noted about group decision making are the potential for premature decisions, individual domination, and disruptive conflicts (Veninga, 1982).

Premature Decisions

The disadvantages of group work include the fact that decisions can result from pressure. Once a majority vote is taken, there is an element of pressure on the minority as a result of psychological dynamics related to subtle pressure for group acceptance and conformity. It may be difficult to be a "devil's advocate" or to adopt the role of bringing alternative critique points to the group for consideration because of a concern about being personally socially accepted. For example, derision and humiliation can occur if members react with strong negative opinions. This response stifles further input.

Individual Domination

Some of the disadvantages of groups relate to the possible emergence of dominating or argumentative members who obstruct the group process. These members make it an unpleasant experience for all involved. In a sense they sabotage the work of the group. If the group is not functioning well or the members are not adhering to the task of the group because of socializing, avoiding the task, or not preparing themselves, then it becomes costly and time-consuming to work out interpersonal dynamics instead of progressing forward on the group's task.

Disruptive Conflicts

When one position is felt to have an adverse effect on a group member or members, or if people feel threatened, conflicts usually emerge. Conflicts are accelerated in a competitive environment, as members vest in their own position. Conflicts may also occur over personality differences, differences of opinion, or clashes of values. Although it may seem contradictory, conflicts are also a control mechanism in a group and may actually result in far superior outcomes. When group members are comfortable disagreeing and conflicting with each other, this prevents the premature acceptance of decisions and helps ensure that opposing viewpoints are considered. However, group members and leaders must be skilled and comfortable in dealing with conflict. Chapter 24 discusses power and conflict in greater detail.

Group work can be, and typically is, a very slow process. It takes more time for a group to arrive at a decision than if one person makes the decision.

GROUP DECISION MAKING

There is a continuum of decision-making power that may be vested in a group (Figure 26.2). A group or committee has certain powers, tasks, and functions, as well as certain parameters or

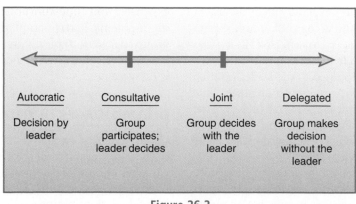

Figure 26.2
Range of decision powers.

latitude in terms of how far to go in making a decision. Thus decision power is a matter of degree. There are four different distinct points on the continuum of authority for decision making.

On one end of the continuum is an *autocratic decision procedure* in which the leader makes the decisions. In this process, majority votes are not honored. There is input, perhaps, but not necessarily a vote. For example, in certain legislative committees the chairperson may or may not be able to put forth legislation or block a bill. It may be the case that there is an autocratic leader who controls the power and the committee exists mainly for the sake of appearance. This type of committee is set up for reasons other than making participative decisions. Hopefully, there are very few of these structures found in the organization as they can generate increased leader and employee cynicism.

A *consultative decision procedure* occurs when decisions involve employee participation but the leader makes the final decision alone. Thus it is one step away from authoritarian or autocratic decision making. The employees may make certain decisions that must then go to the leader, chairperson, or head of the group, who makes the final decision. There is more participation with this type of procedure, but the ultimate decision is not under the control of the group members.

Some decision procedures result in *joint decision making*. In this approach the entire group decides, whether by a two-thirds vote, simple majority, consensus, or some other process. In a joint decision procedure the employees have as much influence as the leader. The leader has one voice, one vote. The leader can use persuasion, but when it comes down to the final vote, the leader's vote is equivalent to any other member of the group. This is fundamentally different from the leader making the decision with group input.

Finally, at the other end of the decision continuum is the *delegated decision procedure*. This occurs when the committee chair or group head allows participants to make the decision. For example, in true self-scheduling, the leader may set up the basic parameters, but the staff members actually decide what schedule they work. The true test of a delegation decision procedure is whether or not the committee head or group leader overrides the followers' decision. Technically, the leader would not have the authority to veto or override. If it is truly a delegation situation, the leader would go forward with the approach that the decision is the choice of the group. The leader becomes the advocate and the spokesperson but not the decision maker. Hersey and colleagues (2001) labeled these same four procedures as authoritative, consultative, facilitative, and delegative decision-making styles. They related these styles to their situational leadership theory.

During participation in groups, it is advisable for the followers to determine who has the authority to make decisions. Knowledge about what type of group it is and what delegation or decision procedures can be anticipated is critical to participation. A leadership or conflict moment may occur when a group assumes that delegation is the decision procedure rule in effect. Anger is a by-product that occurs when a committee assumes that a delegated decision is *its* to make, yet the leader has a different idea. Clarity before beginning work on an issue avoids unnecessary conflict.

WORK TEAMS

Sovie (1992) noted that care and service teams are the new imperative in health care, as a matter of survival. High-performance teams are essential to an organization's efficiency and effectiveness. Previously, teamwork was not an explicit performance expectation or organizational value. However, it seems clear now that collaboration and teamwork are essential to achieving high-quality work outcomes and cost control in client care.

Three types of teams found in health care are (1) primary work teams, (2) executive or management leadership teams, and (3) ad hoc teams. Primary work teams include all forms of client care teams such as an emergency department trauma team. In the operating room there are often teams based on the specialty, for example, a cardiovascular or an orthopedic team. The top executive team is an example of an executive or management leadership team. At the department level there may be a leadership team that is composed of the nurse manager, the charge nurses, and perhaps an educator. Continuous quality improvement teams, project teams, and problem-solving teams are examples of ad hoc teams. Specific problem-solving teams in departments are other examples of ad hoc teams. The chief characteristic of these teams is that they are created to perform a very specific piece of work. When that work is completed, the team dissolves. Among all types of teams, any team may become a self-directed work team. This is a group that accepts increasingly higher levels of authority for its responsibility. A self-directed work team is fully responsible for delivering a well-defined segment of a finished product or service (Manion et al., 1996). It has the requisite capacity and authority for the work undertaken.

Designing, building, and implementing effective work teams requires a specific methodology and process. A primary work team fails if it behaves like a collection of individuals operating from narrowly defined jobs; if it is composed of the wrong mix of members, size, structure, responsibility, or expertise; or if it cannot fluidly shift activities and adapt to changes. The following four steps are key to designing a highly effective health care team (Manion et al., 1996):

1. Define the total pool of work for the team
2. Differentiate responsibilities within the pool
3. Narrow the design options to attractive alternatives
4. Identify the single best design to implement

These principles apply regardless of the type of team being formed. After the team has been carefully designed for the work it is to accomplish, the next step is to build the team by incorporating the essential elements needed to function. These elements are meaningful purpose, consistent membership, specific performance goals, commitment to a common approach, complementary and overlapping skills, and mutual accountability for outcomes.

Managing this development process is a key leadership function. This means that the leader guides the team in the development of its purpose statement. The team members are more likely to coalesce into a strong team if they have been given the time and opportunity to carefully reflect on their purpose and come to agreement about what they do and for whom they do it. The team becomes a true team by doing its work. Specific performance goals give it direction and also provide evaluative criteria by which the team's success can be measured. Although it is simplistic to say that the team has common working approaches, this is an area where unnecessary conflict occurs if the leader and team members have not established these key processes. There needs to be agreement about how things are going to be done. This ranges from the establishment of team behavioral norms to agreement on procedural issues. This step usually requires a significant amount of time and continues to be addressed throughout the lifetime of the team. By laying a foundation carefully, effective teams can emerge (Manion et al., 1996).

The dynamics of interdisciplinary teams create some unique issues. Regrouping people into multidisciplinary groups can create anxiety and fear. A lack of common vocabulary and understanding about other disciplines' practices may become apparent. It has been said that professionals simply do not know how to work together in teams (Sorrells-Jones, 1997). Other perils and pitfalls occur when teams are assigned, not designed. Additional errors may include the following: confusion occurs about the team's work, the team lacks real authority, structural team building is not done, dysfunctional behavior occurs, or team-based outcome measures and coaching are lacking (Manion et al., 1996). Trust and communication are critical elements of building effective work teams.

It is not enough to simply structure the team. Team members need to work collaboratively and interdependently first before striving to work synergistically. Key to moving away from independent action and toward synergistic work teams is to change the use of power among team members toward finding synergistic solutions that address divergent needs (Gage, 1998). An infrastructure of open communication with an emphasis on information sharing enables team members to understand and believe in the team's strategies. Teams benefit from a communication critical path and the valuing of individual accountability for communication (Page, 1998).

Team performance and effectiveness are important managerial concerns. Dysfunctional team behaviors can occur. Teams form, grow through stages, and mature. The team dynamics change throughout this process. Teams benefit from team building and developmental training. Articulating and negotiating expectations for healthy interpersonal behavior benefits team development. For example, active listening and demonstrating mutual respect promote an open environment. Direct communication and honest feedback, addressing conflict, and negotiating for win-win solutions facilitate healthy interpersonal dynamics in teams and enhance their productivity and performance (Manion et al., 1996; Page, 1998). A key characteristic of an emotionally intelligent team is one that has established norms that guide team member behaviors (Cherniss & Goleman, 2001).

Team norms are best established when the team initially forms. They are continually revisited, modified, and expanded throughout the lifespan of the team. The process for developing norms is usually leader-initiated and begins with a conversation within the team about how it expects members to behave and contribute. The norms are usually developed during a group meeting where ideas are shared, refined, and finally negotiated with all team members. Appropriate topics for behavioral norms include, but are not limited to, expectations around the following:

- Communication, both at the individual and group levels
- How team members treat each other
- How support is to be demonstrated
- Decision-making processes
- How conflict is to be handled

For example, one team developed the following expectations of each other:

I expect you to:

- Communicate in an open, honest, and direct manner with me.
- Give me feedback when my behavior creates a difficult or uncomfortable situation for you.
- Persist and work with me on difficult issues until we reach a mutually agreeable resolution.
- Pitch in gladly, provide help when asked, and look for ways to help each other out.
- Respect confidences and not share sensitive information we discuss with others without my knowledge or permission.
- Be trustworthy as evidenced by honoring and meeting commitments made, being loyal to absent team members, and by presenting me in the best light to others.

Many times these norms are referred to as the *team operating agreement*, *the code of conduct*, or *articulated expectations*. In many teams, once they are identified, team members sign them, indicating agreement, and they often are posted in sight in the workplace. These norms are more than just a paper exercise, and signing them indicates that the team member agrees to live by the expectations and, just as important, agrees to address other team members who do not live up to the expectations.

Katzenbach and Smith (1993) plotted the following five discrete points along a team performance curve:

1. A working group in which there is no incentive to form a team
2. A pseudoteam that has no common purpose or set of goals
3. A potential team in which significant incremental performance is needed
4. A real team that fits their definition
5. A high-performance team that outperforms other teams and has members deeply committed to one another's growth and success

The greater the performance, the greater the advantage to the group and the organization.

Performance in teams is linked to productivity, but the direct applicability to the delivery of nursing care remains a complex challenge (Sheafor, 1991). For example, Schmeiding's (1990) research indicated that many staff nurses may prefer dependence on those in higher hierarchical positions. Clearly some nurses were not motivated, prepared, or inclined to assume a high level of personal responsibility for decision making in client care coordination and work group administration. This has implications for leadership and management of professional nurses and for decentralization and shared governance. Furthermore, it is not known whether these attitudes are still valid or have shifted with time.

Nurse leaders need to learn how to manage in a team-centered environment; staff nurses must learn how to be effective team players (Sovie, 1992). Interactive leadership is needed to create a group identity. Participatory management; sharing power and information; and generating trust, mutual respect, and enhanced self-worth are seen as key elements in successful performance teams. Teamwork begins with members who are well prepared and personally competent. Teamwork then includes shared ownership and decision making (Sovie, 1992). Nurses often begin with experiences on client care teams and ad hoc problem-solving teams or continuous quality improvement teams, moving later to senior leadership and interdisciplinary teams (Farley & Stoner, 1989).

Group process is a framework by which to understand team development (Farley & Stoner, 1989). Sovie (1992) identified four essential components of high-performing teams: roles, activities, relationships, and the environment. This means that highly effective teams establish positive roles among the members, who are able to focus their activities toward productivity. To become highly effective, the relationships of the team members need to become cohesive. The team requires a facilitative and supportive environment in which to work through the task and relationship elements. Management of team building and team performance includes skill in the process of conflict management. Diverse backgrounds and varying views result in the potential for differences, conflicts, turf battles, and office politics.

The leader's repertoire must include strategies of conflict resolution, empowerment, collaboration, and coordination. Sovie (1992) called the manager "a gatekeeper at the critical boundary of team and organization" (p. 97) who has to keep communication, objectives, and needs flowing both ways. Diplomacy, negotiation, and power-based strategies or alliances may be employed in team building (Farley & Stoner, 1989).

The complementary skills that are needed, in the right mix, to do the team's task fall into at least three categories: technical or functional expertise, problem-solving and decision-making skills, and interpersonal skills. To assess and strengthen team performance, Katzenbach and Smith (1993) recommended an analysis of each of their six basic elements of teams: small in number, adequate levels of complementary skills, a truly meaningful purpose, specific goal(s), clear working approach, and sense of mutual accountability (Box 26.1). The characteristics of highly effective teams include a common purpose or clear, elevating goal; agreed-on performance goals or results-driven structure; competent members; a common approach for the work; a unified commitment; complementary skills; a collaborative climate; mutual accountability; standards of excellence; external support and recognition; and principled leadership (Katzenbach & Smith, 1993; Manion et al., 1996).

Box **26.1**

Team Performance Checklist

✓ Small in number
✓ Adequate levels of skills
✓ Meaningful purpose
✓ Specific goal(s)
✓ Clear working approach
✓ Sense of mutual accountability

Data from Katzenbach, J., & Smith, D. (1993). *The wisdom of teams: Creating the high-performance organization.* New York: Harper Collins.

COMMITTEES

An essential part of any nurse's role is to be involved in committee and group work. Work is accomplished through people, and the coordination of care is furthered through committee actions. Previously, the nurse manager or the nursing administrator provided the primary participation in most committees. This type of arrangement did not necessarily provide the highest-quality input because the nurses at the caregiver level often are the ones with reliable information about a given problem, especially regarding client care problems. With the changes in health care delivery, it is becoming essential that the staff participate in groups and committees. It also is important to the nurses' job satisfaction and autonomy to have an avenue of involvement and participation in which to actively solve problems.

Some people react negatively to committees because they dislike the time involved and because they are frustrated with the psychodynamics of group process and decision making. However, committees are a mainstay of organizations and can be an important way to make changes in clinical practice. Understanding committee workings facilitates the process of being a more effective nurse.

Committee structures are preferable in the following two kinds of situations:

1. *When each member's input is needed to attain a certain goal:* For example, a committee may be set up to implement self-scheduling or to start a new program to benefit clients. If the work cannot be done alone or if there is a need to have everyone's agreement, then a committee is probably appropriate.
2. *Situations in which diverse representation facilitates implementation of proposed activities:* To have a diverse group of people provide input in order to get the job done, a committee should be created. For example, a multidisciplinary products committee could be established to develop a process in which there would be a review of products before a large amount of purchasing was done. This approach avoids having the nurses at the bedside finding

themselves using products that are potentially unsafe, unusable, and thus costly.

Several types of committees are found in organizations. One kind is the standing committee, which, as the name implies, is a constant, ongoing part of the organizational mission, performing critical and essential functions that must be done. For example, policy committees are standing committees because there always are policies to write and review. The same is true for quality assurance/improvement committees because quality improvement activities are ongoing and continuous.

Contrasted to a standing committee is the task force, also called a *project team* or *ad hoc committee.* This is a committee that is developed in response to some emergent or immediate need. A need arises, and a group is formed. A task force is not part of the organizational core mission. It is formed in response to a specific circumstance that arises or to study a specific problem. The committee is expected to disband when the issue is resolved. An example is a search committee to replace an advanced practice nurse or a problem-solving group dealing with an issue such as patient flow issues in the emergency department.

There are some groups or committees that are structured to gather together members based on organizational position or job position. For example, all the nurse managers may belong to a group of nurse managers or staff nurses to a staff nurse council. By holding the position of nurse manager, the person belongs to that committee. This provides an opportunity for peer interaction, support, and problem solving.

There are multidisciplinary interdivisional committees. A multidisciplinary committee includes participants from several divisions or specialties. The participants may all be from within the institution or from both inside and outside the organization. These committees often are used to coordinate and eliminate boundary conflicts. Some examples are a products committee, a risk-management committee, or a medical liaison committee in which nurses and physicians work together to reduce interprofessional conflicts.

In some cases multidisciplinary teams are formed using a committee structure, for example, to develop a critical pathway.

Within organizations, committees perform a central role in the implementation of the strategic plan. A committee is a group that can assume accountability for planning, implementing, and evaluating the outcomes of a strategic goal translated to the operational level. Committees accomplish some departmental activities and provide a mechanism for increasing staff participation in decision making. In an environment characterized by complex work, committees become a major vehicle for resolving issues related to the organization's mission. Two elements promote efficient and effective committee decision making: appropriate representation (by including people affected by changes) and delegation of an appropriate level of authority to the committee (Wilson et al., 1999).

Committees evolve over time. To remain vital, committees need to be evaluated regularly for congruence with organizational mission and contribution to outcomes. Occasionally, environmental changes or internal restructuring create a situation forcing reexamination of the coordination and focus of committees. Both restructuring and revitalization of committees can be accomplished through strategic planning, multidisciplinary forums, enhanced communication, a phased process, and evaluation of the changes (Deveau & McCabe, 1996; Wilson et al., 1999).

If asked to be on a committee as a unit representative, it is advisable for the nurse to explore the nature and characteristics of the committee. The nurse needs to determine the authority level delegated to this particular committee, remembering that this delegation may be formal or informal. Another factor involves assessing who is on the committee and whether the nurse has a positive or negative relationship with the other members. Other factors include whether the people on the committee are highly motivated, whether they are task- or relationship-oriented people, and what committee politics exist. The feedback mechanisms and the committee's productivity are key characteristics. The track record of the committee is reflected in its output. These characteristics are important for the nurse to understand before deciding to participate. Preparation for followership enhances both personal and committee productivity. It is also helpful to clarify any expectations for the committee role being considered. For example, is the nurse to represent others in the department? This role requires more active solicitation of colleagues' opinions and ideas.

EFFECTIVE MEETINGS

Meetings are common occurrences in health care organizations. Whether a meeting involves a group, a committee, or a team, the leader's role is to maximize the benefits of the meeting. Structuring a meeting for effectiveness requires preparation and effort. To manage effective meetings, the leader should consider the purpose for which they are organized. There are several purposes for meetings (Jacobs & Rosenthal, 1984). The first type of meeting is one held for *information dissemination.* For example, the designated leadership person calls the group together to let the members know that a command has come down to cut the budget by 10% because of fiscal retrenchment. A meeting is called to disseminate information about what is happening and to provide time for questions and answers. Perhaps there has been an organizational change, such as the decision that one unit is going to be consolidating with another unit or that a new building, department relocation, or merger is being planned.

Second, there are meetings held for the purpose of *opinion seeking.* The goal of these meetings is open dialogue to solicit group opinions and ideas on specific topics or issues. This purpose does not imply that decision making is the prerogative of the group. Seeking opinions is an input strategy and may be used only for gathering data or testing group reactions. For example, an opinion-seeking meeting may be called to invite input on equipment purchases for budget requests.

The third type of meeting is held for the purpose of *problem solving.* The meeting is structured to solicit help in clarifying, analyzing, and solving a specific problem. This type of meeting is more action-oriented. Group participation in decision making is encouraged. For example, group problem solving or unit meetings may be called to discuss ways to solve problems related to disruptive or manipulative clients or family members. Meetings for the purpose of problem-solving must follow a methodical structure; otherwise, they are likely to deteriorate into either a complaint session or result in unacceptable recommendations. Effectively leading these groups requires strong facilitation skills and knowledge in problem-solving techniques.

There are several team-related functions of group meetings that can contribute to effectiveness. For example, a meeting provides a structure to facilitate a sense of identity and to help the team more fully achieve its purposes. A meeting is a forum for updating shared knowledge among a team. A meeting reinforces the collective goals and objectives of the team. Furthermore, a meeting can create a sense of commitment to group decisions. It can be an opportunity for a manager to be perceived as a leader. A true team uses their meeting time to accomplish a collective work product as compared with a committee or work group, who uses meeting time to discuss issues and then delegate the work outside of the actual meeting time. However, a meeting is a waste of time for all concerned unless there is a clear understanding of what the meeting is intended to achieve (Jay, 1982).

Beachy and Biester (1986) discussed restructuring meetings toward effective group management. As nursing department meetings became unmanageable, one organization developed a questionnaire to survey the group and evaluate the meetings. Aspects such as the cost/benefit ratio of attending meetings, group process, decision making, and relevancy of agenda items were examined for individual members' feelings about effectiveness. The group then discussed ideas for restructuring the meetings. Active participation was seen as being the essence of effective meetings. Certain elements of time management, group

process, and decision making are related to effectiveness in meetings (Beachy & Biester, 1986).

Jay (1982) outlined guidelines for conducting meetings. For example, in a meeting held to achieve specific objectives, each agenda item can be identified as being for information (e.g., progress reports), for development (e.g., new policy or strategy plan), for implementation (e.g., formulating a detailed action plan), or for change within the organization (e.g., changing documentation forms used by multiple user groups). Identifying on the agenda the category of each item helps to clarify and focus the group discussion. Using a timed agenda can also facilitate the process. This involves identifying on the agenda, next to each item, the anticipated amount of time allotted for discussion. This should serve as a guideline rather than a rigid parameter and must not be substituted for good judgment when a particular discussion is productive but takes longer than anticipated.

The leader of the group can facilitate meeting effectiveness by preparing and dealing with both the task and the people involved. The leader needs to listen carefully, process the interactions, control the flow, and keep the meeting directed toward accomplishing the objectives. The ideal size of a group is 4 to 7 people, with 12 being the upper limit (Jay, 1982). Members should be carefully selected for best input. The leader needs to start on time and be alert to seating positions. The leader can facilitate effectiveness by controlling the compulsive talkers, drawing out the silent members, protecting the junior members, encouraging the clash of ideas, discouraging the clash of personalities, avoiding the squashing of creative ideas, and closing on a note of achievement (Jay, 1982). The leader also needs to attend to careful meeting wrap-up. Being sure to summarize at the end the group's accomplishments and verify task assignments going forward are important leader responsibilities. Box 26.2 presents a checklist for leading effective meetings.

Without thought and preparation, people go into a meeting with their own biases and perspectives; they may not be tuned in to how to be productive

Box 26.2

Effective Meetings Checklist for Leaders

✓ Identify the purpose of the meeting:
  - Information dissemination
  - Opinion seeking
  - Problem solving
✓ Prepare an agenda and related materials
✓ Identify the category of each agenda item:
  - For information
  - For development
  - For implementation
  - For change in the system
✓ Set the size at four to seven people
✓ Carefully select members (based on skill and expertise)
✓ Distribute agenda well in advance of meeting
✓ Start on time
✓ Listen carefully
✓ Process the interactions
✓ Control the flow of interactions
✓ Keep the meeting directed toward accomplishing objectives

Data from Jay, A. (1982). How to run a meeting. *Journal of Nursing Administration, 12*(1), 22-28.

within the meeting. However, even in a negative situation, individuals may choose to participate in a way that assists or enhances the process by making constructive suggestions about how things could be done better. This is an ideal situation—one to be encouraged, structured, and facilitated by the leader.

The duties of chairperson include preparation of the physical environment. Comfort and convenience engineering is part of the leader's responsibility in terms of preparing an environment that is conducive to people being satisfied, productive, positive, and working together. The worst-case situation occurs when members have to sit in an uncomfortable chair in a room that is too cold, too hot, or too noisy because of construction; when members cannot hear or talk to other people; or when the technology does not work. Consider how to facilitate group work through hosting functions related to breaks, food, and beverages. It is human nature for members to be more relaxed and productive in comfortable surroundings.

As all nurses are pressured to do more with less under severe time and travel constraints, conducting meetings assisted by technology has become a major strategy. Speaker phones, videoconferencing, Internet hook-ups, real-time (synchronous) discussion boards, and related audio or video technology strategies are commonly employed. They become useful ways to save time by eliminating travel to an in-person site. However, specific problems may occur such as technology incompatibility, speed of transmission, hook-up failures, micro delays in transmission that result in people talking over one another or hesitancy in speaking, a lack of interpersonal modulation due to absence of body language, or a tendency to forget about people who are not actually in the room. Despite these known issues, nurses in the future will increasingly experience meetings assisted by technology.

A leader has a responsibility to prepare and motivate participants. The participants' responsibility is to read and be prepared, show up on time, and attend to the task at hand. The leader needs to prepare an agenda with handouts and background materials and distribute this to the members with enough time to read it. The better-prepared the members are, the more they can participate, increase the quality of decisions, and be more effective.

The leader's preparation activities include reviewing the status of agenda topics as part of preparing the agenda. Questions to ask include the following:
- Where are we?
- What else needs to be done?
- What supporting materials might help the committee?
- Who should be invited?

A leader who comes to the meeting and distributes a handout for a quick look before a vote violates the participants' ability to think through what is being presented. This may be done as a tactic to avoid thorough deliberation by pressuring for the immediacy of a vote, but more often this behavior results from disorganization or lack of attention to leader responsibilities.

CONSTRUCTIVE GROUP MEMBERS

People in groups assume a variety of roles. Lancaster (1981) identified both group building roles and group maintenance roles as being a part of group interactions. Group building roles include initiator, encourager, opinion giver, clarifier, listener, and summarizer. Group maintenance roles include tension reliever, compromiser, gatekeeper, and harmonizer. The group building roles concentrate on relationship functions more than task functions; the group maintenance roles focus more on task functions than relationship functions.

One positive way to handle meetings is to identify a facilitator. Often this is the formal group leader, but it does not have to be. If this is a true team, the role of facilitator may rotate between team members. In a committee, the facilitator is most likely the committee chairperson. A facilitator conducts the meeting, ensuring that everyone has the opportunity to speak, maintains the focus of the meeting, and ensures that group dynamics remain positive.

Also needed is a group recorder. The task of taking minutes may need to be delegated to a clerical support person (if possible) if group members are averse to taking on the task of recording outcomes. However, a recorder who is a group member technically can do far more than just take minutes. This person should be in tune with the group processing and with the inputs and roles of group members and help keep the group on time. The recorder can provide feedback to the facilitator in terms of how to improve the process. One key tip is to construct a standardized meeting record (or minutes) form to facilitate the process and flow documentation. It is helpful to decide in advance the level of detail required in the minutes to avoid lengthy minutes and potentially

unnecessary effort. In some cases a laptop computer is used to directly enter draft minutes.

Finally, group members are needed. *Group members,* in this instance means active participants, each with equal status in the meeting. The three components of facilitator, recorder, and group members contribute to the design of a positive working group.

DISRUPTIVE GROUP MEMBERS

Another role that the group leader assumes is that of process facilitator. The leader must be observant about group member actions and be prepared to control or redirect disruptive behaviors. Following are common types of disruptive group members encountered (Jacobs & Rosenthal, 1984), with strategies for the leader to use in managing dysfunctional members.

Compulsive Talkers

The leader needs to identify individuals who are compulsive talkers and consider how their behavior can be modified. One suggestion is to thank them for their input and then ask to hear from others on that same topic before they are given permission to speak again, as a way of guiding and opening up the meeting to be more effective.

Nontalkers

The nontalkers are the quiet ones. The leader can ask them to write down and submit their ideas or ask to hear their thoughts on the matter at hand. The leader can specifically ask them questions to draw them out and thereby open up a broader range of group input.

Interrupters

The leader has to control the interrupter because this person is demonstrating a lack of self-control. The interrupter can be a problem in groups because the person who is interrupted feels violated and wonders why he or she is not given the courtesy of finishing a thought and having his or her full input considered. The leader needs to halt the interruption and control and redirect the interrupter.

Squashers

These people try to squash an idea before it is even developed. Suggestions about processes or procedures that have not been proven or even tried are much easier to criticize than are facts or opinions. Persons who are averse to change may have a litany of reasons why a potential solution would never work or why this proposed project simply cannot or should not happen. These are often people who do not want to take a personal risk or undergo the personal effort of making a change, so it is easier to squash everything and maintain the status quo. Especially during brainstorming sessions, the leader must be alert to and have a method for containing the squasher. An easy way to influence this is to set the expectation at the beginning of the session by saying, for example, "No analyzing or saying anything negative about the ideas until we have them all identified." The leader may choose to handle the negative input for a certain amount of time and then move the group beyond it. One method to move the group is to direct an equal amount of time to exploring the positive benefits and potentials of the proposal. The leader may need to express a vision or ideal future and challenge the group to take up the opportunity.

Busybodies

These are people who really are not committed to the group's work. They frequently arrive late, leave early, take personal messages or cell phone calls during the meeting, never read the agenda, are passive-aggressive, and simply want to show up for a few minutes for the purpose of appearances but do not contribute any effort. They are meeting their needs by showing up, but they are not contributing to the ongoing group work or the task at hand; nor are they invested in the group's goals. The leader needs to find creative mechanisms to engage the busybodies, perhaps by giving them a concrete assignment with accountability. If this does not work, they may need to be released from the group or placed in an advisory role.

A key way the group leader can control disruptive group behavior is to take advantage of several creativity techniques to heighten both the content and the process of group work. Since perceptions and biases may cloud individuals' ability to generate creative ideas or solutions, the techniques of brainstorming, Delphi survey, or nominal group technique (NGT) can be employed (Van de Ven & Delbecq, 1974). Brainstorming is the encouragement of the generation of large numbers of diverse ideas, free from critique or labeling in regard to practicality or feasibility. A Delphi survey technique employs sequential rounds of questionnaires to collect the judgment and consensus of opinion of experts on a topic. It often is used for prioritization purposes.

The NGT (Van de Ven & Delbecq, 1974) avoids social exchange contamination by following a process of silently gathering ideas in writing, using round-robin feedback from group members to identify ideas, clarifying and evaluating each identified idea, and individually voting on priority ideas. The group decision is derived mathematically. An example of NGT would be when a nurse leader of a nursing unit calls a staff meeting to address issues of group conflict. The first step is to have group members write down key causes of conflict silently and independently. Then, going around the group, the ideas about key causes of conflict that were identified by group members are written on a flip chart, one at a time. Next, each recorded idea is discussed by the group to obtain clarification and evaluation. Then group members vote privately in the form of ranked priorities of which cause is the most fundamental. Individual priority rankings are displayed. A group decision is made about the top key cause based on these ratings, and an action plan is then developed. The structure provided by using these creativity techniques often serves to influence negative group behavior.

Thus the nurse leader can take an active role in structuring group work for positive processing and effective outcomes. It is important to control the flow to modulate disruptive group members without humiliating them. Another way is to structure positive and constructive group roles among members. The leader also may choose to involve the group in managing dysfunctional members. This can be done by agreement on behavioral norms (such as respect for all persons' input) and on how the group collectively will enforce them. Peer pressure also is a powerful group behavior modification tactic. The leader's vision, enthusiasm, interpersonal relationship skills, and empowerment of followers all facilitate group effectiveness.

LEADERSHIP AND MANAGEMENT IMPLICATIONS

The leadership and management role in groups, teams, and committees includes strategically considering the work to be accomplished, determining the structure most suited to doing the work, putting the structure in place, and facilitating the work process. This requires a leader who understands the basic differences between work groups and teams, committees, and informal groups. The leader also must be able to think carefully about the work to be accomplished and determine whether it is primarily collective or individual work.

The leader's role includes inspiring members to participate, preparing critical questions, developing agendas and background materials, and guiding the long-range strategy. Leaders and managers address questions such as the following: What is the task? What is the best way for this task to be accomplished? Is there collective work involved? Do we need a team, or will a good work group or committee suffice? How many meetings will it take? How much effort is required? How can the tasks be divided? How can they be delegated? This is a planning, coordinative, and tracking function.

In planning for meetings, a good leader puts in the time and effort to get all the members prepared, so that when they come to the meeting, they know what the issues are and they are familiar with the background of the task to be accomplished. The leader facilitates the group coming to some agreement about norms for decision making, length of discussion, when to vote, and the process through which the task is completed efficiently and effectively. This is done as a deliberate agenda item that the leader initiates, opens for discussion, and brings to consensus. Nurses may find that the group leader role challenges them to plan, organize, coordinate, and evaluate the work of the group.

An effective leader understands that there is a process involved in creating effective work teams,

◤ LEADERSHIP & MANAGEMENT **BEHAVIORS**

Leadership Behaviors

- Enables group members to participate
- Communicates enthusiasm and vision of group goals
- Motivates followers to accomplish group goals
- Models constructive group participation
- Inspires team collaboration
- Facilitates constructive group roles
- Monitors group process

Management Behaviors

- Plans committee agenda and task accomplishment
- Organizes a team

- Delegates group work and assigns tasks
- Arranges support services
- Communicates through reporting structure
- Handles conflict situations

Overlap Areas

- Communicates to further the group's productivity
- Monitors the group's movement toward goal accomplishment

highly functioning groups, and committees. The process requires facilitation and a significant amount of coaching from the leader. The leader's style must fit the development stage of the group, with the leader providing more extensive structure and direction in early stages and minimal structure and direction in later stages. Coaching involves the transfer of responsibility to the team or the group. Skill, capability, and readiness of the group must be assessed.

CURRENT ISSUES AND TRENDS

Workforce Shortages

Workforce shortage issues are a primary concern in this decade and promise only to worsen in the future as retiring Baby Boomers decimate the current workforce. Organizations are struggling with approaches to attract qualified individuals into nursing, but just as important are the strategies for retaining them. Unless the workplace

Research Note

Source: Kuhar, P., Miller, D., Spear, B., Ulreich, S., & Mion, L. (2004). The meaningful retention strategy inventory: A targeted approach to implementing retention strategies. *Journal of Nursing Administration, 34*(1), 10-18.

Purpose

Nurses' values often determine whether they remain working with an organization or not. The purpose of this study was to explore retention strategies that are meaningful for staff nurses.

Discussion

The authors developed, tested, and implemented a tool, the Meaningful Retention Strategy Inventory, in a multihospital system to determine which retention strategies would be of most interest to staff nurses. Both staff nurses and nurse leaders were surveyed. The instrument consisted of 59 items related to job satisfaction that were elicited from an extensive literature review. Among all staff nurses (n = 971), the top three strategies included the following:
1. Teamwork-staff members' ability to work together to get the job done, 79.6%
2. Periodic increases in salary, 78.5%
3. Support from coworkers, 77.0%

Nurse leaders ranked the following top three strategies:
1. Teamwork, 84.6%
2. Support from coworkers, 80.2%
3. Periodic salary increases, 76.9%

When these factors were compared across various age groups of staff nurses, teamwork and coworker support were the most highly rated strategies by all nurses over 36 years of age. Younger nurses rated these two strategies in their top four picks.

Application to Practice

The findings of this study support the basic premise of this entire chapter. Not only do nurses work interdependently in the workplace, in groups and teams, but they highly value teamwork. They identified it as one of the most meaningful retention strategies that could be implemented. Closely related and valued is coworker support. Although coworker support can come in a variety of ways, one very effective mechanism is through working together collectively in groups or teams. Thus any managerial or leadership intervention that focuses on developing good healthy working relationships, strengthening effective group processes, and obtaining meaningful outcomes of group work has a direct impact on reducing turnover rates and increasing the retention of staff nurses.

environment is positive and affirming, many new practitioners leave all too quickly (Manion, 2005). A key aspect of a positive work environment includes the relationships one has with colleagues and coworkers. Groups and teams with healthy interpersonal relationships help foster a strong sense of connection and community among people (Manion & Bartholomew, 2003; Manion, 2004). Another aspect of a positive workplace related to groups has to do with people's need to see problems solved and difficult aspects of work resolved so that things become better over time. Effective problem-solving groups are a crucial aspect of making this happen.

Interdisciplinary Teams

Interdisciplinary teams are considered to be essential for the effectiveness of health care organizations. Consequently, students need to have exposure to interdisciplinary teams and be integrated into them for experiential skill building. Hansen and Hays (1998) described one approach to integrating students into interdisciplinary teams. Strategies were used to build relationships through shared knowledge, practices, and values. This helps prepare future caregivers for collaborative practice.

New Methods of Compensation

As health care organizations restructure, reorganize, and implement team-based collaborative practice, new methods of employee compensation are needed. Compensation programs that reward employees only for individual effort become counterproductive to the rewards and incentives needed for effective work teams. Innovative approaches to pay and rewards are needed. A compensation program sends an inherent message to employees. The old system of compensation used pay-for-performance or step/grade systems. Emerging forms of compensation include competency-based pay, group variable pay, and individual awards. A menu of compensation offerings is recommended that addresses both individual and team successes (Barksdale, 1998).

Innovation Groups

Groups and committees are used as vehicles to promote innovation and change in organizations. One example in nursing is the institution of research-based nursing practice by using a planned change process and a research utilization committee to facilitate the process of incorporating evidence-based practice in nursing. Groups that are skilled in creativity techniques and understand the process of innovation can be very effective in disseminating and implementing evidence-based practice changes.

Other examples of innovation groups and committees are total quality management (TQM) initiatives in organizations. Continuous quality improvement (CQI) methods such as TQM are used as ways of addressing problems related to cost and quality (Sovie, 1992). Total quality management is a concept that comes from the work of Deming (Aguayo, 1990; Darr, 1989), who emphasized moving decision making to the worker level. The worker who is closest to actually producing the work is the one with the greatest knowledge and the greatest potential for solving production problems. Deming further recommended work group problem-solving teams. Problems, in Deming's methodology, are defined as systems problems. By contrast, a common way of thinking about problems is to look for an individual to blame. The result of systems thinking is to capture the energy of teams to tackle systems problems.

Following the Institute of Medicine's report *To Err Is Human: Building a Safer Health System* (Kohn et al., 2000), the entire health care delivery system has been challenged to focus on systems problems and review and improve processes and procedures. This work is often done in groups and committees. The overall focus on quality has led to adoption of business management concepts such as Lean and Six Sigma. These are customer-focused and data-driven approaches to deriving best practices. The focus is on reducing process variation and then on improving process capability. Lean focuses on process speed; Six Sigma focuses on process quality.

Whether CQI, TQM, or Six Sigma, staff nurses are expected to participate more actively in multidisciplinary teams. In an organization that looks at problems as systems problems, the next step is to acknowledge that anyone involved in that part of the system is engaged in solving the problem. Therefore coordinating client care and solving problems through interdisciplinary committees and groups with people of equal status is the strategy best suited to solving systems problems. It is thus important for nurses to be prepared for multidisciplinary group or team work and to be skilled in team participation and leadership.

The basic strategy behind each of these systems-based approaches is to bring together interdisciplinary collaborative groups. This means that if there is a problem in client care, the physicians, nurses, ancillary staff, and any other direct caregivers are involved. They get together and collaborate about problems with the client care delivery system and discuss how these problems can be fixed. The facilitator does not have to be a content expert or the person with the most expertise in that problem area. In fact, having the most expertise in a problem area can actually be problematic when functioning as a facilitator because it becomes too tempting to take over the process. More important are that individual's facilitation skills.

Establishing coequal peers regardless of status and using expertise and responsibility result in a different way of looking at work, which has implications in terms of how nursing practice may change. It also means nurses are going to be involved more substantially in groups, committees, and teams. To increase effectiveness, a current trend is to address the serious issue of professionals not knowing how to work together in teams (Sorrells-Jones, 1997). For example, one study demonstrated the positive outcomes, including improved physician/nurse communication, by the use of a collaborative approach to standardized protocol development and implementation (Lassen et al., 1997).

Nursing Organizations

An example of a nationwide group approach to problem solving in nursing is the American Nurses Association's Tri-Council. For a long time one of the problems of organized nursing has been the fact that nurses have not spoken with one unified voice. Despite the fact that there are more than 2 million people licensed as RNs in this country, nursing previously had not unified to speak on issues of health care policy, acquiring resources for nursing, or responding to the larger profession's needs and directions. There are four core groups that comprise the Tri-Council: the American Nurses Association (ANA), the National League for Nursing (NLN), the American Organization of Nurse Executives (AONE), and the American Association of Colleges of Nursing (AACN). Several states have actually employed this same model to increase the collaboration among these key groups at the local level. The Tri-Council is a network of groups in which representatives of large nursing organizations link together to tackle national professional nursing issues and problems. It is a good example of how the group process can be used positively and constructively and how much clout can be generated by working together and speaking in unity.

There is also an organization of specialty groups in nursing called the Alliance, which brings together the interests of all nurses in the various specialties. Formed in 2001 by the Nursing Organizations Liaison Forum (NOLF) and the National Federation of Specialty Nursing Organizations (NFSNO), the Alliance includes a broad range of membership. It allows for joint efforts between associations and nursing groups who have aligned interests. Clearly, the profession of nursing is working to capitalize on the positive synergy and power of collective action that groups and teams provide.

Summary

- Nurses are involved in and accomplish their work through participation in a variety of groups.
- There are many types of groups in health care organizations, including informal groups, work groups, teams, and committees.

- Group interactions are composed of process, standards, problem solving, communication, and roles.
- Groups tend to go through a series of developmental stages that are predictable.
- People join groups to fulfill primary needs and psychological drives.
- There are both advantages and disadvantages to the use of groups in organizations.
- Meetings can be structured for effective group participation.
- The purpose of a group meeting may be for information dissemination, opinion seeking, or problem solving.
- Decision-making power in groups is delegated along a continuum from none to all.
- A group may be formally structured into a committee, a relatively stable group, to accomplish an organizational goal.
- The committee leader has certain tasks and responsibilities to perform in managing the group toward productivity.
- One leadership role is to control disruptive group members.
- Group participation has become an increasingly large part of the nurse's role in practice because of team-building strategies and the development of multidisciplinary work groups in complex organizational structures.
- True teams require a great deal of developmental time and effort but are capable of moving the collective performance of a group to a higher level than a work group.

Study Questions

1. Where in nursing are the most appropriate uses for teams? For work groups? For committee structure?
2. What motivates an individual to join a group?
3. What are the significantly different elements between a work group and a team? What elements are similar? How do you determine whether you need a team?
4. How is leading a group like the nursing process? The management process?
5. What team-building strategies are most useful when trying to develop a team?

CASE STUDY*

Instituting a Nurse-Managed Clinic

The changes in health care require proficient utilization of resources. Nurses today must actively seek out opportunities to make changes in ways that favorably affect their work and patient care. Although we do not always have a say in whether or not to change the way we work, we have a choice in the way we respond to change. The use of groups to solve efficiency problems is one manner in which to bring about effective and efficient change.

One treatment option for advanced prostate cancer patients is monthly hormone therapy. This treatment blocks the body's utilization of testosterone, thereby "starving" the prostate of testosterone and stopping cancer growth. These patients require monthly treatment for the rest of their lives. The population of these patients in our clinic had grown such that the volume was unmanageable. It was evident that a change was required.

Each nurse had his or her own case load of patients seen each month. The norm was that no matter what the nurse was doing when his or her patient arrived for an appointment, the nurse would quit what he or she was doing and proceed to see the patient. This method of patient care management was adequate until more physicians were added to the department and there was an extraordinary increase in all areas of clinic activity. There was a large increase in procedures, treatments, and clinic visits. The fact that the patient's primary nurse would "drop" whatever he or she was doing when the patients arrived became incredibly disruptive to patient flow in all areas of the clinic. It was obvious that a new method of patient care management was needed.

---

*Case study provided by Lynne A. NezBeda, BSN, RN, CURN, Nurse Manager, Urology, Cleveland Clinic Foundation, Cleveland, Ohio.

There was a long history of "each nurse has his or her own patients" to overcome; it was the norm for years. Resistance was expected in changing this norm and instituting a new one. Although most nurses realized the difficulties with the current system, some had fears. In order for the change to be effective, these fears had to be addressed, and all had to participate in the process of defining and implementing the change.

A series of staff meetings was held to address the problem. It was important that the entire staff was present so that each person could participate, voice opinions, and identify fears and uncertainties. With everyone joining in with suggestions, more ideas with which to work were produced. A clinical nurse specialist (a nurse with a master of science in nursing degree) in urological oncology was invited to attend the meeting. She had a long history of working with the group when there were difficult patient situations. She also was a former nurse manager, and her management experience was invaluable. She supported the need for a change.

The manager presented the idea of the need for a change and asked the group for suggestions. Ideas were voiced and were augmented by other members until the concept of an innovative nurse-managed clinic, where the bulk of the 90 patients would be seen on a single day, came about. Monday, the day of least patient activity in the clinic, was chosen. The entire concept was a direct result of seeking member involvement; the finalized idea was better than any one person's individual idea. Now that the basic concept of a nurse-managed clinic had been identified, it was time to address the nurses' concerns about this clinic. These fit into three main categories: adequate patient follow-up, decreased patient satisfaction, and the loss of the nurse-patient relationship. All these concerns involved giving up "control" of the patient care and trusting other staff to maintain the quality of care each nurse gave. In the past each nurse maintained his or her own caseload and had direct control over the patient's care. Each nurse also enjoyed close interpersonal relationships with patients in her caseload.

The group discussed the fact that adequate follow-up was crucial because if the patient missed a dose of his or her medication, the cancer could spread. Each nurse had previously used his or her own method of scheduling follow-up, and it became obvious that standardization was now essential. This was addressed by standardizing what was documented each visit, including follow-up appointments, by use of a rubber stamp.

Decreased patient satisfaction was another concern. It was evident that patients enjoyed having one nurse to call with questions and that a rapport had developed. This concern, however, also contained the fact that nurses might lose relationships with patients and their families that had developed. It was feared that patients would be deeply dissatisfied if they had a different nurse at each monthly visit. As one group member said, "After all, these are cancer patients and they have special needs." The group discussed these fears and agreed that, if at all possible, patients should have only two or three nurses that they see in hopes of maintaining rapport and trust. This concern was addressed by assigning each nurse a day of the week to see patients. Because the hormone injection was given every 28 days, patients had the opportunity to schedule their visit on the same weekday each month. This compromise also allowed nurses to maintain some of their relationships with patients and their families.

Implementation took about 6 months. Nurses had to change their concept of patient care, but so did the patients. It was each nurse's responsibility to discuss the new care management system with his or her patients and move their appointments to Monday, the chosen day of the new clinic. Surprisingly, few patients resisted.

A standardized documentation and assessment system removed the concern of poor follow-up and standardized the tracking of worrisome patient systems.

Patients are more educated about their disease because the same assessment questions are asked each visit. Patients call with early changes in status, preventing permanent sequelae. Patients usually see one of three nurses when they come for the

CRITICAL THINKING EXERCISE

Organize into a small group; then select a leader. Take a few minutes to do this, then select or appoint a process recorder. The leader's role is that of a nurse manager at Our Lady of Sorrow Community Hospital. The leader has just been informed that she must cut two nurse jobs immediately. This is part of an immediate RIF (reduction in force) at the hospital to meet some very serious financial reversals. To accomplish the task, the leader has called together your group (the nurses of the unit). The leader has the task of deciding how to cut the nursing personnel budget and must now lead your group to develop a plan while preserving a sense of teamwork. The process recorder is to prepare a summary of the group's work and report as requested.*

1. Observe the process the group uses to select its own leader. Did anyone try to avoid selection? Was someone an enthusiastic volunteer? How long did the process take? Were the selection criteria discussed? What were the selection criteria?
2. What method was used to select/appoint a process recorder? What power strategy was used to make this decision?
3. What is the problem identified in the task?
4. What did the group leader do to handle the situation?
5. What should the group leader do to handle the situation?
6. How did group members respond to the task?
7. What leadership and management strategies might be effective?
8. What could the leader and followers consider changing in the situation?
9. How did group members feel about what happened?

*Follow up this exercise with one that tackles a similar problem: this time the leader has just been informed of a serious staffing crisis. Nurse turnover during this time of nursing shortage has created a serious coverage problem. Some nurses who have been working 80 hours per week in double shifts are now threatening to quit. A plan for safe coverage needs to be developed.

---

monthly visit. Some physicians have changed their follow-up of these patients from twice a year to once a year, evidencing their trust in the nursing staff's ability to assess patients and identify problems. A file card system has been implemented to give the nurse immediate access to patient symptoms and information when patients telephone and the patient record is not available. Patient satisfaction has been monitored in a quality assurance study with the result of 100% of patients being "satisfied" or "very satisfied" with their nursing care. This study is repeated biannually.

Involving members in change helps both members and management. Members benefit because they are involved in what affects their work. Management benefits because involvement tends to reduce resistance and increase ownership of the change.

References

Aguayo, R. (1990). Dr. Deming: *The American who taught the Japanese about quality.* New York: Carol Publishing Group.

Barksdale, G.T. (1998). Changing reward systems for team-based systems. *Seminars for Nurse Managers, 6*(4), 199-204.

Beachy, P., & Biester, D. (1986). Restructuring group meetings for effectiveness. *Journal of Nursing Administration, 16*(12), 30-33.

Blegen, M. (1993). Nurses' job satisfaction: A meta-analysis of related variables. *Nursing Research, 42*(1), 36-41.

Book, C., & Galvin, K. (1975). *Instruction in and about small group discussion.* Falls Church, VA: Speech Communication Association.

Brown, B. (1998). 10 trends for the new year: Nurse managers predict the skills, technology, and mind-set you'll need to prosper in 1999. *Nursing Management, 29*(2), 33-36.

Cherniss, C., & Goleman, D. (2001). *The emotionally intelligent workplace: How to select for, measure, and improve emotional intelligence in individuals, groups, and organizations.* San Francisco: Jossey-Bass.

Dabney, D. (1995). Workplace deviance among nurses: The influence of work group norms on drug diversion and/or use. *Journal of Nursing Administration, 25*(3), 48-55.

Darr, K. (1989). Applying the Deming method in hospitals (Part 1). *Hospital Topics, 67*(6), 4-5.

Deveau, B.J., & McCabe, D.U. (1996). Results-oriented committee restructuring. *Journal of Nursing Administration, 26*(10), 35-46.

Drucker, P.F. (1993). *Post capitalist society.* New York: Harper Business Publishers.

Farley, M., & Stoner, M. (1989). *The nurse executive and interdisciplinary team building. Nursing Administration Quarterly, 13*(2), 24-30.

Gage, M. (1998). From independence to interdependence: Creating synergistic healthcare teams. *Journal of Nursing Administration, 28*(4), 17-26.

Hansen, M.C., & Hayes, P.A. (1998). Integrating students into interdisciplinary teams: Extending the caring circle. *Seminars for Nurse Managers, 6*(4), 214-218.

Hersey, P., Blanchard, K.H., & Johnson, D.E. (2001). *Management of organizational behavior: Leading human resources* (8th ed.). Upper Saddle River, NJ: Prentice-Hall.

Jacobs, B., & Rosenthal, T. (1984). Managing effective meetings. *Nursing Economic$, 2*(2), 137-141.

Jay, A. (1982). How to run a meeting. *Journal of Nursing Administration, 12*(1), 22-28.

Katzenbach, J., & Smith, D. (1993). *The wisdom of teams: Creating the high-performance organization.* New York: Harper Collins.

Kohn, L.T., Corrigan, J.M., & Donaldson, M.S. (Eds.). (2000). *To err is human: Building a safer health system.* Washington, DC: National Academies Press.

Lancaster, J. (1981). Making the most of meetings. *Journal of Nursing Administration, 11*(10), 15-19.

Laramee, A. (1999). The building blocks of successful relationships. *The Journal of Care Management, 5*(4), 40, 42, 44-45.

Lassen, A.A., Fosbinder, D.M., Minton, S., & Robins, M.M. (1997). Nurse/physician collaborative practice: Improving health care quality while decreasing cost. *Nursing Economic$, 15*(2), 87-91, 104.

Leppa, C.J. (1996). Nurse relationships and work group disruption. *Journal of Nursing Administration, 26*(10), 23-27.

Manion, J. (2004). Strengthening organizational commitment: Understanding the concept as a basis for creating effective workforce retention strategies. *The Health Care Manager, 23*(2), 167-176.

Manion, J. (2005). *Create a positive healthcare workplace: Practical strategies to retain today's workforce and find tomorrow's.* Chicago: AHA Press.

Manion, J., Lorimer, W., & Leander, W.J. (1996). *Team-based health care organizations: Blueprint for success.* Gaithersburg, MD: Aspen.

Manion, J. & Bartholomew, K. (2003). Community in the workplace: A proven retention strategy. *Journal of Nursing Administration, 34*(1), 46-53.

Page, C. (1998). Pathway leadership: A mature framework for teams. *Seminars for Nurse Managers, 6*(4), 195-198.

Ponte, P.R., Fay, M.S., Brown, P., Doyle, M., Perron, J., Zizzi, L., et al. (1998). Factors leading to a strike vote and strategies for reestablishing relationships. *Journal of Nursing Administration, 28*(2), 35-43.

Schmeiding, N. (1990). A model for assessing nurse administrators' actions. *Western Journal of Nursing Research, 12*(3), 293-306.

Sheafor, M. (1991). Productive work groups in complex hospital units: Proposed contributions of the nurse executive. *Journal of Nursing Administration, 21*(5), 25-30.

Sorrells-Jones, J. (1997). The challenge of making it real: Interdisciplinary practice in a "seamless" organization. *Nursing Administration Quarterly, 21*(2), 20-30.

Sorrells-Jones, J., & Weaver, D. (1999). Knowledge workers and knowledge-intense organizations. I. A promising framework for nursing and healthcare. *Journal of Nursing Administration, 29*(7/8), 12-18.

Sovie, M. (1992). Care and service teams: A new imperative. *Nursing Economic$, 10*(2), 94-100.

Spitzer, R. (1998). Teams and teamwork. *Seminars for Nurse Managers, 6*(4), 169.

Van de Ven, A., & Delbecq, A. (1974). The effectiveness of nominal, Delphi, and interacting group decision making processes. *Academy of Management Journal, 17*(4), 605-621.

Veninga, R. (1982). *The human side of health administration: A guide for hospital, nursing, and public health administrators.* Englewood Cliffs, NJ: Prentice-Hall.

Wilson, R.D., Mateo, M.A., & Brumm, S.K. (1999). Revitalizing a departmental committee. *Journal of Nursing Administration, 29*(3), 45-48.

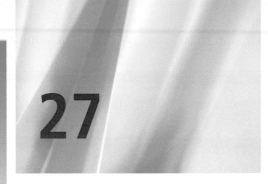

27

Confronting the Nursing Shortage

Amelia McCutcheon

CHAPTER OBJECTIVES

- Define nursing shortage
- Profile the history of nursing shortage and surplus
- Critically analyze factors that contribute to a nursing shortage
- Link leadership and management concepts to strategies to confront the nursing shortage
- Use critical thinking to conceptualize and analyze possible solutions to a practice exercise

The nursing shortage is a major phenomenon affecting nurses and the provision of patient care. According to the National Center for Health Workforce Analysis (2002) of the U.S. Department of Health and Human Services, there are more than 2.3 million licensed registered nurses in the United States. However, a projected 275,000 more nurses will be needed by 2010. At the same time, enrollment in nursing schools is falling. The American Association of Colleges of Nursing (2003) estimated that enrollment in nursing programs must increase by 40% to meet the projected demand for nurses.

Nursing shortages have been cyclical over the past few decades; however, the current shortage may last longer because of a variety of factors. For example, the National Center for Health Workforce Analysis (2002) found that the average age of registered nurses is 44 years old. This "graying" factor makes the nursing shortage an even greater issue in light of the fact that between 1980 and 2000, the proportion of RNs under the age of 30 decreased from 25% to 9%.

To confront the nursing shortage, the following three strategies must be examined and implemented:

1. Education-related strategies aimed at increasing nursing school enrollments
2. Work environment initiatives designed to retain staff
3. Health delivery system–related strategies aimed at reducing the demand for nursing services

An overarching strategy is the need to build stronger partnerships and alliances with colleges and universities, professional associations, other health care employers, government, community organizations, corporations, foundations and the public.

DEFINITIONS

A nursing shortage is a condition in which the delicate balance of nurse supply and nurse demand is not at equilibrium. A **nursing shortage** is defined as a situation in which the demand for employment of nurses (how many nurses employers would *like* to employ) exceeds the available supply of nurses willing to be employed at a given salary. A nursing shortage is not just a matter of understaffing; in fact, understaffing can occur in conditions of shortage, equilibrium, or surplus, depending on local factors such as tight budgets or poor working conditions. The hallmark of a nursing shortage

⚠ LEADING & MANAGING **DEFINED**

Nursing Shortage

Situation in which the number of nurses that employers would *like* to employ (demand) exceeds the number of nurses willing to be employed at a given salary (supply).

Span of Control

The number of staff reporting directly to a manager.

Transformational Leader

A leader who inspires and transforms followers.

Turnover

Termination of membership in an organization.

---

is the discrepancy between the supply and demand for RNs.

A nursing shortage can be identified by opinions of nurses, the public, or experts. Nurses or the public may believe there is a shortage based on a variety of factors. Experts generally use indicators such as employer reports, vacancy rates, turnover, recruitment difficulty, staffing levels, RN supply per population, or forecasting models to determine a nursing shortage.

Definitions of other factors surrounding a nursing shortage are as follows:

- **Span of control:** The number of persons who report directly to a single manager; affects the functions of planning, organizing, and leading (Hattrup & Kleiner, 1993).
- **Transformational leader:** A leader who inspires and transforms followers by raising their sense of the value of the task and their sense of importance (Bass, 1998). Bass outlined four components of transformational leadership: (1) charisma or idealized influence, (2) inspirational motivation, (3) intellectual stimulation, and (4) individualized consideration.
- **Turnover:** The termination of membership in an organization. Turnover rate is derived by dividing the total number of nurses who left a unit in 1 year by the total number of nurses employed on that unit.

BACKGROUND

Registered nurses make up the largest health care occupation, holding about 2.3 million jobs in 2002,

with about 1 in 5 working part time (Bureau of Labor Statistics, 2004). Despite large numbers, the supply of RNs has not been in balance with demand or stable over time. Since the early 1900s, U.S. nursing has undergone repeated cycles of shortage and surplus. Although the length of each phase varies, clearly the alternation between shortage and surplus has been more frequent since the mid-1960s. Shortage phases have lasted longer, with only brief periods of surplus. Figure 27.1 shows the cycles of nursing shortage and surplus from 1901 to 2005.

These cycles are interrelated with social and economic forces, shifts, and changes. For example, the nursing shortage from about 1915 to 1920 resulted from the inability to recruit qualified and suitable students, since students provided most of the service on hospital wards (King, 1989). A little more than a decade later, in the context of the Great Depression (1929-1932), a surplus prevailed (Carlson et al., 1992). The 20 years after World War II (1945-1965) saw yet another nursing shortage (Carlson et al., 1992; Grando, 1998). The availability of financial aid via the Nurse Training Act of 1964 increased nursing enrollments, and wage increases triggered increased labor force participation, thus lowering job vacancy rates during the next cycle (1965-1970). During the 1970s nurse job vacancy rates climbed steadily, and a chronic shortage existed from 1970 to 1980 (Carlson et al., 1992). The recession in 1981 again converted the cycle to one of surplus until about 1985, when the results of implementing diagnosis-related groups (DRGs) passed and more

	Nursing Shortage	Nursing Surplus		Nursing Shortage	Nursing Surplus
1901			1954		
1902			1955		
1903			1956		
1904			1957		
1905			1958		
1906			1959		
1907			1960		
1908			1961		
1909			1962		
1910			1963		
1911			1964		
1912			1965		
1913			1966		
1914			1967		
1915			1968		
1916			1969		
1917			1970		
1918			1971		
1919			1972		
1920			1973		
1921			1974		
1922			1975		
1923			1976		
1924			1977		
1925			1978		
1926			1979		
1927			1980		
1928			1981		
1929			1982		
1930			1983		
1931			1984		
1932			1985		
1933			1986		
1934			1987		
1935			1988		
1936			1989		
1937			1990		
1938			1991		
1939			1992		
1940			1993		
1941			1994		
1942			1995		
1943			1996		
1944			1997		
1945			1998		
1946			1999		
1947			2000		
1948			2001		
1949			2002		
1950			2003		
1951			2004		
1952			2005		
1953					

Figure 27.1
Nursing shortage and surplus cycles. (Copyright Diane L. Huber, 2005.)

ill patients were housed in hospitals. A shortage again was noted from about 1986 to 1992, marked by an increase in the hospital RN vacancy rate at a national average of 11% (Buerhaus et al., 2005). By 1992, managed care, capitated reimbursement, cost containment, and downsizing hit the hospital industry only 5 years later, and nurses once again experienced a surplus. However, this cycle again reversed by 1998, when the beginning of a shortage was once again in evidence. By 2001, the hospital RN vacancy rate was at a national average of 13% and ranging up to 20%. This cycle of shortage entered its eighth year in 2005 (Buerhaus et al., 2005).

Clearly the cycling through surplus and shortage increased in frequency in the last quarter of the twentieth century. Such rapidity of change disrupts individual nurses' lives and careers and makes the economic welfare of nurses precarious. Policies and practices related to recruitment into nursing as a career, recruitment and attraction to specific jobs, and retention in both job and career swing with the immediate crisis. This robs nursing of stability and long-term growth. Both historical indicators and research on nursing shortages have indicated that the basis of the problem relates to the nature of the work, low wages, poor working conditions, and hospital administrators' desire to keep nursing costs down and prevent salaries from increasing (Carlson et al., 1992; Grando, 1998; King, 1989). Clearly, as the shortage/surplus cycles have increased in cycle time, planning change in the nurse labor force has become more difficult. Projecting the future demand for nurses requires careful attention to social and economic forces.

The future projected demand for nurses is tied to an increase in chronic illnesses and an increasingly geriatric population. Salaries in nursing have been increasing, although compensation is sensitive to economic and political forces. Salary compression occurs over a work career in nursing. The demographics of the workforce are changing. There are new configurations of nurse extenders, ancillary workers, and unlicensed assistive personnel, reflecting a struggle with what is the proper balance of

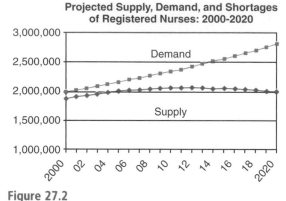

Figure 27.2
Projected supply, demand, and shortages of registered nurses: 2000-2020. (From National Center for Health Workforce Analysis. [2002]. *Projected supply, demand, and shortages of registered nurses: 2000-2020.* Rockville, MD: U.S. Department of Health and Human Services, Health Resources and Services Administration. Retrieved May 21, 2004, from *www.bhpr.hrsa.gov/healthworkforce/reports/rnproject/report.htm*)

staff mix. There is a common assumption that an all-RN staff is too costly, but beyond that the "ideal mix" is unknown. On the other hand, research suggests that the greater the RN mix, the less care outcomes are negative (Kovner & Gergen, 1998).

The year 1998 marked the beginning of the current shortage. Unlike some previous shortage cycles, the current shortage is not resolving quickly (Buerhaus et al., 2003; Huston, 2003; O'Neil & Kimball, 2002). Figure 27.2 shows the results of the National Sample Survey of Registered Nurses (National Center for Health Workforce Analysis, 2002), projecting the following RN shortage numbers:

- 149,000 in 2004
- 275,000 in 2010
- 507, 000 in 2015
- 808,000 in 2020

All states are expected to be affected by the current shortage. However, the predictions for some states are especially grim. For example, Nevada has the lowest proportion of working RNs per 100,000 population, and California will need at least 25,000 more RNs in the next 5 years than will be available (United States General Accounting Office, 2002).

The shortage of nurses is reflected in nurse vacancy rates. According to a commissioned report on health workforce shortages, U.S. hospitals had average nurse vacancy rate of 13%, with over one in seven hospitals reporting a severe RN vacancy rate of more than 20% (First Consulting Group, 2001). Nurse vacancy rates in hospitals or other agencies are one measure of nursing shortage. Leaving a job is not equal to leaving the profession, although both may occur.

The U.S. nurse shortage is made more dramatically pronounced by the fact that many other countries are experiencing similar shortages. The International Council of Nurses (2003) reported the following statistics. In the United States in 2002, there were 126,000 vacant nursing positions (12% of the total workforce requirements). The projected shortfall by 2016 in Canada is 113,000; a similar shortage is expected in Europe when the difference in population size is considered. Projected shortfalls in European countries include the following: United Kingdom—22,000; Denmark—22,000 (by 2025); Germany—13,000; Netherlands—13,000; Switzerland—3,000. In France, 6% of the nursing workforce left the public sector in 2001, compared with 4% in 1997; 18,000 nurses leave public hospitals every year, and the private sector reports a worse situation. Another 33 countries, most of which are in Oceania, Africa, Central America, and the Caribbean, also reported nursing shortages, worsened by the outflow of nurses to richer countries. The exceptions are Spain, Hong Kong, Korea, Taiwan, and the Philippines. The Spanish government stated that 13,000 nurses are unemployed, and it was working to find jobs for them in the UK. Spain's national nursing associations are challenging this figure. They reported a reduction in demand as a result of hospital downsizing. Hong Kong, Korea, and Taiwan reported a surplus of nurses. The Philippines has a unique situation, reporting a balanced supply and demand while thousands of Philippine nurses continue to be recruited by the international market, particularly the United States.

The nursing shortage is complex and is acknowledged to be the result of a combination of multiple factors. Just as numerous factors contribute to the nursing shortage, multiple possible solutions are needed to resolve it.

CURRENT ISSUES AND TRENDS

Health workforce dynamics are a current issue for leadership and management in nursing. Nurse leaders and managers have the responsibility for managing scarce resources, including the human capital resources related to nursing service delivery. Chief among these resources is the adequate and appropriate mix of RNs and assistive personnel. Because the RN workforce has not been stable, workforce dynamics are an ongoing issue in clinical practice. Therefore the current nurse shortage (one that is projected to continue) becomes one of the preeminent current issues in nursing leadership and care management.

Cycles of nurse shortage and surplus have been the focus of study and discussion over the years. Many factors contribute to these phenomena. An analysis of the supply and demand for RNs will highlight the nurse shortage as a current and future issue. Then leadership and management implications will be discussed.

Factors that Contribute to the Nursing Shortage

The nursing shortage is a national and international phenomenon. The causes are complex and interactive. There is no one simple, quick fix. To best understand the main factors that contribute to the nursing shortage, factors that affect both the supply of and the demand for nurses must be examined separately.

Supply

Factors that affect supply include the following:
- *Nursing education factors:* Those affecting the number of new graduates

- *Work environment factors:* Those affecting the ability of the workplace to attract and retain nurses
- *Demographic factors:* Those affecting the nature of the RN workforce, thus the number of practitioners who can continue to work

Nursing education

The ability of the education system to produce new graduates is affected by low enrollment, a shift from associate degree to baccalaureate-prepared RNs, and a shortage of nursing school faculty. First, enrollment in nursing schools is not growing quickly enough to meet the projected demand for nurses. The American Association of Colleges of Nursing (AACN, 2003) found that enrollments in entry-level baccalaureate programs decreased for 6 straight years, 1995 to 2001; yet enrollment must increase by 40% to meet the projected demand for nurses. Buerhaus and colleagues (2000) reported that women graduating from high school in the 1990s were 35% less likely to become nurses than women who graduated in the 1970s. Women now have more career opportunities and are increasingly entering medicine, business, engineering, and other careers traditionally chosen by men. Nursing has become less attractive (O'Neil & Kimball, 2002).

Second, the shift from associate degree to baccalaureate-prepared RNs has also affected the growth in supply. Baccalaureate-prepared RNs need twice as long to complete their education and enter the workforce than those graduating from associate degree programs. The number of new licenses in nursing is projected to be 17% lower in 2020 than in 2002 (National Center for Health Workforce Analysis, 2002).

Third, a shortage of nursing school faculty is limiting enrollments. In 2002, U.S. nursing schools turned away over 5,000 applicants. In 2003 almost 16,000 applicants were denied entry to entry-level baccalaureate nursing programs (AACN, 2003). Lack of faculty was the stated reason two-thirds of the time. Fewer than 1% of nurses hold earned doctoral degrees and only 10% have master's degrees (Chitty, 2001). To further confound the shortage, the average age of nursing faculty is 50 years old

(Buerhaus et al., 2000), posing a potential large surge of retirements in the near future.

Work environment factors

One in five nurses is considering leaving nursing for reasons other than retirement within the next 5 years (Letvak, 2002). Several work environment factors have been cited as reasons for increased turnover (Buerhaus et al., 2000; Laschinger et al., 2001a; Tri-Council for Nursing, 2004), including workload, autonomy, relations with managers, and compensation. Such factors influence job stress, in turn leading to job satisfaction or dissatisfaction (Moos, 1994). Job satisfaction is a strong predictor of turnover and intent to stay (Blegen, 1993; Davidson et al., 1997; Irvine & Evans, 1995; Larabee et al., 2003; Shader et al., 2001). For example, in a meta-analysis of 18 studies (16 were nursing), Irvine and Evans found a strong negative relationship between job satisfaction and intent to stay, suggesting that the more unhappy staff members are, the more likely they are to leave the organization.

Workload. One of the findings of a study by Aiken and colleagues (2002) is that nurses with the highest nurse-to-patient ratio were more likely to describe feelings of burnout, emotional exhaustion, and job dissatisfaction than nurses with lower ratios. In addition, 43% of nurses who reported high levels of burnout and dissatisfaction intended to leave their jobs within a year. In contrast, only 11% of nurses who did not complain of burnout or dissatisfaction expressed intent to leave their current jobs.

Autonomy. Professional autonomy, or control over the practice environment, was identified as the strongest predictor of nurses' identification with the organization (Apker et al., 2003). Nurses who did not believe their jobs provided sufficient freedom were less likely to experience feelings of affiliation and loyalty toward their employers. In a study of magnet hospitals, high levels of autonomy increased nurses' job satisfaction, managerial trust, and nurses' assessment of the quality of patient care (Laschinger et al., 2001b).

Relations with managers. The manager's leadership style was found to be a significant predictor

Figure 27.3

Comparison of actual earnings for RNs and elementary school teachers and "real" earnings for RNs for the years between 1983-2000. (From National Center for Health Workforce Analysis. [2002]. *Projected supply, demand, and shortages of registered nurses: 2000-2020.* Rockville, MD: U.S. Department of Health and Human Services, Health Resources and Services Administration. Retrieved May 11, 2004, from www.ftp://ftp.hrsa.gov/healthworkforce/ reports/rnproject/report.htm)

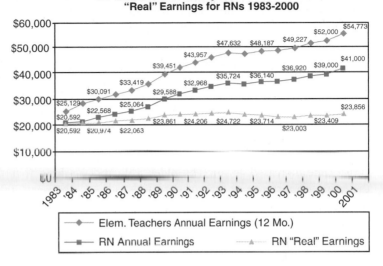

Comparison of Actual Annual Earnings for RNs and Elementary School Teachers and "Real" Earnings for RNs 1983-2000

of nurses' job satisfaction (Bakker et al., 2000; Loke, 2001; McCutcheon, 2004) and retention of nurses (Irvine & Evans, 1995; Leveck & Jones, 1996; Medley & Larochelle, 1995; Shader et al., 2001).

Compensation. The National Center for Health Workforce Analysis (2002) reported that on average, RNs have seen no increase in purchasing power over the last 9 years. Conversely, the average salary for elementary school teachers has always been greater than that for RNs and is growing at a faster pace. For example, in 1983, the average elementary school teacher earned $4,400 more than the average RN; and in 2000 elementary school teachers earned about $13,600 more (Figure 27.3).

Demographic Factors

Understanding the demographic nature of the RN workforce requires an examination of the number of practitioners who may continue to work, the aging of the RN workforce, and the changing composition of the RN workforce. Demographic factors help to highlight trends and flows nationally. These factors have implications for human resource initiatives.

Aging of the RN Workforce

The aging of the RN workforce is affected by the following two factors:

1. The higher average age of recent graduating classes
2. The aging of the existing pool of licensed nurses

The data from the National Center For Health Workforce Analysis (2002) were used in this section (unless otherwise indicated). Graduates of associate degree programs, the largest source of new RNs, are on average 33 years old, considerably older than in 1980, when the average age was 28. The result has been a significant decline in the proportion of RNs under the age of 30. Between 1980 and 2000, the proportion of RNs in the licensed pool who were under the age of 30 declined from 25% to 9%. The second factor is the "graying" of the existing licensed pool who were of nurses. The average age of the working nurse today is 44 years (Buerhaus et al., 2000), and about half of RNs are projected to be over age 50 by 2010 (Buerhaus et al., 2003). Nurses appear to be leaving the RN license pool, through death or retirement, at a faster rate than ever, with an average retirement age of 49 years. Between 1988 and 1992, 30,000 RNs left the license pool; 23,000 left between 1992 and 1996. The loss of RNs between the 1996 and 2000 surveys increased six- to seven-fold, to nearly 175,000, which points to a critical situation. The "graying" factor makes the nursing shortage an even greater issue, as the RN loss is projected to be 128% higher in 2020 than in 2002.

Changing Composition of the RN Workforce

Of the more than 104,000 total estimated increase in hospital RN employment in 2002, about two-thirds were RNs over age 50, and the remaining one-third were foreign-born RNs (Buerhaus et al., 2003). The increased reliance on older RNs and the rising importance of foreign-born RNs is the result of a fundamental shift occurring in the RN workforce. This shift is the decline in younger women choosing nursing as a career during the past two decades. If a dramatic increase in enrollment does not occur, there will be an increased need for foreign-born RNs. However, there are ethical implications to foreign nurse recruitment, given a coexisting international nurse shortage.

Demand

The recent increase in demand for RNs is projected to continue as a result of population growth, a rising proportion of people over age 65, economic growth, and advances in technology. Demand for RNs is projected to increase 40% over the next two decades, with the majority of employment growth occurring in hospitals (National Center For Health Workforce Analysis, 2002).

To explore the factors contributing to the increase in demand, a discussion of the changing demographic nature of the population and the health delivery system follows.

Changing demographic nature of the population

Population growth and aging Baby Boomers are the major factors changing the demographic nature of the population, which in turn are affecting the demand for RNs. The National Center For Health Workforce Analysis (2002) reported the following statistics. Recent projections (Figure 27.4) show that the U.S. population will grow 18% between 2000 and 2020, which equates to an additional 50 million people requiring health care.

Increased life expectancy resulting from advances in science and medicine account for most of this population growth, as well as the increase in the proportion of the population over the age of 65. The subgroup of people 65 years old and older will grow 54% between 2000 and 2020, which equates to an additional 19 million people in this age group. Individuals over 65, particularly those 85 and over, have the greatest per capita demand for health care, and thus the greatest need for the services of RNs. These individuals tend to have (1) a higher incidence of chronic conditions such as arthritis (50%), hypertension (36%), and heart disease (32%); and (2) a higher occurrence of multiple conditions requiring more regular care. As a result, this population visits physicians twice as often as those under 65, accounts for 38% of hospital discharges

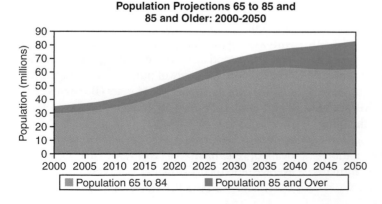

Population Projections 65 to 85 and 85 and Older: 2000-2050

Figure 27.4

Population projections for ages 65 to 84 and 85 and older, 2000-2050. (From National Center for Health Workforce Analysis. [2002]. *Projected supply, demand, and shortages of registered nurses: 2000-2020.* Rockville, MD: U.S. Department of Health and Human Services, Health Resources and Services Administration. Retrieved May 21, 2004, from www.bhpr.hrsa.gov/healthworkforce/reports/rnproject/report.htm)

(they represent 13% of the population), and has annual per capita health care expenditures of $5,400 compared with $1,500 for those under age 65.

Health delivery system

Health delivery systems form the structure around how care is delivered, where it is delivered, and how it is paid. For example, Medicare and Medicaid reimbursement, along with regional and local customs and culture, influence the demand for nursing services (Tri-Council for Nursing, 2004). It is commonly known that socioeconomic determinants such as culture, income, educational level, and age affect an individual's health practices, which in turn affect the person's health status and subsequent use of and access to health care services. Thus the demand for nurses may be more or less intense depending on local health system characteristics. For example, a General Accounting Office report (GAO-03-460) (2003) on emergency department overcrowding found waiting times to be longer in communities with more uninsured people. In rural areas, services or specialists may not be available without long-distance travel, which could result in delays in diagnosis, treatment, and care. Such delays could adversely affect outcomes, resulting in patients becoming more ill. Increased acuity of patients puts more demand on critical care services such as emergency and intensive care areas, thereby increasing the need for nurses. A combination of increased demand and decreasing supply creates a serious nursing shortage.

LEADERSHIP AND MANAGEMENT IMPLICATIONS

Linking Leadership and Management Concepts to Strategies for Confronting the Shortage

Just as multiple factors contribute to the nursing shortage, multiple possible solutions may exist to resolve it. Leadership is needed at all levels, in both the profession and in organizations. Several initiatives have been developed by hospitals, other health organizations, and health professional associations in response to the factors contributing to the nursing shortage. These initiatives include formal recruitment and retention programs, collaboration between education and practice settings to recruit more people into nursing, sign-on

◢ LEADERSHIP & MANAGEMENT **BEHAVIORS**

Leadership Behaviors

- Creates and communicates a sense of purpose
- Discovers and creates possibilities to recruit and retain nurses
- Motivates nursing staff's sense of value and importance
- Builds and sustains trust and commitment
- Develops leaders
- Transforms followers
- Makes decisions

Management Behaviors

- Communicates objectives
- Administers, maintains, focuses on work environment systems, and controls

- Sets staffing budgets, monitors progress
- Develops schedules
- Organizes the group
- Implements the plans
- Thinks critically
- Takes appropriate risks
- Measures performance
- Delegates tasks
- Makes decisions

Overlap Areas

- Communicates purpose and objectives
- Makes decisions

bonuses and other types of hiring incentives, and actions to improve the work environment of nurses (American Hospital Association [AHA], 2002).

The strategies that are most likely to provide for a stable nursing workforce now and in the future cluster into the following three areas:

1. Education-related strategies aimed at increasing nursing school enrollments
2. Work environment initiatives designed to retain staff
3. Health delivery system–related strategies aimed at reducing the demand for nursing services

Most of the proposed solutions are primarily derived from the following three sources:

1. The Bureau of Health Professions (2002), which outlined the Nursing Reinvestment Act
2. The Joint Commission on Accreditation of Healthcare Organizations (JCAHO, 2002)
3. The Tri-Council for Nursing (2004)

The Tri-Council consists of the American Association of Colleges of Nursing (AACN), the American Nurses Association (ANA), the American Organization of Nurse Executives (AONE), and the National League for Nursing (NLN). An overarching strategy is collaboration. Nursing needs to partner and network with the public colleges and universities, professional associations, and the various stakeholders of health care services.

Education

The following strategies are designed to increase enrollment in nursing programs:

- Advocate for increased nursing education funding under publicly funded initiatives to improve the capacity and resources for nursing education
- Encourage younger, more diverse population of nursing students
- Enhance image of nursing
- Articulate a clear vision of nursing that includes career progression

Advocate for increased nursing education funding

In 2002 the U.S. Congress drafted legislation to address the nursing shortage (Bureau of Health Professions, 2002). The Nurse Reinvestment Act, priced at 250 million dollars (as yet still unfunded),

is a reinvestment in nursing and offers funds to do the following:

- Provide scholarships to increase the number of students in nursing programs
- Finance the education of the next generation of teachers
- Project a new image of nursing
- Establish a National Nurse Corps to provide nurses for shortage areas
- Develop strategies to address workplace factors, including demonstration projects to enhance communication, mentoring young nurses through internships and residencies, and implementing best practices in nursing care, leadership, and management practices

JCAHO (2002) recommended the establishment of the federal funding of a graduate nursing residency program.

Encourage a younger, more diverse population of nursing students

Two examples of national media campaigns launched to attract young people into nursing were reported by Ulrich (2003). The first one was the "Nurses for a Healthier Tomorrow" campaign, led by a coalition of 40 nursing and health care organizations working together to raise interest in nursing careers among middle school and high school students. The campaign conducted nationwide focus groups with students ages 6 to 15 years, raised more than $600,000 in sponsorship, launched a website, and created a televised public service announcement. The second campaign is the "Campaign for Nursing's Future" launched by the Johnson & Johnson Company to promote careers in nursing. The campaign consisted of paid television commercials, a recruitment video, a website, and brochures mailed to schools across the country. A related need is to encourage gender, racial, and ethnic diversity. This need occurs throughout all nursing care settings, not just in hospitals.

Enhance the image of nursing

To attract younger people into nursing, the profession must be communicated as a positive, satisfying, and inspiring career. Nursing must provide for a balanced work life, offer leadership opportunities in which nurses may hone their management skills, and create an environment in which young nurses may plan to move toward higher pay and better hours. Wieck (2003) recommended expanding the image of nursing from caring and caregiver to opportunities and outcomes. Young people want opportunities to succeed and outcomes against which they can measure their success. Nursing must be advertised by focusing on such specialties as operating room nursing and emergency nursing, which are outcome driven and meet many young people's desires for a fast-paced, high-intensity work environment. Nursing must learn from Drucker's (1999) model of productivity—that is, young people value productivity and want to be rewarded for it. If the nursing profession is not able to adapt to this model, the emerging workforce will pursue other careers that do.

Communicating the significant contributions of nursing and important nursing practice innovations and discoveries enhances the image of nursing. Nurses need to reach out to the media and seek their help in increasing the public's awareness of the relationship between nursing and patient outcomes, that is, the relationship between nursing variables and quality of care. For example, lower hospital mortality rates have been associated with higher RN skill mix (Hartz et al., 1989). This important research is an example of rigorous evidence of the significant contribution of nurses to health care that can elevate the prestige and image of nursing, thus attracting people to careers in nursing.

Articulate a clear vision of nursing

For long-term solution, there is a need to formulate and articulate where the nursing profession is going. Wieck (2003) discussed having a nursing vision so that young people may see opportunities for great rewards and experiences. A lifelong nursing practice path, which includes a series of value-added steps (such as the nurse as a doer, a thinker, a practitioner, and a researcher), is recommended. Nursing needs to recruit outstanding students and appropriately educate the nursing workforce.

Part of this effort needs to be directed at making nursing attractive to the next generation of nurses. Tuition funding and scholarships, enhanced image in society, career paths, attractive compensation, and employee-friendly work environments are strategies to be considered. The challenge is to find the unique combination of attractors that will entice youth into nursing. Clearly, residency and mentorship programs need to be expanded to help new RNs settle into beginning practice. Both from social policy (government funding) and organizational perspectives, these guided experiences make sense. They are the principal method used to avoid "eating the young." Nurse leaders can use these strategies to attract and retain nurses, decrease the costs of turnover, and create a nurturing work environment.

Work Environment

One way to address the current nursing shortage and prevent future crisis would be to create and maintain Centers of Excellence in leadership and management aimed at advancing the profession and practice of nursing through the following strategies:

- Establishing appropriate leadership and management structures
- Providing nurses with sufficient autonomy
- Ensuring adequate nurse staffing
- Implementing appropriate compensation and benefit programs

Establish appropriate leadership and management structures

The manager's leadership style is one of the factors influencing the retention of nurses (Irvine & Evans, 1995; Leveck & Jones, 1996; Medley & Larochelle, 1995) and nurses' job satisfaction, which subsequently affects turnover (Bakker et al., 2000; Loke, 2001; McCutcheon, 2004; Stordeur et al., 2000; Stordeur et al., 2001). McCutcheon (2004), for example, found that the higher the nurses rated their manager as having a transformational leadership style, the higher the nurses' job satisfaction and the lower the unit turnover rate. Similar findings were reported by Medley

Research Note

Source: McCutcheon, A.S. (2004). Relationships between leadership style, span of control and outcomes (Doctoral dissertation, University of Toronto, Canada). *Dissertation Abstracts International, DAI-B65/05*, 2344 (Pub No AAT NQ91797).

Purpose

The purpose of this study is to examine the relationships between leadership style, span of control, and outcomes using a conceptual model linking concepts from three theories: Transformational Leadership Theory, Span of Control Theory, and Contingency Theory. The sample consisted of 717 nurses, 41 nurse managers, and 51 patient care units drawn from four types of units (medical, surgical, obstetrics, and day surgery) and seven hospitals. Hierarchical linear modeling and multiple regressions were used to test the study hypotheses.

Discussion

The study findings support the theoretical relationships between leadership style, span of control, and outcomes. Results of the study supported the argument that transformational leadership matters—the higher the nurses rated their manager as having a transformational leadership style, the higher the nurses' job satisfaction and the lower the unit turnover rate. Transactional leadership style had a similar effect on nurses' job satisfaction, although to a lesser extent. Management-by-exception leadership style, on the other hand, decreased nurses' job satisfaction.

The study findings also supported the argument that span of control matters—the wider the span of control, the higher the unit turnover rate. A very important and interesting finding is the significant moderating influence of span of control on the effects of leadership on nurses' job satisfaction. Span of control decreased the positive effects of transformational and transactional leadership styles on nurses' job satisfaction while increasing the negative effects of management-by-exception and laissez-faire leadership styles on nurses' job satisfaction. These findings demonstrated that no leadership style may overcome a wide span of control.

Application to Practice

Recommendations for practice include designing and implementing management education programs that focus on effective leadership, such as a transformational style of leadership and the development of guidelines regarding the number of staff a nurse manager may effectively supervise and lead. Recommendations for theory and research include further testing of the proposed relationships in the study's theoretical model and continued examination of how various organizational factors affect leaders, staff, work groups, and organizations.

and Larochelle (1995) and Stordeur and colleagues (2000). When managers with high transformational leadership scores were compared with managers who had high transactional leadership scores, transformational managers were more likely to have staff nurses with higher job satisfaction scores. Transformational leaders exert a significant positive impact on staff satisfaction by providing support, encouragement, positive feedback, and individual consideration and promoting open communication. These leadership behaviors tend to generate a favorable climate on the unit, characterized by increased cooperation and teamwork and fewer interpersonal conflicts. Nursing needs to recruit and train managers in supportive and participative leadership styles, such as the transformational leadership style (Bass, 1998).

Another factor that affects turnover is span of control (McCutcheon, 2004), defined as the number of staff reporting directly to the manager (Hattrup & Kleiner, 1993). McCutcheon (2004) found that the turnover rate increases by 1.6% for any increase of 10 in the size of the manager's span of control. For example, a manager with a span of control of 50 is predicted to have a unit turnover rate of 8%. The wider the manager's span of control, the higher the unit turnover. Possible explanations for this effect may be found in the findings of Green and colleagues (1996) and Gittell (2001). Green and colleagues found that when the work unit increases in size, relationships between managers and staff become less positive. Managers are not able to develop close relationships with staff and provide support and individual consideration, while at the same time seeing to the daily operations of their unit. Similarly, Gittell found that small supervisory spans have positive effects on group process; that is, managers with smaller spans tend to relate better with the staff. Managers with smaller spans work with, and provide, intensive coaching and feedback to their staff.

In addition to the effect of the manager's span of control on turnover, McCutcheon (2004) found that span of control influenced the relationship between the manager's leadership style and nurses' job satisfaction. The positive effect of transformational leadership style on nurses' job satisfaction is significantly reduced in units where managers have wider spans of control.

The results of a review of literature on span of control support the importance of the manager's span of control in creating a positive work environment (McCutcheon, 2005).

Increase autonomy

Apker and colleagues (2003) stressed the importance of developing nursing jobs and management practices that increase nurses' professional autonomy in their practice. For example, nurse leaders may establish organizational structures such as shared governance, continuous learning, and nursing research. These structures encourage nurses to take part in making decisions that influence patient care and nursing practice, and they encourage greater participation in clinical decision making with physicians and the interdisciplinary team. Nurse leaders also need to extend professional autonomy into quality-of-work-life issues such as promotion and advancement, flexible scheduling, and organizational culture that promotes respect and collaboration.

Ensure adequate competent staff

To ensure adequate competent staff, nurse leaders need to increase their participation in decision making, retain older RNs, and develop a policy on recruitment of foreign-born RNs. There is a need for nurse leaders to be part of the senior management team. Nurse leaders must have a strong voice in executive decisions that affect the ability of managers to ensure the provision of adequate competent staff.

Experienced RNs have a wealth of clinical expertise, nursing knowledge, skills, and judgment. Initiatives that may help retain older RNs include clinical ergonomic adaptations to minimize the physical strain in the work environment, flexible scheduling and part-time work, new roles (such as mentorship and internship), and economic incentives.

It is probable that foreign-born RNs are likely to play an increasingly important role in providing nursing care in the United States. The use of foreign-born RNs in the United States may not be favored by the following groups: unions, because of a possible negative impact on wages; patient advocates, because of possible effects on quality of care; and other associations and foreign governments, because of possible worsening of shortages in their own countries. Conversely, the use of foreign-born RNs may be supported by provider and payer groups because of possible reductions in labor costs and by foreign governments because of possible benefits for foreign-born RNs, namely, the opportunity to work in the United States and send money home. Policymakers must encourage debate and the formulation of policies in the use of foreign-born RNs.

Implement appropriate compensation and benefit programs

After years of almost zero salary growth for nurses, nursing needs to implement appropriate compensation and benefits commensurate with nurses' contributions to health care. Although pay often is not listed as a major factor motivating nurses, clearly society judges value, esteem, and image through compensation.

Health Delivery System

As mentioned above, the creation of Centers of Excellence would be a positive step in addressing the nursing shortage. By focusing on prevention, as well as the use of technology, research, and innovation, Centers of Excellence could highlight strategies specific to the health delivery system, with an emphasis on reducing the demand for services.

Strengthening primary prevention

Programmatic changes for reimbursement are needed to strengthen primary health care and increased access to health care services for specific populations. Primary prevention is a nursing function that nurses need to reclaim and build into autonomous practice. There is a need as well for nurses to participate actively in the policy process and in making policy decisions. Grassroots information and lobbying efforts are effective in increasing government support. Examples of primary prevention efforts that have been effective include campaigns such as mandatory seatbelt use, legislation on driving under the influence of alcohol, and prohibiting smoking in the workplace and indoor public places. Nurses play a major role in advocacy and in motivating clients toward positive health behaviors.

Technology, research, and innovation

Technology, research, and innovation can reduce the demand on services and enhance the capacity of a reduced nursing workforce. For example, technological advances in surgery, such as laparoscopic and minimally invasive surgeries, have made it possible to do major surgical procedures as outpatient day surgery or as inpatient surgery with significantly shorter lengths of stay.

Nurses have a responsibility for creating a positive and productive work environment. Although this is a leadership and management issue, all nurses play a part. Factors related to the nursing shortage play a part in the atmosphere of work environments. Nurses at all levels need to be a part of the solution. Each nurse embodies and reflects the image of nursing and contributes to strategies of collective activism. Nurse leaders and managers allocate scarce resources and manage the shortage. Organizations make strategic decisions about recruitment and retention. The nursing profession has a responsibility for education, collective political action, and influence. Society needs to direct health workforce configuration and funding. Thus at all levels, a nursing shortage is a concern in need of targeted interventions.

Summary

- The nursing shortage is a major national and international phenomenon.
- Nursing shortages have been cyclical over time.
- The current shortage is predicted to continue into the future, partly because of the "graying" of America.
- A nurse shortage is a condition in which demand and supply are not in equilibrium.
- The nursing shortage is complex and the result of multiple factors.
- Demographic factors highlight trends and suggest strategies.
- Supply and demand are major parameters.
- Strategies to confront the nursing shortage include those aimed at education, work environment, and health delivery systems.
- At all levels, nurses need to develop creative responses to a nursing shortage.

Study Questions

1. What creative strategies can the average nurse consider to tackle one or more factors contributing to the nursing shortage?
2. What would make nursing attractive to the next generation of nurses?
3. How can mentorship help alleviate the nursing shortage? Who should do this? How?
4. How and in what ways can the image of nursing be enhanced?
5. How can technology be of use in a nursing shortage?
6. Describe how demand affects the health care delivery system and nursing.
7. Give examples of policies that would address the nursing shortage at the nursing unit level, hospital level, and national level.

8. What research questions would increase our understanding of the causes and effects of nursing staff shortage?

Nurse Manager Rebecca Jones' 80-bed surgical unit has been suffering from a severe nurse shortage. She recognizes the following problems: lack of staff involvement, high turnover rate, high sick time, and low patient satisfaction. Nurse Jones wants the opportunity to work with the staff in developing a vision that will empower the staff and improve staff satisfaction, recruitment and retention, thereby improving patient care and outcomes. She knows she must use both leadership and management skills to accomplish this important goal. First, she begins with a clear articulation of her vision.

Nurse Jones knows she needs to develop strategies that will help her team achieve this vision. The strategies need to be consistent with organizational priorities, which include patient satisfaction, staff satisfaction and empowerment, and improved performance outcomes, such as recruitment and retention, improved patient, and organizational outcomes. Her first strategy is to create a small interdisciplinary team to lead the development and implementation of several specific strategies. The initial step is the identification of program, unit, and staff needs, key issues, and challenges. This is achieved by conducting a survey and focus groups.

Second, she organizes a retreat for teambuilding, discusses the results of the survey and focus groups, and crafts a consensus-based vision and a plan to achieve the vision. Third, she determines a strategy to implement the plan, which includes the development of a shared governance structure that promotes staff participation in decision making.

The governance structure includes three subcommittees reporting to the main unit committee. The three subcommittees are the Quality of Care and Clinical Outcomes Subcommittee; the Healthy Worklife Subcommittee; and the Research, Education, and Innovation Subcommittee. The Quality of Care and Clinical Outcomes Subcommittee's responsibility includes the development, implementation, and evaluation of standards of care, clinical pathways, patient/family satisfaction, and patient/family education. The Healthy Worklife Subcommittee is responsible for the following items: working relationships, clarification of roles, staff satisfaction, equipment, and physical space. The Research, Education, and Innovation Subcommittee leads the planning, implementation, and evaluation of staff education, research and utilization, and innovation. After implementing her grassroots-based interdisciplinary teambuilding strategies, a self-sustaining and effective interdisciplinary team is created. Positive performance outcomes—patient, staff, unit, and organizational—are being achieved through the governance structure and process.

Rebecca Jones is the manager of an 80-bed surgical unit, which is split into two units, one located on the 9th floor of Building A and the other located on the 14th floor of Building B. Nurse Jones started 2 weeks ago. She has noticed that most of the staff are pleasant but quiet. The staff tends to come to her for small things on a regular basis. Although there are numerous hospital committees, there are no committee representatives from this unit. In addition, there are no existing unit-based committees. Nurse Jones is the third manager on this unit in the last 2 years. Her colleagues mention that her unit has had difficulty recruiting and retaining not only managers but staff as well. The unit has a high absenteeism rate and a very high agency nursing usage. These rates suggest that an underlying nurse shortage is occurring. The unit's patient satisfaction scores are the lowest in the hospital.

1. What are the problems that need to be addressed?
2. How will the unit's functioning be improved once the problems are addressed?
3. What strategies need to be implemented to address the problems?
4. To what extent are these strategies consistent with solutions to a nurse shortage?
5. What outcomes should Nurse Jones aim to achieve?

REFERENCES

Aiken, L.H., Clarke, S.P., Sloane, D.M., Sochalski, J., & Silber, J.H. (2002). Hospital nurse staffing and patient mortality, nurse burnout, and job dissatisfaction. *Journal of the American Medical Association, 288*(16), 1987-1993.

American Association of Colleges of Nursing (AACN). (2003). *Faculty shortages in baccalaureate and graduate nursing programs: Scope of the problem and strategies for expanding the supply.* Washington, DC: AACN. Retrieved May 21, 2004, from *www.aacn.nche.edu*

American Hospital Association (AHA). (2002). *In our hands: How hospital leaders can build a thriving workforce.* Chicago: American Hospital Association.

Apker, J., Zabava Ford, W., & Fox, D. (2003). Predicting nurses' organizational and professional identification: The effect of nursing roles, professional autonomy, and supportive communication. *Nursing Economic$, 21*(5): 226-233.

Bakker, B., Killmer, C., Siegriest, J., & Schaufeli, W. (2000). Effort-reward imbalance and burnout between nurses. *Journal of Advanced Nursing, 31,* 884-891.

Bass, B. (1998). *Transformational leadership: Industrial, military, and educational impact.* Mahwah, NJ: Lawrence Erlbaum Associates, Inc.

Blegen, M. (1993). Nurses' job satisfaction: a meta-analysis of related variables. *Nursing Research, 42,* 36-41.

Buerhaus, P.I., Donelan, K., Ulrich, B.T., Norman, L., & Dittus, R. (2005). Is the shortage of hospital registered nurses getting better or worse? Findings from two recent national surveys of RNs. *Nursing Economic$, 23*(2), 61-71, 96.

Buerhaus, P.I., Staiger, D., & Auerbach, D. (2000). Implications of an aging registered nurse workforce. *Journal of the American Medical Association, 283*(22), 2948-2954.

Buerhaus, P., Staiger, D., & Auerbach, D. (2003). Is the current shortage of hospital nurses ending? *Health Affairs, 22*(6), 191-200.

Bureau of Health Professions. (2002). *Authorizing legislation: Nursing workforce development, Public Health Service Act, Title VIII.* Rockville, MD: U.S. Department of Health and Human Services, Health Resources and Services Administration. Retrieved May 21, 2004, from *http://bhpr.hrsa.gov/nursing/about.htm*

Bureau of Labor Statistics. (2004). *U.S. Department of Labor, Occupational Outlook Handbook, Registered Nurses* (2004-2005 ed.). Washington, DC: U.S. Bureau of Labor Statistics. Retrieved May 21, 2004, from *www.bls.gov/oco/ocos083.htm*

Carlson, S.M., Cowart, M.E., & Speaker, D.L. (1992). Perspectives of nursing personnel in the 1980s. In M.E. Cowart, & W.J. Serow (Eds.), *Nurses in the workplace* (pp. 1-27). Newbury Park, CA: Sage.

Chitty, K. (2001). *Professional nursing: Concepts and challenges* (3rd ed.). Philadelphia: Saunders.

Davidson, H., Folcarelli, P., Crawford, S., Duprat, L., & Clifford, J. (1997). The effects of health care reforms on job satisfaction and voluntary turnover among hospital-based nurses. *Medical Care, 35,* 634-645.

Drucker, R. (1999). *Management challenges for the 21st century.* New York: HarperBusiness.

First Consulting Group. (2001). *The healthcare workforce shortage and its implications for America's hospitals.* Long Beach, CA: First Consulting Group. Retrieved January 8, 2005, from *www.aha.org/aha/key_issues/ workforce/resources/Content/FcgWorkforceReport.pdf*

General Accounting Office report (GAO-03-460). (2003). *Hospital emergency departments: Crowded conditions vary among hospitals and communities.* Washington, DC: U.S. General Accounting Office.

Gittell, J. (2001). Supervisory span, relational coordination and flight departure performance: A reassessment of post-bureaucracy theory. *Organization Science, 12,* 468-483.

Grando, V.T. (1998). Making do with fewer nurses in the United States, 1945-1965. *Image, 30*(2), 147-149.

Green, S., Anderson, S., & Shivers, S. (1996). Demographic and organizational influences on leader-member exchange and related work attitudes. *Organizational Behavior and Human Decision Processes, 66,* 203-214.

Hartz, A., Krakauer, H., Kuhn, E., & Young, M. (1989). Hospital characteristics and mortality rates. *New England Journal of Medicine, 321*(25), 1720-1725.

Hattrup, G., & Kleiner, B. (1993). How to establish the proper span of control for managers. *Industrial Management, 35,* 28-30.

Huston, C.J. (2003). Quality health care in an era of limited resources: Challenges and opportunities. *Journal of Nursing Care Quality, 18*(4), 295-302.

International Council of Nurses. (2003). *Global issues in the supply and demand of nurses. SEW news January- March 2003.* Geneva, Switzerland: International Council of Nurses. Retrieved on May 21, 2004, from *www.icn.ch/ sewjan-march03.htm*

Irvine, D., & Evans, M. (1995). Job satisfaction and turnover between nurses: Integrating research findings across studies. *Nursing Research, 44,* 246-253.

Joint Commission on Accreditation of Healthcare Organizations (JCAHO). (2002). *Health care at the crossroads: Strategies for addressing the evolving nursing crisis.* Oakbrook Terrace, IL: JCAHO. Retrieved January 8, 2005, from *www.jcaho.org/about+us/public+policy+ initiatives/health+care+at+the+crossroads.pdf*

King, M.G. (1989). Nursing shortage, circa 1915. *Image, 21*(3), 124-127.

Kovner, C., & Gergen, P.J. (1998). Nurse staffing levels and adverse events following surgery in U.S. hospitals. *Image, 30*(4), 315-321.

Laschinger, H., Finegan, J., & Shamian, J. (2001a). Promoting nurses' health: Effect of empowerment on job strain and work satisfaction. *Nursing Economic$, 19,* 42-52.

Laschinger, H., Shamian, J., & Thomson, D. (2001b). Impact of magnet hospital characteristics on nurses' perceptions of trust burnout quality of care, and work satisfaction. *Nursing Economic$, 19*(5), 209-219.

Larabee, J., Janney, M., Ostrow, C., Withrow, M., Hobbs, G., & Burant, C. (2003). Predicting registered nurse job satisfaction and intent to leave. *Journal of Nursing Administration, 33*(5), 271-283.

Letvak, S. (2002). Retaining the older nurse. *Journal of Nursing Administration, 32,* 387-392.

Leveck, M., & Jones, C. (1996). The nursing practice environment, staff retention, and quality of care. *Research in Nursing & Health, 19,* 331-343.

Loke, J. (2001). Leadership behaviours: Effects on job satisfaction, productivity and organizational commitment. *Journal of Nursing Management, 9,* 191-204.

McCutcheon, A.S. (2004). Relationships between leadership style, span of control and outcomes (Doctoral dissertation, University of Toronto, Canada). *Dissertation Abstracts International, DAI-B65/05,* 2344 (Pub No AAT NQ91797).

McCutcheon, A. (2005). Span of control. In L. McGillis Hall (Ed.), *Quality work environments: For nurse and patient safety* (pp. 93-104). Toronto, Ontario, Canada: Jones & Bartlett Publishers.

Medley, F., & Larochelle, D. (1995). Transformational leadership and job satisfaction. *Nursing Management, 26*(9), 64JJ-LL.

Moos, R. (1994). *Work environment scale manual: A social climate scale: Development, applications, research* (3rd ed.). Palo Alto, CA: Consulting Psychologists Press.

National Center for Health Workforce Analysis. (2002). *Projected supply, demand, and shortages of registered nurses: 2000-2020.* Rockville, MD: U.S. Department of Health and Human Services, Health Resources and Services Administration. Retrieved May 21, 2004, from *www.bhpr.hrsa.gov/healthworkforce/reports/rnproject/ report.htm*

O'Neil, E., & Kimball, B. (2002). *Health care's human crisis: The American nursing shortage.* Princeton, NJ: The Robert Wood Johnson Foundation.

Shader, K., Broome, M., Broome, C., West, M., & Nash, M. (2001). Factors influencing satisfaction and anticipated turnover for nurses in an academic medical center. *Journal of Nursing Administration, 31,* 210-216.

Stordeur, S., Vandenberghe, C., & D'Hoore, W. (2000). Leadership styles across hierarchical levels in nursing departments. *Nursing Research, 49,* 37-43.

Stordeur, S., D'Hoore, W., & Vandenberghe, C. (2001). Leadership, organizational stress, and emotional exhaustion between hospital nursing staff. *Journal of Advanced Nursing, 35,* 533-542.

Tri-Council for Nursing. (2004). *Strategies to reverse the new nursing shortage: A policy statement from tri-council members.* New York: National League for Nursing. Retrieved May 24, 2004, from *www.nln.org/aboutnln/ news_tricouncil2.htm*

Ulrich, B. (2003). The nursing shortage and potential solutions: An overview. *Nephrology Nursing Journal, 30*(4), 364-369.

United States General Accounting Office (GAO). (2002, July). *Nursing workforce. Emerging nurse shortages due to multiple factors.* July 2001:2. GAO-01-944. Washington, DC: GAO. Retrieved May 21, 2004, from *www.aarn. nchc.edu/Media/shortageresource.htm*

Wieck, K. (2003). Faculty for the millennium: Changes needed to attract the emerging workforce into nursing. *Journal of Nursing Education, 42*(4), 151-159.

28

Cultural and Generational Workforce Diversity

G. Rumay Alexander

CHAPTER OBJECTIVES

- Develop an awareness of the full spectrum of cultural diversity issues in the workplace
- Define cultural relativism, cultural competence, corporate culture, and race
- Analyze generational challenges and their impact in the workplace setting
- Recommend strategies to become effective in the workplace
- Evaluate the impact of biases, stereotypes, and prejudices on collegial care provider interactions, particularly nurse to nurse
- Use critical thinking to conceptualize and analyze possible solutions to a practice exercise

Diversity from all fronts has come to have an impact on businesses nationwide. Being in touch with the realities of the changing nature of society is critical not only to surviving but also to thriving in both organizational life and the life of professions vital to society, such as nursing. Managing diversity in the workforce, as in life, is about acknowledging differences instead of ignoring them. The advantages of doing so can bring tremendous yields, such as the following:

- Provide more supportive work environments, maximizing discretionary effort and consequently enhancing performance
- Improve retention of the best people, which directly affects costs of recruitment, selection, training, and start-up, as well as productivity and "brain drain"
- Fortify team effectiveness and take advantage of the wealth of skills available for the organization's maximum impact
- Capitalize on the likelihood that people from nontraditional environments, who often seem to push organizations to out-of-the-box thinking, can help address today's problems
- Capture the interest of more consumers and relate to more customers' needs, thereby increasing market share by means of a workforce that not only reflects the same market composition but also understands what only those who are members of the representative cultures can articulate
- Lay the groundwork and provide the appropriate contexts for future growth in business opportunities at a time when differences in race, culture, language, customs, and styles have become essential considerations

Diversity is a basic component of a strong team. Valuing team members creates synergistic relationships, which translate into a higher quality of production. Ignoring diversity inhibits full participation and may even disrupt the workings of an effective team (Caver & Livers, 2002).

Over the last 30 years, five major socioeconomic developments have helped to define American society and will continue to do so for the foreseeable future: (1) the emergence of a global economy,

(2) **technoshrink**, which is the diffusion of information and telecommunications technology, (3) the maturation of the Baby Boom generation, (4) the continued rise of individualism at the cost of collective responsibility, and (5) the deterioration of principles of economic justice. All of these factors have special implications for the nursing profession.

The world population is expected to double by 2050, with 85% of the increase occurring in developing countries. The mean age of the global population is declining, with 50% of the world's current population younger than 20 years of age. Conversely, industrialized nations are "going gray," with a rising median age and a declining ratio of active workers to retired persons (Kotlikoff & Burns, 2004).

The demographic face of America is changing radically in the areas of age and ethnicity; accompanying these changes is a shift in "who is large and in charge." In less than a century, the United States will move from being "forever young" to "forever old." The largest part of this change will occur in the next 30 years as Baby Boomers retire (Health Resources and Service Administration [HRSA], 2003). Experts expect this change to exact a fiscal toll that will shake the economy. All of the forces capable of enlarging the retired elderly population are in overdrive.

The distribution of the four major U.S. population groups (White, Black, Hispanic, and Asian American/Pacific Islander) is shifting as well. At the turn of the twentieth century, only one in eight Americans was non-White. By 2001, one in four Americans was non-White. This trend, based on data projections, is likely to continue. Latinos account for 12.5% of the population, now surpassing Blacks as the largest ethnic minority in the United States. Growth in the Hispanic population is the major contributor to growth in the minority population. The 2002 U.S. Census allowed for 66 different categories of racial and ethnic combinations. By 2050, an estimated one in three Americans will be Black, Hispanic/Latino, Native American, or Asian/Pacific Islander. The following changes are implications of increasing age and growing ethnicity:

- More chronic illness
- Generational workforce issues
- Language and cultural challenges
- Issues around the use of resources
- Ethical issues

Because ethnic minorities constitute a growing percentage of the working age population, their representation in the professional health workforce will naturally rise. The United States will rely increasingly on ethnic minority caregivers.

With this change come cultural factors that affect every facet of life from the clothes we wear, the food we eat, the art forms and entertainment we prefer, and who marries whom—to issues of education, housing, and census reporting. Also affected are how we think; how we look; our preference for doing things the way we do; and the systems in which we move, live, and experience our being. In an attempt to keep pace, health care institutions have joined with other business, social, educational, and economic endeavors to recognize the importance of workforce diversity. This growing appreciation for the global community not only has raised the awareness of differing values within other cultures, but also has heightened an awareness of differing values in subcultures in the local community. It is no longer acceptable to presume that the current predominant Eurocentric culture in the United States is more right or more appropriate in all situations, nor is it to be expected as the majority view.

The increased emphasis on individualism can be traced to a rise in the standard of living since the 1950s in this country. With this has also come a rise in fragmentation of the family, crumbling of the public school system, and growing mistrust of government, business, and the professions. Over the last 27 years, the distribution of both income and wealth has shifted to the advantage of the affluent. Income for the wealthiest 5% rose 54%, and the top 20% enjoyed a 35% increase; the bottom 20% advanced only 1.5% (Hacker, 1997). This shift gives credence to the statement so often heard these days that this country no longer has a middle class. More and more, people are either in the "haves" or "have nots" category. For those living in poverty, the prospect of escaping it has become an elusive dream. According to *USA Today* (2004), older adults have fared better and children worse during this period. Since the enactment of Medicare in 1965, the distribution of federal health dollars has shifted from a 50-50 balance between adults and children to a 90-10 distribution, favoring seniors.

There is a growing need to approach all relationships, whether with patients or colleagues, with full respect for the many dimensions of culture that, in varying degrees, exert a strong influence on any kind of encounter. Demographic changes mean there will be diverse approaches to work and diverse meaning to the work itself, which may affect who should do what work and why some interventions are done at all. For example, nurses from a socialized medicine system have difficulty seeing health care as a business. Yet the public now clearly demands value, accountability, and customization. Signals ignored, decisions deferred, and changes postponed all have an impact on the future. The aggregate consequences of choices, actions taken, and actions deferred also set a course for the evolving future.

In today's workplace the ability to work with all health care personnel and their patients, including those who speak English as a second language or English as a new language, is a must. In fact, as of 2006, the Joint Commission on Accreditation of Healthcare Organizations' (JCAHO) Information Management Standard requires hospitals to collect information on patients' language and communication needs (JCAHO, 2005). Nurses can ill afford to ignore the fact that the place where health care professionals received their provider education or where they had prior work experiences must also be considered. Nursing education outside of the United States is more focused on clinical skills and less on the psychosocial needs of patients or nursing theory. Such cross-cultural comparative perspectives influence behaviors in the workplace. From this awareness has emerged the understanding that the more each of us knows about these aspects of our patients' and co-workers' culture, the better

able we will be to provide culturally competent care, facilitate meaningful communication between the nurse and the client, engage families in efficacious health practices, and partner with colleagues in our day-to-day work. To understand, respect, and provide the best choices for the multitude of human responses to health and illness or the vicissitudes of life, the nurse must also recognize the multifaceted ways in which culture affects and morphs perspectives and outcomes.

DEFINITIONS

Cultural competency and cultural diversity are not two sides of the same coin, but they are intricately related. Equating diversity with inclusion has inhibited our ability to see it beyond race and gender. **Cultural diversity** refers to the variations among groups of people with respect to the habits, values, preferences, beliefs, taboos, and rules for behavior determined to be appropriate for individual and societal interaction. This refers not only to the idea that persons are unique but also to the notion that organizations are unique and possess a **corporate culture**, which is a way or manner in which business is conducted, often based on written and unwritten rules. Metaphors are often used to capture the nature of such cultures—for instance, a business or place of employment might be referred to as a circus, a minefield, a roller coaster, a puzzle, a rat race, or a zoo. In the context of **culture**, "values and beliefs" encompass what deserves attention, what gets rewarded, what things mean, and which reactions are acceptable in a given situation and which are not. An organization is defined by accountabilities.

There are often disconnections between the values espoused and those that actually guide daily interaction—that is, between the *de jure* and *de facto* cultures. **Diversity**, stripped of its cultural and political baggage, is about differences that make a difference. For example, **people of color** is a positive, politically correct term of inclusivity to describe all non-Whites. A frequent mistake is to give the bulk of attention to race and gender in societal groupings in the definitions used to capture the meaning of

▲ LEADING & MANAGING **DEFINED**

Technoshrink

Diffusion of information and telecommunications technology.

Cultural Diversity

Refers to the variations among groups of people with respect to the habits, values, preferences, beliefs, taboos, and rules for behavior.

Corporate Culture

A way or manner of doing business.

Culture

Beliefs, behaviors, actions, values, communication, perceptions, traditions, and customs common to a population.

Diversity

A broad range of differences.

People of Color

A positive, politically correct term of inclusivity to describe all non-Whites.

Racism

Any type of action or attitude, individual or institutional, which prescribes and legitimizes a minority group's subordination by claiming that the minority is biogenetically or culturally inferior.

Prejudice

An emotional categorical mode of mental functioning involving rigid prejudgment and misjudgment of human acts.

Stereotypes

Fixed and/or distorted views, whether positive or negative, toward all members of a group of people.

Cultural Relativism

Maintaining a sense of objectivity and holding multiple perspectives without judgment.

Bias

A mental preference or inclination.

Cultural Competence

Having the capacity to function effectively as an individual and an organization within the context of the cultural beliefs, behaviors, and needs presented by consumers and their communities.

Ethnicity

Shared origins and shared culture.

Health Disparity

Population-specific difference in the presence of disease, health outcomes, or access to care.

---

inclusivity while giving only minor, if not negligible, attention to the other dimensions. Race is not biological. It is a political construct, and to that extent, it is a latent force of our existence, both visible and invisible, to be considered when issues of diversity are at hand. Racism and its related elements of biases, stereotypes, and prejudices need to be understood as well. **Racism** is discrimination based on race or color. It is often accompanied by inferences of inferiority or subhumanism. It affects factors that in turn affect outcomes (IOM, 2003) (Figure 28.1).

Prejudice is an emotional categorical mode of mental functioning involving rigid prejudgment

(stereotypes) and misjudgment of human acts. Prejudices bring a mixture of exploitative gains such as economic advantage, social snobbery, or a feeling of superiority. The building blocks of prejudice are generalizations or preconceived notions about a group of people. They can be negative or positive, but seldom are they neutral. They provide a rationale for putting people in boxes, which keeps the real person from being seen and known. **Stereotypes** are fixed and/or distorted views, whether positive or negative, toward all members of a group of people. Stereotypes that are a part of society encircle and cloud view points and perceptions,

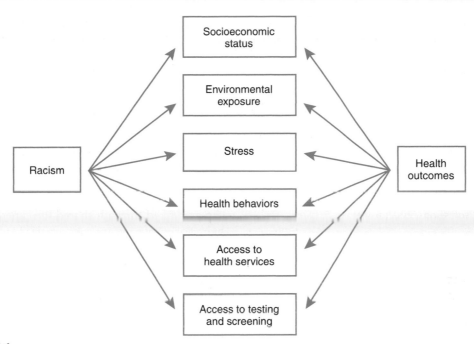

Figure 28.1
Racism as a precursor model. (From Institute of Medicine [IOM]. (2003). *Unequal treatment: Confronting racial and ethnic disparities in health care.* Washington, DC: National Academies. Retrieved May 14, 2004, from *www.nap.edu/books/030908265X/html/*)

even though an individual may actively disagree or not consciously hold that stereotype.

The concept of **cultural relativism** requires that individuals not judge but rather that they consider the actions, beliefs, or traits within their own cultural contexts in order to better understand them. It involves maintaining a sense of objectivity and an appreciation for the values of other cultures, not judging whether they are "good" or "bad" by external standards (Loustaunau & Sobo, 1997). Emotions have a way of manifesting themselves, and when the emotion is prejudice, the resulting manifestation is a **bias** or preference. Mix a strong preference or emotion with power and the means by which to use it, and the stage is set for resultant acts such as disparity in health care outcomes due to a provider's views being influenced by his or her culture.

Providing care effectively to persons from a multiplicity of cultures is called *cultural competence*. **Cultural competence** includes recognizing the importance of integrating persons who are nondominant to the culture and the consideration of their values in the process of organizational operations. There are many definitions for cultural competence, but transcending those definitions is the sense of a dynamic, evolving process. The Federal Civil Rights legislation and the 2001 National Standards for Culturally and Linguistically Appropriate Services (CLAS) in Health Care (Betancourt et al., 2002; Office of Minority Health, 2001) use an expanded definition of cultural competency:

Cultural and linguistic competence is a set of congruent behaviors, attitudes, and policies that come together in a system, agency, or among professionals that enable effective work in cross-cultural situations. Culture refers to integrated patterns of human behavior that include the language, thoughts, communications, actions, customs, beliefs, values, and institutions of racial, ethnic, religious, or social groups. (Center for the Health Professions, 2002, p. 49)

Ethnicity is tied to notions of shared origins and shared culture. It should be acknowledged that cultural identities are simultaneously inclusive and exclusive. At times this works as an advantage on which to capitalize; at other times it is a disadvantage with challenges requiring attention.

Competence implies having the capacity to function effectively as an individual and an organization within the context of the cultural beliefs, behaviors, and needs presented by consumers and their communities. (Center for the Health Professions, 2002, p. 49)

BACKGROUND

What difference does difference make? Apparently a great deal, particularly in the workplace. Differences in time orientation, communication patterns, value systems, perceptions of staff responsibilities or nursing roles—along with differences in educational preparation—are common sources of conflict. Disagreements such as conflict between two or more parties can also occur when the parties perceive the same event differently based on differences not only in race, ethnicity, gender, or sexual orientation but also in the generations in which the parties were born and the subsequent attitudes, beliefs, values, or needs that are exhibited. It has been estimated that supervisors spend as much as 29% of their time resolving employee personality clashes and

relationships issues. Eighty-five percent of the people fired in 2003 were fired because of relationship problems (The Murphy Leadership Institute, 2004). Those who are different are often seen or labeled as the problem.

Generational Workforce Diversity

A growing issue in nursing leadership and management is the problem of generational workforce diversity. Sociologists categorize generational groups into what they call *cohorts* (Alexander, 2001). These cohorts are members of a generation who are linked through shared life experiences in their formative years. As each new cohort matures, it is influenced by what sociologists call *generational markers*. Individuals are all products of their environment. Generational markers are events that have an impact on all members of the generation in one way or another. Thus, being aware of generational differences is essential for every organization's leadership in managing a multi-age workforce. Each generation possesses unique characteristics and often deems the values and behaviors of another as character flaws instead of cultural differences (Table 28.1).

The Baby Boomers, born between 1946 and 1964, have entered the leadership chairs of many executive suites, including those in health care organizations. Boomers present a striking contrast and replace members of the previous generation, those born between 1925 and 1945, often referred to as the Mature Generation or the

Table 28.1

Generational Characteristics			
Matures	*Baby Boomers*	*Generation X*	*Millennials*
Hard work	Personal fulfillment	Uncertainty	What's next?
Duty	Optimism	Personal focus	On my terms
Sacrifice	Crusading causes	Live for today	Just show up
Thriftiness	Buy now/pay later	Save, save, save	Earn to spend
Work fast	Work efficiently	Eliminate the task	Do exactly what's asked

Source: Center for Generational Studies, Aurora, CO.

Silent Generation. Members of the Silent Generation grew up in a period of strong military and political leaders, a time when respect for authority was expected, conformity was the characteristic most treasured and exhibited, and children were to be seen but not heard.

Boomers, historically the second largest generation in the workforce, have dominated U.S. society for many years. Beginning in January of 1996 and continuing for the next 18 years, a Baby Boomer will turn 50 every 18 seconds, and their preferences in every facet of American life are affected by their sheer numbers alone (U.S. Census Bureau, 1996). Efficiency, teamwork, quality, and service have thrived under their leadership. Boomers grew up in a period of unprecedented economic growth during which the United States had virtually no strong economic competitors. They grew up thinking they were special and that they could ignore or break rules and still be successful. They love convenience and brought true meaning to "charge it" when it comes to debt management. Financial security will remain a central issue for many. Consequently, many Boomers will work past the age of retirement. They have questioned traditional authority structures, blurred gender roles, and made vigorous attempts to push systems towards their ideas of perfection. During the Vietnam War, the Civil Rights confrontations, and Watergate, Baby Boomers saw clearly the vulnerability of authority; and they have been reluctant to accept formal authority since. Their preference is for a more participative and less authoritarian workplace.

Support for such a workplace environment comes also from members of Generation X, born between 1965 and 1980, who share with Boomers an aversion to authority, but with a decided preference for a balanced life. X'ers are the first generation of latchkey kids; as such, they found the need to be resourceful at an early age. Their childhood years have been marked with economic uncertainty, and thus they are skeptical of traditional practices and beliefs. In their view, employment contracts are agreements that either side can cancel at will, which means that placing their future in the hands of employers makes them extremely uneasy and is thus highly unlikely. The length of time spent with an organization is less relevant to X'ers than how to protect themselves from the capriciousness of business challenges (Wendover, 2002). Trust imposes its own constraints and has its own rules.

Both the youngest group in the workplace and the largest group in U.S. history are the Millennial workers, those born between 1981 and 1999. This group is known by several other monikers, including *Generation* Y, *Generation Why?, Nexters,* and the *Internet Generation.* The common marker of their developmental years is technology. This group is the most demographically diverse generation in this country's history. These workers have astonishing multitasking skills. They also tend to have a positive outlook and a desire to improve the world.

Many believe that Millennials are shallow on basic skills; but, because they grew up with computers, they can create solutions that other generations could not have imagined. Technology guides their every move. They are problem solvers who grew up in a flourishing economy. Millennials matured in a world where short cuts, manipulation of rules, and situational ethics seem to have reigned. They got the message somehow that the final word is not the final word. They do not live to work; they work to live. Thus they have a different set of expectations about the world of work. Most enjoy the liberty of working on their own in a style that favors their work ethic. Millennials have learned that their presence is in demand. To thrive, they need clear definitions of outcomes, resources to do what needs to be done, and a deadline.

Nurses recognize that cultural diversity, awareness, and unconditional positive regard for people are critical core concepts (Habayeb, 1995). Yet somehow cultural diversity is not seen as a powerful variable in how nurses communicate and interpret behaviors or mediate conflict between themselves or patients. There can be a direct impact on how problems, assessments, diagnoses, and intervention strategies are determined. As global trends in mobility, migration, cultural identity importance, and changing roles increase, there is a greater need for awareness (Leininger, 1997). Shifts in the site of care to the community, a rise in moral/ethical issues in health care, and a desire by many, but not all, consumers to control and regulate their own health care—along with a concomitant desire to make it better for others—have created a necessity to know and respect diverse perspectives (Galanti, 1999; Gazmararian et al., 1999).

Awareness of Differences

The meltdown of the "melting pot" resulting from waves of immigration, the inability of the workforce to keep pace with the demands for health care providers, and the subsequent recruitment of foreign nurses from Great Britain, Ireland, Canada, and the Philippines has had the unintended consequence of thrusting cultural diversity onto agendas that had resisted addressing the issue in spite of the fact that U.S. society has historically been characterized by its pluralism. However, the predominant Eurocentric White majority has not come to view all persons, including themselves, as having a valuable cultural heritage. Cultural diversity in many places in health care is being intentionally ignored or benignly neglected or receiving rhetorical lip service.

Without a sense of cultural competence, U.S. health care providers tend to force on people of other cultures the Eurocentric concepts of work rules of engagement, empowerment, and decision making. For example, a staff meeting designed to plan for the future could be seen as a waste of time by those who, because of their generational influence or the locus of control dictated by their cultures, wish to spend company time working on issues and problems of the present. Assumptions about U.S. health care abound for those operating and navigating the health care system—whether they fit their culture or not. Some of these assumptions are as follows:

- Self-determination, autonomy, independence
- Right to know
- "I" make the decisions about my health care

- Moral obligations and medical ethics based on Judeo-Christian beliefs
- Health care providers have the "obligation to tell the truth"
- Duty to give all information to the competent patient (individual) or his or her surrogate
- The institution's written bill of rights for patients and staff are defined as individual rights rather than inclusive of other ways of viewing individuals within a group context
- Informed consent does not include family unless the individual is legally unable to make his or her own decision. In this situation, the individual chooses a family member or someone else or a legal protocol to procure a surrogate to make those decisions (Crow et al., 2000).

These assumptions configure into the health care context, which is always dynamic. The context dictates "where one is coming from" and how information or knowledge is communicated in human transactions or relationships, and it is culturally based. From a global perspective, the cultural context of the Western world is "low context." In low context cultures, the explicit verbal or written message carries the meaning. Low context cultures require extensive detailed explanations and information because they are making up for what is missing in a situation. In high context cultures, often found in the non-Western world, that which is written or stated rarely carries the meaning. The meaning of the message is understood by reading between the lines for what is not written or stated. In high context cultures most of the meaning is assumed to exist by the nature of the situation (i.e., the context). Most nuclear families are high context, relying on high interpersonal interaction and subtle messages. Placing someone from a high context culture in a work place setting dominated by individuals in leadership positions from a low context culture who have the power to define the rules of work and to determine what will be rewarded, who gets promoted, what benefits will be offered, and what values will be define the organization increases the likelihood of perceptions of inequity and workplace conflicts (Hall & Hall, 1990).

Table **28.2**

Low- and High-Context Cultural Differences		
	Low-Context	High-Context
Countries/Regions	United States, Canada, England, Russia, Northwestern Europe	China, Japan, Arabia, Mexico, South America, Pacific Islands
Characteristics	Very verbal	Less verbal or nonverbal
	Individual	Group
	Equality	Individual dignity
	Democracy	Consensus
	Personal freedom	Obligation to others
	Fairness	Fate (karma, joss)
	Achievement	Process/role
	Innovation	Continuous improvement
	Entrepreneurship	Communal
	Competition	Cooperation

Table 28.2 displays countries by low- and high-context characteristics.

Cultural competence, to be properly understood, should be viewed as a process or a journey rather than a destination. It involves an ongoing expansion and updating of an individual's understanding of different cultures. However, it is equally important to remember that culture shapes behavior but does not predict it. A person's identification with a culture does not necessarily mean that that person agrees with all the dominant beliefs in that culture. In fact, cultural diversity involves differences not only between cultures but also within cultures.

Nurses also need to recognize their own cultural values in seeking cultural competence. The expectations, attitudes, and behaviors of nurses are affected by their cultures just as surely as the expectations, attitudes, and behaviors of clients are influenced by theirs. This can be a barrier to gaining cultural competence if the nurse does not exhibit self-awareness and sensitivity to others. In addition, nurses need to examine the culture of nursing itself for opportunities to increase cultural competence and diversity. For example, nursing in the United States has

been overwhelmingly composed of White females.

On the journey toward cultural competence there are road signs that can help define the way. Some are basic common sense, such as stopping to think about others. Others require specific knowledge of the individual with whom you are interacting.

STRATEGIES FOR CULTURAL COMPETENCE

Cultural differences in ways of doing things are learned and transmitted via cultural environments. Because cultural differences are learned, cultural sensitivity and competence, regardless of the setting, also can be learned. A few suggestions are as follows:

- Know your own culture, values, and biases.
- Listen and observe.
- Emphasize the corporate values up front.
- Develop the ability to be a teacher and a learner at the same time.
- Hold up your end of the bargain. Follow through with commitments.
- Give extremely clear directions, provide support and resources, and always give a deadline of completion for projects.

- Delegate the outcomes instead of the individual tasks.
- Give the big picture. Give examples of how to make tenure and success work in a win-win situation for all involved.
- Consider the rules and procedures you implement within the workplace. Be sure they are clear but expect them to be interpreted in ways you had not anticipated.
- Manage your expectations. Be open to ideas and comments.
- Provide straightforward steps for decision making.
- Be courageous, and correct behavior. Take action, document, and follow through.
- Manage according to values and attitudes of the individual's generation.
- Provide the opportunity to grow.

HEALTH DISPARITIES

Germane to this discussion is a connecting of the dots about how the health care system cares for ethnic minority patients and the subtle messages that ethnic minority nurses and other providers receive about how the system does not welcome or respect them. Over the past several decades there have been enormous advances and improvements in health care. No one has benefited more from those advances than Americans. Unfortunately, though, all Americans have not benefited equally (Garcia, 2003).

According to the Institute of Medicine (IOM, 2003) and other recent national health studies, ethnic and racial minorities have not shared the same positive health outcomes as the majority population (Washington, 2003). Demographic changes have also revealed that, in the land that espouses "all men are created equal," all are not equal. There is evidence of racial and ethnic disparities in the one arena that should be a safe haven for all people. Phrases such as "disproportionate burden," "prevalence rates," and "access to quality care" are becoming increasingly familiar as people seek to understand the relationship between being a minority or "other," suffering

from chronic illness, and dying young. Evidence suggests there is a correlation.

The National Institutes of Health described **health disparities** as "differences in the incidence, prevalence, mortality, and burden of diseases and other adverse health conditions that exist among specific populations in the United States" (Washington, 2003, p. 1). According to the Health Resources and Services Administration, "Health disparity is a population-specific difference in the presence of disease, health outcomes or access to care" (Washington, 2003, p. 11). The Center on Health Disparities Research at Johns Hopkins University School of Nursing defined health disparities as "differences in access to care, processes of care, or health outcomes" (Washington, 2003, p. 11). They described underserved populations as those "who have less access to care even though care may be available; those who receive less or different care than the majority of the general population; or those for whom traditional models of care are inappropriate for cultural or other reasons" (Washington, 2003, p. 11). The IOM published a report entitled *Unequal Treatment: Confronting Racial and Ethnic Disparities in Health Care* (IOM, 2003). This report suggested that racial and ethnic disparities are caused by both patient-related and system-related factors, as follows:

Patient-Related Factors
- *Socioeconomic differences:* patient income and education
- *Health-education differences:* patient knowledge of health symptoms, conditions, and possible treatments
- *Health-behavior differences:* patient willingness and ability to seek care, adhere to treatment protocols, trust and work with health care providers

System-Related Factors
- *Discrimination:* health care system and provider bias and stereotyping
- *Language differences:* health care provider's inability to communicate sufficiently with patients and families, taking into account the estimated 329 different languages that are spoken in the United States daily

- *Workforce diversity differences:* poor racial and ethnic match of health care professionals and the patients they serve
- *Cultural competence differences:* insufficient knowledge of and sensitivity to cultural differences
- *Payment/reimbursement differences:* insufficient reimbursement for treating Medicare, Medicaid, and uninsured patients
- *Insurance coverage differences:* inadequate coverage of services provided to certain patients, especially those individually insured and uninsured
- *Data deficiencies:* insufficient information on patients and health by race, ethnicity, and geographic area

The complexities of this issue are becoming abundantly clear. Health disparities are a legislative issue, a social issue, a care-delivery issue, a patient-driven issue, a health care systems issue, and a care provider's issue, particularly for those of the nonmajority.

One of the essential qualities of the clinician is interest in humanity, for the secret of the care of the patient is in caring for the patient.

Dr. Francis Peabody (1926)

Addressing health disparities is integral to the practice of nurses as they strive to work together for the benefit of patients and their families. Having access to medical services is an obvious contributor to good health and to the ability of everyone to reach his or her ultimate potential.

Unequal treatment also extends into the educational system and impacts on future nurse supply issues. Recruitment into nursing is often built on a strong background in science, and increasing minority recruitment will be aided by minorities having access to preparation in the sciences. Science, as its own culture, has traditionally been targeted at the privileged student and used as a portal for advanced study, as well as mental training for increasing processing skills and abstract levels of thinking. If non-privileged students are not prepared in science, math, and other skills

that equip them for college, the disparities in the workplace will continue to exist. The issue of minority performance in science is a preparation problem, not an achievement problem. *Science Highlights 2000,* published by the National Assessment of Educational Progress (NAEP) (Dantley, 2004), provides a current picture of student performance in science by racial/ethnic subgroups. According to this report, science performance at the national level is disaggregated into three content areas—earth science, life science, and physical science for grades 4, 8, and 12—and based on three ability levels: low, middle, and high performance. Upon examination of the most recent high school NAEP data, all percentile scores are declining for each ability level, with the middle, or 50th, percentile decreasing the most. Accordingly, Black high school students performed the lowest in each science area.

Optimal health requires a safe community, a safe home, adequate food and clothing, and access to quality education. Policy decisions at the federal and state levels play a great role in the optimal health equation. Politics determine which schools are funded and which are underfunded, which nurses to hire and which dedicated professionals to ignore. Legislators decide how much money to commit to state universities, thus implicitly deciding who can attend based on tuition rates and other constraints. The terms and conditions of education, affirmative action, rising tuition costs, the lack of financial aid and other issues need focused attention. The best social program is a quality education for all.

Although the majority of poor people in the United States are White, both people of color and recent immigrants are disproportionately represented and therefore more likely to rely on public benefit programs to meet their basic needs. When these programs originated, they categorized people as "worthy" and "unworthy." That system continues today. As a society we tend to distrust the poor and blame them for their poverty, ignoring potentially significant factors such as race, language, or disability. An individual's social status almost always hinges on his or her socioeconomic status.

Public health experts estimate that roughly 50% of a person's health status depends on lifestyle and health behaviors. The environment is responsible for another 30% and genetics for about 20% (Kent, 2000).

The treatment of immigrants is another example of how we as a society contribute to unfair access to assistance. According to Massachusetts General Hospital (Forman, 2003), the Welfare Reform Law of 1996 created two groups of legal immigrants: *qualified* and *unqualified* (also called *special status*). Many state budgets eliminated insurance for special status aliens (who, by the way, pay taxes). This includes immigrants fleeing persecution with pending applications for asylum, immigrants with permission to live in the United States because conditions in their home countries are unsafe, and certain permanent legal residents who are not eligible for federal benefits for 5 years from their date of entry.

Historically, there have been caps placed on the number of entrants allowed from some countries and preferential treatment extended to others, based to some extent on race. Individuals who reside in this country illegally, or as "undocumented" immigrants, are eligible for very little public assistance, such as emergency medical care. They are not eligible for cash assistance.

Unfortunately, the impact of our failure as a society to fully address these issues falls dispro-portionately on communities of color, as do the expectations placed on them to advocate for the rights of the underprivileged. Clearly, improving the health status of ethnic minorities benefits the health of the entire nation and must be vigorously addressed by all. Unless the courage is summoned to put professional core values into practice, an aura of hypocrisy surrounds the discussion of valuing differences, which may be seen as simply talk and no action.

Issues of race, ethnicity, and health disparity help to highlight the fact that nurses need to continue to hone their skills in cultural and linguistic sensitivity and competence as an essential part of practice. Each nurse lives and works within a meld of cultural aspects and values. This includes influences from race, community, ethnicity, lifestyle, professional, and organizational cultures. The nursing leadership and management challenge is to effectively manage diversity.

LEADERSHIP AND MANAGEMENT IMPLICATIONS

Differences per se do not create tensions in the workplace; the judgments people make about one another do. The goal of leadership is to get divergent points of view working for the common good with the outcome being success in accomplishing what needs to be done (Alexander, 2002).

⚠ LEADERSHIP & MANAGEMENT **BEHAVIORS**

Leadership Behaviors

- Envisions holistic care, including cultural competence
- Influences others to be culturally sensitive
- Inspires trust and confidence among culturally diverse people
- Leads others toward cultural competence

Management Behaviors

- Coordinates care to include cultural assessment and planning

- Integrates cultural diversity into the workplace
- Plans cultural sensitivity training
- Organizes teams that include culturally diverse workers

Overlap Areas

- Plans for cultural diversity issues
- Motivates others toward culturally competent communication

It would behoove leaders to consider the knowledge about generations and cultural parameters when putting people together to accomplish the goals of the organization and when choosing communications, messages, and the best modality to fit the recipient.

Data suggest that it will be many years before the profiles of health professionals reflect the population as a whole (HRSA, 2002). This underscores the need for all health care providers in a given community to be culturally competent. Advocates for increased ethnic minority representation in the health workforce argue that increasing the number of ethnic minority providers will improve access to care for ethnic minorities and other vulnerable, underserved populations (AHA, 2002). In fact, these advocates argue that increased representation of minorities in the health workforce not only will increase equity, but also will improve the efficiency of the health care delivery system. The synergy of diverse viewpoints can improve nursing's knowledge base and care strategies. The same issues of communication, interpersonal space, social proscriptions, time sense, and other variations in beliefs and behaviors need to be balanced and smoothed in work groups and teams. The nurse care manager can employ cultural competence principles in leading and managing work groups (Davidhizer et al., 1998).

A related issue is the recruitment of foreign-born registered nurses into the United States to alleviate the current nurse shortage. Although this strategy may be part of the solution to the U.S. shortage, it has ethical ramifications. Given a global shortage of RNs, is this practice ethical? What preparations are made to increase cultural sensitivity once foreign-born RNs arrive?

Estimates from the 2000 Sample Survey of Registered Nurses (HRSA, 2001) indicated that approximately 86.6% of RNs were non-Hispanic White, 4.9% were non-Hispanic Black, 3.5% were Asian; 2% were Hispanic; 0.5% were American Indian or Alaskan Native, 0.2% were Native Hawaiian or Pacific Islander, and 1.2% were of two or more racial backgrounds. These statistics point to the need for nursing to fuel strong cultural competence initiatives. The focus needs to be both on culturally competent client care practices and on a culturally competent workplace environment. Lack of understanding of cultural practices may result in longer hospital stays, noncompliance issues, loss of meaningful nurse-client or provider-to-provider communication, more readmissions to health care facilities, and more ER visits (AHA, 2003).

Learning and showing respect for differences, exploring beyond the comfort zone, withholding judgment of others, emphasizing the positive, and practicing good communication techniques are strategies for success (Grossman & Taylor, 1995). Leaders are urged to develop a human resources strategic plan that outlines how the organization will recruit and retain a diverse staff that reflects the community. A great deal of time and concern is being focused on the supply of workers in the future. A favored formula is known as "$\frac{1}{2} \times 2 \times 3$"— meaning half as many people working twice as hard and paid on average twice as well, yet producing three times as much. This formula makes it poignantly clear that understanding our workforce is not only wise but urgent. Cultural competency standards should be incorporated into all aspects of the institutional strategic plan for such areas as patient care, patient education, staff training, and community outreach. The sharing of data and the provision of cultural competency education is needed at board or trustee level to inform and enlighten those who are making major institutional decisions.

Managers are challenged to examine policies and practices in every phase of the organization within the context of generational differences. Recruiting techniques, communications, human resource policies, and benefit plans must be tailored to these varying groups (who have varying needs) and the values they embrace. In a global economy, the workforce continues to change, challenging generational and racial/ethnic stereotypes. A word is caution is worth noting. Diverse populations do not fall into the same categories as their American counterparts of the same age: "They are more apt to focus on survival" (Alexander, 2001, p. 3).

Research Note

Source: American College of Healthcare Executives (ACHE). (2003). A race/ethnic comparison of career attainments in health care management: 2002. Chicago: ACHE. Retrieved June 10, 2004, from *www.ache.org/pubs/research/research.cfm*

Purpose

The purpose of this cross-sectional study of White, Black, Asian, and Hispanic health care executives was to determine whether race/ethnic disparities in health care management careers still exist and whether they have narrowed since 1997.

Discussion

A 1992 joint study by the American College of Health care Executives, an international professional society of health care executives, and the National Association of Health Services Executives, whose membership is predominantly Black, compared the career attainments of their members. The study found that, although Blacks and Whites had similar educational backgrounds and years of experience in the field, Blacks held fewer top management positions, less often worked in hospitals, earned 13% less, and were less satisfied in their jobs.

In 1997, the study was replicated and included White, Black, Asian, and Hispanic health care executives. That research showed that disparities in the proportions of top-level management positions continued to exist between White women and minority women but that there were no significant differences in the proportion of top positions held by male managers in the various race/ethnic groups. Other measures of career attainment continued to show disparities between Whites and minorities: Whites were more often employed in hospitals and, in general, expressed higher levels of satisfaction with various aspects of their jobs. While the earnings gap grew between White and Black women, it narrowed between White and Black men. Other minority executives' earnings fell between the White and Black averages.

The findings of the third study show that minorities continue to lag behind Whites in several areas, including job satisfaction, winning senior-level jobs, and median total compensation.

Application to Practice

Although the field has made progress in promoting racial and gender diversity in health care management during the past 30 years, evidence shows there is still a long way to go.

Suggested recommendations, which hopefully are important steps toward leveling the playing field, were as follows:
- Establish flexible hiring criteria that allow for judgment relative to talent and potential and avoid limiting positions to those with precise prior experience.
- Identify internal candidates of color who exhibit leadership attributes to assume senior-level executive positions. Through such systematic succession planning, organizations will develop a diverse talent pool to draw from as senior leadership positions become available.
- Promote executives of color to senior-level positions, especially in organizations serving predominantly minority communities.
- Urge senior executives to speak out and advocate for diversity in the organization's leadership team.
- Encourage senior managers to promote managers of color by following guidelines for succession if these have been established; conducting candid, periodic evaluations of such managers; and providing counselors to help bridge cultural differences between minorities and whites on the management team.

The basis for enhancing the work environment for all comes down to trust, respect, shared goals, affirmation of identity, and communications. It is all about relationships. With an increasingly diverse workforce, managers of every age are encouraged to emphasize the values of the organization before their personal values.

CURRENT ISSUES AND TRENDS

There is an old saying: Sticks and stones may break my bones, but words will never hurt me. How easy life would be if only that were true. Race would certainly be a different issue today. Discrimination on every level is still around. Given the proclivity of humans to focus on the physical—those aspects that our eyes tell us are different—and given the fact that people cannot disguise certain features, the dynamics of race continue to this day to be fundamental to the understanding of the existence of health care disparities. Race affects the working relationship issues of an inclusive workforce.

The following excerpt, "10 Things Everyone Should Know about Race," was developed to accompany a three-part PBS series titled *RACE—The Power of an Illusion*. This piece outlines the current thinking that nudges us to question our notions of race.

Our eyes tell us that people look different. No one has trouble distinguishing a Czech from a Chinese. But what do those differences mean? Are they biological? Has race always been with us? How does race affect people today?

There's less—and more—to race than meets the eye:

1. **Race is a modern idea.** Ancient societies, like the Greeks, did not divide people according to physical distinctions, but according to religion, status, gender, class, even language. The English language did not even have the word 'race' until it turned up in 1508 in a poem by William Dunbar referring to a line of kings.

2. **Race has no genetic basis.** Not one characteristic, trait or even one gene distinguishes all the members of one so-called race from all the members of another so-called race.

3. **Human subspecies don't exist.** Unlike many animals, modern humans simply have not been around long enough or isolated enough to evolve into separate subspecies or races. Despite surface appearances, we are among the most similar of all species.

4. **Skin color really is only skin deep.** Most traits are inherited independently from one from another. The genes influencing skin color have nothing to do with the genes influencing hair form, height, blood type, musical talent, athletic ability or forms of intelligence. Knowing one trait, like skin color, does not necessarily tell you anything else about him or her.

5. **Most variation is within, not between, "races."** Of the small amount of total human variation, 85% exists within any local population, be they Italians, Kurds, Koreans or Cherokees. About 94% can be found within any continent. That means two random Koreans may be as genetically different as a Korean and an Italian.

6. **Slavery predates race.** Throughout much of human history, societies have enslaved others, often as a result of conquest or war, even debt, but not because of physical characteristics or a belief in natural inferiority. Due to a unique set of historical circumstances, ours was the first slave system where all the slaves shared similar physical characteristics.

7. **Race and freedom evolved together.** The U. S. was founded on the radical new principle that "All men are created equal." But our early economy was based largely on slavery. How could this anomaly be rationalized? The new idea of race helped explain why some people could be denied the rights and freedoms that others took for granted.

8. **Race justified social inequalities as natural.** As the race idea evolved, white superiority became "common sense" in white America. It rationalized not only slavery but also the extermination of Indians, exclusion of Asian immigrants, and the taking of Mexican lands by a nation that otherwise professed a deep belief in liberty and equality. Racial practices became institutionalized within American government, laws, and society.

9. **Race is not biological, but racism is still real.** Race is a powerful social idea that gives people different access to opportunities and resources. Our government and social institutions disproportionately, albeit often invisibly, channel wealth, power, and resources to the "unmarked" race—white people. This affects everyone, whether we are aware of it or not.

10. **Colorblindness will not end racism.** Pretending race does not exist is not the same as creating equality. Race is more than stereotypes and individual prejudice. To combat racism, we need to identify and remedy social policies and institutional practices that advantage some groups at the expense of others (California Newsreel, 2003, p. 1).*

Culture is a kind of knowledge that all of us in society use and act on and provides a basis for self-evaluation of our "learned humanity." Nurses have an obligation to fulfill their social contracts with society and, above all, to do no harm to those in their care. This means nurses must be prepared to the best of their ability to care for all those in their communities of practice and to work effectively with providers from other cultures and subcultures. Nursing school curricula and continuing education offerings need to be revised in order for this to occur (Campinha-Bacote et al., 1996).

*RACE—*The Power of an Illusion* was produced by California Newsreel in association with the Independent Television Service (ITVS). Major funding was provided by The Ford Foundation and the Corporation for Public Broadcasting Diversity Fund. It is available on videocassette and DVD from California Newsreel (www.newsreel.org).

The nursing profession is projected to be one of the largest job growth areas among professions in the United States. New nursing career opportunities, along with replacement needs as projected retirements occur, provide a significant opportunity to assist the nation's health care systems to respond to these changes and proactively extinguish health care disparities wherever they exist by increasing the presence of persons who can bring with them an understanding of the values of other cultures, an increase in diversity and perspectives, and the ability to implement care that reflects such understanding.

Summary

- Managing diversity is about acknowledging differences.
- Factors of a global economy, diffusion of information, generational issues, the rise of individualism, and the deterioration of economic justice all affect nursing and society.
- The distribution of major U.S. population groups is shifting.
- Cultural diversity refers to variations among groups of people with respect to habits, values, preferences, beliefs, taboos, and rules for behavior.
- Racism is related to biases, stereotypes, and prejudices.
- Cultural relativism requires that individuals consider their own cultural contexts.
- Cultural and linguistic competence is a set of congruent behaviors, attitudes, and policies that enable effective working together.
- Generational cohorts exist and may clash in the workplace.
- Immigration has resulted in cultural diversity.
- U.S. health care providers need to explore the differences between high and low content cultures.
- Health disparities describe differences in the burden of disease and other adverse health conditions that exist among specific populations.
- Racial and ethnic disparities arise from patient-related and system-related factors.

- The nursing workforce does not match the profile of the population in terms of diversity.
- Nurses and nursing leaders need to manage diversity effectively.

Study Questions

1. Why is cultural competence important for nursing?
2. What are the components of cultural awareness?
3. How does the nurse apply cultural competence in the workplace?
4. Where do ideas about race come from? What are the sources of your information?

CASE STUDY

Case 1

"I have had it with the 27-year-old twit I now work for," Charlie said to his wife. "I walked into her office today to discuss the system analysis she wanted me to do, but she had that tribal music going and I couldn't understand half of what she was saying. When I asked her to turn it off, she did. But she looked at me like I was senile. I was working for this company when she was in diapers.

Then there's that tongue stud in her mouth. How can you talk when that thing's banging around on your teeth? She may be a bright kid, but she doesn't have a clue how to work with us."

Questions

1. What can Charlie do to foster his relationship with his supervisor?
2. What parameters would you set around his supervisor's management style?
3. Now reverse the situation. How do you think the 27-year-old supervisor views the aging Boomer Charlie? What parameters would you set around Charlie's interpersonal interactions at work?

CRITICAL THINKING EXERCISE

RELIGIOUS/CULTURAL PROHIBITIONS

Example 1

A female college student from another country sought health care for menstrual pain after arriving in the United States. She went to a physician to obtain a prescription for medication to ease the pain. The physician decided that the woman should have a Pap smear. Being unmarried, the patient could not agree to this for religious prohibition reasons. She tried to explain the situation to both the doctor and the nurse, but neither realized the cultural/religious issue nor seemed to understand the patient's inability to comply. The nurse told the woman, "Whatever your reasons are, you should have the Pap smear first as a diagnostic procedure." The woman refused, left the clinic, and did not return.

Example 2

Ramadan is the holy month of fasting and prayer in the Muslim religious tradition. During Ramadan, Muslims refrain from food and drink from early morning until early evening. Although pregnant women, children under the age of 14, and those who are ill are exempt from the fast, many Muslims will not take medications during the hours when they are fasting. Muslim patients who normally take medication, such as those with diabetes, can benefit from guidance that would help them alter their medication schedules in keeping with their fast.

Questions

1. What is the problem in each example?
2. Whose problem is it?
3. What should the nurse do in each case?
4. How can the nurse be culturally competent in each case?

Case 2

In a disagreement between two employees, one Black and the other a Filipina, a few heated words were exchanged. Wanting to avoid an escalation of the conflict, the Filipina employee walked away. The Black employee, on the other hand, valuing direct confrontation of conflict and wanting to settle the problem, followed her coworker, trying to talk to her. This only caused more anxiety and panic for the Filipina woman, who had been taught to value harmony and smooth interpersonal relationships. Thus she continued to refuse to discuss it. When the Black woman persisted, the Filipina turned and threatened her coworker, telling her if she came any closer, she would hit her. The result was a grievance in which both employees reported physically being threatened by the other.

Questions

1. What perceptions of each employee can be explained by cultural differences?
2. How could this conflict have been avoided or defused?
3. Why is dealing with conflict important?

REFERENCES

Alexander, C. (2001). Understanding generational differences helps you manage a multi-age workforce. *The Digital Edge* (p. 3). Vienna, VA: New Media Federation, Newspaper Association of America. Retrieved June 17, 2004, from *www.digitaledge.org/monthly/2001_07/gengap1.html*

Alexander, G.R. (2002). A mind for multicultural management. *Nursing Management, 33*(10), 30-33.

American Hospital Association (AHA). (2002). *In our hands: How hospital leaders can build a thriving workforce.* Chicago: AHA Commission on Workforce for Hospitals and Health Systems.

American Hospital Association (AHA). (2003). *Unequal treatment: Confronting racial and ethnic disparities in health care.* Chicago: AHA news.com. Retrieved November 12, 2004, from *www.aha.org*

Betancourt, J.R., Carrillo, J.E., & Green, A.R. (2002). Cultural competence in health care: Emerging frameworks and practical approaches. New York: The Commonwealth Fund. Retrieved November 12, 2004, from *www.cmwf.org/tools/tools_show.htm?doc_id=234730*

California Newsreel. (2003). *Race—The power of an illusion.* San Francisco: California Newsreel. Retrieved June 4, 2004, from *www.pbs.org/race*

Campinha-Bacote, J., Yahle, T., & Langenkamp, M. (1996). The challenge of cultural diversity for nurse educators. *The Journal of Continuing Education in Nursing, 27*(2), 59-64.

Caver, K.A., & Livers A.B. (2002). "Dear white boss." In HBR OnPoint (Ed.), *Required reading for white executives* (pp. 7-11). Boston: Harvard Business School Publishing Corporation.

Center for the Health Professions. (2002). *Toward culturally competent care: A tool box for teaching communication strategies.* San Francisco: University of California.

Crow, K., Matheson, L., & Steed, A. (2000). Informed consent and truth telling: Cultural directions for health care providers. *Journal of Nursing Administration, 30,* (3), 148-152.

Dantley, S.J. (2004). Leaving no child behind in science education. *Black Issues in Higher Education, 21*(8), 114.

Davidhizar, R., Bechtel, G., & Giger, J. (1998). Model helps CMs deliver multicultural care. *Case Management Advisor, 9*(6), 97-100.

Forman, E. (2003, October 16). Health disparities from a social work perspective. *Caring Headlines* (pp. 4, 12). Boston: Massachusetts General Hospital.

Galanti, G. (1999). Caring for culturally diverse patients at home. *Home Health Care Consultant, 6*(1), 33-34.

Garcia, R.S. (2003, May 9). The misuse of race in medical diagnosis. *The Chronicle of Higher Education,* p. B15.

Gazmararian, J.A., Baker, D.W., Williams, M.V., Parker, R.M., Scott, T.L., Green, D.C., et al. (1999). Health literacy among Medicare enrollees in a managed care organization. *Journal of the American Medical Association, 281*(6), 545-551.

Grossman, D., & Taylor R. (1995). Cultural diversity on the unit. *American Journal of Nursing, 95*(2), 64-67.

Habayeb, G.L. (1995). Cultural diversity: A nursing concept not yet reliably defined. *Nursing Outlook, 43*(5), 224-227.

Hacker, A. (1997). *Money: Who has what and why.* New York: Scribner.

Hall, E.T., & Hall, M.R. (1990). *Understanding cultural differences.* Yarmouth, ME: Intercultural Press, Inc.

Health Resources and Services Administration (HRSA). (2001). *The registered nurse population: Findings from the 2000 national sample survey.* Rockville, MD: HRSA, U.S. Department of Health and Human Services. Retrieved May 14, 2004, from *www.bhpr.hrsa.gov/healthworkforce/reports/rnsurvey/default.htm*

Health Resources and Services Administration (HRSA). (2002). *Projected supply, demand, and shortages of registered nurses: 2000-2020.* Rockville, MD: HRSA, U.S. Department of Health and Human Services. Retrieved May 14, 2004, from *www.bhpr.hrsa.gov/health-workforce/reports/rnproject/*

Health Resources and Service Administration (HRSA). (2003, Spring). *Changing demographics: Implications for physicians, nurses, and other health workers.* Rockville, MD: HRSA, U.S. Department of Health and Human Services. Retrieved May 14, 2004, from *www.bhpr. hrsa.gov/healthworkforce/reports/changedemo/content. htm*

Institute of Medicine (IOM). (2003). *Unequal treatment: Confronting racial and ethnic disparities in health care.* Washington, DC: National Academies. Retrieved May 14, 2004, from *www.nap.edu/books/030908265X/html*

Joint Commission on Accreditation of Healthcare Organizations. (2005). JCAHOnline. *New requirement for language, communication needs.* Oakbrook Terrace, IL: JCAHO. Retrieved May 10, 2005, from *http://www. jcaho.org/about+us/news+letters/jcahonline/jo_05-05.htm*

Kent, C. (2000). Perspectives. Disparities: A shadow on U.S. health landscape. *Medicine & Health*, *54*(Suppl 35), 1-4.

Kotlikoff, L.J., & Burns, S. (2004).The perfect demographic storm: Entitlements imperil America's future. *The Chronicle of Higher Education*, *LI*(3), B6-B10.

Leininger, M. (1997). Transcultural nursing research to transform nursing education and practice: 40 years. *Image*, *29*(4), 341-347.

Loustaunau, M.O., & Sobo, E.J (1997). *The cultural context of health, illness, and medicine* Westport, CT: Bergin & Garvey.

Office of Minority Health. (2001). *Assuring cultural competence in health care: Recommendations for national standards and an outcomes-focused research agenda.* Rockville, MD: Office of Minority Health, Public Health Service, U.S. Department of Health and Human Services. Retrieved October 24, 2004, from *www.omhrc. gov/clas/cultural1a.htm*

The Murphy Leadership Institute. (2004). *National conference on transforming the work environment of nurses.* The Murphy Leadership Institute, February 25-26, Washington, DC.

USA Today. (2004, October 18). Wealth gap wider after recession. *USA Today*, B1.

U.S. Census Bureau. (1996). *Population projections of the United States by age, sex, race, and Hispanic origin: 1995 to 2050 (Current Population Reports, Series P25 1130).* Washington, DC: U.S. Census Bureau, U.S. Department of Commerce. Retrieved October 19, 2004, from *www.census.gov:80/population/www/projections/ natproj.html*

Washington, D. (2003, October 16). Disparities in health care: The challenge for the new millennium. *Caring Headlines* (pp. 1, 11). Boston: Massachusetts General Hospital.

Wendover, R.W. (2002). *The corrosion of character.* Aurora, CO: The Center for Generational Studies. Retrieved June 17, 2004, from *www.gentrends.com/articles.html*

29

Staff Recruitment and Retention

Linda L. Workman

CHAPTER OBJECTIVES

Recruitment and retention of registered nurses in health care services has never been such an imperative as it is today. The nation is facing a critical nursing shortage. This nursing shortage is unlike either of the immediately prior two shortages (Buerhaus et al., 2000; Prescott, 2000). According to Prescott, this shortage is driven by supply-side economics (the amount of labor available to work), not just misdistribution of nurses or demand-side economics (employers' willingness to hire nurses). Causes related to this shortage are numerous and include, but are not limited to, the following:

- Decrease in the U.S. birthrate since the 1950s
- Increase in number of nurses approaching retirement
- Decrease in the number of students entering into nursing in the 1980s
- Increase in the number of students in their 30s who enrolled in associate degree programs during the 1980s
- Inability of schools of nursing to currently accommodate the number of students applying for nursing

- Discuss why organizations need to perceive and treat the human resources (health care employees, including nurses) within the organization as their primary business asset
- Examine internal and external health care processes that have affected the nursing shortage
- Differentiate factors that contribute to staff nurse shortage versus managerial nurse shortage
- Evaluate turnover rates and related costs
- Analyze the impact of generational differences on worker expectations and practices
- Address the role of the registered nurse in the delivery of quality health care services
- Describe major factors that affect registered staff nurses' and managerial nurses' recruitment and retention
- Explore the relationship between Senge's concept of "learning organization" and the organization's ability to recruit and retain nursing and other health-related staff
- Analyze recruitment and retention strategies used by managers and/or organizations that have had a positive impact on nurse recruitment and retention
- Examine the positions professional organizations have taken relative to the nursing shortage, recruitment, retention, and strategies for management
- Exercise critical thinking to conceptualize and analyze possible solutions to a practice exercise

- Decrease in the number of qualified faculty available to teach the students
- Increase in the number of positions available to nurses in the workplace
- Increase in the need for nurses in hospitals to manage the high-acuity patient populations
- Increase in patient volume in acute, specialty, and long-term care facilities related to the increased aging population (Buerhaus et al., 2000)

The number and percentage of nurses preparing for retirement in the next 15 years is of significant concern, since this group accounts for approximately 40% to 50% of the current workforce (Buerhaus et al., 2000; The HMS Group, 2002). If the projections of Buerhaus and Associates and the HMS Group are true, by the year 2020 the nursing workforce will remain at about its current size, which will be nearly 20% below the required need. This means that the nursing workforce, even at more than 2 million strong, will be short approximately 400,000 nurses. Others have projected the deficit in the U.S. registered nurse workforce to range from 500,000 to 808,416 (Cohen et al., 2003; Upenieks, 2003; U.S. Department of Health and Human Services [USDHHS], 2002). This shortage is of particular concern because of the 78 million Baby Boomers who will be retiring by the year 2015, a factor expected to cause health care demands to soar.

DEFINITIONS

Issues surrounding the nursing shortage have highlighted the important leadership and management interventions related to recruitment and retention of nursing personnel. **Recruitment**, defined as replenishment, is the process used by organization to seek out or identify applicants for potential employment (Dictionary.com, 2004a). The impact is to ensure that an adequate number and quality of workers is available for selection and employment. **Retention** is the act of retaining. It is defined as the ability to continue the employment of qualified individuals, that is, nurses and/or other health care providers/associates who might otherwise leave the organization (Dictionary.com, 2004b). The impact of this action is to maintain stability and enhance quality of care while reducing cost to the organization. **Selection** is defined as the job of determining the most qualified candidate for a job. This process includes reviewing, sorting, ranking, and offering of candidates recruited for a job. **Staff vacancy** is defined as an employee position full time or part-time equivalent that is budgeted but not filled. **Turnover** is defined as the loss of an employee due to transfer, termination, or resignation. **Transfer** is the movement of an employee whose performance is satisfactory from one area to another within the same institution or corporation; **termination** is the discharge of an employee who is performing at a less than satisfactory level or is not a good match for the organization; and **resignation** is the failure

---

⚠ LEADING & MANAGING **DEFINED**

Recruitment

The process used by organizations to replenish employees.

Retention

The ability to continue the employment of qualified individuals.

Selection

Determination of the most qualified candidate for a job.

Staff Vacancy

A budgeted but not filled employee position.

Turnover

Loss of an employee due to transfer, termination, or resignation.

Transfer

Movement of an employee whose performance is satisfactory from one area to another within the same institution.

Termination

Discharge of an employee who is performing at a less than satisfactory level or is not a good match for the organization.

Resignation

Failure to retain an employee who is performing at or above satisfactory level.

to retain an employee who is performing at or above satisfactory level. Although all turnovers have an associated cost to the organization, the most costly are those dealing with the last two components of turnover.

THE NURSING SHORTAGE

According to Atencio and colleagues (2003) the changes in the nursing workforce are already being felt in acute care institutions. The national vacancy rate in 2000 was 21.3%, while acute care hospital vacancy rates nationally were at 10.2%. The vacancy rate by services within acute care hospitals ranged from 14.6% (critical care), 14.1% (medical/surgical), and 11.7% (emergency department), with the lowest rates in the OR/perioperative (9.4%) and obstetric areas (9.65%). Vacancies and turnover varied by region across the United States. Overall, the vacancy range was 9.3% to 12.2%, and the turnover range was 17.4% to 24%. The Western and Southern regions had both the highest vacancy and turnover rates, with vacancy rates at 12.2% and 11.0% and turnover rates at 22.2% and 24%, respectively. The region with the lowest vacancy rate was the Midwest (8.95%), and the lowest turnover rate was in the Northeast (17.4%). The Western region, however, reported having the largest proportion of RNs in the age range of 50 to 59 years, whereas the Southern region reported having the largest proportion of RNs in the age ranges of 20 to 29 years and 30 to 39 years. During this same time period the national vacancy rate for RN managers was 6.5%, with the Western and Southern regions having the largest rate at 8.5% and 8.2%, respectively. Urban and suburban hospitals reported higher vacancy rates than did rural hospitals, and individual and multihospital systems reported higher average RN vacancy rates than did integrated delivery systems. The percentage of facilities that used temporary staff such as agency staff or travelers to compensate for vacancies was approximately 54%. Range of usage (53% to 24%) varied by specialty service with critical care, medical/surgical, and emergency departments requiring the most and obstetrics and OR/perioperative areas requiring the least.

The impact of the shortage and use of higher-paid agency or traveler workers was a significant financial expense for 69% of the organizations. In addition to the cost, 51% of the organizations reported overcrowding in the emergency area, and 26% reported going on diversion for an average of 4 hours per week. Other impacts included restriction in admissions, increased waiting time for surgery, and reduced or eliminated services. Approximately 17% of the organizations reported that the shortage had a serious impact on nurse staffing and staff, including increased overtime usage, higher stress, restricted expansion, changes in recruiting and hiring practices, decreased quality of care, and increased difficulty in scheduling coordination.

This shortage is further being fueled by the international demand for nurses. According to Daniel and colleagues (2000) and Gamble (2002), international recruitment of nurses has once again surfaced as a way of addressing the nursing shortage, specifically in the United States, United Kingdom, Canada, and Western Europe. Given the global magnitude of this shortage, few countries have nurses in excess; as a result, recruiting nurses internationally often creates an even more severe shortage in their home country. Nurses have identified two major reasons for leaving their home country: (1) economic security and (2) professional opportunity, although personal safety/security in the workplace and/or country has also been noted.

INTERNATIONAL RECRUITMENT

International recruitment has been of major concern to the International Council of Nurses (ICN), given the magnitude of the global nursing shortage. The ICN (1999) released a position statement, "Nurse Retention, Transfer and Migration." In this document the ICN linked the nursing shortage (inadequate supply of nurses) to lack of quality in health care. The statement addressed the individual nurse's rights, as well as positive and negative issues related to migration. It also delineated roles that national nurses associations should take in order to raise nurse awareness of potential constraints and ensure that countries seeking to recruit nurses had policies and practices relative

---

Box 29.1

ICN Ethical Nurse Recruitment Principles

1. Effective human resources planning and development
2. Credible nursing regulation
3. Access to full employment
4. Freedom of movement
5. Freedom from discrimination
6. Good faith contracting
7. Equal pay for work of equal value
8. Access to grievance procedures
9. Safe work environment
10. Effective orientation/mentoring/supervision
11. Employment trial periods
12. Freedom of association
13. Regulation of recruitment

ICN, International Council of Nurses

---

to fair and humane treatment of nurses. The ICN supports the migration of nurses as a short-term strategy for addressing the nursing shortage, viewing nurse migration as a way of increasing the nurse's career opportunities and personal self-interests. Nurse migration is further viewed by the ICN as a way of increasing multicultural practice and learning opportunities within the nursing profession. Concerns related to recruitment practices, however, led the ICN in 2001 to issue a position statement on ethical nurse recruitment. In this document 13 key principles specific to the recruitment of international nurses were identified as needing to be addressed (Box 29.1).

These principles are relevant because they address changes that need to take place to ensure that nurses are treated fairly and equably in the international market place. Unethical recruitment of nurses in the past has led to nurses being exploited and misled into accepting job responsibilities and work conditions incompatible with their qualifications, skills, and experiences. The ICN further condemns the recruitment of nurses into countries where authorities support human rights violations.

AMERICAN NURSES ASSOCIATION'S CALL TO ACTION

In September 2001, the American Nurses Association (ANA, 2001)—in conjunction the American Organization of Nurse Executives (AONE), Sigma Theta Tau International (STTI), and 60 other professional nursing organization and 19 steering committee organizations—held a summit meeting to begin to analyze the nursing shortage problem and to develop a strategic plan entitled *Nursing's Agenda for the Future: A Call to Action* (ANA, 2002). The outcome of this meeting was a vision statement and 10 domains for action. The vision statement was as follows:

> Nursing is **the** pivotal health care profession, highly valued for its specialized knowledge, skill and caring in improving the health status of the public and ensuring safe, effective, quality care. The profession mirrors the diverse population it serves and provides leadership to create positive changes in health policy and delivery systems. Individuals choose nursing as a career and remain in the profession because of the opportunity for personal and professional growth, supportive work environments and compensation with roles and responsibilities. (p. 7)

The 10 domains that emerged from this summit were derived from the research literature and the Institute of Medicine's study *Crossing the Quality Chasm: A New Health System for the 21st Century,* published in 2001. The domains are as follows:

1. Leadership and planning
2. Delivery systems
3. Legislative/regulatory/policy
4. Professional/nursing culture
5. Recruitment/retention
6. Economic value
7. Work environment
8. Public relations/communication
9. Education
10. Diversity (p. 7)

In addition to the vision and domains, a short-term plan was developed that outlined the desired future state, strategies for achieving the desired state, objectives to support the primary strategy and the co-champions for each. The project was extremely comprehensive given that the nursing shortage and its impact on health care are not linear. On the contrary, the problem is extremely complex. The group recognized that in order to actualize the *Nursing's Agenda for the Future: A Call to the Nation* by 2010, extensive partnerships would be required to bring about strategic change, and change would have to occur in health care leadership, health care organizations, academic programs, health care policy, governmental agencies, health care and professional regulatory agencies, governmental and private funding, professional practice groups, consumer groups, etc.

The ANA (2002) as part of the *Nursing's Agenda for the Future: A Call to the Nation* developed a "Desired Future Statement (Vision)" for each of the 10 domains. The statement for the domain of "Recruitment and Retention" clearly delineated the comprehensiveness of the undertaking, as follows:

> Nursing is comprised of a diverse body of individuals committed to promoting and sustaining the profession through addressing diversity, image, education, funding, practice models and environments, and professional development. (p. 17)

The vision was derived from the nursing research literature and incorporated the recurring themes related to recruitment and retention. Five strategies were formulated to achieve this vision. The strategies also addressed the two-pronged recruitment issue of the shortage (supply-side economics) and recruitment of (1) students for nursing education programs and (2) qualified nurses for health care agencies. The strategies also targeted retention issues to be addressed within health care agencies and academic programs focusing on the development of career-based opportunities within health care, development and funding of creative educational initiatives, creating a desirable and appealing image for nursing as a career choice, formulation and implementation of professional practice models, work environments that ensure career satisfaction, and development of comprehensive recruitment and retention strategies that will appeal to a diverse customer group/population (ANA, 2002). These global strategies were then broken down for the primary strategy in each

Table **29.1**

Student- and Faculty-Related Strategies for Recruitment and Retention		
Recruitment Strategies	Students	Faculty
Develop professional mentoring models	✗	
Create a specific curriculum to address diversity	✗	✗
Obtain funding to support minority enrollment	✗	
Develop and distribute promotional and recruitment materials to attract individuals from diverse backgrounds into nursing	✗	
Recruit retired nurses to form professional mentoring corps		✗
Provide joint educational and service standardized internships and residencies	✗	✗
Co-op program/SCA program	✗	
Negotiate professional paid development opportunities with employers		✗
Create a website for leadership development that can be used by education, service, and professional organization members	✗	✗

of the domains, with work on the remaining strategies to be developed. The ANA also identified strategies that could be used to enhance student and faculty recruitment and/or retention (Table 29.1).

The multifaceted approach undertaken by the organizations that participated in the Nursing Professional Summit called by the ANA in 2001 addressed issues that were consistent with the findings identified by Goodin (2003). Goodin's findings were based on a comprehensive, integrative review of the nursing shortage literature in the United States from 1999 to 2001. The findings of this analysis revealed that the major contributors to the nursing shortage and factors effecting recruitment and retention were directed at four major themes. The themes and examples of the related intervention approaches are listed in Box 29.2.

In order to meet the demand for nurses now and in the future, actions need to be taken that are directed at what drives young people and career switchers to choose nursing as a career. Erickson and colleagues (2004) reported on an initiative undertaken by Partners Healthcare in Boston. The goal was to gain insights into the dynamics of career selection by young people and career switchers. In order to determine this information, a consulting firm was hired to conduct focus groups and telephone interviews. Specific questions used in this qualitative approach focused on the following: How were decisions made relative to choosing a career? How did significant influences in one's life affect career choice? What was the individual's perception and image of nursing? As a result of this study, vital information was identified reflecting differences in the two groups. Outcomes of the study included two major marketing strategies that would promote the image of nursing as a career choice: "Be Somebody" and "Valuable Partner." In addition, the following nine strategies for promoting nursing as a career were identified:

1. Classroom ambassadors program
2. Job-shadowing experiences
3. Bring your child to work day
4. Volunteer health care settings opportunities for students and adults

5. Part-time employment opportunities for students and adults need to be developed
6. Presentation to clubs/organizations regarding nursing
7. Participation at community health fairs
8. Advertising campaigns directed at job satisfaction, making a difference in people's lives, flexible scheduling, and competitive salary and benefits
9. Advertising that directs people to dynamic, comprehensive web sites that offer positive, motivating information about nursing and its reward (Erickson et al., 2004, p. 86)

RECRUITMENT

As identified by the above studies and actions, recruitment has taken on a whole new perspective. It has always been about the replacement of non-retained staff and the hiring of staff to fill newly created and/or expanded positions. With the changes that have occurred in health care over the last two decades, the concept of recruitment has begun to focus more and more on the identification and development of pre-employment hires. This means marketing the agency to potential pre-nursing students and active nursing students. Recruitment, therefore, has become more complex and more linked to partnerships than ever before. These partnerships are not only with schools of nursing but also with elementary and secondary schools and other community agencies. Co-op programs and/or student clinical assistant (SCA) programs (Henriksen et al., 2003) and other related preceptor programs create a model for attracting and retaining new graduates. These and other student-related activities create a blending of the student-employee role, thus changing recruitment to a retention strategy once the student gets linked in a nursing capacity to the health care facility. These linkages in the form of precepting and mentoring activities have also been shown to have a positive impact on job satisfaction among experienced RNs (McClure et al., 1983).

Based on the above, it is clear that recruitment has both a long-term and short-term directive. Although the long-term directive is one that is extremely important, most of the organization's

Box 29.2

Themes and Related Intervention Strategies

Aging Workforce

- Strive to minimize work demands on older nurses
- Find ways to increase reimbursement or salary equity for experienced nurses
- Develop care management approaches that increase health and decrease physical injury of nurses
- Find ways to increase use of nurse expertise as workload burdens increase
- Develop strategies for retaining older nurses

Declining Enrollment

- Target younger students in elementary and junior high
- Target nontraditional students—males, minorities, etc.
- Continue to develop diverse tracks for varied entry levels into nursing
- Continue to develop methods for bringing nonpracticing nurses back into the workforce and foreign nurses into the workforce
- Work to ensure that there are adequate faculty to teach students
- Provide career opportunities and lifelong learning opportunities for nurses

Changing Work Climate

- Work to ensure that nurses have the opportunity to practice care delivery versus managing the system
- Provide opportunity for ongoing education that will allow nurses to move within specialty areas of care
- Organizationally support ongoing education
- Develop new approaches for relieving nurses in times of high patient care demands
- Increase flexibility
- Promote assignments/workload that is reasonable and achievable
- Avoid use of mandatory overtime
- Develop strategies for accommodating lifestyle needs of new graduates

Poor Image of Nursing

- Work to change the image of nursing among young potential nurses through Career Days for middle school students and Shadow Days for junior and senior high school students
- Develop web-based career information
- Involve practicing nurses in recruitment initiatives and school activities
- Provide community programs and individual activities that address the rewarding challenges of nursing
- Continue to work with the TriCouncil and external organizations such as Johnson and Johnson to develop targeted campaigns
- Reform educational and credentialing mechanisms in order to empower nurses in the workplace
- Lobby Congress to pass legislation that promotes nursing as a career and provides funding of students—scholarship, loan forgiveness, retention grants, elder care

resources are going to the short-term directive—the filling of vacant and/or newly created positions. The recruitment focus of this chapter will be directed at the short-term directive.

RECRUITMENT OF PROFESSIONAL NURSES

In 1983 a study was conducted to identify variables in hospital organizations and their nursing services that create a magnetism which attracts and retains professional nurse staff as well as to identify particular combinations of variables that produce nursing practice models within hospitals in which nurses receive professional and personal satisfaction to the degree that recruitment and retention of qualified staff are achieved (McClure et al., 1983). The study included 41 out of 165 hospitals from 10 geographic regions (designed by the Bureau of Labor Statistics). The hospitals were nominated by Fellows in the American Academy of Nursing (AAN). Each AAN Fellow was asked to nominate 6 to 10 hospitals of varying size in their region of the country that demonstrated success in recruiting and retaining staff. The final selection of the institutions for inclusion in the study was done after a review and ranking of the top 10 choices in each region based on established criteria and recruitment and retention data provided by each institution. Originally, 46 hospitals were chosen, but 5 were unable to participate. The results of the study clearly showed three major variables of administration, professional practice, and professional development and related attributes that positively affect hospitals' ability to recruit and retain registered nurse staff. These variables and related attributes are listed in Box 29.3.

This study was one of the first to describe organizational and leadership factors that are important to the recruitment and retention of nurses in the workplace. As noted by the variables above, the nurses specifically wanted leadership and organizational structure that supported participatory involvement, as well as flexibility for work scheduling and personal/professional development. In addition, nurses wanted to work in an institution that had a clearly defined professional practice model that used the skills and knowledge of the professional nurse. Nurses were also interested in working in an organization that allowed them to be "able to practice nursing." Managerial visibility and support were viewed as strengths in promoting autonomy. Nurses also wanted to have control over their practice (autonomy) and

---

Box 29.3

Organizational and Nursing Service Variables of Magnetism that Attract and Retain Professional Nurses

1. Administration
  a. Management style
  b. Quality of leadership
    i. Nursing managers
    ii. Nursing directors
  c. Organizational structure
    i. Decentralization
    ii. Committees
  d. Staffing
  e. Personnel policies
    i. Work schedules
    ii. Promotion opportunities

1. Professional practice
  a. Quality of patient care
    i. Professional practice models
    ii. Autonomy
    iii. Consultation and resources
  b. Teaching
  c. Image of nursing

1. Professional development
  a. Orientation
  b. Inservice/continuing education
  c. Formal education
  d. Career development

collaborative relationships with physicians relative to care management. This study and the follow-up study conducted by Kramer and Hafner (1989) five years later were the basis for the ANA's Magnet Recognition program.

Recruitment initiatives in the last several years have used strategies targeted at nurse satisfiers as reported in the nursing and health care literature. Satisfiers have included strategies such as professional practice model usage, preceptor/mentorship opportunities, increased flexibility in work scheduling, low patient-to-RN ratios, collaborative practice environment, Magnet Recognition status, environment of respect and value, and a competitive compensation model. Strategies commonly used related to nurse recruitment of new and experienced nurses are identified in Box 29.4.

Human Resources, Managerial, and Staff Roles Associated with Recruitment

In the context of a nurse shortage, recruitment is a major human resources strategy. Because the organization needs to find and hire the best qualified nurses who also "fit" with the culture and are willing to work for a specific salary and work conditions, both recruitment and retention are important. Both managers and staff contribute to successful recruitment and retention. A complex and detailed process is followed in effective recruitment and retention. The nine major processes or phases of recruitment are as follows:

1. Position posting
2. Advertising
3. Screening
4. Interviewing
5. Selecting
6. Orienting
7. Counseling/coaching
8. Performance evaluation
9. Staff development

Position Posting

Position posting for recruitment begins following determination of vacancies based on position controls developed for each of the clinical/service areas. The vacancies are identified based on the

---

Box 29.4

Recruitment Strategies

Flexible hours
Competitive salaries
Bonus pay
Relocation pay
Fixed shifts
Weekend option program
Part-time pay with bonus hours
Flexible benefits packages
Scholarships for BSN or graduate studies
Tuition benefit plan
Educational loan repayment
RN specialty internships
Professional development opportunities
Career opportunities
Specialty certification reimbursement
Low nurse-to-patient ratios (workload staffing)
Shared governance/leadership models
Care delivery model that promotes professional care at the bedside
Clinical ladder/career ladder
Free parking
Magnet recognition
Culture of safety: zero tolerance for incivility
Research/evidence-based practice
NCLEX review course
Qualified managerial support
Clinical support: staff educators, clinical nurse specialists
Workforce diversity
Interdisciplinary collaboration opportunities

---

full-time equivalent (FTE) status for each of the positions. Once the positions have been identified and the shift/holiday schedules are determined, the first step is to post them internally for staff review and selection. The length of this posting time is determined by each organization and/or respective collective bargaining contracts. Positions not filled within a defined time period are then posted externally to the organization. Based on the need and/or limited number of nurses in a given specialty, recruitment agencies may be contacted

Research Note

Source: Curran, C. (2003). Nurse recruitment: A waste of postage, paper, and people. *Nursing Economic$, 21*(1), 5, 32.

Purpose

The purpose of this research was to determine the effectiveness of organizational recruitment initiatives, using a recruitment scorecard approach.

Discussion

Study was conducted of 100% of hospitals in two states (N = 150) using a fabricated resume of a seasoned "perfect nurse" applicant who was interested in relocating. Letters were sent out with the resume to the human resources director/vice president requesting employment information about the institution for consideration by the applicant. The letters included personal information, including telephone number and e-mail address. A recruitment scorecard of 100 possible points was created for measuring predetermined attributes, including, but not limited to, the following: response time, personalization, distinctiveness, application sent, ease of application completion, and follow-up by the organization. Results indicated that the average score was in the 30s and the highest score was 58. Overall, hospitals were found to have slow response time, using primarily a paper mail system versus electronic messaging (e-mail); responses lacked personalization; information provided about the organization failed to address the distinctiveness of the organization or address the role of nursing in the system; applications were sent as hard copies rather than online; website referral to provide the candidate with additional information about the organization was provided by only 10% of the sample group; follow-up with the candidate was lacking in approximately 75%.

Application to Practice

The author pointed out the blatant disregard hospitals demonstrated in their attempt to recruit a highly qualified new nurse who was planning to move into the community. Such a message suggests that money spent on recruitment might better be used elsewhere in the organization, since responses at this level will not yield the results desired or needed by health care organizations. This study is a wake-up call for organizations to evaluate the true message that is being sent to potential candidates and the likelihood of the human resources program attracting qualified, interested candidates. Is it any wonder that nurse administrators are frustrated with the candidates they receive or the feedback provided by the candidate about the obstacles they had to endure while seeking employment? In addition, is it any wonder that nurses seek to work as entrepreneurs or go through private recruiters rather than spend personal time job seeking? If organizational recruitment is to be truly effective, the process needs to be revamped using evaluation data from candidates' employee surveys in order to ensure that the strategies used match the candidates' expectations.

---

at this time to conduct a regional, statewide, or national search for the position.

Advertising

Advertising includes the development of an institutional advertisement outlining the position(s) or job opportunities within an organization. The advertisement addresses the area of need and specific information that would be likely to attract an employee (RN) to the position. The Human Resources (HR) Department determines distribution sites, with input from the specific departments. Sites may include professional journals or newspapers, local or regional newspapers, radio, or the organization's website. An advantage of online advertisement is that the application process can be made available at the same time, making it a one-stop process for the person seeking employment.

If the recruiter is planning to attend special events, information about the position will be taken for posting along with the employee applications. In addition, information about the organization and related benefits and specialty strengths will be highlighted. A shortcoming that needs to be addressed related to advertising is that organizations often spend an enormous amount of money on advertising only to miss the most important aspect, that of a quick, effective, courteous follow-up with potential candidates (Curran, 2003). All of the positive effects that the expensive advertising and recruiting efforts have engendered in candidates for a position can be lost in how the institution follows-up with candidates. For example, if potential candidates for a positon have been encouraged to apply through advertising and recruitment efforts and then log on to an institution's website to find that they cannot complete an application for the job, they may in frustration decide not to pursue the job further (Curran, 2003). In addition, if candidates are unable to obtain a response about the status of their application after submitting it, they may decide that this institution is not the kind for which they wish to work. If recruitment and advertising efforts are to be productive, these kinds of flaws in the system must be avoided.

Screening

Screening is the process in which applications are reviewed prior to determining whether or not the nurse meets the preestablished criteria for the position. During this activity the reviewer makes a selection about who should be interviewed. It is important to remember that if an organization is classified as an equal opportunity employer, the reviewers are required to follow the guidelines established by the federal government.

Interviewing

Interviewing is the time for clarification of information presented in the application and dossier submitted by the applicant. The job description is the basis for a hiring interview. The interview can be conducted in person or over the telephone, in a group/committee or one-on-one meeting. For best results, predefined questions should be used to interview all candidates for the position. Also, questions should be directed at the work expectations outlined in the position description and/or practices. Open-ended questions and follow-ups are recommended. For example, the following questions or discussion points can be posed:

- *Tell me about your current position.*
- *What do you like least about it?*
- *What do you like best about it?*

To get at more in-depth responses and to determine behavior-specific examples, questions can be framed as follows:

- *Think of a time in your experience when X was needed and describe how you did X.*
- *How did you handle X?*

It is appropriate to ask the candidate about aspects of his or her practices related to the job, such as the following:

- *Given the varied work hour requirements, how would you handle this?*
- *What problems do you see the work hour requirements presenting?*
- *Based on the work requirements relative to lifting, how would you go about transferring a patient whose body weight is more than 350 pounds?*

The information obtained through this process will help the committee or manager assigned to the recruitment process determine the applicant's "fit" with the unit and/or organizational culture, as well as consistent data for comparison of candidates. Use of formalized questions is often referred to as a structured interview or targeted selection process (DDI, 1997, 2004; Lipsey, 2004). The targeted selection process is built on analysis of work per job, organizational values, clear identification of competencies for key positions, and development of interview skills and confidence of the interviewers. Using the targeted interview ensures that all candidates are interviewed based on the same criteria. In addition, during the targeted interview process, the interviewer asks questions that are directed at having the candidates describe typical situations that they have encountered in previous jobs. Use of the targeted interview method allows the interviewers to gain data from the candidates to more fully evaluate their values and practice patterns. It further allows for objective comparison of candidates based on their responses, and it decreases personal biases and assumptions. Questions that should be avoided during the interview relate specifically to personal information about the candidate, such as the following: age, marital status, living arrangements, children, limitation or disabilities, religion, substance abuse, and membership in professional organizations.

Selecting

Selecting is the determination of who will be offered an opportunity for employment (termination of the recruitment process). A committee or manager may complete the selection process. For best results, data used in the screening and interviewing phases should be used when comparing candidate responses and other related data. The selection process also involves the formal activity of making an offer to the candidate. Who does this activity varies according to institutional policy, but it usually involves either the manager or HR personnel. At the time the job offer is made, the employee is informed of the position/job being offer, the FTE allocation (FT or PT) for the position, and the salary offer and benefits. Regardless of who makes the final offer, HR pays a role in determining the salary range.

Selection of an employee who is a match with the core values of an organization has been shown to have important implications. It facilitates ease of employee transition into the new role and fit with staff within the unit and organization. Employee fit and related retention has also been shown to have an impact on cost savings within the organization. According to Lipsey (2004), return on investment of hiring the right versus the wrong person (poor performer) is more significant than just the costs of simple replacement of an employee. The costs of hiring the wrong person are associated not only with the recruitment, replacement, and hiring expenses,

but also with secondary costs. Secondary costs of hiring a poor performer include increased dollars wasted on training and development, decreased productivity and increased errors, lost opportunities to improve processes and/or outcomes, decreased or poor staff morale that results from staff struggling to pick up slack of the poor performer, and dissatisfied customers. The secondary costs have a significant impact on the organization and workers and are often much greater than those associated with the initial recruitment process.

Orienting

Orienting is an important activity for bringing new employees into the organization, department, and unit. It is the employee's introduction to the culture and values of the organization and discipline. It provides new employees with background information needed to execute their role, as well as an introduction to the social milieu and culture in which they will be working (Jernigan, 1988). Orientation provides new employees with an introduction to the philosophy, mission, and goals of the organization and department. It also provides them with knowledge related to the practice of nursing within the organization and resources available for their further use. Progressive organizations have expanded the concept of orientation from a 1-week review of forms, policies, and procedures to an interactive process built around self-learning and renewal. Preceptorship or mentorship programs exist in many institutions to provide employees with consistent ongoing support and a colleague relationship. Changes in orientation format and content have occurred as a result of study outcomes that have shown the relationship between job satisfaction and staff retention.

Counseling and Coaching

Counseling and coaching are strategies used to promote a sense of community for new and ongoing employees. These strategies create a professional and social network for new employees, an attribute identified in Magnet-status institutions. Use of these strategies also creates a sense of a nonpunitive culture in which staff can learn and grow. Senge (1990) described a "learning organization" as a place "where people continually expand their capacity to create the results they truly desire, where new and expansive patterns of thinking are nurtured, where collective aspiration is set free, and where people are continually learning how to learn together" (p. 3). Although counseling and coaching is just one aspect of a learning organization, it has been shown to have a significant impact on staff satisfaction.

Performance Evaluation

Performance evaluation is a mechanism for giving feedback to employees—new and experienced. New employees usually are expected to receive their initial performance evaluation within the first 60 to 120 days, depending on the policies of the organization. This feedback is directed at the individual employee's progress relative to orientation (formative evaluation). During this evaluation, the employee and managerial staff also should take the time to evaluate the employee's "fit" with the organizational and departmental culture (summative evaluation). Strategies to address further needs and/or employment status should be decided at this time. A full performance evaluation then occurs at the end of the orientation period and annually thereafter. Feedback regarding ongoing performance should be provided to employees on a regular basis. Performance evaluation should focus on the employee's achievement toward defined goals, with feedback directed at the individual's contribution to the development of peers, and clinical and/or leadership practices. The meeting can be conducted using a formal or informal process, one-on-one or in a group.

Staff Development

Staff development has been identified in the literature as an important factor in job satisfaction. It provides employees with an opportunity to improve their practice, level of competency, or other areas of self-interest. Programs for staff development are usually determined based on staff surveys conducted annually. Programs developed are usually posted for staff selection, and the institution provides scheduling flexibility and funding for employees to participate.

Staff development, as defined in the Magnet study (Kramer & Hafner, 1989; McClure et al., 1983), identified four areas of professional development beyond orientation. The four areas included in-service education, continuing education, formal education, and career development. Professional development was valued for its economic potential. However, other attributes identified were personal and professional growth opportunities, career advancement opportunities, and preceptor skill development. Nurses also reported that the variety of programs available provided increased flexibility, as did the instructional methods used. Nurses in these institutions viewed education as being valued. Administrative support was provided and available, as were clinical and managerial resources. Professional development opportunities overall were shown to have a positive influence on nurse satisfaction.

RETENTION: NEW GRADUATES AND QUALIFIED EXPERIENCED REGISTERED NURSES

Renewed attention has been directed at retention of nurses over the last 10-15 years (Upenieks, 2003). Retention initiatives have been aimed at promoting job satisfaction and establishing a culture of safety and respect. The primary focus of this culture is nurse autonomy, including professional practice models, interdisciplinary collaboration, and professional care delivery models that address specialty population needs and related staffing requirements. In addition, compensation models are being considered or put in place that provide nurses with options that promote a sense of financial security and personal choice (Kramer & Hafner, 1989; McClure et al., 1983)—for example, investment opportunities in 401Ks, gains sharing, and IRAs (Nursing Executive Center, 2001). The Nursing Executive Center (2001) identified three categories and nine subcategories of reasons that nurses had given for remaining at a Destination Hospital. These categories and their related subcategories are listed below in the order of greatest importance:

1. High-Quality Care
   1.1 Hospital's commitment to providing high-quality patient care
   1.2 Hospital's reputation as outstanding setting for clinical care
2. Strong Nurse Leadership
   2.1 Quality of direct manager
   2.2 Quality of overall nursing leadership
3. Meeting the Baseline
   3.1 Salary
   3.2 Scheduling options
   3.3 Benefits package
   3.4 Hospital's reputation for assigning nurses lower numbers of patients
   3.5 Location/Convenience (Nursing Executive Center, 2001, p. 23)

Nurses are also becoming more actively involved in creating an organizational climate and developing change strategies such as participating in the surveying of staff to determine needs and target "dissatifiers" within the organization and/or its practices (Upenieks, 2003). Nurses are further involved in CQI projects at all levels of the organization and development of change strategies to improve the overall performance of organizational and patient outcomes. Organizations that have been successful in their communication and work with staff have been shown to have increased stability and retention in the workforce, higher job satisfaction, higher quality patient outcomes, and fewer nurse injuries (Aikin et al., 1997; Laschinger & Wong, 1999). Decreased cost has also been associated with effective recruitment strategies, consistent with the Magnet program (Upenieks, 2003).

It should be noted that generational differences have been identified as factors that affect staff perception and selection of retention and recruitment strategies. Age-related cohorts appear to hold divergent perceptions, needs, and attitudes toward work that may be challenging to manage or fulfill. Both retention and recruitment can be affected if clashes or conflict ensue.

Generational workforce diversity refers to the differences in employee perspectives of the job security, work behaviors and related skills, work expectation associated with the job, value placed on employer versus personal/family needs, etc., as associated with the generation/period of the employees' birth. Generational workforce group and related periods usually include the following categories:

- Mature/Silent Generation: 1909-1945
- Baby Boomers: 1943-1964
- Generation X: 1965-1981
- Generation Y/Next Generation/Millennium Generation: 1982 to date

With four generational groups now in the workplace, it is important that managers and staff consider differences when developing strategies for change or rewards. Each generation has its own perspective, and there is diversity even among each generation. Therefore it is imperative that generational groups have representation or opportunity for input in planning and decision making. In addition, it is important to develop a variety of alternatives from which employees can select rather than targeting a single approach. Strategies commonly used for nurse recruitment of new and experienced nurses are identified in Box 29.5.

TURNOVER: COST AND MANAGEMENT STRATEGIES

Turnover of qualified staff is not only disruptive to the care community (Manion & Bartholomew, 2004) in which the nurse works; it is also extremely costly to the organization. Kuhar and colleagues (2004) suggested that a single nurse replacement cost could be as low as $44,000, but its impact on customer satisfaction is not included in this cost. According to Atencio and colleagues (2003), the cost of replacement is approximately two times the nurse's annual salary. Thus the average replacement cost for a medical-surgical nurse is approximately $92,442 (based on a national average salary of $46,832), whereas replacement of a critical care nurse is almost $145,000. Expenditures include a variety of costs—advertising and marketing, human

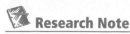
Research Note

Source: Kuhar, P.A., Miller, D., Spear, B.T., Ulreich, S.M., & Mion, L.C. (2004). The meaningful retention strategy inventory: A targeted approach to implementing retention strategies. *Journal of Nursing Administration, 34*(1), 10-18.

Purpose

The nursing shortage has driven administrators to begin to evaluate new and creative strategies for retaining qualified experienced nursing staff. With this need in mind, the authors sought to develop an inventory to be used with staff nurses and managers to identify issues that could be addressed. The purpose of this study was to determine retention strategies perceived as meaningful to nurses and to design and implement interventions directed at resolving issues that were of greatest importance.

Discussion

As part of this study the authors developed a valid and reliable instrument, the Meaningful Retention Strategy Inventory (MRSI). This inventory was used to measure staff nurse and nurse manager perceptions of retention strategies and overall level of importance. Data were collected on nursing and managerial staff at eight of the Cleveland Clinic Health System hospitals. The results of the study indicated that staff nurses from three different age groups were able to agree on 9 of the top 10 ranked retention strategies selected. One difference among the staff nurse groups was related to "pay increase" and "differential pay," with nurses under 36 years selecting pay increase and those nurses over 36 years and under 56 years selecting differential pay among their most preferred choices. Another difference was associated with nurses over 56 years, who included "respect from physicians," "respect from administration" and "educational opportunities" among their preferred choices. The results of the staff nurse and nurse manager groups also indicated consistency relative to 9 of the top 10 preferred choices. The only difference noted was that staff nurses included "shift of choice" as a preferred choice, whereas managers ranked this strategy as twenty-fifth.

Major concerns identified relative to job satisfaction and retention were in the areas of teamwork, compensation/benefits, staffing flexibility, and equipment. The retention items with the highest mean scores were categorized into three groups—people, process, and technology—for the purpose of strategy development. Activities related to each of these three categories were described, along with the impact observed and related outcomes. Each of the hospitals used institution-specific nurse/manager data to devise and implement retention strategies. Some examples of the retention strategies used per category included the following:

- *People:* flexible staffing options, development of a new compensation structure, addition of new role to support the nurse at the bedside
- *Process:* redesigned transportation processes, changes in dietary services support, forms revision
- *Technology:* increase in use of wireless technology on pilot units, electronic medical record, new tracking systems in the ED and OR, ergonomic care devices

Implementation of these retention strategies was reported to have had a positive impact on nurse satisfaction and nurse retention, as well as achievement of the Magnet Recognition award.

Application to Practice

Because nothing can be done to alter the aging of nurses, it is important to identify ways of positively affecting nurse retention. The availability of an instrument that is institutionally sensitive and can be used by nurse administration to objectively determine the retention strategies nurses prefer will greatly add to the development of a retention plan that is likely to bring about the positive results in a more cost-effective manner. Use of the MRSI and the structural design of this study provide an objective method for positively affecting retention within a given organization. In addition, the methods can be evaluated over time and/or replicated by other institutions to determine strategies that are most effective in influencing nurse satisfaction and retention. The inventory developed in this study also provided a valid and reliable measure for future research in nursing administration. The strategies designed and their effectiveness over time will provide useful data for future planning within nursing and health care agencies. Certainly, the use of this approach to planning is grounded in performance improvement.

Box 29.5

Retention Strategies Used to Retain New Graduates and Experienced Nurses

Flexible hours/schedules
Bonus pay
Fixed shifts
Creation of autonomous self-managed units
Part-time pay with bonus hours
Scholarships for BSN or graduate studies
Professional development opportunities
Leadership and clinical support for ongoing professional development and decision making
Financial support associated with credentialing
Mentoring/precepting program opportunities
Provision for sabbatical
Initializing of new technology into practice
Realignment of salary structure/compression management
Bonus pay for recruitment of employees
Profit/gains sharing program
Shared governance/leadership models
Career advancement program
Clinical ladder/career ladder
Magnet recognition
Free parking
Concierge services
Culture of safety
Physician-nurse collaborative partnership
Creation of a community culture
Child/elder care

costs associated with the review, interview, and selection process. Based on the projected medical-surgical nurse replacement costs identified by Atencio and colleagues, the loss of 21.3% (which represents the national average) from a staff of 100 could cost an organization as much as $1,969,014.

The replacement cost of turnover can be determined using the formula for cost per RN hire (Figure 29.1) presented by Hoffman (1984). Other related costs associated with turnover and a nurse shortage are decreased patient outcomes. These include longer lengths of stay, increased risk for falls, medication errors, infections, gastrointestinal bleeding, and failure to rescue (Aiken et al., 2002; Needleman et al., 2002). Intrinsic costs associated with the remaining nurses are increased dissatisfaction and burnout when staffing ratios increase for sustained periods of time (Aiken et al., 2002). Increased dissatisfaction in nurses has also been directly linked with nurses' intent to leave, which has been shown to be the greatest predictor of whether a nurse will leave the job (Atencio et al., 2003). Loss of experienced, qualified nurses has had a major impact on the care delivery within a unit of service and is a hard to quantify indirect cost. As noted earlier, changes in the community of care have negative implications and should be avoided if at all possible. Factors shown to have a negative impact on retention include overload due to increased patient assignments related to too few staff or too many patients, as well as exhaustion and nurses' associated fears of making mistakes under those conditions.

Analysis of turnover is an important continuous quality improvement process because it provides the data needed to identify and address trends and patterns related to staff retention. The HR department usually provides turnover data

resource salary costs, travel expenses for nurses interviewing, temporary replacement costs for per diem nurses, overtime usage, terminal payout, orientation costs, as well as employee and managerial

$$\frac{\text{Total cost (recruitment, training, coverage, etc.)}}{\text{Total RNs hired}} = \text{Cost per RN hired}$$

Figure 29.1
Cost-per-RN-hire formula.

$$\frac{\text{Number of terminations per year}}{\text{Average workforce per year}} \times 100 = \% \text{ Turnover}$$

Figure 29.2
Turnover formula.

because it is the repository for employee records. Turnover data are primarily reported quarterly, but that depends on organizational and/or managerial needs. Managerial staff can calculate their own unit-based turnover using the formula in Figure 29.2, presented by Hoffman (1984).

When calculating turnover data, the manager should confer with HR to verify employee numbers (resignations and terminations) that have occurred during the specified timeframe. Failure to do so may result in discrepancies between HR and managerial data sets. These discrepancies may call the data into question and decrease their value at the organizational level. It should also be pointed out that transfer data are not included in turnover because the employee is not "lost" to the organization. Tracking and trending transfer data are important, however, because these steps may alert the manager to unit-based issues that need to

be addressed. Tracking and trending these data can also alert the administrative team to managerial leadership issues that need to be evaluated.

LEADERSHIP AND MANAGEMENT IMPLICATIONS

Whether more registered nurses are needed is an issue that needs to be further addressed. Using an economic model (supply and demand), history would suggest that with increased labor available in the workforce (supply), opportunities and pay will diminish (Prescott, 2000). If this happens, nurses will once again begin to withdraw from the marketplace, recreating a nursing shortage. There is no disputing the fact that there is a correlation between the number of registered nurses available on nursing units and quality patient outcomes. However, although nursing and health care

▲ LEADERSHIP & MANAGEMENT **BEHAVIORS**

Leadership Behaviors

- Motivates followers to lifelong learning
- Inspires staff education efforts
- Ensures access to education and training opportunities
- Enables higher-quality staff recruitment and selection
- Models lifelong learning and professional development
- Selects highly qualified candidates
- Mentors employees

Management Behaviors

- Plans for lifelong learning when formulating employee benefits
- Manages human resource processes

- Establishes a staff development department
- Monitors orientation, inservice, and continuing education
- Evaluates staff development needs
- Conducts educational and orientation sessions
- Coaches employees
- Determines employees competence

Overlap Areas

- Provides leadership and management in human resource development
- Makes recruitment and selection decisions
- Establishes and manages a comprehensive human resource system

organizations are moving forward to address the current shortage, efforts also need to be directed at the development of new practice models and changes in organizational systems, processes, and practices that enhance nurses' ability to successfully perform nursing work. Changes in health care and nurse reimbursement systems will also need to be addressed. According to Parsons and Stonestreet (2004), factors that have been closely linked with nurse retention "coalesce into two categories: the quality of administrative management systems and quality of relationships with physicians, managers, peers, and administrators" (p. 111). Bower and McCullough (2004) suggested that the development and use of technology will have to be expanded if nurses are to be used to their fullest.

According to the literature, in order to truly address and effectively manage the changes needed relative to this current nurse shortage, partnerships will have to be formed among health care organizations, educational programs, professional organizations, and collective bargaining groups (ANA, 2002; AHA, 2001; Nevidjon & Erickson, 2001; Prescott, 2000). In order to achieve the outcomes desired, extensive data analysis, strategy design, and policy changes will be required.

In addition, administration will need to evaluate its organizational structure and scope of assignment for managerial staff, as nurses repeatedly report that lack of managerial presence and support is a significant dissatisfier (Peterson, 2001). Managerial staff, specifically, need to be aware of the ongoing support and development requirements of new nurse graduates. Managers need to work with experienced staff to develop mentorship and/or preceptor models that promote the development of new graduates. Managers further need to work with support staff (staff educators and clinical specialists) to develop unit-based registered nurse staff with skills and knowledge about how to manage workload and be accountable for outcomes while promoting growth of nonnurse caregivers and other support staff (Nevidjon & Erickson, 2001).

To meet the current and future demand for nurses and to create stability in the workplace, greater efforts will have to be directed at recruiting minorities, including males, into the profession. Nurse managers need to explore all opportunities to fill vacant positions. Special attention will need to be directed at retention of qualified, experienced staff. This can be accomplished in a number of ways. One approach that is strongly supported in the literature is to survey staff and to plan institutionally-based recruitment and retention strategies jointly with staff (Kuhar et al., 2004).

Numerous strategies shown to be effective in both recruitment and retention have been outlined in the literature. It is therefore imperative that the nurse manager has a working knowledge of these strategies and uses them in the work setting. It is also important that the culture within an organization is one that supports and promotes professional nursing practice, nursing autonomy, quality patient care, and interdisciplinary collaboration as a means of achieving organizational outcomes. Another strategy is the recruitment of foreign nurses. Although recruitment of foreign nurses provides a nurse to fill a permanent position, care must be taken in this endeavor, since it is not without its drawbacks (Daniel et al., 2000). Recruiting a foreign nurse takes time, approximately 2 years, and it is an expensive process (Gamble, 2002). There are several countries that produce an abundance of nurses, for example, the Philippines. Although many of the Filipino nurses speak English, their understanding of the language and of U.S. culture is often limited (Daniel et al., 2000). Clearly, the addition of any new employee brings about a change in the culture or sense of community; adding a nurse from a different culture increases the stresses in the work environment while at the same time enhancing cultural diversity (Flynn & Aiken, 2002; ICN, 2001). Bringing in a foreign nurse into an organization can be quite successful, but adequate planning and development of staff is required. According to Flynn and Aiken (2002) "increased recruitment of international nurses, without fundamental changes in the practice environment, will not help to solve the nursing shortage" (p. 68) or necessarily decrease nurse burnout.

Job dissatisfaction has been linked with nurse turnover or intent to leave (Aiken et al., 2001). Upenieks (2003) and Flynn and Aiken (2002) recommended that, in light of the nursing shortage, nurse administrators and managerial staff work to ensure that organizational attributes and professional nursing practice environments are as consistent as possible with practices identified by the Magnet studies and Magnet hospitals. According to AHA (2001), in order to maintain an adequate workforce, hospitals will have to actively address issues related to work design and the work environment.

Finally, nurse managers must work closely with their HR department to ensure effective and timely recruitment of nurses and to develop incentive programs that will assist in retaining and recruiting nursing staff. Managers can expect support from the HR department relative to turnover data, demographic information of nursing staff per unit/division, compensation information, job classification, work analysis, personnel management, and leadership and management education. Working with physician groups is another important partnership because nurses have consistently identified concerns over lack of perceived value by physicians as a major dissatisfier (Kuhar et al., 2004; Rosenstein, 2002). As McClure and colleagues (1983) reported in the Magnet study, nurses value a collaborative relationship with physicians and expect to be recognized and consulted by physicians for the contributions they bring to the management of patients.

CURRENT ISSUES AND TRENDS

The current nursing shortage is driven by a number of factors, such as lack of an adequate supply of students, increased aging of the registered nurse workforce, increased demand for nurses within and outside of health care, and generational differences in nurses related to their intention to stay in nursing (AHA, 2001;

Buerhaus et al., 2000). In addition to the shortage of nurses, health care is facing a reduction in all health care workers, both professional and nonprofessional (AHA, 2001). The overall shortages of health care workers are driving organizations to use higher-cost contractual labor. The costs associated with contractual labor, as well as changing reimbursement, increased higher consumer demand for and use of technology, increased numbers of chronically ill aging patients, and the high intensity of care services required are significantly affecting the cost, quality, and demand for health care service. Nursing care has been strongly linked to both quality and cost; yet organizations are struggling to establish an environment and culture that promotes job satisfaction and retention of nurses (Parsons & Stonestreet, 2004). Many of the recruitment practices within hospitals have proven to be counterproductive to nurse satisfaction, such as sign-on bonuses (Gamble, 2002); therefore greater attention will need to be given to nurse preferences if organizations plan to stabilize the workforce in the future.

As identified in the literature, nurse managers play a key role in both retention and recruitment of staff. The nurse manager's leadership style plays a major role in setting the tone for the unit and/or establishing a culture of retention. Manion (2004) defined a culture of retention as "an environment where people want to stay . . . or that meets peoples' needs" (p. 30). Manion, based on her research with nurse managers, described five themes and associated activities relative to the manager's role that contribute to the establishment of a culture of retention. These themes and related activities are as follows:

1. Put the staff first
  1.1 Listen and respond
  1.2 Appreciate and recognize
  1.3 Support
2. Forge authentic connections
  2.1 Get to know them
  2.2 Create a sense of community
  2.3 Hire the right people
  2.4 Have fun together

3. Coach for—and expect—competence
    3.1 Set high standards
    3.2 Support development
    3.3 Model behavior
    3.4 Manage performance
4. Focus on results
    4.1 Solve problems
    4.2 Empower and involve staff
    4.3 Provide adequate resources and a pleasing physical environment
5. Partner with staff
    5.1 Visibility
    5.2 Accessibility
    5.3 Set clear boundaries
    5.4 Communicate openly (pp. 30-39)

These themes were also supported in research related to retention conducted by Parsons and Stonestreet (2004) with staff nurses. It is clear from the literature that considerable work needs to be done within nursing services and health care administration in order to establish a community/culture of caring and safety/security for nurses and other health care providers. People, for the most part, want to be able to go to work each day with a sense of pride and respect for their contributions. In return, they expect to be treated with respect and have a sense of security within the job and work environment. It is projected that this area of study and the application of related strategies will be a major thrust in the future. This approach is consistent with the Magnet Recognition Program by the ANA (2003), the AHA report *In Our Hands* (2002), and the IOM report *Crossing the Quality Chasm* (2001).

Summary

- Nursing retention issues are strongly associ-ated with job satisfaction and an aging work force.
- The nursing shortage has long-term implications for quality patient care and hospitals' ability to provide services.
- In order to meet future nursing demands, changes will have to occur at the supply side, as well as policy formulation at the state and national levels.

- Recruitment processes are clearly defined and amenable for use by both management and staff.
- Nurse recruitment is driven predominately by staff turnover rates.
- Nurse retention strategies based on the Magnet studies have proven to be successful.
- Retention rates to be effective must be multi-faceted.
- Use of sign-on bonuses for the new employee as incentives for recruitment has resulted in an unstable and often unretained staff.
- Foreign nurse recruitment is a way of stabilizing staff turnover, but it is not without its own set of problems.
- The Philippines is one country that actively promotes, for its own economic benefit, nurses as expatriates.
- Staff turnover and related costs can be calculated by the nurse manager or reported by the HR department as a way of tracking and trending issues at the unit level.
- Nurse managers need to work closely with the HR department to ensure an adequate flow of candidates for selection and hire.
- Instruments and methods for measuring staff concerns or perceptions relative to job satisfaction and/or intent to leave are available for use by the nurse manager.
- Partnerships among health care organizations, schools of nursing, and industry/private business sector that have focused on changing the image of nursing as a career are having a positive impact on students and career switchers.
- Nurse managers and physician relationships play major roles in retention of nurses.
- Culture of retention and community have been repeatedly reported by nurses to be of value relative to intent to leave and staff retention.

Study Questions

1. What are the common recruitment practices in your community? Which entice you?
2. Which retention strategies are most effective? Do these vary by cohorts of nurses?
3. Who are the logical partners for nurses in recruitment and retention initiatives?

4. What areas of the country have the greater vacancy rates and/or turnover of staff and what impact does this have on the delivery of services within the region, community, and/or institution?

5. What are the strengths and weaknesses related to hiring of international nurses as a means of addressing the nursing shortage in the United States?

6. What is the view of the ANA and ICN relative to the use of international nurses within the United States?

7. What are the major factors/domains that affect quality care as defined by the Institute of Medicine and American Nurses Association?

8. What are some of the recruitment and retention strategies developed/posed by the ANA to address quality-of-care concerns?

9. What impact has the delineation of Magnet characteristics and the movement toward Magnet Recognition had on recruitment and retention of nurses within organizations?

10. What is the role of human resources relative to recruitment and retention of nurses?

11. What influence (positive or negative) do nurse managers and RN peers/colleagues have relative to recruitment and retention of nurses?

12. Why is it important to understand generational difference relative to recruitment and retention of RNs?

13. What are some of the strategies that have been shown to have the greatest impact on positive recruitment and retention of RNs?

14. What impact have the reports on the current and future nursing shortage had on legislative decisions and public awareness?

CASE STUDY

Todd Samuelson, the nurse director (ND) for the intensive care unit, is reviewing the annual (FY2006), vacancy and turnover data for the four units that he manages: (1) Cardiac Care (CCU), (2) Cardiac Stepdown (CSU), (3) Medicine Intensive Care (MICU), and (4) Medical Stepdown (MSU).

The data reveal a vacancy rate of 30% and a turnover rate of 46% in the last two quarters for the MICU and MSU, respectively. The vacancy and turnover rates for the CCU and CSU are 8% and 10% in both of these units. Further review of the data from the previous fiscal year (FY2005) indicated that both the MICU and MSU have been increasing volume 4% to 6% incrementally for the past 18 months. In addition, the personnel costs have increased exponentially over the last 12 months, and medication error rates and staff injury are at an all-time high for the two units. Physician complaints have also increased. Prior to meeting with Alicia Stone, the nurse manager (NM) responsible for two of the units, Nurse Samuelson arranged a meeting with Jody George, the nurse recruiter (NR) in the Human Resources Department.

At the meeting with Ms. George, Nurse Samuelson carefully reviewed the number and types of full-time (FT) and part-time (PT) RN positions open in the MICU and MSU, as well as the turnover data for each job classification. The information obtained showed that 7.6 positions, 4 FT and 8 PT, are open in the MICU; and 3.8 positions, 3 FT and 3 PT, are open in the MSU. During the discussion Nurse Samuelson paid careful attention to the role of both Ms. George and Nurse Stone in the recruitment and retention processes. Ms. George reported that 35 RN applications were forwarded to Nurse Stone to review and request for interview. To date, only 12 RNs had been interviewed, and only 6 (4 in MICU and 2 in MSU) have been hired in the last 6 months.

During this same period three nurses had resigned or transferred from each of the two units. Nurse Samuelson's dialog with Ms. George also revealed that the NM responsible for these two units, Nurse Stone, had been making the decisions for interview and hire without input from the staff on either unit and that the application review process took at least 4 weeks before a decision regarding the interview was made. This delay had resulted in numerous RNs withdrawing their application and/or obtaining another job prior to being contacted for interview. Ms. George also reported that agency nurses and travelers have expressed frustration and dissatisfaction with the care on the unit and the way they are being treated by staff. Nurse Samuelson queried Ms. George to determine whether this information had been shared with Nurse Stone on the units. The response was yes. Review of retention strategies implemented on the units by Ms. George and/or Nurse Stone revealed that food had been provided on occasion when staffing was extremely tight, but no proactive actions (e.g., staff survey to identify needs and concerns, recognition activities for outstanding staff performance or contributions, staff involvement in the recruitment process, preceptor usage, or mentorship offerings) have occurred. Nurse Samuelson asked Ms. George to put together a table outlining the recruitment and retention activities that have occurred over the past 2 years for a meeting in the next week with Nurse Stone and the staff members.

Nurse Samuelson next met with the NM of MICU and MSU, Nurse Stone, to discuss the issues related to high vacancy and turnover rates. At the meeting Nurse Samuelson inquired about the level of concern Nurse Stone had related to these statistics and asked her to discuss strategies that have been put into place to increase the hiring and decrease the turnover on both of these two units. Nurse Stone reported that she is getting poor response from Ms. George relative to the specialty requirements for critical care nurses. She also reported that the relationship between her and Ms. George is less than positive, noting that interviews are not set up quickly and that salary offerings are late in coming. This makes it difficult to get back with the RN applicant in a timely manner. Nurse Stone reported that staff involvement in the recruitment and retention process has been limited due to the high staffing needs and overtime worked. Staff attitudes have been less than positive of late, and from Nurse Stone's perspective, asking staff members to be involved in addition work responsibilities would further inflame them. In addition, extensive use of agency nurses and travelers has already resulted in a negative personnel budget variance.

Nurse Stone further stated that she did not bring this problem to Nurse Samuelson because she was hoping to have it resolved in the near future.

After the meeting with both Ms. George and Nurse Stone, Nurse Samuelson next approached the staff to determine their concerns and responses to the nurse vacancy and turnover rates on the units. The staff revealed that although there were a number of open positions, Nurse Stone had been good about giving them time off when requested and that agency nurses and travelers were filling in for the most part. However, use of supplemental staff often cut into their ability to work overtime, something that they all did as a way of increasing their monthly salary. Several of the staff blamed the agency nurses and travelers for the increase in error rates, noting that they were too busy to monitor everything that happened on the units. The staff also indicated that many of the new RNs who had joined the staff were not a "good fit" and left within a few weeks or months of hire. When asked about their role in precepting the new RNs, only one nurse indicated that she had taken an active role as both a preceptor and mentor with three of the new RNs, only one of whom decided to stay. Staff attitude and lack of support was reported by this nurse preceptor as the major reason for decreased retention of new hires. Another reason given for the high rate of turnover was a lack of training support for nurses with limited medical intensive care experience and/or knowledge. Staff reported that developing staff took time away from care giving and suggested that it needed to be provided off-unit by staff educators or clinical nurse specialists.

After the interviews, Nurse Samuelson formulated an analysis outlining the strengths, weaknesses, opportunities, and threats (SWOT) on each of the units relative to the recruitment and retention of staff. To implement change, Nurse Samuelson established a unit-based work group on each of the units because an action and implementation plan with defined outcome goals and timeline was needed.

CRITICAL THINKING EXERCISE

As a nurse manager of a cardiac critical care unit (CCCU), Maria Gonzales is struggling to retain qualified experienced nurses who are being recruited to work at a new cardiac care hospital that has just recently opened in the community. She has been asked to present a retention plan to the chief nurse officer (CNO). In preparation for the plan, Nurse Gonzales becomes aware that more then 65% of the registered nurse staff in the CCCU have 15 or more years of experience and employment at the current institution. However, these nurses are at the top of the pay scale in their job classification. In addition, 25% of the RNs have less than 1 year of experience. The complexity of the patient population is continuing to change, requiring greater use of technology, so traditional continuing education is no longer an option for staff. Based on this and other information available, Nurse Gonzales develops a plan that she believes will maximize retention and ensure stabilization of the unit.

1. How would Nurse Gonzales go about determining staff perceptions relative to job satisfaction and preferred retention strategies?
2. What department would Nurse Gonzales work with to determine common retention practices used in the community and RN pay scales for experienced CCCU nurses in the community/region?
3. Where would Nurse Gonzales go to get data relative to the CCCU patients—populations served, year-to-date volume, complexity of care requirements, treatment requirements, etc?
4. Who else in the organization could Nurse Gonzales partner with in addressing this issue?
5. What do you think might be Nurse Gonzales' final recommendations to the CNO?

REFERENCES

Aiken, L.H., Sloan, D.M., & Klocinski, J.L. (1997). Hospital nurses' occupational exposure to blood: Prospective, retrospective, and institutional reports. *American Journal of Public Health, 87*(1), 103-107.

Aiken, L.H., Clarke, S.P., Sloane, D.M., Sochalski, J.A., Busse, R., Clarke, H., et al. (2001). Nurses' reports on hospital care in five countries. *Health Affairs, 20*(3), 43-53.

Aiken, L.H., Clarke, S.P., Sloane, D.M., Sochalski, J., & Sibler, J.H. (2002). Hospital nurse staffing and patient mortality, nurse burnout, and job dissatisfaction. *Journal of American Medical Association, 288*, 1987-1993.

American Hospital Association (AHA). (2001, January 23). *Workforce supply for hospitals and health systems: Issues and recommendations*. Chicago: AHA. Retrieved June 28, 2004, from *www.hospitalconnect.com/ahapolicyforum/ resources/workforce010123.html*

American Hospital Association (AHA). (2002). *In our hands: How hospital leaders can build a thriving workforce*. Chicago: AHA.

American Nurses Association (ANA). (2001). *Nursing organizations to hold summit to address quality of care, staffing issues and the emerging shortage* [ANA press release]. Washington, DC: ANA. Retrieved June 28, 2004, from *www.nursingworld.org/pressrel/2001/pr0907a. htm*

American Nurses Association (ANA). (2002). *Nursing's agenda for the future: A call to the nation*. Washington, DC: ANA.

Retrieved June 20, 2004, from *www.nursingworld.org/ naf/indexb.htm*

American Nurses Association (ANA). (2003). *Magnet recognition program: Recognizing excellence in nursing service*. Washington, DC: American Nurses Credentialing Center.

Atencio, B.L., Cohen, J., & Gorenberg, B. (2003). Nurse retention: Is it worth it? *Nursing Economic$, 21*(6), 262-268, 299.

Bower, F.L., & McCullough, C. (2004). Nurse shortage or nursing shortage: Have we missed the real problem? *Nursing Economic$, 22*(4), 200-203.

Buerhaus, P., Staiger, D., & Auerbach, D. (2000). Why are shortages of hospital RNs concentrated in specialty care units? *Nursing Economic$, 18*(3), 111-116.

Cohen, J.A., Palumbo, M.V., & Ramur, B. (2003). Combating the nursing shortage: Vermont's call to action. *Nursing Leadership Forum, 8*(1), 3-12.

Curran, C.R. (2003). Nurse recruitment: A waste of postage, paper, and people. *Nursing Economic$, 21*(1), 5, 32.

Daniel, P., Chamberlain, A., & Gordon, F. (2000). Expectations and experiences of newly recruited Filipino nurses. *British Journal of Nursing, 10*(4), 256-265.

DDI. (1997). *LearningLinks: Your guide to using DDI technology to enhance performance*. Pittsburgh: Development Dimensions International, Inc.

DDI. (2004). *Targeted Selection^R: Access^R*. Pittsburgh: Development Dimensions International, Inc. Retrieved November 29, 2004, from *www.ddiworld.com/products_ services/targetedselectionaccess.asp*

Dictionary.com. (2004a). *Recruitment* definition. Los Angeles: Lexico Publishing Group LLC. Retrieved May 24, 2004, from *www.dictionary.reference.com/search?q=recruitment*

Dictionary.com/retention. (2004b). *Retention* definition. Los Angeles: Lexico Publishing Group, LLC. Retrieved, January 8, 2005, from *www.dictionary.reference.com/search?q=retention*

Erickson, J.I., Holm, L.J., & Chelminiak, L. (2004). Keeping the nursing shortage from becoming a nursing crisis. *Journal of Nursing Administration, 34*(2), 83-87.

Flynn, L., & Aiken, L.H. (2002). Does international nurse recruitment influence practice values in U.S. hospitals? *Journal of Nursing Scholarship, 34*(1), 67-73.

Gamble, D.A. (2002), Filipino nurse recruitment as a staffing strategy. *Journal of Nursing Administration, 32*(4), 175-177.

Goodin, H.J. (2003). The nursing shortage in the United States of America: An integrative review of literature. *Journal of Advanced Nursing, 43*(4), 335-350.

Henriksen, C., Page, N.E., Williams, R., II, & Worral, P.S. (2003). Responding to nursing's agenda for the future: Where do we stand on recruitment and retention? *Nursing Leadership Forum, 8*(2), 78-84.

Hoffman, F.M. (1984). *Financial management for nurse managers.* Norwalk, CT: Appleton-Century-Crofts.

Institute of Medicine (IOM). (2001). *Crossing the quality chasm: A new health care system for the 21st century.* Washington, DC: National Academies Press.

International Council of Nurses (ICN). (1999). *Nurse retention, transfer and migration.* Geneva, Switzerland: ICN. Retrieved June 21, 2004, from *www.icn.ch/psretention.htm*

International Council of Nurses (ICN). (2001). *Ethical nurse recruitment: Position statement.* Geneva, Switzerland: ICN. Retrieved May 23, 2004, from *www.icn.ch/psrecruit01.htm*

Jernigan, D.K. (1988). *Human resource management in nursing.* Norwalk, CT: Appleton & Lange.

Kramer, M., & Hafner, L. (1989). Shared values: Impact on staff nurse job satisfaction and perceived productivity. *Nursing Research, 38*(3), 172-177.

Kuhar, P.A., Miller, D., Spear, B.T., Ulreich, S.M., & Mion, L.C. (2004). The meaningful retention strategy inventory: A targeted approach to implementing retention strategies. *Journal of Nursing Administration, 34*(1), 10-18.

Laschinger, H.K.S., & Wong, C. (1999). Staff nurse empowerment and collective accountability: Effect on perceived productivity and self-rated work effectiveness. *Nursing Economic$, 17*(6), 308-316.

Lipsey, J. (2004). *Targeted selection.* Omaha, NE: Leadership Solutions, LLC. Retrieved June 28, 2004, from *www.leadsolutions.com/ts_article.htm*

Manion, J. (2004). Nurture a culture of retention. *Nursing Management, 35*(4), 29-39.

Manion, J., & Bartholomew, K. (2004). Community in the workplace: A proven retention. *Journal of Nursing Administration, 34*(1), 46-53.

McClure, M.L., Poulin, M.A., Sovie, M.D., & Wandelt, M.A. (1983). *Magnet hospitals: Attraction and retention of professional nurses.* Kansas City, MO: American Nurses Association.

Needleman, J., Buerhaus, P., Mattke, S., Stewart, M., & Zelevinsy, K. (2002). Nurse-staffing levels and the quality of care in hospitals. *New England Journal of Medicine, 346,* 1715-1722.

Nevidjon, B., & Erickson, J.I. (2001, January 31). The nursing shortage: Solutions for the short and long term. *Journal of Issues in Nursing, 6*(1), Manuscript 4. Retrieved June 28, 2004, from *www.nursingworld.org/ojin/topic14/tpc14_4.htm*

Nursing Executive Center. (2001). *Destination nursing: Recommitting to health care's greatest profession.* Washington, DC: The Advisory Board Company.

Parsons, M.L., & Stonestreet, J. (2004). Staff nurse retention: Laying in groundwork by listening. *Nursing Leadership Forum, 8*(3), 107-113.

Peterson, C. (2001, January 31). Nursing shortage: Not a simple problem-No easy answer. *Journal of Issues in Nursing, 6*(1), Manuscript 1. Retrieved June 28, 2004, from *www.nursingworld.org/ojin/topic14/tpc14_1.htm*

Prescott, P. (2000). The enigmatic nursing workforce. *Journal of Nursing Administration, 30*(2), 59-65.

Rosenstein, A.H. (2002). Nurse-physician relationships: Impact on nurse satisfaction and retention. *American Journal of Nursing, 102*(6), 26-34.

Senge, P. (1990). *The fifth discipline: The art and practice of the learning organization.* New York: Currency and Doubleday.

The HMS Group. (2002). Acute care hospital survey of RN vacancy and turnover rates in 2000. *Journal of Nursing Administration, 32*(9), 437-439.

Upenieks, V. (2003). Recruitment and retention strategies: A magnet hospital strategies prevention model. *Nursing Economic$, 21*(1), 7-13, 23.

U.S. Department of Health and Human Services (USDHHS). (2002). *Projected supply, demand, and shortage of registered nurses: 2000-2020.* Rockville, MD: USDHHS, Health Resources and Services Administration, Bureau of Health Professional & National Center for Health Workforce Analysis. Retrieved June 28, 2004, from *www.bhpr.hrsa.gov/healthworkforce/reports/rnproject/report.htm*

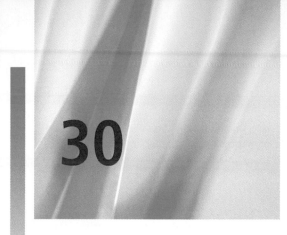

30

Performance Appraisal

Lynne S. Nemeth Kimberly Y. Harris-Eaton Karen Weaver

CHAPTER OBJECTIVES

- Define and describe performance appraisal
- Explain factors that drive the need for effective nursing performance
- Describe how organizational culture can catalyze changes in performance
- Discuss the roles and expectations of interdisciplinary team members in the process of performance appraisal
- Review performance appraisal criteria critically, considering reliability and validity in measurement
- Relate the role of leadership in performance appraisal, contrasting the need for effective staff development with the process for performance appraisal
- Exercise critical thinking to conceptualize and analyze possible solutions to a practice exercise

anaging the performance of people is an important organizational strategy designed to exceed expectations of consumers in today's competitive health care environment. Many complex processes and strategies are involved in managing employee behavior. Managers need to be clear in defining the roles and expectations that are needed in the variety of settings in which individuals provide their efforts in return for compensation. Managers need to be actively engaged in several performance management activities that will enable the staff they employ to achieve goals, such as providing a sustainable source of motivation; communicating the important issues that affect performance; being available to problem-solve issues that arise for the individual who may experience conflict or difficulty following established procedures; and using critical skills in providing a fair appraisal of the individual's abilities, talents, and opportunities for improvement.

DEFINITIONS

Performance is defined as the execution of an action; something accomplished; the fulfillment of a promise, claim, or request (*Merriam-Webster's Collegiate Dictionary*, 1997). Leading staff to accomplish the goals and responsibilities inherent in a specific position requires clear communication, effective observation and feedback in a concurrent manner, coherent performance criteria, and the ability to reflect organizational mission, vision and values.

Performance appraisal means evaluating the work of others. Albrecht (1972) defined **conventional performance appraisal** as a systematic, standardized evaluation of an employee by the supervisor, aimed at judging the perceived value of the employee's work contribution, quality of work, and potential for advancement. The employee's work is measured against standards, and in

▲ LEADING & MANAGING **DEFINED**

Conventional Performance Appraisal

A systematic, standardized evaluation of an employee by the supervisor, aimed at judging the value of the employee's work contributions, quality of work, and potential for advancement.

Peer Review

The examination and evaluation of practice by the employee's associate.

Self-Evaluation

A self-assessment of employee's own perceptions regarding performance according to stated expectations.

that sense it is very much like the quality assessment process. Standards, whether explicit or not, are applied to what ought to be or to what is superior, excellent, average, or unacceptable performance. **Peer review** in nursing is defined as the examination and evaluation of practice by a nurse's associates (Christensen, 1990). **Self-evaluation** is the aspect of performance appraisal whereby employees do self-assessments of their own perceptions about their performance as compared with stated objectives and expectations.

PERFORMANCE APPRAISAL PROCESS

Performance appraisal is a required process in organizations to ensure that the quality of care is met and to provide a fair human resources management process. Feedback is needed by all staff

employed in a designated role. Performance appraisal uses formal and informal methods to provide staff members with the information necessary to determine whether they are meeting expectations or can do better to improve their performance to the level that is required.

The process of performance appraisal includes assessing needs and setting goals, establishing the objectives and the time frame, assessing the progress and evaluating the performance, and then starting over again (Figure 30.1). At the start of a new job, an employee is assessed as to knowledge and skills. In the orientation program, progress will be assessed and tracked and then evaluated periodically throughout employment.

Performance appraisal is cyclical. It begins when the employee is hired and ends when the employee leaves. Job analysis should identify

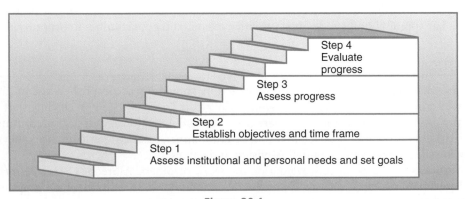

Step 4
Evaluate progress

Step 3
Assess progress

Step 2
Establish objectives and time frame

Step 1
Assess institutional and personal needs and set goals

Figure 30.1
Four steps of a performance appraisal.

competencies required for job performance. Next, the job description should specify work standards and the knowledge, skills, and abilities necessary for the job. The performance appraisal then identifies behaviors and employee traits deemed critical by management and compares job performance to critical criteria. A variety of measurement methods may be used. Performance appraisal using interview and goal setting are conducted, corrective action may be taken, or training needs may be identified. Cyclical processing and iterative improvements enhance the functioning of the system. Outcome criteria include equitable rewards and recognition that are objectively administered using valid tools (Frank, 1998).

The performance appraisal process is both informal and formal. The informal process includes day-by-day supervision or coaching to moderate, modulate, or refine small parts of performance. Coaching is an approach to developing people in an organization that falls somewhere between preceptoring and mentoring. The term *coach* invokes a sports metaphor. Every team relies on a coach to help the athlete(s) reach full potential. Coaching as a management tool is ongoing, face-to-face collaboration and influence to improve skills and performance. By contrast, the formal performance appraisal should include written documentation and a formal interview with follow-up.

The employee's work is measured against some standard for the purposes of determining the level of quality of the job performance. The guides to evaluation criteria include governmental standards, such as Medicare/Medicaid regulations, professional standards published by the American Nurses Association or other specialty organization, nursing care audits, opinion polls, client feedback in various forms, and departmentally developed standards. Ideally, a performance appraisal measures performance and motivates the person. However, performance appraisal is not the only or major source of motivation for most nurses. Measuring performance is not at all easy, and motivating someone else is an art. To combine those things in a performance appraisal that may have negative connotations is a challenging endeavor.

There are integral components of a comprehensive performance appraisal system that provide an overarching framework for the process. The tools and methods for a comprehensive performance appraisal system involve a clear determination of the abilities required for the position (job description); a match of the key requirements for the position with the individual's capabilities (personnel selection); development of the abilities of the employee (staff development); and using a motivational reward system to enhance employee performance (reward system) (Nauright, 1987). Box 30.1 outlines the key components of the performance appraisal process.

Performance attributes of an individual are determined by two elements: ability and motivation. Ability is made up of a collection of physical and mental capacities that enable a person to exhibit a skill or set of skills. Knowledge, experience, and skill form the ability to successfully complete a task (Hersey et al., 2001). Thus ability is an innate capacity that is molded by experience and training. Motivation is a willingness to work and a desire to achieve. Motivation influences the vigor and diligence with which an individual applies his or her capability to a task (Nauright, 1987).

Performance management includes processes of human resources management. There are several purposes for this system. For the employee, these include job productivity, compensation, job performance recognition, and planning for professional development. For the organization, they include worker requirements, job analysis, compensation

---

Box **30.1**

Components of a Comprehensive Appraisal System

- Determine the ability required (job description)
- Match abilities of the employee with job requirements (personnel selection)
- Improve employee's abilities (staff development)
- Enhance employee's motivation (staff development and reward system)

administration, training needs analysis, and employee promotion or discipline evaluation. Performance management is focused on the job, involves continual evaluation, and is participative. As a major component of the system, performance appraisal is done for evaluation purposes (Frank, 1998).

Organizational Culture as a Catalyst to Improving Performance

Given the national concerns about patient safety and quality of care, examination of the concept of organizational culture as a factor influencing performance appraisal for change and improvement can add value toward such efforts. The change of an error-prone health care system involves leadership and organizational learning, which requires significant strategic commitment and administrative direction. An environment that values and creates shared vision and purpose can lead to reflection and learning, that then enables and strengthens organizational culture toward creative and effective solutions in health care delivery (Carroll & Edmondson, 2002).

Culture consists of shared norms, behaviors and values. Schein (1992) defined the culture of a group as "a pattern of shared basic assumptions that the group learned as it solved its problems of external adaptation and internal integration, that has worked well enough to be considered valid and, therefore, to be taught to new members as the correct way to perceive, think, and feel in relation to those problems" (p. 12). Culture is "the integrated pattern of human knowledge, belief and behavior that depends on man's capacity for learning and transmitting knowledge to the succeeding generations; the set of shared attitudes, values, goals and practices that characterizes a company or corporation" (*Merriam-Webster's Collegiate Dictionary*, 1997, p. 282). Culture consists of "the predominating attitudes and behavior that characterize the functioning of a group or organization" (*The American Heritage Dictionary of the English Language*, 2000, online). The learning that occurs within the system over time influences organizational culture.

The quality of care and the quality of work life are driven by the culture within a health care organization (Gershon et al., 2004). Culture is reflected in "the way things are done" in an organization (Stetler, 2003), and it surrounds all individuals and influences leadership. Characteristics of the culture are manifested differently in subgroups and by the various stakeholders within the organization, which warrant more in-depth assessment to fully understand (Nemeth, 2005).

Subcultures and Stakeholders

Socialization of new members into an organization is an important way to learn the rules and norms of a group. New members need to learn the assumptions of the group, which are not always transparent. Group behaviors and perceptions may reveal some elements of the culture, and some of the rituals and processes undertaken within the organization may reflect the assumptions that are held. Groups that are stable and have a history of shared learning are likely to have developed some degree of culture, but groups with significant turnover of members and leaders may lack shared assumptions (Schein, 1992). Organizational culture has been referred to as the social glue that binds the organization, in which the deeper meanings of the way things are done in the organization are learned (Cameron & Quinn, 1999; Detert et al., 2000).

Evaluation of organizational culture should consider both the larger organization and the smaller unit within which a member belongs. Exploring the microsystem within a health care system reveals the unique disciplinary focus of each department and treatment setting (Donaldson & Mohr, 2000). The performance characteristics of academic departments, clinics, and hospital units and departments highlight the different functions and shared assumptions that members bring to the patient care setting. These varying perspectives enrich the mix of the organization by enabling diverse contributions, attitudes, and skills to be developed.

Members of a larger organizational culture may also belong to subcultures within that organization, whose group learning over time may have generated very different sets of basic assumptions. Behavior and language of organizational members are subject to interpretation through the cultural biases of the subgroup. Conflict may be experienced when members of the subculture do not understand the biases within the larger culture or vice versa. Using an organizational cultural approach to conflict management would enable subcultures to examine the assumptions that underlie the behavior and reinterpret such conflict as the result of diverse experiences. Problem-solving issues that are based on different assumptions, with the intent to evaluate the utility of such differences, demonstrates an effective learning process (Nemeth, 2005).

The criteria for performance appraisals should include measures of key performance indicators that reflect the values of the organizational culture. With these characteristics embedded within appraisal tools, managers can craft the culture within the unit. If there is not an explicit organizational mission, vision, or value statement, managers must translate their vision and values into a clear framework that all can understand. This framework should provide the structure for staff to operationalize the required behaviors for successful performance. The scoring of the performance appraisal tool indicates the weight that these organizational culture characteristics contribute toward performance, which communicates the importance of those to the overall appraisal.

Goals for Performance Appraisal

The most direct goal of any performance appraisal system is the improvement of performance. Considering the process of performance appraisal systems, the outcome for the system should lead to positive organizational outcomes. Used effectively, the performance appraisal offers the opportunity for numerous organizational goals to be achieved. Box 30.2 provides an overview of the goals of the process of performance appraisal.

Roles and Expectations of Team Members

There are numerous stakeholders within the process of performance appraisal of nurses. Most important, the voice of the patient, who is

---

Box 30.2

Goals of Performance Appraisal

- Improve performance
- Improve communication
- Reinforce positive behavior
- Communicate about and, ultimately, correct negative or less-than-optimal behaviors
- Provide a basis for rewards, which also is a basis for motivation
- Provide a basis for termination if necessary
- Identify learning needs and develop personnel

---

the end consumer of the care provided, must be considered within the overall process that is used to evaluate the performance of nurses. The patient's voice can be obtained from patient satisfaction data that are formally used within the organization. Often, the patient or family member will offer direct verbatim comments that can be used to provide constructive support to individuals or groups. Nurse managers should seek out the comments of the patient regarding the patient's experience of care. Through this proactive process, the manager may find that the voice of the patient regarding specific exceptional staff members or those who may need to improve can provide useful input for managing staff behavior.

The peers of the nurse, who are coworkers in the setting where the nursing care is delivered, are individuals who have the opportunity to know firsthand how well the individual meets patient care needs and how well the individual is able to meet his or her responsibilities as a member of the team. These peers include the staff members who may work on the same shift or alternate shifts or the nurses who may interact with the individual from the perspective of another unit's function. Those nurses generally have the experience of direct communication about the patient's status, and they know the specific expectations of care that are required in the individual setting. For example, a nurse may work on a unit that receives patients frequently from the emergency department or the recovery room, and there are bilateral communications and expectations that these staff members have of one another. These are key individuals who interact with the nurse and may be in an excellent position to provide input related to performance. Although this may not be a customary source of performance appraisal input, it may be a worthwhile source to consider.

The interdisciplinary team members who count on the nurse also have expectations for the nurse to communicate and collaborate regarding the plan of care and inform key members of the need to become involved in assisting the patient. For example, social workers or therapists may rely on referrals from the nurse who has made an initial assessment of the patient's needs. If key criteria for referrals are clearly identified but not implemented, then the interdisciplinary care plan for the patient may not be developed as effectively as is needed. Interdisciplinary team members need to work together on behalf of the patient's needs, not within their own disciplinary silos. Nurse managers need to think about acquiring input from the perspective of the key interdisciplinary team members that provide services within the specific unit or department.

Physicians also have expectations that the nurse will follow through on the orders that are prescribed for patient care, observing the patient for critical changes in condition and communicating any changes that warrant more intensive physician interventions. Physicians thus can provide feedback in the process for performance appraisal of staff. There are multiple levels of physicians and other medical staff members in the hierarchy. The most effective clinical areas seek to establish a collaborative and inclusive process so that all clinical care can be guided by a strong base of supportive relationships. To develop this level of support requires the mutual trust and respect among the physician teams that provide care within the specific area. This would include ongoing communication regarding opportunities for improved performance by staff and physicians alike.

Administrative members have expectations that are more global in nature, but essentially they require that individual staff have the knowledge of policies and procedures that must be implemented in the care of patients. With numerous stakeholders, it is important that systematic processes guide the nursing management function of performance appraisals. With data being collected from numerous sources in a systematic way, a more meaningful performance appraisal process can be achieved.

Manager's Role

The management style of the person in charge is frequently cited by nurses when asked why they are leaving the nursing profession (Parse, 1997). The performance appraisal process provides the opportunity for managers to articulate and identify individual staff values and talents that bring them to the team. Parse identified reverence for others as an essential concept that differentiates managers from leaders. *Reverence* is defined as "honor or respect felt or shown" (*Merriam-Webster's Collegiate Dictionary*, 1997, p. 1002). The manager, who has learned to lead with reverence, respects the talents of others and is proud to offer opportunities for others to advance without fear of being overshadowed (Parse, 2004).

The nursing population is growing older. In 2003, the average age of a nurse was 44.5, and some predict the average age will be 50 by the year 2020 (Letvak, 2003). The nursing profession must develop new leaders, and a powerful tool to accomplish this is the performance appraisal. Nurse managers who have learned to lead with reverence use the performance appraisal process as an opportunity to mentor and coach their staff into new experiences.

Ideally, upon filling a nursing position, the manager meets with the employee during a planning stage to discuss the tasks, objectives, competencies, and performance characteristics. The preparation of the planning stage is an integral step in the performance management process because it allows the manager to clearly communicate what is expected of the employee (McKirchy, 1998). Clarity is essential in the performance appraisal process, and the manager has the duty to provide this to all staff members.

This process allows the individual to talk specifically about his or her performance goals and to come to agreement with the manager on reasonable performance expectations.

Many managers will include staff self-appraisal as an important component in the appraisal process. This is a valued aspect of the process because it promotes individual input, personal responsibility, and feedback regarding job performance. Appraisal is a structured process of facilitated self-reflection, which allows individuals to review their professional activities comprehensively and to identify areas of real strength and need for development (Conlon, 2003).

It is imperative to provide staff members with adequate time to participate in the performance appraisal process. A schedule for conducting performance appraisals must be consistent and clear. Managers who create a healthy work environment offer adequate time for feedback and input. If the concept of reverence is important for mangers in the performance appraisal, the concept of self-esteem may shed some light on the perspective of the staff member. Audit and feedback are important mechanisms to provide objective data to the nurse regarding the quality of care provided. To improve clinical practice and motivate nurses to learn from the audit experience, individual self-esteem must be at a level that promotes motivation (Ward, 2003). The imperative for nurse managers is to recognize that the use of feedback in the performance appraisal process may influence an individual's self-esteem, which may affect practice. Providing feedback is a delicate art of nursing management, which should be managed to encourage and motivate the individual to improve his or her individual care provision.

Melding Multiple Sources of Input

Incorporating the input of peers also must be handled carefully because the opinions of peers often substantially influence a person's self-esteem (Ward, 2003). Many organizations include the input of peers in the performance appraisal process. This allows managers to determine whether there are consistent opinions regarding the employee's job performance. Objectivity cannot ever be presumed in reviewing the input of others, and when there are differences of perceptions, the manager is in the position of determining the final score for the performance appraisal. This process must be used judiciously to avoid creating conflict among staff members and management (Arnold & Pulich, 2003).

Individual self-appraisal, as well as peer and other stakeholder input, provide a mechanism for a 360-degree performance appraisal that enables a wider perspective beyond what the individual manager can provide to the staff member. Organizational cultures that encourage the use of 360-degree feedback do so to provide a learning opportunity for the individual. Financial rewards are not necessarily tied to 360-degree reviews, but development opportunities are to be gained through this method, which is a more important outcome. A key decision in the process of using 360-degree feedback is whether to keep the process as a confidential process or have it be one in which the person being evaluated knows or selects peers and subordinates to participate in the review.

Performance Appraisal Criteria and Retention

Performance-based career advancement systems provide a means to recognize and reward clinical expertise in direct patient care roles. Differentiated practice models enable employee development and higher performance at a level consistent with individual interest and motivation. For those nurses who seek a higher level of professional contribution, these systems can provide a mechanism for compensation that is based on additional performance and effort. The Vanderbilt Professional Nursing Practice Program is an example of a program that was designed to attract, retain, and reward nurses (Robinson et al., 2003).

A supportive environment is one of the key factors related to the success of professional nursing practice models. In the 1990s, large system redesign and reengineering occurred in many hospital systems, which decreased the numbers of full time equivalent employees (FTEs) in many institutions.

Research Note

Source: Drach-Zahavy, A. (2004) Primary nurses' performance: Role of supportive management. *Journal of Advanced Nursing, 45*(1), 7-16.

Purpose

Few studies have evaluated the outcomes of staff performance in primary nursing systems and the role of supportive management practices in primary nursing systems. This study evaluated how the role of the manager impacts the performance of primary nurses, conducted in a hospital in Haifa, Israel.

Discussion

A cross-sectional survey was designed to examine the impact of primary nursing on the performance of nurses and to evaluate the impact of supervisor support and the perceived costs of seeking support. The study aimed to develop a predictive model regarding the performance of primary nurses. Surveys (n = 520) were distributed in 56 nursing units from six major hospitals in Israel. Returned surveys totaled 368, indicating a response rate of 71%. Primary nursing was rated using a 5-point Likert scale, with the items representing different types of support. Supervisors rated nurses' performance using a 7-item measure to provide an overall evaluation of performance and professional competence. A moderating model was used in which the independent variable (primary nursing) was used to examine the effect of the dependent variable (nurses' performance), along with the moderating variables of supervisor support and the costs of seeking support. A hierarchical regression analysis was used to compute the predictors regarding nursing performance in primary nursing environments. Primary nursing was not associated with nurses' performance, but supervisor support was seen to be positively associated with it. The highest levels of primary nursing practice were seen in areas where the supervisor's support was the highest.

Application to Practice

The study highlighted a model that used structure, process, and outcome variables to predict performance of nurses in a primary nursing professional model. The structure is the primary nursing model of care delivery, the processes are supervisor support and nurses' perceptions regarding the costs of seeking such support, and outcomes are nursing performance in such a system. Supervisor support was seen as efficient in improving the performance of primary nurses. A social exchange framework helps to explain the bilateral commitments that are made by both employees and supervisors in such a system. With the supervisor's support, stress can be reduced and the increased responsibility and accountability that is needed to be effective in a primary nursing system can be seen. When nursing models are changed, supportive interactions by nurse managers can lead to higher performance by nurses. This suggests that more autonomy and support provided by the nurse manager can lead to higher motivation and performance levels by nurses. Empowerment and support can be combined to augment the performance levels of the nurse.

Many systems merged several units under the scope of responsibility of one nurse manager (NM), who often had to manage more than 80 employees. Nurse managers had a mixed reaction to this movement. On the one hand, they were flattered that the organization had increased the importance of the NM role. However, the overall result to the nurse manager was a feeling of being pulled away from the bedside to focus on staffing issues and management problems. NMs believed that they should be more visible on the units to set direction and address issues and concerns for the staff members to come together as a team. Although nurse managers believed they were needed on the unit by their staff, their increased responsibilities made it difficult to be visible at the bedside. To address this issue, many institutions have decreased the scope of responsibility of the nurse manager to enable a more consistent presence on the unit. This has enabled nurse managers to have the time to work with their staff and be able to evaluate staff members' performance in a more effective manner.

Performance Appraisal Criteria

It is essential to set expectations regarding job criteria and performance as soon as the nurse begins employment. The organization should have the employee sign the performance tool as a planning stage for the performance criteria that are to be met and provide a copy for the employee to refer to throughout the year. Armed with clear expectations, the employee should understand how he or she will be rated at the end of the evaluation year.

It is a challenge for a manager to maintain objectivity when conducting performance appraisals. Because of the wide variety of individuals in the workforce and increased diversity of cultures, there may be instances of personality conflicts with the manager and the employee. Employees may feel that the manager dislikes them and therefore is biased about their performance (Arnold & Pulich, 2003).

There are potential problems that may impede a manager from performing a fair evaluation on an employee. Arnold and Pulich (2003) described the following potential problems, called *sources of error,* related to perception that may incorrectly influence managerial ratings on performance appraisals:

- *Recent behavior bias:* Occurs when the rater remembers behavior primarily from the most recent period of the employee's performance period as opposed to the entire rating period
- *Horn effect:* Occurs when a manager perceives one negative aspect about an employee or his or her performance and generalizes it into an overall poor appraisal rating
- *Halo effect:* Occurs when a manager perceives one positive characteristic about an employee or his or her performance and generalizes it into an overall high rating
- *Similar-to-me effect:* Occurs when a manager rates the employee performance higher when a person is accurately or inaccurately perceived to have the same characteristics as the manager

Developing skill in assessment and interview techniques is a key to effective performance appraisal. Asking questions can elicit important evaluative data. Using a coaching process means studying present behavior and developing planned, purposeful change strategies or intermediate multiple small steps to bring performance closer to what is desired. Coaching uses constant communication and clear consequences. Coaching becomes the management of consequences by praising, reprimanding, and redirecting (Hersey et al., 2001). A process of the employer and employee establishing mutual goals contributes to improved performance.

A distinction can be made between counseling, coaching, and mentoring. *Counseling* addresses problem performers such as employees whose work is consistently substandard, those who regularly miss deadlines, or those who are uncooperative, insubordinate, absent, or tardy. The problem needs to be brought to the employee's attention, the employee given time to respond, and specific actions to improve performance agreed on. *Coaching* involves all employees in improving their ability to do their job and increase future potential. Activities include role modeling, hiring carefully, encouraging growth, creating a positive environment, using praise, and encouraging stretch goals. *Mentoring* is for employees who show promise and is used to shorten learning curves and increase productivity. Developmental needs demand a greater commitment. The closer the link between the employee's needs and the mentor's competencies, the more likely it is that the mentorship will be productive. Mentoring requires mutual trust and respect (Stone, 1999).

The more explicitly the performance criteria are stated, the less conflict is generally experienced in the scoring. Reliability of scoring on an institutional basis can be enhanced by stating the extent of the performance required to achieve specific ratings. In specific position descriptions, the behaviors that are needed to score a rating of "meets expectations," "exceeds expectations," or "substantially exceeds expectations" can be elaborated. This methodology sets a standard that is institution-wide and provides clarity and consistency among nurse managers on different units.

An example of evaluation criteria associated with each job task is shown in Figure 30.2 for the Clinical Nurse Coordinator employed in the Operating Room at the Medical University of South Carolina. These criteria were developed to enable a new hire or an employee transferring to a unit to have a clear understanding of the expectations and what the employee will need to do to reach each level.

ALTERNATIVE TYPES OF PERFORMANCE APPRAISAL

To minimize factors of bias in the performance appraisal, the manager should utilize other methods to perform a fair evaluation of performance on each employee. Some of these alternative methods include the following:

- *360-degree evaluation:* The 360-degree evaluation can be obtained by seeking input from approximately four sources: (1) a peer, (2) a physician, (3) a subordinate, and (4) a self-evaluation. Once all the input is obtained, the evaluating manager adds his or her input and merges the feedback to develop the final score. The 360-degree evaluation tends to be more applicable in evaluating advanced practice roles or a management positions because of the diverse interactions that staff in these roles have. For evaluation of the staff nurse role, this may not be as effective because the expectations may be for a more uniform standard of performance.
- *Peer review:* In this process, employees rate the performance of others in the same job classification, utilizing objective criteria that have been established. Input is provided to the manager by a Peer Review Committee. The manager then incorporates the feedback into the person's evaluation along with the manager's comments. The negative aspect of this process is that staff may feel that members of the Peer Review Committee are not fair in their assessment of other staff members' abilities. Peer review is

most applicable for evaluating staff positions in which a common set of expectations and performance standards exists, because the staff members who work with one another are best suited at having the core knowledge about the quality and nature of the work performed by the individual. An effective peer review system may offer the individual honest and specific feedback that allows that person to make specific adjustments in his or her role to better meet objectives and performance standards.
- *Management by objectives:* In this method, the employee and manager establish performance goals for the upcoming appraisal year. This process is difficult and not effective for evaluating the entry-level nurse. As the nurse develops and gains more experience this process, management by objectives may be helpful in defining goals and objectives for the next year and providing the manager with a specific set of goals to follow up with the individual on at regular intervals.

RELIABILITY AND VALIDITY IN MEASUREMENT

Reliability and validity are important considerations in any system of measurement. Tools must be constructed so that the score one rater would give would be consistent with another person's rating. If the criteria are developed in a manner that is clear and observable, they are more likely to lead to increased interrater reliability. Performance appraisal tools should be tested by several raters who, using the same criteria on the same person, would rate observable performance consistently. If two raters were recording their observations on the same person using the same tool, there should be equivalence of the results. This would indicate a highly reliable tool.

To test the reliability of a tool involves examining the amount of random error. The characteristics of the tool must be dependable, consistent, accurate, and comparable (Burns & Grove, 2001). Stability of the performance criteria demonstrates consistency with repeated measures of the same tool.

Job Purpose:		
Clinical Nurse Coordinator (CNC)		
The CNC on the _____ Unit reports to the Manager. Under general supervision, the CNC provides individualized, goal-directed patient care to families and patients at the competent level utilizing the principles and practices of the nursing process, delivers safe and effective care, and interacts with other members of the health care team to achieve desired results.		
Part A **JOB TASKS** **Job Tasks and Objectives (optional)** account for 70% of the performance evaluation rating.	 **% weight**	**Performance Level** S(4) E(3) M(2) B(1) **weight × rating = score** **(use whole number not percentage weight in this calculation)**
1. Job Task (E): **Clinical Practice (Assessment)** Manages comprehensive nursing care for patients (within specialty area) whose needs range from uncomplicated to complex and rapidly changing. **Success Criteria:** a. Based on holistic assessment, identifies relevant aspects of the situation and determines the appropriate course of action and reports abnormal findings to appropriate members of interdisciplinary team. b. Assesses subtle changes in patient status; anticipates problems before they occur and implements measures to minimize risk. c. Begins to become a resource person	20%	**Evaluation Criteria:** **1a.** 4. Always coordinates and follows through on completion of Perioperative Record. Demonstrates greater individualization of plans of care. 3. Demonstrates greater individualization of patient care. Regularly recognizes exceptions/additions; consistently revises plan of care. 2. Completes admission assessment and consistently updates plan of care. Prioritizes and follows through on patient needs. 1. Inconsistently completes assessment. Fails to identify all patient needs. Does not implement a complete standard of care. Cannot prioritize patient needs. **1b.** 4. Adapts to rapidly changing complex needs and takes appropriate action. Consistently tailors plans to meet complex patient needs and follows through

Figure 30.2   *Continued*

Clinical nurse coordinator (CNC) evaluation criteria. (Courtesy Medical University of South Carolina, Charleston, SC.)

Nurse managers who are comfortable with a performance appraisal tool should be able to measure the same person at multiple intervals in a stable and consistent manner. This is referred to as *test-retest reliability.*

Establishing equivalence is a more complex process that involves direct observation of specific processes at the same time by different individuals. The percentage of agreement is computed to derive interrater reliability. Perfect interrater reliability would be demonstrated if two individuals rated all performance criteria consistently. The lowest acceptable coefficient for reliability would be 0.80 (Burns & Grove, 2001).

for case-specific procedures, positioning devices, sterilizers, and equipment.

d. Actively reports and troubleshoots discrepancies in patient care, equipment, and instruments.

e. Exhibits knowledge of sterilizers and functions.

f. Understands, implements, and monitors patient safety guidelines.

to desired outcomes.

3. Demonstrates greater age-appropriate individualization of plans; regularly notes exceptions/additions; consistently revises needs list.

2. Patient needs list developed; reflects both patient/family needs.

1. Does not implement standards of care.

1c.

4. Independently works with interdisciplinary team. Documents all personal and positioning devices. A resource person.

3. Assists others to work with interdisciplinary team. Documents all personal and positioning devices.

2. Provides, identifies, and uses proper equipment, instruments, and positioning devices for case-specific procedures.

1. Consistently fails to identify, use, and provide proper equipment, instruments, and positioning devices for case-specific procedures.

1d.

4. Excels in patient care and immediately recognizes any discrepancies and antici-pates needs of team members to take corrective action. Knows the operation of most pieces of equipment/instruments in the operating room and can be a resource to others.

3. Monitors the patient and recognizes problems immediately and takes corrective actions. Consistently advocates for patient. Able to troubleshoot pieces of equipment/instruments within specialty and be a resource for others.

2. Recognizes discrepancies in patient care and reports to proper team member. Checks and/or tests equipment/instruments before time of use.

Figure 30.2—Cont'd

Clinical nurse coordinator (CNC) evaluation criteria. (Courtesy Medical University of South Carolina, Charleston, SC.)

The validity of a tool is the determination of the extent that the tool is measuring the construct that is under evaluation. Evaluation tools must capture the critical behaviors and outcomes that result from effective nursing care. The term *construct validity* is used to establish that the criteria are appropriate, meaningful, and useful in measuring what they are intending to measure. There is no guarantee of perfect validity, and to define validity in a specific tool often takes many years.

To provide objective measures to ensure that staff members are evaluated fairly, both the reliability and validity of the evaluation tool must be established. Drawing from recent research regarding performance appraisal and variance in measurement, generalizability theory (GT) has been

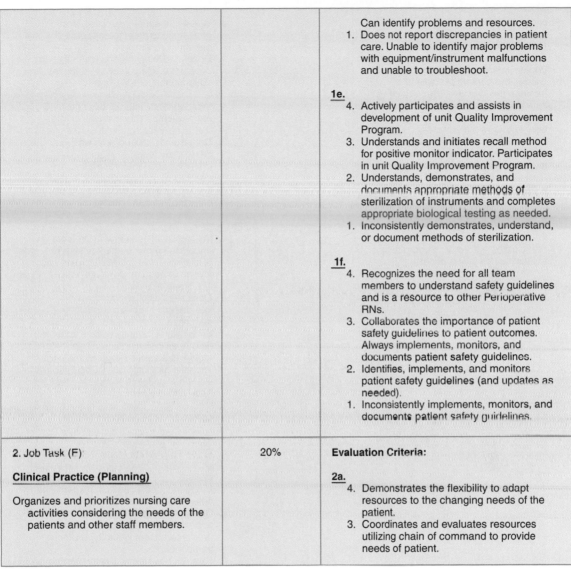

| | | Can identify problems and resources.
1. Does not report discrepancies in patient care. Unable to identify major problems with equipment/instrument malfunctions and unable to troubleshoot.

1e.
4. Actively participates and assists in development of unit Quality Improvement Program.
3. Understands and initiates recall method for positive monitor indicator. Participates in unit Quality Improvement Program.
2. Understands, demonstrates, and documents appropriate methods of sterilization of instruments and completes appropriate biological testing as needed.
1. Inconsistently demonstrates, understand, or document methods of sterilization.

1f.
4. Recognizes the need for all team members to understand safety guidelines and is a resource to other Perioperative RNs.
3. Collaborates the importance of patient safety guidelines to patient outcomes. Always implements, monitors, and documents patient safety guidelines.
2. Identifies, implements, and monitors patient safety guidelines (and updates as needed).
1. Inconsistently implements, monitors, and documents patient safety guidelines. |
| **2. Job Task (F)**

Clinical Practice (Planning)

Organizes and prioritizes nursing care activities considering the needs of the patients and other staff members. | 20% | **Evaluation Criteria:**

2a.
4. Demonstrates the flexibility to adapt resources to the changing needs of the patient.
3. Coordinates and evaluates resources utilizing chain of command to provide needs of patient. |

Figure 30.2—Cont'd

Continued

used to describe the variability that is associated with multisource ratings (Greguras et al., 2003). As more employment settings undertake the use of multiple raters providing feedback for performance appraisal systems, it is important to understand the nature of the feedback and consider the reliability of the sources used to provide this feedback. It has been demonstrated that when ratings are used for administrative purposes, the scores have tended to be less reliable than those scores used for development of the person being rated.

Generalizability theory provides a framework for examining the dependability of behavioral measurement of the rater. As the information that has been obtained for the performance appraisal is compiled, the final rater must take into

Success Criteria:

a. Provides leadership to develop, analyze, integrate complex data, and update individualized plan of care.
b. Utilizes the nursing process to facilitate the individualized plan of care using time and resources efficiently, and assumes accountability for plan's effectiveness. Coordinates care with the interdisciplinary members consistent with roles and responsibilities.
c. Designs, implements, and evaluates a comprehensive, culturally sensitive, patient plan of care.
d. Uses professional judgment to appropriately delegate and follow through.
e. Participates with service coordinators to individualize plans of care.

2. Utilizes personnel, supplies, and equipment to meet the needs of the patient.
1. Does not identify needs completely or does not utilize personnel, supplies, and equipment appropriately.

2b.

4. Independently intervenes, follows through, and evaluates effectiveness of interdisciplinary team.
3. Consistently collaborates with interdisciplinary team.
2. Identifies and facilitates referral for services of other disciplines.
1. Fails to address needs of the patient and impedes function of other disciplines.

2c.

4. Initiates inservices and/or projects to (increase) improve efficient staff resource utilization. Takes initiative to plan and follows through on complex patient needs in a timely manner.
3. Consistently collaborates with interdisciplinary team to evaluate patients plan of care with regards to Cultural Sensitivity. Efficiently utilizes suitable resources including people and materials.
2. Identifies appropriate problems and implements a care plan. Documents and evaluates patient's progress in the intraoperative setting.
1. Inconsistently plans and implements a comprehensive patient care plan.

2d.

4. Takes appropriate action related to failure of team members to perform delegated tasks.
3. Delegates and follows up on activities delegated to ensure plan is carried out.
2. Consistently able to delegate safely and appropriately to other members of the health care team including assistive personnel.
1. Fails to consistently delegate and/or uses

Figure 30.2—Cont'd
Clinical nurse coordinator (CNC) evaluation criteria. (Courtesy Medical University of South Carolina, Charleston, SC.)

consideration the variance due to the person being evaluated, the items being evaluated, and the interaction of the rater with the person being evaluated. For peers and subordinates there may be a substantial amount of variance (Greguras et al., 2003).

When compiling the information that is used to complete the performance appraisal, the rater must take into account the following factors affecting the reliability and validity of the ratings:

• The way the information is communicated, either verbally or in writing
• How the information is organized
• The potential influence of the relationship the rater has with the person being rated
• The cognitive ability of the rater

		ineffective interpersonal skills to delegate.
		2e. 4. Participates in identifying needs, creating tools, or revising existing tools to enhance knowledge and improve patient care. 3. Actively utilizes teaching/learning tools to improve patient outcomes. 2. Documents individualized plan of care. 1. Fails to participate with Service Coordinator to coordinate the individual plan of care.
3. Job Task (E): **Clinical Practice (Intervention)** Makes age-appropriate interventions based on individual patient needs. **Success Criteria:** a. Competently performs technical skills in area of practice. Demonstrates practice based on knowledge of hospital policies, procedures, nursing standards, and legal issues in areas of specialty. b. Coordinates and manages care by applying analytical reasoning, reflection, problem-solving skills, using age-appropriate information, and incorporating patient safety initiatives. c. Participates in shared decision making and problem solving to promote effective collaboration with interdisciplinary partners and to enhance own practice.	20%	**Evaluation Criteria:** **3a.** 4. Consistently performs technical skills with little or no supervision and functions as a clinical resource in the specified area of practice. 3. Practice consistently reflects awareness of hospital and departmental policy changes as well as "Current Standards and Recommended Practices" of AORN. 2. Completes and demonstrates in practice unit-specific competencies. 1. Inconsistent compliance with policies and procedures. **3b.** 4. Develops and implements a plan of care utilizing and coordinating appropriate resources. 3. Participates in plan of care and makes suggestions to enable a positive patient outcome utilizing appropriate resources. 2. Carries out plan of care consistently and safely. 1. Unfamiliar with patient problems and needs. Requires additional assistance with implementing plan of care.

Figure 30.2—Cont'd

Continued

LEADERSHIP AND MANAGEMENT IMPLICATIONS

Developing Staff Members Through Performance Appraisal

For managers, the performance appraisal process is an opportunity to gather insight about their staff. This is more than just a piece of paper that is addressed yearly; it is a process in discovering the individual's perception of his or her job. Managers who are leaders consider the performance appraisal as an opportunity to identify what motivates their staff members and also identify their values and interest.

Managers use the performance appraisal process as a way to translate organizational goals into concrete objectives for the individual employee to fulfill. Through a process of communication, coaching and development, employees are provided with feedback regarding how their performance fits

Text continued on p. 667.

		3c.
		4. Active member of committee or task force, participating in development of tools for improvement of patient care. 3. Uses critical thinking and appropriate resources to identify and/or anticipate problems. Regularly provides input to Manager and colleagues to improve departmental concerns and/or positive patient outcomes. 2. Consistently obtains patient care data from multiple data sources to generate and implement feasible patient care solutions. Regularly attends and participates in staff meetings and other unit meetings. 1. Does not participate in data gathering. Inconsistently attends staff and unit meetings.
4. Job Task (E): **Clinical Practice (Evaluation)** Uses established outcome measures to evaluate effectiveness of care. **Success Criteria:** a. Promotes effective and efficient use of Perioperative Standards of Care to promote achievement of best clinical outcomes that are targeted to age-specific populations.	15%	**Evaluation Criteria:** 4a. 4. Verbalizes and identifies all Perioperative Standards of Care, including criteria. Serves as a resource to other team members. 3. Utilizes all Standards of Care and documents appropriate outcomes. 2. Utilizes Standards of Care in daily practice. 1. Fails to utilize Standards of Care in daily practice.
5. Job Task (E): **Professional Development** Assumes personal responsibility for quality patient care, environment, and professional development.	10%	**Evaluation Criteria:** 5a. 4. Obtains formal education including conferences, workshop attendance, formal classes and presents to staff, service groups, and/or orientees. On self-evaluation lists strengths, weaknesses, and goals. Utilizes Employee Performance Management System (EPMS) as a professional growth tool. Attends 100% of all staff and educational offerings.

Figure 30.2—Cont'd
Clinical nurse coordinator (CNC) evaluation criteria. (Courtesy Medical University of South Carolina, Charleston, SC.)

Success Criteria:

a. Identifies own learning needs and seeks out resources to meet those needs, utilizing EPMS and self-evaluation. Demonstrates the insight and self-awareness necessary to recognize own impact on others and to change behavior accordingly. Accepts constructive feedback and uses it to improve performance. Attends and participates in staff meetings and Continuing Education opportunities.

b. Shares knowledge with interdisciplinary team to improve patient care and to contribute to overall unit functions.

c. Assists in the orientation of new staff members and students.

d. Demonstrates effective use of computer-based information for decision support, continuous quality improvement, and professional development.

e. Annually obtains six Continuing Education Units (CEUs) and provides documentation.

f. Able to communicate by hospital-based e-mail system.

3. Obtains formal education including conferences, workshop attendance, and formal classes. Completes self-evaluation and lists strengths, weaknesses, and goals. Attends 95% of all staff and educational offerings.

2. Identifies and follows through with additional educational opportunities. Completes self-evaluation and goals in a timely manner. Accepts constructive feedback and develops appropriate objectives to improve practice. Attends 85% of all staff and educational offerings.

1. Does not complete self-evaluation and/or provide goals. Does not seek out learning needs. Does not accept constructive feedback. Fails to attend 85% of all staff educational offerings.

5b.

4. Presents information or inservices on a yearly basis to staff and interdisciplinary team members.

3. Presents information at unit inservice.

2. Knows unit resources and administration personnel. Communicates problems and suggestions to appropriate personnel. Utilizes appropriate tools to document issues and concerns. Routinely participates in unit staff meetings. Arrives to staff meeting in a timely manner.

1. Fails to follow chain of command. Communicates problems to inappropriate persons and/or uses inappropriate manner.

5c.

4. Actively assists in orientee assignments to meet learning needs of specific service group. Assists with learning needs of students related to aseptic technique and patient safety.

3. Seeks out learning needs for new employees. Actively evaluates orientee performance. Assists students in meeting learning needs and goals.

Figure 30.2—Cont'd   *Continued*

<table>
<tr><td></td><td></td><td>

2. Demonstrates a positive attitude. Explains interdisciplinary team member roles and functions. Acts as a preceptor for new employees.
1. Demonstrates lack of a positive attitude in educating new staff members and students.

5d.
4. Utilizes additional computer resources to identify additional patient care resources (i.e., Oasis, PACS)
3. Notifies appropriate coordinator if changes are needed to computer-based preference cards/pick sheets. Utilizes computer programs to increase knowledge base.
2. Utilizes appropriate computer programs in daily practice, hospital-based e-mail and intranet, and CATTS. Updates surgeon preference books as necessary.
1. Does not utilize computer programs in daily practice.

5e.
4. Obtains greater than 9 CEUs.
3. Obtains 7-8 CEUs.
2. Obtains 6 CEUs.
1. Fails to obtain 6 CEUs.

5f.
4. Consistently communicates with interdisciplinary team by offering constructive unit improvements.
3. Communicates with interdisciplinary team members.
2. Utilizes hospital-based e-mail to check for education and/or unit updates.
1. Fails to communicate with hospital-based e-mail system.

</td></tr>
</table>

Figure 30.2—Cont'd

Clinical nurse coordinator (CNC) evaluation criteria. (Courtesy Medical University of South Carolina, Charleston, SC.)

◣ LEADERSHIP & MANAGEMENT BEHAVIORS

Leadership Behaviors

- Enables high level performance
- Inspires high performance in individuals
- Models desirable performance characteristics
- Evaluates performance
- Counsels followers with performance problems
- Motivates followers to improve knowledge and skills

Management Behaviors

- Evaluates performance
- Conducts performance appraisals

- Coaches subordinates
- Analyzes performance problems
- Corrects performance problems
- Disciplines employees
- Validates clinical competence

Overlap Areas

- Evaluates performance
- Takes corrective actions

6. Job Task (E):	10%	Evaluation Criteria:
Leadership Actively and effectively assumes leadership role in unit. **Success Criteria:** a. Demonstrates high standards of patient care and is a role model for others. b. Knows the roles of the inter-disciplinary team members and delegates appropriately to provide effective patient care c. Communicates with team members, service coordinators, and charge nurse in proactive manner, orally and in writing, to promote patient care. d. Promotes teamwork by facilitating positive group relationships. e. Demonstrates a spirit of service and cooperation in responding to needs of patients and co-workers, including ability to deal with stressful situations in a mature, positive manner. f. Participates in unit development by supporting change and offering suggestions; actions and decisions reflect an awareness of unit budget. g. Demonstrates a professional commitment to patients and staff by adhering to unit procedures, rules, and policies (including attendance and call). h Follows through on meeting patient needs and requests by using appropriate mechanisms.		**6a.** 4. Serves as a resource for staff, coaches others in decision making and actively serves on a committee. 3. Follows through on issues and concerns. 2. Adheres to the standards of nursing practice. 1. Fails to practice according to standards of nursing practice. **6b.** 4. Prioritizes/delegates well in stressful situations. Able to function as a nurse coordinator. 3. Sets appropriate priorities, holds others accountable for their actions. 2. Delegates appropriately to others. 1. Delegates reluctantly and/or inappropriately. **6c.** 4. Discusses issues and identifies problem solving solutions with appropriate surgical team members, utilizing communication skills. 3. Assertive communication, independent problem solving, through documentation. 2. Demonstrates ability to communicate effectively. Utilizes resources to problem solve. 1. Ineffective communication. **6d.** 4. Confronts barriers to positive group relationships. 3. Acknowledges, utilizes, and promotes the abilities of others. 2. Positive team player. 1. Creates barriers to teamwork.

Figure 30.2—Cont'd   *Continued*

with the expectations for the organization and the manager's vision regarding the culture of the individual microsystem. The manager identifies the strengths and weaknesses of the employee and provides recognition and support of positive behavior, as well as encouragement and specific recommendations regarding opportunities for improvement. The appraisal should show both the employee and the manager what the employee's possibilities for growth and development are.

All of the developmental activities that a manager provides to an individual employee should be aimed at helping the individual to better utilize his or her skills and improve performance on the current position or develop toward desired future opportunities for advancement. Leaders, supervisors, and managers who model preferred organizational behaviors, identified through the performance appraisal process, inevitably motivate staff to adapt desired outcomes.

i. Addresses problems and systems issues in a timely manner by contacting appropriate personnel through the proper chain of command.
j. Demonstrates and practices fiscal accountability for one's own practice while providing quality care.

6e.
4. Helps others effectively deal with stressful situations; demonstrates initiative and willingness to respond to the needs of others.
3. Proficient in stressful situations (i.e., codes, multiple admissions, staffing issues, interpersonal conflicts); collaborates/delegates effectively, positively.
2. Handles stress appropriately; helps without hesitation.
1. Unable to function effectively under stress, unwilling to help others.

6f.
4. Takes initiative to implement and facilitates positive change.
3. Identifies need for change; supports it.
2. Adapts to change with a positive, cooperative attitude.
1. Creates barriers to change.

6g.
4. Demonstrates exceptional flexibility with own schedule to meet unit needs.
3. Willingness to make adjustments to meet unit needs.
2. Adheres to unit Policies and Procedures expectations.
1. Noncompliant with policies and schedule.

6h.
4. Evaluates effectiveness; changes strategies as needed.
3. Makes extra effort to ensure follow through.
2. Meets patients needs in timely manner.
1. Fails to follow through on patient needs.

6i.
4. Evaluates and reassesses problems for a new plan of action.
3. Takes steps to develop a plan of action to resolve problems.

Figure 30.2—Cont'd
Clinical nurse coordinator (CNC) evaluation criteria. (Courtesy Medical University of South Carolina, Charleston, SC.)

The prevailing purpose of performance appraisal is to improve and motivate the staff, which in turn will enhance organizational effectiveness. This clearly identifies the performance appraisal process as a means to addresses institutional needs, as well as individual staff needs and abilities. The manager who uses the performance appraisal process effectively will become more capable in supporting, coaching, and managing the development of his or her staff members.

CURRENT ISSUES AND TRENDS

The appraisal of performance occurs at multiple levels. There appears to be a hierarchy of performance evaluation targets. At the individual level, performance is measured by a performance

		2. Addresses issues and problems by utilizing the proper chain of command. 1. Fails to contact appropriate personnel to address problems. **6j.** 4. Researches, implements, and evaluates ideas for cost-saving changes in practice. 3. Demonstrates a heightened awareness of costs to patient and institution. Formulates cost-saving measures. 2. Provides quality patient care while demonstrating fiscal accountability. 1. Inconsistently demonstrates fiscal accountability for practice.
7. Job Task (E): **Research and Evaluation** Participates in Performance Improvement/Research activities designed to improve patient care, and/or organizational processes. **Success Criteria:** a. Knowledgeable of Unit's Performance Improvement Projects/Research Activities. b. Actively contributes and participates in Unit-Based Performance Improvement Projects. c. Demonstrates spirit of inquiry through ongoing and systematic evaluation of care given to patients.	5%	**Evaluation Criteria:** **7a.** 4. Leads and evaluates Process Improvement Project/Research Activity. 3. Uses individual and unit data to make changes in patient care delivery systems. 2. Independently completes required hospital/unit audits, mandatories, computer-based competencies, and license. 1. Fails to complete required hospital/unit audits, mandatories, computer-based competencies, and license. **7b.** 4. Assists committee member/chair; promotes Continuous Quality Improvement (CQI) to colleagues. Identifies and seeks resources for study. 3. Willingly participates in unit/hospital studies. Completes 95% of assigned monitors. 2. Adheres to clinical protocols in ongoing studies. Completes 85% of assigned monitors.

Figure 30.2—Cont'd   *Continued*

appraisal. At the unit level, performance may be estimated using budget or quality criteria. At the organizational level, performance is appraised by accreditation review such as a Health Plan Employer Data and Information Set (HEDIS) or Joint Commission on Accreditation of Healthcare Organizations (JCAHO) accreditation. In turn, the JCAHO has been evaluated by the Inspector General of the Department of Health and Human Services (USDHHS), who criticized the JCAHO's oversight system. Thus performance review ranges from individual employee evaluations through unit and organizational quality reviews to the level of political accountability performance appraisals such as that done by the USDHHS. In fact, the analysis can be carried on to include performance appraisal of the USDHHS and its Inspector General by the President of the United States and the Congress. Ultimately, their performance is appraised by the U.S. voters.

	= 100%	1. Fails to consistently adhere to research protocols. Completes less than 85% of assigned monitors and chooses not to participate in projects and monitors. **7c.** 4. Initiates area for study; seeks resources, challenges effectiveness of treatment/care based on investigation and evaluation. 3. Identifies a need for investigation of chosen specific project (specify) and willingly participates in unit/hospital-wide studies. 2. Adheres to clinical protocols of ongoing projects/studies and explores reasons for perioperative care. 1. Fails to consistently adhere to clinical protocols, does not question perioperative care for its cause and effect.
	SECTION III, Part A Sum of Tasks (and OBJECTIVES SCORES) ÷ 100 = Total Tasks Score _____	

Figure 30.2—Cont'd

Clinical nurse coordinator (CNC) evaluation criteria. (Courtesy Medical University of South Carolina, Charleston, SC.)

Within an organization, performance appraisal of individuals and teams forms the core of management process control.

Performance appraisal is an activity that individuals do informally all the time. For example, restaurants and hotels solicit client feedback. For employees in an organization, part of a manager's job is to formally appraise the performance of employees. The process of managerial control includes doing evaluations. These are done for multiple purposes. For example, managers need to assess and determine the competency of staff personnel as one element of quality care. It is not sufficient to assume that because nurses are licensed, they are competent. Certainly to payers and consumers, the quality of caregivers is an issue. Regulatory agencies also are requiring proof of competency assessment. They look for evidence of staff in-service and the range of nursing

skills attained. The overall reason for the management step of evaluating and controlling is to measure the quality and effectiveness of nursing activities.

The current processes for appraising staff performance in health care environments need to be revisited. With the increased concern for patient safety exposed within the past 5 years (Institute of Medicine [IOM], 2000, 2001, 2003, 2004), the drive for a blame-free culture of safety, and current research regarding nursing-sensitive outcomes and nurse staffing (Aiken et al., 2002; IOM, 2004; Needleman et al., 2002), nursing managers and administrators have much to consider regarding how this process can be best crafted.

Considering the multitude of system errors that have been exposed during the last several years and the current emphasis by regulatory agencies for improvements in system performance and patient safety (JCAHO, 2004), nurses are in an extremely visible position at the forefront of health care delivery. The 44,000 to 98,000 deaths per year in American hospitals that were presented as evidence in *To Err Is Human: Building a Safer System* (IOM, 2000) provide the impetus for health care leaders to redesign safer systems of care. Errors occur when planned actions fail or when wrong plans are used to achieve unintended outcomes. Adverse events occur when health care interventions cause injury to the patient and are considered preventable (IOM, 2004).

Health systems managers and administrators need to consider that, in order to reduce errors that cause patient harm, a systems approach is needed. Recognition of the fact that human error is to be expected in all organization (Reason, 2000), combined with diligence to uncover the root causes of events that result in patient harm, is a management responsibility. Multiple factors in health care systems increase the vulnerability of the nurse to errors. The experience and educational background of the nurse, the supervision and feedback that the individual nurse receives daily in the process of care, and the maturity of the nurse to raise issues in the environment that pose a risk to safe patient care are factors to be considered. Nursing performance can be enhanced in an environment in which open and honest feedback to individuals is valued, shared leadership and decision making are encouraged, and a system is created whereby errors are discussed or risky situations are revealed by all participants. Nurse managers and leaders need to develop their staff members as critical "systems thinkers" who explore issues that negatively affect patient outcomes as well as job satisfaction. Critical "systems thinkers" are able to see the bigger context than their individual perspective within the subculture to which they belong. Individual goals and performance should be viewed within the context of how one interacts within a system, but clearly the competencies of the individual, as well as the behaviors that are enacted, must be developed and strengthened for optimal performance. Performance appraisal is one component of a performance management system used by organizations to motivate employees.

Summary

- Conventional performance appraisal systems are designed to measure performance and motivate personnel.
- Peer review is an examination and evaluation of practice by a nurse's associates.
- Performance is determined by two elements: (1) ability and (2) motivation.
- The most direct goal of any performance appraisal system is the improvement of performance.
- In health care, performance appraisal is done as a part of overall quality assessment.
- Performance appraisal may be conducted through personal, peer, or administrative/managerial evaluation.
- The process of performance appraisal includes assessing the needs and setting goals, establishing the objective and the time frame, assessing the progress and evaluating the performance, and then starting over again.
- Performance appraisal can have positive outcomes.
- Performance is measured from collected data. There are various methods and tools used.
- There are a number of evaluator rating errors.
- To be effective, a performance appraisal system needs to provide objective assessment of the knowledge, skills, and abilities of employees and also must enhance staff development.

Study Questions

1. What experiences have you had in the past with performance appraisals? Have those experiences been positive or negative? Why?
2. Why does the handling of the performance appraisal process leave an aftermath of feelings?
3. Think about those times when you were evaluated in a positive and constructive manner. Why was that a good experience?

4. How do you feel when you are expected to evaluate others? Why?

5. How are performance appraisal and quality improvement related?

6. How should pay, promotions, and other rewards be tied to performance and its evaluation?

7. How do you evaluate the performance of a team?

Interactive Group Discussion Exercise

A useful method to promote creative group interaction and discussion is role playing. Role playing allows participation in actual challenging situations. For this exercise, the readers are asked to conduct a mock performance appraisal. One participant will portray the role of employee and one will portray the role of manager. In preparation for this exercise, the employee will complete a self-evaluation and the manager will complete an evaluation. (Figure 30.2 can be used for this exercise.) Role playing will provide participants the opportunity to present different employee and management styles in a creative manner. This interaction should occur in a setting that promotes open dialogue regarding the performance appraisal process.

CASE STUDY

Julie Henderson, RN, BSN, was a nurse manager of PICU/Pediatrics at the Cleveland Clinic Foundation Children's Hospital in Cleveland, Ohio. She described her techniques for managing staff performance appraisal:

For a nurse manager, annual staff evaluations are a natural part of the job. Nurse managers, however, cannot always identify the positive and negative attributes of all members of the staff. I found this out in my first year as a nurse manager, when I had to write the annual evaluations for the entire staff.

The difficulty I encountered was in being able to describe the individual's performance throughout the year. I kept a log in which every 2 to 3 weeks I would write down my observations of

staff members' performance. I would also note any comments from patients or families and feedback from peers. Nurses, however, can sometimes be overly critical of their coworkers. Whenever something went wrong, as when a nurse did not follow a doctor's order, someone would make sure I was the first to know. If something positive happened, as when a nurse acted as a patient advocate or handled a difficult situation, I was usually the last to be informed. Thus, when it came time to write the evaluation, I had the data to write constructive criticism but was unable to include positive feedback or cite that special incident with a patient or family. Pointing out where a nurse excels is necessary so that the positive feedback can promote a healthy and hopeful work environment.

The following year I tried a different approach, peer evaluation, which I found to be more reliable. I gave each staff member two blank evaluations with a peer's name on each, so that each nurse evaluated two other nurses. Each nurse also received a blank evaluation form for self-evaluation. Guidelines for evaluation were provided and posted in the unit. Performance ratings were Exceeds Expectations, Achieves Expectations, or Needs Improvement. Staff members were instructed to cite examples of their peer's performance to support one of the three ratings. Matching up those being evaluated with those doing the evaluation required much planning on my part to avoid the bias that might arise from two nurses who were close friends.

As the staff turned in the evaluations, I reviewed the self-evaluation along with the two peer evaluations. I also continued to maintain my own log of observations and incidents. I used these to write my final evaluation for each staff member for the annual performance appraisal. Confidentiality was essential for the peer evaluations and self-evaluations, so that the feedback could be as honest and constructive as possible.

In the administration of the annual evaluations, the staff would ask me what others thought of their performance. This would give me the opportunity to relay the positive qualities that their

CRITICAL THINKING EXERCISE

Nurse Linda Gero has completed her first year as a nurse on a 17-bed orthopedic floor. During her first year she has worked 40 hours per week at a day-night position and has began to assume charge nurse duties. She arrives to work in a timely fashion and completes her tasks. Because she is shy, she avoids personal conversations. Her co-workers described her as quiet and a bit distant.

One evening Nurse Gero's nurse manger hands her a performance appraisal form and asks her to complete it by the end of her shift. Her nurse manager will be back in the morning to discuss the performance appraisal with her. Two of Nurse Gero's coworkers, picked by her manager, have already completed peer evaluations. This is the first time Nurse Gero had seen or heard about a performance appraisal. She attempts to finish her evaluation but is unclear about how to complete the form. In the morning, at the end of Nurse Gero's shift, her nurse manager asks her to come to her office to discuss her performance appraisal. During their discussion, her manager identifies that Nurse Gero has been described as distant and unapproachable by her coworkers. The manager continues by telling Nurse Gero that immediate improvement is necessary for her to remain in her position. Nurse Gero is stunned. She has never had a conversation with her manager regarding job performance before this moment. She signs the appraisal at her manager's request because she does not want to appear difficult. Nurse Gero leaves her unit distraught and confused.

1. What is the problem?
2. Why is it a problem?
3. Whose problem is it?
4. What should Nurse Gero do?
5. How should the problem be handled?
6. Describe the management and leadership style of Nurse Gero's nurse manager.
7. What parts of the performance appraisal process could be improved? How?

peers identified, which really helped to create a better team by clarifying everyone's expectations. Peer evaluations also helped identify suggestions for improvement and strategies for achieving it, such as a seminar on how to deal with difficult people.

The self-evaluations and peer evaluations often had similar comments. For example, one nurse had difficulty communicating with physicians. Both the nurse herself and her peers identified this problem, and her peers suggested how she might improve this skill. Together the nurse and I set goals for the upcoming year and focused on her communication skills. Throughout the year the rest of the staff and I worked with this nurse and noticed a marked improvement.

Peer and self-evaluations seem to have been successful in our unit by giving the staff a chance to think about the quality of performance and to critique their peers on a professional level.

REFERENCES

Aiken, L., Clarke, S., Sloane, D., Sochalski, J., & Silber, J. (2002). Hospital nurse staffing and patient mortality, nurse burnout, and job dissatisfaction. *Journal of the American Medical Association, 288*, 1987-1993.

Albrecht, S. (1972). Reappraisal of conventional performance appraisal. *Journal of Nursing Administration, 2*(2), 29-35.

The American Heritage Dictionary of the English Language. (2000). Boston: Houghton Mifflin. Retrieved February 7, 2004, from *www.bartleby.com/61/11/C0801100.html*

Arnold, E., & Pulich, M. (2003). Personality conflicts and objectivity in appraising performance. *Health Care Manager, 22*(3), 227-232.

Burns, N., & Grove, S.K. (2001). *The practice of nursing research: Conduct, critique & utilization* (4th ed.). Philadelphia: W.B. Saunders.

Cameron, K.S., & Quinn, R.E. (1999). *Diagnosing and changing organizational culture: Based on the competing values framework.* Reading, PA: Addison-Wesley.

Carroll, J.S., & Edmondson, A.C. (2002). Leading organizational learning in health care. *Quality and Safety in Health Care, 11*, 51-56.

Christensen, M. (1990). Peer auditing. *Nursing Management, 21*(1), 50-52.

Conlon, M. (2003). Appraisal: The catalyst of personal development. *British Medical Journal, 327*(7411), 389-391.

Detert, J.R., Schroeder, R.G., & Mauriel, J.J. (2000). A framework for linking culture and improvement initiatives in organizations. *Academy of Management Review, 25*(4), 850-863.

Donaldson, M.S., & Mohr, J.J. (2000, November 3). *Exploring innovation and quality improvement in health care microsystems: A cross-case analysis.* Washington, DC: Institute of Medicine, National Academies Press. Retrieved November 25, 2004, from *www.nap.edu/openbook/NI000346/html/65.html*

Frank, B. (1998). Performance management. In J.A. Dinenemann (Ed.), *Nursing administration: Managing patient care* (2nd ed.) (pp. 461-484). Stamford, CT: Appleton & Lange.

Gershon, R.R.M., Stone, P.W., Bakken, S., & Larson, E. (2004). Measurement of organizational culture and climate in health care. *Journal of Nursing Administration, 34*(1), 33-40.

Greguras, G.J., Robie, C., Schleicher, D.J., & Goff, M. (2003). A field study of the effects of rating purpose on the quality of multisource ratings. *Personnel Psychology, Inc., 56*, 1-21.

Hersey, P., Blanchard, K.H., & Johnson, D.E. (2001). *Management of organizational behavior: Leading human resources* (8th ed.). Upper Saddle River, NJ: Prentice-Hall.

Institute of Medicine (IOM) (Ed.). (2000). *To err is human: Building a safer system.* Washington, DC: National Academies Press.

Institute of Medicine (IOM) (Ed.). (2001). *Crossing the quality chasm: A new health system for the 21st century.* Washington, DC: National Academies Press.

Institute of Medicine (IOM) (Ed.). (2003). *Priority areas for national action: Transforming health care quality.* Washington, DC: National Academies Press.

Institute of Medicine (IOM) (Ed.). (2004). *Keeping patients safe: Transforming the work environment of nurses.* Washington, DC: National Academies Press.

Joint Commission on Accreditation of Health care Organizations (JCAHO). (2004). *National patient safety goals.* Oakbrook Terrace, IL: JCAHO. Retrieved May 16, 2004, from *www.jcaho.org/accredited+organizations/patient+safety/npsg.htm*

Letvak, S. (2003). The experiences of being an older staff nurse. *Western Journal of Nursing Research, 25*(1), 45-46.

McKirchy, K. (1998). *Powerful performance appraisals: How to set expectations and work together to improve.* Franklin, NJ: The Career Press.

Merriam-Webster's Collegiate Dictionary. (10th ed.). (1997). Springfield, MA: Merriam-Webster, Inc.

Nauright, L. (1987). Toward a comprehensive personnel system: Performance appraisal—Part IV. *Nursing Management, 28*(2), 29-32.

Needleman, J., Buerhaus, P., Mattke, S., Stewart, M., & Zelevinsky, K. (2002). Nurse-staffing levels and the quality of care in hospitals. *The New England Journal of Medicine, 346*, 1715-1722.

Nemeth, L. (2005). *Implementing change in primary care practice.* Unpublished doctoral dissertation. Medical University of South Carolina, Charleston, S.C.

Parse, R.R. (1997). Leadership: the essentials. *Nursing Science Quarterly, 10*(3), 109.

Parse, R.R. (2004). Power in position. *Nursing Science Quarterly, 17*(2), 101.

Reason, J. (2000). Human error: Models and management. *British Medical Journal, 320*(7237), 768-770.

Robinson, K., Eck, C., Keck, B., & Wells, N. (2003). The Vanderbilt Professional Nursing Practice Program: part 1: Growing and supporting professional nursing practice. *Journal of Nursing Administration, 33*(9), 441-450.

Schein, E.H. (1992). *Organizational culture and leadership* (2nd ed.). San Francisco: Jossey-Bass.

Stetler, C.B. (2003). Role of the organization in translating research into evidence-based practice. *Outcomes Management, 7*(3), 97-103.

Stone, F.M. (1999). *Coaching, counseling & mentoring: how to choose & use the right technique to boost employee performance.* New York: AMACOM.

Ward, D. (2003). Self-esteem and audit feedback. *Nursing Standard, 17*(37), 33-36.

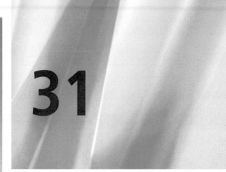

31

Prevention of Workplace Violence

L. Jean Henry   Gregory O. Ginn

CHAPTER OBJECTIVES

- Explain why violence in the workplace is a particular concern for nurses.
- Define the various terms associated with workplace violence.
- Discuss the legal, ethical, and economic costs of workplace violence in health care organizations.
- Identify the sources of and risk factors for violence.
- Give an overview of regulatory actions and NIOSH and OSHA recommendations to prevent workplace violence.
- Explain the relationship of various management frameworks and leadership in mitigating and preventing workplace violence.
- Explain the role of Human Resource Management policies and procedures in preventing workplace violence.
- Identify the legal issues concerning workplace violence.
- Discuss management actions necessary to provide a legal defense against claims arising from workplace violence.
- Exercise critical thinking and inquiry to conceptualize and analyze possible solutions to a practice exercise.

Violence in the workplace is a salient issue for nurses and others in the health care industry. The Department of Labor reported a workplace violence rate of 38 cases per 10,000 workers for nursing and personal care facilities. This is much higher than the rate of 3 cases for every 10,000 workers in private industry. The majority of nonfatal assaults that were reported occurred in service industries such as health care. Of those assaults, 27% occurred in nursing homes, 13% in social services, and 11% in hospitals. Health care and social service workers have the highest incidence of injuries from workplace assaults (National Institute for Occupational Safety and Health [NIOSH], 1996).

Assaults and threats of violence against nurses are prevalent throughout the world. Studies in the United Kingdom, Canada, and Australia also reported high rates of violence against nurses. The Australian Institute of Criminology cited the health care industry as the most violent industry in Australia (Henry & Ginn, 2002).

Violence in hospitals is due to a combination of internal and external factors. External conditions include an increasingly violent society, the availability of handguns, and high-crime neighborhoods. Many health care facilities are located in inner cities where crime rates are higher than average. Internal factors include inadequate staffing levels, larger numbers of dangerous patients, poor security for drugs and money, staff members working alone, poorly lit facilities, and unsecured, continuous access to health care facilities. Furthermore, the turbulent nature of the health care industry makes working conditions increasing stressful. Health care workers are often required to work in shifts that result in their coming and going at odd hours of the day when they are more vulnerable to crime (Bruser, 1998). The very nature of the jobs that nurses perform places them at high risk for workplace violence, and circumstances inherent in health care work increase workers' susceptibility to homicide or assault. Nurses often deal with people who are ill or injured. Nurses often infringe on patents' personal space, removing their sense of personal control. Many patients are in pain, emotionally disturbed, or cognitively impaired. Often, their families are experiencing strong emotions brought on by grief, catastrophic injuries, criminal victimization, or severe psychiatric disturbances (Edwards, 1999; Smith-Pittman & McKoy, 1999). Thus for a number of reasons, violence in the workplace is a particular concern for nurses.

From a public health perspective, it makes sense to approach workplace violence prevention in much the same way as other types of illnesses or injuries. However, from the perspective of an organization, the connection between workplace violence prevention and the attainment of broader organizational objectives such as financial performance may seem very tenuous. At the same time, the organization is uniquely situated to exert a powerful influence over the environment of the workplace, and because of its position, has far more ability to effectively reduce both the incidence and severity of incidents of workplace violence. Thus the issue is to convince organizations that (1) they can be effective in accomplishing a public health objective such as workplace violence prevention and (2) that the attainment of broader organizational objectives is very much facilitated by success in workplace violence prevention programs (Ginn & Henry, 2002).

DEFINITIONS

Violence may be defined narrowly to include only obvious acts of violence such as assault, battery, manslaughter, or homicide. NIOSH (1996) defined **workplace violence** as violent acts, including physical assaults and threats of assault, directed toward persons at work or on duty. The Center for Violence Prevention and Control (1996) identified violence as the intentional use of physical force that results in or has a high likelihood of resulting in injury or death.

Violence may be defined broadly to include verbal abuse, threats, and harassment (Carroll & Morin, 1998). Speaking in a hostile manner or adopting a threatening posture can be considered an assault. For workplace policy and procedures, it is important to define violence broadly (Elliot, 1997).

The cost of violence is significant. When broadly defined, violence can be enormously dysfunctional to an organization in terms of lost productivity due to absenteeism, low morale, emotional pain, anxiety, and turnover (Murray & Synder, 1991; Smith-Pittman & McKoy, 1999). One source estimates that the eradication of bullying in the workplace may increase productivity and profits by as much as 10% ("Violence Threatens the Workplace," 1998). When combined with other costs, such as lawsuits, lost productivity, higher insurance costs, and workers' compensation claims, the bottom line of workplace violence is an estimated $36 billion annually (Jossi, 1999).

Sources of violence vary. One source of violence is from criminals who have no other connection with the workplace but simply intend to commit a crime. A second source of violence is from customers, clients, patients, or students. A third source is from a current or former employee. A fourth source of violence is from someone who is not employed at the workplace but has a personal relationship with an employee, such as a spouse or domestic partner (Rugala & Isaacs, 2004).

Risk factors for violence in health care organizations include working with volatile people, understaffing, long waits, poor environmental design, lack of training, inadequate security, substance abuse, access to firearms, poor lighting, and unrestricted access by the public (NIOSH, 2002). Working in hospitals may be dangerous because of the availability of drugs or money in the pharmacy area, the necessity of working evening or night shifts in high-crime areas, and the availability

Violence

Narrowly defined: assault, battery, manslaughter, or homicide; broadly defined: ranging from verbal abuse, threats, and unwanted sexual advances to physical assault and homicide.

Workplace Violence

Violent acts directed toward persons at work or on duty.

Sources of Violence

Violent acts committed by (1) criminals who have no connection with the workplace; (2) customers, clients, patients; (3) current or former coworkers; or (4) persons not employed at the workplace but who have a personal relationship with an employee.

Risk Factors for Violence

Things that predispose a workplace to violence, including interpersonal elements, environmental characteristics and design, and organizational culture.

Environmental Designs

Provisions that include signaling systems, alarm systems, monitoring systems, security devices, security escorts, lighting, and architectural and furniture modifications to improve worker safety.

Administrative Controls

Measures that include adequate staffing patterns to prevent personnel from working alone and reducing waiting times, controlled access, and development of systems to alert security personnel when violence is threatened.

Behavior Modifications

Changes in behavior that provide all workers with training in recognizing and managing assaults, resolving conflicts, and maintaining hazard awareness.

Violence Prevention Programs

Programs that are available to all employees, track progress in reducing work-related assaults, reduce severity of injuries sustained by employees, decrease the threat to worker safety, and reflect the level and nature of threat faced by employees.

Violence Prevention Written Plans

Plans that demonstrate management commitment by disseminating a policy that all types of violence will not be tolerated, ensure that no reprisals are taken against employees who report or experience workplace violence, encourage prompt reporting of all violent incidents, and establish a plan for maintaining security in the workplace.

Worksite Analysis

A common-sense look at the workplace to find existing or potential hazards for workplace violence.

Hazard Prevention and Control

The implementation of work practices to prevent and control identified hazards.

Safety and Health Training

Education designed to make all staff members aware of security hazards and ways to protect themselves through established policies, procedures, and training.

Recordkeeping and Evaluation of Programs

Systems designed to provide the data to track progress in reducing work-related assaults.

Risk Management

An integrated effort across all disciplines and functional areas to protect the financial assets of an organization from loss by focusing on the prevention of problems that can lead to untoward events and lawsuits.

Total Quality Management (TQM)

The general processes of setting standards, collecting information, assessing outcomes, and adjusting policies; and evaluation of all systems to improve the quality of goods or services by reducing costs in ways that ensure customer satisfaction.

Threat Assessment

The evaluation of the threat itself and an evaluation of the threatener.

Threat Management

The course of action to be taken after conducting a threat assessment.

Continued

of furniture or medical equipment that could be used as weapons (Occupational and Health Administration [OSHA], 2003).

Managerial factors have implications for workplace violence. Organizations that are perceived as unjust, unfair, or unethical are thought to be more prone to violence. Organizations with a high degree of centralization are thought to make employees feel alienated and more prone to violence. Similarly, organizations that take a scientific management approach to employees are thought to dehumanize employees and possibly predispose them toward violence (Ginn & Henry, 2002).

REGULATORY BACKGROUND

Workplace violence has received increasing attention over the last three decades as a substantial contributor to occupational injury and death. NIOSH reported that homicide has become the second leading cause of occupational injury death. Assaults represent a serious safety and health hazard for American workers, and violence against employees continues to increase (NIOSH, 1996).

Acknowledging that workplace violence was a pervasive and growing problem, the Occupational Safety and Health Act of 1970 declared that employers had a general duty to provide safe and healthy working conditions. Through this act, NIOSH was charged with drafting and recommending occupational safety and health standards (OSHA, 2003).

OSHA followed up on the general duty requirement in 1989 with voluntary, generic safety and health program management guidelines for all employers to use as a foundation for their safety and health programs. The guidelines were not regulations; however, under the OSHA act, employers face fines if an incident of workplace violence occurs. The agency made it clear that safety and health programs could include workplace violence prevention programs (OSHA, 2003).

In 1998, OSHA built on the 1989 generic workplace safety and health guidelines by announcing guidelines specifically targeted at the health care and social services industry. The new guidelines identify common risk factors and include policy recommendations and practical corrective methods to help prevent and mitigate the effects of workplace violence (OSHA, 2003).

In summary, managers of health care organizations have an ethical obligation to protect the safety of workers. Managers also have a general legal duty to prevent workplace violence. Last, given the significant economic costs of workplace violence and the potential legal liability, managers have a fiscal responsibility to prevent workplace violence.

NIOSH Recommendations

NIOSH is located within the Centers for Disease Control and Prevention (CDC). NIOSH recognizes that workplace violence is a particular issue in the health care industry and recommends the following violence prevention strategies for employers: environmental designs, administrative controls, and behavior modifications. **Environmental designs** include signaling systems, alarm systems, monitoring systems, security devices, security escorts, lighting, and architectural and furniture modifications to improve worker safety. **Administrative controls** include adequate staffing patterns to prevent personnel from working alone and reducing waiting times, controlled access, and development of systems to alert security personnel when violence is threatened. **Behavior modifications** provide all workers with training in recognizing and managing assaults, resolving conflicts, and maintaining hazard awareness (NIOSH, 2002).

OSHA Guidelines

The Occupational Safety and Health Administration (OSHA) is an agency in the United States Department of Labor. OSHA suggests that all health care organizations should have a violence prevention program. Ideally, **violence prevention programs** are available to all employees, track progress in reducing work-related assaults, reduce severity of injuries sustained by employees, decrease the threat to worker safety, and reflect the level and nature of threat faced by employees. (OSHA, 2003). The main components in a violence prevention program are (1) a written plan, (2) worksite analysis, (3) hazard prevention and control, (4) safety and health training, and (5) recordkeeping and evaluation of program (Box 31.1 and Figure 31.1). **Violence prevention written plans** demonstrate management commitment by disseminating a policy that all types of violence will not be tolerated, ensure that no reprisals are taken against employees who report or experience workplace violence, encourage prompt reporting of all violent incidents, and establish a plan for maintaining security in the workplace. **Worksite analysis** is a common-sense look at the workplace to find existing or potential hazards for workplace violence. **Hazard prevention and control** implements work practices to prevent and control identified hazards. **Safety and health training** makes all the staff aware of security hazards and how to protect themselves through established policies, procedures, and training. **Recordkeeping and evaluation of programs** provide the data to track progress in reducing

work-related assaults (see Leading & Managing Defined box).

LEADERSHIP AND MANAGEMENT IMPLICATIONS

Management Frameworks

The implications for management of the threat of workplace violence vary depending somewhat on the source of violence. With regard to the first source of violence (criminals with no connection to the employer), a risk management approach is appropriate. With the second source of violence (patients), a total quality management approach may be effective. In regard to the third source of violence (current or former workers), good human resource management policies are essential. In dealing with the fourth source of violence (someone who has a personal relationship with an employee), employee assistance programs can be especially useful.

Risk management is an integrated effort across all disciplines and functional areas to protect the financial assets of an organization from loss by focusing on the prevention of problems that can lead to untoward events and lawsuits. A wide variety of measures are appropriate in order to prevent violence from criminal activity. Among these measures are the posting of security guards, the restriction of access to the general public, adequate lighting, escort services for those coming or going from parking lots, and the installation of alarm systems and systems to call for emergency assistance. These actions can be helpful in preventing or mitigating losses from actions by criminals with no connection to the workplace.

Total quality management (TQM) comprises the general processes of setting standards, collecting information, assessing outcomes, and adjusting policies. TQM and risk management share the goals of problem elimination, performance enhancement, and eliciting total organizational commitment (see Leading & Managing Defined box). Under TQM, the organization uses all available resources available, builds long-term relationships

Box **31.1**

Environmental Analysis

Hazard Prevention and Control

Identify hazards found in the worksite analysis and then provide administrative and work practice controls to make hospitals a safer workplace. For example, the following measures may increase safety:

- Provide better visibility and good lighting, especially in high-risk areas such as the pharmacy or isolated treatment areas.
- Implement safety measures to deter handguns inside facility—for example, using metal detectors.
- Install Plexiglas in the payment window in the pharmacy area.
- Use security devices such as panic buttons, beepers, surveillance cameras, alarm systems, two-way mirrors, card-key access systems, and security guards.
- Place curved mirrors at hallway intersections or concealed areas.
- Control access to work areas.
- Provide training for staff in recognizing and managing hostile and assaultive behavior.
- Provide adequate staffing even during night shifts. Increase staffing in areas where assaults by patients are likely (e.g., emergency department).
- Increase worker safety during arrival and departure by encouraging car pools and by providing security escorts and shuttle service to and from parking lots and public transportation.
- Ensure accurate reporting of all violent behavior.
- Make patients aware of zero-tolerance policy for violence.
- Establish liaison with police authorities and contact them when indicated.
- Obtain previous records of patients to learn of any past violent behaviors.
- Establish a system to chart or track and evaluate possible assaultive behaviors, including a way to pass on information from one shift to another.
- Implement a violence prevention plan to develop strategies to deal with possibly violent patients.

A safer room for a possibly violent patient features the following:

- Has furniture arranged to prevent entrapment of staff; furniture should be minimal, lightweight, without sharp corners, and/or affixed to the floor
- Is free from clutter, with nothing available on countertops to throw at workers or use as weapons
- Is provided with a secondary door for escape in case main door is blocked by patient
- Is one entered with a buddy; do not be alone with patient

Modified from Occupational Safety and Health Administration [OSHA]. [2003]. *Guidelines for preventing workplace violence for health care and social service workers* [rev. 2003]. Washington, DC: OSHA, U.S. Department of Labor. Retrieved December 9, 2004, from *www.osha.gov/SLTC/etools/hospital/hazards/workplaceviolence/checklist.html*

with both employees and patients, and remains open to ways in which processes can be improved to enhance the quality of operations. Teamwork is an integral part of TQM, along with establishment and tracking of violent incidents (Smith, 2001; Wagner et al., 2001). All levels of the organization are expected to be involved in decision making and employee training. Training topics should

impart skills that support the strategic goals of the organization and could include the following: prevalence, incidence, and warning signs of violence; policies and procedures; critical incident response; and availability of services associated with violence in the workplace (Smith-Pittman & McKoy, 1999). Health care organizations can expand the team concept to include providers

Workplace Violence Checklist

The following items serve merely as an example of what might be used or modified by employers to help identify potential workplace violence problems.

This checklist helps identify present or potential workplace violence problems. Employers also may be aware of other serious hazards not listed here.

Designated competent and responsible observers can readily make periodic inspections to identify and evaluate workplace security hazards and threats of workplace violence. These inspections should be scheduled on a regular basis; when new, previously unidentified security hazards are recognized; when occupational deaths, injuries, or threats of injury occur; when a safety, health and security program is established; and whenever workplace security conditions warrant an inspection.

Periodic inspections for security hazards include identifying and evaluating potential workplace security hazards and changes in employee work practices which may lead to compromising security. Please use the following checklist to identify and evaluate workplace security hazards. **TRUE** notations indicate a potential risk for serious security hazards:

_____ T _____ F   This industry frequently confronts violent behavior and assaults of staff.

_____ T _____ F   Violence has occurred on the premises or in conducting business.

_____ T _____ F   Customers, clients, or coworkers assault, threaten, yell, push, or verbally abuse employees or use racial or sexual remarks.

_____ T _____ F   Employees are **NOT** required to report incidents or threats of violence, regardless of injury or severity, to employer.

_____ T _____ F   Employees have **NOT** been trained by the employer to recognize and handle threatening, aggressive, or violent behavior.

_____ T _____ F   Violence is accepted as "part of the job" by some managers, supervisors, and/or employees.

_____ T _____ F   Access and freedom of movement within the workplace are **NOT** restricted to those persons who have a legitimate reason for being there.

_____ T _____ F   The workplace security system is inadequate—i.e., door locks malfunction, windows are not secure, and there are no physical barriers or containment systems.

_____ T _____ F   Employees or staff members have been assaulted, threatened, or verbally abused by clients and patients.

_____ T _____ F   Medical and counseling services have **NOT** been offered to employees who have been assaulted.

_____ T _____ F   Alarm systems such as panic alarm buttons, silent alarms, or personal electronic alarm systems are **NOT** being used for prompt security assistance.

_____ T _____ F   There is no regular training provided on correct response to alarm sounding.

_____ T _____ F   Alarm systems are **NOT** tested on a monthly basis to assure correct function.

_____ T _____ F   Security guards are **NOT** employed at the workplace.

_____ T _____ F   Closed circuit cameras and mirrors are **NOT** used to monitor dangerous areas.

_____ T _____ F   Metal detectors are **NOT** available or **NOT** used in the facility.

_____ T _____ F   Employees have **NOT** been trained to recognize and control hostile and escalating aggressive behaviors and to manage assaultive behavior.

_____ T _____ F   Employees **CANNOT** adjust work schedules to use the "Buddy system" for visits to clients in areas where they feel threatened.

_____ T _____ F   Cellular phones or other communication devices are **NOT** made available to field staff to enable them to request aid.

_____ T _____ F   Vehicles are **NOT** maintained on a regular basis to ensure reliability and safety.

_____ T _____ F   Employees work where assistance is **NOT** quickly available.

Figure 31.1

Checklist for violence in the workplace. (From Occupational Safety and Health Administration [OSHA]. [2003]. *Guidelines for preventing workplace violence for health care and social service workers* [rev. 2003]. Washington, DC: OSHA, U.S. Department of Labor. Retrieved December 9, 2004, from *www.osha.gov/SLTC/etools/hospital/hazards/workplaceviolence/checklist.html*)

⚠ LEADERSHIP & MANAGEMENT **BEHAVIORS**

Leadership Behaviors

- Envisions a violence prevention program
- Creates a zero-tolerance environment
- Inspires the commitment to a safe work environment
- Collaborates to secure the work environment

Management Behaviors

- Plans a worksite analysis of threats
- Analyzes workplace security trends
- Takes action to modify areas of concern

- Collaborates on strategies to minimize violence
- Manages violence risks
- Develops systems of documentation and reporting
- Structures a violence prevention policy

Overlap Areas

- Takes prompt and appropriate action regarding potential and actual violence
- Collaborates with others for safety and security

---

outside the organization by engaging staff with local police in security planning and education (Hoag-Appel, 1999).

Essential to establishing a safe working environment is the development of systems for reporting and documenting incidents of assaults and acts of aggression, as well as taking prompt action when a report is made. The reporting system should include the creation of special forms to report violent incidents, as well as the establishment of a hotline and confidential procedures for employees, to encourage timely and accurate reporting of all forms of violence (McKoy & Smith, 2001; Smith-Pittman & McKoy, 1999). The principles of TQM are manifest in OSHA's guidelines for violence prevention programs in health care; Henry and Ginn (2002) illustrated and discussed this relationship in more depth.

Human Resource Management Policies

A comprehensive violence prevention policy and procedural manual should be developed to guide organizational violence prevention efforts. A number of management policy recommendations in the literature can be applied to the prevention of violence. In the area of personnel, some suggest that organizations have policies to require thorough screening of applicants to weed out those who may have a propensity for violence. Such procedures may eliminate some violence from coworkers because a

history of violence is the best indicator of future violence (Corbo & Siewers, 2001). Other procedural approaches recognize that violent acts at work are often triggered by an employee being fired, receiving a termination notice, or some similar event. Some literature suggests that managers can avoid violence by suspending or terminating employees with the proper technique, such as walking a terminated employee out the back door instead of the front door in order to avoid humiliation. Other articles suggest that employees be terminated on a Monday instead of a Friday (Karl & Hancock, 1999). Thorough employee screening and appropriate termination policies will, at the very least, contribute to a legal defense that reasonable action to prevent violence has been taken.

The importance of securing the work environment, organizational policies, employee training, and personal survival skills are also stressed in the literature (Coco, 1998). Health care organizations should have policies about bringing weapons onto company property and reporting alcohol or drug use (Cantarella, 1996). In a similar vein, the literature suggests the formulation of policies to facilitate the reporting and elimination of bullying, verbal threats, harassment, intimidation, pushing, shoving, slapping, kicking, and fist fights (Atkinson, 2001). Some suggest training in the warning signs of potential violence and intervention techniques and the use of good communication concerning

---

Box 31.2

Online Resources about Violence

American Nurses Association (ANA)
Preventing workplace violence [Brochure].
Available from *www.nursingworld.org/osh/
violence.pdf*

**Occupational Safety and Health
Administration (OSHA)**
*Guidelines for preventing workplace violence for
health care & social service workers.* Available
from *www.osha.gov/Publications/osha3148.pdf*

**Occupational Safety and Health
Administration (OSHA)**
*Hospital eTool: healthcare wide hazards—workplace
violence.* Available from *www.osha.gov/SLTC/
etools/hospital/hazards/workplaceviolence/
viol.html*

**U.S. Department of Justice, Federal Bureau of
Investigation (FBI)**
Rugala, E.R., & Issacs, A.R. (Eds.) (2004). *Workplace
violence: Issues in response.* Available from
www.fbi.gov/publications/violence.pdf

Box 31.3

Questions to Ask in a Threat Assessment

1. Is there evidence of substance abuse or mental illness/depression?
2. Has the subject shown an interest in violence through movies, games, books, or magazines?
3. Is the subject preoccupied with violent themes; interested in publicized violent events; or fascinated with and/or recently acquired weapons?
4. Has the subject identified a specific target and communicated with others his thoughts or plans for violence?
5. Is the subject obsessed with others or engaged in any stalking or surveillance activity?
6. Has the offender spoken of homicide or suicide?
7. Does he have a past criminal history or history of past violent behavior?
8. Does the offender have a plan for what he would do?
9. Does the plan make sense; is it reasonable; is it specific?
10. Does the offender have the means, knowledge, and wherewithal to carry out his plan?

From Rugala, E.R., & Issacs, A.R. (Eds.) (2004). *Workplace violence: Issues in response.* Washington, DC: U.S. Department of Justice, Federal Bureau of Investigation (FBI). Retrieved July 19, 2004, from *www.fbi.gov/publications/violence.pdf*

---

downsizing and rightsizing status and activity (Moore, 1997). Box 31.2 lists useful online resources.

In dealing with potential violence from coworkers, threat assessment and threat management are important concepts to consider. **Threat assessment** consists of the evaluation of the threat itself and an evaluation of the threatener. Health care managers must make some effort to determine whether the person making threats was serious about inflicting harm or just verbalizing frustration; however, this is not to diminish the seriousness of verbal assaults. **Threat management** refers to the course of action to be taken after conducting a threat assessment (see Leading & Managing Defined box). Health care managers might want to investigate the person making threats and admonish, reprimand, counsel, or terminate the employee, as well as providing postincident counseling for the victim of the threats (Rugala & Isaacs, 2004). Still another procedural approach is to circulate generalized information such as typical profiles of workplace killers (violent employees), characteristics of disgruntled employees, motivations for violent actions, and factors that contribute to the problem. Furthermore, established disciplinary responses should be flexible enough to take situational circumstances into account (Litke, 1996) (Boxes 31.3 and 31.4).

An essential issue for human resource management is accurate reporting of violent incidents. Nurses often fail to report threats or other verbal

Box 31.4

Threat Assessment: A True-Life Example

The following is an account of a threat assessment conducted jointly by a criminal investigator and a mental health professional as reported at the NCAVC's Violence in the Workplace Symposium.

During a training session, the 46-year-old subject made comments regarding his alcoholism, causing such a disturbance that he was subsequently referred to the Employee Assistance Counseling Program. On two other occasions, he displayed inappropriate behavior by storming around the office, cursing, and throwing objects. In another training workshop, he made verbally abusive comments, disturbing the class.

After a month's leave, he had a verbal outburst during a meeting on his first day back in the office and requested a transfer due to stress. The request was denied. He then requested more leave, which was granted. The subject was noticeably withdrawn and his performance declined. Supervisors documented a pattern of unusual agitation over minor issues, unreasonable complaints, unacceptable work, and allegations that coworkers were conspiring against him. The subject was voluntarily hospitalized twice for homicidal ideations. He was treated for psychosis and suicidal and paranoid delusions associated with his coworkers. His physician recommended a disability retirement.

A month before his disability pension was approved, he began to leave harassing voice-mail messaged on a coworker's telephone. An example of the message is: "Hi Darlene, it's Stan, Just wanted to say Happy Thanksgiving. And, you give this message to Yvonne. Tell her if she had been off the property the day she hollered at me, I would have beat her [obscenity deleted]. Bye Darlene." He was diagnosed with delusional disorder, paranoid type. This information was also provided to law enforcement during the investigation.

His retirement papers contained disturbing comments. For example, recalling a meeting with a Human Resources staff member, he said: "I started to grab her by the throat and choke her, until the top part of her head popped off. Then I was going to step on her throat and pluck her bozo hairdo bald. Strand by strand . . ."

Some months later, the subject told a former coworker that he was following a former supervisor and her family. He provided specific information, stating that he knew where some of the targets lived and the types and colors of vehicles they drove. The subject also made comments about the target's family members and stated that he had three guns for each of his former supervisors.

At this point, law enforcement was notified. While the police investigation was under way, the subject made threats against five former female coworkers. A threat assessment was conducted analyzing letters, voice mails, reports from EAP, and interviews with various individuals. The subject's communications were organized and contained specific threats. For example, he wrote "Don't let the passage of time fool you, all is not forgotten or forgiven," and "I will in my own time strike again, and it will be unmerciful." The material suggested that he was becoming increasingly fixated on the targets and his communications articulated an action imperative that suggested that the risk was increasing. After obtaining additional information, the investigators informed the subject of specific limits and consequences that would occur if he continued his threatening behavior and communications.

The subject assured law enforcement agents that his intent was to pursue legal reparations. Four months later, however, he mailed letters to his five targets stating that he wanted to "execute" one of them. The letters indicated that he was close to committing an attack. Based on the foregoing assessment and insight into his thinking and behavior over several months, the threat assessment team, consisting of an investigator and a mental health professional, initiated a conference call with the district attorney. In the conference, the mental health professional provided an assessment of the subject's potential for violence, and the investigator presented evidence regarding the laws violated and law enforcement actions taken to date.

The threat assessment report, along with other evidence, was used by the district attorney in obtaining an arrest warrant and a search warrant. The final recommendation by the team was that the subject should be arrested and held without bond. Six months later, he was found not guilty by reason of insanity.

From Rugala, E.R., & Isaacs, A.R. (Eds.) (2004). *Workplace violence: Issues in response.* Washington, DC: U.S. Department of Justice, Federal Bureau of Investigation (FBI). Retrieved July 19, 2004, from *www.fbi.gov/publications/violence.pdf*

assaults because institutional policies fail to classify them as violence (Harulow, 2000). Nurses frequently encounter acts of intimidation—an implied threat when someone hits a wall, throws an object, or glares at someone in the immediate area—as a form of violence (Carroll & Morin, 1998). Unfortunately, the toleration of hostile or threatening behavior can result in escalation that results in physical harm (Hoag-Apel, 1999). Training programs should emphasize the broad definition of violence and the importance of reporting all incidents of violence.

Human resource management policies are essential for the prevention of violence from current or former workers in health care organizations. Policies on hiring, discipline, counseling, training, threat assessment, threat management, and reporting can prevent or mitigate loss due to violence from coworkers.

Employee assistance programs (EAPs) provide a range of services to help employees cope with stressors that occur at home and at work (see Leading & Managing Defined box). Family counseling might be useful in reducing domestic violence that can spill over into the workplace. Programs that counsel both the victim and the abuser could be instrumental in initiating needed interventions to defuse domestic violence situations that could impact the worksite. Furthermore, individual counseling can help employees cope with personal stressors that might contribute to unpredictable or violent behaviors. In short, EAPs can be very useful in preventing or mitigating loss due to domestic violence that spills over into the workplace.

Leadership

It is important to establish and maintain a corporate culture that is serious about protecting employees from violence. Employees often perceive the failure of management to prevent violent incidences or to respond quickly and appropriately when incidents do occur as lack of organizational commitment and loyalty. Ensuring a nonviolent workplace may require culture change, and alterations in practice may be necessary in such areas as labor relations, injury management, and other human resource

procedures (McKoy & Smith, 2001). Consistent with the principles of quality improvement, leadership for such tasks as worksite analysis, threat assessment, and development of organizational policies and procedures would be provided by multidisciplinary teams, composed of representatives of all aspects of the organization.

Legal Implications

Several *legal issues* surround workplace violence, as follows (Dolan, 2000):

- Employers may be faced with paying higher workers' compensation rates after injuries sustained from workplace violence.
- Employers may be subject to claims that they were negligent with regard to the security provided.
- Employers may also be subject to claims concerning negligent hiring, retention, and supervision.
- Employers may be subject to claims that they failed to warn subsequent employers about the criminal propensities of former employees.
- Threat management is complicated in that disability discrimination legislation restricts employers from taking action against employees solely because of their psychological disabilities and requires that action be taken only when the employee poses a direct threat.
- Sexual discrimination laws make employers liable in some instance for sexual harassment.
- Employers may be liable for citations, fines, and even criminal penalties.

Legal defense can be based on a variety of proactive actions by management, including conducting a risk assessment to determine what would be reasonable and appropriate action (Egger, 2000). Developing written antiviolence policies and procedures is the first step in reducing workplace violence. Policies should address factors such as employees, patients, non-hospital employee providers, and visitors (Smith-Pittman & McKoy, 1999). The following policies and procedures are useful in both preventing workplace violence and providing a legal defense if violence should occur: policies forbidding weapons, alcohol, drug use, bullying, and sexual harassment; and policies requiring preemployment screening and appropriate termination procedures. Similarly, policies clearly defining violence, requiring the reporting of violent acts, and specifying appropriate disciplinary actions for committing violence are essential (Ginn & Henry, 2002). Although no program can guarantee violent acts will not occur, the existence of a program can provide evidence in court that the health care organization has taken appropriate and reasonable action.

Last, there is **damage control** if all prevention efforts fail. The literature suggests specific steps to respond to workplace incidents such as the following (Litke, 1996) (see Leading & Managing Defined box):

- Remaining calm
- Evaluating facts objectively
- Calling in additional resources

Furthermore, after a violent incident, employers must address the emotions of employees and notify family members. Employers must also take steps to preserve the company image, quash rumors, prepare for ancillary incidents, ward off lawsuits, and return to normal operations (Botting, 2001). EAPs can also serve as a valuable tool in debriefing of employees after involvement in a violent incident, reducing the potential negative impact on both the employees and the organization.

CURRENT ISSUES AND TRENDS

Violence appears to be inherent in modern society and increasing in all aspects of society. Thus it is understandable that violence will continue to be present in the nursing profession. Reducing the impact of violence on the profession will require an expansive view of the problem that objectively explores all potential factors and pursues broad-based, collaborative efforts at resolution. In recent years, violence in the workplace has come to be viewed in the same light as other occupational hazards, allowing some measure of controllability by health and safety professionals.

Publicized violent incidents against nurses and the evidence in the literature that violence against

nurses continues to rise have prompted increased emphasis on prevention of violence in the health care workplace. In response, government agencies have published voluntary guidelines for preventive measures, the health care community has launched several initiatives aimed at prevention, and some states have passed legislation requiring training in prevention. The following violence prevention topics have been determined in the literature to warrant discussion as critical or new perspectives: improving prediction of violence, environmental design, collaboration among organizations and agencies, and increasing government oversight.

Prediction of Violence

An ideal way to reduce violent incidents would be to accurately predict who might become violent. Improving the prediction of violence is a common recommendation found in the literature; however, studies show that predicting violence in patients is very difficult, even when using thorough and validated nursing assessments. Among the difficulties of research is that violence is a very complex phenomenon, and knowledge about one kind of violence and its predictors cannot be generalized to other forms. Additionally, most research efforts are field-based, and there are myriad confounding variables and biases in the research design. However, these challenges should not deter ongoing attempts to improve predictions of violence. Current research on the prediction of inpatient violence has been designed to determine statistical predictors or to test the accuracy of predictors. Steinert (2002) suggested that exact predictions are not possible and that accepting a lower level of confidence of prediction would be appropriate for research in this area. Continued work in this area is warranted, because avoidance of violent incidents is far preferable to the necessity of intervention or response to violence.

Environmental Design

An occupational hazard approach to violence prevention looks at violence in the context of the

Research Note

Source: Lowe, T., Wellman, N., & Taylor, R. (2002). Limit-setting and decision-making in the management of aggression. *Journal of Advanced Nursing, 41*(2), 154-161.

Purpose

Previous research has suggested that inpatient aggression toward nursing staff is influenced by characteristics of the nurse-patient interaction. This study examined the structure of mental health nurses' judgments in conflict situations by obtaining measurement of nurses' perceptions of the relative importance of different aspects of intervention.

Discussion

The rise in incidence of violence and aggression by patients is a growing concern in the nursing profession and is of particular note in mental health nursing. Nurses experience considerable internal conflict in making decisions regarding interaction with patients in potentially aggressive situations. This study used a case scenario approach, presenting nurses with 10 conflict situations and 10 possible nursing responses to each event. Nurses were asked to rate the response statements for appropriateness. The results suggest that imposing limits and boundaries in patient behavior (limit-setting) and giving clear guidelines and expectations of patients (use of structure) are regarded as highly important; however, these must be considered concurrently with a sense of respect for patients and their autonomy (confirming). The relative importance of confirming interventions suggests that moral judgments are being made and that assumptions about blame or accountability are involved. Results showed that nurses with the most experience tended to make less restrictive judgments. Among the proposed explanations for this are the following: mental health training could have an effect on individual judgments about the appropriateness of interventions; greater understanding of mental illness leads to less blaming of patients, increased knowledge leads to greater confidence and a more relaxed view of patient behaviors. Clearly, there is evidence of a need for more research and discussion regarding effective nurse response in potentially critical situations, as well as the role of the organization in eliciting and reinforcing particular responses.

Application to Practice

The management of patients in potentially aggressive situations clearly presents a challenge to nurses. Many nursing practices are firmly based in history and law; thus nurses find it difficult to see alternatives to traditional modes of intervention. The results of this study carry implications for nursing administration and policy in terms of standardizing procedures for dealing with potentially aggressive patients, emphasizing nurse training in recognition and management of violence, establishing postincident reviews, and reviewing ethical dilemmas and dimensions of decision-making among nurses.

---

total environment, a systems approach to address prevention. The high rates of assault on health care workers can be attributed to a variety of causes, including issues related to design of the physical environment and to organizational culture, such as policies, procedures, and actual response, or lack of response, to violent incidents.

In responding to violence, it is easy to focus attention strictly on individual responses and behaviors; however, there is growing emphasis on evaluation of the contribution of the physical environment. Clearly, there are physical aspects that could enable or contribute to the perpetration of violent incidents. NIOSH (2002) presented a variety of suggestions for designing a safe work environment, including the following: emergency signaling alarms and monitoring systems; metal detectors at entrances and security cameras in hallways; appropriate design of waiting areas for patients and families; adequate lighting and security escorts in parking lots; design of triage and other public areas to minimize risk for assault.

Organizational culture is also considered an aspect of environment in a systems approach. The current health care delivery environment is turbulent and marked by a rapid pace of evolution (Kreitzer et al., 1997). In order to evolve, the U.S. health care industry is experiencing substantial restructuring through ownership consolidation and development of new forms of interorganizational relationships (Bazzoli et al., 2000). Organizational changes, such as restructuring, mergers, and downsizing create significant levels of uncertainty and anxiety in employees, which can eventually lead to stress-related consequences, possibly including violence.

Among the recommendations of OSHA and TQM approaches in the area of environmental design is to have a worksite analysis conducted by a threat assessment team or similar taskforce or coordinator. Such an effort analyzes records, trends, workplace security, physical characteristics, operating policies, and screening surveys of staff to provide an overview of the work environment. Based on the results of this assessment, direct action should be taken to resolve any identified areas of concern.

Collaboration

Nursing care occurs in many different settings, involves both professionals and laypersons, and exposes nurses to unacceptably high levels of many different types of violence. Thus there is the potential for various organizations and agencies to work together to develop strategies to minimize violence against nurses. Within health care, professional organizations, industrial unions, worksite management teams, and key nursing bodies can work together to ensure that nurses are provided with adequate support and resources to change the face of violence in the nursing profession. When necessary, advice and assistance should be sought from resources outside the health care facility, such as threat-assessment psychologists, psychiatrists and other professionals, social service agencies, and law enforcement agencies. Rugala and Isaacs (2004) offer a number of suggestions for strengthening the relationship between health care organizations and local law enforcement for preventing workplace violence.

Increased Government Oversight

OSHA is the only regulatory agency that directly oversees the safety and health of health care workers although several health care oversight agencies attempt to provide industry self-regulation of the safety of health care workers. At this time, OSHA's guidelines are voluntary, thus lacking in power of enforcement. The Joint Commission on Accreditation of Healthcare Organizations (JCAHO) provides clear standards for support of patient safety but does not offer the same guidance in regard to the safety of health care workers. The American Nurses Association supports the establishment of the OSHA recommendations as mandatory requirements.

New perspectives are also offered in the literature to shed light on the problem of violence in nursing, including horizontal violence (nurse against nurse), the potential impact of terrorism on nursing, and postincident response. In addition, one nursing setting that was noted in the literature as becoming of more concern in regard to violence is that of schools.

Horizontal Violence

The literature reveals that nurses are the most common perpetrators of some forms of violence, such as bullying. Some researchers (McMillan, 1995) suggested that the workplace environment and nursing culture allow this horizontal violence to occur unimpeded and actually accept it as a normal part of workplace culture. This seems to be particularly evident in regard to nursing experience; bullying is most often reported to be directed toward new nurses by more seasoned nurses. This type of violence usually manifests as psychological harassment rather than physical aggression, involves a series of incidents, and often creates hostility and discomfort among staff. These acts often seem to be precipitated by staffing shortages and increasing workloads.

The impact of horizontal violence is in some ways greater that that of other types. In addition to dealing with the violent episode itself, the victim also has to deal with the ramifications of poor working relationships—a situation that affects all coworkers, as well. A number of consequences have been found to accompany horizontal violence, including demoralization, feelings of vulnerability, a negatively changed attitude to work, loss of confidence, and impaired work performance (McKenna et al., 2003). Some nurses report that such incidents have led to consideration of leaving the profession (Wheeler, 1998). Violence in the form of bullying and harassment may be so endemic that it is taken for granted and dismissed as inconsequential. Nurses are urged to confront this underreported form of workplace violence, become a source of support for colleagues, and work as change agents in calling for managerial support for workplace safety.

Terrorism

The threat of terrorism has captured the attention of the world, and the workplace is no exception. The most notable terrorist attacks in the United States have occurred in settings that qualify them as occupational violence: the World Trade Center and the Oklahoma City Federal Building. Since the attack on the World Trade Center, America's workplaces have recognized the need to be prepared to handle not only the traditional threats of violence, but also the external threat of terrorism. Terrorist activity can be motivated by political, social, issue-oriented, and religious views. For some militant groups, Western civilization represents evil, and thus anything in Western civilization could be a target. However, some organizations may have characteristics that make them particularly salient to terrorists. By considering the motivations of some terrorist groups and attempting to view one's organization through the eyes of a potential terrorist, one may conclude that the profile of an organization should be altered in subtle ways to make it a less egregious symbol to terrorists (Brown, 1998). Certainly, health care providers will be pivotal responders in the event of major terrorist incidents, and the violence itself may spill into the health care workplace.

Postincident Response

Postincident response is becoming recognized as a critical element in reducing both the short- and long-term impact of workplace violence. Health care workers who do not receive adequate support following an incident may quit or be fearful of returning to work. Failure to respond quickly and appropriately to violent incidents is perceived by employees as lack of management commitment and concern for the workforce. OSHA (2003) and the Federal Bureau of Investigation (FBI) (Rugala & Isaacs, 2004) have recommended that employers set up trained response teams and provide postincident response that includes such measures as prompt medical treatment, psychological evaluation, counseling, support groups, stress debriefing, trauma crisis counseling, and employee assistance programs. The first responsibility of the response team is to ensure the safety and well-being of the victim(s) of violence. Response team members may be called in at any stage of a violent incident—to defuse an escalating situation, intervene in an event, or respond to the aftermath of a traumatic event. Consequently, response teams should receive special training in evaluation, threat assessment, and conflict resolution, as well as procedures to monitor, document, and respond to situations. Teams should also have plans for dealing with other issues, such as news media and public reaction to a major incident. Postincident response should involve an integrated system of services and procedures to reduce the potential impact of a1 violent incident on employees. Incident debriefing should be offered to all employees, not just those involved in the event (Henry & Ginn, 2002).

Clearly, violence in the workplace has an impact that goes beyond what is done to a particular victim. It damages trust, community, and the sense of security that every employee has a right to feel while at work. Employing agencies need to show a commitment to safety for nurses, providing protection against acts of violence in all clinical areas, but especially in high-risk settings. Educational institutions and employers need to share responsibility for properly preparing nurses to deal with potentially violent situations.

Summary

- Employers have legal and ethical obligations to promote a work environment free from violence.
- Workplace violence exacts an economic cost through lost productivity, low morale, increased workers' compensation, medical claims, and possible lawsuit and liability costs.
- The four sources of violence include (1) person with no connection to the organization, (2) patients or family of patients, (3) current or former employees, and (4) someone with a personal relationship with an employee.
- Management philosophy and practice influence the potential for violence in an organization.
- NIOSH recommended three violence prevention strategies: environmental design, administrative controls, and behavior modifications.
- The main components of a violence prevention program as set forth by OSHA are a written plan, worksite analysis, hazard prevention and control, safety and health training, and record-keeping and evaluation.
- Human resource departments should develop comprehensive violence prevention policies and procedures manuals to include such issues as preemployment screening, threat assessment, and threat management.
- EAP programs can help employees and their families cope with stressors that might contribute to unpredictable or violent behaviors.
- Leadership should be provided by multidisciplinary teams composed of representatives of all areas of the health care organization and appropriate community representatives.
- Legal defensibility should be grounded in proactive actions by management, starting with written antiviolence policies and procedures.
- Research is warranted in improving the prediction of violence, including consideration of lowering the level of confidence for statistical prediction.
- Efforts at environmental design should include both the physical environment and organizational culture.
- Horizontal violence has a greater impact on the organization than other types and contributes to reduced morale, increased turnover, and nurses leaving the profession.
- Effective violence prevention collaborations will include representatives from within and outside of the health care organization.
- The first responsibility of the postincident response team is to ensure the safety and well-being of the victims of violence.

Study Questions

1. Why should nurses be vigilant regarding the potential for violence from coworkers?
2. When is a threat important enough to report?
3. How do you know when an incident has a potential for violence?
4. What can nurses do about verbal abuse from physicians?
5. What laws apply to workplace violence?
6. What steps should nurse administrators take to secure a safe workplace?

CASE STUDY

Nurse Juanita Evans is in her first nursing job. She was assigned to the emergency department (ED) 4 months ago, as a last-minute assignment, without any prior ED training. Ms. Amy Jones has been waiting in the ED for 3 hours to receive care for abdominal pain. Amy's brother, John, becomes agitated, begins to pace the waiting area, and chastises several staff members as they pass by. As Nurse Evans passes, John tries to grab her arm; she pulls away and tells him there are other people in worse shape, and he will just have to wait his turn. He continues to chastise and to make verbal threats of retaliation against the hospital and staff if his sister is not cared for soon. The staff ignore him and dismiss his threats as just the stress of the situation. Amy eventually receives the care she needs and is released. Four days later, Nurse Evans is walking to her car in a far corner of the parking garage when she is attacked by John and left unconscious on the ground.

CRITICAL THINKING EXERCISE

Nurse Millie Adams is a nursing administrator at Good Care Hospital, a facility that serves as an educational training hospital. Nurse Adams has noticed several trends recently: nurse turnover has been higher than usual; sick leave has increased; student nurses frequently request transfers to other facilities. In searching for answers, she hears a lot of talk about nurses being threatened or verbally confronted by other nurses; however, there has been no increase in reports of violent incidents.

1. What are the problems?
2. What are the potential sources for these problems?
3. What are some possible explanations for the problems?
4. What information does Nurse Adams need, and how should she gather this information?
5. What could be done to resolve the problems?

1. What are the warning signs of a potential problem?
2. Why is each a problem?
3. Apply the five components of OSHA's Violence Prevention Plan to identify what should be done to ensure that such a situation does not happen again.
4. How could Nurse Evans have handled the situation differently?

REFERENCES

Atkinson, W. (2001). Keeping violent employees out of the workplace. *Risk Management, 48*(3), 12-21.

Bazzoli, G.J., Chan, B., Shortell, S.M., & D'Aunno, T.M. (2000). The financial performance of hospitals belonging to health networks and systems. *Inquiry, 37*(3), 234-252.

Botting, J.M. (2001). Picking up the pieces. *Security Management, 45*(1), 26-39.

Brown, H. (1998). Armed against terrorism. *Occupational Health & Safety, 67*(10), 172-176.

Bruser, S. (1998). Workplace violence: Getting hospitals focused on prevention. *The American Nurse, 30*(3). Retrieved July 19, 2004, from *http://nursingworld.org/tan/98mayjun/violence.htm*

Cantarella, A. (1996). Increase your personal security at work. *Professional Safety, 41*(11), 32.

Carroll, V., & Morin, K. (1998). Workplace violence affects one-third of nurses: Survey of nurses in seven SNAs reveals staff nurses most at risk. *American Nurse, 30*(5), 1. Retrieved July 19, 2004, from *www.nursingworld.org/tan/98sepoct/violence.htm*

Center for Violence Prevention and Control. (1996, August). *A guide to courses that include content pertinent to violence prevention and control.* Minneapolis, MN: University of Minnesota. Retrieved July 19, 2004, from *www1.umn.edu/cvpc/pub_coursedir.html*

Coco, M. (1998). The new war zone: The workplace. *S.A.M. Advanced Management Journal, 63*(1), 15-20.

Corbo, S.A., & Siewers, M.H. (2001). Hazardous to your health: Don't get burned when tempers ignite. *Nursing Management, 32*(3), 44C-44F.

Dolan, J.B. (2000). Workplace violence: The universe of legal issues. *Defense Counsel Journal, 67*(3), 332-341.

Edwards, R. (1999). Prevention of workplace violence. *Aspen's Advisor for Nurse Executives, 14*(8), 8-12.

Egger, E. (2000). Reasonable and appropriate action important in preventing violent crime. *Health Care Strategic Management, 18*(10), 13-14.

Elliot, P.P. (1997). Violence in health care. *Nursing Management, 28*(12), 38-41.

Ginn, G.O., & Henry, L.J. (2002). Addressing workplace violence from a health management perspective. *S.A.M. Advanced Management Journal, 67*(4), 4-10.

Harulow, S. (2000). Ending the silence on violence. *Australian Nursing Journal, 7*(10), 26-29.

Henry, L.J., & Ginn, G.O. (2002) Violence prevention in health care organizations within a TQM Framework. *Journal of Nursing Administration, 32*(9), 479-486.

Hoag-Apel, C.M. (1999). Smart safeguards for the ED. *Nursing Management, 30*(5), 31-33.

Jossi, E. (1999). Defusing workplace violence. *Business & Health, 17*(2), 34-49.

Karl, K.A., & Hancock, B.W. (1999). Expert advice on employment termination practices: How expert is it? *Public Personnel Management, 28*(1), 51-62.

Kreitzer, M.J., Wright, D., Hamlin, D., Towey, S., Marko, O., & Disch, J. (1997). Creating a healthy work environment in the midst of organizational change and transition. *Journal of Nursing Administration, 27*(6), 35-41.

Litke, R. (1996). Defusing the workplace time bomb. *Journal of Property Management, 61*(4), 16-21.

McKenna, B.G., Smith N.A., Poole, S.J., & Coverdale, J.H. (2003). Horizontal violence: Experience of Registered Nurses in their first year of practice. *Journal of Advanced Nursing, 42*(1), 90-96.

McKoy, Y.L., & Smith, M.H. (2001). Legal considerations of workplace violence in healthcare environments. *Nursing Forum, 36*(1), 5-14.

McMillan, I. (1995). Losing control. *Nursing Times, 91*, 40-43.

Moore, L.R. (1997). Preventing homicide and acts of violence in the workplace. *Professional Safety, 42*(7), 20-23.

Murray, M.G., & Synder, J.C. (1991). When staff are assaulted. *Journal of Psychosocial Nursing and Mental Health Nursing, 29*(7), 24-29.

National Institute for Occupational Safety and Health (NIOSH). (1996). *National Institute for Occupational Safety and Health, current intelligence bulletin 57. Violence in the workplace: Risk factors and strategies.* Washington, DC: NIOSH, Centers for Disease Control and Prevention, U.S. Department of Health and Human Services.

National Institute for Occupational Safety and Health (NIOSH). (2002). *Violence: Occupational hazards in hospitals.* Washington, DC: NIOSH, Centers for Disease Control and Prevention, U.S. Department of Health and Human Services. Retrieved July 19, 2004, from *www.cdc.gov/niosh/2002-101.html*

Occupational Safety and Health Administration (OSHA). (2003). *Guidelines for preventing workplace violence for health care and social service workers. OSHA publication 3148* (rev. 2003). Washington, DC: OSHA, U.S. Department of Labor.

Rugala, E.R., & Isaacs, A.R. (Eds.) (2004). Workplace violence: issues in response. Washington, DC: U.S. Department of Justice, Federal Bureau of Investigation (FBI). Retrieved July 19, 2004, from *www.fbi.gov/publications/violence.pdf*

Smith, A.P. (2001). Removing the fluff: The quality in quality improvement. *Nursing Economics, 19*(4), 183-185.

Smith-Pittman, M.H., & McKoy, Y.D. (1999). Workplace violence in healthcare environments. *Nursing Forum, 34*(3), 5-13.

Steinert, T. (2002). Prediction of inpatient violence. *Acta Psychiatrica Scandinavica, 106*(s412), 133-141.

Violence threatens the workplace. (1998). *The Internal Auditor, 55*(5), 13.

Wagner, C., Groenewegen, P.P., de Bakker, D.H., & van der Wal, G. (2001). Environmental and organizational determinants of quality management. *Quality Management in Health Care, 9*(4), 63-77.

Wheeler, H. (1998). Nurse occupational stress research 5: Sources and determinants of stress. *British Journal of Nursing, 7*, 40-43.

32

Collective Bargaining

Harriet Forman

CHAPTER OBJECTIVES

- Formulate an understanding of collective bargaining and how it relates to nursing professionalism
- Define and describe terms relative to collective bargaining and nursing management/leadership
- Chronicle the history of U.S. collective bargaining legislation and its impact on nursing
- Examine the tension that often develops between unionized nurses and their managers
- Analyze ways and means to lessen the tension between unionized nurses and their management/leadership team
- Exercise critical thinking to conceptualize and analyze possible solutions to a practice exercise

Collective bargaining consists of negotiations between the management of an organization and a collective of employees, typically represented by a labor union. Management and employees negotiate over terms and conditions of employment, attempting to reach agreement on items that the employees feel provide fairness to them and which management feels they can live with in terms of financial and managerial needs in organizational operations. Collective bargaining is a large and complex topic. Collective bargaining encompasses negotiations between an employer and a group of employees. Those negotiations determine the conditions of employment for the employees and are spelled out in what is called a *collective bargaining agreement*. The collective bargaining process that occurs is governed by federal and state laws, administrative agency regulations, and judicial decisions. Where there is an overlap between the federal and state law, federal laws usually prevail (Legal Information Institute [LII], 1999a, 1999b).

Employees shall have the right to self-organization, to form, join, or assist labor organizations, to bargain collectively through representatives of their own choosing, and to engage in other concerted activities for the purpose of collective bargaining or other mutual aid or protection, and shall also have the right to refrain from any and all such activities except to the extent that such right may be affected by an agreement requiring membership in a labor organization as a condition of employment as authorized in section 8(a)(3), the Section of the National Labor Relations Act (NLRA) that makes it illegal to discriminate against employees to encourage or discourage membership in a union (National Labor Relations Board [NLRB], 1997, 2004).

Federal law gives employees the legal right to unionize; yet registered nurses (RNs) struggle with the question, "Does professionalism and unionization go together, or is unionization better left to blue-collar workers?" Accompanying with this concern is the tension that often exists between unionized staff and their management. This latter issue is of particular concern as nursing moves more deeply into the twenty-first century. This is a century of health care personnel shortages, especially nurses and nurse faculty; globalization, along with its concomitant spread of exotic diseases; and terrorism and the stress-related conditions resulting from threats of terrorism.

DEFINITIONS

The lexicon of terms associated with collective bargaining is long and specific. Some of these terms have a precise meaning that is defined by law and specific to the rules and regulations surrounding collective bargaining activities. For example, the NLRB provides a glossary of terms (NLRB, 2004). The following definitions are provided to further clarify and provide specificity to collective bargaining terminology:

- *Arbitration (interest):* The use of an impartial third party(s) to arrive at a solution to a dispute between parties concerning the contents of a collective bargaining agreement. The decision of the arbitrator(s) is usually, but not always, binding on the parties at interest.
- *Arbitration (grievance):* The use of an impartial third party(s) to settle a dispute between the parties to a collective bargaining agreement as to the meaning and application of certain language in the bargaining agreement. The decision of the arbitrator(s) is usually, but not always, binding on the parties to the collective bargaining agreement.
- *Bargaining agent/representative:* The organization that the employees in a bargaining unit select, under regulations of the appropriate labor agency, to represent exclusively the employees in that unit in all negotiations with their employer. This pertains to all parts of the employment relationship mandated by the applicable state or federal statutes. There frequently will be a local bargaining agent/ representative who is affiliated with a national or international bargaining agent/representative.
- *Bargaining unit:* The employees or jobs that are joined together as a group by the authorized agency (NLRB or a state labor agency) for purposes of bargaining collectively with the employer. The appropriate labor agency determines that certain employees or jobs have a commonality that supports the negotiation of one contract agreement to cover their employment relationships with the employer.
- *Certification:* The official designation by the appropriate labor agency of a bargaining agent/representative as the exclusive representative of employees in a bargaining unit concerning matters of employment that are required to be negotiated between management and that agent/representative.
- *Collective bargaining:* The process used by representatives of an employer and the certified bargaining agent/representative for a group of employees to reduce to writing and sign an agreement covering terms of employment that are either mandated or allowed by applicable state or federal law.
- *Contract:* The written agreement between the employees in a bargaining unit and the employer concerning some or all of the conditions of employment applicable to any or all of the employees in the bargaining unit.
- *Good faith bargaining:* The performance of the mutual obligation of the employer and the representative of the employees to meet at reasonable times and confer in good faith with respect to wages, hours, and other terms and conditions of employment specified under the applicable state or federal law. This obligation does not compel either party to agree to a proposal or to make a concession.
- *Grievance:* The allegation by an employee or employees or certified bargaining agent/representative that management has violated the collective bargaining agreement (contract) between the parties.
- *Grievance procedure:* A written plan outlining the actions to be taken by both employees and their certified bargaining agent/representative and the employer to adjust a grievance. This plan usually involves progressive steps through the employer's administrative structure that end with external arbitration (if agreement is not reached internally).

▲ LEADING & MANAGING **DEFINED**

Collective Bargaining	**Collective Action**
The process used by representatives of an employer and the certified representatives for a group of employees to negotiate and sign an agreement covering terms of employment.	Action, such as mass resignations, taken by employees or professional organization groups in order to bring about changes in terms of employment.

- *Impasse:* A deadlock in negotiations between management and employee representatives over the terms and conditions of employment specified by the appropriate state or federal law.
- *Management rights:* Policies or practices that the applicable national or state collective bargaining law says are not subject to negotiation.
- *Mandatory bargaining items:* Policies or practices that the applicable national or state collective bargaining law says management *must* negotiate with its employees' agent/representative.
- *Mediation:* The use of a neutral third party to facilitate negotiations between management and the bargaining agent/representative.
- *Nonmandatory bargaining items:* Policies or practices that the applicable national or state collective bargaining law says management *may* negotiate with its employees' agent/representative.
- *Prohibited bargaining items:* Policies or practices that the applicable national or state collective bargaining law, or other law, says management *may not* negotiate with its employees' agent/representative.
- *Unfair labor practice:* An allegation made by an individual, an employer, or a labor organization of a violation of the applicable state or federal law concerning bargaining.

BACKGROUND

A look back in history is always useful to understand the present and successfully plan for the future. In the early industrial age, prior to federal legislation directed at protecting workers, child labor, unhealthy and often dangerous working conditions, and repressive management were often the norm. Some workers suffocated to death in mine accidents. Women and children were burned to death in sweatshop fires. Industrial unions were the only hope of relief for downtrodden workers who marched in the streets, singing and chanting in their efforts to unionize. At the same time, RNs were trained in hospital apprenticeship systems where they were assigned to staff wards on all three shifts for no pay while also attending classes during the day. Hospitals had a ready source of unpaid labor. Support staff such as aides, orderlies, maids, porters, and others were poorly paid and often poorly treated.

Recognizing that workers needed protection, Congress enacted the Wagner Act, known as the National Labor Relations Act (the NLRA), in 1935 under its constitutional power to regulate interstate commerce. It was signed into law by President Franklin D. Roosevelt. Since then, labor's relationship with management has been governed by federal law. State laws have also increasingly played a role. The labor-management relationship is further governed by rules and decisions from regulatory agencies both at the state and federal level, such as Occupational Safety and Health Administration (OSHA) and The Department of Health (DOH).

When the NLRA was passed, not-for-profit hospitals were excluded from the law. Because Congress came to believe the provisions of this act were too heavily weighted in favor of labor, they amended it in 1947 (the Taft-Hartley Act). In 1974, Congress passed another amendment extending the coverage of the Act to private not-for-profit hospitals and nursing homes. For the first time, these employees, including RNs, could engage in federally protected labor union activity.

Under the NLRA, procedures were established for the selection of a union or other labor representative for employees who wished to engage in collective bargaining. An employee unit is created based on an old industrial model linking like with like. Following is one definition:

> The bargaining unit is a group of employees with common interests who are represented by a labor union in their dealings with agency management. Prior to an election, representatives from management, the union, and the Federal Labor Relations Authority meet to define the scope of the unit. One factor in defining the scope of the unit is that it must ensure employees the fullest freedom in exercising the rights guaranteed under the Federal Service Labor-Management Relations Statute. Furthermore, a unit will be considered appropriate only if it will ensure a clear and identifiable community of interest among the employees in the unit and will promote effective dealings with, and efficiency of the operations of, the agency involved (Army CPOL, 2004).

Essentially, a unit is determined based on community of interest concerning wages, hours, and conditions of employment. The NLRB has found that RNs should occupy their own bargaining unit based on a community of interest. The law prohibits employers from interfering with the employees' selection of the representative (labor union) and requires that the employer bargain with the representative that is selected. The law establishes guidelines for *good faith* bargaining but does not require that either side make concessions or agree to any proposal. The law also places certain restrictions on the tactics that either side may use in bargaining (i.e., strikes or lockouts). The NLRA prohibits employers and unions from engaging in unfair labor practices (ULPs) (LII, 1999a, 1999b).

State laws frequently provide guidelines for those employers and employees who are not covered by the NLRA, such as employees of state and local government and agricultural laborers. Federal employees and agencies are governed in their collective bargaining by the Federal Service Labor-Management Relations Act (FSLMRA), administered by the Federal Labor Relations Authority. The Railway Labor Act covers labor relations in the railway and airline industries (LII, 1999a, 1999b).

In the private sector, employees are typically under the jurisdiction of the NLRA, with the NLRB being the governing agency responsible for administering the law. The NLRB conducts representation elections and certifies the results and serves as a deterrent to ULPs by either side. The processes of the NLRB are begun only when requested. ULPs will be addressed later in this chapter.

In the public sector, employees are routinely under the jurisdiction of a state labor agency. State laws and agencies are frequently patterned after the federal approach, but many states have adopted a narrower view of the employment relationship, which must be bargained by employers with their organized employees. Most of the state statutes permitting collective bargaining for public employees have been enacted since the late 1970s. One exception to the rules for public sector employees is the Veterans Administration (VA). These employees, along with other federal public sector employees, are governed by the Federal Service Labor-Management Relations Authority (FSLMRA), which is administered by the Federal Labor Relations Authority.

Although federal protection was not available, there were many states in which employees in not-for-profit hospitals and nursing homes had organized for purposes of collective bargaining. In many of these facilities, RNs, including the RN managers, were incorporated into the bargaining units—often under the auspices of state nurses associations.

In the years immediately following 1974, when the second amendment to the NLRA was made by Congress, many of these not-for-profit hospitals filed unit clarifications or decertification petitions. They asked the NLRB to decertify RN managers and supervisors from the union. The union, on the other hand, insisted that these individuals did not meet the definition of supervisors under the statute and should remain under the protection of the collective bargaining contract.

Supervisors and managers are exempt from protection under the NLRA. To meet the definition of statutory supervisor, there must be evidence that an employee spends a *reasonable* amount of time in the following activities: hiring, firing, assigning, directing, evaluating, approving transfers, promoting, addressing grievances, suspending, laying off workers, or effectively recommending such action. (In this context, "effectively recommending" means that the individual recommends the action and that the action takes place.)

A decertification hearing occurs in a courtroom-like setting. An NLRB administrative law judge hears the case. Lawyers for each side present evidence. Witnesses are sworn. There is a lot at stake for both sides. Management must present evidence without alienating its own staff. Staff members recognize that they, too, are stakeholders regardless of the outcome.

Emotions run high on both sides of the issue. In fact, emotions tend to run high on both sides of most issues in the arena of collective bargaining. This would include collective bargaining and professionalism, collective bargaining and nursing, or collective bargaining and negotiating.

For the emerging nurse manager and the seasoned nurse leader, it is of great importance to remember that unions do not create the groundswell movement to install unions—management does. Why would staff feel the need for third-party intervention if they have open and trusting communication and professional relationships with their leadership?

For the most part, the age of cigar-chomping, tough-talking, street-cursing union organizers is over. Union organizers of today tend to be recruited from the same colleges and universities that graduate nurses, physicians, and attorneys come from. They are a new breed who understand organizational psychology, the power of persuasion, and communication theory. It is therefore important that nurse leaders and nurse managers are also experts in the same fields. They need expertise in communication theory and management, including collective bargaining, leadership, and nursing, in order to provide the best these

disciplines have to offer. This way, staff members either come to believe that they do not need third-party representation, or if the staff is already unionized, management is able to work with the staff and the union most productively. The key question is this: Just what is collective bargaining, and why does it raise such high emotion?

COLLECTIVE BARGAINING

Collective bargaining is basically a method of mutually determining wages, hours, and terms and conditions of employment through negotiation. During this process, the employer and the union representatives work out a collective bargaining agreement.

Subjects

What specific elements of work life may be included in the subjects of collective bargaining remains a source of confusion. For example, nurses may believe that they can bargain collectively over nurse staffing ratios. In each case, it is imperative that the applicable laws be reviewed and understood. For nurses who are covered by the Fair Labor Standards Act (FLSA) for purposes of collective bargaining, there is a broad category of items that the employer must bargain over once an employee organization has been certified to represent the nurses.

Employees covered by FLSA include all employees of an enterprise that is engaged in the operation of a hospital (Department of Labor, 2004). There are three general categories of aspects of work life that may be included as subjects of collective bargaining. These are mandatory, permissive, and illegal subjects (NLRB, 1997).

Mandatory

Mandatory subjects are those that the law requires must be addressed. These include wages, overtime, discipline, grievance, seniority, promotion, safety, layoff, recall, discharges, sick leave, and leaves of absence. Other matters covered include pensions for current employees, bonuses, group insurance, grievance procedures, safety practices, seniority, procedures for discharge, layoff, recall, or discipline, and union security. Certain managerial decisions such as subcontracting, relocation, and other operational changes may not be mandatory subjects of bargaining, even though they affect employees' job security and working conditions. The issue of whether these decisions are mandatory subjects of bargaining depends on the employer's reasons for taking action. Even if the employer is not required to bargain about the decision itself, it must bargain about the decision's impact on unit employees.

Permissive

Permissive subjects are those that may be bargained for but are not obligatory. They are employee rights, management rights, and benefits for retired union members. On "nonmandatory" subjects—matters that are lawful but not related to wages, hours, and other conditions of employment—the parties are free to bargain and to reach agreement. However, neither party may insist on bargaining on such subjects over the objection of the other party.

Illegal

Illegal subjects are unlawful by statute. Major issues in this category are a "closed shop" (employers will only hire union members), discriminatory treatment, and the "hot cargo clause" (employees will not be required to handle work during a strike).

STATE LABOR LAWS

For nurses covered by state labor laws covering collective bargaining, categories of mandatory bargaining items may differ. Requirements for employer bargaining vary from state to state. The following list provides a few examples of state bargaining scope requirements:

- *Alaska:* Alaska Statute 23.40.070 (2) requires public employers to negotiate with and enter into written agreements with employee organizations on matters of wages, hours, and other terms and conditions of employment.

- *Iowa:* Iowa Code 1997: Section 20.9 calls for negotiating in good faith with respect to wages, hours, vacations, insurance, holidays, leaves of absence, shift differentials, overtime compensation, supplemental pay, seniority, transfer procedures, job classifications, health and safety matters, evaluation procedures, procedures for staff reduction, in-service training, and other matters mutually agreed on. Negotiations shall also include terms authorizing dues check-off for members of the employee organization and grievance procedures for resolving any questions arising under the agreement. All retirement systems are excluded from the scope of negotiations.

- *Oregon:* Oregon Revised Statute 243.650 (7)(A) pertains to matters concerning direct or indirect monetary benefits, hours, vacations, sick leave, grievance procedures, and other conditions of employment. Oregon excludes from bargaining certain items in various professions, such as class size for teachers.

HISTORY OF UNIONIZATION OF NURSES

Nurses participated in strikes and demonstrations early in the twentieth century (Forman, 1989). However, in 1911, the American Nurses Association (ANA) released a statement in the October issue of the *American Journal of Nursing* (AJN) deploring nurses' involvement in work stoppages and job actions. In the 1930s, nurses' work environments shifted from private homes to hospitals, a shift that precipitated a unionization movement because nurses were subjected to the same poor working conditions that befell other service workers. The first recorded nurses' union was formed in 1937 in New York City. It was composed of nurses working for the city (Forman, 1989).

The ANA originally opposed the formation of nurses' unions. It believed that through membership in the professional association, and working through its state chapters, RNs could achieve improvement in every phase of their professional lives. The ANA reiterated this policy in 1983, but RNs continued to organize, most prominently in

Research Note

Source: Brewer, C.S. (1998). The history and future of nursing labor research in a cost-control environment. *Research in Nursing & Health, 21*(2), 167-177.

Purpose

Nursing shortages stimulate research about the labor supply behavior of registered nurses. The purpose of this article was to overview and critique three generations of nursing labor research. Methodological issues affecting labor predictions were discussed, and future directions were indicated.

Discussion

Since the first comprehensive study of the labor market for nurses (Yett, 1970), understanding nurses' labor supply response to changes in wages has been a crucial factor for accurately predicting response to market demand. RN wages were stagnant from 1992 to 1996, whereas health care as a percentage of GNP continued to grow. Flat wage growth for nurses during explosive managed care growth indicate shifts in underlying conditions affecting nurses. Although this article was framed in the context of the predicted surplus of RNs by the 1995 Pew report, it is important to understand and analyze nursing labor research. This research will be used for policy recommendations. Brewer divides the research into three generations, roughly appearing in the 1970s, 1980s, and 1990s. Variability in results and wage elasticity calculations are due to differences in methods, samples, model specification, selection bias, lack of accurate wage data, and changes in the population participation rates over time.

Application to Practice

Determining rational policy responses to the labor market for nurses is a critical human resources management issue. Nurses collectively organize and bargain over issues of wages and working conditions. Understanding the labor supply response of nurses to changes in wage rates is important for labor supply economics and recommendations for wage issues. Although the nurse supply is projected to grow, it is not clear how the supply will interact with demand and the extent to which RNs will respond to changes in wages and working conditions. Better econometric models and better data are needed. Regional workforce studies, investigation of time and money costs for women (RNs are 92.9% female), and research into labor preferences of various subgroups will help indicate practical applications for labor issues in nursing.

New York, New Jersey, California, Washington, Oregon, Kentucky, Massachusetts, and West Virginia.

The late 1960s was productive for collective bargaining, with a major impetus having come from President John F. Kennedy in 1962. He issued an executive order protecting the collective bargaining rights of nurses and others employed in federal hospitals. Large numbers of nurses, especially those working in VA hospitals, organized. By 1969, the numbers of RNs under contract jumped from 8,000 to more than 30,000. It again tripled in the next 5 years, jumping to 90,000. Contracts were negotiated by professional nursing associations (Forman, 1989).

Over and above collective bargaining, which is regulated by law, nurses as a group are able to take **collective action** (see Leading & Managing Defined box). There have been several instances of collective action taken by RNs, all serving to prove to hospital hierarchies and to nurses themselves that hospitals cannot run without nurses. These actions occurred in New York City in 1966.

Problems began when negotiations stalemated. As a result of a greater than 50% vacancy rate of RNs, working conditions at city hospitals were horrible. The remaining nurses decided to resort to an en masse resignation to become effective after a 30-day notice period. RNs at one of the hospitals submitted their resignations first. Word spread and soon nurses at another hospital submitted their resignations. The nurses readily found employment in the private sector. Before any more nurses were lost to the city system, negotiations resumed and a settlement was reached (Forman, 1989).

Similar tactics were used in Chicago, and strikes have occurred in San Francisco and Idaho. Further organizing activity continued throughout the 1970s and 1980s, and strikes became a routine form of protest among nurses. There no longer was a question as to *whether* nurses would organize. Instead it was a matter of which group would represent them: a professional organization or a trade union?

Because nurses work so closely with physicians, a word about MDs and collective bargaining is in order. MDs started to organize in the 1970s, when health maintenance organizations began to erode their right to make independent decisions on behalf of their patients. The Union of Physicians and Dentists was formed in 1972; however, of the 26 unions that emerged during the 1970s, none managed to survive except the Union of American Physicians and Dentists, which currently is the union representing practicing physicians. The personality traits that tend to bring people into medicine—independence and self reliance—may account for general resistance to unions. Just as some nurses thought unionization was inconsistent with professionalism, so too, did physicians. Just as some nurses thought strikes anathema to patient care commitments, so did physicians. However, during the Reagan years there was a shift in the public's attitude toward a free market economy in health care thus making the idea of a union more acceptable.

Since the spread of managed care in the 1990s and heavy-handed cost-containment measures, many physicians have looked to unions for protection. Currently, of the 775,000 physicians nationwide, about 50,000 are unionized. Furthermore, the Professional Employees International Union and the Service Employees International Union have begun new efforts to recruit physicians. Time will tell whether this trend continues (Fine, 2003-2004).

SETTING THE SCENARIO

Collective bargaining occurs through a series of processes. For example, assume that a group of RNs working at Anyplace General Hospital feels dissatisfied with wages, benefits, and conditions of employment. Based on this scenario, discontent is generated. (It should be noted that the issue of conditions of employment differs from working conditions. For example, *conditions of employment* may refer to vacation, sick time, or flex time, whereas *working conditions* may refer to lighting, access to locker rooms, or cleanliness of the facility.) The nurses at Anyplace General are being asked to do mandatory overtime, they are not involved in a meaningful way in nurse practice committees, and they believe they are understaffed. The nurses have tried to resolve their problems through discussions with management, to no avail. A local union organizer has contacted one of the RNs and has offered to arrange a meeting at a local coffee shop. A few of the RNs accompany her and hear how this health care union *will* obtain better wages, no mandatory overtime, better staffing, and a list of other things the nurses believe they need to give better care to their patients. They have been unable to obtain these improvements through management. In fact, they have not even been granted a meeting with management. And, to make things worse, there were rumors that the chief executive officer, whom they never see, was just given a huge raise in salary.

Steps to Union Organizing

Before long, the inevitable happens and a major union organizing campaign is under way. The entire hospital has taken sides. Unionizing—as well as everything that goes along with it—is adversarial by nature, because of the way the law is written. This is not to imply that a mature management team cannot create and maintain good working relationships with its own staff or even with the union representatives. However, it takes much maturity, maximum effort, and strong patient focus to do so (Forman & Powell, 2003d).

In order to file for an election with the NLRB, the union must obtain the signatures of one-third of the eligible employees on show-of-interest cards. These are then presented to the NLRB, which calls for an election, which it will supervise, within 42 days. The union wants to keep secret the fact that it is attempting to organize a facility for as long as possible. On the other hand, administration wants to know as soon as possible so that a counter-campaign can be mounted. Often, administration will call in a consultant to assist in that campaign to avoid falling into the many pitfalls that exist under the law. For example, there are unfair labor practices (ULPs) that management wants to avoid.

Unfair Labor Practices

Once nurses, or any other group, begin the process of formally organizing, the NLRA becomes an operative federal law and the rules of the NLRB apply. It is important for nurses, whether they are employees or management, to read, know, and understand the specific laws and applicable regulations. For example, the NLRA forbids management and labor to refuse to bargain in good faith. Furthermore, it forbids an employer to do any of the following:

> … interfere with, restrain, or coerce employees in the exercise of the rights guaranteed in section 7. Any prohibited interference by an employer with the rights of employees to organize, to form, join, or assist a labor organization, to bargain collectively, to engage in other concerted activities for mutual aid or protection, or to refrain from any or all of these activities, constitutes a violation of this section. This is a broad prohibition on employer interference, and an employer violates this section whenever it commits any of the other employer unfair labor practices. (NLRB, 1997, pp. 27-28)

The acronym *TIPS* helps in remembering these ULPs, as follows:

- *T*—**Threatening** employees with loss of jobs or benefits, or interfering with, restraining, coercing, or retaliating against employees if they join or vote for a union or engage in union activity. (For example, management cannot dominate a labor organization or threaten to close down the entire employment operation.)
- *I*—**Interrogating** employees about their opinion, current activity, or future intentions pertaining to union activity if this is intended to restrain or coerce the employees.
- *P*—**Promising** wage increases or benefits to employees to discourage their union support.
- *S*—**Spying** on employees by having "friendly" employees attend meetings and report back.

Remembering these rules and avoiding them are two different things in the heat of a union organizing campaign when emotions can override good sense. Often, a good labor management consultant is worth his or her weight in gold if a labor/management environment can be created in which staff members begin to believe they do not need a "middle man."

ULPs also are defined for the labor side; these are practices that the union may not legally commit. Labor unions must abide by the rules designed to impose order and fairness into the process. Prohibited union actions include the following:

- Threats to do bodily injury to nonstriking employees
- Acts of force or violence on the picket line, or in connection with a strike
- Mass picketing in such numbers that nonstriking employees are physically barred from entering the premises
- Threats to employees that they will lose their jobs unless they support the union's activities
- Telling employees who oppose the union that they will lose their jobs if the union wins a majority
- Entering into an agreement with an employer that recognizes the union as the exclusive bargaining representative when it has not been chosen by a majority of the employees
- Fining or expelling members for crossing a picket line that is unlawful under the NLRA or that violates a no-strike agreement

- Fining employees for crossing a picket line after they resigned from the union
- Fining or expelling members for filing ULP charges with the board or for participating in an investigation conducted by the board
- Unfair representation
- Coercing or restraining employees in the exercise of their union rights
- Charging discriminatory or excessive membership fees
- Refusing to bargain in good faith (NLRB, 1997, p. 40)

Some union organizing campaigns involve informational picketing. This happens when eligible employees join a picket line (e.g., those RNs who are interested in joining and who are working with a union to convince fellow employees to do likewise). These picketers hand out flyers and other information to people entering and leaving the premises. This is usually done in a businesslike manner. It is geared toward eliciting sympathy and support.

During the campaign, labor will lobby eligible employees, telling them why they should vote for the union. Management will lobby the staff and explain why employees are better off voting against the union. Among the reasons management will present are increased costs to the employee by way of union dues and the fact that they will have to go through a middleman (a union delegate) instead of having direct dialogue with management. As Pamela Thompson, executive director of the American Organization of Nurse Executives (AONE), said: "When you bring in a third party, you relinquish the ability to solve problems through open dialogue and common problem solving" (Bilchik, 2000, p. 41).

The fact that staff members have brought in a union usually indicates high levels of dissatisfaction. This should encourage management to have an outside specialist conduct a vulnerability audit to ascertain the areas of weakness in its own labor-management relationships. Armed with this information, management can immediately start to strengthen relationships, communication, and management/leadership behaviors. It is never too late to improve. Management also should communicate these efforts to staff, being certain to remain within legal boundaries.

Neutrality Agreements

There has been a recent trend in the health care industry toward neutrality agreements. A *neutrality agreement* is a contract between a union and an employer under which the employer agrees to remain neutral during a union's attempt to organize its workforce. Generally, a union officer approaches a health care administrator and offers to conduct a campaign among a selected group of employees such as RNs. Management agrees to not mount a counter-campaign. In other words, it agrees to remain neutral. In return, the union agrees to bargain a long-term labor contract favorable to the employer. For a health care administrator under pressure in today's volatile health care marketplace, this may seem like a very attractive offer. Neutrality agreements are relatively new in the marketplace and have not been called on to withstand challenges before the NLRB or the test of time.

The Election

Returning to the scenario at Anyplace General Hospital, the 42 days since the NLRA certified the election have gone by. It now behooves management to "get out the vote." Every vote is important. Generally, a non-vote is a vote for the union; often, RNs who favor management but fail to vote are disappointed to find they are represented by a union when they preferred to remain union-free.

Sometimes management and labor agree to use a *card check mechanism* to count the votes. This is common practice when a neutrality agreement has been signed. Both parties agree to have a neutral third party, such as a clergyman or justice of the peace, count the votes and compare them with a full-time employee roster. When a majority is reached, the third party declares a winner. This may be faster and easier for the union, but it denies the employee the privacy ensured by a secret ballot election guaranteed in a procedure overseen by the NLRB.

NURSING AS A PROFESSION

A major issue to consider is that of nursing professionalism, both as an entity unto itself and as it interrelates with collective bargaining. This issue has threaded through the context of collective bargaining in nursing.

There are many definitions of the term *profession*. Elements often cited are a discrete body of knowledge, altruism, lifelong learning, autonomy, and peer review. Nursing has a discrete body of knowledge, requires lifelong learning, and relies on altruism for its practitioners to discharge its responsibilities in a humane manner. However, it falls short in the areas of autonomy and peer review. Until there is one consistent source of educational entry into the profession, nursing will continue to be lacking in these areas. Also, because nursing is dependent on following physicians' orders, autonomy presents a thorny conundrum. Is a practitioner (nurse) who follows the orders of another discipline (physician) dependent, or can that practitioner (nurse) create a patient care plan that is consistent with the medical regimen and therefore be autonomous?

Currently, in some instances the master's-prepared advanced nurse practitioner makes and carries out autonomous decisions. In venues such as home care, independent decision making among RNs may be the norm. However, in the acute care setting, nurses at the bedside often have all they can do to complete the myriad tasks that confront them. The more medical students, interns, and residents there are on staff, the fewer independent decision-making opportunities there are for nurses.

Peter Senge's (1990) work on learning organizations states that professionals draw strength from working in a learning organization in which the leadership lives by the following principle: people at all levels, individually and collectively, are continually increasing their capacity to produce results they really care about.

REGISTERED NURSES: WHO ARE THEY?

A national sample survey of RNs reported by Spratley and colleagues (2000) showed pre- and posteducational patterns of RNs. Of nurses nationwide, 23% hold diplomas, 34.3% hold associate degrees, and 32.7% have baccalaureate degrees. Approximately 10.2% of RNs hold graduate degrees. Between 1997 and 2002, 55.4% of RNs obtained degrees from associate degree programs, 38% from baccalaureate programs, and 6% from diploma programs (Spratley et al., 2000).

There are approximately 2.6 million licensed RNs in the country. They became RNs by sitting for the National Council Licensing Examination-RN (NCLEX) examination. That is where consistency ends, as the above statistics show. All who pass the exam become registered as nurses in their state and become recognized as RNs. It is only at their place of employment that differentiated practice may take place, and this often is recognized only through small educational salary differentials. Sometimes practice models fail to recognize differences in basic education at all. Entry into the practice of nursing in the United States has a long and tumultuous history.

Entry into Practice

In 1965 the American Nurses Association (ANA) presented its *First Position on Nursing Education,* in which it proposed a two-tiered system of technical and professional education for nurses. The ANA recommended that all future education of nurses take place in colleges or universities, thus phasing out hospital-based diploma programs. According to those recommendations, individuals interested in a beginning technical role would earn an associate degree after a 2-year course of study. Those interested in a professional role would pursue a baccalaureate degree after a 4-year course of study. The licensed practical nurse would be replaced by the associate degreed nurse (Donley & Flaherty, 2002).

These recommendations were not well received in many circles. In 1965, hospitals had been in the business of educating or training nurses for nearly a century. They had been accustomed to using students as staff, providing hospitals with a ready source of newly graduated nurses who required little or no orientation to join the staff and also act as instructors and supervisors. Also, this was the era of the Great Society, the age of Medicare and Medicaid, with the promise of more patients coming into the acute care setting. This did not create a supportive environment for hospitals who wished to close hospital-based schools of nursing. It was not a good time for even the best of ideas to be made public (Donley & Flaherty, 2002).

Moving through successive decades, increasing numbers of consumers came to the acute care setting demanding care. In addition, ambulatory centers, clinics, home care, skilled nursing and assisted living facilities, hospices, and a myriad of other care centers competed for RNs at a time when other career options opened for women and enrollment in nursing programs declined. Shortages of RNs recurred in frequent cycles. Eventually, managed care and reorganization entered the scene, and layoffs of RNs spread across the country. In such an environment, union activity among RNs reenergized.

Union Activity among Registered Nurses

The mission statement of the United American Nurse (UAN), the union that is a branch of the American Nurses Association, is as follows:

> The United American Nurses, AFL-CIO, is the premier union for registered nurses, by registered nurses. The UAN works to shape the future of all staff nurses and the health care system for the better by improving the economic and general welfare of nurses, providing a quality work environment, protecting nurse and patient safety and influencing nursing practice standards. (UAN and ANA, 2004, p. 1)

The UAN is just one of many unions that represent RNs in their work. The other major health care workers' union is Service Employees International Union (SEIU) Local 1199, which originally started as a union to represent pharmacists and then health care workers other than RNs. It now also

represents RNs through its League of Registered Nurses in many of its constituent organizations. There are also non-health care unions representing RNs. For example some RNs are represented by traditional trade unions such as the Teamsters, the United Auto Workers, a grocery workers union, or even a meat packers union. This may occur when a disgruntled RN has a spouse, sibling, or close friend who is happy with the union's representation at his or her place of employment and encourages the RN to speak with that union's representative. Sometimes, this is all it takes for unrelated unions to come to represent health care workers. In other cases, a union may launch a deliberate organizing campaign.

The ANA and its state nurses associations promote economic and general welfare for nurses and deem collective bargaining as beneficial to nursing as a profession. They believe that nurses can use the collective bargaining process to "protect their professionalism" (ANA, 1999, p. 4). However, there are nurse executives who consider it a conflict of interest to belong to these associations. They understand the adversarial nature of collective bargaining. They also may consider it to be *their* job as nurse leaders to protect and promote the professionalism of the RNs on their staff.

Just what is it that makes the collective bargaining process so adversarial? The easy answer is that long years of poor labor/management relationships culminate in contentious union organizing campaigns, fractious elections, and forced negotiations. By the time both sides get to the bargaining table, trust is gone and nerves are frayed.

NEGOTIATIONS

The union's negotiating team usually consists of a professional negotiator and a cadre of delegates who also are employees. These generally are the members of the staff who were proactive in bringing the union into the organization. The management team will also have a professional negotiator—the labor attorney and members of the nursing management team. Often the chief of human resources will attend as well.

A wide range of issues will be presented by the union. These will include professional concerns such as staffing ratios, the establishment of employee-dominated nurse practice committees, nonnursing functions, continuing education, and staff development. Nonprofessional subjects may be introduced as well, such as specific items of attire (e.g., sneakers or scrubs). When a union wins an election, everything is subject to bargaining, including wages, benefits, policies, working conditions, and more. There is no limit to how long bargaining can go on. The longer it continues, the more apt RNs are to feel let down by their employers and by the unions they turned to for assistance. Employers hire agency and other temporary personnel and conduct business as usual. RNs may walk informational or adversarial picket lines and work per diem shifts or as agency nurses in neighboring hospitals. This strange dance can go on for months, and sometimes for years, as tempers flare and RNs seek other opportunities for employment. The nurses generally suffer the most. Wages, benefits, and conditions of employment freeze at what was in place at the time of the election and remain frozen while the collective bargaining process proceeds at a snail's pace.

Management will present counterproposals. Neither side will expect to obtain everything it proposes. Generally, each side will know what is most important to the other side. For management, it is important to know what issues are most likely to cause the union to strike. A health care strike is not something to be taken lightly. It is extremely disruptive. Because it involves patient care, the NLRA requires a 10-day notice of a union's intent to strike. Prepared management should always have a strong strike-contingency plan in place at the start of every negotiation (Forman & Powell, 2003a).

POINTS OF VIEW

The New York State Nurses Association (NYSNA), which has a long history of collective bargaining activity, described collective bargaining as a bilateral process of determining the terms and conditions of employment through negotiation. The process is one used to enhance the quality of client care, advance professional growth, achieve satisfactory compensation agreements, and establish effective communication channels with employers. The NYSNA listed the benefits of collective bargaining as the ability to negotiate enforceable contracts that spell out specific working conditions important to nurses and adding voice to legislative initiatives (NYSNA, 2004).

However, there are other ways to achieve similar goals. As an example, Porter-O'Grady and Finnigan (1984) proposed a shared governance model to do this. A current concept is collaborative governance: "Collaborative governance is the decision making process that places the authority, responsibility, and accountability for patient care with the practicing clinician" (Erickson et al., 2003, p. 96.). These models are viable alternatives under specific circumstances. All professional leadership/management models that empower staff nurses to be involved in decision making require a professional, well-educated, self-assured leadership team headed by a well-educated, self-assured leader with concomitant power, authority, and the respect of his or her boss.

Just as critical care and emergency care are specialties, management is a specialty, but it is often not treated as such. Nurse managers can be moved into their positions without proper credentials. In such cases, staff nurses are left with no choice but to turn to a union for leadership and protection. When a supervisor treats a staff nurse unfairly and shouts, "I don't care how tired you are, you have to do another shift," where is that staff nurse to turn? When a physician calls a nurse "stupid" and nothing is done about it, what is the nurse to do?

For nurses, job satisfaction lies at the heart of unionization. Frustration, disillusionment, limited career growth opportunities, poor working conditions, diminished professional autonomy, feelings of powerlessness, lack of respect, and limited access to information, resources, and support underlie unionization. Unionization is seen as a means of taking collective action, with protection, to attain conditions that allow nurses to provide quality care. Unions often state they will solve all the problems presented to them. In reality, they cannot do so. If this is not recognized up front, the nurses who voted for the union, especially in a neutrality agreement scenario, might find themselves once again dissatisfied. Indeed, once a union is on board, the status quo is bound to prevail for a period of time, and nurses may feel let down, frustrated, and saddled with union dues. Furthermore, union officials, once in place, do not always accomplish the promises they made during a campaign, especially with regard to obtaining raises, eliminating mandatory overtime, decreasing patient ratios, or improving the food provided to staff.

LEADERSHIP AND MANAGEMENT IMPLICATIONS

Collective bargaining issues among nurses were prominent in the 1970s, but with the strike of the air traffic controllers (PATCO) and resultant union breakup in the early 1980s, labor union influence in the United States diminished. As with many trends, the prominence of unions is cyclical. Beginning in the 1990s, unionization of nurses experienced a strong up-swing because of managed care, externally driven redesign of the work, and nurse leaders who in many cases had no choice but to go along with the programs set up by administrators and fiscal consultants. This was a manifestation of nurses' conflicts with employer organizations over economic and nursing welfare, including staffing ratios, mandatory overtime, and governance.

Connected to work redesign are the dual issues of a dramatic alteration in staff mix to drastically reduce the number of RNs and a corollary rise in the use of nonnurse assistive personnel. Nurses argue that such externally induced rapid changes compromised patient safety. Administrators and consultants argue that nurses merely want to save their jobs, not assist the fiscal needs of the organization.

Until recently, there were no data to support nurses' allegations that substituting RNs with unlicensed assistive personnel was dangerous to patients. Now there is. The research conducted by Linda Aiken and her colleagues (Aiken et al., 2002) clearly and rigorously demonstrated the link between low RN staffing and poor patient outcomes. The study examined 10,000 nurses and 230,000 patients in 168 Pennsylvania hospitals from 1998 to 1999. Some of the findings are as follows:

- Each additional patient assigned to a nurse resulted in a 7% increase in 30-day patient mortality.
- Failure-to-rescue rate increased by 7%.
- Odds of nursing dissatisfaction increased by 15%.
- Odds of nurse burnout increased by 23%

Furthermore, when nurses had eight patients instead of four, their patients had a 31% higher chance of dying within 30 days of admission. Of the nurses surveyed, 43% were "burned out" and emotionally exhausted. Nurses who experienced burnout were four times more likely to report that they were leaving their jobs in the next year.

From the evidence base, it is clear that RNs at the bedside equate with better patient outcomes. However, there is also a dire shortage of RNs, one that will not abate any time soon. Although many unions promise to mandate favorable staffing ratios, and in some states staffing ratios have been legislated, no one has mandated or legislated an increase in the numbers of RNs in the employment pool. The challenge to both staff members and management RNs is to perform the following:

- Work together to create patient delivery paradigms that differentiate the practice levels of RNs based on education and skills and to develop pay models that recognize those levels.
- Set up some form of shared governance model that empowers the staff nurse through the work of councils led by staff nurses.
- Eliminate mandatory overtime and other unacceptable practices identified by staff nurses. This can be done through the work of the staff nurse council. Work-life balance is a key goal of this millennium.

▲ LEADERSHIP & MANAGEMENT **BEHAVIORS**

Leadership Behaviors

- Creates unit and organizational climate that values nurses
- Guides nurses in conflict resolution strategies
- Creates a vision of professionalism and collectivity
- Inspires professional autonomous behavior
- Communicates relevant work-related information
- Leads others to value and respect the work of nurses
- Advocates for nurses' values and needs
- Inspires trust and respect and pushes the envelope

Management Behaviors

- Plans career growth opportunities
- Structures the work environment for professional autonomy
- Manages work-related conflicts
- Organizes the flow of work-related communication
- Acquires specific state and federal collective bargaining rules, regulations, and information

- Administers the collective bargaining contract fairly and equitably
- Ensures that management's rights and employee's rights are respected

Overlap Areas

- Leads and manages the unit and organizational climate for nurses
- Manages the flow of communication
- Enhances organizational respect for nurses
- Serves as a role model at all times
- Applies critical thinking skills and serves as a mentor and team builder
- Keeps the patient as the central focus and uses patient-centered language as a problem solving technique

---

- Ensure adequate numbers of well-trained, unlicensed assistive personnel (UAPs) and availability of supplies and wholesome nourishment for staff 24/7.
- Provide professional leadership and management around the clock.
- Reward positive performance and eliminate punitive thinking and action.
- Work toward a cooperative labor-management relationship, keeping the focus on the patient.
- Develop and use patient-focused language.

If some staff members are represented by a labor union, management still retains its rights to run its business. Be wary of the phrase "the union doesn't let us do that." Most collective bargaining agreements (contracts) have a management rights clause. The clause asserts management's right to run its business. Box 32.1 lists items typically contained within an RN collective bargaining agreement (Forman & Powell, 2003b, 2003c).

CURRENT ISSUES AND TRENDS

In a labor relations development of the 1990s, the U.S. Supreme Court ruled that nurses who oversee lower-level personnel are supervisors and, as such, are not protected by federal laws on collective bargaining under the NLRA. This was a reversal of the traditional holding of nurses under the NLRA. The decision narrowed the definition of who can participate in an RN collective bargaining unit. Eligibility was to be decided locally. The ANA's argument that there is a distinction between an RN's direction of other employees in the exercise of professional judgment in the care of clients and the exercise of supervisory authority in the interest of the employer was not upheld. The question then became, When does a professional become a supervisor? (Ketter, 1994). Although the answer may lie with the NLRA, the interpretation and reinterpretation of the NLRA through subsequent

Box **32.1**

Items Typically Covered in a Collectively Bargained RN Labor Agreement

- Scope of agreement
- Union security (determines how all eligible employees must establish a relationship with the union)
- Dues checkoff (union financial obligations are withheld from employees' paychecks and forwarded to the union)
- Union representatives' number and access to the premises
- Union bulletin board
- Local union representatives (employees called *union stewards*) and rules for their release with or without loss of pay for such things as arbitrations, off-premises meetings, grievances on premises, and negotiations
- Professional status issues, including nonnursing functions, committee on nursing practice, staff development, continuing education, staffing, staffing committee
- Probationary period
- Seniority
- Layoff and recall
- Low census: call-off procedure
- Employment security
- Definitions of full-time, part-time, and per diem employees
- Posting of positions
- Job descriptions
- Personnel file review by employees
- Postprobationary discharge
- Work time, including hours, work day, work week, weekends, overtime, flex time, weekend work shifts, fixed or rotating shifts
- Floating
- Development of and posting of schedules
- Time-recording procedure
- Break periods
- Zipper clause (contract is complete and final; nothing can be added to it or taken away.)
- Practices regarding pay for time not worked
- Monetary benefits, including base rate, regular rate (including all differentials), premium rate, overtime, pay period, wages, paycheck errors, holidays and personal days, vacation, sick leave, jury duty, bereavement days, marriage days, birth or adoption leave, shift, education, on call pay, charge pay, experience, longevity, degree, certification and preceptorship differentials
- Unpaid (by the employer) leaves of absence: disability, personal, workers' compensation, family and medical leave act, and military leave
- Monetary benefits: health insurance and pension, uniforms, tuition reimbursement, meal allowance, etc.
- No-strike clause
- Management-rights clause
- Dispute resolution, grievance and arbitration procedures
- Labor management meetings
- Successors
- Subcontracting procedures
- Duration and termination

rulings has a local and national impact on nurses and nursing.

In 1996 the NLRB ruled that RNs, including charge nurses, were not automatically statutory supervisors. Therefore, they are protected by federal labor law and have the right to organize for collective bargaining purposes. According to the ANA (1996), some hospitals used the 1994 Supreme Court decision to fight nurses' attempts to organize for collective bargaining. Others tried to decertify units or refused to include them in the group of employees for whom they were negotiating. The NLRB ruling removed employer tactics designed to impede union organizing by RNs (ANA, 1996). The job description and the actual work performed by the employee form the nexus of decision making. If reasonable people sit down and have reasonable discussions, problems diminish. Unfortunately, as previously discussed, collective bargaining is adversarial by its very nature. However, there are other ways to lessen the tension. The resurgence of the Magnet Recognition Program is an example of a program that makes a difference in job satisfaction (Upenieks, 2002).

The roots of the Magnet Recognition Program stretch back to 1983 (McClure et al., 1983), when the ANA published results of a study conducted by the American Academy of Nursing, an ANA subsidiary. It identified variables that created an environment to attract and retain well-qualified nurses who promote quality patient care. It was the ability to attract and retain professional nurses that deemed a number of hospitals as "magnets."

Subsequently, in 2004 Congress passed the Nurse Reinvestment Act, which among other measures, included grants to encourage facilities to implement Magnet criteria for excellence in nursing services. Just days after President Bush signed that legislation into law in 2004, the Joint Commission on Accreditation of Healthcare Organizations (JCAHO) released a report on the nursing shortage that recommended facilities adopt the characteristics of Magnet hospitals to foster a workplace that empowers employees and is respectful of nursing staff (JCAHO, 2004).

There is no question that patients need quality nursing care. In order for nurses to provide high levels of safe care, they need to be supported by management. In addition, they need to be respected and to have input into matters that affect their work life. If they do not trust their management, they will invariably turn to a third party to represent them. Unions are at the ready to provide that intervention and will quickly establish a social bond with nurses who believe management has failed them.

Just as collective bargaining agents are educated in their field of labor relations, so too should nurse managers be educated in their field of leadership and management with a strong component in collective bargaining. Both patients and the staff that care for them deserve no less.

Summary

- Collective bargaining consists of labor and management negotiations.
- Unionization in nursing has steadily increased over the last quarter of the twentieth century.
- Unionization is governed by federal and state legislation and administrative rules and regulations.
- Unionization versus professionalism is a continuing issue in nursing.
- Nurses need to be aware of the structure and scope of collective bargaining in nursing.

Study Questions

1. What are the attributes of a profession?
2. Does nursing meet these criteria? If not, why not?
3. Is it unprofessional to join a labor union? Why or why not?
4. What is the NLRA? The NLRB? Why are they important?
5. Should nurses be allowed to strike? Why or why not?
6. What other options besides unionizing are available for labor-management conflict resolution?

CASE STUDY

Monica Hendricks, a master's-prepared RN educator, has recently been hired as the director of nursing education in a unionized acute care hospital. She has had past experience in unionized organizations and understands managing in a collective bargaining environment. One of the responsibilities outlined to her by her new employer is to upgrade the management team so that everyone is at least at a basic level of management expertise with knowledge and skill in collective bargaining. Eventually, she is to upgrade them further from there.

Nurse Hendricks thought she would have some time to get to know the staff and set up her schedule and curriculum, but shortly after her arrival, she became aware that supervisors were using the phrase "Oh, the union won't let us do that." She also noticed that staff members often extended their breaks and that the units seemed unusually disorganized. As she made her rounds, she asked the same question of all management personnel in the department: "Do you have a copy of the union contract?" No one did.

Nurse Hendricks had sufficient copies of the union contract printed for all managers and set up her classes so that every manager could attend. Then, using the clauses of the contract as a roadmap, she immediately started discussion groups to review the contract line by line. It was not long before management personnel from other departments started to wander in to her classes, where they received a warm welcome.

CRITICAL THINKING EXERCISE

It has been 42 days since the NLRB certified a trade union as eligible to attempt to organize the nurses in registered Nurse Janet Hargrove's hospital. At first she was in favor of the union because RNs had been laid off. Staffing ratios were very high, and staff nurses such as Nurse Hargrove had to do mandatory overtime. They were expected to orient and direct unlicensed assistive personnel, as well as newly hired, newly graduated nurses. Supplies were often short, especially on the off-shifts and weekends. In addition, although the nurses had not been given a salary raise in more than 2 years, pharmacists had received substantial pay increases because they were in such "short supply." Often, RNs were treated disrespectfully by physicians, family members, patients, and even within their own hierarchy.

What was making Nurse Hargrove question her original decision to vote for the union was that, right after the NLRA certified the campaign, a new chief nurse executive (CNE) had come on board. The new CNE immediately moved her office from the insular location it had always been in to a central location with an open door. She had started around-the-clock group meetings and instituted what she called *MBWA*,

or "management by walking around" on every nursing unit, during all three shifts. The CNE quickly began to get to know staff members by name. She asked staff members for input in identifying three priority problems (excluding those that involved money or structural repair) that could be solved quickly. Then, by working with a volunteer staff nurse committee, the CNE solved those problems almost immediately.

Nurse Hargrove, along with other RNs, were very happy with the CNE and her new approach, but union reps warned them that goodwill by management would end unless they voted for the union. They brought in nurses from other unionized hospitals to reinforce this message and to "talk up" the union. Nurse Hargrove and her colleagues were confused. They did not know what to do.

1. What critical thinking techniques might Nurse Hargrove use to come to a decision?
2. How might Nurse Hargrove weigh the pros and cons of voting for the union or for management?
3. What is the significance of 42 days in the first paragraph?
4. What is the significance and value of MBWA?

The phrase *knowledge is power* was actualized. Nurse Hendricks was careful to alert human resources (HR) to her activities, and HR had appropriate conversations with union leadership. Over time, patients became the central focus, but not without some difficulty. After all, when you change an existing paradigm, there is bound to be some resistance. However, persistence and goodwill eventually overcame resistance. Patient focus, patient-focused language, and carefully staying within the confines of the collective bargaining agreement were Nurse Hendricks' winning strategies.

REFERENCES

Aiken, L.H., Clarke, S.P., Sloane, D.M., Sochalski, J., & Sieber, J.H. (2002). Hospital nurse staffing and patient mortality, nurse burnout, and job dissatisfaction. *Journal of the American Medical Association, 288*(16), 1987-1993.

American Nurses Association (ANA). (1965). *First position on nursing education. Kansas City, MO: ANA.*

American Nurses Association (ANA). (1996). ANA applauds NLRB ruling on RN status. Silver Spring, MD: ANA. Retrieved November 24, 2004, from *www.nursingworld. org/pressrel/1996/nlrb.htm*

American Nurses Association (ANA). (1999). *Workplace issues: Organizing and collective bargaining.* Silver Spring, MD: ANA. Retrieved November 24, 2004, from *www. nursingworld.org/dlwa/barg/index.htm*

Army CPOL. (2004). *Bargaining unit.* Washington, DC: U.S. Department of Defense. Retrieved November 24, 2004, from *www.cpol.army.mil/library/permiss/411.html*

Bilchik, G.S. (2000). Norma Rae, RN. *Hospital & Health Networks, 74*(11), 40-44.

Department of Labor. (2004). *Handy reference guide to the Fair Labor Standards Act.* Washington, DC: U.S. Department of Labor. Retrieved November 24, 2004, from *www.dol.gov/esa/regs/compliance/whd/hrg.htm*

Donley, R., & Flaherty, J. (2002, May 31). Revisiting the American Nurses Association's first position on education for nurses. *Online Journal of Issues in Nursing.* Retrieved April 5, 2004, from *www.nursingworld.org/ ojin/topic18/tpc18_1.htm*

Erickson, J.I., Hamilton, G.A., Jones, D.E., & Ditomassi, M. (2003). The value of collaborative governance/staff empowerment. *Journal of Nursing Administration, 33*(2), 96-104.

Fine, S.D. (2003-2004). *Emergence of unionization: A threat or salvation for physicians?* Arlington Heights, IL: American College of Osteopathic Family Physicians. Retrieved December 1, 2004, from *www.acofp.org/ member_publications/busmar_02.htm*

Forman, H. (1989). *Descriptive analysis of the effects of union and non-union affiliation on perceived role conflict, conflict resolution modes, leader behavior styles, and leadership effectiveness of head nurses.* New York: Columbia University Teachers College.

Forman, H., & Powell, T.A. (2003a). Effective labor relations managing during an employee walkout. *Journal of Nursing Administration, 33*(9), 430-433.

Forman, H., & Powell, T.A. (2003b). Effective labor relations management rights. *Journal of Nursing Administration, 33*(1), 7-9.

Forman, H., & Powell, T.A. (2003c). Effective labor relations living with a union contract. *Journal of Nursing Administration, 33*(1), 611-614.

Forman, H., & Powell, T.A. (2003d). Effective labor relations union-management cooperation *Journal of Nursing Administration, 33*(12), 621-623.

Joint Commission on Accreditation of Healthcare Organizations (JCAHO). (2004). *Health care at the crossroads: Strategies for addressing the evolving nursing crisis.* Oakbrook Terrace, IL: JCAHO.

Ketter, J. (1994). Ruling questions NLRA protection for nurses. *The American Nurse, 26*(6), 10, 13.

Legal Information Institute (LII). (1999a). *Collective bargaining and labor arbitration: An overview.* Ithaca, NY: LII, Cornell University Law School. Retrieved November 24, 2004, from *www.law.cornell.edu/topics/collective_ bargaining.html*

Legal Information Institute (LII). (1999b). *Labor: An overview.* Ithaca, NY: LII, Cornell University Law School. Retrieved November 24, 2004, from *www.law.cornell. edu/topics/labor.html*

McClure, M.L., Poulin, M.A., Sovie, M.D., & Wandelt, M.A. (1983). *Magnet hospitals: Attraction and retention of professional nurses.* Kansas City, MO: American Nurses Association.

National Labor Relations Board (NLRB). (1997). *A guide to basic law and procedures under the National Labor Relations Act.* Washington, DC: U.S. Government Printing Office.

National Labor Relations Board (NLRB). (2004). *Fact sheet on the National Labor Relations Board.* Washington, DC: NLRB. Retrieved November 24, 2004, from *www.nlrb. gov/nlrb/press/facts.asp*

New York State Nurses Association (NYSNA). (2004). *Why do RNs need a union?* Latham, NY: NYNSA. Retrieved November 24, 2004, from *www.nysna.org/programs/ egw/faqs.htm*

Porter-O'Grady, T., & Finnigan, S. (1984). *Shared governance for nursing: A creative approach to professional accountability.* Rockville, MD. Aspen.

Senge, P.M. (1990). *The fifth discipline: The art and practice of the learning organization.* London: Random House.

Spratley, E., Johnson, A., Sochalski, J., Fritz, M., & Spencer, W. (2000). *The registered nurse population: Findings from the national sample survey of registered nurses.* Washington, DC: U.S. Department of Health and Human Services.

UAN and ANA (United American Nurses and American Nurses Association). (2004). *Mission statement.* Silver Spring, MD: UAN, ANA. Retrieved November 24, 2004, from *www.nursingworld.org/uan/mission.htm*

Upenieks, V.V. (2002). Assessing differences in job satisfaction in magnet and nonmagnet hospitals. *Journal of Nursing Administration, 32*(11), 564-576.

Yett, D.E. (1970). Causes and Consequences of salary differentials in nursing. *Inquiry, 7,* 78-99.

33

Staffing and Scheduling

Diane L. Huber

CHAPTER OBJECTIVES

- Define and compare staffing and scheduling
- Describe staff mix
- Differentiate nursing resources, nursing workload, acuity, and intensity
- Construct four essential elements of a staffing program
- Formulate suggested steps for developing staffing patterns
- Critique workload measurement and patient classification systems
- Analyze staffing issues and economic pressures
- Exercise critical thinking to conceptualize and analyze possible solutions to a practice exercise

S taffing is a human resources function that is targeted at creating the personnel and favorable work conditions for optimal productivity and the professional practice of nursing. Staffing and scheduling are complex, multifaceted responsibilities that are central to nursing efforts to effectively integrate organizations and systems. Staffing and scheduling affect the jobs, positions, workload, personal lives, and morale of nurses. Staffing and scheduling decisions impact the organization or unit's financial management plan, impinge on productivity, and affect patient outcomes. These activities are both frustrating and time-absorbing for nurse managers. In addition, issues of safety and quality of client care may arise due to specific staffing and scheduling decisions. "One of the most critical issues confronting nurse executives today is nurse staffing" (Abdoo, 2000, p. 459). Staffing is a universal and perennial concern of human resource management in nursing. A study by Sullivan and colleagues (2003) noted, "In discussing challenging aspects of the leadership role, all participating nurse managers, nurse administrators, and chief nurse officers universally identified staffing as the most burdensome responsibility. Managers described making 'phone calls begging . . .' and discussed being 'mired in staffing'" (p. 546). According to Abdoo, "Staffing policies and needs affect the nursing department budget, staff productivity, quality of care provided to clients, nursing staff morale, and even nurse retention" (2000, p. 459).

Nursing care is a major component of health care. Registered nurses (RNs) are the critical input to the process of nursing care. Nursing care delivery is a service industry whose products are client care and client outcomes. A service industry relies on service providers. For nursing, this means RNs, LPNs, and the assistive personnel who work with them. Whether in hospitals, community nursing organizations, long-term care, or other settings, the delivery of nursing services to clients is founded on having the right skill mix of providers in the right numbers at the right place and properly prepared to render care. Regulatory agencies such as the Joint Commission on Accreditation of Healthcare Organizations (JCAHO) have a standard that calls for a sufficient number of qualified registered nurses to be on duty at all times to give clients nursing care that requires the specialized skill and judgment of an RN. JCAHO's standard HR.2 requires that "… the hospital provides an adequate number of staff members whose qualifications are consistent with the job responsibilities" (JCAHO, 2004a, p. 1). In 2002, JCAHO implemented its new hospital staffing effectiveness standard HR.2.1: "The organization uses data on clinical/service indicators in combination with human resource indicators to assess staffing effectiveness" (JCAHO, 2004b, p. 2).

Registered nurses can be considered a scarce human resource critical to the provision of health care because the availability of RN services to clients may be limited by financial, reimbursement, or political decisions. "There is little question that personnel is the single greatest cost in health care" (Finkler & Kovner, 2000, p. 7). Health care organizations limit the number of RN positions and overtime use when they tightly control labor budgets. Thus nurses are a human resource that may be sparsely deployed despite being fundamental to achieving client outcomes. Because of this, nurse staffing has been described as a barometer for health care (Beyers, 2000). It is an indicator of the challenges and issues in health care, often reflecting hidden aspects of the organization's structure, such as available resources, support services for client care, and devotion to education and professional development for nurses. There is less controversy over staffing decisions under good economic conditions, but staffing becomes contentious when resources are less available. According to Beyers, "Staffing is one of the outcomes and indicators of the effectiveness of nursing management practices" (2000, p. xxii).

DEFINITIONS

The major goal of staffing and scheduling systems is to identify the need for and provide the number and type of personnel required to deliver care (Smith, 1994). **Staffing** is defined as human resources planning to fill positions in an organization with qualified personnel. Nurse staffing has three main components: planning, scheduling, and allocation. Planning refers to determining the number of nursing personnel needed over a long-term period. Scheduling is assigning nursing staff for specific time periods by shift. Allocation refers to making adjusted assignments or reallocations on a daily or shift-by-shift basis (Abdoo, 2000). The staffing plan is a written plan that specifies the number and classification type of staff personnel who are needed to implement a care delivery model for each unit on a shift-by-shift basis (Smith, 1994). The care delivery model organizes processes of care, associated workload, and assignment of caregiver roles. Short-term plans involve filling existing positions. Long-term plans are concerned with determining the gap between the present and a desired future human resources status (Jernigan, 1988). The determination of how many and what types of personnel will be needed for a given unit or program should be made based

⚠ LEADING & MANAGING DEFINED

Staffing

Human resources planning to fill positions in an organization with qualified personnel.

Scheduling

The ongoing implementation of the staffing pattern by assigning individual personnel to work specific hours and days in a specific unit or area.

Fixed Staffing

Builds around a fixed projected maximum workload requirement.

Variable Staffing

Staffs units below maximum workload conditions and then supplements as needed.

on production requirements: client needs, program goals, and/or set standards. A reliable database that provides real-time accurate data is critical to staffing decision making. Unruh (2003) stated, "RN staffing is usually evaluated by assessing RN/patient and RN/nursing staff ratios" (p. 201). A *staffing strategy* is a set of actions undertaken to determine the organization's future human resources needs, recruit qualified applicants, and select the best of the applicants as new employees. Staffing activities need to mesh with other organizational strategies and the mission (Fried & Johnson, 2002).

Scheduling is defined as the ongoing implementation of the staffing pattern by assigning individual personnel to work specific hours, days, or shifts and in a specific unit or area (Barnum & Mallard, 1989). The schedule covers a specified period (Smith, 1994). Scheduling generally means the actual preparing of work hour assignments according to the staffing plan and mix. *Self-scheduling* is defined as the process of all nurses on a work unit together constructing their schedules for the coming time period, rather than accepting schedules constructed by management (Hung, 2002).

Staff mix is defined as the skill level of individuals delivering the required care (Kirby & Wiczai, 1985). Staff mix in nursing includes RNs, LPNs, nursing assistants, and unlicensed assistive personnel (UAPs). *Skill mix* is the proportion of RNs to total nursing staff. It is usually expressed as RN/total nursing personnel (Unruh, 2003).

The term *nursing resources* refers to the number and types of employees designated to provide nursing services to clients (Brett & Tonges, 1990). There are many ways to distribute resources within any organization. *Workload* is defined as the volume of work for a unit or department (Finkler & Kovner, 2000). *Nursing workload* is defined as the nursing care needs of clients. It refers to the nursing resources required for delivering nursing services to individuals or groups of clients. Beyers (2000) stated, "The real driver of nurse staffing is patient demand for care.... staffing in practice is all about nurses taking care of patients and families" (p. xxii).

Nursing workload is a measurement of the nursing work activities and the dependence of the clients on nursing care. Thus both direct and indirect nursing care activities are a part of nursing workload (O'Brien-Pallas et al., 1997). Nursing workload in a hospital is a function of two variables: the number of patient days and the hours of nursing care required per patient day (Kirby & Wiczai, 1985). Workload is the use of time, and time is the basis of nursing workload measurement.

Acuity is defined as the severity of illness or client condition. Acuity can translate into volume (census, visits, or encounters) or severity or intensity. Patient classification systems have been used since the 1960s to measure in some fashion clients' needs for care and care activities and assign acuity scores. They have become the basis for workload systems that determine staffing (Prescott & Soeken, 1996).

Nursing intensity is defined as both the amount of care and the complexity of care needed by patients in hospitals. Werley and Lang (1988) operationalized intensity as nursing care hours and staff mix. Prescott (1991) identified four major dimensions to nursing intensity (Box 33.1). The four components of severity of illness, client dependency on nursing, complexity, and time are related to each other and have been combined into a 10-item nursing intensity scale, called the Patient Intensity for Nursing Index (PINI)

Box **33.1**

Four Major Dimensions of Nursing Intensity

1. *Severity of illness:* The medical condition and how ill the person is in relationship to abnormality and instability of physiological parameters
2. *Client dependency:* Need for assistance with activities of daily living
3. *Complexity of nursing care*
4. *Time:* The hours of direct and indirect care received by a client

(Soeken & Prescott, 1991). Prescott and Soeken (1996) have developed a companion measure for ambulatory care called the Patient Intensity for Nursing Ambulatory Care (PINAC). Three PINI conceptual components of complexity, dependency, and severity were modified for PINAC to severity of illness, patients' psychosocial needs, and complexity of care. Type of visit also was included as a descriptor. Intensity is usually a composite measure of the amount of work or time involved with a level of complexity of the care required (Detwiler & Clark, 1995). Nurse staffing intensity, which is expressed as the ratio of RNs to patient census in hospitals, has been associated with lower mortality in hospitals (Aiken et al., 2002; Mitchell & Shortell, 1997).

BACKGROUND

The nurse leader and manager will find staffing and scheduling to be a critical, core function. The decisions have broad impact. Staffing and scheduling are a fine balance of competing interests and needs. There are predetermined standards, budget constraints, personal preferences, legal aspects, and individuals to please. Tenure versus equity may need to be balanced. For example, nurses may need to confront individual and collective philosophies about whether experience and time in a job are the decision factors in staffing and scheduling or whether experience and tenure are weighted with or replaced by a balance of needs of both newer and longer employed unit members. Shared governance may include self-staffing as an aspect of autonomy. Legal or regulatory changes such as the Family Medical Leave Act may create challenges to ongoing staffing and scheduling at the specific unit level because of the constraints to wide flexibility that may be imposed.

Staffing and scheduling are two aspects of the allocation of scarce and expensive personnel resources. To increase the chance of successful and appropriate allocation of resources, the administrative function of planning is involved in staffing and scheduling. The planning may be simple or complex. It may be as simple as deciding what is wanted (e.g., an all-RN staff) and then as complex as determining what must be done to obtain it (e.g., budgeting, recruitment, and retention). Staffing methodology needs to be based on quantifiable and measurable data. The following three variables are central to the staffing methodology (Abdoo, 2000):

1. Assessment of patient needs for care (patient classification)
2. Assessment of required nursing time to meet needs (workload determination)
3. An algorithm that uses the first two variables

Staffing and scheduling have obvious budgeting and costing implications. This linkage of an expensive labor supply to the fluctuations in client care needs and revenue income absorbs considerable managerial time and effort in nursing. The effort is especially intense under conditions of diminished levels of reimbursement, tight budgets, and cost-containment pressures.

Staffing, scheduling, resource pool use, information management, and unit workload interact to compete for the time and attention of managers as well as for top priority. Especially where manual systems are in use, these functions may reach chaos and crisis levels. Sometimes the crisis mode becomes a chronic way of managerial operating. Thus, for example, a staff nurse may not be able to know the work schedule enough in advance in order to determine the possibility of taking a college class or attend a family event. In one hospital, a resource management plan was developed to switch from crisis mode to a proactive system for staffing and scheduling. The resultant detailed plan provided direction for responding to resource needs under conditions both of service demands (high volume) or deficit demands (lower-than-needed staffing). The core foundation of the plan involved stabilizing the unit core staffing. Five design teams were developed to address scheduling, daily staffing, nursing resource pool, workload variability, and management information (Kirkby et al., 1998). Because of manual computational complexity, many health care organizations have contracted with vendors for informatics-based staffing and scheduling systems. In some cases, sophisticated analytical tools are used to derive staffing models.

Staffing may be based on research results. The typical model is based on trend data or fitting a staffing mix into a preset budget.

Principles for Nurse Staffing

The American Nurses Association (ANA) has been concerned about the impact of nursing care on patient outcomes and the professional well-being of nurses (ANA, 2000). Previous work, such as the ANA's report card for nursing and the Institute of Medicine's *Nursing Staff in Hospitals and Nursing Homes: Is it Adequate?* (Wunderlich et al., 1996), highlighted the need for research evidence to determine whether differences across acute care hospitals in nurse staffing could be shown to be related to measurable differences in important patient outcomes. The ANA's social policy statement (1999) noted that "adequate nurse staffing is critical to the delivery of quality patient care" (p. 1). However, identifying and maintaining the appropriate number and mix of nursing staff is a real problem. Thus the ANA (1999) formulated *Principles for Nurse Staffing*. Its policy statements emphasized the need for nurse staffing patterns and level of care provided to be independent of payor type and for staffing to be based on achieving quality-of-care indices, meeting organizational outcomes, and ensuring appropriate quality of nurses' work lives.

Using an expert panel, the ANA (1999) identified nine principles to guide nurse staffing, grouped into three categories of (1) patient care unit–related, (2) staff-related, and (3) institutional/organization-related. The nine principles are as follows:

I. Patient Care Unit–Related
  A. Appropriate staffing levels for a patient care unit reflect analysis of individual and aggregate patient needs.
  B. There is a critical need to either retire or seriously question the usefulness of the concept of nursing hours per patient day (HPPD).
  C. Unit functions necessary to support delivery of quality patient care must also be considered in determining staffing levels.

II. Staff-Related
  A. The specific needs of various patient populations should determine the appropriate clinical competencies required of the nurse practicing in that area.
  B. Registered nurses must have nursing management support and representation at both the operational level and the executive level.
  C. Clinical support from experienced RNs should be readily available to those RNs with less proficiency.

III. Institution/Organization-Related
  A. Organizational policy should reflect an organizational climate that values registered nurses and other employees as strategic assets and exhibit a true commitment to filling budgeted positions in a timely manner.
  B. All institutions should have documented competencies for nursing staff, including agency or supplemental and traveling RNs, for those activities that they have been authorized to perform.
  C. Organizational policies should recognize the myriad needs of both patients and nursing staff. (ANA, 1999, p. 2)

In addition, the ANA (1999) displayed a matrix for staffing decision making to emphasize the serious concern about using the concept of nursing hours per patient day (HPPD) as a one-size-fits-all formula. Rather, "staffing is most appropriate and meaningful when it is predicated on a measure of unit intensity that takes into consideration the aggregate population of patients and the associated roles and responsibilities of nursing staff" (ANA, 1999, p. 2). The simple quantification of the needs of the "average" patient is not useful or reliable for staffing. Instead, "a distinct standardized definition of unit intensity must be developed" (ANA, 1999, p. 5). To evaluate staffing, the ANA (1999) noted that ongoing evaluation and benchmarking are necessary. Collection and analysis of nursing-sensitive indicators need to be done. Changes in staffing levels, numbers, and mix should be based on analysis of effects of alterations in staffing on outcomes of standardized, nursing-sensitive indicators.

STAFFING AND SCHEDULING DECISIONS

To determine appropriate staffing, the ANA (1999) presented a matrix for staffing decision making composed of the following four critical factors:

1. The number of patients, including elements of patient characteristics and the number of patients for whom care is being provided
2. The levels of intensity of the unit and care, including individual patient intensity; across-the-unit intensity; variability of care; admissions, discharges and transfers; and volume
3. Contextual issues, including architecture, geography of the environment, available technology, and same unit or cluster of patients
4. Level of expertise and preparation of those providing care, including learning curve; staff consistency, continuity and cohesion; cross-training; control over practice; involvement in quality-improvement activities; professional expectations; preparation; and experience

Thus decisions about appropriate staffing levels for any patient care unit need to reflect the analysis of both individual and aggregate patient needs, as well as unit functions necessary to support quality patient care delivery.

Staffing and scheduling decisions contain unique factors, depending on the care delivery setting. Much of the literature is focused on acute care hospitals. However, staffing and scheduling for a home health agency, community program, long-term care facility, or ambulatory clinic will require different approaches. Even within acute care, needs vary. For example, staffing an operating room requires different considerations based on schedule, space, time, coordination of personnel, and special skills or equipment needs. The staffing and scheduling similarities include ensuring safe, cost-effective care, dealing with workload fluctuations, using a variety of caregivers, and maximizing and maintaining resources in a responsible way (Barratt & Schutz, 1997).

Considerable preliminary work precedes staffing and scheduling decisions. The following four elements are essential to a staffing program (Ramey, 1973):

1. A statement of philosophy for the unit, department, and institution that defines values and beliefs
2. Objectives—general for the department and specific for each unit
3. Job descriptions for each type and level of personnel
4. A determination of the frequency with which nursing care is to be provided and who will provide it

It is thought that the quality of a staffing program is related to the philosophy and objectives of the department of nursing. Staffing and scheduling by patient census in a hospital may ignore nursing's philosophy, objectives, and job descriptions in predicting staffing requirements and scheduling needs. When this happens, it complicates efforts to evaluate or measure progress based on patient safety, quality of care, and RN professional judgment.

Staffing and scheduling decisions usually are based on some measure of volume and/or time. Staffing and scheduling may be the result of methods of time sampling, work sampling, continuous sampling of time or work, or self-report. The measurement of the staff's workload in many instances is not done through an ongoing compilation of what actually occurs. Rather, a workload measure is devised as a proxy. For example, the mean direct care time can be determined for an "average client." Averages, or means, are sensitive to outliers. This means that unusually high or low numbers throw the mean value off from the typical case. Thus changes in average direct care times or shifts within severity of illness categories may have a substantial impact on staffing. Averages do not allow individualization to a client's care experience and subsequent linkage to outcomes at the level of an individual client. Staffing and scheduling decisions need to be setting-specific and based on some combination of minimum external standards; review of trend data; outcomes for clients, staff, and the organization; risk factors; and organizational revenue.

An intense focus on measuring and quantifying the time spent in nursing activities, usually by means of time-and-motion studies, can make nurses uncomfortable. This is because of the similarity to models of industrial efficiency. Discomfort is further generated if nursing's psychosocial work aspects and values related to spending time being with and interacting with clients and families are not taken into account. It is difficult to justify the reduction of professional nursing care to repetitive tasks and procedures.

Nurse staffing and scheduling in some settings may be based on standardized volume measures (Table 33.1). For example, a home health agency may set a minimum of six visits per day as the norm for determining staffing. In a small community hospital's labor and delivery unit, the staffing pattern may be two RNs as a standard. These and other forms of staffing ratios based only on volume measures such as patient census or client encounters ignore important factors related to planning nurse staffing. Other factors include amount of travel or downtime, type of equipment available to facilitate the staff's work,

ease of communication, the physical design of a unit, proximity to related resources, the availability of specialists, and individual client complexity. The complexity and variability of patient conditions partially create the demand for nursing care and influence the intensity of care. Four key concepts better describe variations in the intensity of nursing work: patient nursing condition, medical condition, caregiver characteristics, and the environment (O'Brien-Pallas et al., 1997).

Knowledge of the nursing time needed to care for different types of clients is fundamental in determining staffing and scheduling. However, simplistic workload measures and many patient classification systems do not yield the type of data needed to make the leap between workload data and staffing plans. The numbers may be calculated, but they are not enough to make nurses comfortable about perceived workable staffing decisions. The lack of an easy fit between workload data and staffing plans creates a level of stress and tension in the work of nursing. An alternative approach is to use an expanded staffing formula based on a nurse workload calculation that incorporates staff expertise, patient acuity, MD availability, work intensity, support staff and unit physical layout. Seago (2002, p. 53) presented the following formula:

$$\text{Nurse workload} = f(\text{RN staff expertise} + \text{Patient} \\ \text{acuity} + \text{MD availability} \\ + \text{Work intensity} + \text{Support staff} \\ + \text{Unit physical layout})$$

STAFFING METHODS

Nursing provides a service to clients, which is the use of expertise to solve health problems, provide direct care, and assist with self-care management. The common denominator for identifying and measuring activities for quality and quantity is the unit of service. The unit of service is a volume measure and may be patient days, treatments, visits, encounters, births, operations, exercise sessions, or client contact. Time is measured in "hours per . . ."—for example, hours per patient day (HPPD). Averages or standards may be derived and entered into staffing planning and

Table 33.1

Standardized Volume Measures	
Volume Measure	Setting
Number of visits	Home health agency
Core staff	Emergency department
Patient days or occupied beds	Inpatient hospital unit
Client encounters	Ambulatory care clinic
Covered lives	Capitated reimbursement system in a health maintenance organization (HMO)
Births	Labor and delivery
Operations	Operating room surgical services
Exercise sessions	Wellness program

calculations (Kirk, 1988). Activities related to client care are evaluated in relation to the consumption of staff labor per hour. For example, inpatient nursing units may calculate the HPPD as a productivity measure. If a generic productivity equation divides work inputs by work outputs, then the nursing application of this productivity standard divides nursing hours required by the unit of service (such as patient days) to result in HPPD (Soule & Dobson, 1992). Calculating the HPPD is an example of a direct method of patient classification-related staffing (DeGroot, 1994). Using HPPD alone as a productivity system assumes a direct relationship between HPPD and salary expense per patient day (SEPPD), a measure of cost. Research indicates that HPPD alone is insufficient for either accurate staffing and scheduling projections or for monitoring and controlling labor budgets (DeGroot, 1994; Soule & Dobson, 1992). This is because many factors affect time requirements, and averages do not describe or account well for outlier cases.

Two general methods of nurse staffing are the traditional fixed staffing and controlled variable staffing. With **fixed staffing**, staffing is built around a fixed projected maximum workload requirement, and the plan is based on maximum workload conditions. With **variable staffing**, units are staffed below maximum workload conditions and staff then supplemented as needed. Supplementation may be done by creating a "float pool" or by using supplemental staffing agencies. This is a system of flexible resource management (Bennett, 1981). Fixed staffing based on historical census trend data and projections results in predictable staffing and scheduling that are handy for budgeting. However, real world occurrences of workload fluctuations, both high and low, result in overtime, short staffing, or periods of idleness, all with budget and staff morale implications. Kirk (1988) listed a semiflexible system as a third type of nurse staffing system. In this system, about 10% to 15% of staff members are fixed, whereas the rest are flexible and the volume is adjusted to match the need.

If variable staffing is to be used, then a system is needed that accurately measures workload. In an accurate system, effective staffing would result from matching resources to the workload. The system needs to be responsive to fluctuations in workload, simple to use, and credible with both nurses and administration (Kirby & Wiczai, 1985). Although there are various calculations and ways to determine nurse staffing and scheduling, no completely satisfactory method has been identified. Kirby and Wiczai (1985) noted that the credibility of nursing leadership and management may be tested, because staff nurses question the appropriateness and fairness of the distribution of resources, and hospital administration questions nursing's ability to manage costs. An added challenge is to balance workload fluctuations with specialization requirements in large, complex, or specialized organizations. An application of systems thinking to staffing and scheduling helps direct solutions through an analysis of inputs, organizational goals, unit goals, the staffing and scheduling system, and outputs (Smith, 1994).

STEPS IN DEVELOPING A STAFFING PATTERN

Nurses need to know how staffing assignments are made and how client acuity data are used. This includes each unit's staffing plan, the relationship of the acuity system to the staffing plan, and the mechanism used to facilitate changes in the acuity system (Smith & Zuel, 1998). The staffing pattern is based on a plan that quantifies the total number and number-by-category of staff to be scheduled for each day or each shift. Ramey (1973) suggested the following eleven steps for developing hospital staffing patterns:

1. Select criteria to classify clients into severity of illness categories. Survey the unit at intervals to establish percentages.
2. Record all direct and indirect activities, the number of times performed, and the total time needed for performance for a specified period.
3. Collect data on a representative number of clients to determine valid averages by classification.
4. Collect data in several ways.

5. Average the number of minutes required to accomplish each nursing activity to equal an average performance time.

6. Determine the average performance time for new functions to be instituted.

7. Note the skill level of personnel required to perform each nursing activity per severity of illness category.

8. Calculate the average amount of nursing time required by each client in each severity of illness category by the percentage of time devoted to them by both professional and nonprofessional nursing personnel by shift.

9. Obtain the projected patient days on the unit for the year.

10. Calculate the total number of nursing hours needed annually for the unit. Compute the hours worked in a year by professional and nonprofessional staff, discounting time off.

11. From the average amount of nursing time required and the total number of nursing hours needed annually, derive the number of persons required on each shift. An additional calculation is needed to determine the number of personnel needed to cover inservicing, unit administration, orientation, and research or professional development activities.

A consensus-building process is recommended when using a systems framework to build a staffing and scheduling model targeted toward meeting hours of care and financial standards (Smith, 1994).

The American Organization of Nurse Executives (Fralic, 2000) compiled a text on nurse staffing that discussed a clinical labor resource management system (RMS). The four components of an RMS are budgeting, scheduling, daily staffing, and management information (McKinley & Cavouras, 2000).

Staffing-related budget components are full-time equivalent positions (FTEs), unit of service (UOS) as a workload volume indicator, average daily census (ADC) as a template for the skill mix and number of workers needed for the core

staff, and the hours per patient day (HPPD) as an indicator of hours of care given to patients. HPPD is calculated by tallying the hours staff worked at patient care for a 24-hour period, divided by the patient midnight census (or other measure such as visits or procedures). The formulas are as follows:

$$\frac{\text{Hours worked per day}}{\text{Midnight census}} = \text{Hours worked per patient per day}$$

$$\frac{\text{Total hours worked}}{\text{Number of days in reporting period}} = \text{Hours worked per day}$$

Related expense budget calculations include patient classification/acuity rankings of patients, occupancy rate, and productive and nonproductive hours. Because common hospital nurse staffing measures such as nurses or hours of nursing care divided by patients or patient days of care do not take into account the fact that staffing needs vary with the amount and type of care delivered to each patient, Unruh and Fottler (2004) suggested that an ideal measure of nursing staff adequacy would consider intensity. It would indicate the number of nurses of a certain skill level that are necessary for the given number of patients given the intensity of nursing care required. This formula is as follows:

$$\text{Adequate Nursing Staff} = \frac{\# \text{ RNs}}{\# \text{ Patient days} \times \text{Intensity of RN care for those patient days}}$$

SCHEDULING

The daily work schedule is a short-range plan for human resource management. It establishes the needed human resources for a unit or area. The number of shifts per day and the number of FTEs need to be calculated, and this information needs to be converted into the specific positions needed (Finkler & Kovner, 2000). Figure 33.1 illustrates an example of a spreadsheet for FTEs by type and shift for a hospital. A table listing all positions by title and showing shift worked, number of positions,

STAFF	7AM-3PM shift	3PM-11PM shift	11PM-7AM shift	TOTAL
Fixed Positions				
Nurse Manager				
Secretary				
Staffing Clerk				
Subtotal				
Variable Positions				
RN				
LPN				
Aide				
Subtotal				
TOTAL				

Figure 33.1

Sample spreadsheet for full-time equivalent (FTE) positions in a hospital.

FTEs, and hours also can be constructed to help track and analyze positions.

Once the average or minimum number of staff needed to meet patients' needs is determined, personnel scheduling follows. This is not as simple as it seems because weekend and holiday off- time plus sick time and vacation time taken need to be factored into daily coverage. Each unit or organization needs to develop guidelines and scheduling policies to maintain order and fairness. One specific area needing attention is changes to the schedule after posting. This normally should be done through exchanges (McKinley & Cavouras, 2000).

There are a variety of types of time-scheduling systems: block, unstructured, skeleton, cyclical, and master. A block schedule is fixed until revised yearly. Requests are not accommodated. An unstructured schedule is created weekly and fluctuates based on staff's needs. This decreases predictability. A skeleton schedule starts with a basic skeleton staffing and fixes only a portion of the schedule, usually weekends. There is less predictability and greater time consumed in preparing the schedule. A cyclical schedule sets a pattern for each staff person's days on and days off. Shifts are rotated. This is more predictable and less time-consuming to prepare. A master schedule is a cyclical repetitive schedule, covering an entire area for a long period such as a 4-week block (McKinley & Cavouras, 2000).

Daily Staffing and Management Information

Factors such as fluctuating demands for nursing care, highly variable census or volume, and staff turnover make delivering the level of needed daily staffing resources a challenge. RN staff may be supplemented by float, agency, or traveler nurses. Computerized nurse scheduling may be used to integrate patient classification, workload calculations, staffing, and scheduling. Graf and colleagues (2003) described the use of one vendor's software suite to make informed, data-driven staffing and scheduling decisions.

Self-Scheduling

As Hung (2002) stated, "Scheduling of nurses is a major operational challenge in hospitals" (p. 37). Because the schedule needs to satisfy staffing needs while meeting individual needs of nurses, it become a constant challenge. Self-scheduling is an alternative method whereby nurses on a unit work together to construct their schedules for the upcoming timeframe rather than having schedules constructed by management (Hung, 2002). Once the number of nurses needed per shift for the timeframe is determined, nurses sign up for any shifts they want to work, within guidelines and contractual bounds. An upper limit is placed on the number allowed to sign up in each time block. In the case of conflicts, adjustments are made based on consensus (Bard & Purnomo, 2004). Generally, a worksheet is posted, with guidelines and requirements. Nurses have a specified time frame to post preferences. Then the manager examines the worksheet and either approves it or reposts for nurses to negotiate changes (Hung, 2002). There are advantages to self-scheduling,

such as reduced nurse manager time and frustration and increased predictability and nurse control over work schedules. However, it may be difficult to implement or not be perceived as fair.

Another related alternative is preference scheduling. This is a system in which nurses sign up for shifts prior to the timeframe and submit a list of requests. The nurse manager compiles requests and generates the final roster. Bard and Purnomo (2004) described the use of an operations research application using a computerized algorithm to identify attractive nurse schedules.

LEADERSHIP AND MANAGEMENT IMPLICATIONS

Workload Measurement and Patient Classification Systems

Patient classification means grouping patients or clients according to a standard assessment of their nursing care requirements over a specified period of time (Reitz, 1985). Patient classifications systems provide a quantified measure of the nursing time and effort required to care for clients (Giovannetti, 1979). Nurse managers seek ways to quantify nursing resource requirements. Three ways to accomplish this quantification are by time-and-motion techniques, work-sampling techniques, and acuity estimation or patient classification systems.

Time-and-motion studies are aimed at developing time standards for specific nursing activities. In time-and-motion studies, nurses are observed to determine actual activities performed and the amount of time devoted to each task. Average or mean times are derived per task, and a uniform standard time per task is established. Many patient classification systems use this information in deriving standard times for the average client. Although the practice of nursing is central to a health care organization's products, no generally accepted universal standards of nursing time exist (Mowry & Korpman, 1986). Some benchmarks may be generated internally, and external benchmarks may be available from databases of like users.

▲ LEADERSHIP & MANAGEMENT **BEHAVIORS**

Leadership Behaviors

- Integrates philosophy, values, and beliefs in staffing plan
- Enables followers to self-schedule
- Communicates the need for the staff mix
- Collaborates with others in staffing and scheduling
- Encourages discussion of workload issues

- Allocates labor resources
- Determines job descriptions
- Matches client needs to available staff
- Negotiates staff coverage
- Evaluates workload data
- Communicates the staffing method

Management Behaviors

- Develops a staffing plan
- Makes out a schedule

Overlap Areas

- Plans staffing
- Communicates about staffing and scheduling

Work sampling is used to capture work activities by observation at regular intervals over random times. Activities are classified by types, and probability and statistics are used on the work activities observations to generalize to all nursing care. The information needed to classify activities, however, may not be clear or distinct. The concepts of time-and-motion and work sampling became the foundation for systems of patient classification based on nursing time requirements and labor costs. The various patient classification systems have been used to project staffing and scheduling (Mowry & Korpman, 1986).

Patient classification systems are developed to group or categorize clients. There are a variety of patient classification systems that differ in terms of their degree of specificity and comprehensiveness of scope. Patient classification systems have been designed to tackle the management problems of the proportion of RNs to unlicensed assistive personnel, the proper use of nursing resources under cost containment, and realizing improvements in the delivery of care (Mowry & Korpman, 1986). Research in nursing has indicated that medical care-based systems such as diagnosis-related groups (DRGs) do not reflect nursing care intensity and, therefore, like standard hours of care based on census, do not become useful to categorize clients according to nursing care requirements.

The medical care-based systems are not workable to bridge the gap between client categorization and nursing resource consumption prediction. Advanced efforts focus on categorizing clients according to their anticipated and actual requirements for nursing care.

There are three broad types of patient classification systems, as follows (Mowry & Korpman, 1986; Reitz, 1985) (Box 33.2):

1. *Prototype systems* are based on average care times for groups of clients defined by broad categories and typical characteristics. Categories are hierarchical (such as low-medium-high) according to the amount of care required. Clients are classified by being compared with the described prototype. Prototypes are often called *subjective systems* whose reliability is questioned.

2. *Factor systems* use critical indicators to describe individual elements of direct care requirements. For example, time-and-motion studies may be conducted to derive those elements of the job that are critical to work accomplishment. Adjustments are added for indirect care. The indicators are each rated, relatively valued or weighted, and combined to determine a score and category. Factor systems are heavily based on tasks and specific activities. Their ability to capture the full scope of the nursing process is questioned.

Types of Patient Classification Systems

Prototype

Prototype is based on average care times for groups of clients defined by broad categories and typical characteristics.

Factor

Critical indicators are used to describe individual elements of direct care requirements. Adjustments are made for indirect care. Each indicator is rated, relatively valued or weighted, and the combination of these ratings determines the score and category.

Computerized Real-Time Factor

Actual times of all direct and indirect nursing care activities are recorded. These time computations and acuity ratings are automatically calculated and updated in real time.

3. *Computerized real-time factor systems* record the actual times of all direct and indirect nursing care activities. Time computations and acuity ratings are automatically calculated and updated in real time. If all activities are documented, the computer captures actual activity performed for the client, rapidly and automatically calculates data, and determines acuity and staffing while avoiding subjectivity and information delay. In some systems, nursing diagnoses, interventions, and outcomes form the basis of the care activities documentation. Standardized languages and classification systems are used in order to generate comparable data.

Overall, patient classification systems attempt to identify acuity, which can approximate workload and become the basis for staffing and budgeting. The systems have been criticized for reliability, validity, and comparability across settings. Some are not practical; some do not lend themselves to evaluation. The need for nationwide standardized definitions and classifications for comparable input data has been suggested to avoid "managing without facts." Acuity systems may be of use to nurses but ignored by organizational financial administration (McManus & Pearson, 1993). Because nurses devote considerable time and energy into developing and maintaining patient classification systems, it is important to analyze whether the time is well spent. Are valid and reliable data generated that are useful to nurses and nursing? Should the effort be abandoned because political decisions allocate resources, not data-based decisions? Nurses need to assess and analyze their work settings to determine the best way to manage acuity and workload.

CURRENT ISSUES AND TRENDS

Management of human resources is one of the most important components of a health care service. Personnel costs have been described as the single largest health care expense item, variously estimated at 35% to 40% of the total budget of the average hospital (Halloran, 1985). In a typical hospital, about half of the personnel are employed in nursing service. However, the extent to which nursing care costs are accurately ascribed and contribute to hospital costs is open to debate. Some nurse researchers have estimated that nursing costs account for only 20% to 25% of total hospital costs (Phillips et al., 1992). Labor expenses are a logical target for cost containment, and nursing service becomes the visible and obvious area to cut in poor economic times (Mowry & Korpman, 1986). This issue remains a very real concern for nursing as nurse leaders seek to develop workforce stability, alleviate the effects of the nurse shortage, and address patient safety issues.

Two cycles of economic pressures have occurred in the recent past: the mid-1980s with the implementation of DRGs and prospective reimbursement, and the mid-1990s with health care reform and restructuring. The immediate responses were to slash budgets and lay off nursing personnel. Many nursing positions became in effect part-time jobs as forced time off occurred. Staff mix rapidly changed. As acuity rose and lengths of stay were reduced in hospitals, the RN role also changed. Workload measurement standards and acuity systems came under review. The roles and functions of advanced practice nurses were reviewed and revised (Mowry & Korpman, 1986).

Several general issues were triggered. Layoffs and downsizing created short-term economic gains for employers, but these actions caused threats to job security and resultant low morale. They established a difficult climate for recruitment and retention when the inevitable nursing shortage cycled around again. A predisposition to unionization was sparked by employers' actions. Nursing's roles, functions, and skill mixes were affected in ways that appeared to follow fads instead of research knowledge. Thus over time, nursing practice appeared to be driven more by employer-determined job descriptions and positions than by nursing-determined parameters of practice. It was not clear what the most effective and efficient mix of RNs, LPNs, and unlicensed assistive personnel is or should be. Thus the role of the nurse was unclear. Staffing and scheduling became more complicated without clear standards and guidelines. As the number of RNs in the skill mix dropped, however, a backlash of concern over patient safety emerged. A series of reports from the Institute of Medicine (IOM), beginning with *Nursing Staff in Hospitals and Nursing Homes: Is it Adequate?* (Wunderlich et al., 1996) and including *To Err Is Human* (Kohn et al., 2000), stimulated a national impetus for a variety of patient safety initiatives, including examining nurse staffing and scheduling.

Minimum Staffing Ratios

Although the profession of nursing had been dealing with surplus and shortage cycles throughout the 1900s, by the mid-1990s the chaos and trauma of hospital redesign and downsizing had reached an unbearable point for nurses. Staffing issues had become a major patient safety issue (Wunderlich et al., 1996) and a critical workplace dissatisfier as nurses were forced to work mandatory overtime when the subsequent nurse shortage hit. Despite strong evidence of increased RN

staffing being related to positive patient outcomes (Aiken et al., 2001), there was a lack of research evidence regarding adequate nurse staffing levels in general and optimal staffing for specific patient populations (Seago et al., 2003).

Under conditions of tight financial resources, hospital administrators and nurse executives try to reduce the amount of money spent on RN salaries because this is a large and visible budget item. A leaner RN skill mix (RNs to total nursing staff) was tried by Kaiser Permanente Northern California in the early 1990s (to 55%) and in 1995 (to 30%) (Robertson & Samuelson, 1996). Ways to change skill mix include work redesign, downsizing, or different care modalities. Changes in skill mix led to real or perceived increases in RN workload, patient safety concerns, and/or nurse and consumer complaints (Seago et al., 2003).

Despite complaints and reports of nurse dissatisfaction, little was done until 1999, when the California legislature passed Assembly Bill 394 (AB394), after several years of effort by the California Nurses Association to legislatively mandate minimum nurse staffing ratios. AB394 mandated that the California Department of Health Services establish minimum, specific, and numerical nurse-to-patient ratios by licensed nurse classification and hospital unit. The range of tasks performed by unlicensed personnel also was specifically limited (Seago et al., 2003).

The purpose of AB394 was to improve the quality of care. However, this law passed and required a determination of minimum nurse staffing ratios at a time when there was little research evidence to rely on to establish "safe" staffing levels. The following variety of issues arose:

- What should the minimum ratio be?
- How can rural hospitals come into compliance, given cost and nurse shortage pressures?
- How will costs be covered?
- How will hospitals adjust actual RN staffing?
- How will lunch and breaks be covered?

Clearly more research is needed about the relationship of RN staffing and quality of care. It is not clear that more is better. It has been suggested that a staffing formula might be a better

Research Note

Source: Unruh, L. (2003). The effect of LPN reductions on RN patient load. *Journal of Nursing Administration, 33*(4), 201-208.

Purpose

The 1990s saw downsizing of RNs and nursing personnel and then a nurse shortage. A concern arose that the numbers of skilled nursing staff are not adequate to meet patients' needs. There is not enough research to understand RN patient load and skill mix issues. The purpose of this study was to examine changes in RN and LPN numbers together, using data from Pennsylvania hospitals from 1991 to 2000, to explore changes in skill mix effects on RN patient load.

Discussion

This study examined the percentage of change in the number of RNs, LPNs, nursing assistants (NAs), and total nursing staff in Pennsylvania hospitals from 1991-2000. Changes in patient load, acuity-adjusted patient load, and skill mix were also explored. Numbers of staff were measured in FTEs. Patient load was measured by adjusted patient days of care (APDC), calculated as follows:

Yearly number of patients $\times$ Length of stay (LOS) for each patient + Estimated number of outpatient days = APDC

Nursing staff patient load equals the ratio of nursing staff to 1000 APDC (RN/1000 APDC). A lower value indicates a higher load. Acuity adjusted patient load (AAPL) was based on a vendor's patient acuity system. A hospital level index was derived from adding patient acuity scores in each hospital and dividing by the number of patients:

$$\frac{(\text{Sum of individual patient acuity})}{\#\ \text{Patients}} = \text{Hospital level index}$$

Then the AAPL was calculated as follows:

$$\frac{\text{RN/1000 APDC}}{\text{Hospital level acuity score}} = \text{AAPL}$$

The number of hospitals included in the study varied from year-to-year (n = 185-215). Data analyses were yearly and overall changes in mean nursing staff categories and paired t tests of difference.

For the 10-year period, the number of FTE RNs (247 of 283) rose 5%, the number of FTE LPNs (36 out of 283) fell 29%, and the number of nursing assistants (54 out of 337) rose 14%. Total nursing staff increased by 2%. Of all categories, only LPNs experienced a significant decline. However, because they are a small proportion of all licensed nurses, the level of licensed nurses (RNs + LPNs) remained about the same. Growth of RN staff slowed. There was an actual reduction in licensed staff and lowering of skill mix. When adjusted for patient acuity, the patient load increased significantly for all staff categories. When there was no increase in number of patients, the intensity of their care did increase. Because of deep and continuing LPN reductions, both RNs and LPNs experienced an increase in the number of patients in some years. Both also experienced an increase in the intensity of care. Licensed nurses had more supervisory tasks as a result of the substitution of nursing assistants for LPNs.

Application to Practice

These results help explain perceptions that hospitals are understaffed, especially with regard to skilled nurses. More supervision of NAs increases the RNs' workload beyond intensity of care increases due to sicker patients. Differences in results from prior studies may be due to differences in chosen severity measures. Measuring and evaluating changes in all categories of nursing staff gives a more complete understanding of RN staffing. The fall in LPN numbers has only a small impact on the skill mix of nurses when RNs and LPNs are counted together as licensed nurses to total nursing staff. However, substitutions in the skill mix directly affect RNs' workload. Therefore, economizing by using fewer LPNs may have a more negative impact than expected. It is important to maintain an adequate RN staff and evaluate fully changes to skill mix, patient acuity and workload.

alternative to staffing ratios (Seago, 2002). The mandating of minimum nurse-to-patient ratios has been controversial. In other states that have explored taking the same action, ratios were negotiated into some collective bargaining agreements. Mandated ratios are one alternative to address a real nursing practice concern. It is not yet clear whether this is the best alternative. However, the bold action of California's state legislative mandate stimulated focused attention on addressing nurse staffing issues.

RN Staffing, Patient Outcomes, and Ratios

The relationship between RN staffing levels and patient outcomes is a current issue receiving intense focus since the late 1990s. The government, regulatory agencies and researchers have concentrated efforts on identifying the evidence base for the relationship of nurse staffing to patient outcomes. For example, the IOM's (2004) *Keeping Patients Safe: Transforming the Work Environment of Nurses* addressed issues of staffing levels and work hours in relation to patient safety. The Health Resources and Services Administration (HRSA), Health Care Financing Administration (HCFA), Agency for Healthcare Research and Quality (AHRQ), and the National Institute for Nursing Research (NINR) jointly sponsored a study titled *Nurse Staffing and Patient Outcomes in Hospitals* (Needleman et al., 2001). This study found "strong and consistent relationships between nurse staffing variables and important patient outcomes in acute care hospital inpatient units in the following" (HRSA, 2005, p. 1):

- **Medical Patients**
  Urinary tract infections
  Pneumonia
  Shock
  Upper gastrointestinal bleeding
  Length of stay
- **Major Surgical Patients**
  Failure to rescue (defined as the death rate among patients with sepsis, pneumonia, shock, upper gastrointestinal bleeding, or deep vein thrombosis) (HRSA, 2005, p. 1)

An AHRQ-funded evidence-based practice center reviewed 26 studies on the relationship between nurse staffing levels and measures of patient

safety (Stanton & Rutherford, 2004). These studies found that "lower nurse-to-patient ratios were associated with higher rates of nonfatal adverse outcomes," both at the hospital and nursing unit levels (Stanton & Rutherford, 2004, p. 3). For example, in hospitals with high RN staffing, medical patients had lower rates of five adverse patient outcomes (Needleman et al., 2001). Specifically, "three AHRQ-funded studies found a significant correlation between lower nurse staffing levels and higher rates of pneumonia" (Stanton & Rutherford, 2004, p. 4).

Clearly, research evidence has converged to indicate a strong relationship between RN staffing levels and selected patient outcomes. Stanton and Rutherford (2004) concluded the following:

> Research findings indicating what minimal nurse staffing ratios should be either within the hospital or within its various subunits are not available. Researchers believe that more accurate and consistent measures of acuity and quality and more complete data on staffing for all types of nursing personnel are needed to explain the complex relationship between nurse staffing and the quality of care. (p. 8)

However, in an integrated review of the research done on nurse staffing and patient outcomes, Curtin (2003) concluded that research indicates that RN staffing has a real and measurable impact on patient outcomes, medical errors, length of stay, nurse turnover, and patient mortality. She noted that researchers are now providing the information needed to help determine what is appropriate staffing.

> Ratios are important—a consensus seems to be emerging supporting a range of from 4 to 6 patients per nurse in most hospital inpatient settings, with no more than one to two patients per nurse in high-acuity settings. However, ratios must be modified by the nurses' level of experience, the patients' characteristics (e.g., acuity level or debility), and the quality of clinical interaction between and among physicians, nurses, and administrators. (Curtin, 2003, p. 8)

Armed with evidence-based benchmark data, knowledge about the relationship between nurse staffing and patient outcomes can be used to better manage nursing resources and thereby optimize the delivery of patient care. The decisions influencing nursing staffing and deployment are best served by being data-driven (Potter et al., 2003).

Summary

- Delivery of nursing services is founded on staffing, scheduling, and skill mix determinations.
- Staffing is a process of planning to fill positions with qualified personnel and allocate scarce resources.
- Scheduling is implementing the staffing plan by preparing work hours.
- Nursing workload is the time determination of the nursing care needs of clients.
- Acuity and intensity measure the volume of care and the complexity of care needed.
- Staffing decisions are complex and based on volume and/or time.
- Methods of time sampling, work sampling, continuous sampling, or self-report are used to decide on staffing.
- Standardized volume measures may be used for staffing.
- Staffing systems may be fixed, controlled variable, or semiflexible.
- Patient classification systems group clients according to nursing care requirements of time and effort.
- The three types of patient classification systems are prototype, factor, and real-time factor.
- Economic pressures have altered RN staffing and created patient safety issues
- Research has shown a relationship between RN staffing to patient outcomes
- Mandatory nurse-to-patient ratios are controversial

Study Questions

1. Should nursing services be staffed to the minimum, maximum, or mean? Why?
2. What is the influence of the budget on staffing and scheduling?
3. To what extent should staff preferences determine staffing and scheduling? Explain.
4. What is the role of the patient classification system for staffing and scheduling? Does this vary by setting of care?
5. Should a manager do the schedule, or should staff schedule themselves?
6. What is the "right" mix of RNs, LPNs, and assistive personnel?
7. Should nurse-to-patient ratios be mandated? Why or why not?

CASE STUDY

Sira Habibu is the new head nurse in a large emergency department with many overlapping shifts. When she began her new job, she found that the unit was facing productivity problems, along with high absentee rates, low morale, and a lack of organizational loyalty among the nursing staff.

Nurse Habibu set about gathering some information from colleagues and the professional literature about different approaches that she could use to try to improve the unit's operations. She found that self-scheduling had been shown to have many organizational and personal benefits, including increased unit productivity, decreased absenteeism, increased organizational loyalty, and the promotion of professional autonomy. She also found that at a number of hospitals, self-scheduling had been used as a recruiting tool and as a way to improve staff retention.

Nurse Habibu decided to capitalize on these advantages by initiating self-scheduling in the emergency department. As she planned for the implementation and discussed her plans with the department staff, she found that adjustment would have to be made so that the advantages of self-scheduling could be realized. Self-scheduling had some inherent problems. The major issue encountered was the inequitable distribution of desirable shifts that resulted when individual staff members put personal needs ahead of unit needs. The literature showed that many units, in an attempt to equitably distribute shifts, created guidelines for the order in which staff were allowed to sign up for shifts. These guidelines either allowed those with seniority to sign up first or specified some type of rotating sign-up arrangement.

Other units formed staffing committees or appointed staffing liaisons to supervise the completion of the schedule.

Nurse Habibu found that although these methods produced workable schedules, they often came at a high price. Staffing committees and liaisons were labor-intensive and costly to the organization. Although the rotating sign-up method was more cost-effective, it did not provide a consistent work schedule template to address these problems. Nurse Habibu decided to establish unit staffing requirements based on patient volume. On the basis of those requirements, the department began with a blank schedule and used numbers to represent individual staff positions. Depending on which shift(s) a particular position was designated to cover, Nurse Habibu plotted a schedule that met unit needs and equitably distributed both desirable and undesirable shifts among each position. She believed that at this point it was important to look at positions and not consider individual staff members or vacation time.

Once this task was complete, Nurse Habibu replaced each position number with the name of the staff member who was hired into that position. She then took individual preferences into consideration whenever possible. The result was the master schedule template that served as the guideline for future schedules.

When it was time to prepare the next schedule, Nurse Habibu recorded any requested vacation time onto the master schedule and adjusted staffing as equitably as possible to provide coverage consistent with the established guidelines. The schedule was then posted, and staff members were allowed to make any desired changes to their schedule using red ink. This forced staff to consider unit coverage when making changes to their schedules. It also provided a way to monitor schedule changes. Staff soon began to negotiate between themselves when schedule changes adversely affected unit staffing.

Many of the benefits cited in the literature became reality. Having input into their personal schedule improved shift-to-shift cooperation and collaboration. It positively affected morale and improved cooperation between staff and leadership. Using the master template provided visual guidelines for scheduling that allowed staff to make informed decisions and provided leaders a tool for monitoring schedule changes. Self-scheduling evolved into a satisfying method for managing the complexities and hassles of nurse scheduling.

Based on original data from Irvin, S.A. (2000). Unit-friendly self-scheduling. In D.L. Huber (2000). *Leadership and nursing care management* (2nd ed.) (p. 579). Philadelphia: Saunders.

CRITICAL THINKING EXERCISE

Much has been changing at We-Care Hospital. Inpatient care has become more complex and high-acuity. Lengths of stay have dropped. New technology has been introduced. Restructuring has occurred to create differentiated and patient-centered practice, but bad will has been generated by layoffs. Nurse Sean Danielson has managed a unit through all these changes and was hoping to have a period of tranquility. Now, however, the rumors of an impending nursing shortage have become a reality and hit home. Turnover has created a shortage. Nurse Danielson has five openings for RNs that urgently need to be filled, and no applications are pending. In the meantime, the staff nurses are disgruntled about working short-staffed and being forced to work when they want time off. Trying to put out the next schedule has become fraught with tension.

1. What is the problem?
2. Why is it a problem?
3. What should Nurse Danielson do first?
4. What information does Nurse Danielson need? What variables should be measured?
5. What staffing issues are involved?
6. What scheduling issues are involved?
7. What further actions should Nurse Danielson take?

REFERENCES

Abdoo, Y.M. (2000). Nurse staffing and scheduling. In L.M. Simms, S.A. Price, & N.E. Ervin (Eds.), *Professional practice of nursing administration* (3rd ed.) (pp 459-480). Albany, NY: Delmar.

Aiken, L.H., Clarke, S.P., Sloane, D.M., Sochalski, J.A., Busse, R., Clarke, H., et al. (2001). Nurses' reports on hospital care in five countries. *Health Affairs, 20*(3), 43-53.

Aiken, L.H., Clarke, S.P., Sloane, D.M., Sochalski, J.A., & Silber, J.H. (2002). Hospital nurse staffing and patient mortality, nurse burnout, and job dissatisfaction. *Journal of American Medical Association, 288*(16), 1987-1993.

American Nurses Association (ANA). (1999). *Principles for nurse staffing.* Silver Spring, MD: ANA. Retrieved January 4, 2005, from *www.nursingworld.org/readroom/stffprnc.htm*

American Nurses Association (ANA). (2000). *Nurse staffing and patient outcomes in the inpatient hospital setting: Executive summary.* Silver Spring, MD: ANA. Retrieved January 4, 2005, from *www.nursingworld.org/pressrel/2000/st0504.htm*

Bard, J.F., & Purnomo, H.W. (2004). Preference scheduling for nurses using column generation. *European Journal of Operational Research, 164,* 510-534.

Barnum, B., & Mallard, C. (1989). *Essentials of nursing management: Concepts and context of practice.* Rockville, MD: Aspen.

Barratt, C.C., & Schultz, M.K. (1997). Staffing the operating room: Time and space factors. *Journal of Nursing Administration, 27*(12), 27-31.

Bennett, T. (1981). Operations research and nurse staffing. *International Journal of Bio-medical Computing, 12,* 433-438.

Beyers, M. (2000). *Foreword.* In American Organization of Nurse Executives (AONE) (Ed.), *Staffing management and methods: Tools and techniques for nursing leaders* (pp. xxi-xxii). San Francisco: Jossey-Bass.

Brett, J., & Tonges, M. (1990). *Resource allocation in managing the nursing shortage* (Monograph 3). (Pub #154182). Chicago: American Hospital Association.

Curtin, L.L. (2003, September 30). An integrated analysis of nurse staffing and related variables: Effects on patient outcomes. *Online Journal of Issues in Nursing.* Retrieved January 4, 2005, from *www.nursingworld.org/ojin/topic22/tpc22_5.htm*

DeGroot, H. (1994). Patient classification systems and staffing: Part 1, problems and promise. *Journal of Nursing Administration, 24*(9), 43-51.

Detwiler, C., & Clark, M. (1995). Acuity classification in the urgent care setting. *Journal of Nursing Administration, 25*(2), 53-61.

Finkler, S.A., & Kovner, C.T. (2000). *Financial management for nurse managers and executives* (2nd ed). Philadelphia: W.B. Saunders.

Fralic, M. (Ed.). (2000). *Staffing management and methods: Tools and techniques for nursing leaders.* San Francisco: Jossey-Bass.

Fried, B.J., & Johnson, J.A. (2002). *Human resources in healthcare: Managing for success.* Washington, DC: AUPHA Press.

Giovannetti, P. (1979). Understanding patient classification systems. *Journal of Nursing Administration, 9*(2), 4-9.

Graf, C.M., Millar, S., Feilteau, C., Coakley, P.J., & Erickson, J.I. (2003). Patients' needs for nursing care: Beyond staffing ratios. *Journal of Nursing Administration, 33*(2), 76-81.

Halloran, E.J. (1985). Nursing workload, medical diagnosis related groups, and nursing diagnosis. *Research in Nursing and Health, 8,* 421-423.

Health Resources and Services Administration (HRSA). (2005). *Nurse staffing and patient outcomes in hospitals.* Washington, DC: HRSA. Retrieved January 4, 2005, from *www.bhpr.hrsa.gov/nursing/staffstudy.htm*

Hung, R. (2002). A note on nurse self-scheduling. *Nursing Economic$, 20*(1), 37-38.

Institute of Medicine (IOM). (2004). *Keeping patients safe: Transforming the work environment of nurses.* Washington, DC: National Academies Press.

Jernigan, D. (1988). *Human resource management in nursing.* Norwalk, CT: Appleton & Lange.

Joint Commission on Accreditation of Healthcare Organizations (JCAHO). (2004a). *Hospital standards for staffing effectiveness.* Oakbrook Terrace, IL: JCAHO. Retrieved January 4, 2005, from *www.jcrinc.com/subscribers/perspectives.asp?durki=3116&site=10&return=2897*

Joint Commission on Accreditation of Healthcare Organizations (JCAHO). (2004b). *Accreditation process improvement (API): Staffing effectiveness standards.* Oakbrook Terrace, IL: JCAHO. Retrieved January 4, 2005, from *www.jcrinc.com/subscribers/perspectives.asp?durki=2506&site=10&return=2897*

Kirk, R. (1988). *Healthcare staffing & budgeting: Practical management tools.* Rockville, MD: Aspen.

Kirby, K., & Wiczai, L. (1985). Budgeting for variable staffing. *Nursing Economic$, 3*(3), 160-166.

Kirby, M.P., Dost, P., Holdwick, C.C., Poskie, M., Glaser, D., & Sage, M. (1998). Improving staffing with a resource management plan. *Journal of Nursing Administration, 28*(11), 25-29.

Kohn, L.T., Corrigan, J.M., & Donaldson, M.S. (Eds.). (2000). *To err is human: Building a safer health system.* Washington, DC: National Academies Press.

McKinley, J.W., & Cavouras, C.A. (2000). Evolving staffing measures. In M. Fralic (Ed.), *Staffing management and methods: Tools and techniques for nurse leaders.* (pp. 1-33). San Francisco: Jossey-Bass.

McManus, S., & Pearson, J. (1993). Nursing at a crossroads: Managing without facts. *Health Care Management Review, 18*(1), 79-90.

Mitchell, P.H., & Shortell, S.M. (1997). Adverse outcomes and variations in organization of care delivery. *Medical Care, 35*(11 Suppl), NS19-NS32.

Mowry, M., & Korpman, R. (1986). *Managing health care costs, quality, and technology: Product line strategies for nursing.* Rockville, MD: Aspen.

Needleman, J., Buerhaus, P.I., Mattke, S., Stewart, M., & Zelevinsky, K. (2001). *Nurse staffing and patient outcomes in hospitals.* Boston: Harvard School of Public Health.

O'Brien-Pallas, L., Irvine, D., Peereboom, E., & Murray, M. (1997). Measuring nursing workload: Understanding the variability. *Nursing Economic$, 15*(4), 171-182.

Phillips, C.Y., Castorr, A., Prescott, P.A., & Soeken, K. (1992). Nursing intensity: going beyond patient classification. *Journal of Nursing Administration, 22*(4), 46-52.

Potter, P., Barr, N., McSweeney, M., & Sledge, J. (2003). Identifying nurse staffing and patient outcome relationships: A guide for change in care delivery. *Nursing Economic$, 21*(4), 158-166.

Prescott, P. (1991). Nursing intensity: Needed today for more than staffing. *Nursing Economic$, 9*(6), 409-414.

Prescott, P.A., & Soeken, K.L. (1996). Measuring nursing intensity in ambulatory care part I: Approaches to and uses of patient classification systems. *Nursing Economic$, 14*(1), 14-21, 33.

Ramey, I. (1973). Eleven steps to proper staffing. *Hospitals, 47*(6), 98-104.

Reitz, J. (1985). Toward a comprehensive nursing intensity index: Part 1, development. *Nursing Management, 16*(8), 21-30.

Robertson, R., & Samuelson, C. (1996). Should nurse patient ratios be legislated? Pros and cons. *Georgia Nursing, 56*(5), 2.

Seago, J.A. (2002). The California experiment. Alternatives for minimum nurse-to-patient ratios. *Journal of Nursing Administration, 32*(1), 48-58.

Seago, J.A., Spetz, J., Coffman, J., Rosenoff, E., & O'Neil, E. (2003). Minimum staffing ratios: The California workforce initiative survey. *Nursing Economic$, 21*(2), 65-70.

Smith, M. (1994). Staffing and scheduling: A systems approach. In R. Spitzer-Lehmann (Ed.), *Nursing management desk reference: Concepts, skills & strategies* (pp. 178-197). Philadelphia: Saunders.

Smith, M.S., & Zuel, S.A. (1998). From staff nurse to charge nurse-Introducing a management viewpoint. In J.A. Dienemann (Ed.), *Nursing administration: Managing patient care* (2nd ed.). (pp. 452-459). Stamford, CT: Appleton & Lange.

Soeken, K., & Prescott, P. (1991). Patient intensity for nursing index: The measurement model. *Research in Nursing & Health, 14*(4), 297-304.

Soule, T., & Dobson, J. (1992). SEPPD and HPPD: More effective control of nursing care costs. *Nursing Economic$, 10*(3), 205-209.

Stanton, M.W., & Rutherford, M.K. (2004). Hospital nurse staffing and quality of care. *Research in Action, 14*, 1-9.

Sullivan, J., Bretschneider, J., & McCausland, M.P. (2003). Designing a leadership development program for nurse managers: An evidence-driven approach. *Journal of Nursing Administration, 33*(10), 544-549.

Unruh, L. (2003). The effect of LPN reductions on RN patient load. *Journal of Nursing Administration, 33*(4), 201-208.

Unruh, L., & Fottler, M.D. (2004, June 6-8). *Patient turnover and nursing staff adequacy.* San Diego: Academy Health Annual Research Meeting. Retrieved January 4, 2005, from *www.academyhealth.org/2004/ppt/unruh. ppt#257,1,PatientTurnoverandNursingStaffAdequacy*

Werley, H.H., & Lang, N.M. (Eds.). (1988). *Identification of the nursing minimum data set.* New York: Springer.

Wunderlich, G.S., Sloan, F.A., & Davis, C.K. (1996). *Nursing staff in hospitals and nursing homes: Is it adequate?* Washington, DC: National Academies Press.

34

Legal and Ethical Issues

Robert W. Cooper

A major advantage of being viewed as a profession is the societal grant of autonomy in practice. In professional terms, autonomy means that the occupational group has control over its own practice. The American Nurses Association's (ANA) original *Nursing: A Social Policy Statement* (1980) identified two mechanisms that frame autonomy: the legal regulation of nursing practice via state licensure laws and the professional regulation of nursing practice via standards and ethical codes of practice.

Although some laws can be unethical, laws generally provide minimum standards of acceptable conduct that are binding on individuals, groups, and businesses in dealing with other members of society. There are many situations, however, that are either not covered by specific laws or involve issues so complicated that, although the law can provide general guidelines for conduct, the issues cannot be fully resolved by the legal system alone. In these cases, ethical codes for a profession provide standards of conduct that serve as guidelines for decision making by the members of the profession.

CHAPTER OBJECTIVES

- Explain how the law and professional codes of ethics confer autonomy—both authority and accountability—on nurses and nurse managers
- Identify and describe the grounds on which nurses, nurse managers and health care organizations can be found legally liable for harm caused to others by civil wrongs
- Compare the sources of legal liability to which nurses and nurse managers are exposed in clinical practice to those encountered in carrying out their responsibilities related to delegation and supervision
- Describe the various steps nurse managers can take to protect themselves, the staff nurses reporting to them, and their facilities from legal liability and its related costs
- Define judicial risk and explain its potential effects on the litigation process
- Identify the key sources of ethical conflict encountered in clinical health care and describe the resources available for use in deciding how to resolve the resulting dilemmas
- Describe the conflict faced by nurse managers due to the clash between clinical and organizational ethics
- Explain the various steps nurse managers can take to prepare themselves and the staff nurses reporting to them for dealing effectively with the dilemmas arising from the clash between clinical and organizational ethics
- Exercise critical thinking to conceptualize and analyze possible solutions to a practice experience

By the very nature of their work, nurses and nurse managers are decision makers constantly faced with making choices in personal, clinical, and organizational situations. These decision-making situations are commonly fraught with legal and ethical issues that often become entwined. As members of a profession, nurses and nurse managers are guided by both legal and ethical considerations in making decisions.

LEGAL ASPECTS

There are extensive legal aspects to both nursing practice and nursing management. For example, nurse practice acts exist for each state and govern the legal practice of nursing, including delegation and supervision. The legal regulation of nursing via nurse practice acts and related administrative rules arises because society needs to have safeguards that protect the health and safety of citizens. In regard to health care, the public demands assurance that health care providers, including nurses, are properly prepared and competent to deliver needed services. Thus to practice nursing, the person must hold a valid license issued by the state. Therefore it is illegal to practice nursing without a license. State licensure confers autonomy on nurses to the limit of legal standards of practice.

Autonomy involves accountability, as well as authority, for one's decisions and actions. As professional autonomy and responsibility increase, so does the level of accountability and liability. To the extent that nurses are subject to malpractice lawsuits and carry malpractice insurance, nurses are held accountable (Aiken, 2004).

The legal aspects of nursing management center around decision making and supervision. Because all nurses retain personal accountability for their own acts and the use of knowledge and skills in the provision of care, personal accountability cannot be assumed by another. Nurse managers keep their own personal accountability for their own specific acts, but they are also accountable for their acts of delegation and supervision. Nurse managers carry the major responsibility for

developing and upholding the standards of care for the staff.

Nurses and nurse managers carry the accountability for the supervision of others, who are often unlicensed assistive personnel. Supervision includes monitoring the tasks performed, ensuring that functions are performed in an appropriate fashion, and ensuring that assigned tasks and functions do not exceed competency or require a license to perform.

Nurse managers use their autonomy to make decisions about practice situations. They are accountable for carrying out supervisory responsibilities; proper notification; assessing the competency of staff; training, orientation, and evaluation of staff; reasonable staffing decisions; and monitoring and maintenance of professional treatment relationships with clients, called *nonabandonment* (Aiken, 2004; Guido, 2001).

DEFINITIONS

In addition to law included in the federal and state constitutions, United States law is composed of **statutory law** (law enacted by the U.S. Congress, state legislatures, and local government bodies), **administrative law** (regulations promulgated and adopted by federal or state agencies to implement statutory law adopted by Congress or state legislatures), and **common law** (decisions of courts setting precedents to be followed, at least in that court's jurisdiction, until overturned by a higher court). The law recognizes two classes of wrongful acts that may cause harm. These are **criminal acts** (conduct that is offensive or harmful to society as a whole) and **civil acts** (wrongs that violate the rights of individuals by tort or by breach of contract). Persons found guilty of crimes are generally fined and/or jailed, whereas persons who commit civil wrongs are usually required to pay monetary damages to those who are wronged.

Nurses, nurse managers and health care facilities are all subject to being found **legally liable**—that is, legally responsible—for harm caused to others by civil wrongs. More specifically, liability is created when the law imposes a civil obligation

⚠ LEADING & MANAGING **DEFINED**

Statutory Law Law enacted by the U.S. Congress, state legislatures, or local government bodies and signed (approved) as required by the President, Governor, or local equivalent such as a mayor. **Administrative Law** Rules and regulations adopted by federal or state agencies to implement statutory law adopted by Congress or state legislatures. **Common Law** A system of laws or principles based on court decisions and on customs and usages rather than on statutory written laws. **Criminal Acts** Conduct that is offensive or harmful to society as a whole and violates statues prohibiting such conduct; persons found to have committed criminal acts are typically fined or jailed.	**Civil Acts** Conduct that violates the rights of individuals by tort or by breach of contract; there may or may not be in existence statues prohibiting such conduct; persons who have committed civil wrongs are usually required to pay money damages to those who were wronged. **Legally Liable** When the law imposes a civil obligation on a wrongdoer to compensate an injured party for the consequences of a wrongful act. **Negligence** Failure to exercise the proper degree of care required by the circumstances. **Malpractice** Failure of a professional person to act as other prudent professionals with the same knowledge and education would act under similar circumstances.

on a wrongdoer to compensate an injured party for the consequences of a wrongful act. As shown in Figure 34.1, there are two sources of legal liability—torts and contracts.

The most common source of legal liability for nurses and nurse managers is a *tort*—that is, a wrongful act (other than breach of contract) committed against another person or organization or their property that causes harm and can be remedied by a civil (rather than criminal) lawsuit. Although torts most commonly give rise to *personal* (or *direct*) liability for the person committing the wrongful act, in some cases, another person or organization may also be held *vicariously* liable for the same wrongful act they did not commit. For example, when a nurse commits a tort, the nurse may be found to be directly liable, and the nurse's employer may also be found to be vicariously liable for the nurse's wrongful action.

As indicated in Figure 34.1, determination of legal liability as a result of a tort depends on more than just the various technical elements of the tort that must be proved by the injured party (plaintiff), the presentation of various available defenses by the defendant, and the formal rules of the judicial system regarding the litigation process. In the case of torts, the legal outcomes are often also influenced by what may be termed *judicial risk*—various aspects of the litigation process that can introduce further uncertainty and additional cost into the determination of legal liability. As will be discussed later in this chapter, judicial risk can result in findings with respect to legal liability that are not based solely on the merits of the case nor on the rules of law applicable to the case.

There are three categories of torts: negligence, intentional torts, and strict liability torts. **Negligence** is the failure to exercise the proper

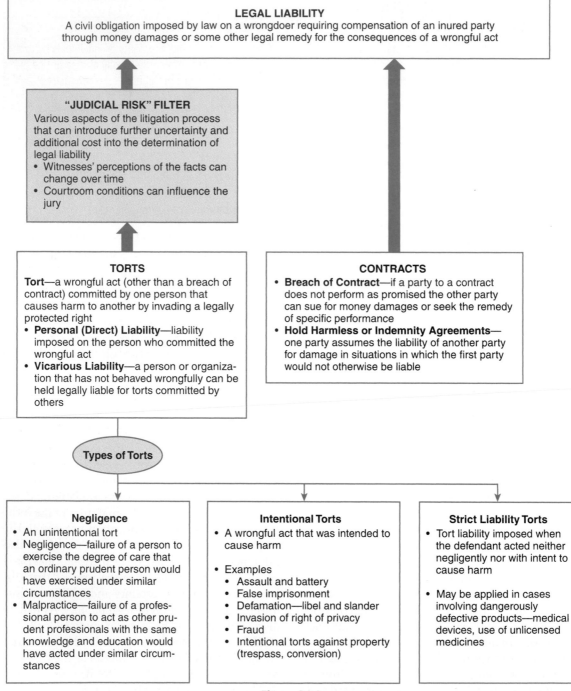

Figure 34.1
Sources of legal liability.

degree of care required by the circumstances. In general, the standard of care is defined as that which a reasonably prudent person would exercise under the circumstances to avoid harming others. **Malpractice** is a special type of negligence that applies only to professionals and employs a higher standard of care than ordinary negligence. Malpractice is the failure of a professional person to act as other prudent professionals with the same knowledge and education would act under similar circumstances. Depending on the nature of the situation involved, nurses and nurse leaders may be subject to either ordinary negligence or malpractice. An example of ordinary negligence would be a situation in which a nurse saw that food had been spilled on a client's floor but failed to have it cleaned up, and as a result, the client slipped and broke her hip. Since this is an act not requiring the exercise of professional judgment, the standard of care in determining negligence would be the degree of care that an ordinary prudent person would exercise under the circumstances. However, if the client had fallen and broken her hip because a nurse had failed to raise the side rails on the client's bed, the standard of care in determining malpractice would be the degree of care other prudent professionals with the same knowledge and education could be expected to exercise under similar circumstances.

Although negligence involves unintentional wrongful acts that harm another person or their property, *intentional torts* are voluntary and willful acts intended to cause harm by interfering with another person's rights. Common intentional torts occurring in the health care field include, among others, assault and battery, medical battery (surgical procedures performed without patient consent), false imprisonment, trespass to land, conversion of property, and intentional infliction of emotional distress.

In some cases, tort liability can be imposed without the defendant acting either negligently or with intent to cause harm. *Strict liability* requires that the responsibility for some accidents automatically rests with the defendant. With strict liability, anyone who engages in an activity known to endanger others assumes responsibility for any resulting damages. In general society, situations requiring strict liability include such activities as blasting, keeping dangerous animals, and selling dangerously defective products. In the health care field, the concept of strict liability has been applied in some cases involving harm caused by, among other things, the use of unlicensed medicines, defectively designed medical devices, tainted or contaminated drugs, and the prescription of dangerous combinations of drugs without obtaining a sufficient medical history to ensure that problems do not occur.

As shown in Figure 34.1, contracts are also a source of legal liability. In most states, employment of nurses generally follows the employment-at-will doctrine in which there is no written contract specifying the term of employment. However, in some cases, nurse managers, especially those at higher levels in an organization, negotiate written employment contracts. In addition, a few courts have ruled that contracts existed on the basis of language used in advertisements and statements made during the interviewing process. Courts also have held that contracts may arise after employment based on statements made in employee manuals and handbooks. With an increasing number of nurses negotiating various types of consulting arrangements with facilities, working as independent contractors and operating their own privately owned businesses, contracts are playing an even greater role in nursing.

Legal liability based on contracts can arise in two ways: breach of contract or an agreement to assume another party's liability. The most common is *breach of contract*, in which one party to the contract fails to perform as promised in the contract. In this case, the injured party can either sue for monetary damages or seek the remedy of specific performance in which the court orders the party that caused the breach to do what was promised by the contract. For example, if a nurse has an employment contract stating that he or she can be discharged only for incompetence but then is discharged for another reason, the nurse can bring a suit for wrongful discharge under contract law due to breach of contract. Less likely to be encountered by nurses is legal liability arising from *an agreement to assume another party's liability.* An example of such an agreement is a "hold harmless" agreement commonly found in leases. For example, in signing a lease for property needed to carry on his or her privately owned business, the nurse likely would be agreeing to assume responsibility for all injuries occurring on the premises, including any caused by the owner of the property.

LAW AND THE NURSE MANAGER

The managers of any health care organization are responsible to the policy-making body of the organization. The managers also hold an obligation to comply with the laws of society at local, state, and national levels. Managers are responsible for ensuring that laws are adhered to in the actions of management itself and also in the actions of those employees who assist the managers in carrying out the mission of the organization. Concern for the law involves three general areas: personal negligence in clinical practice, liability for delegation and supervision, and liability of health care organizations.

Personal Negligence in Clinical Practice

Activities of clinical client care involve corresponding legal accountability and risk. Errors do happen. Some lead to injury to a client. At minimum, nurses have an ethical obligation to nonmaleficence, or to do no harm to clients. This duty is discharged in part by remaining competent in knowledge and skills and the standards of practice. Nursing negligence/ malpractice occurs when the nurse's actions are unreasonable given the circumstances or fail to meet the standard of care or when the nurse fails to act and causes harm. In nursing, harm related to clinical practice commonly arises from negligent acts or omissions (unintentional torts) and a variety of intentional acts (intentional torts) such as invasion of privacy or assault and battery (Aiken, 2004).

To establish legal liability on the grounds of malpractice (professional negligence), the injured client (plaintiff) must prove the following four elements:

1. A duty of care was owed to the injured party.
2. There was a breach of that duty.
3. The breach of the duty caused the injury (causation).
4. Actual harm or damages were suffered by the plaintiff.

Critical in determining liability for malpractice (professional negligence) is the definition of the duty (standard) of care owed by the nursing professional to the client. The standard of care, the minimal requirements that define an acceptable level of care, is "the average degree of skill, care, and diligence exercised by members of the same profession under the same or similar circumstances" (Aiken, 2004, p. 39). Standards of care can be found in the state nurse practice act, standards published by the American Nurses Association, other professional organizations and specialty practice groups, federal agency guidelines and regulations, and the facility's policy and procedure manuals. In malpractice cases, the standard of care owed to the injured client is commonly introduced into evidence by expert witnesses, and the impact of that evidence is ultimately determined by the jury after receiving instructions from the judge on the law applicable to its use.

Common clinical practice areas that give rise to allegations of malpractice include the general areas of treatment, communication, medication, and the broad category of monitoring/observing/ supervising/surveillance. Examples of common negligence allegations in nursing malpractice suits include patient falls, use of restraints, medication errors, burns, equipment injuries, retained foreign objects, failure to monitor, failure to ensure safety, failure to take appropriate nursing action, failure to confirm accuracy of physicians' orders, improper technique or performance of treatments, failure to respond to a patient, failure to follow hospital procedure, and failure to supervise treatment (Aiken, 2004).

Because intentional torts differ in nature from negligence (unintentional torts), establishing legal liability for these intentionally harmful acts is based on different elements than those used in proving malpractice. To establish liability on the grounds of an intentional tort, the injured client (plaintiff) must prove that a voluntary and willful act by the nursing professional (defendant) was intended to interfere with the plaintiff's rights and was a substantial factor in doing so. Unlike negligence, intent is necessary in proving intentional torts. However, proof of actual injury or damage is not required, because intentional torts interfere with another person's rights. Also, there is no need to determine duty or standards of care in proving intentional torts.

Liability for Delegation and Supervision

Over and above personal liability for clinical practice, nurses and nurse managers have accountability and liability for their acts of delegation and supervision. The ethical and legal aspects of delegation and supervision liability are discussed in Chapter 25. Nurses and nurse managers both carry an obligation to report incompetent practice that occurs at any point in the care delivery process. Nurse managers have a duty to train, orient, and evaluate the ability of nursing staff to perform specific functions and tasks. Health care organizations have a duty to monitor the competence and ability of nursing and medical professionals and to inquire about their credentials (Aiken, 2004).

Both nurses and nurse managers have a duty to follow policies and procedures when reasonable. Nurse managers are advised to review policies and procedures carefully, including the language used, in order to adhere to legal and ethical parameters more closely. Clearly, management in nursing practice means that nurses must fulfill obligations and duties both to clients and to the organization. This means using knowledge, skill, and decision-making abilities to reduce the incidence of negligence and malpractice by employees as a way to reduce harm to clients and legal risk to the organization. As primary care coordinators, nurses need to manage the environment of care delivery. Ensuring staff competence and reporting incompetent practice are key activities. For example, in nursing, legal and

ethical issues arise when a nurse is impaired by substance abuse. The overall consideration is protecting the client from harm. Confronting suspected abuse must be done carefully. However, when an incident occurs, the nurse manager has a responsibility to intervene.

Liability of Health Care Organizations

In addition to the liability faced by nurses and nurse managers arising out of malpractice in clinical practice and negligence in the process of delegating and supervising, health care facilities face extensive exposure to legal liability from several sources such as negligence of their employees, negligence of independent contractors, corporate negligence arising out of the facility's responsibilities to hire qualified employees and monitor and supervise their activities, and failure to comply with numerous laws and regulations, especially those related to employment issues. Nurse managers have important roles to play in helping their organizations to control facility liability arising from each of these sources.

Under the doctrine of *respondeat superior* (meaning "let the master answer"), an employer may be held vicariously liable for the negligent act or omission of an employee. In order for the employer to be found vicariously liable, the employee's act or omission must occur both during the course of employment and while the employee was acting within the scope of employment. For example, if a nurse negligently injured a client during the course of and within the scope of employment, not only would the nurse be directly liable for damages, but also the health care organization would be vicariously liable. Due to their "deep pockets" (their ability to pay larger settlements or judgments) and the concept of vicarious liability, health care facilities are almost always named as defendants in malpractice suits. Nurse managers can play a key role in assisting facilities to avoid payments for vicarious liability by ensuring that the nurses they supervise deliver competent care to clients while following facility policies and procedures (Guido, 2001).

Under the doctrine of ostensible authority (or apparent agency), facilities may also become liable for the negligence of an independent contractor if it would appear to a reasonable client that the independent contractor is a facility employee. For example, a hospital might be held liable for the negligence of an agency nurse who appeared to a client to be a nurse employed by the hospital. Guido (2001) recommended that when dealing with agency or temporary personnel, nurse managers should, among other things, do the following:

- Consider their skills, competencies, and knowledge when delegating tasks and supervising their actions
- Ensure that they are made aware of facility policies and procedures, resource materials, and documentation procedures
- Assign a resource person to each temporary staff member to serve in the role of mentor and help prevent potential problems from occurring because of a lack of familiarity with institution routine or where to turn for assistance.

A relatively new area of law being created by the courts, the doctrine of corporate liability, holds health care organizations themselves legally responsible for "ensuring that competent and qualified practitioners will deliver quality heath care to consumers" (Guido, 2001, p. 304). Under this doctrine, facilities can be held liable for a variety of activities that are beyond the control of any single employee such as failure to check references, educational credentials, license status, disciplinary actions and criminal record for applicants; failure to protect the clients from health care providers who can cause harm; failure to monitor the quality of care provided by all medical and nursing personnel within the facility; failure to periodically review staff competency; and failure to terminate an employee who has harmed a client and then injures another client (Aiken, 2004). Nurse managers can help the facility avoid corporate liability by, among other things, ensuring that those who report to them remain competent and qualified and have current licensure. Nurse managers should also report to appropriate managers dangerously low staffing levels or incorrect mixes of staff for effectively meeting the

health care needs of clients as well as report incompetent, illegal, or unethical practices to appropriate authorities (Guido, 2001).

In addition to facility liability arising from vicarious liability, the doctrine of ostensible authority and the doctrine of corporate liability, health care organizations are constrained by specific laws related to employment issues. Although the various health care providers and their employing organizations have specific legal and ethical obligations to clients, such as executing informed consent and following the Patient Self-Determination Act of 1990, organizations carry specific legal and ethical obligations toward employees. The employer has an obligation to provide a safe and secure care delivery environment (Aiken, 2004).

Management policies and procedures must be in compliance in the areas of hiring, performance appraisal, management of employees with problems, and termination (Aiken, 2004). Lawsuits also have formed the basis for the standards to be met for the termination of employees. Discharges may occur for lack of adherence to employer-established policies or standards, "good cause" per institutional policy, illegal activity, assault, insubordination, or excessive absenteeism. Written notice and the reasons for termination avoid misunderstandings and show justice through due-process procedures. Careful documentation is important. If the employee is a member of a protected group, the employer may be required to submit formal justification for the termination (Aiken, 2004).

The various legal and ethical considerations of nursing management span client, provider, and employer rights and obligations. Nurses and their employing organizations are responsible for knowing and following the various applicable laws and regulations. Inservice education can increase knowledge and awareness. Nurse managers will need to manage the environment of nursing care to ensure client safety, provider justice and safety, and organizational compliance with the law.

LEADERSHIP AND MANAGEMENT IMPLICATIONS

As indicated previously, nurses, nurse managers and the facilities that employ them face legal liability from a wide array of sources. Although it is not possible to avoid legal liability in all cases, nurse managers can take a number of steps to protect themselves, staff nurses reporting to them, and their facilities where possible. The first step is summed up in a statement often attributed to football coach Vince Lombardi: *The best defense is a good offense.* There are a number of things that nurse managers can do in applying this strategy of using a good offense to defend against problems leading to legal liability. First, since problems generally can be dealt with more effectively if anticipated in advance, nurse managers should see that both they and the staff nurses who report to them are knowledgeable concerning the most common problem areas related to malpractice and the other sources of legal liability, especially new ones that have not yet been experienced within the unit. Providing this information to staff nurses and using examples will probably improve both recognition and retention. In addition to the previous brief discussion of the sources of legal liability faced by nurses and nurse managers, extensive information, including examples, is available from numerous sources including books (e.g., Aiken, 2004; Guido, 2001), nursing journals (e.g., Eskreis, 1998; Frank-Stromborg & Christensen, 2001a; Miller & Glusko, 2003; Trott, 1998), and a variety of websites (e.g., Croke, 2003; Nurses Service Organization [NSO], 2003; Wetter, 2004).

Next, nurse managers should ensure that both they and their staff nurses are aware of the many prevention activities that can aid them in avoiding these legal liability problems. In addition to facility guidelines, numerous ideas for reducing potential liability are available to the nurse manager and staff nurses in a variety of books that focus on legal and ethical issues in nursing (e.g., Aiken, 2004; Guido, 2001), articles in nursing journals (e.g., Frank-Stromborg & Christensen, 2001b; Miller & Glusko, 2003), and a number of websites that present articles and continuing education materials providing recommendations for avoiding

▲ LEADERSHIP & MANAGEMENT **BEHAVIORS**

Leadership Behaviors

- Serves as spokesperson to the media on legal and ethical issues
- Guides others toward safe, legal, and ethical decision making
- Role-models ethical behavior
- Empowers followers to apply ethical decision-making models
- Facilitates autonomy
- Inspires multidisciplinary teams to discuss and resolve legal or ethical issues

Management Behaviors

- Assesses degree of implementation of laws governing practice
- Interprets the meaning of laws

- Revises policies and procedures following legal and ethical principles
- Establishes an ethics committee
- Manages violations of the law per procedure

Overlap Behaviors

- Scans the environment for trends and new laws
- Disseminates information to others about legal and ethical nursing practice
- Establishes mechanisms to handle legal and ethical issues

Research Note

Source: Eskreis, T.R. (1998). Seven common legal pitfalls in nursing. *American Journal of Nursing, 98*(4), 34-41.

Purpose

Malpractice is a type of negligence for which nurses have been sued. The purpose of this article is to present and analyze legal case studies in seven areas of malpractice allegations commonly brought against nurses.

Discussion

The seven common legal pitfalls in nursing are patient falls, failure to follow physician's orders or established protocols, medication errors, improper use of equipment, failure to remove foreign objects, failure to provide sufficient monitoring, and failure to communicate. The author presents and discusses actual cases arising under each category. Analysis of the actions that lead to a breach of practice includes tips for avoiding problems. In addition, a box of legal definitions of terms is provided. Most useful is a display box titled "Tips for Avoiding Common Legal Pitfalls" in which nursing actions for prevention and risk reduction are presented.

Application to Practice

A negligent professional act that causes injury is known as malpractice. For a successful lawsuit the injured party must prove that the nurse's conduct lacked due care. Knowledge of the most common problem areas, the use of examples, and the display of prevention tips aid the nurse in avoiding problems. A caring nurse-client relationship is an important preventive measure.

---

malpractice (e.g., Croke, 2003; NSO, 2003; Wetter, 2004).

Because many, if not most, of the lawsuits seeking to determine legal liability involve the alleged failure of nurses to meet appropriate standards of care, especially those reflected in the policies and procedures of their facility, nurse managers must not only ensure that they and their staff nurses know the standards of care that apply to them and are competent to satisfy them, but also actively participate in facility committees as well as those at the state, national, and even international level that make decisions as to the standards of care to which nurses will be held.

Although the first step in defending against problems of legal liability involves taking positive action in an effort to prevent them from arising, it is not possible for nurses, nurse managers, and health care facilities to avoid legal liability in all cases. This is so, if for no other reason than the existence of what might be termed *judicial risk.* Judicial risk can result in findings with respect to legal liability that are not based solely on the

merits of the case or on the rules of law applicable to the case. In the case of torts, aside from all the lists of elements that must be proved by injured plaintiffs, all the legal defenses available for attempting to block their arguments for damages and the formal rules of the judicial system regarding the litigation process, legal outcomes are also often influenced by judicial risk—that is, various aspects of the litigation process that can introduce further uncertainty and additional cost into the determination of legal liability. The following are some examples:

- Any client can sue a staff nurse, nurse manager, and/or health care facility for a tort, and if no response is filed within the legal time frame, the court will enter a default judgment against the defendant. Thus, at a minimum, regardless of the apparent validity of the grounds for the lawsuit, the defendant must incur defense costs or lose.

- Given the typical lengthy period between the defendant's act or omission and the introduction of evidence into the trial, many things can happen that will alter the perception of the facts. Witnesses, for example, may be questioned repeatedly, coached, or simply forget exactly what they witnessed (see Case Study 1).

- Conditions in the courtroom can also influence the jury. Some jury members may be influenced by the dress or behavior of the defendant's attorney and form subsequent opinions despite the facts (e.g., a high-priced lawyer with an arrogant attitude may elicit feelings such as "We'll show him"). Or the appearance of the plaintiff may influence jurors (e.g., "How could a little old man like that be partly responsible for his own injuries, and besides, who cares anyway since the defendant has liability insurance?").
- Often there is more than one principle of law that applies to a case, and the outcome may be influenced by which one the judge uses in giving his or her instructions to the jury.
- In suits such as those alleging malpractice in providing or failing to provide proper end-of-life care, juries and even judges can be sufficiently influenced by their emotions so as to rationalize a finding of legal liability against the defendant, especially when, as is generally the case, there is liability insurance available to pay the judgment. In fact, in some cases, a jury can actually change the law of a jurisdiction in making its decision. (See Case Study 2 for an example.)

In some cases, the elements of judicial risk make even one's best efforts to prevent legal liability from being imposed on them and/or their facility impossible. Thus all nurses, whether staff or managers, should carry adequate professional liability insurance to protect themselves against defense costs and liability judgments (or settlements). Although often covered as employees under a facility's professional liability policy, there are a number of reasons why nurses should also carry their own individual professional liability insurance. An employer can sue a nurse found guilty of malpractice for reimbursement (indemnification) of any damages the facility was required to pay as a result of vicarious liability. In addition, because a facility's professional liability insurance

protects a nurse only while acting within the scope of employment or the nurse practice act, individual liability coverage would be required by private-duty nurses and off-duty nurses providing volunteer services. Although a facility's policy may only provide a single attorney to represent the different interests of the facility and the nurse, an individual policy will provide an attorney to specifically represent the nurse's interests. An individual policy will also provide funds to cover a nurse's defense costs and a portion of the judgment (or settlement) in the event that the total judgment exceeds the limits of liability of the facility's coverage. Individual policies generally provide coverage for personal injuries such as libel, slander, assault, battery, and violation of privacy, which may not be covered for employees in facility policies. Despite the large size of potential judgments and thus the high limits of liability required to adequately protect against them, many nurses can obtain individual coverage with limits of $1 million per claim and $6 million aggregate for an annual tax-deductible premium of less than $100 (less than $50 if within 12 months of graduation).

ETHICAL ISSUES

In addition to potential legal concerns, nurses and nurse managers are often faced with ethical dilemmas in connection with decision making. Ethical dilemmas require that decisions be made about what is right and wrong in situations where an individual has to make a choice between equally unfavorable alternatives. Traditionally, nurses, like other health care professionals, have faced ethical dilemmas arising primarily out of clinical practice. These dilemmas have involved conflicts among principles and/or rules attributable to common morality (socially approved norms of human conduct), standards articulated in professional codes of ethics, public policies promulgated by government agencies, and in some cases, the personal values of the health care professionals themselves (Beauchamp & Childress, 1994).

More recently, ethical dilemmas faced by nurses and nurse managers have increasingly involved clashes between the principles, rules, values, and standards of clinical/professional ethics and those of organizational/business ethics.

Although the domain of clinical ethics is the care of clients, the domain of organizational ethics is a facility's business-related activities, including among others, marketing, admissions, transfer, discharge, billing, and the relationship of the facility and its staff members to other health care providers, educational institutions, and payers. These are activities that all directly affect the care of patients (Spencer, 1997). Organizational ethics reflect a health care facility's basic values that serve as guides for proper and acceptable behavior in decision making and thus help ensure that the facility "conducts its business-patient care practices in an honest, decent, and proper manner" (Joint Commission for the Accreditation of Healthcare Organizations [JCAHO], 1996, p. 95). Together, clinical and organizational ethics reflect a health care facility's concern that, whether related to the continuum of care or the continuum of services related to that care, ethical dilemmas should be resolved based on principles of right action (Blake, 1999).

ETHICAL DECISION MAKING IN CLINICAL HEALTH CARE

Many of the decisions nurses and nurse managers make on a daily basis have an ethical component and may involve conflicts among ethical responsibilities. These conflicts may involve clashes between two ethical duties to the client (such as duty to respect autonomy and duty to benefit the client), between the client rights and benefits (such as withholding or withdrawing treatment in respect for a client's right to die by forgoing treatment at any time and treating or continuing treatment that is expected to produce more good for the client), between duties to self and duties to the client (such as a nurse's desire to remain on the same shift because of parental responsibilities and the need to advocate for better treatment of the

clients by some health care practitioners on that shift), and between professional ethical provisions and religious ones (such as a professional code requiring the recognition of the client's right to self-determination and a nurse's religious beliefs prohibiting abortion).

When ethical dilemmas are encountered in dealing with clinical matters, health care professionals commonly refer to various principles, rules, and standards for guidance in making moral decisions. Principles and rules are normative generalizations that provide guidance in ethical decision making. Although rules are more specific in content and restricted in scope than principles, neither can fully guide action, but rather must be complemented by judgment in order for a decision to be made (Beauchamp & Childress, 1994; O'Neill, 2001).

Definitions

Like other health care practitioners, nurses apply four fundamental morality principles and a number of related rules in dealing with ethical dilemmas encountered in clinical practice on a daily basis. The four principles that form the cornerstone of biomedical ethical decision making are (1) autonomy, (2) beneficence, (3) nonmaleficence, and (4) justice. **Autonomy** refers to the client's right of self-determination and freedom of decision making. **Beneficence** means doing good for clients and providing benefit balanced against risk. **Nonmaleficence** means doing no harm to clients. **Justice** is the norm of being fair to all and giving equal treatment, including distributing benefits, risks, and costs equally (Aiken, 2004; Beauchamp & Childress, 1994; Guido, 2001).

Biomedical ethics also recognizes a number of rules that are related to the four fundamental principles and, likewise, provide guidance in dealing with ethical dilemmas (Beauchamp & Childress, 1994). Examples of commonly applied rules are fidelity, veracity, confidentiality, and privacy. **Fidelity** means being loyal and faithful to commitments and accountable for responsibilities. **Veracity** is the norm of telling the truth and not intentionally deceiving or misleading clients.

⚠ LEADING & MANAGING **DEFINED**

Autonomy	**Fidelity**
An individual's right of self-determination and freedom of decision making.	Being loyal and faithful to commitments and accountable for responsibilities.
Beneficence	**Veracity**
Doing good for clients and providing benefit balanced against risk.	Telling the truth and not intentionally deceiving or misleading clients.
Nonmaleficence	**Confidentiality**
Doing no harm to clients.	The prohibition of some disclosures of information gained in certain relationships without the consent of the original source of the information
Justice	**Privacy**
Being fair to all and giving equal treatment, including distributing benefits, risks, and costs equally.	A right of limited physical or informational inaccessibility.

Confidentiality prohibits some disclosures of some information gained in certain relationships to some third parties without the consent of the original source of the information. **Privacy** is a right of limited physical or informational inaccessibility (Aiken, 2004; Beauchamp & Childress, 1994; Guido, 2001).

Code of Ethics

In addition to these basic moral principles and rules of biomedical ethics, nurses are also provided standards of conduct by professional codes of ethics. For example, the ANA's *Code of Ethics for Nurses: With Interpretive Statements* (2001) provides nonnegotiable standards as to the ethical obligations and duties of those who enter the nursing profession. The ANA (2001) indicated that the Code "provides a framework for nurses to use in ethical analysis and decision-making" (p. 3).

As with the principles and rules discussed above, the Code's provisions and accompanying interpretive statements, for the most part, do not focus on giving precise answers to specific ethical problems but rather provide general guidance as to how to act when faced with ethical dilemmas. The Code does, however, identify and provide somewhat more specific advice related to several currently unresolved ethical problems such as those involving practitioner decisions surrounding a client's right to die, the introduction of incentive systems to decrease spending, responding to questionable and impaired practice, handling situations in which a client's needs are beyond a nurse's qualifications and competencies, and the existence of organizational barriers to ethical practice.

Decision-Making Model

Although a number of decision-making models and processes have been proposed for use in resolving ethical dilemmas encountered in clinical practice (Aiken, 2004; Guido, 2001), they are all essentially modified versions of the six-step problem-solving model traditionally used in business, as follows:

1. Define the problem.
2. Develop alternative courses of action.
3. Evaluate each alternative course of action.
4. Select the best course of action.
5. Implement the selected course of action.
6. Monitor the results.

Because an ethical dilemma is merely a type of problem, specifically one that involves conflict, the six-step problem-solving model provides a process for making a decision when a moral dilemma arises in clinical practice. The ethical principles, rules, and standards discussed above are moral resources that can be used along with practitioner judgment to evaluate the alternative courses of action in step 3 of the problem-solving process to provide a basis for selecting the most appropriate course of action for resolving the dilemma.

THE CLASH BETWEEN CLINICAL AND ORGANIZATIONAL ETHICS

In today's rapidly changing health care environment, the traditional clinical ethical principles of autonomy, beneficence, nonmaleficence, and justice are being severely tested as they find themselves competing with demands for financial performance (Mohr & Mahon, 1996) arising out of the reliance of health care facilities on market competition as a vehicle for cost control, a goal demanded by social policy (American Medical Association [AMA], 2000). By the very nature of their work, nurse managers play two very different, and often conflicting, roles: a professional caregiving role and an organizational role involving responsibilities associated with the management of nursing care or other aspects of a health care facility. Harvey Fineberg, former dean and professor at the Harvard School of Public Health, observed the following:

> These two roles, joined together in a single person, require a constant balancing and juggling act that requires coming to grips with the tensions and pulls between putting the patient first in the tradition of nursing and caretaking, versus the responsibilities and obligations of institutional leadership, which bring into play other human, financial, and institutional forces and needs. (Buerhaus et al., 1997, p. 13)

Dilemmas arising from the clash between clinical/professional ethics and organizational/ business ethics are experienced daily by nurses and nurse managers. Unfortunately, despite the passage of time, they continue to present major challenges

to the delivery of professional nursing care in many, if not most, health care facilities (Cooper et al., 2004; Cooper et al., 2002). Specific examples of nurses' ethical dilemmas include the practice of pulling or floating nurses to areas in which they are not cross-trained, an action that also increases the client-to-nurse ratio to greater and greater limits. Nurse managers may be asked to reduce expenditures by leaving specialty areas, such as labor and delivery, uncovered when no clients are present. Organizations may refuse to purchase equipment or provide support services on off-shifts. Home visits may be refused if reimbursement cannot be captured. Time for teaching and counseling clients may be denied via staffing practices. Nurses may experience responses of "there is no money" for nursing care needs while the hospital takes over the office space occupied by nursing services to renovate for a new physicians' lounge and private dining room. A nurse manager may be presented with a request from a physician to deploy a hospital nurse to the physician's private practice office to help with clients. Along with their ethical concerns, most, if not all, of these dilemmas also have the potential to give rise to unfavorable legal consequences if resolved improperly.

CURRENT RESEARCH

Two recent studies provide some evidence as to the perceptions of staff nurses (Cooper et al., 2004) and nurse managers (Cooper et al., 2002) regarding the importance of the clash between clinical ethics and organizational ethics and its key effects on the delivery of quality health care. In each study, randomly selected participants were presented with a list of ethics-related statements that were referred to as ethical issues for simplicity (33 issues for staff nurses and 40 for nurse managers). Participants were asked to rate each issue on a 5-point scale, with 5 meaning that the issue was a major ethical problem for heath care organizations and 1 meaning that it is not a problem. The high positive correlation coefficient for the group means of staff nurses and nurse managers for the 32 ethical issues common to both studies was 0.9023, which suggests that the order of the 32 issues in terms of the extent to which they present problems for health care facilities is quite similar for the two studies.

Another area of similarity is reflected in four of the eight ethical issues rated in the top 10 by both staff nurses and nurse managers. Both the 325 responding staff nurses and 295 responding nurse managers identified failure to provide service of the highest quality (defined by both groups of respondents as service that is inconsistent with both the standards of the nursing profession and the ANA Code of Ethics) as a major problem facing health care facilities. Moreover, the respondents to both studies indicated that this disappointment with the quality of service was felt not only by those in the nursing profession and the clients for whom they care, but also by other health care providers employed by the organization.

Three other ethical issues rated in the top 10 by both the staff nurses and the nurse managers suggest a potential cause of this purported widespread disappointment with the quality of service provided by health care facilities in general. In both studies, the ethics-related statement rated first in terms of the extent to which it causes problems for health care organizations was the failure to provide service of the highest quality due to economic constraints determined by the organization. This issue is a direct reflection of the conflict between clinical ethics, with its primary focus on the delivery of high-quality client care, and organizational ethics, which has been heavily influenced in recent years by cost constraints imposed by the market. Both the staff nurses and nurse managers also rated quite high an ethics-related statement pointing even more directly at the ongoing ethics clash, that of conflict between organizational and professional philosophy and standards (Cooper et al., 2004; Cooper et al., 2002). Finally, in rating department closings and layoffs among the top-10 issues in both studies, staff nurses and nurse managers identified an important problem stemming directly from the conflict between clinical ethics, with its focus almost exclusively on health care needs of individual clients,

and organizational ethics, with its focus on the responsibility of facilities to provide health care to patient populations by responding to market pressures to remain competitive through cost control (AMA, 2000). These findings appear to suggest that the yet unbridled conflict between clinical and organizational ethics may be a major, if not the key, cause contributing to the perceived failure of many health care facilities to provide service of the highest quality as anticipated by the standards and codes of ethics of professional nursing.

LEADERSHIP AND MANAGEMENT IMPLICATIONS

Nurse managers have a responsibility to prepare themselves and those reporting to them to deal effectively not only with the yet unresolved issues of clinical ethics, such as full disclosure and end-of-life care, but also with the many unresolved dilemmas arising from the ongoing conflict between clinical and organizational ethics. A recent study of nurse managers (Cooper et al., 2003) provided suggestions of where the emphasis should be placed to be most productive. The study found that, after their own personal moral values and standards, nurse managers tend to find several aspects of their organizational environment to be more helpful in dealing with ethical dilemmas than they find resources related to the professional environment such as the current ANA Code of Ethics (which was rated least helpful among 17 personal, organizational, and professional resources), professional publications/resources on ethics, literature on ethics/professionalism, and professional meetings where ethical issues can be discussed.

Within the organizational resources, informal factors related to organizational climate were viewed as being more helpful in dealing with ethical dilemmas than formal organizational resources such as a facility's statement on ethics, the organization's policy for identifying and resolving ethical issues, a contact person within the organization to which unethical activity can be reported, and ethics training provided by the organization (which was rated next to last out of 17 possible resources). Involving merely the *absence* of pressure to compromise one's own ethical standards, the two top-rated factors—the fact that your boss does not pressure you into compromising your ethical standards and an organizational environment/culture that does not encourage you to compromise your ethical values to achieve organizational goals—suggest that an important way health care facilities and their managers can assist nursing professionals in resolving ethical dilemmas effectively is by neither explicitly nor implicitly pressuring them to go against their own ethical values (Cooper et al., 2003). Other informal organizational factors rated as being more helpful in dealing with ethical dilemmas than the formal resources provided by one's facility included the organization's culture and management philosophy, management's clear communication of appropriate ethical behavior, and the ability to go beyond one's boss, if necessary, for information and advice on ethical issues. These are all factors that, despite any personal risk involved, nurse managers at all organizational levels can, and must, continually work to improve and maintain if a culture that encourages and supports ethical behavior is to exist within their facility.

In addition to the need for nurse managers to prepare staff nurses and others working for them to identify and otherwise deal effectively with ethical issues encountered in their health care facilities (Porter-O'Grady, 2003), in recent years, the nursing ethics literature has called on nurse managers to encourage participation by staff nurses, as well as increase participation themselves, on facility ethics committees, especially those dealing with issues of organizational ethics and conflicts between clinical and organizational ethics (ANA, 2001; Guido, 2001). Even more directly, the ANA's *Code of Ethics for Nurses: With Interpretive Statements* stated, "Nurse administrators must ensure that nurses have access to and inclusion on institutional ethics committees" (2001, p. 7). The ANA Code continues, "Nurses must bring forward difficult issues related to patient care and/or institutional constraints upon ethical practice for discussion and review" (2001, p. 7). In their role of responsible

representation, nurse managers should also ensure that "the clinical and ethical concerns of nurses are heard at the highest levels of organizational decision making" (Curtin, 2000, p. 12).

To "markedly expand the boundaries of nurses' ethical roles in hospitals" (Dodd et al., 2004, p. 16), nurses have been called on to engage in *ethical activism* in an effort to make facilities more willing to encourage their participation in ethical deliberations, and *ethical assertiveness* to expand their participation in deliberations that shape ethical decisions even when not invited to do so. Finding that "nurses are more likely to employ ethical assertiveness and ethical activism in settings that are already receptive to nursing involvement" and where written protocols mandating nursing involvement in ethics deliberations already exist, Dodd and colleagues (2004) call on nurse managers to "focus on generating administrative support for nursing involvement" and "to make efforts to ensure that nurses experience their setting as receptive to their participation in ethical deliberations" (pp. 25-26).

Although increased and improved training would undoubtedly contribute to better preparing staff nurses and nurse managers to carry out these activities, the key factor for success is an organizational culture that encourages, supports, and rewards ethical behavior (Goodstein & Carney, 1999; Lachman, 2002; Pentz, 1999; Upenieks, 2003). In this context, organizational culture can be defined as a set of shared core values that members of an organization have reflected on, articulated, and accepted as normative (Silverman, 2000). As principles of right action, these shared core values serve as guides for proper and acceptable behavior in making decisions within the organization. Creating an organizational culture that will serve as a resilient base for a successful organizational ethics initiative requires that the core values not only be identified and effectively communicated to the organization's members but also be championed and demonstrated by the organization's top managers (Goodstein & Carney, 1999; Pentz, 1999).

Because in reality the organizational cultures of health care facilities are arrayed along a continuum ranging from those based on letter-of-the-law compliance with regulatory and accrediting requirements to those that encourage, support, and reward ethical behavior, nurses and nurse managers will face varying types and degrees of challenge in their efforts to carry out the activities related to knowledge, participation, disclosure, activism, and assertiveness mentioned above. In many cases, it will take pressure from nurse managers to encourage senior management to recognize the need, and provide their support, for these activities of staff nurses and nurse managers. In facing this challenge, nurse managers should remember that, among other things, leaders are expected to have courage and to take risks in constantly challenging the status quo. Nurse managers should also encourage risk taking among the nurses reporting to them by defending and supporting them when they do (Porter-O'Grady, 2003).

CURRENT ISSUES AND TRENDS

In view of the significant degrees of change and uncertainty associated with the legal and ethical aspects impacting decision making in nursing care management, there is certainly no shortage of current issues and trends in this area. A major current issue, of course, is the nursing shortage and the disturbing expectation of its continuation and growth in the future. This issue gives rise to a number of legal and ethical challenges for nurse managers and staff nurses. Resulting largely from increases in cost-cutting measures and other financial constraints, as well from deterioration of working conditions (American Hospital Association [AHA], 2002; Cornerstone Communications Group [CCG], 2001; O'Neil & Seago, 2002), the nursing shortage has resulted in a major problem called *short staffing*. This refers to the use of an insufficient nursing staff on a unit or in a facility for the number of patients requiring care at various acuity levels (Aiken, 2004; Guido, 2001). Consequences commonly attributed to short staffing (Cooper et al., 2004) include deterioration of patient outcomes in terms of increased mortality and failure-to-rescue rates (Aiken et al., 2002), a general decline in the quality of patient care

(CCG, 2001), deterioration of nurse outcomes resulting from increased burnout and greater job dissatisfaction (Aiken et al., 2002), and increases in organizational costs resulting from increased turnover (AHA, 2002) and legal liability. In an effort to deal with short staffing, nurse managers are often required to do the following: float nurses to areas in which they are not cross-trained, an action that also increases the client-to-nurse ratio closer and closer to staffing requirements; use agency (temporary) personnel; and use unlicensed personnel. Staff nurses, nurse managers, and health care facilities all face numerous possibilities of legal liability, as well as dilemmas involving conflicts between clinical and organizational ethics as a result of short staffing and actions taken in an effort to temporarily solve this problem.

Potential legal and ethical problems are also encountered in connection with unresolved issues of clinical practice such as decisions about withholding or withdrawing life-support systems. Just as the AMA's Code of Medical Ethics (AMA, 1994) provides physicians with guidance in dealing with issues related the withholding or withdrawing of life-sustaining medical treatment, the ANA's Code of Ethics provides guidance for nurses regarding the responsibilities they may face in dealing with key issues associated with end-of-life care, such as respecting the client's right of self-determination, which is consistent with the ethical principle of autonomy, ensuring that the client is fully informed and understands his or her options, enlisting the use of a surrogate if the client's comprehension is questionable, and handling conflicts between the moral standards of the profession and the nurse's own moral values.

Despite this guidance and the best efforts to apply it to end-of-life care, claims of legal liability against a nurse, nurse manager, and/or the facility that employs him or her (not to mention the physician) can arise from a variety of alleged torts related to the withholding or withdrawal of life support. For example, economic, noneconomic (emotional distress), and/or punitive damages might be claimed for negligence (including malpractice) arising out of failure to adequately inform the client in a manner that facilitates an informed judgment, failure to obtain proper consent for an organ donation, provision of life-prolonging treatment against the client's wishes, failure to provide life-sustaining treatment when it is requested by the client, failure to recognize that the client's standardized advance directive document did not deal with CPR even though the client was a candidate for a DNR order, failure to properly interpret the client's advance directive document due to its unreadable legal language, denial of proper medical care, or failure of a nurse to make timely arrangements for another nursing practitioner to take over a particular client's care when the nurse's own moral values conflict with those of the profession.

Damages might also be sought on the grounds of intentional torts such as medical battery for tissue burns, broken bones or other harm arising out of resuscitation, or intentional infliction of emotional distress. A nurse may also be named in a lawsuit filed primarily as a result of a physician's alleged malpractice or intentional tort. Being named in this lawsuit would at least give rise to costs associated with the nurse's defense. Finally, even when the basic rules to avoid negligence or intentional tort have been closely followed, a nurse, nurse manger, and/or facility may still be found legally liable for payment of damages as a result of judicial risk. As mentioned earlier, in some cases, juries and even judges can be sufficiently influenced by their emotions so as to rationalize a finding of legal liability against the defendant, especially when, as is generally the case, there is liability insurance available to pay the judgment. Nurses need to focus on their use of expert judgment in practicing the highest legal and ethical standards in the quest for high-quality care and services.

Summary

- As members of a profession, nurses and nurse managers are guided by both legal and ethical considerations in making decisions.
- Most commonly, nurses and nurse managers are subject to legal liability arising from malpractice and intentional torts they personally commit in clinical practice, from negligence in their acts of delegation and supervision, from failure to follow policies and procedures when reasonable, and from breach of contract.
- Critical to the determination of legal liability for malpractice (professional negligence), standards of care can be found in the state nurse practice act, standards published by the American Nurses Association, other professional organizations and specialty practice groups, federal agency guidelines and regulations, and the facility's policy and procedure manuals.
- Health care facilities can be held legally liable for malpractice or intentional torts committed by nurses and nurse managers they employ under the doctrine of respondeat superior, for malpractice and intentional torts committed by independent contractors (e.g., agency personnel) under the doctrine of ostensible authority, and for failing to ensure that competent and qualified practitioners are hired and that they deliver quality health care to clients under the doctrine of corporate liability.
- Judicial risk can result in findings with respect to legal liability that are not based solely on the merits of the case or on the rules of law applicable to the case.
- The four principles of autonomy, beneficence, nonmaleficence, and justice; several closely related rules of biomedical ethics; and standards of conduct provided by professional codes of ethics provide guidance to nurses and nurse managers when faced with ethical dilemmas arising in the course of clinical practice.
- Many ethical dilemmas encountered in today's health care environment involve a conflict between clinical ethics with its primary focus on the delivery of high-quality client care and organizational ethics reflecting a number of other human and financial considerations, including the reliance of health care facilities on market competition as a vehicle for cost control.
- In preparing themselves and those reporting to them to deal effectively with yet unresolved dilemmas of either clinical ethics or the conflict

between clinical and organizational ethics, nurse managers should work toward the establishment of an organizational culture that encourages, supports, and rewards ethical behavior in both their own area of responsibility and the entire health care facility.

Study Questions

1. What governs the practice of nursing?
2. Why do nurses and nurse managers need to understand how legal liability relates to both their clinical practice activities and their responsibilities in delegating and supervising?
3. What are the various grounds on which nurses, nurse managers, and health care organizations can be found legally liable for injuries to others?
4. What actions can nurse managers take in an effort to protect against legal liability?
5. What resources are available to nurses and nurse managers for dealing with ethical dilemmas encountered in clinical practice?
6. How do the ethical dilemmas encountered as a result of the clash between clinical and organizational ethics differ from those encountered in clinical practice?
7. What responsibilities do nurse managers have to prepare themselves and those reporting to them for dealing effectively with ethical dilemmas?

CASE STUDY

Case 1

This strange case was personally experienced by the author in Las Vegas, a city with high population turnover. It provides an even more extreme example of what complications can occur because of the long delay that is typical between an accusation of negligence and the actual trial. In this case, the individual who showed up in court claiming to be the plaintiff was not of the same race as the injured individual who had actually filed the lawsuit 2 years earlier. The obvious error regarding who was the injured person was not

even recognized by the defense attorney, who was assigned the case shortly before the trial. Had the defendant not pointed the situation out to the judge, who appeared annoyed at having to recognize the defendant at the beginning of the trial, the trial would have continued.

Case 2

In another example, the author served as foreman on a jury in a contributory negligence state. The jury was instructed by the judge that if the plaintiff (a very elderly man who would be spending the rest of his life in some type of health care facility as a result of injuries caused by an auto accident) was even partially at fault for his own injuries, the jury had to find in favor of the defendant and the plaintiff would be awarded no damages. During 6 hours of deliberation, feeling sympathy for the plaintiff, all jury members except the foreman repeatedly ignored the fact that the testimony of witnesses had indicated that the elderly man was completely at fault and voted continually to find that the plaintiff's injuries were completely the fault of the defendant (a trucking company and its driver) who had insurance and thus could afford to pay. Because the foreman was concerned that the viewpoint of the other jurors was not consistent with the judge's instructions regarding the state's law, and thus not faithful to legal instructions, he held out until the issue essentially became one of whether the jury should return and continue deliberations the next day. In the next round of voting, the entire jury properly applied the state's contributory negligence law and found for the defendant. This case illustrates two aspects of judicial risk. First, the radical change in the jury members' votes was clearly not based solely on the merits of the case, but rather on their desire to not have to return the next day for further deliberations. Second, if instead the jury foreman had changed his vote to provide a unanimous verdict for the plaintiff, the jury would have essentially changed the state's law in reaching its verdict by not applying the contributory negligence doctrine to the facts of the case.

CRITICAL THINKING EXERCISE

Ms. Anna vanDahm, one of the wealthiest and most influential people in town, was placed in the hospital's intensive care unit (ICU) after undergoing kidney replacement surgery. Because of the inability to deliver high-quality care as a result of financial constraints and a high turnover rate due to nurse discontentment with the dictatorial leadership styles of ICU nurse managers, the ICU was regularly short of qualified staff nurses. As a solution to this problem of short staffing, nurses from other units with lower levels of client acuity were routinely floated to the ICU, often without regard to whether or not they were cross-trained to take on ICU responsibilities.

Abigail Friendly, an RN without prior training or experience in caring for ICU clients, was floated to the ICU, where she was assigned to provide care for Ms. vanDahm, who had responded very poorly to her surgery and was put on a life-support system by a physician just prior to Nurse Friendly's arrival. While Nurse Friendly was caring for her, Ms. vanDahm said, in the presence of her oldest son, that she did not want to be resuscitated in the event of cardiopulmonary arrest.

When her shift ended a few minutes later, Nurse Friendly, exhausted and overwhelmed by what she had just experienced, left for home. Shortly thereafter, Ms. vanDahm sustained a cardiopulmonary arrest; however, in the absence of proper documentation and notification, she was resuscitated. Subsequently, the son, angry that his mother's request had not been followed, consulted an attorney, who promptly contacted the hospital's CEO. The next day, Nurse Friendly, who had always received highly positive performance evaluations over the 5 years she was employed by the facility and also was subject to protection under the provisions of an antidiscrimination statute, was told by the manager of her unit that she was being fired effective immediately.

Questions for Analysis

1. Nurse Friendly
   a. On what grounds could Nurse Friendly be found legally liable for malpractice?
   b. What actions should have been taken by Nurse Friendly to prevent malpractice in this type of situation?
   c. What ethical dilemma(s) did Nurse Friendly face in this situation?
   d. What factors should have been considered by Nurse Friendly in dealing with the ethical dilemma(s) encountered in this situation?
2. Manager of Nurse Friendly's unit
   a. On what grounds could the nurse manager be found legally liable?
   b. What actions should have been taken by the nurse manager to prevent legal liability in this type of situation?
   c. What ethical dilemma(s) did the nurse manager face in this situation?
   d. What factors should have been considered by the nurse manager in dealing with the ethical dilemma(s) encountered in this situation?
3. Nurse manager of the ICU
   a. On what grounds could the nurse manager be found legally liable?
   b. What actions should have been taken by the nurse manager to prevent legal liability in this type of situation?
   c. What ethical dilemma(s) did the nurse manager face in this situation?
   d. What factors should have been considered by the nurse manager in dealing with the ethical dilemma(s) encountered in this situation?
4. Hospital
   a. On what grounds could the hospital be found legally liable?
   b. What actions should have been taken by the hospital to prevent legal liability in this type of situation?

REFERENCES

Aiken, L.H., Clarke, S.P., Sloane, D.M., Sochalski, J., & Silber, J.H. (2002). Hospital nurse staffing and patient mortality, nurse burnout, and job dissatisfaction. *Journal of the American Medical Association, 288*(16), 1987-1993.

Aiken, T.D. (2004). *Legal, ethical, and political issues in nursing* (2nd ed.). Philadelphia: F.A. Davis.

American Hospital Association (AHA). (2002). *In our hands: How hospital leaders can build a thriving workforce.* Chicago: AHA.

American Medical Association (AMA). (1994). *Withholding or withdrawing life-sustaining medical treatment. Opinion on social policy issues E-2.20.* Chicago: AMA. Retrieved March 24, 2004, from *www.ama-assn.org/ama/pub/category/8457.html*

American Medical Association (AMA). (2000). *Organizational ethics in health care.* Chicago: AMA.

American Nurses Association (ANA). (1980). *Nursing: A social policy statement.* Kansas City, MO: ANA.

American Nurses Association (ANA). (2001). *Code of ethics for nurses: With interpretive statements.* Washington, DC: ANA. Retrieved November 28, 2004, from *www.nursingworld.org/ethics/code/ethicscode150.htm*

Beauchamp, T., & Childress, J. (1994). *Principles of biomedical ethics* (4th ed.). New York: Oxford University Press.

Blake, D.C. (1999). Organizational ethics: Creating structural and cultural change in health care organizations. *Journal of Clinical Ethics, 10*(3), 187-193.

Buerhaus, P.I., Clifford, J., Erickson, J.I., Fay, M.S., Miller, J.R., Sporing, E.M., et al. (1997). Executive nursing leadership: Summary of the Harvard Nursing Research Institute's follow-up conference. *Journal of Nursing Administration, 27*(4), 12-20.

Cooper, R.W., Frank, G.L., Gouty, C.A., & Hansen, M.C. (2003). Ethical helps and challenges faced by nurse leaders in the health care industry. *Journal of Nursing Administration, 33*(1), 17-23.

Cooper, R.W., Frank, G.L., Gouty, C.A., & Hansen, M.C. (2002). Key ethical issues encountered in health care organizations: Perceptions of nurse executives. *Journal of Nursing Administration, 32*(6), 331-337.

Cooper, R.W., Frank, G.L., Hansen, M.M., & Gouty, C.A. (2004). Key ethical issues encountered in health care organizations: The perceptions of staff nurses and nurse leaders. *Journal of Nursing Administration, 34*(3), 149-156.

Cornerstone Communications Group (CCG). (2001). *Analysis of American Nurses Association staffing survey.* Warwick, RI: CCG.

Croke, E.M. (2003). Nurses, negligence, and malpractice. *American Journal of Nursing, 103*(9), 54-63. Retrieved March 13, 2004, from *www.nursingcenter.com/prodev/ce_article.asp?tid=423277*

Curtin, L.L. (2000). The first ten principles for the ethical administration of nursing services. *Nursing Administration Quarterly, 25*(1), 7-13.

Dodd, S., Jansson, B.S., Brown-Saltzman, K., Shirk, M., & Wunch, K. (2004). Expanding nurses' participation in ethics: An empirical examination of ethical activism and ethical assertiveness. *Nursing Ethics, 11*(1), 15-27.

Eskreis, T.R. (1998). Seven common legal pitfalls in nursing. *American Journal of Nursing,* **98**(4), 34-40.

Frank-Stromborg, M., & Christensen, A. (2001a). Nurse documentation: Not done or worse, done the wrong way-part I. *Oncology Nursing Forum, 28*(4), 697-702.

Frank-Stromborg, M., & Christensen, A. (2001b). Nurse documentation: Not done or worse, done the wrong way-part II. *Oncology Nursing Forum, 28*(5), 841-846.

Goodstein, J.D., & Carney, B. (1999). Actively engaging organizational ethics in health care: Four essential elements. *Journal of Clinical Ethics, 10*(3), 224-229.

Guido, G.W. (2001). *Legal and ethical issues in nursing* (3rd ed.). Upper Saddle River, NJ: Prentice-Hall.

Joint Commission for Accreditation of Healthcare Organizations (JCAHO). (1996). *Standards for organizational ethics. 1996 Comprehensive Accreditation Manual for Hospitals.* Oakbrook Terrace, IL: JCAHO.

Lachman, V.D. (2002). Organizational ethics need not be an oxymoron. *Patient Care Management, 18*(3), 1, 4-5.

Miller, J., & Glusko, J. (2003). Standing up to the scrutiny of medical malpractice. *Nursing Management, 34*(10), 20.

Mohr, W.K., & Mahon, M.M. (1996). Dirty hands: The underside of marketplace health care. *Advances in Nursing Science, 19*(1), 28-37.

Nurses Service Organization (NSO). (2003). *Nursing malpractice: Understanding the risks.* Hatboro, PA: NSO. Retrieved January 3, 2005, from *www.nursingcenter.com/prodev/ce_article.asp?tid=405770*

O'Neil, E., & Seago, J.A. (2002). Meeting the challenge of nursing and the nation's health. *Journal of the American Medical Association, 288*(16), 2040-2041.

O'Neill, O. (2001). Practical principles and practical judgment. *Hastings Center Report, 31*(4), 15-23.

Pentz, R.D. (1999). Beyond case consultation: An expanded model for organizational ethics. *Journal of Clinical Ethics, 10*(1), 34-41.

Porter-O'Grady, T. (2003). A different age for leadership. Part 2. *Journal of Nursing Administration, 33*(3), 173-178.

Silverman, H. (2000). Organizational ethics in health care organizations: Proactively managing the ethical climate to ensure organizational integrity. *Hospital Ethics Committee Forum, 12,* 202-215.

Spencer, E.M. (1997). A new role for institutional ethics committees: Organizational ethics. *Journal of Clinical Ethics, 8*(4), 372-376.

Trott, M.C. (1998). Legal issues for nurse managers. *Nursing Management, 29*(6), 38-41.

Upenieks, V. (2003). Nurse leaders' perceptions of what compromises successful leadership in today's acute care inpatient environment. *Nursing Administration Quarterly, 27*(2), 140-152.

Wetter, D. (2004). *The best defense is a good documentation offense* [Online course]. Wilmington, DE: Corexcel. Retrieved March 14, 2004 from *www.corexcel.com/html/documentation.title.ceus.htm*

VI

FISCAL MANAGEMENT

35

Financial Management

Diane L. Huber

CHAPTER OBJECTIVES

- Define and describe financial management
- Outline the four phases of financial management
- Discuss strategic financial planning
- Differentiate charges from costs
- Analyze cost awareness as related to nurse decision making
- Analyze ethical and legal financial management considerations
- Exercise critical thinking to conceptualize and analyze possible solutions to a practice exercise

Health care services continue to be costly, and the pressure to control costs continues to grow. Nurses are urged to become more knowledgeable and sophisticated in financial management. This is because the accuracy of resource-need projections and the efficiency of care provision are crucial to hospitals' and other health care organizations' viability. There is little operating margin to act as a buffer. At minimum, nurses need to develop and justify budgets, use computerized information systems and technology, and economize staff and supply use while ensuring that safe and appropriate care is delivered in nursing services. Under managed care and capitated reimbursement, the financial risk management imperative becomes strong at all levels of the delivery system. Financial management of a unit, program, department, or organization is a major nonclinical managerial task (Finkler & Kovner, 2000).

Financial management is targeted at the allocation of scarce resources. Money is the primary medium, although personnel, time, and tangible goods can have a corresponding monetary value affixed. A major concern of nursing and health care organizations is how to allocate scarce resources efficiently and effectively. Some issues in financial management relate to who (or what level of management) decides how much of an organization's resources will go to staffing, who makes decisions about staff mix and levels, and who decides how many nursing care hours each client receives. Does shared governance mean shared control over financial resources? Can there be split responsibility, with nursing deciding client care hours but management controlling the resources to pay for those hours? Other financial management issues arise over the use of acuity systems for staffing, mechanisms for nurse compensation, costs of technology infrastructure, measurement of the cost of nursing care, and nurse recruitment and retention strategies (Finkler & Kovner, 2000).

DEFINITIONS

Financial management is defined as a series of activities designed to allocate resources and plan for the efficient operation of an organization. It occurs in four phases: (1) budgeting, (2) recording,

(3) reporting, and (4) evaluating. Organizations need to manage financial resources efficiently; the overall goal of financial management is to meet the total financial needs of an organization.

There is uncertainty and risk associated with cash flow and other forces that impact on the ability to meet the organization's financial needs. Thus the managerial process of planning is linked closely with financial management. Operational plans, or programs and plans for the day-to-day provision of services, are based on an assessment of the organization and its environment. Then a plan for the future provision of services and long-range survival is derived. **Strategic planning** is a process of assessing the organization and its departments or divisions (see Chapter 14). Strengths and weaknesses are explored and analyzed. Opportunities and external threats are identified and critiqued. External forces are considered, and their impacts are projected in relationship to the organization. A strategic plan results in strategy formulation. For example, a hospital may need to consider analyzing length-of-stay trends. Rural hospitals may need an analysis of reimbursement sources. A community health agency may need to plan for shifts in federal health policy that would threaten their heavily Medicare-based income stream and the result on service delivery, such as the shift from fee-for-service to prospective payment. Strategic management is the process of setting goals and objectives, then determining and obtaining the resources allocated to goals (Finkler & Kovner, 2000).

BACKGROUND

The financial management of any health care unit or organization is just one piece of a larger context. The environment surrounding a health care organization has a strong impact on and implications for its financial management (Finkler & Kovner, 2000). For example, the number, type, and location of competitors influences potential volume and subsequent revenue streams. The demographic profile of the surrounding population affects the use of services. Payor and provider types and numbers also influence financial management. Employer groups exert considerable influence when they negotiate health care for large blocks of employees. The legal and regulatory environment also influences health care service delivery. The key factors to assess in any community evaluation are the major employers, provider groups, and health care facilities in the area. In the planning of services, population characteristics are important.

Other important factors in financial management are the structure of the health care organization, economic principles, accounting, and finance.

▲ LEADING & MANAGING **DEFINED**

Financial Management

A series of activities designed to allocate resources and plan for the efficient operation of an organization.

Strategic Planning

A process of assessing an organization and its departments or divisions.

Charge

The price asked for services or goods.

Cost

The amount of money required to cover direct production inputs.

Economics is founded on principles related to the finite and limited nature of resources coupled with competing demands. The attempt is to allocate resources in an optimal manner. Resource allocation and the actions of individuals are intimately intertwined. Motivation and incentives play a role in achieving efficiency (Finkler & Kovner, 2000).

The two major financial statements for the overall organization are (1) the balance sheet and (2) a statement of revenues and expenses (nonprofit organizations) or an income statement of profit and loss (for-profit organizations). Both are used to understand and analyze the organization's financial status. Operational decisions follow, as do reports to controlling or interested bodies such as boards of directors or trustees, banks, investors, and the federal government.

Although nurses often do not see balance sheets or statements of revenue and expenses, they need to know they exist. Furthermore, nurses need to become more savvy about the financial "health" of the organization. Resources and jobs may be at stake. One measure of the cultural aspect of "openness" is whether such documents are shared with staff at the operations level (bedside). Balance sheets often are a single page that follows a fairly standard form. Figure 35.1 displays a balance sheet template. Filled in with line items and dollar amounts, the balance sheet presents a snapshot of the status of the organization on a given date. It shows what is owned (assets) and what is owed to others (liabilities). The amount in a line item may be important (e.g., high capital debt may constrict flexibility or new program initiatives), and comparing current and prior time periods indicates higher and lower absolute amounts as they change over time.

The revenue and expenses report is a summary financial report of activity within an accounting period. Figure 35.2 illustrates a revenue and expense template. Note the three timeframes for this comparative operating statement. Line items would be filled in, with dollar amounts in the comparative columns. Thus trends can be identified and analyzed. The result is a reasonable surface understanding of financial trends and events for last year, as well as how this is unfolding in the current year. Just like any person's personal finances, the bottom line is maintaining enough

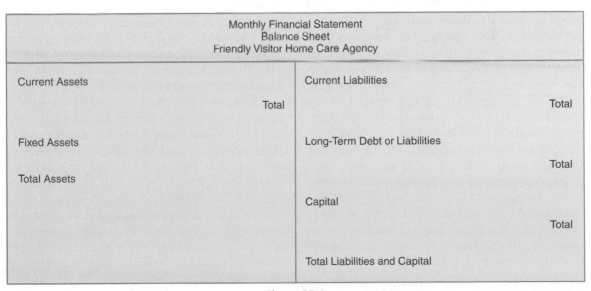

Figure 35.1
Balance sheet template.

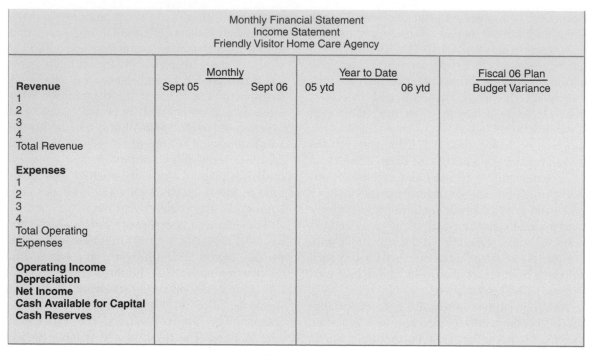

Figure 35.2
Revenue and expense template.

cash flow to remain solvent. Both income and outgo contribute to the bottom line.

Operating finances include revenues and expenses. Although these basic elements of finance apply across many organizations, health care service delivery has some unique features. Health care organizations face special issues related to the cost of regulation; cost containment, avoidance, and reduction; and allocating costs to maximize reimbursement. In addition, concerns about Medicare fraud and abuse have heightened vigilance over health care reimbursement strategies.

Financial accounting is a core aspect of financial management. Accounting is divided into managerial accounting and financial accounting. Managerial accounting is focused on the generation and evaluation of financial information needed by managers to manage parts or all of the organization. Financial accounting is targeted toward

providing information to external sources of investment, money lending, or control. Managerial accounting is designed for internal users; financial accounting is targeted toward external constituents. Managerial accounting results in a wide variety of statements and financial information forms that vary from organization to organization. Financial accounting statements include the income statement (activity, revenues, and expenses), the balance sheet (financial position), the cash flow statement, and the statement of changes in fund balances (Finkler & Kovner, 2000; Finkler & Ward, 1999).

Cost accounting, or cost analysis, focuses on cost measurement and cost reporting. The profit/surplus or loss/deficit each year depend on revenues and costs, both of which require managerial involvement. Cost measurement is a complex endeavor. Calculations differ depending on the object of the analysis and the intended use of the information. For example, calculating the cost to treat each client is different from the marginal cost calculation of treating one more client. Cost information often is based on the unit of service. The unit of service is a defined basic measure of the product or service being produced. For nursing this unit may be visits, treatments, client days, hours of operation, counseling or teaching sessions, or hours of nursing care time. The unit of service becomes the volume measure. Costs may be averaged by dividing the full cost by the volume of the unit of service (Finkler & Kovner, 2000; Finkler & Ward, 1999).

Costs may be fixed (not changing as the volume changes), variable (varying directly with volume changes), or marginal (extra cost of one more unit of service). The volume of the unit of service affects the cost: average costs decline as volume increases; therefore higher volume is preferable to lower volume. This affects profit and loss (Finkler & Kovner, 2000; Finkler & Ward, 1999).

Cost accounting is a major managerial tool. It can be used for planning, control, inventory valuation, income determination, and nonroutine decision making. Planning encourages deliberation and assessment of impact before action is taken. Managerial control attempts to ensure the achievement of objectives by controlling operations to keep to the plan. Planning and control efforts are central to the success of any organization. Strategic planning, budgeting, and the control of operating results form the core of organizational financial planning and control (Finkler & Kovner, 2000; Finkler & Ward, 1999). Nurses at all levels can contribute to the determination of cost accounting definitions, determination of health care costs and rates, planning and control, and analysis of financial information.

Strategic management in nursing includes financial planning, vision, goal setting, identification of opportunities and analysis of risks. Managerial strategies, strategic planning, and cost-containment efforts add value to and affect financial performance outcomes such as net income and operating margin. Thus nursing services are strategically critical to hospitals (Smith et al., 1993).

Demonstration of these effects strengthens nursing's position in any complex bargaining over scarce resources.

HEALTH CARE FINANCIAL STRATEGIES

Health care is a service industry whose product is a service delivered by expert clinicians. Medications, treatments, technologies, and provider compensation all are costly. Americans have been consuming more and more of these costly services. There is great pressure to hold down costs yet maintain high quality and availability of services. Time and money are scarce resources. To understand financial management, managers must learn more about the field of economics, or how scarce resources are allocated among alternative uses. The behavior of individuals and organizations is important. Key concepts are utility, marginal cost, supply and demand, elasticity, incentives, market efficiency, and redistribution of resources (Finkler & Kovner, 2000).

Financial resources are either short-term or long-term. Financing of the health care delivery system is important for nurse managers and leaders to understand. Political savvy can be augmented by understanding the key stakeholders, the basics of insurance and payment to providers and organizations, and methods used to control payments for care. Internally, important financial management concepts are related to both finance and accounting. Finance focuses on the next several years and what might pay off in the longer-run. Accounting has a 1-year time horizon. Thus with accounting, it is difficult to justify programs that do not return gains on investment in less than a year.

Accounting fundaments include the balance sheet and operating statement, assets, equities, revenues and expenses, recording and reporting processes, and fund accounting. Financial statements reflect methods for presenting financial data for analysis, planning and management reporting (Finkler & Kovner, 2000).

Cost management is the analysis and control of costs. In health care, revenues are important, but the control and management of costs is more

Research Note

Source: Murray, M.E., Brennan, P.F., & Moore, S.M. (2003). A model for economic analysis. *Nursing Economic$, 21*(6), 280-287.

Purpose

Technology and other health care innovations are costly. Responsible allocation of resources decisions need to be based on economic assessments. The purpose of this article was to display and discuss a model for the economic assessment of patient care innovations. A production process model was used to define the costs of resources used to produce a specific amount of output. This allowed the derivation of the average cost per unit for the innovation.

Discussion

A production process is a relationship between inputs used and outputs that result. Outputs in health care can be a patient education program, a critical pathway, or a treatment procedure. Characteristics of the production process include economic efficiency, economics of scale, marginal productivity, and the influence of time on short-term and long-term production costs. A cost analysis strategy was used to specify the inputs to the production process and determine total costs and average cost per case. The first step was specifying and defining costs. Less obvious costs, such as fringe benefits, consultation fees, printing costs, out-of-pocket expenses incurred by patients, and training time for staff, needed to be considered. The second step was developing a detailed listing of the costs involved. Using the model, the cost per unit of innovation metric was displayed and discussed using an example from a clinical trial involving the use of a computer-based home care program for postsurgical cardiac patients. The example used was an economic analysis of HeartCare, a home-based self-care technology research project. Four production processes were presented: design, pilot implementation, maintenance, and completion.

Application to Practice

Economic assessments of innovations clearly are crucial steps for nursing administrators. However, methods and measurements are difficult and complex. Selecting the best methodology is a challenge. The production process model, as a way to guide the economic analysis of health care programs, is a good strategy for answering important economic questions.

important to profit/surplus because increasing revenue is more difficult to accomplish. Important concepts are direct and indirect costs, fixed versus variable costs, marginal costs, the impact of volume on cost per patient, and break-even analysis. Beyond understanding costs is the nurse manager and leader's understanding of how health care charges and prices are determined. Setting prices and rate-setting approaches are finance-type decisions that nurses may be able to influence with powerful data. Other cost management areas are traditional cost-finding methods, measuring productivity, activity-based or product-line costing, and costing out nursing services. There are a variety of computerized tools for forecasting and

related financial decision making (Finkler & Kovner, 2000).

Cost containment, avoidance, and reduction strategies are employed to prevent further escalation in the overall costs of health care. Typical problems faced by health care organizations include cash shortages, understaffing, poor deployment of present staff, low productivity, and equipment breakdowns. Strategies employed to tackle these problems include paperwork improvements, productivity enhancements, scheduling alternatives, recruitment programs, and training. Organizations also focus on better planning, coordination of personnel actions, and developing and maintaining standardized systems and processes as a way to increase efficiency. The budgetary process is one system for planning and controlling resource allocation.

Research has shown that customers rate the reliability of service as the single most important feature in judging service quality (Berry, 1999). A service organization's competence and fairness contribute directly to a sense of trust. Trust is fundamental and powerful for organizations that depend on credibility of service to survive (Berry, 1999). Financial management strategies can be used to engender an environment in which high-quality services are reliably produced. When the tools of managerial, financial, and cost analysis are used, data can be constructed to measure the workload accurately and distribute it fairly, to plan and predict staff mix and staffing requirements, to determine direct care actualized per client, to manage human resources through recruitment and retention, to enhance volume through marketing, to influence financial incentives, and to analyze the cost impact of various models of nursing care. Financial evaluative data contribute to more precisely targeted resources and facilitate innovation and creative strategies.

Nurses will continue to struggle with how to allocate scarce nursing resources effectively and efficiently. Financial compensation (pay and benefits) remains an issue for all nurses. Shift work and the consolidation of multiple nursing units in hospitals under one nurse manager are work stresses for nurses. Alteration of staff mix affects the financial bottom line and also morale, recruitment, and quality of reliability of service delivery. These and other issues in the dynamic health care environment press nurses to augment and enhance their skills and abilities in financial management.

In one institution a cost-effectiveness analysis was used to evaluate the cost impact of a new model of care (Gaynor, 1999). A decision-evaluation cost model was used to explore alternatives and evaluate options during planning and budgeting processes. The cost per case under various circumstances was determined in consultation with an economist. Appropriate data were identified. Specific, detailed costs were identified for each subcomponent of the new care delivery model: materials, supplies, personnel, recruitment, training, and on-unit orientation. The previous care delivery model was used to construct a base case. The new skill mix was then substituted to develop scenarios that showed changes in staffing costs per patient day. Interview, financial, and productivity data were collected for each cost element. Alternative scenarios were developed to test the impact of changes in skill mix and turnover rates on the staff costs per case. Sensitivity and "what if" analyses also were conducted to test impacts on the salary cost per patient day. Unit nurse managers used the cost models to test their specific unit data. Criteria for staffing plans for direct caregivers were derived. This enhanced the precision of targeted recruitment efforts for the most cost-effective skill mix to meet outcomes (Gaynor, 1999).

LEADERSHIP AND MANAGEMENT IMPLICATIONS

With a trend toward decentralization of decision making, the nurse manager's role includes increasing accountability for financial management of the work unit. With a trend toward consolidation and the elimination of middle managers, individual nurses begin to assume more of this accountability and responsibility.

The smallest functional unit that generates revenues and expenses is called a *cost center*. Some units generate direct revenue or charges, whereas others (e.g., administration) generate expenses but no direct revenue. A charge is generated for the purpose of acquiring income for the health care organization. There is a difference between the charge and the actual cost, just as there is when purchasing a piece of clothing from a department store. The **charge** is defined as the price asked for services or goods. The **cost** is the actual amount of money required as payment to cover direct production inputs used in producing the service (see Leading & Managing Defined box). *Profit* is defined as the money gained as excess of charges over outlay costs in producing a service.

◢ LEADERSHIP & MANAGEMENT **BEHAVIORS**

Leadership Behaviors

- Determines financial contributions of the group
- Guides a visionary identification of costs and resources
- Analyzes nursing costs and benefits
- Uses creativity to strategize and negotiate for the group's resource needs
- Motivates the group to increase financial knowledge
- Influences the group to find innovative ways to increase revenue
- Develops new resource streams
- Creates a financially savvy work environment

Management Behaviors

- Plans for financial management
- Organizes the needed resources

- Organizes financial data
- Implements the unit budget and financial processes
- Controls expenses
- Determines resource requirements within organizational constraints
- Evaluates technology
- Motivates subordinates to learn about financial elements

Overlap Areas

- Determines resource requirements
- Motivates expanded knowledge about financial aspects
- Manages expenditures

For example, a health care facility may bill a client for $5 for the use of a vial of sterile saline when it cost the hospital $1 to purchase and process the purchase. The difference is profit.

Traditionally, nursing was included as part of the hospital room charge and not separated from hospital-based hotel functions such as housekeeping, support services, and dietary. Thus the actual costs of care and the revenue captured from nursing effort were in effect "invisible." This approach hurt nursing by attributing costs incurred by the operations of other departments to nursing. Nursing was then seen as the costliest item in the organization's budget and was targeted first for budget reductions, restructuring, and layoffs. Research in the 1980s placed nursing's actual contributions to the costs of hospital care at 25% to 35% of the budget at a time when conventional wisdom put this figure at about 60%. A study of for-profit hospitals showed that on average, they spent 31.8% of their budgets on administration in 1990. This figure rose to 34% by 1994. The figures were lower for nonprofit hospitals

(24.5%) and public hospitals (22.9%) in 1994 but varied widely from state to state (Woolhandler & Himmelstein, 1997). Averaging across all types of agencies, administration counted for 31% of U.S. health care expenditures in 1999 (Woolhandler et al., 2003). The costs of administration traditionally have not faced the scrutiny that the costs of nursing have, nor have these cost centers been faced with proportional personnel cuts.

Research also showed that physicians often billed for—and were reimbursed for—services provided by nurses. Ott and colleagues (1989) found that nurses performed many of the services for which physicians were being reimbursed. An examination of the Current Procedural Terminology (CPT) codes revealed that nurses performed many of the services listed; yet the CPT coding system acknowledged only physicians as providers of all the coded services. Nursing services were not a factor in payment review fee schedules, except as a part of a physician's practice costs (Griffith & Fonteyn, 1989; Griffith et al., 1991).

Consequently, nurses were encouraged to identify explicitly the value of the nursing component involved in each physician service, since others appeared to be capturing revenue for what nurses actually did. Nurses perform and coordinate client service delivery. Therefore they contribute to both costs and charges. Nursing needs to examine ways to capture its contribution to revenues and profit and then communicate and negotiate on this basis. The perception of nursing's value in an organization may be affected in subtle ways, including from data on cost effectiveness.

Because most nurses traditionally did not capture fee-for-service as reimbursement, but rather were employees, nursing was considered to be a cost rather than a revenue source. When nursing captures its cost data and can identify the actual cost contribution of nursing services, then a different form of negotiation over needed financial resources can occur. Unless nursing can accurately capture its costs, nurses will not know the actual costs of nursing care. Nurses need this information to better manage care resources regardless of the type of reimbursement structure. Demonstrating the actual cost conservation contributed by nursing can be a powerful negotiating tool for managed care and other contracts.

Overall, both nurses and nurse managers have seen their role expand in scope and importance as empowerment, innovative change, shared governance, and cost containment have occurred. The nurse's role in financial management has grown in concert with these changes. Jones (1993) noted that nurse managers' financial management efforts are directed at determining resource requirements, being able to justify resources, evaluating technology, and holding down expenses for staff, supplies, and equipment. Similarly, staff nurses' financial management efforts can be directed at contributing data and rationale for resource needs and practicing cost awareness in nursing care delivery. Thus nurses at all levels need awareness and knowledge about the basics and techniques of financial management. Leaders and managers can motivate personnel to expand their knowledge base and can model

savvy financial management while planning, organizing, implementing, and controlling money and resources.

ETHICAL AND LEGAL ISSUES

Budgeting and financial management involve intensive decision making about the allocation of scarce resources. Conflicts and ethical dilemmas easily arise in the balancing of competing needs and wants. For example, the institution has an advantage if labor budgets are tightly restricted. However, clients may incur greater wait times or diminished direct care time if nurses and other care providers are not readily available and accessible. Furthermore, nurses experience greater stress when workloads rise and clients' care needs are difficult to meet in the time available. Chronic stress saps nurses' energy and is reflected in their ability to deliver client-oriented service. In severe cases, patient safety is jeopardized and medical errors increase.

Money, personnel, space, and time are scarce resources in organizations; and they become the focal points for power, politics, and conflict. Ethical and moral problems occur as values clash. Ethical obligations of fidelity can be interpreted as promise keeping, an obligation to act in good faith, fulfilling agreements, maintaining relationships, and upholding trust and confidence. In law or business the parallel ideas are contracts, trust, or fiduciary relationships (Beauchamp & Childress, 1994). Ethical dilemmas arise over conflicts of loyalty or conflicts of interest.

Professional fidelity or loyalty means upholding the clients' interests as a priority over the professional's self-interest or others' interests in any conflict. This is also called *advocacy*. Divided loyalties arise from the organizational and financial structures of health care. For example, issuing orders, assignment of duties, or allegiance to other providers, employing agencies, funding sources, corporate structures, or governmental agencies may compel an ethical choice. It is unclear what a health care provider or institution "owes" a client beyond reasonable or "due care."

Because of the structure of health care delivery and nursing's traditions, nurses report pervasive moral conflicts among obligations related to fidelity. This means that nurses may face choices among obligations to clients, physicians, and employing institutions (Beauchamp & Childress, 1994). Some examples arise over privacy rights versus disclosure of information, physicians' orders, respect of clients' wishes, aggressiveness of treatment, impact of teaching and research functions in care delivery, and conflicts of interest with payor restrictions or denial of coverage when care needs still exist.

The ethical value of stewardship relates to the obligation to oversee and use expertise to decide about the appropriate allocation of resources. Stewardship means that nurses will need to make frequent choices among competing values of client needs balanced with organizational financial survival (Reiser, 1994). The overall effects of nurses' decisions related to budgeting and cost containment affect clients and organizations. Managed care systems reward restricted or nonintervention care and frugality by using economic incentives for clinical decisions. Thus providers and organizations may acquire economic gain by rationing care to clients. Other incentives such as job security may conflict with obligations to clients as financial management decisions are made (Beauchamp & Childress, 1994).

Box 35.1 illustrates a type of legal and ethical dilemma that may result from the changing structure of health care financing. The scenario described in the chart is simplified; in reality the issues would probably be much more complex. The purpose of this example is to show the ethical and legal challenges that may be faced by nurses and other health care providers as they decide whether to provide specific interventions for a client. The example given could affect the financial solvency of the neonatal intensive care unit within the larger institution. It is possible, if not likely, that there will be financial sanctions against the department or health care providers who work there when the department overspends its budget because of a decision to provide the additional

---

Box 35.1

Ethical Factors Created by Health Care Financing Restructuring

Scenario: An attending physician in the neonatal intensive care unit (NICU) of a major research hospital has determined that a premature infant (21 weeks' gestation) is of questionable viability. Because of the infant's underdeveloped lungs and other complications, the physician is considering issuing an order to not provide basic life support, including feeding, to the newborn. With the astronomical costs associated with prolonged NICU care and the likely reimbursement level, cost burdens become a consideration. Before finalizing the order, the physician consults with the NICU nurse in charge of the infant.

---

services to the client even when there will be no reimbursement for them. With costs of care so high and reimbursement often capitated, profits are made by for-profit hospitals by laying off nurses and then hiring consultants and bureaucrats to determine how to avoid costly outliers and unprofitable clients as a way of maximizing revenues (Woolhandler & Himmelstein, 1997).

Loyalty to the organization may constrain moral principles and create a tension between the nursing ethic of caring and the profit orientation in corporations (Corley & Raines, 1993). Nurses resolve ethical dilemmas by the bending of rules, responsible subversion, creating meaning from difficult situations, denial, burnout, quitting, remaining silent, choosing self-interest or organization-interest above the client's interest, or facilitating values clarification (Corley & Raines, 1993). Nurse managers have identified three aspects of an ethical practice environment as autonomy, trust, and communication. Complementary nurse manager characteristics, institutional supports, and organizational values are necessary to create autonomy, trust, and communication orientations that promote ethical professional practice (Corley & Raines, 1993). These aspects of value-driven leadership are further emphasized in the literature on business success in service industries. Berry (1999) analyzed labor-intensive service industries to identify the drivers of sustainable success. Three values of control of destiny, trust-based relationships, and investment in employee success were among the nine structural and process drivers that were common across different service businesses. Great service companies build a humane, ethical, and values-driven community.

Employment arrangements create legal as well as ethical rights and obligations. Financial and budgeting implications arise from legal obligations. Malpractice and negligence place nurses and employers at financial risk. Both the nurse and the employer can be held liable under the doctrine of *respondeat superior*, in which the employer is named a defendant in a malpractice claim because the employer is responsible for the acts of its employees. Under the doctrine of corporate negligence, health care organizations have a responsibility to monitor or supervise all personnel, including the quality of care given, and to investigate physicians' credentials (Aiken, 1994).

Although there are clear organizational liabilities for employment issues, the legal risks related to deployment issues are less clear. Short staffing, leading to inadequate care and medical errors, remains a major nursing management ethical problem (Corley & Raines, 1993). The requirement of the law is that the nurse's actions be reasonable under the circumstances. Reasonable in relationship to short staffing is a matter of judgment. Client safety, accepted professional standards and guidelines, and the language of organizational policies and procedures are major considerations. Budgeting and financial management are managerial decisions fraught with both ethical and legal ramifications.

Summary

- Financial management is a major nonclinical managerial task for nurses.
- The allocation of scarce resources is the focus of financial management.

- Financial management aims to facilitate the efficient operation of an organization.
- The four phases of financial management are budgeting, recording, reporting, and evaluating.
- Strategic planning in nursing affects financial outcomes.
- A *charge* is the price asked for services; the *cost* is the amount required to cover direct production inputs.
- Nurses at all levels have a role in participating in financial management efforts.
- Financial management decisions may create legal and ethical dilemmas for nurses.

Study Questions

1. How does financial management relate to leadership? To management and control?
2. How much effort should nurses place on financial management activities?
3. What strategies can nurses use to influence financial decision making?
4. How can nurses gauge the financial effectiveness of their practice?
5. In what ways can nurses address legal or ethical issues arising in financial management?

CASE STUDY

Fiscal accountability begins at the individual provider level. Too often providers are unaware of basic financial management and their individual and collective impact on the cost of delivering patient care. Simple things such as not using preprinted forms for scratch paper or expensive sterile pads to wipe up a spill can incrementally add to the cost of care, thereby diverting resources, through waste, away from needed care delivery. At another level, many practice patterns such as ordering routine (but not evidence-based) vital signs soak up scarce nursing resources and divert them from alternative needs. Yet providers tend to use routine behaviors such as these without conscious analysis or thought. A related issue occurs when nurse managers are responsible for a nursing unit and its supplies, but nonnursing

CRITICAL THINKING EXERCISE

Nurse Hiroshi Watanabe has been the director of a home health agency for 15 years. The agency has experienced some difficult times but has managed to survive. Now, however, with increased competition, rising client acuity, an increase in uncompensated care, and a drop in the major volume indicator (number of visits), the agency is seriously threatened. Furthermore, the Centers for Medicare & Medicaid Services (CMS) have decided to adopt new rules that will severely reduce payments for Medicare home health visits. A close scrutiny of the financial projections indicates impending deficits. Nurse Watanabe has developed the following two options to present to the board of directors:

• Merge with the agency's largest competitor

• Reduce nursing staff and switch employees' health care benefits to a managed care contract that limits the choice of physicians and providers

1. What is/are the problem(s)?
2. How should Nurse Watanabe handle the situation?
3. What should Nurse Watanabe do first?
4. What financial management strategies might work?
5. What creative strategies might be best suited to the situation?
6. What would motivate others to assist in this situation?

---

providers (such as physicians or residents) order or use those supplies without accountability.

One teaching hospital addressed these issues by funding a multidisciplinary education team that developed a project to improve the integration of fiscal knowledge into the practice of nurses, resident physicians, pharmacists, and nursing students (Krugman et al., 2002). A pre- and posttest method was used to evaluate whether the project improved hospital financial outcomes of increased capture of patient charges, improved documentation of services, reduced inventory use, and decreased materials loss/waste. Implementation strategies included educational information in the hospital newsletter, a new employee orientation video, self-learning modules, and a discharge supply review group that used multiple interventions such as compiling a resource guide. Results showed improved awareness of and knowledge about financial aspects of care delivery. Targeted educational interventions were the most successful. The multidisciplinary aspect helped pave the way for increased standardization related to fiscal accountability.

REFERENCES

Aiken, T. (1994). *Legal, ethical, and political issues in nursing.* Philadelphia: F.A. Davis.

Beauchamp, T., & Childress, J. (1994). *Principles of biomedical ethics* (4th ed.). New York: Oxford University Press.

Berry, L.L. (1999). *Discovering the soul of service: The nine drivers of sustainable business success.* New York: The Free Press.

Corley, M., & Raines, D. (1993). An ethical practice environment as a caring environment. *Nursing Administration Quarterly, 17*(2), 68-74.

Finkler, S.A., & Kovner, C.T. (2000). *Financial management for nurse managers and executives* (2nd ed.). Philadelphia: Saunders.

Finkler, S.A., & Ward, D.M. (1999). *Essentials of cost accounting for health care organizations* (2nd ed.). Gaithersburg, MD: Aspen.

Gaynor, S. (1999). Cost studies/value outcomes. *Journal of Child and Family Nursing, 2*(1), 72-73.

Griffith, H., & Fonteyn, M. (1989). Let's set the payment record straight. *American Journal of Nursing, 89*(8), 1051-1058.

Griffith, H., Thomas, N., & Griffith, L. (1991). MDs bill for these routine nursing tasks. *American Journal of Nursing, 91*(1), 22-27.

Jones, K. (1993). The ins and outs of financial management: An introduction. *Seminars for Nurse Managers, 1*(1), 4.

Krugman, M., MacLauchlan, M., Riippi, L., & Grubbs, J. (2002). A multidisciplinary financial education research project. *Nursing Economic$, 20*(6), 273-278.

Ott, B., Griffith, H., & Towers, J. (1989). Who gets the money? *American Journal of Nursing, 89*(2), 186-188.

Reiser, S. (1994). The ethical life of health care organizations. *Hastings Center Report, 24*(6), 28-35.

Smith, H., Mahon, S., & Piland, N. (1993). Nursing department strategy, planning, and performance in rural hospitals. *Journal of Nursing Administration, 23*(4), 23-34.

Woolhandler, S., Campbell, T., & Hummelstein, D.U. (2003). Cost of health care administration in the United States and Canada. *New England Journal of Medicine, 349*(8), 768-775.

Woolhandler, S., & Himmelstein, D.U. (1997). Costs of care and administration at for-profit and other hospitals in the United States. *New England Journal of Medicine, 336*(11), 769-774.

36

Budgeting

Diane L. Huber

CHAPTER OBJECTIVES

- Define and describe a budget
- Categorize general types of budgets
- Define and differentiate a traditional budget from a zero-based budget
- Distinguish between direct and indirect costs
- Outline the stages of a typical budgetary process
- Critique costing out nursing services
- Exercise critical thinking to conceptualize and analyze possible solutions to a practice exercise

The management of client care involves coordinating and integrating clinical care delivery, quality of care, human resources management, and financial management. Budgeting is focused on money as a strategic resource. The control over money significantly affects the control over nursing practice and nursing care delivery by posing opportunities and constraints. Because nurses carry responsibility and accountability for care management, program management, and service delivery, they will need concurrent expertise in and control over budgeting decisions.

Nurses are front-line implementation personnel. Their jobs entail close and ongoing client contact in the direct provision of health care services. As professionals, nurses have some degree of discretion and decision making inherent in their work. Actual implementation decisions, including the use of supplies and equipment, are made by individual nurses. These decisions have a direct financial impact on health care organizations.

Budgeting concepts are important but little emphasized in nursing practice. For a long time nursing has focused its attention on clinical client care. Yet at all levels of care the allocation of scarce resources is an important client care consideration. Nurses play a major role in the implementation-level decisions about care provision and supplies and equipment usage that have financial ramifications. They evaluate equipment for purchase and use. They manage large supply allocations. Nurses comprise a major element of the personnel budget of a health care facility. A basic working familiarity with budgeting concepts can help nurses make better decisions, communicate with financial management staff, and bargain more effectively for scarce resource allocation for nursing.

DEFINITIONS

Budgeting is a major aspect of an organization or unit's planning processes (Figure 36.1). A budget is a plan that is specified in dollar amounts. Expressed in written or computerized form and quantified in dollar amounts, this plan becomes a guiding framework for organizational activities.

⚠ LEADING & MANAGING **DEFINED**

Budget

A written financial plan aimed at controlling the allocation of resources.

Expenses

The costs of activities undertaken in an organization's operations.

Revenues

Income or amounts owed for purchased services or goods.

Operating Budget

The plan for the unit's or organization's daily operating revenues and expenses.

Capital Budget

Plan that tracks purchases of capital assets (i.e., buildings, land, and equipment).

Cash Budget

Plan that tracks cash receipts and cash disbursements.

Expense Budget

Plan that tracks expenditure of resources or costs paid (i.e., wages, benefits, and maintenance costs).

It expresses management's intentions and financial expectations regarding revenues and expenditures. An organization-level budget compares expected revenues with expected expenses to forecast profit (surplus) or loss (deficit). Budgeting is a continuous process of preparing projections, implementing current budgets, and evaluating outcomes and performance. Preparing a budget entails forecasting the future (usually 1 year ahead) and anticipating the impact of trends and how many units of service will need to be provided. However, a specific budget timetable should be constructed to outline the activities and timelines of the annual budgeting decision process.

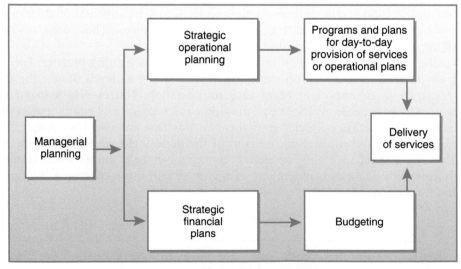

Figure 36.1
Process of managerial and strategic planning.

A budget can be thought of as a roadmap. It is used as a guide to avoid crises, achieve goals and objectives, anticipate potential problems or develop potential solutions, encourage communication and coordination, and evaluate unit and managerial performance (Finkler & Ward, 1999).

A **budget** is defined as a written financial plan aimed at controlling the allocation of resources. It functions as both a planning instrument and an evaluation tool useful for financial management. A budget is used to manage programs, plan for goal accomplishment, and control costs. **Expenses** are defined as the costs or prices of activities undertaken in the organization's operations. **Revenues** are defined as income or amounts owed for purchased services or goods. *Total operating expenses* are the result of summing the costs of all resources used to produce services. *Total operating revenues* are the result of multiplying the volume of services provided by the charges (rate) for the services. *Income* is the excess of revenues over expenses, or revenues minus expenses, for a given time (Johnson & Carpenter, 1990) (Box 36.1). A *variance* is the difference between the budgeted and the actual amounts. A budget becomes a financial timetable and plan for the organization that is translated into monetary terms. However, an alternative viewpoint sees a budget as a political document that results from a complicated bargaining process. The output is a financial document, although the budgetary process varies among organizations. Expenses, for example, may be program-based or itemized

individually, on a separate expense line, as line items.

Organizational budgets actually include a variety of different types of budgets. The master budget is a set of all the organization's budgets for individual purposes. It is important to realize that there are multiple types of budgets in simultaneous operation. Finkler and Kovner (2000) identified the following seven general types of budgets:

1. The **operating budget** is the plan for the unit's or organization's daily operating revenues and expenses and usually applies to a single year. The operating budget for a unit is the budget in which nurse managers tend to have the most intensive involvement. Extensive information is needed to prepare the operating budget. Elements included in operational budgeting are (1) a workload budget with activity reports, units of service, and workload calculations; (2) expense budgets with personnel and staffing requirements and labor costs; (3) expense budgets for supplies, equipment, and overhead; and (4) a revenue budget.

2. A *long-range budget* is a plan, often called *a strategic plan*, that looks at goals and purposes over a span of 3, 5, and sometimes 10 years.

3. A *program budget* analyzes a specific program, one that is planned for the future or one that is in existence and requires evaluation. A budget often cuts across departments and years.

4. The **capital budget** tracks the acquisition of capital assets, or long-term investments, such as buildings, land, or equipment. Capital budget items provide useful service beyond the year they are first acquired or put in use. Expensive equipment generally is procured and replaced through the capital budget.

5. *Product-line budgets* look at the revenues and expenses associated with a defined group of clients, such as those with a common diagnosis. Product lines often are associated with disease groups or medical diagnoses, such as congestive heart failure or heart disease.

6. The **cash budget** tracks the monthly cash receipts and cash disbursements.

Box **36.1**

Calculating Total Operating Expenses, Revenues, Income

Total operating expenses = Cost of resources (1) + Cost of resources (2) + ...

Total operating revenues = Service provided (1) × Charge + Service provided (2) × Charge + ...

Income = Revenues − Expenses

7. A *special purpose budget* is prepared for a program or activity that was not previously planned or budgeted.

In addition, a well-managed organization will have a set of all the major budgets in an organization, called the *master budget.*

BACKGROUND

Budgets and the budgeting process may be approached from a variety of strategies or perspectives. Two basic types of budget formats are the traditional and the zero-based budget.

Traditional budgets identify expenses to be tracked. In nursing the most common expense items are salaries, benefits, supplies, and equipment. Traditional budgets may be called *incremental budgets.* Other expenses include overhead, administrative, and educational costs. Often negotiations are centered around the appropriate amount to increase the budget each year.

Zero-based budgeting is a form of budgeting in which the entire budget is rebuilt from zero each year or each budget cycle. The traditional approach takes the previous year's budget as the status quo and builds up from there. With zero-based budgeting, all expenses are rejustified each year. This process uncovers exactly how money is being spent and avoids budgets becoming bloated over time. Zero-based budgeting emphasizes the consideration of alternative means of providing the same service or program. It provides a method for a sophisticated analysis of these alternatives (Finkler & Kovner, 2000).

For nurses, the primary budgets related directly to the delivery of nursing services are the capital budget and the operating budget. The capital budget is the plan specific to major purchases that meet or exceed the organization's particular definition of a capital expense. The operating budget covers a specific period, called a *fiscal year,* and is the budget plan for day-to-day service delivery operations. It includes historical or trend data, expenses, and revenues. The operating budget is the most time-consuming aspect of financial management for most nurse managers. To prepare the annual operating budget, a variety of information is needed. Nurse managers prepare three major aspects of the operating budget: (1) the expense budget for personnel, (2) the expense budget for costs other than personnel, and (3) the revenue budget. Not all hospital nursing units prepare revenue budgets (Finkler & Kovner, 2000).

For **expense budgets**, the first step is forecasting the volume of work for the coming year. The workload aspect often is measured in units of service. Key units of service need to be identified, the number of units predicted, and expenses and staffing calculated accordingly. Activity reports, such as census and average length of stay, identify trends related to volume of activity. The unit of service often needs to be adjusted to the case or patient mix, which is a proxy for severity of illness or need (Finkler & Kovner, 2000).

With a workload forecast, the manger can proceed to determine the personnel services (or staffing budget) portion of the expense budget. Calculation of staffing is more complex than the total number of hours of care to be delivered per patient day on average. First, the average daily census and occupancy (or utilization) rate are calculated. Then the number of full-time equivalents (FTEs)—that is, the mix of full-time and part-time staff—needed to provide care for the expected number of hours is determined by type and shift. Adjustments need to be made for benefits and downtime, called productive versus nonproductive hours. Next, staff mix (RN, LPN, aide, clerical) is considered and calculated. Administrative and other fixed staff members need to be included. To determine labor costs, straight-time versus overtime, differentials and premiums, and fringe benefits are added in (Finkler & Kovner, 2000).

The operating budget also includes an expense budget for costs other than personnel. Clinical and office supplies, books and publications, training, education and travel, noncapital equipment, brochures, and depreciation may be line items in the other-than-personnel budget. Expenses may be fixed or variable. In some cases a revenue budget also is calculated and managed. Patient revenue (gross) is the number of units of service multiplied by the price per unit. Contractual allowances (discounts), bad debt, and indigent care all become reductions of gross revenue and are generally not under the nurse manager's control (Finkler & Kovner, 2000).

Budgeting Basics

Nurses will be involved in budgeting for nursing services in different ways and to different degrees not only depending on their position within an institution but also based on the institution where they are working. Institutions vary significantly concerning the level of budgetary involvement that nurse managers are expected or allowed to perform.

Usually the nurse's involvement will be for a specific time period (e.g., the accounting time frame of 1 year, broken down into 12 monthly periods) and for a specific level (e.g., unit or department). The two major types of budgets to prepare are capital and operating.

The capital budget is prepared for large equipment, long-term investments, physical plant, or program expenditures. Examples of capital expenses are fixed assets, new or replacement equipment (e.g., new informatics technology),

building renovation or unit relocation, or adding a new program (e.g., endoscopy suite). A spreadsheet is prepared with line item requests and vendor quotes for costs of purchase, installation, and staff education or training. In some cases, a project will be completed in a multiyear timeframe, and projected costs would be broken out for each year.

The operating budget is the more complex and detailed of the two types of budgets nurses will manage. Although there may be variations in the process and forms used, the data available, and the scope of the budget, nurses generally focus on volume, personnel, and supplies and services elements.

Volume is a critical variable. It is important to know whether unit volume is dependent on another department or service. The capacity (e.g., number of inpatient beds) needs to be determined. Volume then becomes, for example, 20 beds × 365 days = 7,300 bed days. Table 36.1 shows a sample volume budget flow sheet. Historical trend data are needed (e.g., occupancy percentages by timeframes such as weekly or monthly) to determine growth projections. The volume of services delivered for a year may be expressed as patient days, visits, procedures, or other units of service. Other effects on volume are

Table **36.1**

Volume Budget Flow Sheet		
Month	Patient Days Budgeted	Patient Days Actual
January	268	272
February	310	315
March		
April		
May		
June		
July		
August		
September		
October		
November		
December		

Table 36.2

Budgeted Salary Expense Flow Sheet		
Expense Item	Budgeted	Actual
Salaries		
Regular		
Overtime		
On-call		
Vacation		
Holiday		
Illness		
Other		
TOTAL SALARIES		

environmental effects such as reimbursement changes, new programs, process improvements, new technology, and marketing. After forecasting volume, the resources (such as labor and supplies) required to provide services need to be forecasted.

After volume is determined, revenue and expense budgets are detailed. Revenue budgets are a set of calculations that determine gross amounts that come from charging patients for services. Nurses have not necessarily been involved in generating or analyzing these budgets. Because the focus in nursing is on expense budgets, nursing is viewed as an expense (to be cut) rather than a revenue-generating department.

Expense budgets include personnel or labor budgets (with fixed and variable components) and nonlabor (supplies, utilities, and depreciation

and leases). Nurses focus on labor and supplies budgets. Because labor costs are the overwhelming proportion of nursing services costs, these budgets become the target of intense scrutiny. Table 36.2 displays a sample budget expense sheet for salaries, whereas Table 36.3 demonstrates how personnel budgets might be displayed. Salary increases might also be included as another column.

Supply budgets are another area of major responsibility in nursing. Supply items such as office supplies, IV solutions, instruments, linen replacement, medical/surgical supplies, drugs, leases, maintenance contracts, and books and subscriptions might be line items that are budgeted for. Dollar amounts would be assigned and compared with actual expenses. It is important for nurses to have line items and appropriate amounts

Table 36.3

Personnel Budget Sheet				
Position	Name	FTE	Hourly Wage ($)	Yearly Salary ($)
RN	Smith	1.0		38,000
RN	Jones	1.0		38,000
LPN	Roe	0.5		29,000
NA	Ash	1.0		22,000
Clerk	Oak	1.0		20,000

RN, Registered nurse; *LPN,* licensed practicing nurse; *NA,* nurse assistant.

for necessary expenditures, such as staff education and travel. It also is important that nurses have authority over supplies and equipment purchases if they have accountability for these budgets.

All organizations have a budgeting cycle, using annual budgets to set parameters for the upcoming year. Regular budget analyses (e.g., quarterly or monthly) are used for monitoring, feedback, and managerial control. Just as with personal finances, the focus is on revenue (income) and expenses (outgo). The variance (difference) between budgeted and actual expenses is determined to identify problem areas, enhance control, and make timely adjustments. The variance difference between actual and budgeted (planned) performance needs to be analyzed to determine the cause so that nurses can take the appropriate action. Variances can be favorable or unfavorable. Causes of variance can be from a change due to a single cause (e.g., volume, rate such as salary, usage, or price) or from a combination of causes. The mathematical calculations vary depending on cause determination.

There also will be variance in some expenditures based on the time of the year. As an example, some expenditures are relatively level throughout the year whereas others will peak and valley at different times (e.g., heating costs will be high in the winter and low or nonexistent in the summer). Comparing current year expenditures at the end of each month, quarter, or other established time period with expenditures from several previous years at the same time will show whether there is a pattern of such differences throughout the year. If patterns can be seen, then lower or higher expenditures may be found to be normal and not a cause of adjustment in expenditure plans. Budgeting is a basic process of managing financial resources. Forecasting and decision analysis are more advanced management tools that add to the organization's overall financial management.

Costs

Nurses are concerned with cost control; thus they manage direct, indirect, and supply costs. Some costs are controllable by the nurse manager, whereas others are outside of the nurse manager's control (such as the organization's salary policy).

Direct costs are all costs that can be traced to a specific unit or activity. Direct costs relate to direct nursing care provision. They may be computed as the amount of time spent with the client times a salary and fringe benefit factor. Direct costs include elements such as nursing time. Such costs are those incurred by the unit and activities for which the manager has responsibility. In nursing, direct costs are the costs of resources used in direct care of a client (Finkler & Kovner, 2000).

Indirect costs are those assigned to a unit from elsewhere in the organization or those costs within a unit not incurred in the direct care of a client (Finkler & Kovner, 2000). Indirect costs relate to miscellaneous costs secondary to direct care provision. Indirect costs may be computed to include all the overhead costs, for example, lights, administrative costs, and building maintenance.

In a review of 73 studies on costing out nursing services, Eckhart (1993) found that there was no consistency in the definitions of direct and indirect nursing costs. Authors frequently did not clearly define the activities being included in direct nursing care. For example, the placement of overtime, orientation, education, and nursing administration costs varied among methods of calculation. Eckhart's recommended standardized definition for direct nursing care is the hourly wages for only the personnel providing "hands on" client care. Indirect costs should be a constant value generated specifically for each facility and should include all supportive services required to provide direct nursing care. Total nursing costs include both direct and indirect nursing costs. Eckhart's opinion was that overhead, housekeeping, and dietary costs are not nursing costs; therefore they should not be figured in nursing expenses. A standardized definition of nursing costs is still needed and would aid in the calculation of costs for comparison purposes.

Taking a cost-accounting perspective, Jones (1994) defined direct costs as "those costs that can be identified with the production of a specific product or service" (p. 4). This would include all costs traced directly to the objective of delivering care to clients. Thus salaries, supplies, and pharmaceuticals would be considered direct costs. Jones (1994) defined indirect costs as "costs that cannot be traced to a specific cost objective" (p. 4). Indirect costs include costs allocated from support services (e.g., housekeeping, dietary) and general hospital overhead (e.g., utility costs, insurance, and administrative salaries). Full costs mean direct costs plus allocated indirect costs. Full costs are used in setting rates and negotiating with third-party reimbursers.

Jones (1994) noted that the nurse manager's two major issues in relation to indirect and overhead costs are accuracy and control. Accuracy relates to whether specific costs included in the total amount of indirect costs may actually belong to specific services or departments. Thus the indirect costs figure may be inaccurate. The control issue relates to the nurse's ability to control the total unit budget while having the responsibility to meet cost control goals. Parts of the budget, such as indirect costs, may not be under the nurse's control. Thus nurses need to be alert to whether the aspect of the budget they do not control is expanding faster than the aspects under their direct control. If the areas they do not control are expanding rapidly, those areas need to be identified and strategies employed for specific cost control in the targeted areas.

Nurses need accurate information about how costs are allocated and what specific costs go into their own budgets. One element that often is missing is accurate and reliable data. Lack of standard definitions robs nurses of reliable data for cost comparisons. Yet data form the basis of many management decisions. The data need to be accurate and reliable and attached to the costs incurred in the delivery of care to a specific client.

One factor to take into account when estimating costs and budgets is how intensely a client absorbs nursing time. This factor is called intensity. For example, there is a difference in the intensity of direct care needs between a client who is comatose and one who is ambulatory. Consequently, the direct cost generated by the client should be greater for a comatose or highly dependent client.

Supply costs also are not standardized, although generally there is an attempt to charge for discrete supply and equipment use. For example, each time a specific piece of equipment, topper sponge, alcohol swab, catheter, or a piece of IV tubing is used, it may be attributed to an individual client. Sometimes the supplies and equipment are directly charged to the client. Other times they are considered to be general supplies. Often, small incidentals such as alcohol swabs, topper sponges, and tape are the kinds of general supplies for which there would be a unit budget; in that situation each client would be charged a certain flat percentage of the total yearly budget, which is broken down and divided by the number of clients as an overhead cost. When supplies are allocated as a general unit budget, there is a danger of large costs due to lack of accountability and the "leaking" of small items that can amount to appreciable costs. Managerial programs to monitor supply chain processes are yielding significant results (Maurano, 2004). The nurse needs to know how the organization allocates supply costs to be able to make budgetary and financial management decisions.

THE BUDGETARY PROCESS

Each institution will establish standard budgetary formats and processes. The budgeting process can become complex and time-consuming. The collection of necessary data and completion of documents or computerized spreadsheets is an involved process. One useful device is to construct a budget timetable with columns for tasks and activities, responsible person, and deadlines for completion. Since the budget is actually implemented by all employees, the involvement of all employees in all aspects of budgeting is recommended (Finkler & Kovner, 2000). Some organizations carefully guard all financial information and restrict access to upper levels and others on a "need to know" basis. Other organizations hold the philosophy that knowledgeable employees are

Research Note

Source: Huang, S., Chen, P., Yang, M., Chang, W., & Lee, H. (2004). Using a balanced scorecard to improve the performance of an emergency department. *Nursing Economic$, 22*(3), 140-146.

Purpose

Emergency departments (EDs) play a crucial role in revenue streams in hospitals in Taiwan because 45% to 70% of hospitalized patients are admitted via EDs. However, EDs are complex and crowded and receive many patient/family complaints. Performance improvement was needed. The balanced scorecard (BSC) was selected in order to simultaneously examine operational and financial measures of performance. The purpose of this study was to develop an approach for implementing BSC in one ED in Taiwan and describe the effectiveness of the BSC's performance indicators.

Discussion

The process to derive the BSC included choosing performance indicators, defining parameters, identifying data sources, and determining relative performance. The BSC had nine indicators, as follows:

- Two for learning and growth
- Four for internal business processes
- One financial indicator
- Two customer measures

Data were collected from staff, patients, and old records. Significant differences occurred before and after program implementation on one learning and growth measure, three internal business measures, and one customer measure. Revenues did increase (the financial measure) but this was not significantly different.

Application to Practice

Expenses were invested up-front; however, after subtracting the Investment costs, profit still increased after implementing BSC. In addition, Information related to costs became available to enhance decision making. Patient satisfaction improved. Both financial and nonfinancial benefits accrued. Other emergency departments can use the findings in implementing balanced scorecards and other outcomes measurement and management.

empowered and motivated employees. They engage creative planning by open communication and full dissemination of financial information.

The budgeting process begins with statements and specifications that form the foundation of budget preparation. These include statements of mission, position, goals, objectives, and policies. Organization-wide assumptions and program priorities also may be included to provide guidance in budget preparation. The budget will need to be in alignment with strategic plans.

With this guidance, unit or department managers prepare an individual budget for each operating unit or program. The individual unit budgets are used to compile a cash budget. When budget requests exceed the available resources (a common occurrence), a round of negotiation and revisions follows the initial budget preparation phase. This continues until the budget is approved. Then managers work to monitor the budget plan during implementation and control results as closely as is possible (Finkler & Kovner, 2000). Because the budget reflects and constrains the allocation of money in an organization, issues of equity and fairness are important. In some cases, if a budget cannot be achieved and failure is probable, a manager's or employee's motivation to work hard may decrease. The budgeting philosophy needs to strike a balance between being an empowering and motivating incentive to work hard (yet involves some risk) and being too tightly controlled and stingy that it creates discouragement from built-in failure (but is lucrative).

The budgeting process is complex and requires the completion of several complicated documents. A typical budget process ties into overall strategic and managerial planning. The multiple steps of a budget process need to be outlined but can be grouped into the following three phases (Finkler & Kovner, 2000):

1. *Establishing the basis for budget preparation:* Strategic plans and program budgets need to be prepared. Other data need to be gathered from an environmental scan; general goals, objectives and policies; budget assumptions; program priorities; and a list of specific and measurable operating objectives.

2. *Preparing the first draft:* Unit and department managers use the gathered data to prepare budget documents for their areas. These documents are used at the organizational level to prepare cash budgets.

3. *Reviewing and re-budgeting:* As budget documents go through serial review and flow to top administration, requests tend to exceed the available resources. This necessitates review, adjustment, and appeal. There may be multiple iterations of re-budgeting before the final budget is approved.

It is at stage 3—review and re-budgeting—that the art of negotiation is employed. At the top levels of management, budgetary requests are collated, thinned, and coordinated. In many organizations the final budget must be approved by the governing board or board of directors. Therefore a strong defense for any item or program may need to be prepared.

Nurse managers may find that budgeting involves the use of multiple separate financial forms or computerized spreadsheets. These include forms designed to display and track the following items:

- Cash budget
- General expense (operating) budget

- Labor or personnel budget
- Capital equipment budget

The two key components for budgeting are (1) a *volume measure* and (2) a *cost measure.* The volume measure is an activity standard based on the unit of service or workload measure adopted by the institution. This may be bed occupancy (per day), acuity level, number of visits, number of deliveries, or nursing care hours per patient day. For a hospital the traditional measure was the census or the number of patient days. The cost measure may be a salary figure, such as the nurses' average salary or wage rate.

The various component statistics used for budgeting have both advantages and disadvantages. For example, an average value reduces a large volume of data to a representative number, but it is skewed by outliers and does not tie activity to an individual client. Thus individual client variability may be lost in the aggregate. Some fine but important discriminations may be lost or distorted by the size of the group being aggregated. Volume measures are only one indicator of activity and may not capture aspects important to the delivery and management of nursing services. The question is: what variables are critical and basic for nurses to have to manage nursing care? These would comprise a Nursing Management Minimum Data Set (NMMDS) (Huber et al., 1997).

LEADERSHIP AND MANAGEMENT IMPLICATIONS

Nursing services comprise the single largest expense aggregate in most health care organizations because they represent a large personnel component and control a large share of supplies and equipment. This is both a strength and a weakness. It is a strength because nurses clearly manage the organization and system, especially at the operational unit level. With powerful and accurate data and analysis support, unit level management becomes effective and efficient. However, many organizations simply do not provide a nurse-friendly support structure. It is a weakness to be the largest aggregate expense

▲ LEADERSHIP & MANAGEMENT **BEHAVIORS**

Leadership Behaviors

- Determines resource requirements for the group
- Guides a visionary justification of resources
- Analyzes expenditures
- Uses creativity to strategize and negotiate for the group's resource needs
- Motivates the group to increase budgetary knowledge
- Influences the group to find innovative ways to do things better
- Finds new sources for resources
- Creates a financially savvy work environment

Management Behaviors

- Plans the budget
- Organizes the needed resources
- Organizes budget justification

- Implements the unit budget and budget processes
- Controls expenses
- Determines resource requirements within organizational constraints
- Evaluates technology
- Motivates subordinates to learn about budgeting

Overlap Areas

- Determines resource requirements
- Motivates expanded knowledge about financial aspects
- Manages expenditures

---

because quick, short-term economic gains can be made by ratcheting down on resources to nursing services. This often occurs at the expense of long-term gains, staff morale, and group cohesion. Because health care generally faces strict fiscal constraints, both staff nurses and nurse managers will need to have knowledge and skill in anticipating financial fluctuations and trends and in making bold decisions based on rapid management information. Staff nurses primarily will be handling day-to-day budgetary decisions. Nurse managers are more involved with strategic or long-range financial planning and decision making.

The budgeting process requires a broad range of leadership and management skills and abilities. Resources are not unlimited. This fact is difficult for some nurses, especially if they believe they should be able to do everything for every client under every circumstance. Some professionals think that their job is to provide the maximum quantity and quality of service and that cost-consciousness should not be a part of service provision. Nurses are familiar with managing clinical

service delivery. These skills can be transferred into the management of money as a necessary adjunct to clinical service provision. However, the management of any scarce resource such as money includes balancing competing interests and making difficult decisions.

Leadership is involved in influencing others to achieve the group's goals within the constraints of scarce resources. Leaders need to be actively involved in setting the vision for how to accomplish goals through budget planning. Ethical considerations, such as fairness and reasonable targets, are part of leadership decision making. Leaders can influence employee morale and organizational culture through role modeling and the decision-making process. Organizational culture can be engaged to diminish the negative tone that is sometimes associated with budgeting.

Budgeting is a managerial responsibility. It involves skills and abilities of planning and projecting, using mathematical analysis, and paying attention to detail in the preparation and interpretation of financial forms. The budgeting process also can be used as a tool for employee motivation, a chance to hone skills in negotiation, and an opportunity for quality improvement or program planning. For example, a break-even analysis was used to investigate the financial viability of a nurse-run community nursing center in the Chicago area. The results pointed to the opportunity for expanding into the market for Medicaid managed care enrollment (Ervin et al., 1998). In another study, activity-based costing and cost-driven analysis were used to develop a care requirements tool and to explore linkages among workflow processes, time requirements, and resource consumption. Data were fed into benchmarking and quality improvement activities (Dodson et al., 1998).

Benchmarking figures are important for both budgeting and staffing. These figures can be generated by both internal and external data. Some external data estimates come from publicly available databases. Comparisons need to be made based on risk-adjusted figures. Resource consumption depends on client case mix and the severity of client illness. Factors such as client type, type of facility, size of facility, services provided, and severity of client illness are important for comparable external benchmarking. For internal benchmarking, actual versus budgeted costs, historical trend data on worked hours, client days, visits, or episodes, activity, and product costs are used. Some intervening factors skew data. These include restructuring, changes in client acuity, new programs or services, changes in physician practices, new therapies or treatments, and large changes in volume or census (Kenny, 1996).

Nurse managers will need to decide which budget-related variables are to be tracked and analyzed. Other leadership and management activities include keeping the boss informed, developing ways to increase revenues, emphasizing the return on the present investment, and looking for creative ways to fund what needs to be done (Starck & Bailes, 1996). Having systems in place to capture important data from a nursing point of view helps to prevent disorganization during a sudden crisis. These systems need to at least capture money in dollars, staff in full-time equivalents, and activity in workload measures. In a successful budget the money, staff, equipment, and materials available need to be sufficient to meet the expected quantity and quality of anticipated and provided services (Bailey, 1996).

COST AWARENESS

Continuous change in the health care system has created a challenge to reduce cost while maintaining or improving the quality of care. Nursing's attention has been drawn to cost-containment efforts. In trying to improve client care by improving managerial and clinical decisions in nursing, there is a need to be cost-conscious. The cost to clients from "what it is that nurses do" is a social and professional concern. The two major themes for nursing practice in the twenty-first century are cost and quality. The questions that will be asked are: What is the cost? Will this provide high-quality care? The cost variable relates to decision making. Cost certainly is not the only consideration to have in decision making, but nurses will need to consciously consider cost as one element. Nurses are motivated by multiple forces including both client care quality and nursing convenience.

Reducing costs and capturing reimbursement are a part of a health care organization's goals that nurses are encouraged to incorporate into their practice. For example, in one facility a cost-containment work group consisting of staff nurses and other nonsupervisory employees was formed to develop cost-reduction strategies. The following five strategies were chosen:

1. Offering education to increase employees' awareness
2. Identifying and eliminating costly habits
3. Making cost-effective decisions
4. Recycling
5. Reducing unnecessary inventory

Specific cost-containment efforts were most effective with managing materials, choosing the least expensive alternatives, and recycling. Developing a unit-based cost-containment program was combined with quality improvement processes

Research Note

Source: Dodson, G.M., Sinclair, V.G., Miller, M., Charping, C., Johnson, B., & Black, M. (1998). Determining cost drivers for pediatric home health services. *Nursing Economic$, 16*(5), 263-271.

Purpose

Cost constraints threaten the financial viability of home health agencies. Capitated reimbursement systems have created financial risks for providers. To manage costs effectively, cost drivers need to be identified. The purpose of this article was to describe the development and implementation of an activity-based costing system for pediatric home health clients.

Discussion

Cost drivers are the causes of costs and the primary factors that influence efficient business performance. They set the costs of key processes and activities. To build a more accurate costing system, one agency chose to develop an activity-based costing system to measure the direct costs of activities and service lines accurately and to allocate indirect costs appropriately among service lines. Cost-driver analysis, activity analysis, and performance analysis were used to construct activity-based management and quality-improvement initiatives. The goals were to deploy resources more efficiently, eliminate unnecessary processes, and improve clinical outcomes by using efficient work processes. Profit enhancement was secondary to value improvements. The first step was to develop an organizational work process activity model. The functions of the agency were highlighted over the structure of the organization. Process modeling software was used to develop a model of agency activities, inputs, controls, outputs, and activity mechanisms. The four core processes identified were intake, first visit, interval visits, and discharge. An activity tracking tool was used to record time requirements. A care requirements tool also was developed to estimate the intensity of nursing resources. The tool was tested and validated. Data were then collected and analyzed for the relationship between care requirements ratings and time expended on interval visit activities. An estimate of projected costs was done.

Application to Practice

The home health care requirements tool could significantly predict resources consumption. It projected costs more sensitively when diagnostic category was factored into the equation. Thus the project resulted in information and cost trajectories for pediatric clients based on care requirements and diagnoses. Useful tools were developed to map work processes, track activities, and identify care requirements. These tools produced information on workflow processes, time requirements, and resource consumption. Internal and external benchmarking, quality improvement, and work redesign efforts were facilitated. Expanded information resource capabilities enhanced staffing and skill mix projections, data for contract negotiations, and cost data for marketing purposes.

to garner significant cost savings (Brady et al., 1998). In another example, a multi-disciplinary financial education research project was undertaken to assess effects on awareness and profit (Krugman et al., 2002).

What cost decisions do nurses control? What can nurses do to reduce costs? The following are suggestions to promote cost control:

- *Do the job efficiently.* The more efficiently the nursing care delivery is organized and run, and the greater the contribution of individuals to the care provided, the less costly that care will be.
- *Time is money.* For example, simple scheduling errors can increase the length of a client's stay. The time element is especially crucial in care coordination activities.
- *Help motivate clients to recover.* This approach improves their health status and reduces dependency costs.

Research Note

Source: Bostrom, J. (1994). Impact of physician practice on nursing care. *Nursing Economic$, 12*(5), 250-255, 286.

Purpose

The purpose of this study was to determine the amount of variation in nursing care hours within a DRG that can be attributed to either severity of illness or variation in physician practice style. Nursing time was measured and related to individual physician practice. The setting was a 600-bed tertiary care hospital. From client discharges over a 5-year period, subjects' data were extracted for 11 DRG categories. The sample was 1,964 subjects and 93 physicians. Data were collected on hours of direct nursing care, severity of illness, client age, DRG, physician code number, total required nursing care hours, and length of stay.

Discussion

The client subjects were analyzed for demographic profiles, lengths of stay, and total required nursing care hours averages. Nursing care hours varied among DRG categories. General linear modeling and analysis of variance (ANOVA) procedures were used to analyze variables related to physicians. Severity of illness accounted for 17% to 49% of the explained variance; physician practice preferences explained 6% to 38% of the variance; and both physician and severity of illness accounted for 34% to 62% of explained variance in the total hours of care.

Application to Practice

The data add weight to previous studies showing a great variation in hours of required nursing care per DRG category. Understanding the causes of the variation in nursing resources contributes to better resource management, stricter cost control for clients, and improved financial management by nurses. Client diagnosis and severity of illness account for a substantial portion of length-of-stay variance. Thus the classification of clients by diagnosis and severity may be useful in predicting resource use, planning care, and allocating costs for reimbursement. Severity of illness does not capture what is needed or overtreatment, only what was done for the client. To some extent, however, severity of illness does capture physician practice. The impact of variation in physician practice style has a direct impact on nursing practice and nursing costs. Both nurse staffing and hospital reimbursement are tied to inpatient census and client diagnosis. In this study a client's nursing care requirements were driven largely by diagnosis, severity of illness, and the individual physician's practice preferences. This raises issues of the efficient use of nursing care as a scarce and costly component of health care.

- *Use supplies carefully.* Know the costs of those supplies. For example, posting a per-unit cost list that would include the cost of an alcohol swab or a roll of tape helps to keep employees aware of the costs of the supplies they are using.

Knowing those costs will facilitate better substitution decisions (Striegel, 1986). For example, Chagares and Jackson (1987) compared price and performance of six pressure-relieving devices, and Smith and Amen (1989) compared the costs of IV drug delivery systems. Their results indicated

alternatives for potential substitution decisions. Such cost comparison projects need to be an ongoing part of practice.

For a client with poor skin integrity, perhaps the most expensive tape should be used because the tape needs to stick and be waterproof. However, in a routine situation, can a lower-cost item be substituted adequately? Nurses cannot contribute to cost reduction unless they know the per-item cost of the supplies they use and then use this information to evaluate substitutions. Large cost savings can accrue to even small (but high-volume) cost reductions. What is noticed immediately is that over time it becomes costly if a topper sponge or sterile pad is used to wipe up spills, a sterile pack is opened to use only one instrument, or preprinted forms are used as scratch pads. There is a convenience versus cost trade-off to consider. For example, bag baths may be convenient or necessary in a staffing shortage, but they also are an expensive supply cost.

Nurses need to participate in organization-wide cost containment and take credit for the cost savings generated by nursing. There needs to be a formal, documented way in which decisions made by nurses and the cost savings that result are visible and rewarded. Knowing the health care organization's charges and what treatments and procedures cost clients gives nursing information with which to advocate for clients. Nurses need nursing cost data for analysis and evaluation, and they need the informatics and information support structure to accomplish this.

There are areas of nursing practice where nurses can begin to identify inefficient or redundant activities and use decision-making abilities. Serving on product committees gives nurses an opportunity to advocate for products that save nursing time and to put pressure on vendors for adaptations to the technology that decreases nursing time. This will assist nurses to work intelligently and efficiently while still enjoying the work of nursing.

In terms of costs and cost awareness, a general finding throughout the literature in the 1980s and 1990s showed that "nursing costs," the actual cost of delivering nursing care, are about 20% to 30% of hospital costs per diagnosis-related group (DRG), depending on the geographic location (Kirby & Wiczai, 1985). In this case, nursing is a reasonably priced service that generates revenue by contributing to the delivery of client care services. Nurses need to contribute to cost control, but this must be balanced by professional decision making. In terms of professional decision making, nurses need to learn to allocate resources when it is appropriate and save money when it does not

need to be spent. This approach is part of professional decision making.

CURRENT ISSUES AND TRENDS

Although nurses will always be engaged in managing costs and handling unit budgeting, two specific aspects will continue to be trends. *First,* the use of a business plan is common for all types of program planning. *Second,* costing out nursing services is an important trend for nurses using data to manage nursing services.

Writing a Business Plan

First used in business and industry for the starting up of a new business venture, the business plan has emerged in health care as a tool for program, project, or service planning. A business plan is a detailed formal document used to assess a proposed venture's financial feasibility and to sell the business to potential backers. It needs to be a complete and honest appraisal of the project and its potential. The proposed project or service needs to fit within the mission and goals of the health care organization and be appraised for whether it will be expected to earn profit to subsidize other operations (Finkler & Kovner, 2000). Used in nursing to propose a new program or service, the formal business plan document needs to be prepared in a fashion similar to those used in business. Books, websites, and software programs can be used to help develop a business plan. The general format is this: front matter, consisting of a cover page and table of contents; and executive summary; detailed descriptions of the proposed program or service, the service (product) to be delivered, the responsible managers and developers, and stakeholders (who benefits); marketing strategies; and a financial prospectus. Attention should be paid to format, layout, and presentation.

Costing Out Nursing Services

Under a fee-for-service reimbursement system, the inequity among provider payment systems was a disadvantage to nursing. Nursing was seen as a cost but not a revenue generator. One strategy proposed to compensate for nursing's revenue disparity was to cost out nursing services. This idea became popular for a while but lost attraction as capitated reimbursement systems gained prominence. With a "per member per month" flat payment structure, conventional wisdom indicated that efforts to cost out for purposes of charging a fee for service were useless. Therefore costing out nursing services was cast aside. However, what was lost was the value of knowing precisely what it costs to deliver nursing services. Whether the purpose is to establish a fee charge or to use the data for other strategic purposes, such as efficiently deploying resources or using data in contract negotiations, accurately determining the costs of nursing service is still an important budgetary function. Nurses need to know their costs to plan better and negotiate more effectively.

Costing out nursing services is defined as the determination of the costs of the services provided by nurses. By identifying the specific costs related to the delivery of nursing care to each client, nurses have data to identify the actual amount of services received. As a result, nursing will be in a much better position to autonomously monitor, justify, and control the costs of nursing care within a cost-conscious environment (Eckhart, 1993). Scherubel (1994) offered a warning, however. If nurses use costing out nursing care services to decrease costs, nursing budget requests may be reduced through decreased resource allocation to nursing departments. Thus it is important to capture incentives in return for cost-control efforts and to ensure that needed resources are actually spent on client service needs.

In reviews of the literature related to costing out nursing services, a variety of variables were examined, such as length of stay, nursing care costs, direct care costs, and DRG reimbursements. Most common was the extrapolation of nursing costs from a specific acuity system. There is a lack of standardization of definitions and elements used to compute direct and indirect nursing care costs (Eckhart, 1993). This lack of standardization impedes comparisons across settings and sites.

The old health care system reimbursed mainly for medical services aimed at curing diseases. Despite reimbursement changes in a managed care environment, nursing costs still need to be determined. The usual model multiplies the amount of nursing time per intensity level (for a DRG) by the average nursing hourly salary and benefits and adds this to the indirect cost amount to arrive at the total nursing cost per DRG or intensity level. Nursing intensity usually is represented by a patient classification measure as a proxy. A serious flaw in this model is the inability to identify what nursing activities actually are delivered to clients. Patient classification or acuity systems tend to measure average or projected care needs, not actual needs and actual services delivered.

Another approach is to calculate nursing cost per nursing intervention or diagnosis. The amount of nursing time per nursing intervention can be multiplied by the average nursing hourly salary and benefits and added to equipment costs to determine direct costs. Direct costs plus indirect costs equal the total nursing cost. As nursing interventions replace intensity in the calculation, the actual nursing care delivered to clients is being measured more accurately. Dodson and colleagues (1998) presented yet another approach to costing by determining the cost drivers for an activity-based costing system. Cost-driver analysis, activity analysis, and performance analysis were employed to create an activity-based management system. The activities of the work processes, inputs, controls, outputs, and activity mechanisms combined to form a model of core processes, time requirements, and resource consumption useful for benchmarking and quality improvement.

Summary

- A budget is a plan designed to control the allocation of resources. It becomes a financial timetable.
- Seven types of budgets within the master budget are (1) operating, (2) long-range, (3) program, (4) capital, (5) product-line, (6) cash, and (7) special purpose budgets.

- Traditional and zero-based budgeting are typical budgetary formats.
- The budgetary process is a financial planning and control system.
- The budget process follows three phases and is displayed on multiple forms.
- The operating budget is a major focus for nurses.
- A volume measure and a cost measure form the basic measurement elements.
- Nurses are concerned with specifying nursing costs, which have been invisible because they have not been identified, standardized, and analyzed.
- Focusing on direct, indirect, and supply costs helps to begin to identify the costs of the services provided by nurses.

Study Questions

1. How does budgeting relate to leadership, control, and management in health care?
2. Do nurses raise health care costs or lower them?
3. How would a nurse manager manage a revenue budget?
4. What leadership roles and activities are important in budgeting?
5. What activities of budgeting are appropriate at the staff nurse level?
6. How can staff nurses best acquire knowledge and skills in budgeting?
7. How is budgeting like balancing a personal checkbook?

CASE STUDY

Helpful Community Hospital was in a tight squeeze. Of all revenue, payment from Medicare comprised 70% of the hospital's income. The state was ranked dead-last in the Medicare payment fee schedule. The result was a squeezed-tight and ever-shrinking hospital operating margin. Hospitals in similar circumstances had closed. However, Helpful Community Hospital was the only acute care facility serving a wide geographic rural area. The Chief Nurse Executive (CNE), Kathryn Gardner, decided to take bold action in

one specific area over which nursing had control: supply chain management.

Nurse Gardner had read about the success of a Visiting Nurse Association (VNA) in patient-specific supply management (Maurano, 2004). Intrigued, she reviewed the supply budgets for the entire hospital. Costs were very high. Next, she met with her managers to discuss the issue. The managers reported high staff dissatisfaction with the "hassle factor" and wasted time hunting down needed supplies. She asked the nurse managers to formally survey staff members. These results highlighted many opportunities for systems improvements.

Next, Nurse Gardner networked with her peers and looked for "best practice" trends in the field. This environmental scan led her to the Supply Sharpies Consulting group. She evaluated their proposal and completed the contract.

The consulting group began with a two-pronged initiative: a detailed analysis of the supply system and an educational initiative with the staff. Over the course of a year, barriers and resistance were overcome or worked through. A dramatic change in the way supplies were distributed and managed was proposed and accepted. A pre- and posttest evaluation design was implemented.

The new system was called *patient-specific supply management*. It involved purchasing and implementing an informatics technology that ordered supplies, tracked inventory, managed use, inserted management controls, and generated billing and other reports and documents. It also involved purchasing high-tech supply carts for each unit. Nurses identified needed supplies for each patient, which were then stocked in the supply cart on a daily exchange basis. Passwords were used to access the carts and remove supplies. If anything else was needed, the order was placed electronically and delivered to the unit.

The system had real-time delivery, individualized supplies, proactive monitoring of supplies, formulary compliance, and nurse convenience. Slippage and wastage, due to such random events as physicians withdrawing supplies from bulk stocks and not using them for patients on that unit, were

CRITICAL THINKING EXERCISE

It's Monday morning, and Nguyet Tran, nurse manager, faces the usual flood of phone calls, e-mails, and staff problems pressing for her attention. She also has a 2 PM appointment to discuss her annual budget with the chief nurse executive. Her capital budget will not be controversial, but Nurse Tran has been working on a proposal to open a new clinical program. She has physician buy-in for the new program, since a related idea was discussed at the physicians' annual professional association's convention. However, she is unsure whether administration will support the program with the necessary financial support.

1. Does Nurse Tran have a problem?
2. If so, what is the problem?
3. How should Nurse Tran handle the situation?
4. What should Nurse Tran do first?
5. What creative strategies might be best suited to the situation?
6. What would motivate others to assist in this situation?
7. What budgeting strategies might work?

greatly reduced. Other positive effects were a dramatic drop in inventory, greater adherence to a standardized product formulary, and decreased waste of nurses' time tracking down and picking up supplies. Significant cost savings to the supply budgets translated into greater operating margin available for new program development. Nurse Gardner was considering using the freed-up resources for a disease management program using nurses to improve patient self-care management.

REFERENCES

Bailey, D. (1996). Budgeting skills. *Nursing Standard, 10*(19), 43-48.

Brady, D.J., Cornett, E., & DeLetter, M. (1998). Cost reduction: What a staff nurse can do. *Nursing Economic$, 16*(5), 273-274, 276.

Chagares, R., & Jackson, B. (1987). Sitting easy: How six pressure-relieving devices stack up. *American Journal of Nursing, 87*(2), 191-193.

Dodson, G.M., Sinclair, V.G., Miller, M., Charping, C., Johnson, B., & Black, M. (1998). Determining cost drivers for pediatric home health services. *Nursing Economic$, 16*(5), 263-271.

Eckhart, J. (1993). Costing out nursing services: Examining the research. *Nursing Economic$, 11*(2), 91-98.

Ervin, N.E., Chang, W., & White, J. (1998). A cost analysis of a nursing center's services. *Nursing Economic$ 16*(6), 307-312.

Finkler, S.A., & Ward, D.M. (1999). *Essentials of cost accounting for health care organizations* (2nd ed.). Gaithersburg, MD: Aspen.

Finkler, S.A., & Kovner, C.T. (2000). *Financial management for nurse managers and executives* (2nd ed.). Philadelphia: Saunders.

Huber, D., Schumacher, L., & Delaney, C. (1997). Nursing management minimum data set (NMMDS). *Journal of Nursing Administration, 27*(4), 42-48.

Johnson, M., & Carpenter, C. (1990). Financial management for nursing executives. In E. Simendinger, T. Moore, & M. Kramer (Eds.), *The successful nurse executive: A guide for every nurse manager* (pp. 91-106). Ann Arbor, MI: Health Administration Press.

Jones, K. (1994). Direct and indirect costs. *Seminars for Nurse Managers, 2*(1), 4-5.

Kenny, M.P.F. (1996). Ask the experts. *Critical Care Nurse, 16*(4), 103.

Kirby, K., & Wiczai, L. (1985). Budgeting for variable staffing. *Nursing Economic$, 3*(3), 160-166.

Krugman, M., MacLauchlan, M., Riippi, L., & Grubbs, J. (2002). A multidisciplinary financial education research project. *Nursing Economic$, 20*(6), 273-278.

Maurano, L. (2004). The results are in: The financial impact of changing supply processes. *Remington Report, 12*(3), 38, 40, 42, 44.

Scherubel, J. (1994). Costing out nursing services: Is it happening? In J. McCloskey & H. Grace (Eds.), *Current issues in nursing* (4th ed.). (pp. 483-489). St Louis: Mosby.

Smith, C., & Amen, R. (1989). Comparing the costs of IV drug delivery systems. *American Journal of Nursing, 89*(4), 500-501.

Starck, P.L., & Bailes, B. (1996). The budget process in schools of nursing: A primer for the novice administrator. *Journal of Professional Nursing, 12*(2), 69-75.

Striegel, E. (1986). Cost-effective use of supplies in the NICU. *Neonatal Network, 4*(6), 46-48.

37

Productivity and Costing Out Nursing

Mary Ellen Murray

CHAPTER OBJECTIVES

- Describe the trends and projections for National Health Expenditures from 1998 to the year 2012
- Analyze productivity in nursing using the production process model
- Use a cost-analysis strategy to determine the cost of a good or service produced by nurses
- Analyze the leadership and management implications of the production process
- Differentiate among cost analysis, cost-effectiveness analysis, and cost-benefit analysis as methods of economic evaluation
- Analyze the challenges of managing a multigenerational workforce
- Exercise critical thinking to conceptualize and analyze possible solutions to a practice exercise

The worldwide nursing workforce shortage, coupled with escalating health care costs, has made it imperative that nurses be concerned with issues of productivity in all settings of clinical practice. Nursing is the largest health profession and the single most costly line item in hospital budgets, the hospital being the most expensive setting of the health care system. Because nursing costs account for a major part of the labor costs in health care organizations, improving nursing productivity is a reasonable strategy for cost savings. However, given the nature of the work of nursing, it is essential to maintain the quality of care and provide for patient safety while simultaneously considering issues of production.

DEFINITIONS

Productivity is a measurement of the output produced using a quantity of inputs. The **production process** is a representation of the relationship between outputs and the inputs used to produce them. The process is characterized by the following five related concepts (Feldstein, 1999):

1. *Marginal productivity:* additional output gained by adding additional input
2. *Economies of scale:* increasing the inputs to the production process resulting in a volume increase such that the average cost per unit is decreased
3. *Short-run distinctions:* time period in which there can be limited change to the inputs to the production process
4. *Long-run distinctions:* the time period in which all of the inputs to the production process can be varied
5. *Substitution:* a strategy of replacing a higher cost input with a lower cost input in the production process

⚠ LEADING & MANAGING **DEFINED**

Productivity

Output produced using a quantity of inputs.

Production Process

Relationships of outputs to inputs.

Costing Out Nursing Services

Methods to determine the actual costs of nursing services.

Economic Evaluation

Evaluating both inputs and outputs and costs and consequences.

Charges

Dollar amount billed to a customer.

Price

Dollar value of each input to the production process.

Total Cost

Dollar value of the production process.

Costing out nursing services refers to methods of determining the actual costs of nursing, in any setting where patients receive care.

Economic evaluation is defined by Drummond and colleagues (1997) as dealing with both the inputs and outputs to the production process or the costs and consequences of activities. This type of evaluation is concerned with the choices people make about the use of scarce resources, in this case, health care resources. Methods of economic evaluation include the following four basic techniques (Table 37.1):

1. *Cost analysis:* determining how much it costs to produce a good or service
2. *Cost-benefit analysis:* measuring the worth of a program in dollars
3. *Cost-effectiveness analysis:* comparing the costs of two (or more) methods of achieving the same outcome
4. *Cost-utility analysis:* considering the preferences of an individual for alternative types of treatment

In all economic analyses, it is important to differentiate between **charges**, which is the dollar amount billed to a customer for a good or service before discounts are taken, and **price**, which is the dollar value of each of the inputs to the production process. **Total cost** is used here as the total dollar value of the production process. In order for any

business to remain viable over time, charges must exceed costs.

BACKGROUND

National Health Expenditures (NHE) are a measure of spending for health care in the United States by type of service delivered (Heffler et al., 2003). In 1998, NHE exceeded 1.0 trillion dollars for the first time. By 2012, NHE are projected to increase to 3.1 trillion dollars. Considered from another perspective, this amount of money, in 1998, represented 13.1% of the gross domestic product (GDP), the value of all the goods and services produced in the United States in 1 year. By 2012, NHE are projected to represent 17.7% of the GDP. Although it is necessary to recognize the uncertainty of these projections, by analyzing the component parts of NHE, an understanding of the reasons for such increases is gained. Experts predict that out-of-pocket expenditures (OOP)—the amount of health care costs not covered by insurance—will grow more rapidly than other sectors because of efforts of employers and insurers to share costs with employees and patients. Hospital spending growth, largely driven by rising labor costs, is expected to remain the most important driver of health spending growth. Hospital spending accounted for 27.1% of the projected increase

Table 37.1

Types of Economic Evaluation	
Type of Study	Answers the Question
Cost analysis	What does it cost?
	Example: What is the cost of having a nurse practitioner conduct preoperative physical examinations prior to elective surgery?
Cost-benefit analysis	Is the program worthwhile, as measured in dollars?
	Example: Intervention A costs $300, has a benefit of $600, and can help 1000 people. Thus the benefit-cost (BC) ratio is 2:1. And the net benefit is $600,000 − $300,000 = Benefit of $300,000
	Intervention B costs $4,000, has a benefit of $12,000, and helps only 10 people. The BC ratio is 3:1. The net benefit is $120,000 − $40,000 = Net benefit of $80,000
	Therefore A is preferred from the perspective of society.
Cost-effectiveness analysis	What is the cost of Method A versus Method B of achieving the same outcome?
	Example: What is the cost of renal dialysis versus renal transplant for 10 years of life gained.
Cost minimization	What is the least costly alternative of two programs?
	Example: Surgery for a modified mastectomy may be performed in an ambulatory surgical center or in the hospital requiring a 1-night stay. Both programs accomplish the same outcome, but which one is accomplished at least cost?
Cost-utility analysis	What are the preferences the individual has for the outcomes of a treatment?
	Example: An individual whose treatment for an illness will require ventilator support may have a different preference for treatment than a person who could be assured confinement to a wheelchair without progressive deterioration.

in health spending in 2002, while prescription drug spending and physician spending accounted for 16.3% and 16.5%, respectively (Heffler et al., 2003).

The magnitude of these projected expenditure increases emphasizes the need for nurses, as members of the largest health care profession, to understand the implications of these data for clinical practice. As early as 1992, Davis (1992) indicated that, as nurses, "we are responsible for assuring that each dollar spent is spent wisely and that supplies and equipment are not wasted. Economic necessity dictates that even if we were

to achieve a consensus about universal access to health care, we would need to couple this with economical nursing practice" (p. 17). Similarly, Hunt (2001) stated that clinical competency is not the only tool that nurses need in an era when economics dominates the health care arena. Nurses also need to have complex business skills.

Understanding the concept of productivity and relating it to the management of professional nursing is a leadership skill that will serve nursing in an era of accelerating health care expenditures. Based on this understanding, the nurse manager will be able to determine the costs associated with providing nursing care.

PRODUCTION PROCESS

The concept of a production process was first used in industrial applications (Murray et al., 2003). For example, in the automotive industry, managers discuss the production process for manufacturing cars. The production process is a relationship between outputs and the inputs used to produce a given quantity of the output. The output of a production process in the automotive industry may be the production of 10,000 cars per month for a certain plant. The inputs would be all the supplies such as steel, rubber, person hours, or technology required to produce those cars. In this example the output is a durable good. However, the output could also be a service, as it is more often in health care. Although the model may seem mechanistic and devoid of the caring that characterizes clinical nursing practice, cost awareness and associated cost-control practices are realities that are integral to the survival of the nursing profession. If nurses understand these concepts, they can participate in the decision making process about the use of health care resources.

Transferring the concept of the production process to health care helps nurses to understand the inputs required to produce the services associated with patient care. In the health care setting, the output of a production process could be as varied as a patient education program, a critical pathway, a specified number of units of family perinatal care, or a wound treatment procedure. Inputs in a health care setting could include laboratory tests, diagnostic procedures, registered nurse time, and medical equipment.

The generic representation of a production process is summarized in the following equation:

$$O_Q = f (I_1, I_2, I_3, Z...)$$

In this equation, the output quantity (O_Q) is a specified amount of a good or service being produced. The output is a function (f) of all the inputs (I) used, beginning with the inception of the process and ending at the completion of the specified output. The inputs $I_1, I_2, I_3, Z...$ represent all the inputs to the production process.

The following example transfers this model to health care:

$$Q_{SNPC} = f \text{ (time of registered nurses, time of licensed practical nurses, time of nursing assistants, computer hardware, equipment, } Z...)$$

In this example, the output (Q) is a quantity of surgical nursing patient care ($SNPC$). The inputs to the production of the care include the time of professional nurses and various assistive personnel, the technology and equipment required, and so forth ($Z...$). Z represents all other inputs to the production process.

There are multiple possible inputs to the production process, which might include things not usually considered, such as pharmacy time, nutritional services, and physical therapy. One approach to identifying the list of inputs to the production process is the use of the line items in the monthly budget reports that are routinely generated as part of the fiscal management process. These reports typically include wage and salary costs, fringe benefits, postage, mileage costs, telephone charges, and supplies that may be helpful in the identification of inputs. Specification of the inputs to the production process is a tedious but essential step that makes it possible to conduct cost analysis.

COST-ANALYSIS STRATEGY

After the inputs have been identified, it is now possible to conduct a cost analysis, the most basic form of economic evaluation that is fundamental to all other forms of economic evaluation. Cost analysis answers the question, "What did it cost to do a certain nursing intervention, to staff a patient care unit, or to produce nursing care for a certain population of patients?" Cost analysis consists of three steps: (1) the identification of the inputs (discussed above), (2) determination of total costs of the production process, and (3) determination of the average cost of each unit of output.

Total Cost of Production Process

To determine the total cost of the production process, it is necessary to know both the price of each input and the amount of each input used. It also is necessary to define what is meant by "price" and "total cost." Price is defined as the dollar value of an input to the production process. "Total cost" is defined as the total dollar value of the production process. The total cost of the production process is equal to the price of the inputs multiplied by the quantity of the inputs used. This is represented by the following equation:

$$TC_{O_Q} = (PI_1 \times QI_1) + (PI_2 \times QI_2) + (PI_3 \times QI_3) + (PZ... \times QZ...)$$

In this equation, the total cost (TC) of the production process is represented by TC_{O_Q}, or the total cost of the output quantity. Next, the cost of the first input (I_1) is calculated by multiplying the price of the input (PI_1) times the quantity of the input (QI_1). For example, if input I_1 is the time spent by the RN to care for a patient having a radical mastectomy, and if 8 hours of time are used, the price of the input is 8 multiplied by the hourly salary of the nurse, which might be $26, for a total of $208.

When using the price of time as an input into the production process, it is necessary to include a proportion of the fringe benefits earned by that staff member. If this is omitted, the total cost calculation will be seriously understated. To add the input of fringe benefits to the cost of the production process, it is necessary to include a proportion of the costs of the benefits of the employee. Typically, an employer determines that fringe benefits are a percentage of salary. It may be, for example, that fringe benefits are 35% of an employee's salary. Thus in this calculation, the cost of the fringe benefits is an additional $72. The prices of all the inputs are added in this manner in order to determine the total cost of the production process.

Average Cost Per Case

In the final step, the average cost per case is determined from the following equation:

$$ACC = \frac{TC}{OQ}$$

where ACC represents the average cost per case, and TC represents the total cost (derived above) divided by the output quantity (OQ). This last step is important because cost per unit of output may well determine the viability of the program or innovation. For example, if a health care system wishes to implement a day treatment program for adults with mental illness and a cost analysis reveals the operational costs to be $500 per day per patient, but reimbursement is only $250 per patient, it is unlikely that the program will be viable.

LEADERSHIP AND MANAGEMENT IMPLICATIONS

Once the production process is defined and the cost analysis is complete, it is possible to use this information to analyze the following five characteristics of the production process:
1. Economic efficiency
2. Substitutability of inputs
3. Marginal productivity
4. Long-run and short-run distinctions
5. Economies of scale

These characteristics are important analysis tools for nurse leaders and managers to use in their clinical practice because they provide economic data to inform decision making.

Economic Efficiency

In the health care environment, the nurse manager is responsible for economic efficiency—that is, producing patient care at the lowest possible cost or, stated differently, minimizing the costs of production. It is essential that, concurrent with cost minimization strategies, nurses maintain high levels of quality of patient care. In fact, poorly

◭ LEADERSHIP & MANAGEMENT **BEHAVIORS**

Leadership Behaviors

- Plans strategy for productive use of resources
- Envisions a productive group output
- Enables followers to be productive
- Influences followers to increase productivity
- Enables release of followers' potential
- Creates a productive environment
- Communicates values that enhance productivity

- Calculates costs and productivity indices
- Monitors cost factors
- Controls resource expenditure
- Communicates the need for productivity
- Evaluates productivity patterns
- Influences subordinates to be productive
- Justifies departmental budget

Management Behaviors

- Plans resource allocation to improve productivity
- Organizes the environment to enhance productivity

Overlap Areas

- Plans for productivity
- Influences others toward productivity

produced patient care is often *more* costly, since it results in adverse outcomes. Therefore although it may be possible to decrease the amount of registered nurse time in producing the output of patient care, this action may not produce the desired outcomes.

A comparison of several production processes that use different inputs may answer the question "What is the least cost method for producing a good or service?" Within each production process, the combinations of inputs and their corresponding costs may be analyzed to determine economic efficiency. The nurse leader selects inputs into the production process with a consideration of the price associated with each input. For example, certified nurse midwives and obstetricians both produce maternity care for low-risk women, but research has shown that midwives produce the care using a lower cost combination of inputs (Oakley et al., 1996).

Substitution

The effect of substitution in the production process is another consideration. Substitution occurs when scarcity drives up the price of one good, or input (Input A). The result is that the quantity used of a second input (Input B) increases, because it is substituted for the more costly input. For example, as the price of registered nurses (Input A) has

increased in the past decade, some hospitals have increased their employment of licensed practical nurses (Input B). This is the substitution of a less costly input (time of LPNs) for a more costly input (time of RNs).

Substitution can be safely done when evidence shows that outcomes remain the same (Murray & Henriques, 2003). However, the manager must consider multiple factors before adopting such a practice. Is there an impact on patient outcomes from this substitution? What are state licensure laws that govern the scope of practice of LPNs? Similar considerations apply when one considers the use of unlicensed assistive personnel such as nursing assistants.

Marginal Productivity

Within the production process, marginal productivity is defined as the additional output achieved by increasing one input, while keeping all other inputs constant. The manager might ask "What would be the effect of adding an additional registered nurse on each of three shifts?" Would such an addition increase the output of the patient care unit? It depends. It may be that the additional nurse will produce an increase in the number of hours available to care for patients who are increasingly acutely ill. In this case, there would be no increase in the output, which is the number of patients cared for,

Research Note

Source: Murray, M.E., & Henriques, J.B. (2003). An exploratory cost analysis of hospital-based concurrent review. *American Journal of Managed Care, 19*(7), 512-518.

Purpose

Most hospitals employ registered nurses to conduct concurrent utilization review (UR), a cost-containment strategy used by the managed care industry. The UR process requires that hospital providers communicate clinical information about patients to payers who make a determination if the planned care is certified for payment. The purpose of the study was to determine the cost to the hospital of conducting the UR process.

This study used time sampling and cost analysis methods to determine the cost to the hospital of the production process for UR, to determine whether differences existed among hospital clinical services, and to see whether differences existed among the types of personnel performing the function.

Discussion

The authors reported that over 12 months, 13,126 reviews were completed at an average time of 15 minutes 41 seconds. Across services, the average total time of each review ranged from a minimum of 11 minutes 18 seconds (medical) to a maximum of 19 minutes 4 seconds (pediatrics). Cost analysis revealed that the cost of the production process for 1 year was nearly $165,000. Four types of personnel completed the reviews at different costs per review: RN, $7.24; MS-prepared clinical social worker, $7.71; MS-prepared nurse, $9.25; and assistive personnel, $4.78. There was no difference in outcomes of reviews associated with the educational preparation of persons doing the review.

Application to Practice

This study illustrates the use of cost analysis in one examination of productivity. The authors demonstrated that, in this institution, four categories of staff completed the reviews with similar results, though at a different cost. This raises the question of the necessity of having registered nurses involved in the process. Given that the United States is experiencing a critical nursing shortage, is this a function that requires the expertise of registered nurses, or could it be delegated to other personnel without a decrease in quality? A second issue is that the cost of having an advanced practice nurse case manager conduct the review is nearly twice the cost of a review completed by an assistive staff person. The question of potential substitution of personnel in the production process might be considered.

---

but the quality of patient care may be improved significantly. In another example in an ambulatory care setting, the manager considers adding additional staff, but the number of examination rooms cannot be increased. It may be that productivity, as measured by patient visits, would not be increased by the addition of staff. In this situation, the manager may consider changing another input to the production process, specifically, additional exam rooms.

Long-Run and Short-Run Distinctions

A nurse manager also needs to consider the time context of the production process. It is not possible at all points in time to simultaneously vary all of the inputs to the production process. The "short-run" is usually defined as that period in which it is possible to vary only some of the inputs; in the "long-run" all inputs may be varied. For example, in the very short term, which might be considered the next 8-hour shift, it may not be possible to hire additional registered nurses or to increase the number of patient rooms on a given unit. But in the long term, both of these options are possible. The manager needs to be aware that when one input is fixed in the short-run, increasing another input may lead to decreased productivity or diminishing returns. This is the case when a hospital may make a decision to increase the number of patient beds in a facility but is then unable to hire the staff to care for the additional patients. This results in a diminished return on the input of additional beds.

Economies of Scale

When there is an increase in all of the inputs to the production process, and the output volume increases by a larger percentage, economies of scale are said to exist. The result is that the average cost per unit of output declines. The basic question becomes, is it less expensive per case to produce a good or service in quantity? For example, when DVD players were first produced, they were quite expensive. With an increase in production, the cost per unit, or cost per DVD, decreased substantially. The same concept applies to the production of nursing care. Many hospitals have chosen to employ diabetes nurse educators and develop extensive programs of care and teaching for patients with diabetes. Nurse managers found that is less costly per patient to increase all of the inputs to the production process for diabetic care (i.e., nurse's time, physician's time, teaching tools, facilities, etc.) and produce this care for a larger number of patients, than to produce the same care for a very small number of patients. This is an example of economies of scale. When considering such a venture, managers may be asked to determine the volume of patients they would have to serve in order to "break-even." The break-even level is the point at which the expense of the program equals the revenue to be generated. In the early implementation of such a project, a break-even level may be acceptable but, at some point, most programs will need to show revenues greater than costs (profit) in order to remain viable.

In general, too little effort has been devoted to determination of the actual costs of nursing and the provision of nursing care. With actual data, nurses will be in a better future position to demonstrate their economic value to health care, and nurse managers will have appropriate information with which to accurately manage nursing services.

Alternative Measures of Productivity

There are various measures of productivity, but all involve relationships between volume of inputs and cost. Nurses' time is the critical input in the production of nursing care. Home health agencies measure their productivity in patient home visits and hours of care; hospitals measure patients days; clinics measure the number of patient visits. The cost measure is the cost of the nursing time required to produce this care. Box 37.1 provides additional methods of calculating productivity.

The oldest method of measuring nursing productivity is the analysis of hours per patient day (HPPD). The input is the nursing hours worked. The number of hospitalized patient days is the output. This index is imprecise because of the wide variation in client acuity, with the result that the measure of patient days is not equivalent across cases.

A variety of data sources and productivity indices can also be considered. In nursing, productivity has been tightly linked to staffing numbers. For example, staffing, calculated as the total number of hours of a given staff for a given

Box 37.1

Measures of Productivity

Productivity (P) = Cost per unit of output

$$P = \frac{Input}{Output}$$

$$P = \frac{Cost}{Unit\ of\ output}$$

$$P = \frac{\$}{Work\ hours}$$

$$P = \frac{Nursing\ hours\ worked}{Number\ of\ hospital\ patient\ days}$$

$$P = \frac{Number\ of\ nursing\ staff}{Census\ or\ patient\ days}$$

time period, can be compared with client volume or census. Using this method, if the output (patient days) increased while staffing remained the same, the productivity, strictly speaking, would be increased. This typically happens in hospitals when the influenza season is severe and a large number of geriatric patients are admitted to the hospital. In this short-term staffing crisis, the same numbers of staff are available to care for the high census, and productivity temporarily increases. However, the gains may be short-lived, in that the short-staffing situation may result in nurse burnout and resignations.

No one measure of productivity adequately measures the knowledge-based work of nursing. Productivity measurement is complex because of the following reasons (Edwardson, 1989):

- Measuring nursing care outcomes is difficult and controversial.
- The relationships among care processes and nursing outcomes are not well understood.
- The most efficient combination of resources for performing care processes is not known.

One solution has been to emphasize outcomes measurement. Research on outcomes measurement is accelerating and provides empirical data to support staffing decision making. Nurse researchers (Cho et al., 2003) demonstrated a relationship between staffing and adverse patient outcomes. They found that an increase in 1 hour worked by registered nurses per patient day was associated with an 8.9% decrease in the odds of patients acquiring pneumonia. These researchers also found that the occurrence of all adverse events (pneumonia, pressure ulcers, wound infections) was associated with a prolonged length of hospital stay, increased mortality, and increased hospital costs. This is an example of outcomes research that will aid managers' decision making in the future.

COSTING OUT NURSING SERVICES

Fundamentally, nurses need to have their own data on actual and specific costs of nursing care. Capturing these data has been difficult. In the era of DRGs and fee-for-service reimbursement in the 1980s, costing out nursing services was seen as a strategy to capture reimbursement for nursing. However, under managed care and capitated reimbursement systems, service costing may need to be done by alternative methods. Activity-based costing is one approach to service costing that is quite different from traditional methods and may be useful in settings such as home health care. It can measure quality improvement efforts in relation to activity costs. The key advantage of activity-based costing is that it reflects what it cost to provide services and identifies why costs were incurred.

There are two steps to the activity-based cost assignment process. *First* is the identification of activities that consume resources, such as provision of client services; the *second* step is to assign activities to cost categories such as service lines or programs. Costs tend to follow a four-level cost hierarchy of unit, batch, business, and enterprise levels. Underlying principles are that activities consume resources and that activities will be different based on payer, product line, program, and positioning in the cost hierarchy. Resource cost is then assigned to activities directly or with resource drivers. Assignment of resource cost to activities is based on actual time spent by activity. Activities with similar attributes can be aggregated. For example, all client care costs related to admission visits in home care would identify the total cost of admission visits. Dividing this figure by the number of clients admitted would result in the average cost of an admission visit, which can be used to benchmark outcomes and performance (McKeon, 1996).

Nursing has been unable to adequately address costs and efficiency insofar as data on the actual costs of nursing services were unavailable to nurses. Yet nurses have become interested in costing out nursing services for the purposes of productivity analysis and for purposes of being acknowledged as a revenue generating component of the institution. Ideas about costing out nursing services arose in the mid-1980s, coinciding with the implementation of DRGs. The importance of determining costs is compelling. The purposes of costing out nursing services are to facilitate health policy and for reimbursement decisions. Costing out nursing services provides data for productivity comparisons. Acuity, or patient classification, is the most frequently used tool for collecting nursing's cost data. A variety of acuity tools are used.

The Medicare Cost Report (MCR) has been suggested as an information resource for costing out nursing services in hospitals. Hospitals being reimbursed by Medicare submit annual data on cost-to-charge ratios. To determine nursing costs, the nursing product needs to be defined in terms of output, process, or a combination. A patient classification system can be used to establish a productivity or relative value unit. Client care hours can be charged on a daily basis, a database developed, and daily charges entered as an outcome measure. Hospital bills can be unbundled and both a cost and price for nursing services set. Services are costed out as direct and indirect expenses, as extracted from the MCR. The costs of nursing care for clients of all acuity types can be calculated from this model (Swansburg & Sowell, 1992).

Two models for costing out nursing services have been identified (McCloskey, 1989). The first model reflects the general trend of the literature: the amount of nursing time per intensity level as related to a specific DRG is multiplied by the nurse's average hourly salary/benefits and added to an indirect cost amount to determine the total nursing cost per DRG. Since the first model has some limitations and lacks an ability to define what nursing activities are provided for the cost, it only yields nursing cost per DRG or intensity level. A second model was developed to yield nursing cost per nursing intervention or nursing diagnosis. In the second model, medical diagnosis and nursing diagnosis both initiate nursing interventions. To measure the costs of nursing interventions, direct costs (nursing time multiplied by average salary, plus equipment) and indirect costs are added to derive total nursing costs. In general, too little effort has been devoted to isolating actual nursing costs. With actual data, nurses are in a better position to demonstrate value and negotiate capitated contracts.

CURRENT ISSUES AND TRENDS

Three major issues related to productivity are the focus of nurse leaders today: (1) a national nursing shortage, (2) integration of economics into the practice of clinical nursing, and (3) a multigenerational nursing workforce.

National Nursing Shortage

Studies by the U.S. Department of Health and Human Services (National Center for Health Workforce Analysis, 2002) predicted a national nursing shortage of 800,000 nurses by the year 2020. A shortage is created when the demand for nurses exceeds the supply. A state-by-state analysis of the nursing shortage places the impact in a personal context. In 2020, for example, California will experience a nursing shortage in excess of 120,000 nurses. Florida will have a shortage of 61,000, and New York almost 45,000. Hospitals will continue to be the major employer of RNs (62%), but there will be an increased need for RNs in nursing homes and home health care. Simultaneous with an increased demand is an increasing rate of nurses leaving the workforce, largely as a result of an aging RN workforce.

These dire statistics point out the need to maximize the productivity of professional nurses. However, this productivity cannot be accomplished by decreasing staffing levels to a level that places patients in jeopardy. The research of Aiken and colleagues (2002) demonstrated that in hospitals with high nurse-patient ratios, surgical patients experienced higher risk-adjusted mortality and higher failure-to-rescue rates. Dr. Aiken also reported that nurses in these hospitals are more likely to experience burnout and job dissatisfaction.

It is possible that increased use of technology will be a partial solution to increasing nursing productivity. Computerized documentation and medication administration systems are widespread applications of technology that have resulted in time savings and subsequent increased productivity for nurses. Information technology is another enhancement to nurses' productivity. Medical records are easily accessed from multiple sites, results of diagnostics tests are communicated instantly, and monitoring devices detect deviations from normal limits and communicate these to the nurse as they occur.

Another responsibility of nurse leaders related to productivity is ensuring a future workforce by participating in the recruitment of future nurses. A telephone survey of 800 youth in grades 7 to 11 and adults ages 19 to 49 revealed disturbing results (Erickson et al., 2004). Only 5% of the students in the sample group stated they would choose nursing; only 29% of the adults (deemed potential career switchers) think nurses are becoming more appreciated and respected in the workplace. Both groups believed that nursing does not offer the economic benefits that they desire. Fewer than 20% of both groups believed that nurses earn $15,000 per year, when in reality nurses earn that much or more. These results indicated that nurse leaders, and all nurses, have a heightened responsibility to present the profession in a favorable and honest way. In a recent conference, a speaker reported that as a colleague leaves her home for work each day, she tells her young children, "Mom is going to go to the hospital to save lives today." Although nursing does not *always* offer that level of drama, it certainly speaks of the importance of the work that nurses do. That importance needs to be communicated to the pool of persons who are potential nurses.

Integration of Economics into Clinical Practice

The incorporation of economic evaluation into clinical practice is important to productivity because health care resources are limited and choices must, and will, be made. In the years preceding managed care, health care providers acted as if health care resources were infinite, with the result that health care costs spun out of control. Today, providers are faced with difficult decisions about "who gets what." Although rationing health

care is inherently unacceptable to most of the population of the United States, it is true that rationing is occurring. Today, rationing is done on the basis of the ability to pay for health care, with the uninsured receiving lesser amounts of health care. Well-educated nurses who understand economics and finance are in a unique position to bring the values of nursing to decision making about the allocation of health care resources.

Cost analysis is the foundation for all economic evaluation. Within the nursing literature, nurse leaders increasingly advocate for "cost-effective nursing practice" without defining what is meant by that term. The term "cost-benefit" is also loosely used without precise definition. It is necessary to make these distinctions in order to utilize appropriately the work of nurse researchers conducting these studies and to be able to conduct similar studies. (See Table 37.1 for definitions and examples of these terms.) On a cautionary note, it is important to remember that these analyses are not intended to be used as the sole tools for decision making. Economic analyses are one factor among many to be considered in decision making about health care programs and policies.

Recognizing the impact of the predicted national health expenditures, the National Institute for Nursing Research, in the summer of 2004, partnered with the Agency for Healthcare Quality and Research and the Institute for Johns Hopkins Nursing to sponsor a workshop on the integration of cost-effectiveness analysis (CEA) into research. The conference brochure pointed out that in a time of constraints on health care resources, CEA studies are tools that help determine which intervention provides the highest health care benefit per dollar. This conference is recognition of the importance of economic evaluation by leaders in nursing. It may be that the study of health care economics will be required coursework in the future curricula of all baccalaureate nursing programs.

Multigenerational Nursing Workforce

For the first time, four generations of nurses are employed at once in the workforce: the Traditional, or Mature, Generation—those born between 1922 and 1943; the Baby Boomers born between 1943 and 1960; Generation Xers born between 1960 and 1980; and the Nexters, born between 1980 and 2000. Gerke (2001) described the impact of a multigenerational workforce in the selection of benefit plans. Boomers wanted generous pension plans whereas Xers wanted salary increases that would enable savings for future educational needs of children. Staff members around the age of 20 (Nexters) wanted similar things but also valued more paid time off. The two younger generations wanted balance between leisure and work. Balancing pay, benefits, and related economic incentives for diverse age cohorts is a major economic challenge, especially in a cost-containment milieu. Nurse managers may need to construct a menu of economic and work-life reward options. Gerke (2001) described new management and motivational skills that will be needed to manage these diverse employees. For example, the Traditional Generation may not desire full-time employment but should be valued for their experience. Generation Xers need to hear in preemployment interviews that the organization wants them to have a life outside of work. Nexters seek connections between their job and their personal goals. Each of these generations contributes to the productivity of nursing, and each is needed in the workforce despite the potential conflicts that might arise from their differing work ethics.

Clearly, raising the productivity of nursing while protecting the quality of patient care will continue to be a major challenge for nurse leaders. The use of the production process is one method to examine the productivity of nurses, comparing the relationship between the output (nursing care) and the inputs used to produce it. The characteristics of the production process (economic efficiency, substitution, marginal productivity, long-/short-run distinctions, and economies of scale) are tools for managers to use in considering changes to the production process. Strategies of economic analysis are presented as ways to compare and evaluate interventions and programs of care.

Summary

- Issues of productivity are important in all clinical practice settings.
- Productivity is the measure of output produced using a quantity of inputs.
- Four basic techniques of economic evaluation are cost analyses, cost-benefit analyses, cost-effectiveness analyses, and cost-utility analyses.
- Charges are different from price and costs.
- Nurses need to understand the concept of productivity.
- The production process applies to the inputs required to produce the services associated with patient care.
- Cost analyses can be performed after inputs are identified.
- Nurse managers need production-process and cost-analysis data to analyze economic decisions.
- Productivity measurement is complex.
- The incorporation of economic evaluation into clinical practice is important to productivity because of limited resources.

Study Questions

1. Why does quality of care suffer when nursing care hours are reduced?
2. Do more-experienced nurses work more productively? Why or why not?
3. Why should nurses worry about productivity?
4. What issues in productivity are most urgent? Why?
5. How do nurses determine whether their care is effective and efficient?
6. Why should nurses cost out their services?
7. How can nurses control health care costs? Nursing costs?
8. What is the ideal ratio of nurses to clients?

CASE STUDY

Nurse Manager Susan Lange, RN, MS, is responsible for an inpatient orthopedic surgical unit and the associated orthopedic surgical clinic.

The inpatient hospital unit cares for an average of 8 patients each week who have had total hip replacement surgery and 12 patients per week who have had total knee replacement surgery. Most of these patients are over 75 years of age and depend on either an elderly spouse or other family caregiver for assistance throughout the surgery and recovery. For elective surgery, patients are admitted to the hospital on the morning of surgery. They have had a preoperative physical and laboratory work within 4 days preceding the surgery.

Nurse Lange is aware of the inconsistency of the quality of the preoperative teaching that the patients receive. Some patients are well prepared, know what to expect, and have practiced ambulation techniques prior to the surgery. Other patients are confused about the plan of care and appear to have had little or no preparation. Nurse Lange has discussed this problem with the registered nurses who work in the clinic. The RNs acknowledge the problem and report that they "do the best that time allows." A second problem in the care of this patient population is the frequent need for temporary nursing home placement after the surgery. The difficulty in finding this type of posthospitalization placement often results in delays in discharge of 1 to 3 days.

Nurse Lange has conducted brainstorming sessions with her staff. They have designed a program whereby a registered nurse would function in the dual role of educator/case manager for this group of patients. The person in the new role would be responsible for designing care plans that would begin in the clinic and follow the patient throughout the surgical experience and even resume in the clinic at postsurgical follow-up. The person would also function as a patient educator. Now, Nurse Lange must "sell" the program to the chief nursing officer and gain funding for the additional position.

1. What data do Nurse Lange need to present to support the request for the new position?
2. What should be the educational requirements of a person in the new position?
3. What should be the experience requirements of the person in the new position?
4. Is any reimbursement possible to offset the costs of the new position? From what source?
5. What outcomes should be measured to demonstrate the impact of the new program?
6. How will the productivity of the person in the position be measured?
7. What other stakeholders in the care of the patient population should be consulted and have input into the program?

CRITICAL THINKING EXERCISE

Bill Ryan is a clinical nurse manager employed at a home health care agency associated with a large teaching hospital. He is frequently called on to provide home care for patients who are ventilator-dependent upon discharge from the hospital. It is a real challenge for the agency to accept these patients because they require registered nurse care for at least 16 hours per day, sometimes 24 hours per day. Nurse Ryan wants to conduct an economic analysis of keeping the patients in the hospital versus caring for them in their homes.

1. What is the economic question Nurse Ryan is asking?
2. What are the programs he is comparing?
3. What are the outcomes of interventions, and what are the units of measurement?
4. What method of economic analysis would you recommend? Why?

REFERENCES

Aiken, L.H., Clarke, S., Sloane, D., Sochalski, J., & Silber, J.H. (2002). Hospital nurse staffing and patient mortality, nurse burnout, and job dissatisfaction. *Journal of the American Medical Association, 288*(16), 1987-1993.

Cho, S., Ketefian, S., Barkauskas, V., & Smith, D. (2003). The effects of nurse staffing on adverse events, morbidity, mortality, and medical costs. *Nursing Research, 52*(2), 71-79.

Davis, C.K. (1992). Who will pay? The economic realities of health care reform. *Scholarly Inquiry for Nursing Practice, 6*(3), 217-219.

Drummond, M.F., O'Brien, B., Stoddart, G.L., & Torrance, G.W. (1997). *Methods of Economic evaluation of health care programmes* (2nd ed.). New York: Oxford University Press.

Edwardson, S. (1989). Productivity measurement. In B. Henry, C. Arndt, M. Di Vincenti, & A. Mariner-Tomey (Eds.), *Dimensions of nursing administration: Theory, research, education, and practice* (pp. 371-385). Boston: Blackwell.

Erickson, I.J., Holm, L.J., & Chelminiak, L. (2004). Keeping the nursing shortage from becoming a nursing crisis. *Journal of Nursing Administration, 34*(2), 83-87.

Feldstein, P.J. (1999). *Health care economics* (5th ed.). New York: Delmar Publishers.

Gerke, M.L. (2001). Understanding and leading in the quad matrix: Four generations in the workplace: The Traditional Generation, Boomers, Gen-X, Nexters. *Seminars for Nurse Managers, 9*(3), 173-181.

Heffler, S., Smith, S., Keehan, S., Clemens, M.K., Won, G., & Zezza, M. (2003, February 7). Health spending projections for 2002-2012 [Online exclusive]. *Health Affairs: The Policy Journal of the Health Sphere.* Retrieved January 3, 2005, from *www.content.healthaffairs.org /cgi/content/full/hlthaff.w3.54v1/DC1?maxtoshow=&HITS =10&hits=10&RESULTFORMAT=&author1=Heffler& andorexactfulltext=and&searchid=1104818054582_4075 &stored_search=&FIRSTINDEX=0&resourcetype=1& journalcode=healthaff*

Hunt, P.S. (2001). Speaking the language of finance. *AORN Journal, 73*(4), 774-787.

McCloskey, J. (1989). Implications of costing out nursing services for reimbursement. *Nursing Management, 20*(1), 44-49.

McKeon, T. (1996). Performance measurement: Integrating quality management and activity-based cost management. *Journal of Nursing Administration, 26*(4), 45-51.

Murray, M.E., Brennan, P.F., & Moore, S.M. (2003). A model for economic analysis. *Nursing Economic$, 21*(6), 280-87.

Murray, M.E., & Henriques, J.B. (2003). An exploratory cost analysis of hospital-based concurrent review. *American Journal of Managed Care, 19*(7), 512-518.

National Center for Health Workforce Analysis. (2002). *Projected supply, demand, and shortage of registered nurses: 2000-2020.* Rockville, MD: U.S. Department of Health and Human Services. Retrieved June 1, 2004, from *www.bhpr.hrsa.gov/healthworkforce/reports/rnproject/ default.htm*

Oakley, D., Murray, M.E., Murtland, T., Hayashi, R., Anderson, H.F., Mayes, F., et al. (1996). Comparisons of outcomes of maternity care by obstetricians and certified nurse midwives. *Obstetrics & Gynecology, 88*(5), 823-829.

Swansburg, R.C., & Sowell, R.L. (1992). A model for costing and pricing nursing service. *Nursing Management, 23*(2), 33-36.

OUTCOMES MANAGEMENT

VII

38

Change and Innovation

Diane L. Huber

CHAPTER OBJECTIVES

- Stimulate thinking about change
- Define and describe change and planned change
- Analyze major areas of rapid change in health care and nursing
- Illustrate the process of planned change
- Distinguish among Lewin's steps in the process of planned change
- Explain a force field analysis
- Associate Rogers's five phases to the adoption of change
- Compare Lippitt's and Havelock's elements of the process of change
- Analyze emotional responses to change
- Define and discuss resistance to change
- Analyze effective change
- Synthesize the concepts of change and innovation
- Exercise critical thinking to conceptualize and analyze possible solutions to a practice exercise

C hange is a pervasive element of society, of today's health care environment, and of life. Many words are used to describe change, including constant, inevitable, pervasive, universal, and powerful.

It is change, continuing change, inevitable change, that is the dominant factor in society today.

Isaac Asimov

In a progressive country change is constant; ... change ... is inevitable.

Benjamin Disraeli

Change is inevitable, but growth is intentional.

Glenda Cloud

Change is the law of life. And those who look only to the past or the present are certain to miss the future.

John F. Kennedy

Some of the following common sayings reflect the pervasiveness of change:
- "Nothing is sure but death and taxes."
- "The more things change, the more they stay the same."
- "Let's go back to the good old days."

On reflection, growth and development can be seen as a process of change: life is a sequential pattern of inevitable change and growing from one stage to another. Professional growth and development also are highlighted by periods of growth and change. Change is a part of nursing today and, if planned, can be used as a leadership and management strategy to accomplish goals.

In this information age, where the economy is fueled by technology and data, the nature of work also has changed. Nurses are now knowledge workers and human capital in a service industry. There are two perspectives on change—positive and negative. Even when it is a positive force, change can contribute to stress, anxiety, and confusion. The negative side is most prominent when people and systems are affected. Both jobs and workplaces feel an impact from dramatic changes. Thus progressive organizations need to be attuned to both the dynamics of change and the needs of employees for a climate of support and assistance as they work through the human aspects of change (Jeska & Rounds, 1996).

DEFINITIONS

Change is defined as an alteration to make something different. This activity of alteration can be either haphazard or planned, obvious or subtle, radical or incremental, left to chance or occurring by drift. *Planned change* is defined as a process of intentional intervention to create something new. In general, it is a process by which new ideas or programs are created and developed, diffused through communication and intervention, and result in consequences of adoption or rejection. Planned change is a leadership strategy that requires planning and action, problem solving, decision making, and interpersonal competence.

From an organizational perspective, planned change is a decision to make a deliberate effort to improve the system. Lippitt and colleagues (1958) added another factor—obtaining the help of an outside agent in making a deliberate effort to improve the system—to the definition of change.

A **change agent** is the outside helper used to plan and implement the change process. The term has come to mean a person who functions as a change facilitator. Rogers (2003) defined a change agent as someone who influences innovation decisions in a direction deemed desirable.

BACKGROUND

Lippitt and colleagues (1958) identified four types of systems that become the focus for change: (1) individuals, (2) face-to-face groups, (3) organizations, and (4) communities. Change can be viewed through the perspective of change in an individual or change in a group. Hersey and colleagues (2001) viewed change from four levels: (1) knowledge, (2) attitudes, (3) individual behavior, and (4) group or organizational behavior or performance as these levels related to participative or directive change cycles (Figure 38.1). These levels of change can be graphed from high to low according to the difficulty and the time involved in making a change. The lowest difficulty and shortest time to make a change occurs with knowledge changes. Attitudes are more difficult to change because of being emotionally charged. Individual behavior is the next most difficult and time-intensive change. Group behavior and performance changes are the most difficult and take the longest time. Participative change uses personal power and is used when new knowledge is made available to a group. Directive change uses position power and when change is imposed.

Nurses use teaching as an intervention to change knowledge as a part of working with clients and managing other people. Changing individual behaviors takes more time and is more difficult.

⚠ LEADING & MANAGING **DEFINED**

Change	Change Agent
An alteration to make something different.	Someone who influences the change process or innovation decisions.

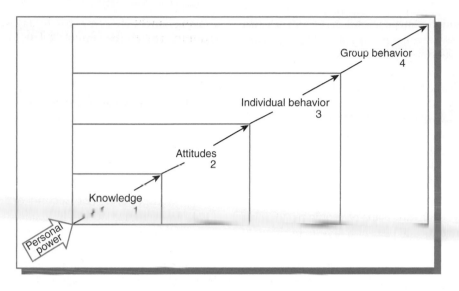

Figure 38.1
Participative change cycle. (From Hersey, P., Blanchard, K.H., & Johnson, D.E. [2001]. *Management of organizational behavior: Leading human resources* [8th ed.]. [p. 391]. Upper Saddle River, NJ: Prentice Hall. Reprinted with permission from the Center for Leadership Studies.)

For example, in working with clients with diabetes, teaching them health principles is easier and takes less time than does effecting a change in their behaviors (e.g., in selecting foods based on size, quantity, and balance of nutrients). It is even more difficult to change group behaviors among staff. This may be partially a function of dealing with two entities simultaneously because the group does not change unless individuals change first. For example, if a group is having communication difficulties and conflict, a change in knowledge can be attempted by an explanation of the destructive behavior. Sensitivity training could be used to change attitudes. The group may understand perfectly, but getting them to actually change their behavior takes more time and is more difficult. Changing individual and group behavior is not impossible, but it involves time and a large investment of effort, persuasion, and surveillance.

Change Strategies

Change occurs on a continuum from haphazard drift at one end to a structured, planned change at the other. Change can occur by drift as things

and people unilaterally change in an uncontrolled way. At the other end of the continuum, change can be deliberate and planned, as occurs when an organization identifies a plan to adopt and implement any new program. This is a conscious decision that is implemented through a planned change process. In the middle are ad hoc or active approaches to change based on strategies of education, emotional arousal, or coercion. These three strategies of organizational change are as follows (Bennis et al., 1976):

1. *Rational-empirical strategy:* Under this strategy the reward and referent power bases are used to motivate change. In other words, the premise is that people will support a change when it is their own self-interest and they can see that the change will result in personal benefit or gain for them. To the contrary, people will resist a change where they will be inconvenienced or will lose something of value. The underlying premise is that people are rational creatures who follow their self-interest.

2. *Normative-reeducative strategy:* Under this strategy the expertise power base is used to motivate change. In other words, the support or

opposition from people will arise from whether they see the consequences of the change having positive or negative impact on important societal norms and values. The underlying premise is that people are committed to maintaining values and norms in society.

3. *Power-coercive strategy:* Under this strategy the legitimate and coercive power bases are used to motivate change. In other words, people will support change that is planned and promoted by powerful figures in powerful positions. The underlying premise is that people are loyal and cooperative with plans of people perceived to be powerful and perceived to be in positions of authority.

An updated view of change strategies was proposed by Tiffany and Lutjens (1998). Change strategies fall into seven categories: educational, facilitative, technostructural, data-based, communication-related, persuasive, and coercive. Education helps adopters to see problems and develop skills. Facilitative strategies provide resources to ease implementation. Technostructural strategies alter the interaction among technology, structure, and physical space. Data-based strategies use the collection and use of data to make social change. Communication strategies spread information through channels in a social system. Persuasive strategies are used to produce change by means of urging, reasoning, and inducement. Coercive strategies control rewards and punishments to threaten and produce change. Coercion may be useful when there is little time and the change must occur rapidly (Tiffany & Lutjens, 1998). Strategies need to be chosen carefully to match the change process and to enhance effectiveness. Strategies need to be congruent and not cancel each other out. Change in an organization may require generating a push for change from the bottom of the organization followed by persuasion of the key leaders at the top of the organization of the need for change.

Models of Organizational Change

There is a rich and extensive literature on organizational change. Lewin's (1947, 1951) unfreezing, moving, and refreezing three stages of change theory is the classic model. Related research and theory development have been done on topics such as strategic planning, adaptive learning, decision theory, management, diffusion of innovations, social-psychological response and adaptation, process improvements, how members manage and achieve change, and weighted factor importance of project selection models (Gustafson et al., 2003).

Hersey and colleagues (2001) discussed two frameworks within which change occurs: (1) first-order change and (2) second-order change. First-order change occurs in a stable system. For an organization, this is adaptation and incremental change based on monitoring the environment and making purposeful adjustments. At the industry level, this is evolution as a response to external forces such as markets. An example in nursing is when a new evidence-based protocol is developed and put into use in clinical practice. This is adaptation and adjustment. Second-order change is discontinuous and radical and occurs when fundamental properties or states of systems are changed. At the organization level, second-order change is described as metamorphosis. The entire organization is transformed, reconfigured, or moved along its life cycle. At the industry level, second-order change occurs when an entire industry is revolutionized or experiences quantum change such as emergence, transformation, or decline. An example in health care is the widespread implementation of computerized physician order entry (CPOE) technology in response to the Institute of Medicine's recommendations for patient safety reforms.

Models for organizational change have proposed a variety of factors to consider in assessing the probability of successful change implementation. Some of these factors are characteristics of organizational management, system users, collaboration between users, the project itself, the project team, the team's approach, the project solution, the organization's readiness to change, level of dissatisfaction with the status quo, a desired future state, first steps needed, and perceived costs of changing (Gustafson et al., 2003).

Research Note

Source: Krejci, J.W. (1999). Changing roles in nursing: Perceptions of nurse administrators. *Journal of Nursing Administration,* *29*(3), 21-29.

Purpose

Both nursing roles and administrative responsibilities have changed over the past 10 years. The purpose of this study was to describe current responsibilities of nurse administrators and to determine their perceptions about role changes in their organizations.

Discussion

Cost-reduction measures in the 1990s resulted in substantive changes in nursing roles and expected competencies. The American Organization of Nurse Executives (AONE) outlined these changes in their evolving role position statements. New competencies were organized under the four categories of clinical processes, leadership, continuous improvement, and critical thinking. The Institute of Medicine identified four changes affecting nurses' roles in the near future: interdisciplinary teamwork, greater intensity of management of care, changing care delivery models, and expanded roles for advanced practice nurses (APNs). To identify the changes occurring in practice, a descriptive survey using a convenience sample of 303 nurse executives was done. The Nursing Role Changes instrument was used to collect data. Participants were asked to identify present roles and those anticipated to increase or decrease. The unlicensed assistive personnel (UAP) role was most frequently projected to increase. The case manager and nurse practitioner roles also were projected to increase. Participants were asked to indicate recommendations for graduate education. The MSN-MBA degree was preferred for nurse administrators.

Application to Practice

Data that identify and track trends are useful for human resource projections and other aspects of workforce planning. The results of this study indicated that administrator roles for nurses are not disappearing, despite a prevalent perception. Nurses are filling systemwide roles, some of which would not necessarily require a nursing background. Case manager and care coordination roles have become established and are projected to increase, despite nursing curricula that prepare direct care providers of episodic illness. There are strong indications of the need for higher education. With the prospect of new roles for nurses, nursing needs to address a dialogue about how to protect a core of traditional staff nurses as direct care providers. Continued research is needed to track changes and monitor and evaluate ongoing nursing role changes for their impact on health care and nursing.

Research by Gustafson and colleagues (2003) resulted in a short survey instrument and a companion statistical model to predict the potential for successful implementation of a health system change. It was shown to be effective in predicting the outcome of actual improvement projects. Called the *Organizational Change Manager* (OCM), it used 18 factors to predict organizational change status in health care (Box 38.1). The factors were displayed on a survey instrument. Each factor is rated for high, medium, or low performance based on definitions of success as rated by the opinions of experts who completed the survey. A Bayesian statistical model was used to predict the probability of success prior to implementation. This model could help in decision making about whether a change is worth it, strengthening critical aspects before implementation, and in evaluating and tracking a change process.

PLANNED CHANGE

The amount of change and the rapidity of change disrupt and disorganize people. Because of the

---

Box 38.1

Factors that Predict Organizational Change Success

1. Mandate/project launch
2. Leader goals, involvement, and support
3. Supporters and opponents
4. Middle manager goals, involvement, and support
5. Tension for change
6. Staff needs assessment, involvement, and support
7. Exploration of problem and understanding customer needs
8. Change agent prestige and commitment
9. Source of ideas
10. Funding
11. Relative advantages
12. Radicalness of design
13. Flexibility of design
14. Evidence of effectiveness
15. Complexity of implementation plan
16. Work environment
17. Staff change required
18. Monitoring feedback

---

rapidity of change in areas such as computer software, it is easy to slip into the perception that history is what occurred 2 years ago and ancient history refers to 5 years ago. Obsolescence occurs before people have had a chance to adapt to the last round of changes. The inevitable result is stress on individuals as they try to cope. These dynamics affect nurses in their roles as care providers and care managers and profoundly influence the profession of nursing through employment and compensation fluctuations. One method to enhance nurses' productivity and decrease stress from turbulence in the environment is to strategically use planned change.

The use of planned change is a nursing management intervention strategy. The nurse uses diagnosis and intervention in clinical practice: the nurse assesses, diagnoses, develops a plan for the client's care needs, and selects an intervention that is matched to that assessment and diagnosis. Managers also assess, diagnose, and plan interventions to meet organizational needs and goals. They look at resource allocation and deployment of people in using planned change as a management intervention. Planned change theories are engineering theories in that they use social science principles to plan change (Tiffany & Lutjens, 1998). Planning and managing the change process may focus on any or all of the following situational elements: organizational structure, people, or resources.

"Two basic kinds of change theories exist—theories that help people watch change and theories that help people cause change" (Tiffany & Lutjens, 1998, p. 15). Planned change refers to deliberately engineered change in groups. A planned change theory is a set of logically interrelated concepts that explain how change occurs, predict forces and effects, and help planners control variables in a change process (Tiffany & Lutjens, 1998). In their review and analysis of the change theory literature, Tiffany and Lutjens (1998) identified three theories popular in nursing and one nonnursing model. The three main theories used in nursing are Lewin's (1947, 1951) planned change theory, writings by Bennis and colleagues (1961, 1976), and Rogers's (2003) theory of diffusion of innovations. One model not used in nursing is Bhola's (1994) configurations, linkages, environment, and resources (CLER) systems model. Lewin's (1947, 1951) theory ranks as the most popular change theory among nurses (Tiffany & Lutjens, 1998).

THE PLANNED CHANGE PROCESS

Lewin's Force Field Analysis

The basic concepts of the change process were outlined by Lewin (1947, 1951). A successful change involves three elements: (1) unfreezing, (2) moving, and (3) refreezing (Figure 38.2).

Lewin's (1947, 1951) theory of change used ideas of equilibrium within systems. Unfreezing, the first stage of change, can be characterized as a process of "thawing out" the system and creating the motivation or readiness for change. An awareness of the need for change occurs. This first stage is cognitive exposure to the change idea, diagnosis of the problem, and work to generate alternative solutions. A change agent needs trust, respect, and rapport to unfreeze individuals and groups effectively. Use of education, motivation, and enthusiasm are leadership strategies. Awareness of the need for change is generated from the following:

- Unmet expectations (lack of confirmation)
- Discomfort about action or inaction (guilt or anxiety)
- Removal of an obstacle to change (psychological safety)

The unfreezing stage is considered to be finalized when those involved in the change process understand and generally accept the necessity of change.

The second change stage is moving. This means proceeding to a new level of behavior, which implies that the actual visible change occurs in this stage. When the individuals involved collect enough information to clarify and identify the problem, the change itself can be planned and initiated. Lewin (1951) observed that a process of "cognitive redefinition," or looking at the problem from a new perspective, occurs. As a first step to launch a change, a pilot test may be done so that the change can be pretested and a transition period launched.

The final change stage is refreezing. In this stage, new changes are integrated and stabilized. Reinforcement of behavior is crucial as individuals integrate the change into their own value systems. It is important to reward change behavior. Leadership strategies of positive feedback, encouragement, and constructive criticism reinforce new behavior. Leaders point the way throughout the process of change.

Lewin's (1947, 1951) planned change process stages can be compared to the nursing process and the generic problem-solving process (Table 38.1). Unfreezing is like assessing in the nursing process and problem identification and definition in the problem-solving process. Moving is similar to planning and implementing in the nursing process and problem analysis and seeking alternative solutions in the problem-solving process. Refreezing is like evaluation in the nursing process and implementation and evaluation in the problem-solving process.

Individuals and systems naturally strive for equilibrium. Lewin (1951) saw this as a balance between driving forces that promote change and restraining forces that inhibit change. Both driving and restraining forces impinge on any situation. The relative strengths of these forces can be analyzed. To create change, the equilibrium is broken by altering the relative strengths of driving and restraining forces. A force field analysis facilitates the identification and analysis of driving and restraining forces in any situation. Unfreezing occurs when disequilibrium is introduced into the system to disrupt the status quo. Moving is the change to a new status quo. Refreezing occurs when the change becomes the new status quo, and new behaviors are frozen.

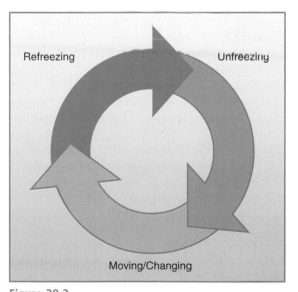

Figure 38.2
Elements of a successful change. (Data from Lewin [1947, 1951]).

Table 38.1

Similarities of Change, Nursing Process, and Problem Solving		
Change	Nursing Process	Problem Solving
Unfreezing	Assessing	Problem identification
Moving	Planning and implementing	Problem analysis and seeking alternatives
Refreezing	Evaluation	Implementation and evaluation

Data from Workman, R., & Kenney, M. (1988). The change experience. In S. Pinkerton, & P. Schroeder (Eds.), *Commitment to excellence: Developing a professional nursing staff* (pp. 17-25). Rockville, MD: Aspen.

The process of change may flow back and forth among stages. It is not a simple linear process in which one step follows the preceding one. The process may move rapidly, or it may stall in any one phase. The goal of planned change is to plan, control, and evaluate the change.

Lewin's (1947, 1951) work forms the classic foundation for change theory. Other change theorists have elaborated further understandings and applications of change theory. Bennis and colleagues (1961) assembled a book of readings on planned change that emphasized planner-adopter cooperation and high levels of adopter participation.

Because actually implementing planned change is more dynamic and complex than Lewin's model, Lippitt (1973) refined and expanded Lewin's (1947, 1951) work on unfreezing, moving, and refreezing to identify the following seven phases of the change process that more fully describe planned change:

1. Diagnosis of the problem
2. Assessment of motivation and capacity to change
3. Assessment of the change agent's motivation and resources
4. Selecting progressive change objectives
5. Choosing an appropriate role for the change agent
6. Maintaining the change once it is started
7. Termination of the helping relationship with the change agent

The first three steps can be compared to Lewin's unfreezing (1947, 1951). Steps 4 and 5 match moving, and steps 6 and 7 are comparable to refreezing. Similar to Lippitt (1973), Havelock (1973) listed the following six elements in the process of planned change:

1. Building a relationship
2. Diagnosing the problem
3. Acquiring relevant resources
4. Choosing the solution
5. Gaining acceptance
6. Stabilization and self-renewal

The first three steps correspond to the unfreezing stage of change, the fourth and fifth are similar to the moving stage, and the last relates to refreezing. The various conceptualizations of the stages of the process of change bear similarity to one another but vary in emphasis (Table 38.2).

Change agents can follow a number of steps in the process of change, as follows:

- Articulating a clear need for the change
- Getting the group participating by leaving details to those people who have to implement the change
- Getting reliable information and the details to those who are to implement the change
- Motivating through rewards and benefits to help the change along
- Not promising anything that cannot be delivered

For example, when implementing a planned change to a new care delivery system, the change agent would need to be clear about the need for and the benefits of the change. This might include greater autonomy for nurses. The details

Table 38.2

Comparisons of the Process of Change Theories			
Lewin	Rogers	Lippitt	Havelock
Unfreezing	Awareness, interest, evaluation	Steps 1, 2, 3	Steps 1, 2, 3
Moving	Trial	Steps 4, 5	Steps 4,5
Refreezing	Adoption	Steps 6, 7	Step 6

of implementation should be left to the group, but only after reliable and detailed information is communicated to them. Rewards and benefits, not threats about performance appraisal, should be the basis of the motivation to change.

Participation itself may be motivating. Promised benefits from the change should be limited to what the change agent can reasonably deliver.

Emotional Responses to Change

Within nursing, Perlman and Takacs (1990) focused on how individuals cope with change and work through the changes that affect them. Although individuals must devote personal resources and energy to accomplish change, organizations tend to overlook the human emotions associated with an organizational change. Using the death and dying literature as a foundation, Perlman and Takacs (1990) described 10 stages in the emotional realm of the process of change (Box 38.2).

Another view of the emotional stages of change was suggested by Manion (1995), who identified the following seven stages people go though during personal transitions:

1. *Lose focus:* Confusion and disorientation abound.
2. *Minimize the impact:* Deny or pretend the change is not significant.
3. *The pit:* Feelings of anger, discouragement, resentment, and resistance arise.
4. *Let go of the past:* Energy returns as the end of the change process is seen.
5. *Test the limits:* More optimism is gained, and the individual tries out new skills or seeks new experiences.

6. *Search for meaning:* The individual reflects on the change process and recognizes what was learned.
7. *Integration:* The transition is completed, and the change is integrated into daily life.

Both Perlman and Takacs' (1990) and Manion's (1995) stages resemble the general grief model. However, Manion's model is more customized to change. Stages 5 through 7 mirror the process of coping that occurs as attitudes reconfigure and individuals work to produce positive outcomes.

Box 38.2

Emotional Stages of Change

1. *Equilibrium:* There is a sense of balance and inner peace before change occurs.
2. *Denial:* Energy is drained by denial of the reality of a change.
3. *Anger:* Energy is used to ward off the change.
4. *Bargaining:* Energy is used in an attempt to eliminate the change.
5. *Chaos:* Energy is diffused, with a loss of identity and direction.
6. *Depression:* No energy is left to produce results.
7. *Resignation:* Energy is expended to accept change passively.
8. *Openness:* Renewed energy is available.
9. *Readiness:* There is willingness to use energy to explore new events.
10. *Reemergence:* Energy is rechanneled, producing empowerment.

Individuals proceed through the emotional stages at various rates. Somewhere between stage 7 (resignation) and stage 8 (openness) the individual begins to heal and cope with the change. Any organizational change process involves continual letting go of the status quo and emotional grief reactions. Change is more successful as the intellectual and emotional issues involved in the change phases are recognized and addressed.

Although most people inherently distrust change, change can be viewed either positively or negatively. Viewing change as an ending entails an understanding of the concept of loss. To help individuals adapt, support needs to be provided along with encouragement that they can control their own response to change. Those who view change as a beginning are more optimistic. The four positive responses to change are uninformed optimism, informed pessimism, hopeful realism, and informed optimism. Communication, open discussion, sharing information, and respect for values and input are helpful strategies (Bonalumi & Fisher, 1999).

The emotional response to change is a psychological process related to an individual's attitude toward change and is one factor over which the individual has control. In times of chaos and stress from change, the ability to manage one's own attitude is a key skill for success.

If you don't like something, change it. If you can't change it, change your attitude. Don't complain.

Maya Angelou

Some people change when they see the light, others when they feel the heat.

Caroline Schoeder

Everyone thinks of changing the world, but no one thinks of changing himself.

Leo Tolstoy

The release of atom power has changed everything except our way of thinking …

Albert Einstein

Spencer Johnson's (1998) book *Who Moved My Cheese?* used the parable of four mice (Snif, Scurry, Hem, and Haw) who look for cheese to eat. Cheese is a metaphor for anything people desire or think will make them happy. When change occurs, individuals suffer trauma if what they want is taken away. There are both simple and complex ways to respond to change. The book helps readers to think about ways of looking at and responding to change and understanding that attitudes and behaviors are choices that can be altered when necessary. So doing reduces stress.

Resistance

Resistance to change should be expected as integral to the whole process of change. Resistance occurs because people are afraid of being disorganized or of having their routines interrupted. Some may have a vested interest in the status quo. Change may diminish the status of some people, or their network of interpersonal relationships may be disrupted.

Almost all changes encounter some resistance as a natural phenomenon. Resistance may be rooted in anxiety or fear. For example, some individuals fear expenditure of the energy needed to cope with change. Some fear a loss of status, power, control, money, or employment. Misconceptions and inaccurate information about what the change might mean and individuals' emotional reactions create resistance to change. Not all resistance is bad. It may be a warning to the change agent to reevaluate the change, clarify the purpose, or increase communication. The change agent needs to anticipate resistance, determine why it is occurring, and decipher what the person who is resisting is trying to protect.

Asprec (1975) identified the following four ways in which resistance to change may be manifested (Figure 38.3):

1. Active resistance through frustration and aggression
2. Organized passive resistance or resisting change collectively
3. Indifference by ignoring or attempting to divert attention elsewhere

4. Acceptance on the surface or by not openly opposing a change

When initiating a planned change, it is advisable to test the waters to see whether individuals or groups are mobilizing organized resistance. There can be a variety of ways in which the resistance surfaces. For example, attendance may drop at meetings. Individuals may withhold information. Individuals or groups may attempt to block the change by refusing to participate or by trying to block, slow down, or stop its implementation. Assessing the quality and character of resistance is helpful in making decisions about how to proceed through the process of planned change by identifying interventions and strategies to use. A key principle in the use of change strategies is to design them to be effective.

Effective Change

Ineffective responses to change do not allow the change process to go forward. They include being defensive, giving advice, and prematurely persuading. The way to deal with emotionality is to allow people to express themselves while avoiding action based on the emotionality. Trying to immediately persuade people cuts off their ability to vent emotions. Without venting, they may not be able to work through the stages. Censuring, controlling, or punishing probably drives resistance underground. The more that a planned change is driven by authoritarian actions, the more that the seeds of future discontent are sown. The most effective managers possess self-confidence, knowledge of the change process, and the interpersonal skill to help participants to accept, allow, and see the process of change as natural, thereby enhancing coping while facilitating planned change.

Change cycles can be either participative or directive. In a participative change, new knowledge is made available to participants to trigger change. Personal power is used to trigger knowledge,

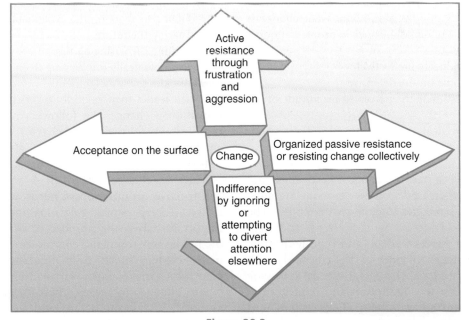

Figure 38.3
Four manifestations of resistance to change. (Data from Asprec [1975].)

attitude, individual behavior, and group behavior change. Directive change occurs when a change is imposed by some external force. Position power is used to trigger group behavior, individual behavior, attitudes, and knowledge change (Hersey et al., 2001).

The probability of effectiveness of the change process can be increased through several techniques, as follows:

- Explain the rationale for a change so that individuals understand it.
- Allow emotions to be worked out.
- Give participants all the information they need.
- Help individuals to cope with change.

The following actions should be avoided when implementing a change within an organization:

- Simply announce a change without bothering to lay a foundation
- Ignore or offend powerful people in the organization
- Violate the authority and communication lines in the existing organization
- Rely only on formal authority in implementing a change
- Overestimate your formal authority
- Make a poor decision about what change is needed and do not be open to people critiquing the decision
- Communicate ineffectively
- Put people on the defensive
- Underestimate the perceived magnitude of the change
- Do not deal with the people's fears about insecurity or change of status

Concerns, insecurities, and resistance are predictable as a part of change. Effectiveness and success are increased as these reactions are anticipated and strategies to cope are developed. The leader's role is to recognize, accept, and help followers to process, adapt, and cope with these emotional stages in order to deal effectively with change. The leader's behaviors are crucial to helping followers with the disruption and reintegration that occur during any change. Thus leaders need

to focus on people, considering factors such as the following:

- The time and effort it takes to adjust
- The possibility of less desirable outcomes
- Fear of the unknown
- Tolerance for change capacity
- Trust levels
- Needs for security
- Leadership skills
- Vested interests
- Opposing group values
- How coalitions form
- Strongly held views
- Existing relationship-dynamics disruptions

Davidhizar (1996) suggested that there are nine common mistakes people make in coping with organizational change. Knowing these areas helps nurses to proactively plan to avoid them and thereby work to ensure effective change processes. These nine mistakes are as follows:

1. Assuming management should keep them comfortable
2. Expecting someone else to reduce the stress
3. Shooting for a low-stress work setting
4. Trying to control the uncontrollable
5. Failing to abandon the expendable
6. Fearing the future
7. Picking the wrong battles
8. Psychologically unplugging from the job
9. Avoiding new assignments

As the leader focuses on followers to help them transition a change, the followers need to take responsibility for their own behavior. The stress of change is felt by both leaders and followers, and both are part of successful outcomes.

How is change effective? A positive and constructive group process needs to be established. Interpersonal relationships are very important. Given the number of changes going on in the environment, empowerment involves using change successfully. Successful change empowers participants. Nurses are empowered when change increases their responsibility, authority, and accountability and gives them the mechanisms to make decisions to be able to affect client care.

Change Management

To ensure that a planned change or new innovation is implemented and used, strategies and tactics are chosen to manage the change. Strategy choice needs to be conscious and deliberate. Both cautious strategy combination and prudent sequencing are essential (Tiffany & Lutjens, 1998).

A variety of strategies and tactics have been proposed. For nurses undergoing reorganization, some strategies that have been suggested as most effective are understanding the change process, encouraging resilience, and developing potential as leaders of change (Bonalumi & Fisher, 1999). O'Connell (1999) indicated the need for action steps, such as maintaining momentum, emphasizing managerial support, encouraging the question "why," emphasizing personal concerns, and exercising tolerance.

Noting that today's most urgent performance challenges demand that a manager learn how to manage people through a period of change, Smith (1996) developed the following 10 change management principles:

1. Keep performance results the primary objective of behavior and skill change.
2. Continually increase the number of individuals taking responsibility for their own change.
3. Ensure that each person always knows why his or her performance and change matters to the purpose and results of the whole organization.
4. Put people in a position to learn by doing, and provide them with the information and support needed in time to perform.
5. Embrace improvisation as the best path to both performance and change.
6. Use team performance to drive change whenever demanded.
7. Concentrate organization designs on the work people do, not the decision-making authority they have.

8. Create and focus energy and meaningful language because they are the scarcest resources during periods of change.
9. Stimulate and sustain behavior-driven change by harmonizing initiatives throughout the organization.
10. Practice leadership based on the courage to live the change you wish to bring about (p. 14).

Smith's (1996) assertion was that by relentlessly focusing on performance and people and by using the 10 management principles, change processes will be successful.

Another useful strategy for preplanning the management of change is to assess readiness for organizational change. One inventory to use is the Organizational Change-Readiness Scale (OCRS) (Jones & Bearley, 1996). The 76-item inventory was designed to analyze the ability of an organization to manage change effectively. The five dimensions of structure, technology, climate, system, and people are assessed for barriers and supportive conditions. The five dimensions tend to influence each other. A Lewin-type force field analysis is applied to the results.

Innovation

An *innovation* is defined as something new: the introduction of a new process or new way of doing something. Kanter (1983) said that innovation refers to the process of bringing any new or problem-solving idea into use. Drucker (1985) defined innovation from an economic perspective as a change in the yield of resources or as "changing the value and satisfaction obtained from resources by the consumer" (p. 23). According to Drucker (1985), change provides the opportunity for new and different things and processes. A purposeful and organized search for change is the basis for systematic innovation. A careful analysis of the opportunities for change is the best hope for successful economic or social innovation. This occurs because successful innovations exploit change. Thus Drucker (1992) came to describe innovation as the systematic use of opportunity from changes in the economy, technology, and demographics. He noted that the challenge today is to make institutions capable of innovation. This can be approached from the viewpoint of innovation as systematic and hard work having little to do with genius and inspiration. Innovation, Drucker (1992) noted, depends on "organized abandonment" (p. 340). This is a process of eliminating the obsolete and the no longer productive efforts of the past. Clearly, there needs to be a willingness to view change as an opportunity.

Drucker (1985, 1992) identified seven sources for innovation opportunities: the unexpected, incongruity, process needs, changes in industry or market structure, demographics, new knowledge, and changes in perceptions or moods. He likened the seven sources to windows on a building in that just as windows let in light and air, innovation can be infused into an organization by these various sources. In an information-based organization where innovation needs to be systematized, the leader or manager will find four skills important: (1) get outside the organization for facts and perspective, (2) take responsibility for one's own information needs, (3) focus for effectiveness, and (4) build learning into the system.

Change and innovation are companion terms. In nursing, theories of planned change and nursing research utilization are used for conceptualization and research on innovations. In one analysis of the nursing literature, Lewin's (1947, 1951) change theory and Rogers's (2003) diffusion theory were the most frequently cited theories (Tiffany et al., 1994). However, popular change theories may be incomplete or inadequate to meet the needs of nurse change agents in practice. This is because popular theories overlook social systems problems or focus on analyzing and watching change rather than being theories of change planning (Tiffany et al., 1994).

Innovation has been differentiated from change. Change is a disruption; innovation is the use of change to provide some new product or service (Romano, 1990). Innovation also has been viewed as the use of a new idea to solve a problem (Kanter, 1983).

Rogers (2003) described a cognitive innovation-decision process through which individuals and groups pass. The five stages of innovation-decision are as follows (Rogers, 2003):

1. First knowledge of an innovation's existence and functions
2. Persuasion to form an attitude toward the innovation
3. Decision to adopt or reject
4. Implementation of the new idea
5. Confirmation to reinforce or reverse the innovation decision.

The innovation-decision process is a series of actions, behaviors, and choices over time as a new idea is evaluated and a decision is made whether or not to incorporate this in practice. The perceived newness and associated uncertainty are distinctive aspects of the innovation decision. knowledge of existence and functions.

According to Rogers (2003), most change agents concentrate on creating awareness-knowledge. However, a more important role could be played by concentrating on how-to knowledge, which adopters need to test out an innovation. Using Hersey and colleagues' (2001) four levels of change concept, the change agent would first work on awareness-knowledge but then move on to address attitudes and emotions and then work on how-to skills in order to create a change in individual behavior.

Individual members of a group or social system will adopt an innovation at a faster or slower rate. This time element of the adoption of an innovation usually follows a normal, bell-shaped curve when plotted over time on a frequency basis. However, if the cumulative number of adopters is plotted, an S-shaped curve appears (Rogers, 2003). The normal adopter frequency distribution was segmented into the following five categories (Rogers, 2003):

1. Innovators
2. Early adopters
3. Early majority
4. Late majority
5. Laggards

Change agents can anticipate these five categories as an expected phenomenon, identify followers as to likely adopter category, and target interventions accordingly. This means that for effective change, nurse leaders can recognize that there will be individual variance in "warming up" to an innovation, plan for this with targeted strategies to decrease resistance, and capitalize on the power of innovations and early adopters.

Individuals need to be interested in the innovation and committed to making change occur. The outcomes of change are either that the change is accepted or adopted or that the change is rejected. If the change is accepted, it can either be continued or eventually dropped. If the change is rejected, it can remain rejected or be adopted later in some other form. Rogers's theory (2003) described change as more complex than Lewin's (1947, 1951) three stages. The following five factors determine successful planned change (Rogers, 2003):

1. *Relative advantage:* The degree to which the change is thought to be better than the status quo
2. *Compatibility:* The degree to which the change is compatible with existing values of the individuals or group
3. *Complexity:* The degree to which a change is perceived as difficult to use and understand
4. *Trialability:* The degree to which a change can be tested out on a limited basis
5. *Observability:* The degree to which the results of a change are visible to others

The *diffusion of innovations* is a term derived from Rogers's work (2003) that is used to discuss the adoption of a new idea or process. Innovations create consequences. To move a new idea to the level of dissemination and adoption requires information, enthusiasm, and authority (Romano, 1990). Four elements to consider in an innovation diffusion are the innovation itself, communication channels, time, and the members of the social system (Romano, 1990).

McCloskey and colleagues (1994) analyzed organizational and management changes in nursing and defined management innovations as "new

strategies, structures, or processes for the organization, delivery, and financing of quality care" (p. 36). They identified five categories of nursing managerial innovations: (1) the introduction of new technology, (2) personnel development, (3) changes in the organization of work, (4) changes in rewards/incentives, and (5) implementation of quality improvement mechanisms. In times of constant change and with pressures for cost containment and quality enhancement, nurses need to be able to evaluate innovations for effectiveness and efficiency. No systematic evaluation method currently exists. Therefore innovations lack the systematic analysis element advocated by Drucker (1985, 1992) and may be adopted primarily according to managerial trends. Because of the energy and resources needed to make a change, careful evaluation is crucial to positive outcomes.

Although health care continues to be enmeshed within a changing environment, nurses can learn to cope with change. Beyond coping, nurses can creatively capture change opportunities to improve client care management and service delivery. The result is greater effectiveness and staff and client satisfaction.

LEADERSHIP AND MANAGEMENT IMPLICATIONS

Because of the complexity and extent of change, systems principles are needed by nurses who are leading and managing change. An organization that is committed to changing itself as required needs continuous learning and adaptation as a systems value. This is referred to as the *learning organization*. These innovative and creative organizations need to build structures and systems that support the commitment to change. Five principles and processes that build a systematic approach to change are as follows (Porter-O'Grady, 1994):

1. No extraneous jobs
2. As few managers as possible
3. Managerial focus on the context of work and the worker's relationship to it

◭ LEADERSHIP & MANAGEMENT **BEHAVIORS**

Leadership Behaviors

- Envisions a changed future
- Enables change to progress constructively
- Models healthy adaptation to change
- Influences followers to change and innovate
- Communicates the need for change
- Plans changes
- Evaluates the impact of change and innovation

Management Behaviors

- Plans changes
- Organizes the group and the environment to implement change

- Directs planned change
- Adapts to change
- Influences subordinates to change
- Evaluates planned changes
- Communicates the need for planned change

Overlap Areas

- Plans changes
- Influences others to change
- Evaluates changes
- Communicates the need for change

---

4. Commitment to change and learning

5. Better and more meaningful use of data

Change is implied in the definition of leadership. If leadership is defined as influencing others, then the activity of influencing is directed toward some change. The ability to envision and communicate a changed future is part of the definition of leadership. Hersey and colleagues (2001) noted that change is an inevitable fact of life, but leaders and managers can cope by developing strategies to plan, direct, and control change. The elements of effectiveness that are needed are good diagnostic skills, adapting the leadership style to the situation, and changing some or all of the situational variables.

Transformational change is a part of organizational transformation and strategic plans. To produce strategic change, transformational leaders act to ignite a vision, change structure and culture, change mindsets and power structures, and empower others (Limerick & Cunnington, 1993). Both leaders and managers can be effective in implementing organizational change. Anyone in the organization can be the focal point for making appropriate and effective change, but the employees at the bottom of the organization need to enlist the cooperation and support of the administrative hierarchy.

Because of constant change, nurses and health care systems have had to learn and adapt. To view the scope of change surrounding nursing in perspective, four areas of major change can be identified. They are organizational structures, nursing labor force, reimbursement, and information systems (Figure 38.4). First, organizational structures have been changing and reconfiguring in response to the environment and financial pressures. For example, population-based care, case management, patient-centered care, and patient safety initiatives are elements reflecting change in regard to client care systems redesign. In health care, bureaucratic systems endured for a long time but were not well suited to the work of professionals. The empowerment of staff to result in outcomes of quality is the goal. Clearly, national health care reform is an issue creating uncertainty and change throughout the health care delivery system and its organizations. Changes also are occurring in health care as integrated networks form and care increasingly is moved into community settings. Changing organizational structures are occurring in the midst of a nurse shortage. The complexion of the nurse workforce is changing; and recruitment and retention, education, and staff deployment alternatives are being explored.

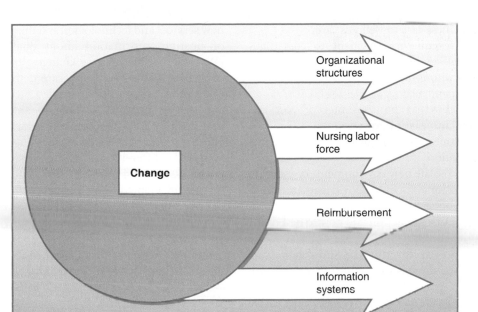

Figure 38.4
Areas of major change in health care and nursing.

Another area of important change in health care is reimbursement. For example, reimbursement (payment) for physicians has been changing, driven by the federal government's relative value units determinations. Reimbursement for nurse practitioners currently is allowed under Medicare/Medicaid. However, managed care, with its capitated reimbursement structure, has changed payment to all forms of health care providers. Payment reforms are likely to continue and change. The cost areas are physician payment, already being ratcheted down, pharmaceutical costs, and equipment and technology costs. The government will continue to review and explore the amount of dollars spent and the way those dollars are spent in an effort to reduce a huge national budget deficit fueled partly by health care costs. An increase in governmental intervention and regulatory control can be predicted in health care.

Present and future changes will bring an increasing use of information systems. A massive increase in computerization is urgent in a managed care environment. For example, there is a national practitioner's data bank that was created from quality concerns. Any physician or nurse who has been party to a lawsuit must have this information reported. Large national databases of all licensed nurses also are being compiled. Powerful computers and sophisticated software programs undergo updates and generational changes within a few years or less, creating challenges of compatibility, archival retrieval, maintaining currency, and staff training.

CURRENT ISSUES AND TRENDS

The character of the changes occurring in health care approach a paradigm shift rather than an adaptation. The following six interconnected transformations compose the major areas of change (Issel & Anderson, 1996):

1. From person-as-customer to the population-as-customer

2. From illness care to wellness care

3. From revenue management to cost management

4. From autonomy of professionals to their interdependence

5. From client as nonconsumer of cost and quality information to consumer

6. From continuity of provider to continuity of information

Nurses can create new environments or establish new organizational forms that will lead and shape the direction of health care. It is a question of which are the best courses of action and how to best direct the transformations.

Change drivers for nursing and health care include cultural diversity, the aging U.S. population, new services and technologies, and the public policy of posting information about quality of care (Wakefield, 2003). These changes have and will continue to alter the health care delivery system. They present both opportunities and challenges, and nurses need to be able to anticipate and monitor trends for their immediate and long-term effects on practice.

It is a different age for leadership (Porter-O'Grady, 2003). This means that leaders need to be able to help followers, colleagues, and others to "live and grow" in the experience of change. "Successful change is always seen in outcomes" (Porter-O'Grady, 2003, p. 173). In order to overcome the major problem of continuing to do the same things when the environment is changing,

Research Note

Source: Sims, C.E. (2003). Increasing clinical, satisfaction, and financial performance through nurse-driven process improvement. *Journal of Nursing Administration, 33*(2), 68-75.

Purpose

One 32-bed progressive care unit was faced with over-budget worked and paid nursing hours, incomplete documentation, falling patient satisfaction, and frenzied and frustrated nurses. Staff requested a decrease in the chaos so they could control their work, not be controlled by it. Employee empowerment was seen as a creative approach to the situation. Process improvement literature was reviewed. The purpose was to identify a method to produce change that would meet key performance targets and retain nursing staff. A staff team was developed to study the issues. The process improvement change selected was to standardize practice across nurses within the unit to improve workflow, efficiency, satisfaction, consistency, met expectations, and the work environment. Rapid-cycle process improvement was chosen as the methodology.

Discussion

Videos were used for education and motivation, a detailed review of work on the unit occurred, and issues/frustrations/barriers were identified. Nominal group technique was used to prioritize issues. The team tackled documentation of the admission assessment; frequency of vital signs; frequency of documentation; the physical environment, supplies and equipment, and paper supplies; communication systems; and mentoring. Changes were made quickly, but the volume and speed overran the education of the rest of the staff. This required creative approaches. Outcomes were positive at 1 month and 3 months post-change.

Application to Practice

The process improvement was deemed successful. The staff were empowered to make changes to improve their direct work processes and environment. Communication with the rest of the staff was critical, as was the leader's role converting to that of coach. Staff can accomplish needed changes if given direction in process improvement methods and support as needed.

one technique used by some nurse managers is rapid-cycle process improvement (Sims, 2003). The focus is on concrete, operational problems, usually process difficulties, that staff can tackle and change in a very short time frame, usually days. This technique facilitates quick implementation of incremental changes and makes results quickly visible in order to sustain the momentum for change.

The health care environment has been described as turbulent because of the rapid rate of change and the perceived constancy of change. However, change can be growth-producing, renewing, and invigorating for individuals and organizations. This occurs as individuals and organizations enlist creativity to derive an innovation that improves the environment or client care delivery. "Leadership *is* the leading of creativity which leads to creative change" (Kerfoot, 1998, p. 99).

An investment in creativity and innovation, with resulting change, provides strategic advantage. Creativity withers in hostile environments where all of the time is spent thinking about survival. Strategies to develop a culture that fosters creativity and change include the following (Kerfoot, 1998):

- Promoting conversations and dialogue
- Providing access to information
- Building relationships
- Teaching rethinking, questioning, and innovation
- Creating a culture of innovation
- Orchestrating and executing

In an organizational context, creativity means producing novel and useful ideas by an individual or a group. It is the basis of invention and innovation. Creativity in organizations is influenced by management practices and creativity-relevant work group skills. Creativity is one important aspect of organizational innovation (Gilmartin, 1999).

Summary

- Change is a pervasive element of society, of today's health care environment, and of life.
- Change is defined as an alteration to make something different.
- Planned change is defined as a process of intentional intervention.
- A change agent is the outside helper used to plan and implement the change process.
- Change occurs on a continuum from haphazard drift to structured planned change.
- The amount of change and the rapidity of the pace of change disrupt and disorganize humans.
- The use of planned change is a nursing management intervention strategy.
- Four systems become the focus for change: individuals, face-to-face groups, organizations, and communities.
- Lewin's theory of change uses ideas of equilibrium within systems.
- A successful change involves Lewin's three elements: unfreezing, moving, and refreezing.
  - Unfreezing is the first stage of change and can be characterized as a process of thawing out the system.
  - The second stage of change is moving to a new level of behavior.
  - The final stage of change is refreezing new changes so that they are integrated and stabilized.
- Both driving and restraining forces impinge on any situation.
- To create change, the equilibrium is broken by altering the relative strengths of driving and restraining forces.
- Rogers identified five phases to the adoption of change and five factors that determine successful planned change.
- Lippitt identified seven phases of the change process.
- Havelock's six elements to the process of planned change are building a relationship, diagnosing the problem, acquiring relevant resources, choosing a solution, gaining acceptance, and stabilization and self-renewal.
- Perlman and Takacs describe ten stages to the emotional voyage of the process of change.
- Almost all changes encounter some resistance.
- Ineffective responses to change do not allow the change process to proceed.

- Change cycles can be either participative or directive.
- Innovation is the use of change to provide some new product or service.
- Rogers' theory of innovation diffusion helps to understand how to create changes in clinical practice and organizational management.
- The ability to envision and communicate a changed future is part of the definition of leadership.

Study Questions

1. How do individuals in organizations get the information resources that they need to effect change?
2. How can informal leaders be used for successful change?
3. What changes need to take place in nursing? Why?
4. How does resistance manifest itself? What should the manager do?
5. How can nurses' perceptions be changed to result in empowerment? Why is this important?
6. How should nursing education change? Why?
7. Do we have too much change? What can be done about this?

CASE STUDY

Nurse Creighton Nau retreated to his office. It had been another "bad day." The long-term care facility he managed was in serious financial trouble. In addition, the staffing situation was in crisis, the staff morale was at rock bottom, and the quality of care was hazardous to dangerous. Things were not working, but change is task-intensive. There just was no extra time. He was at his wit's end. Sinking into his desk chair, he noticed his copy of Spencer Johnson's (1998) *Who Moved My Cheese?* book. He took it down from the shelf. Thumbing through the book, he remembered how much he felt like the character Hem, and then he realized he needed to change himself.

Fortunately, this facility was aligned with a dynamic and successful hospital. Nurse Nau made an appointment with the CNE, who had a reputation for successful turn-around of nursing services. The meeting went well. The CNE was warm and friendly. In the end, the CNE agreed to mentor Nurse Nau. First, Nurse Nau was assigned to read Bradford and colleagues' (2003) article on from survival to success. The he was to outline the relevant points and return for the next meeting.

CRITICAL THINKING EXERCISE

Nurse Lisa Witte works in a large integrated delivery system. The nurses have been dealing with successive waves of change and discontinuity in their practice. Reimbursement changes and mergers have focused attention on methods and processes for "seamless" care coordination and continuity across settings and sites of health care. The decision has now been made to implement an electronic patient record. Nurse Witte has been delegated the task of coordinating the implementation. Although the overall organization has a culture of change (many early adapters), this change would shift order entry from unit secretaries to physicians, require large-scale reengineering, and risk disrupting client care

delivery. Nurse Witte knows the potential benefits in the long run but worries about stressed-out nurses. She is trying to decide what to do first.

1. What is (are) the problem(s)?
2. Whose problem is it?
3. What should Nurse Witte do?
4. What change theory might be useful?
5. How might planned change help implement this innovation?
6. What emotional responses to change might be anticipated?

At the next meeting, Nurse Nau presented the following outline for successful change:

1. A thorough internal assessment is needed.
2. A strategic planning process focusing on governance, mission, vision, and core values is needed next.
3. A review and possible hiring of leadership and staff who are committed and passionate about the organization is needed.
4. It is important to build trust and relationships with staff, patients, and families.
5. A strong image through branding is needed.
6. The reward system needs to be brought into alignment with mission.
7. The needs of community need to be met through programs and services to influence customers.
8. Changes need to be monitored and evaluated.
9. Infrastructure and operating processes need to be efficient and effective.
10. It is critical to move quickly.

Using these 10 points as a guideline, Nurse Nau and the CNE together began to plan for organizational change and transformation. Where possible, rapid cycle process improvement would be used. Nurse Nau and the CNE negotiated an action plan and a mentorship project. Enthused, Nurse Nau got started.

REFERENCES

Asprec, E. (1975). The process of change. *Supervisor Nurse, 6,* 15-24.

Bennis, W.G., Benne, K.D., & Chin, R. (Eds.). (1961). *The planning of change: Readings in the applied behavioral sciences.* New York: Holt, Rinehart & Winston.

Bennis, W., Benne, K., Chin, R., & Corey, K. (1976). *The planning of change.* New York: Holt, Rinehart & Winston.

Bhola, H.S. (1994). The CLER model: Thinking through change. *Nursing Management, 25*(5), 59-63.

Bonalumi, N., & Fisher, K. (1999). Healthcare change: Challenge for nurse administrators. *Nursing Administration Quarterly, 23*(2), 69-73.

Bradford, R.J., Sutton, M.M., & Byrd, N.K. (2003). From survival to success: It takes more than theory. *Nursing Administration Quarterly, 27*(2), 106-119.

Davidhizar, R. (1996). Surviving organizational change. *Health Care Supervisor, 14*(4), 19-24.

Drucker, P. (1985). *Innovation and entrepreneurship: Practice and principles.* New York: Harper & Row.

Drucker, P. (1992). *Managing for the future: The 1990s and beyond.* New York: Truman Talley Books/Plume.

Gilmartin, M.J. (1999). Creativity: The fuel of innovation. *Nursing Administration Quarterly, 23*(2), 1-8.

Gustafson, D.H., Sainfort, F., Eichler, M., Adams, L., Bisognano, M., & Steudel, H. (2003). Developing and testing a model to predict outcomes of organizational change. *Health Services Research, 38*(2), 751-776.

Havelock, R. (1973). *The change agent's guide to innovation in education.* Englewood Cliffs, NJ: Educational Technology Publications.

Hersey, P., Blanchard, K.H., & Johnson, D.E. (2001). *Management of organizational behavior: Leading human resources* (8th ed.). Upper Saddle River, NJ: Prentice-Hall.

Issel, L.M., & Anderson, R.A. (1996). Take charge: Managing six transformations in healthcare delivery. *Nursing Economic$, 14*(2), 78-85.

Jeska, S., & Rounds, R. (1996). Addressing the human side of change: Career development and renewal. *Nursing Economic$, 14*(6), 339-345.

Johnson, S. (1998). *Who moved my cheese?* New York: G.P. Putnam's Sons.

Jones, J.E., & Bearley, W.L. (1996). *Organizational change-readiness scale.* Amherst, MA: HRD Press.

Kanter, R.M. (1983). *The change masters: Innovation and entrepreneurship in the American corporation.* New York: Simon & Schuster.

Kerfoot, K. (1998). Leading change is leading creativity. *Nursing Economic$, 16*(2), 98-99.

Lewin, K. (1947). Frontiers in group dynamics: Concept, method, and reality in social science; social equilibria and social change. *Human Relations, 1*(1), 5-41.

Lewin, K. (1951). *Field theory in social science: Selected theoretical papers.* New York: Harper & Row.

Limerick, D., & Cunnington, B. (1993). *Managing the new organization: A blueprint for networks and strategic alliances.* San Francisco: Jossey-Bass.

Lippitt, G. (1973). *Visualizing change: Model building and the change process.* La Jolla, CA: University Associates.

Lippitt, R., Watson, J., & Westley, B. (1958). *The dynamics of planned change: A comparative study of principles and techniques.* New York: Harcourt, Brace & World.

Manion, J. (1995). Understanding the seven stages of change. *American Journal of Nursing, 95*(4), 41-43.

McCloskey, J., Maas, M., Huber, D., Kasparek, A., Specht, J., Ramler, C., et al. (1994). Nursing management innovations: A need for systematic evaluation. *Nursing Economic$, 12*(1), 35-44.

O'Connell, C. (1999). A culture of change or a change of culture? *Nursing Administration Quarterly, 23*(2), 65-68.

Perlman, D., & Takacs, G. (1990). The 10 stages of change. *Nursing Management, 21*(4), 33-38.

Porter-O'Grady, T. (1994). A systems approach to managing transformation. *Seminars for Nurse Managers, 2*(4), 191-195.

Porter-O'Grady, T. (2003). A different age for leadership. Part 2. *Journal of Nursing Administration, 33*(3), 173-178.

Rogers, E.M. (2003). *Diffusion of innovations* (5th ed.). New York: Free Press.

Romano, C. (1990). Diffusion of technology innovation. *Advances in Nursing Science, 13*(2), 11-21.

Sims, C.E. (2003). Increasing clinical, satisfaction, and financial performance through nurse-driven process improvement. *Journal of Nursing Administration, 33*(2), 68-75.

Smith, D.K. (1996). *Taking charge of change: 10 principles for managing people and performance.* Reading, MA: Addison-Wesley.

Tiffany, C., Cheatham, A., Doornbos, D., Loudermelt, L., & Momadi, G. (1994). Planned change theory: Survey of nursing periodical literature. *Nursing Management, 25*(7), 54-59.

Tiffany, C.R., & Lutjens, L.R.J. (1998). *Planned change theories for nursing: Review, analysis, and implications.* Thousand Oaks, CA: Sage.

Wakefield, M. (2003). Change drivers for nursing and health care. *Nursing Economic$, 21*(3), 150-151.

39

Quality Improvement and Health Care Safety

Luc R. Pelletier   Lecia A. Albright

CHAPTER OBJECTIVES

- Define health care quality
- Identify two industrial models of quality
- Define PDCA
- Propose enhancements to a quality and performance improvement program based on recommendations of recent Institute of Medicine reports
- List and describe two performance measurement selection criteria
- Describe one emerging health care quality model
- Describe the costs of poor quality care
- Define mission and vision
- Propose two core value statements for an organization
- Describe two tools that a nurse can use in a quality improvement activity
- Demonstrate the use of two quality tools/techniques
- Describe the role of quality in accreditation programs
- List two examples of public data reporting systems
- Describe health care safety program components
- Define sentinel events and describe a manager's role in risk management reporting
- Define health care risk management
- Describe the risk management interface with health care safety and performance improvement
- Exercise critical thinking to conceptualize and analyze possible solutions to a practice exercise

Health care quality is an art and science that continues to evolve. Its relevance has been heightened with recent reports from the Institute of Medicine (IOM) and other national organizations related to health care. Well before these reports were published, however, professional nurses have assumed key roles in the business of measuring and monitoring health care quality. The news of health care errors is not a new phenomenon. Nurses have typically taken a leadership role in quality and performance improvement and continue to do so in their roles as executives, quality directors, risk managers, and safety officers. It would be difficult to describe the entire field of health care quality in one chapter. The authors have distilled a large amount of information and emerging trends and have targeted specific content toward nurse managers. This system overview includes industrial, health care, and emerging models of quality, the costs of poor quality, health care quality leadership and planning strategies, resources available to the nurse manager, health care safety, and health care risk management.

DEFINITIONS

Benchmarking is a tool to assist in quality of care decision making. It is defined as the continuous process of measuring what exists against the best in the search for industry best practices

⚠ LEADING & MANAGING **DEFINED**

Benchmarking

A process of measuring what exists against the best.

Best Practice

A service, function, or process that produces superior outcomes.

Continuous Quality Improvement (CQI)

A process of continuously improving a system by gathering data on performance and proposing changes.

Evidence-Based Practice

The conscientious, explicit, and judicious use of current best evidence in making decisions about health care; more recently, evidence-based practices are defined as those clinical and administrative practices that have been proven to consistently produce specific, intended results.

Indicators

Valid and reliable quantitative measures of structure, process, or outcome.

Performance Measurement System

An automated database that generates internal comparisons of organization performance over time.

Quality

Term referring to the characteristics of and the pursuit of excellence.

Quality of Health Care

The degree to which health services for individuals and populations increase the likelihood of desired health outcomes and are consistent with current professional knowledge.

Quality Improvement Program

An umbrella program that provides a continuous, ongoing measurement and evaluation process.

Risk Adjustment

A process in which differences among clients or variables such as age or disease severity are weighted or adjusted for in outcomes analyses.

Risk Management

A process designed to protect the financial assets of the organization and to maintain high-quality medical care.

Risk Management Program

An organization-wide program to identify risks, control occurrences, prevent damage, and control legal liability.

Sentinel Event

An unexpected occurrence involving death or serious physical or psychological injury.

Standards

Written value statements.

Total Quality Management (TQM)

A process to involve all employees in the improvement of the quality of every product or service.

(Katz & Green, 1997). A **best practice** is defined as a service, function, or process that has been fine-tuned, improved, and implemented to produce superior outcomes. Best practices are activities that lead to establishing benchmarks (Hamill & Luchok, 1999).

Continuous quality improvement (CQI) is a process of continuously improving a system by gathering data on performance and using multidisciplinary teams to analyze the system, collect measurements, and propose changes. The four main principles of CQI are (1) a customer focus,

(2) the identification of key processes to improve quality, (3) the use of quality tools and statistics, and (4) the involvement of all people and departments in problem solving (Bohnet et al., 1993; Miller & Flanagan, 1993).

Evidence-based practice is defined by Sackett and colleagues (1996) as "the conscientious, explicit, and judicious use of current best evidence in making decisions about the care of individual patients" (p. 71). More recently, evidence-based practices have been defined as "those clinical and administrative practices that have been proven to consistently produce specific, intended results" (Hyde et al., 2003, p. 15).

Indicators are valid and reliable quantitative measures of structure, process, or outcome that are related to one or more dimensions of performance. Indicators refer to measures of performance. Performance indicators may measure competence (ability) or productivity. Indicators related to clients are called *clinical indicators*. Indicators may be focused on service, practice, or governance. Indicators are the basic criteria specified in "report cards" (Katz & Green, 1997).

A **performance measurement system** is "... an entity consisting of an automated database that facilitates performance improvement in health care organizations through the dissemination and collection of process and/or outcome measures of performance. Measurement systems must be able to generate internal comparisons of organization performance over time, and external comparisons of performance among participating organizations at a comparable time" (Joint Commission on Accreditation of Healthcare Organizations [JCAHO], 1998, p. 1).

Quality refers to characteristics of and the pursuit of excellence. **Quality of health care** is defined as "the degree to which health services for individuals and populations increase the likelihood of desired health outcomes and are consistent with current professional knowledge" (Lohr, 1990, pp. 128-129).

A **quality improvement program** in an organization is an umbrella program that extends into many areas for the purpose of accountability to the consumer and payer. The program is a continuous, ongoing measurement and evaluation process that includes structure, process, and outcomes. The quality improvement process uses pre-established criteria and standards and then follows the evaluation of care with an appropriate change for the purpose of improvement. Thus quality improvement is a process of attaining a new level of performance that is superior to the previous level (Katz & Green, 1997).

Risk adjustment is a process in which differences among clients or variables such as age or disease severity are weighted or adjusted for in outcomes analyses or benchmarking efforts (Maas & Kerr, 1999).

Risk management is defined as "an interdisciplinary process designed to protect the financial assets of the organization and to maintain high-quality medical care" (Velianoff & Hobbs, 1998, p. 91).

A **risk management program** is defined as an organization-wide program to identify risks, control occurrences, prevent damage, and control legal liability; it is a process whereby risk to the institution are evaluated and controlled.

A **sentinel event** is an unexpected occurrence involving death or serious physical or psychological injury, or the risk thereof. Serious injury specifically includes loss of limb or function. The phrase, "or the risk thereof" includes any process variation for which a recurrence would carry a significant chance of a serious adverse outcome. Such events are called "sentinel" because they signal the need for immediate investigation and response (JCAHO, 2005).

Standards are defined as written value statements. These statements form the rules that apply to key processes and the results that can be expected when the processes are performed according to specifications. The three basic types of standards for health care quality are (1) structure, (2) process, and (3) outcome standards (Katz & Green, 1997).

Total quality management (TQM) is a way to ensure customer satisfaction by involving all employees in the improvement of the quality of every product or service. TQM has been defined as a structured system for involving an entire organization in a continuous quality improvement process targeted to meet and exceed customer expectations (Triolo, 1994).

HEALTH CARE QUALITY IN THE TWENTY-FIRST CENTURY

Professional nurses have an obligation to ensure that the care they provide is evidence-based and that work processes are consumer-centric. Providing "quality" health care is "the degree to which health services for individuals and populations increase the likelihood of desired health outcomes and are consistent with current professional knowledge" (Lohr, 1990, pp. 128-129). Nurses, as leaders and managers, have served as health care quality professionals in varied health care settings and have promoted standardization, measurement, and continuous quality improvement in a myriad of delivery settings. Professional nurses have consistently held the practice of quality management in high regard and have the effective care of clients as their primary focus.

Although industry has dutifully explored ways to enhance its business practices, health care has lagged behind and only within the past 20 years or so has embraced improvement concepts. Health care has borrowed and applied models of continuous quality improvement with principles and practices originally developed for the manufacturing industry. As industry has had its quality gurus, so too has the health care quality movement been fostered by professionals who have focused on continuous improvement.

Donald M. Berwick, MD, co-author of the book *Curing Health Care: New Strategies for Quality Improvement* (Berwick et al., 1990), was an early pioneer in identifying how the concepts of industrial total quality management (TQM) programs could apply to health care. In 1991, the National Demonstration Project on Quality Improvement in Health Care was conducted as a collaboration between members of the John A. Hartford Foundation, the Harvard Community Health Plan,

the Juran Institute, the Hospital Corporation of America, and other health care organizations (Institute for Healthcare Improvement, 2004). The goal was to apply the methods and tools of industrial quality improvement in a variety of organizations in order to determine whether they could apply to a service industry. Berwick was a principal investigator for this project. As a result of this endeavor, the Institute for Healthcare Improvement (IHI) was born and became an early advocate for the concepts of process improvement and team problem solving in health care organizations.

In the mid-1990s the Joint Commission on Accreditation of Healthcare Organizations (JCAHO) began incorporating the principles of continuous quality improvement into its revised standards. Starting in 1996, the IOM, through its Committee on Health Care Quality in America, has convened the nation's quality leaders to assess and improve health care for all. These leaders have promoted continuous quality improvement in health care through education, research, and evaluation. Through their dedication and insights, they have defined health care quality for our generation and those ahead of us. Tenets promoted by these health care leaders and organizations, and embraced by health care quality professionals, include the following:

- Processes and systems are the problems, not people.
- Standardization of processes is key to managing work and people.
- Quality can be enhanced only in safe, nonpunitive work cultures.
- Quality measurement and monitoring is everyone's job.
- The impetus for quality monitoring is not primarily for accreditation or regulatory compliance, but a planned part of an organization's culture to continuously enhance and improve its services, based on continuous feedback from employees and customers.
- Consumers and stakeholders must be included in all phases of quality improvement planning.
- Consensus among all stakeholders must be gained to have an impact on quality.

- Health policy should include a focus on continuous enhancement of quality.

A framework for understanding health care improvement has been proposed by the IOM Committee on Quality of Health Care in America (Box 39.1). These six aims for health care quality improvement propose that health care systems ensure that care is safe, effective, patient-centered, timely, efficient, and equitable.

COLLABORATION AND HEALTH CARE QUALITY AS NURSING IMPERATIVES

Collaboration should be a goal of any interaction, regardless of the workplace or situation. Collaboration is an imperative set by the American

Nurses Association (ANA). The ANA, in its release of a revised *Code of Ethics for Nurses with Interpretive Statements* (2001), proposed that, "The nurse collaborates with other health professionals and the public in promoting community, national and international efforts to meet health needs" (p. 23). Collaborative partnerships are part of this imperative and shape the way professional nurses act clinically and how they participate in quality improvement efforts.

Collaboration is about relationships. Conflict is typically the result of a poor interpersonal relationship with a colleague. To overcome conflicts, it is necessary to strengthen, not shy away from, the relationship of the two opposing parties. The Pew Health Professions Commission (PHPC) talked

---

Box 39.1

Institute of Medicine's Specific Aims for Health Care Improvement

- *Safe:* "Patients should not be harmed by the care that is intended to help them, nor should harm come to those who work in health care" (IOM, Committee on the National Quality Report on Health Care Delivery, 2001, p. 47).
- *Effective:* "Refers to care that is based on the use of systematically acquired evidence to determine whether an intervention, such as a preventive service, diagnostic test, or therapy, produces better outcomes than do alternatives—including the alternative to do nothing" (IOM, 2001, p. 49). Evidence-based practice requires that those who give care consistently avoid both underuse of effective care and overuse of ineffective care that is more likely to harm than help the patient (Chassin, 1997).
- *Patient-centered:* "Refers to health care that establishes a partnership among practitioners, patients, and their families (when appropriate) to ensure that decisions respect patients' wants, needs, and preferences; and that patients have the education and support they need to make decisions and participate in their own care" (IOM, Committee on the National Quality Report on Health Care Delivery, 2001, p. 50).
- *Timeliness:* "Refers to obtaining needed care and minimizing unnecessary delays in getting that care" (IOM, Committee on the National Quality Report on Health Care Delivery, 2001, p. 53).
- *Efficient:* "Refers to a health care system where resources are used to get the best value for the money spent" (Palmer & Torgerson, 1999, p. 1136). "The opposite of efficiency is waste; the use of resources without benefit to the patients a system is intended to help. There are at least two ways to improve efficiency: (a) reduce quality waste and (b) reduce administrative or production costs" (IOM, Committee on Quality of Health Care in America, 2001, p. 54).
- *Equitable:* "Providing care that does not vary in quality because of personal characteristics such as gender, ethnicity, geographic location, and socioeconomic status" (IOM, Committee on Quality of Health Care in America, 2001, p. 6).

From Pelletier, L.R., & Hoffman, J.A. (2002). A framework for selecting performance measures for opioid treatment programs. *Journal for Healthcare Quality, 24*(3), 25. Reprinted with permission from the National Association for Healthcare Quality.

about practicing relationship-centered care as one of 21 health profession competencies for the twenty-first century (O'Neil & PHPC, 1998, p. 23). Relationship-centered care in this context surely involves nurse and client/family interactions, but it also stresses the importance of collaborative interdisciplinary relationships. These 21 competencies are necessary ingredients for professional relationships and can become guideposts for successful professional working relationships.

The 21 competencies also include a professional nurse's responsibility and accountability to health care quality. The specific statements related to health care quality include "Take responsibility for quality of care and health outcomes at all levels," and "Contribute to continuous improvement of

the health care system" (O'Neill & PHPC, 1998, pp. 29-43) (Box 39.2).

INDUSTRIAL MODELS OF QUALITY

Industrial models have heavily influenced the way quality is currently understood and measured in health care settings across the continuum. Industry leaders who have influenced nursing's understanding of health care quality include Walter Shewhart, Joseph Juran, Philip Crosby, and W. Edwards Deming. These leaders provided blueprints from which nursing quality management programs have been derived.

Shewhart (Deming, 2000b) explored causes of variation in work processes. He quantified these

---

Box 39.2

Twenty-One Competencies for the Twenty-First Century

1. Embrace a personal ethic of social responsibility and service.
2. Exhibit ethical behavior in all professional activities.
3. Provide evidence-based, clinically competent care.
4. Incorporate the multiple determinants of health in clinical care.
5. Apply knowledge of the new sciences.
6. Demonstrate critical thinking, reflection, and problem-solving skills.
7. Understand the role of primary care.
8. Rigorously practice preventive health care.
9. Integrate population-based care and services into practice.
10. Improve access to health care for those with unmet health needs.
11. Practice relationship-centered care with individuals and families.
12. Provide culturally sensitive care to a diverse society.
13. Partner with communities in health care decisions.
14. Use communication and information technology effectively and appropriately.
15. Work in interdisciplinary teams.
16. Ensure care that balances individual, professional, system and societal needs.
17. Practice leadership.
18. Take responsibility for quality of care and health outcomes at all levels.
19. Contribute to continuous improvement of the health care system.
20. Advocate for public policy that promotes and protects the health of the public.
21. Continue to learn and help others learn.

From O'Neil, E.H., & the Pew Health Professions Commission (PHPC). (1998). *Recreating health professional practice for a new century: The fourth report of the Pew Health Professions Commission.* San Francisco: PHPC.

variations, categorizing variables as common or special cause. His Plan, Do, Check, Act (PDCA) model is probably the most frequently used in health care quality settings today, as follows (Figure 39.1):

- *Plan* (identify an issue and plan a process improvement)
- *Do* (map the current and proposed process, collect data, and analyze the results)
- *Check* (propose a solution and check the results of the new process)
- *Act* (adopt, adapt, or abandon the solution)

Shewhart also provided the industrial community with statistical process control techniques that are used widely today. Deming (2000a, 2000b) adopted his work and refined it.

Juran (1989) defined quality as "fitness for use." Quality, in his work, was defined as freedom from defects plus value and continuously meeting customer expectations. His approach to quality centered around the use of interdisciplinary teams that used diagnostic tools to understand why industrial processes produce a product not fit for use. His framework included a three-pronged approach: quality planning, quality control, and quality improvement. Quality planning is like strategic planning: discovering customer needs, developing products for those needs, and designing processes to produce these products (Carey & Lloyd, 1995; Katz & Green, 1997).

Crosby viewed quality in production terms of zero defects and measured quality in relation to conformance to requirements. He believed that the results or products of a company are made by people. He focused on systems and the consequences of poor quality. He emphasized doing the right thing the first time to prevent waste. Waste and rework were seen as costly, and good managers were those who prevented costly mistakes. Prevention is seen as the key to system quality in Crosby's framework (Bassett, 1998).

In addition to PDCA, Deming focused on statistical process control techniques and on continuous quality improvement through a culture of quality. He is credited as being influential in the success of Japanese industries. He proposed 14 points to help management staff understand and commit to quality. These points are listed in Box 39.3 (Deming, 2000a, 2000b). These 14 points, although created just after World War II, have heavily influenced health care's adoption of quality principles.

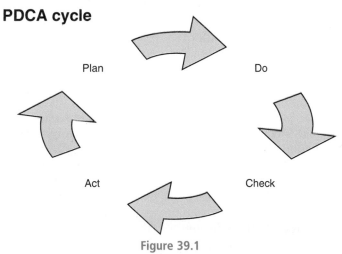

PDCA cycle

Plan

Do

Act

Check

Figure 39.1
PDCA (Plan, Do, Check, Act) cycle.

Box 39.3

Deming's 14 Points for Quality

1. Create constancy of purpose toward improving products and services.
2. Adopt the new philosophy.
3. Cease dependence on inspection to achieve quality.
4. End the practice of awarding business on the basis of cost alone.
5. Improve constantly and forever every process for planning, production, and service.
6. Institute training on the job.
7. Adopt and institute leadership aimed at helping people do their jobs better.
8. Drive out fear by promoting two-way communication.
9. Break down barriers between departments.
10. Eliminate exhortations for the workforce in such forms as posters and slogans; these methods tend to create adversarial relationships.
11. Eliminate numerical quotas for productivity; instead have leaders promote continuous quality improvement (CQI).
12. Permit pride of workmanship by removing the barriers that prevent this.
13. Encourage education and self-improvement for all workers.
14. Define management's commitment to CQI and their obligation to implement these points.

From Deming, W.E. (2000). *The new economics for industry, government, education.* Cambridge, MA: MIT Center for Advanced Engineering Studies; and Deming, W. E. (2000). *Out of the crisis.* Cambridge, MA: MIT Center for Advanced Engineering Studies.

STANDARDS OF QUALITY

Health care quality standards and measures can be grouped in three categories: structure, process, and outcome. Donabedian (1980) developed the initial theoretical model that identified that quality can be measured using these three aspects of a process. Donabedian's (1980) framework of structure, process, and outcomes is the most widely referenced model of quality; professional nurses have used this model to develop quality management programs, conduct improvement studies, and perform research. Standards essentially define quality, against which performance and outcomes are measured. Standards and measures are typically developed from benchmarking activities and reviews of best practices. Therefore the selection of standards and measures are a critical activity in the quality and performance improvement process. In actuality, standards establish the baseline against which measurement and evaluation are conducted.

Therefore it is critical to decide who determines standards and which standards are selected to define quality.

Structure Standards and Measures

Structure standards, or structural measures, focus on the internal characteristics of the organization and its personnel. They answer the questions, "Is an infrastructure in place and tools accessible to allow quality to exist?" and "Is the structure of the organization set up to allow for the effective, efficient delivery of services?" For example, a structural standard for a long-term care facility might be to have an adequate mix of registered nurses and nursing assistants on site to ensure that comprehensive care is delivered. For specialized areas, structure standards may address whether there are enough specialists or "intensivists" to ensure quality care. The presence of certain committees; policy statements; rules and regulations; or manuals, forms, or contracts may be needed. Structure standards regulate the environment to ensure quality. Human, organizational, and physical resources, as well as environmental characteristics, are examples of structure standards.

Process Standards and Measures

Process standards and measures focus on whether the activities within an organization are being conducted appropriately, effectively, and efficiently. Process measures focus on the behaviors of the professional nurse as a provider of care. The interventions recommended in a clinical practice guideline or best practice are examples of process standards. They relate to what the nurse will be doing and the process the nurse should follow to ensure effective, evidence-based care. Process standards look at activities, interventions, and the sequence of caregiving events, sometimes referred to as *work flow*. Typically, processes are assessed by audits, observational studies, or work flow analyses. Examples of process standards include the following: a nursing assessment is completed within 24 hours of admission; client calls are returned within 1 hour of the initial call.

Outcome Standards and Measures

Outcome standards and measures refer to whether the services provided by the organization make any difference: Where they effective? They answer the questions about the services that nurses provide and whether those services make a difference to the clients or to the health status of the population. Outcome standards address physical health status, mental health status, social and physical function, health attitudes/knowledge/behavior, utilization of services, and the client's perception and satisfaction with the care received. *Outcome* refers to a change in the current or future health status attributed to antecedent health care and client attributes of health care. Outcome standards present the possibility of measuring the effectiveness, quality, and time and resources allocated for care. Examples of outcome measures include the following: patient's activities of daily living have improved by 80%; percentage of clients who have stopped smoking after 12 weeks of intensive psychoeducational therapy.

In measuring quality, both structure and process parameters are important, but they are not sufficient in determining whether the care led to an effective outcome or whether the client learned, recovered, or improved his or her health status. Over the years, there has been varying emphasis on structure, process, and outcome aspects of health care. Ultimately, various stakeholders are interested in knowing whether care resulted in a positive, expected clinical outcome, based on objective, measurable criteria.

When developing a quality and performance improvement program, nurse managers are cautioned not to first create new standards and measures. Rather, a literature review will undoubtedly yield hundreds of measures from which to choose. These measures have typically been tested for reliability and validity and have been piloted in the field. Selection criteria can then be adopted and measures chosen for a specific intervention or program. A number of selection criteria guideline statements have been developed over the past few years, including statements from the following (Smith et al., 1997):

- President's Advisory Commission on Consumer Protection and Quality in the Health Care Industry (1998)
- U.K. Department of Health (2002)
- Foundation for Accountability (2002)
- Committee on Using Performance Monitoring to Improve Community Health (Durch et al., 1997)
- JCAHO (1999)
- National Committee for Quality Assurance (2000)
- Committee on Leading Health Indicators for Healthy People 2010, Institute of Medicine (Chrvala & Bulger, 1999)
- National Alliance for the Mentally Ill

The performance measurement attributes common to the above entities' guideline statements have been reported in the set of criteria proposed to be used for a national health care quality report (Institute of Medicine [IOM], Committee on the

National Quality Report on Health Care Delivery, 2001). Common performance measurement selection criteria are listed in Box 39.4 (Pelletier & Hoffman, 2002). The adoption of these performance measurement selection criteria is the first step in developing a comprehensive performance measurement system.

More recently, an international working group on health care quality indicators defined the following as selection criteria (The Commonwealth Fund, 2004), which are similar to those previously cited:

- *Feasibility:* indicators already being collected by one or more countries
- *Scientific soundness:* indicators that are valid and reliable; existing reviews of the scientific evidence and approval by a consensus process in one or more countries

- *Interpretability:* indicators that allowed a clear conclusion (a clear direction) for policymakers
- *Actionability:* measures of processes or outcomes that could be directly affected by the health care entity
- *Importance:* indicators reflective of important health conditions representing a major share of the burden of disease, health care costs, or policymaker priorities

EMERGING MODELS OF HEALTH CARE QUALITY ASSESSMENT AND MANAGEMENT

A number of industry-based models for quality management and measurement have been adopted by the health care industry over the past two decades. These include Six Sigma, Lean Enterprise, the National Malcolm Baldrige Award,

---

Box 39.4

Common Performance Measurement Selection Criteria

- *Relevance:* The measure should address features of the health care system applicable to health professionals, policy makers, and consumers.
- *Meaningfulness and interpretability:* The measure should be understandable to at least one of the audiences. It should help inform them about the important issues or concerns.
- *Scientific or clinical evidence:* The measure should be based on evidence documenting the links between the interventions, clinical processes, and/or outcomes it addresses.
- *Reliability or reproducibility:* The measure should produce the same results when repeated in the same population and setting.
- *Feasibility:* The measure should be specified precisely. Collection of data for the measure should be inexpensive and logistically feasible.
- *Validity:* The measure should make sense (face validity), correlate well with other measures of the same aspects of care (construct validity), and capture meaningful aspects of care (content validity).
- *Health importance:* The measure should include the prevalence of the health condition to which it applies and the seriousness of the health outcomes affected.

Note: Criteria are listed in order of their frequency, with the one mentioned most often listed first. The same label for a criterion can have different meanings depending on the framework, because the criteria are not standardized. The definitions, rather than the labels, were used to construct the figure. Feasibility was used as a category covering several criteria in some of the frameworks and as a single criterion in others. Parts of this figure were adapted from NCQA's list of desirable attributes for HEDIS measures (IOM, Committee on the National Quality Report on Health Care Delivery, 2001, p. 81).

From Pelletier, L.R., & Hoffman, J.A. (2002). A framework for selecting performance measures for opioid treatment programs. *Journal for Healthcare Quality, 24*(3), 26. Reprinted with permission from the National Association for Healthcare Quality.

ISO 9000, and the concept of High-Performance Organizations. These models are briefly described in the following sections.

Six Sigma

A strategy developed by Motorola and implemented successfully at General Electric (GE) and AlliedSignal Companies provided an innovative approach to reduce variation and error rates. Not surprisingly, the Six Sigma approach that these companies utilize is similar to tried and true approaches historically deployed by health care quality professionals, as described previously. In the Six Sigma breakthrough strategy, errors are measured in defects per million opportunities (dpmo). Six Sigma is achieved when the organization reaches an error or defect rate of 3.4 or less per one million. As a result of its implementation and investment of $6 million since 1995, GE boasted financial benefits of over $600 million in 1998 (Harry & Schroeder, 2000). AlliedSignal reported a 1.9% growth in operating margin in the first quarter 1999, and "cumulative impact of Six Sigma has been a savings in excess of $2 billion in direct costs" (Harry & Schroeder, 2000, p. ix). The Six Sigma strategy (Harry & Schroeder, 2000) is remarkably similar to Juran's problem-solving strategy (Plsek & Omnias, 1989), which has been applied to health care. Table 39.1 illustrates these similarities (Pelletier, 2000).

Lean Enterprise

Lean Enterprise is a model of quality measurement that was originally associated with Deming but reintroduced to the United States by Womack in the mid-1990s (Jones & Womack, 2003). The premise of this model is that operational waste needs to be eliminated in the following areas (Martin, 2003):

- Unnecessary processing
- Errors/defects
- Waiting
- Overproduction
- Inventory
- Excess motion by people

- Transportation of product
- Underutilized people

Baldrige National Quality Award

The Baldrige National Quality Award (BNQA) establishes a set of performance standards that define a total quality organization. There are standards in seven areas of excellence: (1) leadership, (2) strategic planning, (3) customer and market focus (focus on patients, other customers, and markets), (4) information and analysis, (5) human resource focus, (6) process management, and (7) business results (organizational performance results). Organizations committed to quality improvement choose to adopt the BNQA approach as another means of defining and improving their organizational processes to achieve quality outcomes. Manufacturing, service, and small business were the original award categories, but in 1999, education and health care were added. With the trend in health care to adopt industry applications and measure sets for quality improvement, it was fitting that the health care industry was recognized as one that could benefit from participating in this program. It is appropriate for health care entities to strive to achieve internationally recognized standards for performance excellence, which enable them to benchmark their "best practices" with others in the field. The first health care organization to apply and be awarded the BNQA in health care was the SSM system in St. Louis in 2002 (White, 2003). Various states have also developed quality awards based on the BNQA criteria.

ISO 9000

The International Organization for Standardization (ISO) is a network of 148 countries that have agreed on an international reference for quality requirements in business and service industries. The ISO 9000 series of standards are those that address quality management, that is, what the organization does to manage its systems and processes. These standards define "what the organization does to fulfill the customer's quality

Table 39.1

Comparison of Six Sigma Breakthrough Strategy and Juran's Problem-Solving Strategy			
Six Sigma Breakthrough Strategy		Juran's Problem Solving Strategy	
Stage	Step (Objective)	Phase	Step
Identification	Recognize Define (Identify key business issues)	Project definition and organization	1. List and prioritize problems 2. Define project and team
Characterization	Measure Analyze (Understand current performance levels)	Diagnostic journey	1. Analyze symptoms 2. Formulate theory of causes 3. Test theories 4. Identify root causes
Optimization	Improve Control (Achieve breakthrough improvement)	Remedial journey	1. Consider alternative solutions 2. Design solutions and controls 3. Address resistance to change 4. Implement solutions and controls
Institutionalization	Standardize Integrate (Transform how day-to-day business is conducted)	Holding the gains	1. Check performance 2. Monitor control system

From Pelletier, L.R. (2000). Editorial: On error-free health care: Mission possible! *Journal for Healthcare Quality, 22*(3), 9. Reprinted with permission from the National Association for Healthcare Quality.

requirements, and applicable regulatory requirements, while aiming to enhance customer satisfaction, and achieve continual improvement of its performance in pursuit of these objectives" (ISO, 2003, p. 1). These standards are applicable to service industries (such as health care) as well as industrial organizations. The appeal of this type of a standard setting system is that the organization is continually evaluating itself against its own consistency in conformance to the standards.

The achievement of an ISO 9000 registration results when a company complies with its own quality system. Again, as many health care organizations are committed to the ongoing pursuit of quality, the ISO 9000 registration process provides another type of assessment and evaluation of an organization's quality systems and sets a benchmark for achievement that is internationally recognized.

High-Performance Organizations

As organizations continue to evolve their quality models, those that are in pursuit of continuous and ongoing improvement are embracing a concept referred to as *high-performance organizations* (HPOs). These are organizations that may already be practicing Six Sigma, Lean Enterprise, or have achieved recognition through ISO 9000 registration or Malcolm Baldrige compliance. HPOs are those that have a culture of "building and sustaining a customer focused, team based organization that pays as much attention to results as it does to process" (Ward, 2004, ¶. 3).

Following are some of the attributes of an HPO:

- Leaders who communicate a strong and clear mission and vision to employees
- Strategic thinking that anticipates customer needs and market changes
- A commitment to ongoing identification of problems and a preoccupation for potential failures
- Resiliency
- Flexibility
- Creative and improvisational problem solving to address failures or "near misses".

HPOs apply the principles learned through study of High Reliability Organizations (HROs). These are organizations that require reliability in order to ensure stable outcomes in the face of variable working conditions.

COSTS ASSOCIATED WITH POOR HEALTH CARE QUALITY

The costs associated with medical errors "in lost income, disability, and health care costs is as much as $29 billion annually" (Quality Interagency Task Force [QuIC], 2000, p. 1) and plagues every sector in the health care industry. The number of medical errors has been described as unacceptable by an IOM report, *To Err Is Human: Building a Safer Health Care System* (Kohn et al., 2000), which has been referenced widely in the professional and consumer press since its release. The IOM report has reached the highest levels in the federal government, but response to its findings and recommendations has been lackluster. The research associated with this report was preceded by other federal initiatives.

The QuIC was established in 1998 in response to the President's Advisory Commission on Consumer Quality in the Health Care Industry to ensure that major federal agencies involved in

purchasing, providing, studying, or regulating health care services are working in a coordinated manner with the common goal of health care quality improvement. The Agency for Healthcare Research and Quality (AHRQ) was given oversight of day-to-day operations (QuIC, 1999). QuIC presented its response to the IOM report to President Clinton in February 2000. Within the structure of a yet-to-be-established Center for Quality Improvement and Patient Safety, the President outlined a commitment of $53 million in funding for the development of the Center and additional funding for medical error and adverse event reporting systems at the Food and Drug Administration. The goal of the funding was to implement recommendations of the IOM report and to cut preventable medical errors by 50% over 5 years (The White House, 2000). A four-tiered approach had been defined by QuIC to include the following:

1. Establish a national focus to create leadership, tools, and protocols to enhance the knowledge base about safety
2. Identify and learn from medical errors through both mandatory and voluntary reporting systems
3. Raise standards and expectations for improvements in safety through the actions of oversight organizations, group purchasers, and professional groups
4. Implement safe practices at the delivery level (QuIC, 2000, p. 4)

Tactics and strategies described in the QuIC report to reduce medical errors were targeted toward 500 federal U.S. Department of Defense military hospitals and 6000 hospitals participating in Medicare.

Both the IOM and QuIC reports defined specific strategies that could inform the development and refinement of health care safety systems nationwide. An important component of these reports is the mention of the error-reduction techniques of other industries. The federal reports provided another opportunity to advocate for patients, families, and populations. They gave health care

Research Note

Source: Anderson, S., & Wittwer, W. (2004). Using bar-code point-of-care technology for patient safety. *Journal for Healthcare Quality, 26*(6), 5-11.

Purpose

Patient safety, in particular medication safety, has become a major issue for health care providers, payers, and patients. Medication errors occur at an alarming rate, and the majority of nonintercepted medication errors originate at the point of care when a nurse mistakenly administers a medication. The 1999 Institute of Medicine report called for increasing the use of information technology to reduce medication errors. Realizing a 59% to 70% decrease in medication administration errors on individual nursing units, this particular hospital demonstrates how bar-code point-of-care medication administration systems successfully track, reduce, and prevent bedside medication errors while having a positive effect on nursing satisfaction.

Discussion

Bar-code technology, which has been used in grocery stores since the 1970s, is currently being adopted by health care organizations to reduce the potential for medication administration errors. Prior to adopting a bar-code point-of-care (BPOC) system, this hospital had already implemented the following safety measures:

- Computerized pharmacy system
- Medication administration records generated by the pharmacy system
- Decentralized pharmacists
- Standard dosing times
- Standard antibiotic dosing
- Restricted purchase of similar-looking drug packages
- Modified storage and labels for "sound alike" medications
- Standardized drip concentrations

With gradual deployment of BPOC, medication error rates fell as much as 70% on some clinical units.

Application to Practice

The adoption of information technology to promote health care safety is an important role for nurse managers. The hospital learned several important lessons in deploying BPOC throughout their enterprise. One important lesson was vendor selection. Software and hardware products should be chosen with the following key elements in mind:

- Real-time, electronic documentation
- Ease of use by clinical nurses and clinical pharmacists
- Decision support characteristics that extend beyond the "five rights"
- Technology that would easily interface with other hospital systems
- User-friendly and expeditious long on/log off features
- Customization features for difference patient care areas
- Cost
- Vendor reliability

The ability of the system to capture "near misses" was another critical feature. Reporting those near misses and educating the staff on their frequency averted future errors. BPOC systems also have an effect on nursing work flow, most often reducing process steps significantly, which in turn reduce the opportunity for error.

quality professionals the evidence and research with which to defend a quality management budget, enhance information systems and technologies to track errors, and further develop quality activities and studies using proven tools and techniques. The reports are also models in defining and describing cost/benefit analyses and return on investment scenarios for quality and performance improvement programs. In essence, they provided a business case for quality.

A technical report published by the IOM identified key characteristics that health care microsystems use to continuously enhance the services that they provide to individuals and communities (Donaldson & Mohr, 2000). After interviewing 43 microsystems, the researchers identified eight common themes, including "integration of information, measurement, interdependence of care team, supportiveness of the larger system, constancy of purpose, connection to community, investment in improvement, and alignment of role and training" (p. 21).

The IOM report *Crossing the Quality Chasm: A New Health System for the 21st Century* (IOM, 2001) recommended that Congress establish a Health Care Quality Innovation Fund "to support projects targeted at 1) achieving the six aims of safety, effectiveness, patient-centeredness, timeliness, efficiency, and equity; and/or 2) producing substantial improvements in quality for the [15] priority conditions" (p. 11). The overall goal of the funding would be to produce a "public-domain portfolio of programs, tools, and technologies of widespread applicability" (p. 11). The report recommended an initial investment of $1 billion over 3 to 5 years to support this goal. Health care organizations could take the lead by either enhancing the current resources dedicated to quality and performance improvement in their organizations or by using the funds to finance regional collaborative health care quality projects. These successes could then be described in the literature for wider application.

The third in a series of IOM quality chasm reports, entitled *Leadership by Example: Coordinating Government Roles in Improving*

Health Care Quality, was released in 2002 (Corrigan et al., 2002). The original charge of the IOM Committee on Enhancing Federal Healthcare Quality Programs (CEFHQP) was to acknowledge that "The current federal quality oversight programs represent a patchwork of requirements and processes that have evolved over the last 30 to 35 years" (IOM, 2002, ¶. 1). The committee was convened "to re-examine the various federal quality improvement and oversight programs to assess whether changes are needed to 1) provide adequate protection to beneficiaries, 2) provide strong incentives to providers to improve quality, and 3) improve the efficiency of the oversight processes by reducing redundancy" (IOM, 2002, ¶. 1). This study was requested by Congress and sponsored by the U.S. Department of Health and Human Services, the California Health Care Foundation, and The Commonwealth Fund. In doing their work, the committee held workshops to obtain perspectives and information from various stakeholders with expertise in the fields of quality measurement, improvement, oversight, and research on ways to improve current federal programs (Medicare, Medicaid, Children's Health Insurance Program, Tricare, and Veterans Affairs).

From his introductory remarks at the press briefing, the committee chair outlined the major findings of the study as follows (Omenn, 2002):

- There is a lack of consistency in performance measurement requirements both across and within these government programs.
- The programs are not using standardized measures.
- There is no well-thought-out conceptual framework to guide the selection of performance measures.
- Medicare, Medicaid, and the State Children's Health Insurance Program lack computer-based clinical data, which is seen as a major impediment.
- There is also a lack of commitment to transparency and openly sharing information on safety and quality (p. 2).

These findings were not a surprise to many nurses and health care quality professionals, who have been burdened with duplicative reporting for years. The positive message was that strong recommendations from this committee were sent to the federal government's leadership, asking them to attack these problems with a good deal of muscle to shape the measurement of performance for the whole health care sector. The charge was clear to the three Secretaries of the U.S. Department of Health and Human Services, Department of Defense, and Department of Veterans Affairs: "work together to establish standardized performance measures, as well as public reporting requirements for clinicians, institutional providers, and health plans in each program. The standardized measurement and reporting requirements should replace the many performance assessment activities currently under way in various programs" (Omenn, 2002, p. 3).

Standardization of protocols and measures is not a new idea (Pelletier, 1998). To reduce administrative burden and duplicative reporting could easily put time back in the hands of clinicians to do what they do best: provide health care services to individuals, families, and communities.

LEADERSHIP AND MANAGEMENT IMPLICATIONS

Planning for Health Care Quality

An organization that adopts and nurtures a continuous quality improvement culture acknowledges that change is an everyday event. One of the ways that change can be managed is to acknowledge it and make it a part of the organization's strategic planning process. Just as an organization defines its mission, vision, and core values, so too must change agents and teams define the purpose of the change (expected outcomes), the mission and vision of the change process, and the core values of the group that will be responsible for managing the change.

An organization's mission is a concise statement that answers the question "What business are we in today?" (Pelletier, 1999a). Some companies refer to their mission as a purpose. Pfizer, a pharmaceutical company, refers to it purpose as follows: "We dedicate ourselves to humanity's quest for longer, healthier, happier lives through innovation in pharmaceutical, consumer, and animal health products" (Pfizer, 2004, ¶. 1). The Mayo Clinic's (2004a, 2004b) mission statement reads: Mayo's mission "... is to provide the best care to every patient every day through integrated clinical practice, education and research" (Mayo Clinic, 2004a, ¶. 1). Some companies and health systems only state their vision. For example, the Yale New Haven Health System states that its vision is, "To be the preferred, comprehensive, integrated health care delivery system recognized for advanced clinical care, quality, service, cost-effectiveness, and commitment to improving the health status of the communities we serve" (Yale-New Haven Health, 2001, ¶. 1).

An organization's vision should accurately depict what the company is striving to become. The vision statement should be able to stand on its own and be understandable to people new to the enterprise. It should be forward-thinking to ensure that it "will resist erosion in a sea of change in the marketplace and in the organization" (Dahlberg et al., 1997, p. 362). In Pfizer's case, they state: "We will become the world's most valued company to patients, customers, colleagues, investors, business partners, and the communities where we work and live" (Pfizer, 2004, ¶. 1).

It is critical for mission and vision statements to be communicated effectively to internal stakeholders (employees and management personnel) and to external stakeholders (investors, clients, patients, vendors, and accreditation agencies). In this way, internal and external stakeholders share "a common basis for action" (Dahlberg et al., 1997, p. 362). Nurse managers should be familiar with the company/organization's mission and vision statements. They should be involved in the development of these core value statements. Mission and vision statements should be reviewed and updated periodically in order to accurately reflect what leadership, staff, and stakeholders believe is

▲ LEADERSHIP & MANAGEMENT **BEHAVIORS**

Leadership Behaviors

- Builds a culture of quality and safety
- Models quality care management
- Encourages use of electronic systems for quality management
- Envisions high-quality care
- Collaborates across disciplines to enhance quality
- Is visible in quality management activities
- Enables interdisciplinary quality improvement
- Evaluates quality of care

Management Behaviors

- Plans for quality in care delivery
- Organizes a quality-driven service

- Directs others to achieve quality
- Monitors quality of care
- Evaluates quality of care
- Participates in ongoing quality management

Overlap Areas

- Evaluates quality of care
- Injects quality into care delivery and management of care

---

the purpose and future direction of the organization. This is important because mission, vision, and values form the foundation for quality and its management and improvement.

Just as a nurse's professional behavior is based on personal values, so too must an organization describe the core values that are the foundation of their enterprise or endeavor. Strategic planning often includes the development of core value statements that are in alignment with the mission and vision statements of the organization. "Value statements become part of an organization's culture; they act as a quick reference or navigation device—just as mission and vision statements do" (Pelletier, 1999b, p. 2). Marcus and colleagues (1995) defined values as "interests that reflect fundamental purpose and integrity: issues to which you hold fast as a matter of principle, with little room for compromise" (p. 430). Furthermore, "Values are operational qualities used by organizations to maintain or enhance performance" (Harmon, 1997, p. 246).

Values consciously and unconsciously guide a professional nurse's personal and professional behavior. His Holiness the Dalai Lama and Cutler (1998) had the following to say about values:

> Higher stages of growth and development depend on an underlying set of values that can guide us. A value system that can provide continuity and coherence to our lives, by which we can measure our experiences. A value system that can help us decide which goals are truly worthwhile and which pursuits are meaningless. Values help us with the challenges of everyday life. (pp. 192-193)

Nurses' personal and professional values come from the experiences they have shared with others in interpersonal exchanges at work and at home. To identify a group's core values, ask and record the responses to these questions: Which three people have had the greatest influence in your personal and professional life? What are the three most important values these influential people taught you? The answers to these questions can help inform the development of mission, vision, and core value statements. An example is a set of core values or "core principles" from the Mayo Clinic, as outlined in Table 39.2.

CURRENT ISSUES AND TRENDS

A Nurse Manager's Health Care Quality Toolbox

With the paradigm shift from quality assurance to organizational performance improvement came

Table 39.2

Mayo Clinic Core Value Statements	
Primary value: The needs of the patient come first.	
Core Value	Description
Practice	Practice medicine as an integrated team of compassionate, multi-disciplinary physicians, scientists and allied health professionals who are focused on the needs of patients from our communities, regions, the nation and the world.
Education	Educate physicians, scientists and allied health professionals and be a dependable source of health information for our patients and the public.
Research	Conduct basic and clinical research programs to improve patient care and to benefit society.
Mutual respect	Treat everyone in our diverse community with respect and dignity.
Commitment to quality	Continuously improve all processes that support patient care, education and research.
Work atmosphere	Foster teamwork, personal responsibility, integrity, innovation, trust and communication within the context of a physician-led institution.
Societal commitment	Benefit humanity through patient care, education and research. Support the communities in which we live and work. Serve appropriately patients in difficult financial circumstances.
Finances	Allocate resources within the context of a system rather than its individual entities. Operate in a manner intended not to create wealth but to provide a financial return sufficient for present and future needs.

Courtesy Mayo Clinic. (2004). *Mayo's mission, primary value, core principles* (¶3). Rochester, MN: Mayo Clinic. Retrieved June 9, 2004, from *www.mayoclinic.org/about/missionvalues.html*

the expectation that accredited organizations become skilled at the art and science of continuous quality improvement. This included the concepts of leadership involvement, a commitment to customers' needs (i.e., patients and families), an understanding of the principle of process versus people, a devotion to data collection and analysis as the foundation for problem solving, and the view that multidisciplinary teams working within the processes under study were the experts and therefore best equipped to drive change and improvement.

Nurse managers in accredited organizations were expected to learn these principles and tools for quality improvement, to educate staff in these tools and techniques, to identify improvement opportunities on their units, and to be able to speak to process changes that occurred as a result of data analysis. They were also tapped to participate in organization-wide improvement teams designed to address overarching problem resolution or process redesign projects. Many of the early quality leaders received training in facilitation and group meeting techniques, in addition to the QI tools. This enabled them to promote the team-based model of cross-functional problem solving that became the standard for most organizations. Skills and expertise in the concepts of team building, conflict resolution, statistical process control, customer service, and process improvement continue to be needed by nurse leaders in the new millennium.

Health care quality professionals and those nurses involved in quality and performance

Table 39.3

A Nurse Manager's Health Care Quality Toolbox	
Data-collection tools	Checksheets and checklists facilitate the gathering of data for eventual analysis and reporting. Good data collection tools can help you count and categorize data (see Figure 39.2).
Control chart	This tool includes data points and their placement on a graph to depict variation. Its purpose is to illustrate whether the process variation is expected ("common cause") or an unexpected or unusual variation ("special cause"). Included are three lines—the mean, an upper control limit (UCL), and a lower control limit (LCL). Generally, a process is considered "out of control" when the data points stray outside of the control limits or a series of data points follow a defined pattern that illustrate lack of control in the process (see Figure 39.3).
Cause-and-effect (or fishbone) diagram	This tool resembles diagramming sentences. The "effect" is illustrated in a box at the end of a midline (or "head" of the fish.) The "causes" are generally four to five categories of elements that might contribute to the effect (e.g., machines, methods, people, materials, measurements) and the specific activities. Under each of these category headings, individual items that might lead to the effect are listed. By diagramming all of the possible contributors, the predominant or root causes may be found more readily (see Figure 39.4).
Detailed flowchart	Using various shapes, this tool is used to depict a work process, from start to finish, illustrating all of the processes' action steps, decision points, hand-offs, or waiting stages. Flowcharts form the cornerstone of process improvement planning and analysis. The entire process must first be accurately defined in order to identify problems or process improvement opportunities (see Figure 39.5).
Pareto chart	This bar graph can help depict the "80/20" rule. In the nineteenth century, it was used to show that 80% of the wealth was held by 20% of the people. In health care, typically 20% of the issues cause 80% of the problems. The use of this tool allows a performance improvement team to focus on the "vital few" causes of the problems in a process under study (see Figure 39.6).
Scatter diagrams	This graph describes the relationship between two variables that are continuous. It is used when the potential causes on effects under study cannot be easily categorized, such as in a Pareto Chart or cause-and-effect diagram. Data points are plotted along the vertical and horizontal axes of the graph, and a correlation between the two variables can either be weak or strong, based on the pattern of the data points (see Figure 39.7).

improvement activities have an enormous set of resources available to them as they plan for an enterprise-wide quality program. Tools and techniques that nurses can readily use are illustrated in Table 39.3. Figures 39.2 through 39.7 illustrate examples of templates and forms to be included in a nurse manager's quality "toolbox."

In addition, the Internet can provide professional nurses with administrative and clinical tools to support a quality and performance improvement program, regardless of the delivery setting. A list of relevant websites can be found in Box 39.5 (see p. 850)

A health care quality glossary can also assist professional nurse managers in navigating the health care quality field. A glossary of frequently used terms is discussed under the definitions section and synopsized in the Leading & Managing Defined box.

HEALTH CARE SAFETY AND HEALTH CARE RISK MANAGEMENT

Accreditation and Regulatory Influences on Quality

Health care organizations have always been required to meet the standards and requirements of federal and state reimbursement regulations (Medicare and Medicaid) and state licensure rules and regulations in order to operate. These regulations have traditionally defined requirements for quality. However, the private accreditation process has probably had the most significant impact on the development of quality improvement systems in health care. It has been through organizations such as the JCAHO, the Commission on Accreditation of Rehabilitation Facilities (CARF), the National Committee for Quality Assurance (NCQA), and others that performance standards have been promulgated and universally adopted. In each of these accreditation processes, the concept of systemwide quality improvement provides the framework for the standards. Although accreditation is not mandatory, eligibility to participate in

Data Collection Sheet

Organization/Unit: _____   Date: _____

Process: _____

MEASURE	DATE	TIME	WHERE	WHEN

Figure 39.2
Sample data collection sheet for a nurse manager's quality toolbox.

and receive reimbursement from managed care organizations or federal and state program funding sources is often tied to the achievement of accreditation by one or more of the voluntary accreditation organizations.

Of all of these voluntary accreditation programs, JCAHO has had the greatest degree of impact on the health care industry. Founded in 1951, it led the way in establishing a set of performance standards for hospitals to follow in order to become accredited. Over the years, it has evolved to reflect the myriad of types of providers that now constitute our health care system and has expanded its role beyond hospital accreditation. Currently, JCAHO sponsors accreditation programs for organizations that provide services in the areas of ambulatory care, assisted living, behavioral health, critical access hospitals, health care networks, home care, laboratory, long-term care, and office-based surgery.

Throughout its evolution over the past 50 years, JCAHO has continually adjusted its performance standards for quality. Initially, the focus was on quality assurance, and JCAHO promoted a "10-Step Process for Quality Assurance" that provided the framework for quality in hospitals throughout the 1980s and much of the 1990s. The "Agenda for Change" was announced by JCAHO, which identified the need to improve the accreditation process itself; in 1994, the accreditation standards manuals were completely revised. The new approach organized the standards into *cross-functional processes of care and services* (such as Patients Rights, Patient Assessment, and Patient Family Education), rather than by separate departmental standards sections as previously published (e.g., Nursing, Physical Therapy, and Dietary). Additionally, a new section entitled "Improving Organizational Performance" was introduced that created standards for quality

Text continued on p. 853.

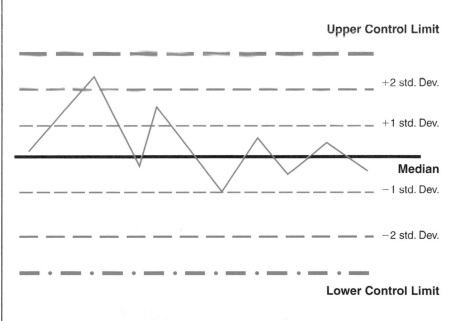

Figure 39.3
Sample control chart for a nurse manager's quality toolbox.

Cause-and-Effect Diagram

Organization/Unit: _____ Date: _____

Process: _____

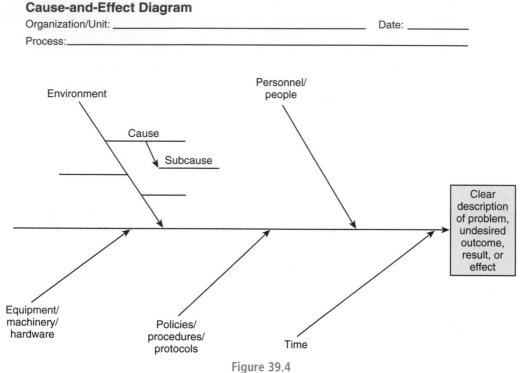

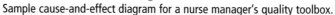

Figure 39.4
Sample cause-and-effect diagram for a nurse manager's quality toolbox.

Detailed Flowchart

Organization/Unit: _____ Date: _____ Process owner: _____

Process: _____

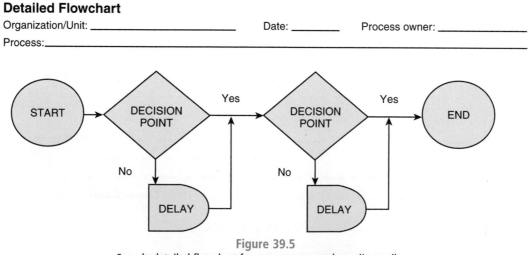

Figure 39.5
Sample detailed flowchart for a nurse manager's quality toolbox.

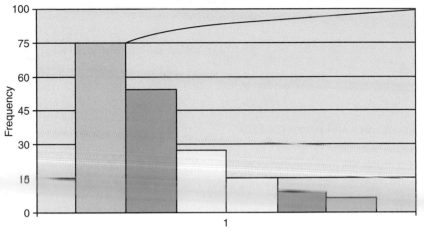

Causal Factors

Figure 39.6

Example of a Pareto chart for a nurse manager's quality toolbox.

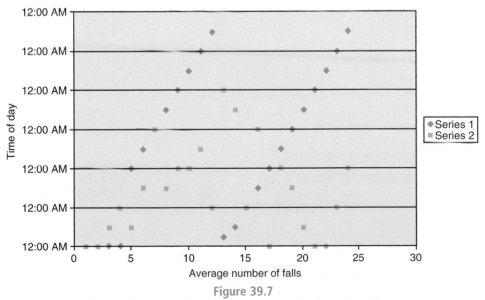

Figure 39.7

Example of a scatter diagram for a nurse manager's quality toolbox.

Box 39.5

Internet Sites Related to Health Care Quality

Agency for Healthcare Research and Quality (AHRQ): Quality Indicators

www.qualityindicators.ahrq.gov/

The AHRQ Quality Indicators (QIs) are measures of health care quality that make use of readily available hospital inpatient administrative data.

AHRQ: Medical Errors and Patient Safety

www.ahcpr.gov/qual/errorsix.htm

A major federal initiative has been launched to reduce medical errors and improve patient safety in federally funded health care programs, and by example and partnership, in the private sector.

AHRQ: WebM&M (Morbidity and Mortality)

www.webmm.ahrq.gov/
WebM&M is the nation's first web-based patient safety resource and journal.

American Productivity & Quality Center (APQC)

www.apqc.org

An internationally recognized resource for process and performance improvement, the American Productivity & Quality Center (APQC) helps organizations adapt to rapidly changing environments, build new and better ways to work, and succeed in a competitive marketplace.

American Society for Healthcare Risk Management (ASHRM)

www.hospitalconnect.com/ashrm/

Established in 1980, the American Society for Healthcare Risk Management is a personal membership group of the American Hospital Association with more than 4,300 members representing health care, insurance, law, and other related professions.

American Society for Quality (ASQ)

www.asq.org

Established in 1946, ASQ has a worldwide membership of 104,000 members. Its goal as a professional association is to create better workplaces and communities worldwide by advancing learning, quality improvement, and knowledge exchange to improve business results.

Association for Quality and Participation (AQP)

www.asq.org/perl/index.pl?g=teamwork

AQP, the Association for Quality and Participation, is an international not-for-profit membership association dedicated to improving workplaces through quality and participation practices, now housed in the ASQ Teamwork and Participation Forum.

Australian Patient Safety Foundation

www.apsf.net.au/
The Australian Patient Safety Foundation (APSF) is a nonprofit, independent organization dedicated to the advancement of patient safety.

Box **39.5**

Internet Sites Related to Health Care Quality—Cont'd

Baldrige National Quality Program

www.quality.nist.gov/

The Baldrige Award is given by the President of the United States to businesses—manufacturing and service, small and large—and to education and health care organizations that apply and are judged to be outstanding in seven areas: leadership, strategic planning, customer and market focus, information and analysis, human resource focus, process management, and business results.

Centers for Disease Control and Prevention (CDC), "Ensuring Patient Safety"

www.cdc.gov/washington/overview/patntsaf.htm

The Centers for Disease Control and Prevention (CDC) is recognized as the lead federal agency for protecting the health and safety of people—at home and abroad—providing credible information to enhance health decisions, and promoting health through strong partnerships.

Foundation for Accountability (FACCT)

www.markle.org/resources/facct/index.php

FACCT's mission was to improve health care for Americans by advocating for an accountable and accessible system, in which consumers are partners in their care and help shape the delivery of care. FACCT (Foundation for Accountability), a national nonprofit organization, closed its operations in 2004 after 9 years of advocacy for an accountable heath care system. David Lansky, president of FACCT, has since joined the Markle Foundation as a director of the Health Program, which has long supported and collaborated with FACCT on health care quality and consumer outreach programs. The Markle Foundation is committed to seeing that FACCT's key health care policy and research documents remain accessible to the public and has agreed to host them on the Markle website.

Institute for Healthcare Improvement (IHI)

www.ihi.org/ihi

The Institute for Healthcare Improvement (IHI) is a not-for-profit organization driving the improvement of health by advancing the quality and value of health care.

Institute for Safe Medication Practices (ISMP)

www.ismp.org/

The Institute for Safe Medication Practices (ISMP) is a nonprofit organization that works closely with health care practitioners and institutions, regulatory agencies, professional organizations, and the pharmaceutical industry to provide education about adverse drug events and their prevention.

International Society for Performance Improvement (ISPI)

www.ispi.org

The International Society for Performance Improvement (ISPI) is the leading international association of professionals who are dedicated to improving individual and organizational performance through a systematic, measurable, and reproducible methodology known as Human Performance Technology.

Continued

Box 39.5

Internet Sites Related to Health Care Quality—Cont'd

International Society for Quality in Health Care (ISQua)

www.isqua.org.au/welcome.html

ISQua, the International Society for Quality in Health Care, is a nonprofit, independent organization with members in more than 70 countries.

JCAHO National Patient Safety Goals

www.jcaho.org/accredited+organizations/patient+safety/index.htm

In July 2002, JCAHO approved its first set of 6 National Patient Safety Goals, with 11 related specific recommendations, for improving the safety of patient care in health care organizations.

The Leapfrog Group

www.leapfroggroup.org/index.html

The Leapfrog Group, a coalition of more than 135 public and private organizations that provide health care benefits, was founded by The Business Roundtable (BRT), a national association of Fortune 500 CEOs.

Managing for Quality

www.erc.msh.org/quality/

Managing for Quality is a collaborative effort between Management Sciences for Health and UNICEF to develop a practical, useful, and interactive resource that managers can use to improve quality in the many different types of health and family planning programs in which they work.

MEDERRORS.com

www.mederrors.com

MEDERRORS.com is intended as a useful link to experts in the fields of medication error and adverse drug event prevention and continuous quality improvement.

USP Medication Errors Reporting (MER) Program

www.usp.org/patientSafety/reporting/mer.html

This nationwide program makes it possible for health professionals who encounter actual or potential medication errors to report confidentially and anonymously, if preferred, to the United States Pharmacopeia (USP).

National Association for Healthcare Quality (NAHQ)

www.nahq.org

The National Association for Healthcare Quality (NAHQ) is the nation's leading organization for health care quality professionals.

The National Quality Forum (NQF)

www.qualityforum.org

The National Quality Forum (NQF) is a not-for-profit membership organization created to develop and implement a national strategy for health care quality measurement and reporting.

Box **39.5**

Internet Sites Related to Health Care Quality—Cont'd

National Quality Measures Clearinghouse

www.qualitymeasures.ahrq.gov/
The National Quality Measures Clearinghouse is a database and website for information on specific evidence-based health care quality measures and measure sets.

U.S. Department of Health and Human Services: Quality Improvement Organizations (QIO)

www.cms.hhs.gov/qio/2.asp
The QIO Statement of Work (SOW) is based on Title XI of the Social Security Act, Part B as amended by the Peer Review Improvement Act of 1902. This legislation established the QIO Program. As a result of legislative mandates and CMS's experience in administering the Program, CMS has identified the following SOW requirements.
(1) improve quality of care for beneficiaries by ensuring that beneficiary care meets professionally recognized standards of health care; (2) protect the integrity of the Medicare Trust Fund by ensuring that Medicare only pays for services and items that are reasonable and medically necessary and that are provided in the most appropriate (e.g., economical) setting; and (3) protect beneficiaries by expeditiously addressing individual cases such as beneficiary complaints, provider-issued notices of non-coverage (HINNs), EMTALA violations (dumping), and other statutory responsibilities.

U.S. Food and Drug Administration (FDA) MedWatch

www.fda.gov/medwatch/index.html
The FDA has the responsibility for ensuring the safety and efficacy of all regulated marketed medical products. MedWatch, the FDA Safety Information and Adverse Event Reporting Program, serves both health care professionals and the medical product-using public.

United States Pharmacopeia

www.usp.org
The United States Pharmacopeia (USP) is a nongovernment organization that promotes the public health by establishing state-of-the-art standards to ensure the quality of medicines and other health care technologies.

U.S. Department of Veterans Affairs, VA National Center for Patient Safety (NCPS)

www.patientsafety.gov/
The National Center for Patient Safety (NCPS) embodies the Department of Veterans Affairs' (VA) uncompromising commitment to reducing and preventing adverse medical events while enhancing the care given their patients.

---

initiatives that were based on the principle of continuous improvement rather than on preestablished thresholds for performance of individual indicators. This change reflected the influence of the industrial quality movement on health care in the early 1990s that was discussed previously in this chapter.

With this major restructuring of the JCAHO standards, the new era of thinking in terms of *process improvement* rather than *quality assurance* began, not only for JCAHO-accredited organizations, but also for other accrediting bodies. The description for this organization-wide programmatic approach, or *performance improvement* (PI), established the expectation that the quality initiatives in the organization were no longer the responsibility of a quality assurance nurse or department, but rather they were the responsibility of the enterprise's leaders. Quality outcomes were to be reviewed by the administrative and clinical leaders of the organization in order to effectively provide oversight to the quality of care being provided to patients and families (customers).

The PI standards delineate specific requirements for data collection in high-risk areas such as medication management and blood transfusions. However, beyond these mandatory indicators, each organization is expected to set its own priorities for measurement that reflect the types of services provided to the various populations served; these priorities must be set by the leaders of the organization. The PI standards also expect that the outcomes of data analysis and the actions taken to address improvement opportunities should be communicated to staff. This is where a nurse manager can essentially make the PI process "come alive" for nursing staff. Rather than simply a cataloguing of percentage of compliance to arbitrarily set indicators, staff can relate to and understand data outcomes that are based on the everyday processes in which they work. The nurse manager can involve staff in identifying relevant and significant data collection measures for the unit/department that will have a direct impact on changing and continuously improving care processes. A sample data collection sheet is displayed in Figure 39.2.

Nurse managers also need to stay abreast of changes in the standards of their organization's primary accrediting and regulatory agencies. A step further would be to participate in local, regional, and national committees that set standards. This can be done through professional associations such as the American Nurses Association and the National Association for Healthcare Quality. As new standards are introduced, policies and procedures must be updated and/or revised. Staff must be educated about the impact of the standards that are applicable to the care they provide.

Documentation requirements may change, and this may have an effect on clinical data measures or reimbursement. Nurse managers must provide leadership in adopting and adapting to ongoing changes in these arenas. Very few organizations enjoy the luxury of having one individual or department solely devoted to accreditation or regulatory compliance issues. At best, in those organizations with such functions, they can only serve as facilitators of the accreditation and licensing processes. As an example, JCAHO completely revised its survey process in 2004, and by 2006 surveys were conducted on an unannounced basis. This requires that managers throughout the organization be in a continual state of readiness (i.e., to have their departments and staff in compliance with all applicable standards at all times). Thus the onus of responsibility and accountability for continuous readiness moved from a single department or a QI Department chief to all leaders and managers in the organization.

Data Collection and Public Reporting of Quality Outcomes

By 1998 JCAHO had developed a requirement for accredited organizations to participate in the ORYX® initiative. This program required participating health care organizations to select six outcome measures that reflected the operations of their organizations and to choose a performance measurement vendor to aggregate and analyze the data and submit them on a quarterly basis to JCAHO. Since 1991 the HEDIS® (Health Plan Employer and Data Information Set) outcomes have been an integral part of the NCQA accreditation process for managed care plans. By contrast, CARF has required both program evaluation and quality outcomes measurement since the 1980s as component of its accreditation process, about a decade before the other accreditors.

The drawback of JCAHO's initial ORYX® process, and that of quality reporting required by most other accreditors, was an inability to compare performance across and among health care organizations. This was primarily due to the variability in selection of measures and reporting systems.

Also, as most organizations that analyzed their ORYX® data discovered, there was a limitation in identifying improvement opportunities with data that were purely outcomes-based. In further refinement of its ORYX® process, JCAHO devised its Core Measures program (JCAHO, 1999). Three measures, initially derived from the Centers for Medicare & Medicaid Services' (CMS; formerly the Health Care Financing Administration or HCFA) 6th Scope of Work, included both outcome and process data. The sets of measures related to these priority conditions: acute myocardial infarction (AMI), community-acquired pneumonia, and heart failure. A measure for pregnancy and related conditions was added after the initial pilot testing. In July 2002, accredited organizations were required to begin collecting data on the Core Measures (with some exceptions, such as pediatric hospitals) and submit the data to JCAHO. Although participation in these data collection programs is mandatory for each organization's accreditation, the results were not initially made public.

Since the 1980s CMS has mandated that the cost and quality of services provided to its Medicare recipients be evaluated through its peer review organizations (PROs). These PROs evolved into state and regional Quality Improvement Organizations (QIOs) that have continued their statutory mandate through the "Statement of Work" projects. At the time of this publication, CMS has just published its "8th Scope of Work." The statutory mission is "... to improve the efficiency, effectiveness, economy, and quality of services delivered to Medicare beneficiaries" (U.S. Department of Health and Human Services [USDHHS], 2004b, p. 1). The previous 6th and 7th Scope of Work projects focused on clinical quality measures in specific diagnostic categories such as heart failure and pneumonia. This new program will integrate with the new national "Quality Initiative" for health care described below.

CMS has also historically mandated data submission requirements for other types of health care organizations to participate in their Medicare programs. For long-term care facilities, CMS has required the submission of data through its Minimum Data Set (MDS) program. For home health care, CMS requires submission of data to the Outcome and Assessment Information Set (OASIS) that include clinical quality, cost, and administrative measures. In all of these initiatives, the results for individual providers were not originally made public.

In fall 2001 the U.S. Secretary of Health and Human Services announced the Bush administration's commitment to ensure quality health care through the publication of consumer information, along with quality improvement support, through CMS's QIOs. Their program, "The Quality Initiative" began in 2002 with the Nursing Home Quality Initiative (NHQI) and continued in 2003 with the Home Health Quality Initiative (HHQI) and the Hospital Quality Initiative (HQI). The future components of this national program will look at Doctor's Office Quality (DOQ) and the management of End-Stage Renal Disease. The components of the Hospital Quality Initiative include the following:

- The National Voluntary Hospital Reporting Initiative (NVHRI), consisting of a starter set of 10 quality measures that will eventually be expanded. (The standardized starter set of measures [Table 39.4] was developed by CMS in collaboration with the National Quality Foundation, the American Hospital Association, JCAHO and its own QIOs [USDHHS, CMS, 2004a.])
- Passage of the Medicare Prescription Drug Improvement and Modernization Act of 2003
- A patient survey designed to collate information on patient perspectives on hospital care
- Partnership with the Connecticut Department of Public Health, the legislature of which has mandated public reporting of hospital data utilizing the same clinical measures and patient perspectives
- The Premier Hospital Quality Incentive, which will provide financial rewards to top-performing hospitals through increases in their Medicare payments

Table 39.4

The National Voluntary Hospital Reporting Initiative: Ten-Measure Starter Set*

Performance Measures	Measure Description
AMI—Aspirin at Arrival	Acute myocardial infarction (AMI) patients without aspirin contraindications who received aspirin within 24 hours before or after hospital arrival
AMI—Aspirin Prescribed at Discharge	Acute myocardial infarction (AMI) patients without aspirin contraindications who are prescribed aspirin at hospital discharge
AMI—ACEI for LVSD	Acute myocardial infarction (AMI) patients with left ventricular systolic dysfunction (LVSD) and without angiotensin-converting enzyme inhibitor (ACEI) contraindications who are prescribed an ACEI at hospital discharge
AMI—Beta Blocker at Arrival	Acute myocardial infarction (AMI) patients without beta blocker contraindications who received a beta blocker within 24 hours after hospital arrival
AMI—Beta Blocker at Discharge	Acute myocardial infarction (AMI) patients without beta blocker contraindications who are prescribed a beta blocker at hospital discharge
HF—LVF Assessment	Heart failure (HF) patients with documentation in the hospital record that left ventricular function (LVF) was assessed before arrival or during hospitalization or is planned for after discharge
HF—ACEI for LVSD	Heart failure patients with left ventricular systolic dysfunction (LVSD) and without angiotensin-converting enzyme inhibitor (ACEI) contraindications who are prescribed an ACEI at hospital discharge
PNE—Initial Antibiotic Timing	Pneumonia patients who receive their first dose of antibiotics within 4 hours after arrival at the hospital
PNE—Pneumococcal Vaccination	Pneumonia patients age 65 and older who were screened for pneumococcal vaccine status and were administered the vaccine prior to discharge, if indicated
PNE—Oxygenation Assessment	Pneumonia patients who had an assessment of arterial oxygenation by arterial blood gas measurement or pulse oximetry within 24 hours prior to or after arrival at the hospital

From Centers for Medicare and Medicaid Services (CMS). (2004). *Hospital Quality Alliance (HQA) ten measure "starter set."* Baltimore: CMS.

*Online references: *www.cms.hhs.gov/quality/hospital/HeartAttack.pdf* and *www.cms.hhs.gov/quality/hospital/Pneumonia.pdf*

- The Robust Measures Project, which will support the efforts of the NVHRI by identifying a "robust" and comprehensive set of measures for public reporting

One of the first actions resulting from this Hospital Quality Initiative has been to require hospitals to submit their quality performance data for the 10 measures in order to comply with Section 501 the Medicare Prescription Drug Improvement and Modernization Act (MMA). Organizations that do not submit these data will receive 0.4% smaller Medicare payments in fiscal year 2005.

Over the past 10 to 15 years, many states also began to require health care organizations to submit data for the purpose of public reporting. Pennsylvania was one of the first states to enact legislation, creating the Health Care Cost Containment Council (HCCCC), whose responsibilities include giving "… comparative information about the most efficient and effective health care providers to the public" (Commonwealth of Pennsylvania, Pennsylvania HCCCC, 2004, ¶. 2) and "to collect, analyze and make available to the public data about the cost and quality of health care in Pennsylvania" (Commonwealth of Pennsylvania, Pennsylvania HCCCC, 2004, ¶. 5).

Initially, health care providers were resistant and concerned about issues such as data integrity and the lack of risk adjustments that would ensure that the results were comparable. They were convinced that without safeguards built into state reporting systems, their organizations might look "bad" to the public. Data-analysis systems have certainly evolved and improved over the years to address these concerns. A majority of states have now enacted legislation requiring public reporting, and with federal reporting requirements linked to reimbursement, providers must participate in data submission for public reporting or risk losing accreditation, income, and community status. Nurse managers need to be cognizant of the variety of measures being collected for state, federal, and accreditation purposes that apply to their units and patients. They often have to participate in the data-collection effort, discuss outcomes at quality improvement committees, and implement corrective action plans to address issues of noncompliance with the indicators (e.g., not documenting education about smoking cessation with AMI patients). In the future, patients and families may inquire about publicly reported data, so it is also imperative for managers to understand the organization's data outcomes and be able to address them.

Health Care Safety and Quality Improvement

A landmark report from the IOM in 1999 (Chrvala & Bulger, 1999) launched a major national focus on the safety of health care systems and processes. In fact, its conclusion that 98,000 deaths in health care organizations were preventable was considered a call to action, not only by health care providers, but by business and government as well. Not surprisingly, health care safety became the focus as a key component of the accreditation process. Soon after the millennium, new standards were established by JCAHO and other accrediting, regulatory, private, and public organizations that addressed the issue of health care safety within health care organizations.

In July 2001, new standards were introduced that required all JCAHO-accredited hospitals to establish and implement a formal Patient Safety Program. Additional requirements for integrated health care safety programs have been added over time. The components of a Health Care Safety Program are listed in Box 39.6.

Those individuals and organizations committed to health care safety initiatives believe that a rigorous, ongoing, and proactive approach to the identification of risks will result in the prevention of errors as well as provide the framework to respond most effectively when errors do occur.

Just as a paradigm shift was required to move from a quality assurance mindset to performance improvement, the new paradigm for health care safety requires that organizations create a non-punitive culture for error reporting. This is the application of the "process or system, not people" philosophy in its truest form. Old systems for singling out caregivers who committed errors must be eliminated. More important, nurse managers must learn the principles of the nonpunitive approach (i.e., that they applaud and commend staff for reporting errors or "near misses"). In fact, in some industrial models, those managers or staff who detect and report errors or system failures in their areas are rewarded. An example of the effectiveness of this approach is reported in a study conducted by Harvard Business School professor Amy Edmondson. She found that the nursing units in one hospital that were considered to be the best performing were those that had higher detected rates for adverse drug events (Hesselbein & Johnston, 2002). Certainly, the

Box 39.6

Components of a Health Care Safety Program

- Leadership commitment as evidenced through the allocation of resources for health care safety
- Assignment of individual(s) to manage the program
- Interdisciplinary (cross-organizational) participation, coordination and communication about safety activities
- Education of patients and families about health care safety issues
- Disclosure of unanticipated outcomes of care to patients and families
- Education of staff on safety-related topics and training in team techniques
- Data collection and analysis in safety-related areas, including the following:
  - Incident reporting
  - Medication errors
  - Infection surveillance
  - Facility/environmental surveillance
  - Staff willingness to report errors
  - Staff perceptions of and suggestions for improving safety
  - Patient and family perceptions and/or suggestions for improvement regarding safety
- Definition of terms related to safety, including sentinel events, "near misses" and what is reportable, and the development of policies and procedures to address each category of event
- Management of sentinel events
- Adherence to JCAHO National Patient Safety Goals
- Establishment of a risk reduction process to include Failure Modes Effects and Criticality Analysis (FMECA)

conclusion was not that more errors were committed on this unit, but the staff's willingness to report errors contributed to the improvement of the unit's overall processes, resulting in a positive reputation within the hospital.

Two examples of organizations that have created health care safety programs and initiatives since the IOM reports were released are the Veterans Affairs (VA) National Center for Patient Safety and the Leapfrog Group for Patient Safety. The VA National Center for Patient Safety (NCPS) is committed to the reduction of error and improvement of quality through proactive approaches to risk reduction (U.S. Department of Veterans Affairs, 2004). This is accomplished through focusing on prevention, creating nonpunitive environments, and conducting safety research through such concepts as human factors analysis and studying High Reliability Organizations (HROs) in other industries such as aviation and nuclear energy. The VA has created numerous educational programs

through the NCPS and freely shares them with all health care providers who want to learn about health care safety tools and techniques. They have taken the lead in adopting the tools and methodology of health care Failure Modes Effects and Criticality Analysis (FMECA) described later in this section.

The Leapfrog Group for Patient Safety was founded by the Business Roundtable (an association of Fortune 500 CEOs) and consists of more than 150 public and private organizations that provide health care benefits (The Leapfrog Group for Patient Safety, 2004). This coalition is committed to the identification of health care risks and the adoption of proven strategies to reduce these risks and improve care. Their purpose is to create an incentive for providers to make "leaps" in improving quality and reducing errors by adopting these proven strategies. Their plan is to reward those that make "leaps" with monetary incentives. The Leapfrog Group has influenced regulators and accrediting bodies in sharpening their focus on health care safety.

Nurse managers can personally create an environment that is devoted to health care safety by doing the following:

- Learning the concepts and tools related to risk identification, analysis, and error reduction
- Adopting and embracing the concept of non-punitive error reporting
- Advocating for the establishment of a non-punitive culture if it is not currently a strong ideal within the organization
- Encouraging staff to be constantly vigilant in identifying potential risks in the environment
- Creating a sense of partnership with patients and families in order to promote communication about safety concerns and suggestions to correct and prevent potential risks
- Becoming a role model for staff and peers in practicing health care safety concepts

Sentinel Events

One element included in the JCAHO standards for both the Leadership and Performance Improvement chapters addresses a key component in health care safety—that of the organizational response to sentinel events. A sentinel event is defined by JCAHO as follows:

> ... an unexpected occurrence involving death or serious physical or psychological injury, or the risk thereof. Serious injury specifically includes loss of limb or function. The phrase "or the risk thereof" includes any process variation for which a recurrence would carry a significant chance of a serious adverse outcome. Such events are called "sentinel" because they signal the need for immediate investigation and response. (JCAHO, 2005, p. 1)

In 1999, JCAHO began requiring health care organizations to respond to sentinel events in a systematic and formal way (i.e., expecting that a Root Cause Analysis [RCA] be conducted by the staff involved with the event). Timeframes for concluding this analysis and guidelines for

conducting a "credible" process were outlined in the standards. Organizations not familiar with the quality tools for conducting RCAs (primarily flow-charting and cause-and-effect diagramming) had to learn them quickly. The purpose of the RCA is to "drill down" to the most common cause(s) for the event and to determine what process improvements can be made to prevent the sentinel event from occurring in the future. Controversy over whether a sentinel event was reportable to JCAHO, and what information could be shared with the accreditor from a risk management and legal perspective, resulted in the creation of a number of alternatives for submission of the required RCAs. The detailed requirements for reporting and submitting RCAs are contained in the Sentinel Event policy and can be found on the JCAHO website (*www.jcaho.org*). Some specific sentinel event outcomes are considered "reviewable" by JCAHO. Reviewable sentinel events are events that have resulted in an unanticipated death or major permanent loss of function, not related to the natural course of the patient's illness or underlying condition, or one of the following events (even if the outcome was not death or major permanent loss of function, not related to the natural course of the patient's illness or underlying condition):

- Suicide of any individual receiving care, treatment, or services in a staffed round-the-clock setting or within 72 hours of discharge
- Unanticipated death of a full-term infant
- Abduction of any individual receiving care, treatment, or services
- Rape
- Hemolytic transfusion reaction involving administration of blood or blood products having major blood group incompatibilities
- Surgery on the wrong patient or wrong body part (JCAHO, 2005, p. 1)

Organizations that have initiated comprehensive and robust health care safety programs are committed to the process of ongoing risk identification and prevention. These organizations will encourage the staff to identify potential errors and report any "near misses" that occur.

They will conduct RCAs on these identified risks in order to prevent a sentinel event from occurring.

The JCAHO accreditation standards also now require that organizations go a step beyond the RCA process in their health care risk reduction and management programs. They expect that, at least annually, a formal process of Failure Modes Effects and Criticality Analysis (FMECA) will be performed on one identified high-risk process. The leaders of the organization are expected to select the process for study and provide the necessary resources for its successful completion. The FMECA is conducted by an interdisciplinary team of professionals who own the process being studied. The FMECA team is facilitated by someone with knowledge and skills in quality improvement tools. The FMECA process starts with flowcharting the steps of the process being studied. The team assesses risk points within the process steps. The key risk points are identified through a ranking of the importance of each step of the process on the potential failure of the system and the corresponding criticality score associated with that failure. The team then "designs out" the most critical of the potential failures and recommends process improvements for prevention of the failures. Once these prevention strategies are identified, action plans for implementing them are reported to the enterprise leaders and endorsed for implementation (see the VA National Center for Patient Safety website for a detailed description of the Healthcare Failure Mode and Effects Analysis [HFMEA™] at *www.patientsafety.gov/HFMEA.html*).

National Patient Safety Goals

Since the late 1990s JCAHO has been collecting data on sentinel events and the outcomes of their RCAs for the purpose of sharing those data with health care organizations in order to prevent similar events from occurring. These were published by JCAHO in a series of newsletters entitled *Sentinel Event Alerts*. These *Sentinel Event Alerts* addressed events such as wrong-sided surgery, infant abduction, infection control issues, fires,

and medication error events, among others. At the time of this publication, 28 *Sentinel Event Alerts* have been published. The original intent of these alerts was for health care organizations to review the "lessons learned" from those facilities that had experienced these sentinel events and to incorporate the recommendations for prevention contained in each alert. This process was entirely voluntary and initially not tied to the accreditation process. However, certain sentinel events continued to plague the health care industry (such as wrong-sided surgery and the frequency of certain deadly medication errors). With the creation of the health care safety accreditation standards, the impact of the IOM report and the industrywide emphasis on error prevention as a backdrop, JCAHO formalized the information contained in their sentinel event database into a new accreditation standard.

In 2002, JCAHO's Board of Commissioners approved an initial list of six National Patient Safety Goals (NPSGs) that comprised the most commonly occurring and/or serious events from the sentinel event database and from the recommendations of an interdisciplinary task force. Each goal had evidence-based or expert-based recommendations to define how to successfully implement the goal. These new NPSGs went into effect in January 2003 and were included as a component of the accreditation process. JCAHO's plan is that the goals will be reevaluated annually by the Board. New goals will be added to the list if necessary, and/or existing goals may be replaced with new goals that have become more relevant (e.g., the list of 2004 NPSGs includes the addition of a goal on Infection Control). Each accredited organization must demonstrate compliance with all applicable NPSG recommendations during the time of their accreditation survey.

Health Care Risk Management

Risk management is defined as "an interdisciplinary process designed to protect the financial assets of the organization and to maintain high-quality medical care" (Velianoff & Hobbs, 1998, p. 91).

Risk management as a leadership and care management concept is different from the client outcomes concept of risk adjustment, in which differences among clients or variables such as age or disease severity are weighted or adjusted for in outcomes analyses or benchmarking efforts (Maas & Kerr, 1999).

Risk management is an integral component of an organization's quality improvement and health care safety programs. A *risk management program* is defined as an organization-wide program to identify risks, control occurrences, prevent damage, and control legal liability; it is a process whereby risks to the institution are evaluated and controlled. The term has been used in health care since the 1970s, triggered by the quality assurance movement and malpractice claims.

Risk management is a process whereby risks to the institution are evaluated and controlled to reduce or *prevent future loss.* Prior to the advent of comprehensive performance improvement and health care safety programs, one of the primary purposes of risk management was to prevent financial loss resulting from malpractice claims. JCAHO has traditionally required a risk management program for the entire organization as a part of its quality improvement efforts. Because a risk management program is structured to identify, analyze, and evaluate risks, these programs have now been incorporated as key components in organization-wide health care safety and PI programs. A risk manager is one of the "first responders" in a serious or sentinel event situation. Risk managers should facilitate the process by which the organization's definition of risk categories is established (i.e., what constitutes a "near miss," what is reportable on an incident report, what is included in the organizational definition of sentinel event). A new concept called "enterprise risk management" addresses the evaluation of all risks confronting an organization in order to maximize safety and risk reduction. The idea is to prevent undesirable events from happening and to minimize the impact of unpreventable risks. This concept dovetails with the overall requirements of a comprehensive approach to health care safety.

Risk management focuses on overall processes to reduce the causes and frequency of untoward or lawsuit-potential events. If an adverse event occurs, risk management personnel work to reduce the severity and impact of a financial loss (Velianoff & Hobbs, 1998). Risk managers are called on to respond to adverse events and perform the following functions:

- Assess the situation for ongoing risk potential and take measures to prevent further risk or damage from occurring
- Ensure that patients and staff are removed from immediate threat
- Secure/sequester any equipment, supplies, documents, or other elements involved with the event and take them out of service as applicable/appropriate
- Investigate the facts and circumstance of the event
- Determine whether the event meets the definition of "sentinel event" or whether it meets another risk category definition
- Make reports as needed/required to appropriate outside agencies or regulators
- Communicate with the patient, family and staff involved in the event
- Communicate with administrative and clinical leaders and legal counsel as appropriate
- If necessary, organize the first meeting of the clinical team to conduct the RCA of the sentinel event
- Ensure that follow-up to recommendations for improvement/prevention are implemented
- Collect data on the event and incorporate it into the organization's risk management database

Risk managers coordinate activities such as administering insurance coverage and risk financing, managing claims, collaborating with legal counsel, administering the risk management operations, analyzing the risk management database, conducting in-service training and education, communicating risk management information, and monitoring ongoing compliance to state, federal, and local regulations and laws (such as the Emergency Medical Treatment and Active Labor Act of 1986 [EMTALA] and the

Health Insurance Portability and Accountability Act [HIPAA]).

As a tool for ongoing risk identification and reporting, *incident reports* form the core of organizational reporting from a risk-management perspective. The purpose of an incident report is to provide a factual accounting of an incident or adverse event to ensure that all facts surrounding the incident are recorded. A successful incident-reporting process is one in which 100% of all appropriate incidents/adverse outcomes are reported to the risk manager. This goal is more apt to be achieved in those organizations that have adopted a nonpunitive culture for reporting errors. The data contained in an incident report also alerts the risk manager about facts and circumstances that may contribute to a potential malpractice or lawsuit claim. The incident-reporting system provides the risk manager with the opportunity to investigate all serious situations immediately. Data from incident reports are collated, analyzed, and utilized by leadership to identify risk areas that have ongoing trends or to point to areas that have emerging risk potential. Aggregated data from the organization's health care risk management program are reported through the performance improvement and health care safety reporting systems in order to coordinate information about overall organizational risks.

Clearly, health care quality has been an accountability of nurses since the profession's inception. Over the years, nurses have assumed roles in various health care settings for oversight of quality and performance improvement, as well as health care risk management. The recent IOM reports only served to bring to public awareness the lack of standardization in processes and public data reporting. These were issues that have challenged health care quality professionals and nurse managers for decades. With a heightened awareness and funding by the federal government, health care organizations are attempting to adopt cultures of quality and safety. Professional nurses, in direct care, managerial, and executive roles, will continue to be at the forefront of continuously enhancing the quality of care and

services provided to patients/clients, families, and communities.

Summary

- Quality and safety are key dimensions of health care.
- Nurses are key players in ensuring the delivery of evidence-based quality health care.
- Health care quality is an art and science that continues to evolve.
- Quality management and performance improvement are an organization's efforts to provide services according to accepted professional standards and in a manner acceptable to various organizational stakeholders.
- Nurses have a professional responsibility to be accountable for quality of care and health outcomes at all levels and contribute to continuous improvement of the health care system.
- Health care professionals can use an identifiable model of Plan, Do, Check, Act (PDCA) to explore causes of variation in work processes.
- Nurse managers are cautioned not to first create new standards and measures; rather, a literature review often will reveal valid and reliable measures.
- Six Sigma and Lean Enterprise are emerging quality measurement models being applied to health care.
- A quality improvement program should pervade the entire organization, and continuous improvement should be a part of everyone's job.
- Performance standards are critically important and are the first step of a quality improvement program.
- Evaluation is based on mutually agreed-on performance standards and goal setting.
- Structure, process, and outcomes are types of performance standards.
- Mission, vision, and core value statements are the foundation on which an organization builds a quality infrastructure.

- Accreditation standards formed the basis for some of the first mandatory requirements for outcome measurement reporting (e.g., ORYX® and HEDIS® measures).
- Public reporting of process and outcome measures are the wave of the future, and all health care organizations will be required to participate in these public reporting arenas.
- Patient safety programs are now a key component and focus of quality initiatives in health care organizations.
- The organization's leaders should establish the expectation that the entire organization, as well as patients and their families, should be involved in the identification of potential or actual errors.
- Risk management is an extension of quality improvement.
- A risk management program is an organization-wide program to identify risks, control occurrences, prevent damage, and control legal liability.
- There are certain known risk-prone areas in health care and known ways of preventing errors.
- High performance organizations (HPOs) employ creative and improvisational problem solving.
- A nonpunitive culture promotes error reporting.

Study Questions

1. Who is responsible for quality management?
2. What are the differences between institutional and professional responsibilities for quality? Why does this occur?
3. How is quality defined? How is it measured?
4. List and describe four tenets embraced by members of the Institute of Medicine's Committee on Quality of Health Care in America. How are these incorporated in nursing practice?
5. Why is it important to have standardized performance measures?
6. Describe JCAHO's National Patient Safety Goals. Pick one safety goal and describe how it has been implemented in your organization.

7. List four ways nurse managers can personally create an environment that is devoted to health care safety.
8. What is a FMECA, and how does it contribute to improving patient safety?
9. Describe strategies that a nurse manager can employ to avoid or prevent a sentinel event from occurring in his or her areas of responsibility.
10. List at least one public reporting system to which your organization submits data. Describe the outcomes from one of these measures.

CASE STUDY

Nurse Katharine Lauren has been asked by senior leadership to spearhead a group to evaluate patient falls in order to decrease their frequency and ideally prevent them from occurring. Based on the risk management data available, she selects nurses and nurse's aides for her team from the four patient care units in which patient falls are most prevalent. She adds a pharmacist and physician to her team to represent the pharmaceutical and medical care aspects of the issue. Nurse Lauren then applies the PDCA process (Plan, Do, Check, and Act) to her project on patient falls.

In the "Plan" phase, she and the team utilize flowcharting to visually illustrate the steps that occur when a patient falls. Next, the team brainstorms a list of all of the problems that are associated with a patient fall. From this list, Nurse Lauren directs the team to categorize these factors into five to six groups, utilizing an affinity diagram. Once the categories are defined, the team uses a cause-and-effect (fishbone) diagram to identify all of the potential causes that lead to the eventual effect of a patient fall. From this fishbone diagram, specific factors are considered as potential root causes—for example, bedrails too high, patient confusion, slippery floors, inappropriate medication dosages, independent ambulation, and the patient trying to use the bathroom alone when the call bell is not answered promptly.

Nurse Lauren suggests collecting more data on each of these potential root causes. She further suggests that the data be stratified by patient age and gender, time of day, patient diagnoses, patient location, and staffing. She and the team design a data collection tool that will allow all of the data to be collected on one form.

After the data are collected, the team uses a Pareto Chart to visually illustrate the most frequently occurring problems in descending order. By using this technique, they find that call bells not answered promptly and bedrails too high are the factors that occur most frequently in patient falls. They also use Pareto Charts to further define the stratification categories. When using this tool, they find that women over 75 years of age with postoperative hip surgery seem most likely to fall on the evening shift. Most of the occurrences are on 4 South (the postsurgical unit).

During the "Do" phase, Nurse Lauren and the team design an assessment tool for the 4 South staff that collects data on all of the key factors identified earlier. As a trial, however, only the rooms of those female post-op hip surgery patients over age 65 are designated with a special symbol created by the team to represent a Fall Risk. Stickers with this symbol are also put on the call bell system lights for these rooms. Staff members are educated to the issue regarding quick call bell response and are requested to be especially vigilant in responding to the rooms with the special stickers. The data are collected for a 4-week trial period.

In the "Check" phase, the team reconvenes to evaluate the data collected in the trial. The data demonstrate a 37% reduction in patient falls from the same month in the previous year (and this was just from addressing call bell response alone).

Because the data on a sole factor demonstrated such a clear improvement, the team proceeds with development of a fall protocol, incorporating action plans to address the other key factors identified earlier. The trial is expanded to another unit. When the data are analyzed for these two units and compared with the two other units with high fall occurrences, it is clear to the team that the protocol is having a positive impact on patient fall reduction. Throughout the process, nursing staff on the two trial units are solicited for feedback on the project, and their recommendations are incorporated into the protocol.

In the "Act" phase, the new Fall Prevention Protocol is adopted. Prior to its official "launch" in the organization, physicians, pharmacists, and nursing personnel are educated on the protocol. Data are collected not only on the outcomes but also on compliance with the steps of the protocol. After 3 months, the data demonstrate that those units with the lowest frequency of falls were those that had adopted the new protocol with enthusiasm and commitment. Nurse Lauren shares the data with the Nursing Leadership group, using control charts to demonstrate the outcomes. Based on the results, and in consultation with the risk manager and the Performance Improvement Council, the group expands the definition of Fall Risk to include those patients who experienced a "near miss" (i.e., a fall in which the patient was assisted when falling and did not reach the floor). Data will now be collected on these patient occurrences and on their contributing factors. In so doing, leadership believes that overall patient safety can be further enhanced. Nurse Lauren and her team receive an award at the hospital's annual Quality Day for contributing to improved patient care outcomes.

REFERENCES

American Nurses Association (ANA). (2001). *Code of ethics for nurses with interpretive statements.* Washington, DC: American Nurses Association.

Bassett, S. (1998). Continuous quality improvement (CQI) principles. In S.A. Price, M.W. Koch, & S. Bassett (Eds.), *Health care resource management: Present and future challenges* (pp. 41-63). St Louis: Mosby.

Berwick, D.M., Godfrey, A.B., & Roessner, J. (1990). *Curing health care: New strategies for quality improvement.* San Francisco: Jossey-Bass.

Bohnet, N., Ilcyn, J., Milanovich, P., Ream, M., & Wright, K. (1993). Continuous quality improvement: Improving quality in your home care organization. *Journal of Nursing Administration, 23*(2), 42-48.

Carey, R.G., & Lloyd, R.C. (1995). *Measuring quality improvement in health care: A guide to statistical process control applications.* New York: Quality Resources.

Chassin, M.R. (1997). Assessing strategies for quality improvement. *Health Affairs, 16,* 151-161.

Chrvala, C.A., & Bulger, R.J. (Eds.). (1999). *Leading health indicators for Healthy People 2010: Final Report.* Washington, DC: National Academies Press.

Commonwealth of Pennsylvania, Pennsylvania Health Care Cost Containment Council (HCCCC). (2004). *About the council: Mission.* Harrisburg, PA: Pennsylvania HCCCC. Retrieved June 30, 2004, from *www.phc4.org/council/aboutthe.htm*

Corrigan, J.M., Eden, J., & Smith, B.M. (Eds.). (2002). *Leadership by example: Coordinating government roles in improving health care quality.* Washington, DC: National Academies Press.

Dahlberg, A.W., Connell, D.W., & Landrum, J. (1997). Building a health company-For the long term. In F. Hesselbein, M. Goldsmith, & R. Beckhard (Eds.), *The organization of the future* (pp. 359-366). San Francisco: Jossey-Bass.

Deming, W. Edwards. (2000a). *The new economics for industry, government, education.* Cambridge, MA: MIT Center for Advanced Engineering Studies.

Deming, W. Edwards. (2000b). *Out of the crisis.* Cambridge, MA: MIT Center for Advanced Engineering Studies.

Donabedian, A. (1980). *Explorations in quality assessment and monitoring: The definition of quality and approaches to its assessment* (Vol. 1). Ann Arbor, MI: Health Administration Press.

Donaldson, M.S., & Mohr, J.J. (Eds.). (2000). Exploring *innovation and quality improvement in health care micro-systems.* Washington, DC: National Academies Press.

Durch, J.S., Bailey, L.A., & Stoto, M.A. (Eds.). (1997). *Improving health in the community: A role for performance monitoring.* Washington, DC: National Academies Press.

Foundation for Accountability (FACCT). (2002). *Supporting quality-based decisions.* New York: FACCT (now The Markle Foundation). Retrieved March 7, 2002, from *www.facct.org/*

Hamill, C.T., & Luchok, J. (1999). Best practices: A necessity in modern health care. *The Case Manager, 10*(5), 23.

Harmon, F. G. (1997). Future present. In F. Hesselbein, M. Goldsmith, & R. Beckhard (Eds.), *The organization of the future* (pp. 239-247). San Francisco: Jossey-Bass.

Harry, M., & Schroeder, R. (2000). *Six sigma: The breakthrough strategy revolutionizing the world's top corporations.* New York: Currency/Doubleday.

Hesselbein, F., & Johnston, R. (2002). *A leader-to-leader guide: On high-performance performance organizations.* San Francisco: Jossey-Bass.

His Holiness the Dalai Lama & Cutler, H.C. (1998). *The art of happiness.* New York: Riverhead Books.

Hyde, P.S., Falls, K., Morris, J.A., Schoenwald, S.A. (2003). *Turning knowledge into practice: A manual for behavioral health administrators and practitioners about understanding and implementing evidence-based practices.* Boston, MA: The Technical Assistance Collaborative.

Institute for Healthcare Improvement (IHI). (2004). *About IHI.* Boston, IHI. Retrieved June 30, 2004, from *www.ihi.org/about/*

Institute of Medicine (IOM), Committee on Enhancing Federal Healthcare Quality Programs, (2002). *Project description.* Washington, DC: National Academies Press. Retrieved October 30, 2002, from *www.iom.edu/iom/iomhome.nsf/pages/Fed+Qual+Home?OpenDocument*

Institute of Medicine (IOM), Committee on Health Care Quality in America (CQHCA). (2001). *Crossing the quality chasm: A new health system for the 21st century.* Washington, DC: National Academies Press.

Institute of Medicine (IOM), Committee on the National Quality Report on Health Care Delivery. (2001). M.P. Hurtado, E.K. Swift, & J.M. Corrigan (Eds.). *Envisioning the national health care report.* Washington, DC: National Academies Press.

International Organization for Standardization (ISO). (2003). *ISO 9000 and ISO 14000—In brief* [Online]. Geneva, Switzerland: ISO. Retrieved June 30, 2004, from *www.iso.ch/iso/en/iso9000-14000/index.html*

Joint Commission on Accreditation of Healthcare Organizations (JCAHO). (1998). *Glossary of terms for performance measurement.* Oakbrook Terrace, IL: JCAHO. Retrieved January 11, 2005, from *www.jcaho.org/accredited+organizations/behavioral+health+care/oryx/glossary+of+terms/glossary.htm*

Joint Commission on Accreditation of Healthcare Organizations (JCAHO). (1999). *Attributes of core performance measures and associated evaluation criteria.* Oakbrook Terrace, IL: JCAHO. Retrieved January 11, 2005, from *www.jcaho.org/pms/core+measures/attributes+of+core+performance+measures.htm*

Joint Commission on Accreditation of Healthcare Organizations (JCAHO). (2005). *Sentinel event policy and procedures updated: March 2005.* Oakbrook Terrace, IL: JCAHO. Retrieved May 5, 2005, from *www.jcaho.org/accredited+organizations/sentinel+event/se_pp.htm*

Jones, D., & Womack, J. (2003). *Lean thinking: Banish waste and create wealth in your corporation, revised and updated.* New York: Free Press.

Juran, J.M. (1989). *Juran on leadership for quality: An executive handbook.* New York: The Free Press.

Katz, J.M., & Green, E. (1997). *Managing quality: A guide to system-wide performance management in health care* (2nd ed.). St Louis: Mosby.

Kohn, L.T., Corrigan, J.M., & Donaldson, M.S. (Eds.). (2000). *To err is human: Building a safer health care system.* Washington, DC: National Academies Press.

Lohr, K. (Ed.). (1990). *Medicare: A strategy for quality assurance, Volume 2.* Washington, DC: National Academies Press.

Maas, M.L., & Kerr, P. (1999). Risk adjustment in nursing effectiveness research. *Outcomes Management for Nursing Practice, 3*(2), 50-52.

Marcus, L.J., Dorn, B.C., Kritek, P.B., Miller, V.G., & Wyatt, J.B. (1995). *Renegotiating health care: Resolving conflict to build collaboration.* San Francisco: Jossey Bass.

Martin, K. (2003). On lean enterprise and its potential health care applications [Editorial]. *Journal for Healthcare Quality, 25*(5), 2, 43.

Mayo Clinic. (2004a). *General information about Mayo Clinic: Mission.* Rochester, MN: May Clinic. Retrieved June 9, 2004, from *www.mayoclinic.org/about/*

Mayo Clinic. (2004b). *Mayo's mission, primary value, core principles.* Rochester, MN: Mayo Clinic. Retrieved June 9, 2004, from *www.mayoclinic.org/about/missionvalues.html*

Miller, S., & Flanagan, E. (1993). The transition from quality assurance to continuous quality improvement in ambulatory care. *Quality Review Bulletin, 19*(2), 62-65.

National Committee for Quality Assurance (NCQA). (2000). *Desirable attributes of HEDIS measures* (HEDIS 2001, Vol. 1). Washington, DC: NCQA. Retrieved January 11, 2005, from *www.ncqa.org/Programs/HEDIS/desirable%20attributes.html*

Omenn, G. (2002). *Public briefing: Opening statement: Leadership by example: Coordinating government roles in improving health care quality.* Presented at the Institute of Medicine, Washington, DC, October 30, 2002.

O'Neil, E.H., & the Pew Health Professions Commission (PHPC). (1998). *Recreating health professional practice for a new century: The fourth report of the Pew Health Professions Commission.* San Francisco: PHPC.

Palmer, S., & Torgerson, D.J. (1999). Definition of efficiency. *British Medical Journal, 318,* 1136.

Pelletier, L.R. (1998). Guest editorial. *Journal of Nursing Care Quality, 13*(1), vii.

Pelletier, L.R. (1999a). Editorial: On strategic planning. *Journal for Healthcare Quality, 21*(3), 2, 17.

Pelletier, L.R. (1999b). Editorial: On values and achievements. *Journal for Healthcare Quality, 21*(6), 2, 10-11.

Pelletier, L.R. (2000). Editorial: On error-free health care: Mission possible! *Journal for Healthcare Quality, 22*(3), 2, 9.

Pelletier, L.R., & Hoffman, J.A. (2002). A framework for selecting performance measures for opioid treatment programs. *Journal for Healthcare Quality, 24*(3), 24-35.

Pfizer. (2004). *Mission statement.* New York: Pfizer. Retrieved June 8, 2004, from *www.pfizer.com/are/mn_about_mission.html*

Plsek, P., & Omnias, A. (1989). *Juran institute quality improvement tools: Problem solving/glossary.* Wilton, CT: Juran Institute, Inc.

President's Advisory Commission on Consumer Protection and Quality in the Health Care Industry. (1998). *Quality first: Better health care for all Americans.* Washington, DC: Government Printing Office.

Quality Interagency Task Force (QuIC). (1999). *Fact Sheet. Quality Interagency Coordination Task Force (QuIC).* Rockville, MD: QuIC. Retrieved June 8, 2003, from *www.quic.gov/about/quicfact.htm*

Quality Interagency Task Force (QuIC). (2000). *Doing what counts for patient safety: Federal actions to reduce medical errors and their impact. Report of the Quality Interagency Task Force (QuIC) to the President of the United States.* Rockville, MD: QuIC. Retrieved June 8, 2004, from *www.quic.gov/report/errors6.pdf*

Sackett, D.L., Rosenberg, W.M.C., Gray, J.A.M., Haynes, R.B., & Richardson, W.S. (1996). Evidence-based medicine: What it is and what it isn't. *British Medical Journal, 312*(7023), 71.

Smith, G.R., Manderscheid, R.W., Flynn, L.M., & Steinwachs, D.M. (1997). Principles of assessment for patient outcomes in mental health care. *Psychiatric Services, 48,* 1033-1036.

The Commonwealth Fund. (2004). *First report and recommendations of The Commonwealth Fund's International Working Group on Quality Indicators.* New York: The Commonwealth Fund. Retrieved June 8, 2004, from *www.cmwf.org*

The Leapfrog Group for Patient Safety. (2004). *About us.* Washington, DC: Leapfrog Group for Patient Safety. Retrieved June 30, 2004, from *www.leapfroggroup.org/*

The White House. (2000). Press Release: *Clinton-Gore Administration announces new actions to improve patient safety and assure health care quality.* Washington, DC: The White House. Retrieved January 11, 2005, from *www.clinton5.nara gov/WH/New/html/20000222_1.html*

Triolo, P. (1994). TQM/CQI: What is it? Does it work? In J. McCloskey & H. Grace (Eds.), *Current issues in nursing* (4th ed.) (pp. 321-326), St. Louis: Mosby.

U.K. Department of Health. (2002). *NHS performance indicators: February 2002.* London: U.K. Department of Health. Retrieved March 7, 2002, from *www.doh.gov.uk/nhsperformanceindicators/2002/index.html*

U.S. Department of Health and Human Services (USDHHS), Centers for Medicare and Medicaid Services (CMS). (2004a). *Hospital quality initiative: Fact sheet: Building on the foundation, hospital measures for public reporting.* Baltimore: CMS. Retrieved June 30, 2004, from *www.cms.hhs.gov/quality/hospital/*

U.S. Department of Health and Human Services (USDHHS), Centers for Medicare and Medicaid Services (CMS). (2004b). *Medicare quality improvement organization program: Summary of proposed 8th scope of work: May 13, 2004.* Baltimore: CMS. Retrieved June 30, 2004, from *www.cms.hhs.gov/qio/2s.pdf*

U.S. Department of Veterans Affairs. (2004). *The VA National Center for Patient Safety.* Ann Arbor, MI: VA National Center for Patient Safety. Retrieved June 30, 2004, from *www.patientsafety.gov/index.html*

Velianoff, G.D., & Hobbs, D.K. (1998). Designing a patient care risk management system. In J.A. Dienemann (Ed.), *Nursing administration: Managing patient care* (2nd ed.) (pp. 91-99). Stamford, CT: Appleton & Lange.

Ward, B. (2004). *The five key facets of high performance leadership,* Edmonton, Alberta, Canada: Affinity Consulting. Retrieved June 30, 2004, from *www.affinitymc.com/Five_Facets_of_Leadership.htm*

White, S.V. (2003). Interview with a quality leader: Sister Mary Jean Ryan on the first Baldrige award in health care. *Journal for Healthcare Quality, 25*(3), 24-25.

Yale New Haven Health. (2001). *About Yale-New Haven Health System: Our vision.* New Haven, CT: Yale New Haven Health. Retrieved June 9, 2004, from *www.yalenewhavenhealth.org/s_about/healthsys.html*

40 Measuring and Managing Outcomes

Diane L. Huber

CHAPTER OBJECTIVES

- Create a framework for understanding outcomes
- Define and describe outcomes, indicators, outcomes measurement, and outcomes management
- Express the need for outcomes studies
- Trace the development of outcomes measurement
- Inventory outcome measurement systems sensitive to nursing care
- Illustrate current trends in outcomes measures for quality health care management
- Exercise critical thinking to conceptualize and analyze possible solutions to a practice exercise

Outcomes research seeks to understand the end results of particular health care practices and interventions. End results include effects that people experience and care about, such as change in the ability to function. In particular, for individuals with chronic conditions—where cure is not always possible—end results include quality of life as well as mortality. By linking the care people get to the outcomes they experience, outcomes research has become the key to developing better ways to monitor and improve the quality of care (Agency for Healthcare Research and Quality [AHRQ], 2004, p. 1).

Nurses have always had an outcomes focus. Although her work is not generally recognized in this way, Florence Nightingale pioneered the systematic use of client outcomes in the form of mortality data that demonstrated the use of interventions to improve health care. Using data collection and analysis and care process improvement techniques specific to nursing care, she reduced the mortality rate in a military hospital in the Crimea from 60% to 1% (Kalisch & Kalisch, 1978). Because of this, Nightingale can be considered to be the founder of nursing outcomes measurement and management.

In today's environment, outcomes measurement and management is an imperative for nurses. This is because it is not sufficient to demonstrate that the proper process was followed in the delivery of health care services. More is demanded. Consumers, employers, and payers expect to see the evidence of appropriate and positive outcomes of care. The measurement and management of care outcomes results in evidence to demonstrate the effectiveness, efficiency, and equity of the efforts and actions of both providers and health systems.

In the 1990s there was a change in the norm for health care and the manner in which nursing care was delivered. The changes resulted from the pressure to control health care costs while still demonstrating that quality care was being provided to health care consumers. The evolving managed care approach in health care delivery generated pressures of cost and competition, which in turn engendered consumer demand for changes in health care industry norms. The measurement of client and family outcomes is one way to satisfy that consumer demand to know whether clients are benefiting from the health care they are provided. At the same time the process allows institutions to measure the quality of care that is being provided: "A focus on patient outcomes may help nurses survive an unstable job market; maintain or improve the quality of the care they provide; better inform health care consumers; and ensure that their perspective regarding outcomes management is represented, both in their organizations and in national studies" (Oermann & Huber, 1999, p. 40).

DEFINITIONS

The key terms related to outcomes and their measurement and management are *outcomes, indicators, outcomes measurement, outcomes management,* and *benchmarking.* A variety of sources exist for defining these terms, from theorists and the literature to governmental and accrediting agencies. A simple definition of an **outcome** is the result or results obtained from the efforts to accomplish a goal (Huber & Oermann, 1998). To most nurses, outcomes refer to the consequences of an intervention or treatment. The term *outcomes* has been defined as "end results, or that which results from something" (Lang & Marek, 1990, p. 158) and as conditions to be achieved (Peters, 1995). Donabedian (1985) described outcomes as changes in the actual or potential health status of individuals, groups, or communities.

Indicators are defined as "valid and reliable measures related to performance" (Oermann & Huber, 1999, p. 41). The observing, describing, and quantifying of indicators of outcomes is the way in which outcomes are measured. Indicators are used as measures of all three of Donabedian's (1985) aspects of quality: structure, process, and outcomes. (Chapter 39 provides further information about Donabedian's framework.)

Because quality is so important yet so elusive to define, a variety of accrediting or regulating bodies and related health care quality assessment organizations have developed standardized health care performance indicator data sets. For example, the American Nurses Association (ANA) (2004) has the National Database of Nursing Quality Indicators (NDNQI) based on their Nursing Quality Indicators initiative (ANA, 1996, 2004). Outcome measures or indicators, according to the ANA, measure how nursing care is affecting clients. The ANA list included elements such as the measurement of urinary tract infection incidents after 72 hours of hospitalization as an indicator of nosocomial infection rate. Furthermore, the ANA suggested the measurement of responses to a uniform series of questions as indicative of client satisfaction. The evaluation of the nature and amount of care provided to clients by nurses can be reviewed through process indicators such as pressure ulcers. Structure indicators such as the mix of registered nurses (RNs), licensed practical

◣ LEADING & MANAGING **DEFINED**

Outcomes

The result(s) obtained from the efforts to accomplish a goal.

Indicators

Valid and reliable measures related to performance.

Outcomes Measurement

Determining the indicators, gathering necessary data, analyzing that data, interpreting the results,

making changes in nursing care, and evaluating effectiveness.

Outcomes Management

A multidisciplinary process designed to provide quality health care, decrease fragmentation, enhance outcomes, and constrain costs.

nurses (LPNs), and unlicensed nurse extenders caring for clients can assess the delivery and organization of nursing care. These can be measured by the full-time equivalent (FTE) ratio of RNs with direct care responsibilities to LPNs and unlicensed assistive staff.

Other national quality indicator databases include the ORYX® initiative by the Joint Commission on Accreditation of Healthcare Organizations (JCAHO, 2004a, 2004b). A part of JCAHO's Agenda for Change was the integration of performance measurement data into the accreditation process through ORYX®. The National Committee for Quality Assurance (NCQA) accredits managed care and other health plans (NCQA, 2004). Its indicator measurement system is the Health Plan Employer Data and Information Set (HEDIS®, 2005). Each data set and its tools are continually being refined and updated. (See Chapter 39 for further information on quality measurement initiatives.)

To evaluate outcomes states as reflected by important indicators, outcomes need to be measured. **Outcomes measurement** can be defined as measuring the results of care (Nadzam, 1997). A more complete definition is "determining the indicators, gathering necessary data, analyzing that data, interpreting the results, making changes in nursing care, and evaluating effectiveness. Through outcomes studies, specific nursing interventions and treatment protocols can be examined and relevant questions answered" (Oermann & Huber, 1999, p. 41).

Measurement involves the utilization of scientific inquiry and problem solving. The process of measuring outcomes involves first determining the key elements or indicators (those measures that are of interest); then, after the appropriate data have been gathered, the data are aggregated and analyzed. Following interpretation of the results, changes are made and the process begins anew with the measurement of the key elements and evaluation of the effectiveness of the changes that were incorporated. Intrinsic to outcomes management is the use of the information gathered from analysis of collected data to improve the

nursing care delivery toward achievement of the ideal (Huber & Oermann, 1998).

A related term is *outcomes monitoring*, which refers to ongoing surveillance. Outcomes measurement, which is data analysis related to indicators, is distinguished from outcomes monitoring, which involves repeated quantification of outcomes data based on trend observation and benchmarking of the indicators.

Outcomes management is a process that is distinct from *outcomes measurement*. Outcomes can be disciplinary or multidisciplinary and can be related to the clinician provider, the client, the system, or some combination of these. However, for outcomes management in health care, the multidisciplinary aspect is emphasized. Since care provision is complex and requires input from many sources, the most comprehensive way to manage outcomes is to adopt the multidisciplinary perspective. **Outcomes management** is defined as "a multidisciplinary process designed to provide quality health care, decrease fragmentation, enhance outcomes, and constrain costs. The core idea of outcomes management is the use of process activities to improve outcomes" (Huber & Oermann, 1998, p. 4). In other words, in outcomes management the care process is what is being managed in order to achieve outcomes. This relies on variance analysis. To understand outcomes, the entire care process also needs to be carefully examined because altering the care process is a major strategy to affect outcomes. The process of managing outcomes includes the following five steps:

1. Data are collected about outcomes.
2. Trends are identified from data analysis.
3. Variances are investigated.
4. Appropriate service delivery changes are determined.
5. Changes are implemented and reevaluated.

In managing outcomes, the information derived from measuring client outcomes is collected, trends are identified, variances are examined, and appropriate care needs are determined in order to improve care to an individual, group, or population. Goals of this process include quality improvement and risk reduction. Variance analysis is one outcomes management tool. A variance is a deviation from what is expected. For nurses, this may mean a departure from the anticipated clinical trajectory. Variances may be positive or negative but are most useful for trends analysis.

The term *benchmarking* comes from the concept of a benchmark, which is a surveyor's mark that indicates a point of known height about sea level. Benchmarking draws on predetermined indicators. These indicators are chosen from experience, clinical practice, relevancy, and the evidence base. There is no "gold standard" set of outcomes indicators. Benchmarks offer one standardized point of comparison. *Benchmarking* is defined as a process of continually measuring what exists in one system against what is determined to be the industry's best practice. Best practices are those processes and services that have been refined to produce superior outcomes. Best practices activities generate the benchmarks on key indicators that are used by others to monitor outcomes.

The determination of nursing care effectiveness in improving client outcomes is accomplished through outcomes measurement. The use of outcomes studies enable nurses to determine how to assist clients and their families to understand the client's health needs and care needs at home. Those studies also enable nurses to determine which interventions are most productive in accomplishing the desired improvement in the client's health status. Identifying these most productive interventions can provide invaluable information to enable clients to manage their symptoms and care for themselves (Oermann & Huber, 1997, 1999).

BACKGROUND

The demand for measurement of outcomes was the result of many factors, including the lack of outcomes studies, the need for quantifiable data concerning health care, and variations within medical practice. There has been significant variation, based on geographical area, in medical treatment (Wennberg, 1990). Significant variation in treatment has also been documented based on the care provider involved. Clients question why such differences exist, including why some providers would not perform less invasive and less costly procedures even though they may be just as effective as more invasive and costly procedures.

> The urgent need for outcomes research was highlighted in the early 1980s, when researchers discovered that "geography is destiny." Time and again, studies documented that medical practices as commonplace as hysterectomy and hernia repair were performed much more frequently in some areas than in others, even when there were no differences in the underlying rates of disease. Furthermore, there was often no information about the end results for the patients who received a particular procedure, and few comparative studies existed to show which interventions were most effective. These findings challenged researchers, clinicians, and health systems leaders to develop new tools to assess the impact of health care services. (AHRQ, 2004, p. 1)

The absence of outcomes studies documenting the effectiveness of many nursing care interventions has also led to the demand for outcomes studies. Outcomes studies provide information on which to base decisions about the most effective interventions. The study of client outcomes in light of nursing interventions differs from the controlled environment of research studies. Nursing outcomes studies are conducted in the client care setting since that is where the interventions and outcomes occur. Nursing outcomes studies can provide answers to questions such as the following:

- To best manage clients' symptoms, which nursing treatment will be most productive?
- Will clients be better prepared for diagnostic tests following an existing or proposed protocol?
- Following surgery, which method for teaching clients and families about postoperative care will be the most effective?
- To achieve the most effective clinical and financial outcomes, which clinical pathway should be followed?

Outcomes studies also are being demanded by employers who provide health benefits for their employees. Employers and other payers want to know not only about the costs of the care provided but also about the client outcomes derived from that payment. The absence of outcomes studies in the past means that it is not yet clear exactly what consumers' expectations are where quality of care is concerned. Just as outcomes need to be studied, it will be necessary to study the type of quality information that consumers need to make informed health care decisions, how the presentation of that information can influence their decisions, and how consumers interpret the information provided to them. What is clear, however, is that both employers and consumers expect the highest possible quality for the lowest possible cost. In order to substantiate nursing contributions to high quality and low cost, reliable data must be obtained (Cleary & Edgman-Levitan, 1997; Oermann & Huber, 1999).

DEVELOPMENT OF OUTCOMES MEASUREMENT

Mortality rates were the mainstay of client outcomes data from the time of Nightingale until the early 1960s. Morbidity rates eventually came into use for measuring quality of care. For many years, outcomes were defined as medical outcomes or the results of medical care in terms of palliation, control of illness, cure, or rehabilitation. The classic list of outcomes was death, disease, disability, discomfort, and dissatisfaction (Lohr, 1988). In the late 1980s, the classic Medical Outcomes Study (MOS) framework for medical outcomes was reported (Tarlov et al., 1989). Clinical end points, functional status, general well-being, and satisfaction with care were identified as the outcomes of physician care. Although this is an important framework, the MOS lacks a multidisciplinary perspective and does not address some outcomes that are important and sensitive to nursing care (Kelly et al., 1994).

In the early 1960s Aydelotte (1962) brought about the inclusion of client welfare as an outcome of nursing care. In this new approach—studying nursing care's impact on outcomes—various measurements of outcomes were used, including the following:

- Number of postoperative days
- Dose of medications
- Instruments to measure the client's behavioral characteristics and physical state of health
- Time spent by the client in certain activities

The activity in defining and developing nursing outcomes measurement increased significantly in the 1970s, influenced by a number of important projects. These early-stage projects provided the underpinning for measuring outcomes in nursing that went well beyond the former measurement standards of mortality and morbidity. Early projects in the 1970s included the following:

- JCAHO recommended the use of outcome criteria in nursing audits, highlighting the importance of outcomes.
- Criteria for measuring quality of services were developed by many health care agencies.
- Hover and Zimmer (1978) put forward the following five outcomes for use in measurement of nursing care quality:
  1. Client's knowledge of illness and treatments to be performed
  2. Medications
  3. Skills
  4. Adaptive behaviors
  5. Health status
- Horn and Swain (1978) developed an extensive set of outcomes measures.
- A patient classification system, including five levels of outcomes from recovery to terminal care, was developed by Daubert (1979).

Also in the 1970s the Visiting Nurse Association (VNA) of Omaha contributed to outcomes measurement advancement with the development of the Omaha System. The original intent of the VNA work was to improve its client record system. As part of this improvement a measurement of three outcomes, known as the Problem Rating Scale for Outcomes, was developed. The scale was created to measure the following:

- *Knowledge:* the client's ability to remember and interpret information

- *Behavior:* observable actions, responses, and activities by the client
- *Status:* the client condition in terms of signs and symptoms

From its beginnings in the 1970s, the Omaha System developed and evolved into a practice, documentation, and information management system that is used by home care and public health nurses, as well as other health personnel (Martin & Sheet, 1992).

The 1980s saw the continuation of emphasis on client outcomes measurement as a means of reviewing quality of care. During the same time frame as criteria were being developed for measuring outcomes, other mechanisms were being developed to control expenditures in health care and to ensure the quality of care. The Healthcare Financing Administration (HCFA), now called the Centers for Medicare & Medicaid Services (CMS), put forward an initiative that would measure both effectiveness and appropriateness of health care services provided to Medicare and Medicaid patients, including the development of a large database to review the outcomes of certain treatments. The Agency for Health Care Policy and Research (AHCPR) was created in 1989 with a goal of reviewing the effectiveness of various treatments for medical conditions. It is now called the Agency for Healthcare Research and Quality (AHRQ). Clinical practice guidelines were developed to assist both clients and their care providers in decision making about responses to specific clinical conditions. Also in the 1980s JCAHO changed its agenda and developed outcome indicators that could be used in evaluating the quality of care provided by health care organizations. Those indicators, developed by expert groups (including nurses), were tested extensively and led to the creation of the Indicator Measurement System (IMSystem) (Huber & Oermann, 1998). This later evolved into ORYX.

The nursing profession has continued since the 1980s to develop increasing interest in the measurement of client outcomes as a way to identify the effectiveness of nursing care. More and more studies have been conducted to identify outcomes that are sensitive to nursing care.

A number of these studies took place in the area of home care. Lalonde (1986) identified seven outcome measures for home care clients, Rinke (1988) attempted to categorize outcomes for home health care into five areas, and an outcome-based home care quality assurance program was developed in Alberta, Canada (Sorgen, 1986) (Box 40.1). Shaughnessy and colleagues (1995) conducted extensive research into outcomes measurement for home care. The result of this work was the standardized Outcomes and Assessment Information Set (OASIS). In work conducted in the 1980s and 1990s, the OASIS project became significant in bringing about a partnership between home care agencies and Medicare. This resulted in Medicare's adopting Conditions of Participation requiring that certified home care agencies collect outcomes data through the use of OASIS.

A study done by Marek (1989, 1997) identified outcomes to measure in reviewing the effectiveness of nursing care. The types of outcomes identified by Marek were physiological, psychosocial, functional, behavioral, knowledge, home functioning, family strain, safety, symptom control, quality of life, goal attainment, client satisfaction, cost and resource utilization, and resolution of nursing diagnoses.

In nursing, the ANA's NDNQI has been underway, but it has not gained widespread acceptance within nursing. Although a consensus still is lacking in the nursing profession about what outcomes to measure, the early studies that began in the 1980s provided the basis for many of the continuing outcomes measurement projects used in nursing. Outcomes measurement continues to be a significant quality-related initiative in nursing.

LEADERSHIP AND MANAGEMENT IMPLICATIONS

The coordination of care to produce cost-minimizing and positive outcomes generating care services for clients and families is an intersection area in health care frequently managed by nurses. It is an area in which nursing has an opportunity to move forward with innovative

Research Note

Source: Adams, C.E., & Short, R. (1999). Rural versus urban home health: Does locale influence OASIS outcomes? *Outcomes Management for Nursing Practice, 3*(1), 26-31.

Purpose

Outcomes management is a visible issue in home health. Home health administrators select performance evaluation measures to meet the benchmarks required by JCAHO and HCFA. The purposes of this study were to describe selected characteristics of clients in rural versus urban locales and to determine whether rural versus urban setting influences outcomes.

Discussion

In 1998, home health accreditors and payers, JCAHO and HCFA, began to require outcomes data and performance measurement systems. The HCFA funded Outcome Assessment and Information Set (OASIS) was the plan chosen by most administrators. The concern now is for risk adjustment. If a risk adjustment process to reduce, remove, or clarify the influence of confounding client factors that differ among groups is not done, comparative data will misrepresent outcomes in home health care. Risk adjustment factors include comorbidity, severity and complexity of illness, functional status, and client demographics (e.g., age and gender). Rural versus urban locale was not on the list developed by JCAHO. However, a priority review panel of the National Institute of Nursing Research (NINR) documented major differences by these two locales, as did some nursing research. To investigate the locale impact, a cross-sectional study was done of 4,546 clients admitted to six home health agencies that were Medicare certified and licensed in Washington state. Data elements were a subset of OASIS, and data collection followed OASIS protocols. Both improvement and stabilization scores were calculated. The results showed differences in rural and urban client characteristics. Overall, more rural clients improved or stabilized on five outcome measures and fewer rural clients failed to improve or deteriorated. However, the size of the relationship was small, and the influence of locale on outcomes was minimal. The overall results were consistent with the NINR report and previous research. More rural clients were male and more immobile.

Application to Practice

The results of this large-sample cross-sectional study indicated that home health administrators do not need to select performance measurement systems or develop indicators that risk-adjust for rural versus urban location. Of interest was the result that on all five chosen outcomes (ambulation, bathing, management of oral medications, frequency of pain, and shortness of breath) proportionately more rural clients improved and stabilized. Client demographics, client diagnosis, or variations in depth of nurse-client relationships might have caused these differences.

---

outcomes management designed for complex care coordination. Despite the tendency to assume and measure outcomes as a simple linear relationship of client, nursing intervention, and an outcome (or a few outcomes), the reality of what happens is more complex, interactive, and multidimensional. The inputs to an episode or experience of health care services include client, family, provider, organization or system, and community environment characteristics. The outcomes that

result occur at multiple levels and can be related to clients, families, providers, organizations or systems, and populations or communities. Complex interactions also occur within, between, and among these factors (Huber & Oermann, 1999a, 1999b).

Leaders and managers in nursing can guide the way toward more complete descriptions of important outcomes and how to measure and manage them. They have a crucial role in

---

Box **40.1**

Home Care Outcomes Studies

Lalonde

Outcomes measures for home care clients:

- Taking prescribed medications
- Symptom distress
- Discharge status
- Caregiver strain
- Functional status
- Physiological indicators
- Knowledge of health problems

Rinke

Areas of outcomes measures for home health care:

- Physical
- Behavioral
- Psychosocial
- Knowledge
- Functional

Alberta, Canada

Client and family outcomes in home care:

- Pain management
- Symptom control
- Physiological status
- Activities of daily living
- Instrumental activities of daily living
- Well-being
- Goal attainment
- Knowledge and ability to apply that knowledge
- Client and family satisfaction
- Family strain
- Home maintenance

---

toward comprehensive outcomes management. Knowing nursing's important data first enables nurses to integrate more fully into multidisciplinary teams for better overall client care.

Leaders in today's health care delivery system are charged with the responsibility of producing quality services that achieve desired outcomes. Outcomes need to demonstrate a value for consumers, and services need to be valued by payers and purchasers of care.

Despite being highly interrelated, outcomes measurement and management do not necessarily equal a perception of quality. This occurs because of the multiple outcomes desired from multiple perspectives. There are at least three major levels of outcomes, as follows:

1. *Individual level:* For example, pain alleviation
2. *Organizational level:* For example, reduced length of stay
3. *Population or community-related level:* For example, decreased incidence of obesity

To reflect the idea of three levels of outcomes, Jennings and colleagues (1999) presented a framework for classifying outcome indicators. Outcome indicators from medicine, nursing, and health services clustered into the following three categories:

1. Patient-focused
2. Provider-focused
3. Organization-focused

Arguing for the use of the full scope of outcomes indicators, they identified the three categories from the literature. They noted that, in concept, a fourth category of population-focused outcomes would be important, but this was not identified in the literature. Some examples of indicators by category are displayed in Box 40.2. A sophisticated indicator system would select indicators across levels to provide a comprehensive collection of outcomes data with which to view the delivery of health care services and evaluate their effectiveness.

Many outcomes frameworks ignore the second and third levels while narrowly focusing on level 1. Other frameworks emphasize providers' perspectives over those of the patient or family. The solution is a broader view of outcomes that is balanced

determining the important outcomes sensitive to nursing care, acquiring computerized data support for nursing-sensitive outcomes, and then participating in leading and managing multidisciplinary teams

⚠ LEADERSHIP & MANAGEMENT **BEHAVIORS**

Leadership Behaviors

- Inspires outcomes thinking
- Enables the identification and use of evidence-based knowledge to drive outcomes
- Describes a vision for both client and systems outcomes
- Enables outcomes measurement using computerization and large nursing databases
- Removes barriers to outcomes improvement
- Articulates the value of nursing outcomes and practice

Management Behaviors

- Identifies outcomes of care and service
- Measures outcomes
- Manages the process of outcomes measurement
- Analyzes variances
- Takes corrective action when variances occur

Overlap Areas

- Determines outcomes to be measured and managed
- Leads and manages outcomes evaluation

Box 40.2

Outcome Indicator Examples

Patient-Focused

Diagnosis-focused: Examples are vital signs and laboratory values.

Holistically focused: Examples are health related quality of life and functional status.

Provider-Focused

Professional provider–focused: Examples are use of an evidence-based protocol and appropriateness of treatment of sentinel events.

Family caregiver–focused: Examples are caregiver burden and caregiver interactions.

Organization-Focused (measures aggregated across patients)

Access
Cost
Length of stay
Morbidity
Mortality
Other rate-based measures

---

and comprehensive. Nurse leaders need to be actively involved in indicator selection and outcomes monitoring, measurement, and management. Lancaster and King (1999) suggested a "spider" diagram as a visual representation for evaluating quality of care from the comprehensive view of structure, process, and outcomes. Figure 40.1 illustrates an example of a spider diagram.

Because outcomes measurement and management are important to leaders and managers for decision making, the quality of data is an urgent issue. Accurate and timely data are the foundation for the best decisions. The first step to quality outcomes is to determine facts. One type of facts that contribute to management decisions are the common causes of variance or variability. Special causes, or sentinel events, usually are readily identifiable. However, common causes are more subtle and difficult to identify. Deming (Walton, 1986) discussed several helpful tools that can be used in organizing and visually displaying data to examine common cause variation. The seven helpful charts are flow charts, cause-and-effect diagrams, Pareto charts, run or trend charts, histograms, control charts, and scatter diagrams. These tools can be used individually or in combination. They form

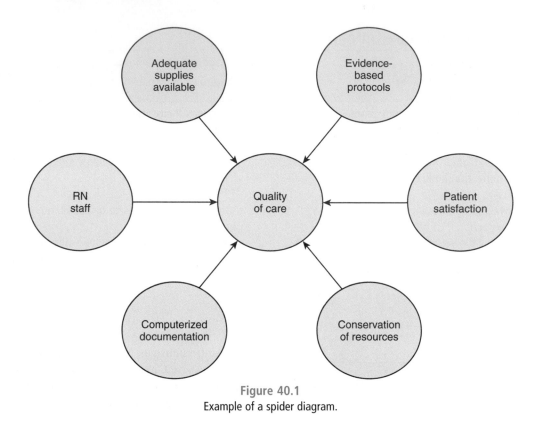

Figure 40.1
Example of a spider diagram.

essential statistical methods designed to understand work processes, bring the processes under control, and help improve them. Leaders and managers find these tools simple and easy to use. Their use requires only basic-level mathematics (Walton, 1986). The combination of outcomes thinking, multidisciplinary teamwork, and statistical data tools provide nurse leaders and managers with a powerful arsenal for managing outcomes in nursing practice.

CURRENT ISSUES AND TRENDS

Outcomes Measures for Quality Health Care Management

The quality of services delivered by health care organizations came under intense review during the 1990s. As part of this increasing attention, competing approaches were developed and aimed

at not only measuring the quality of health care but also reporting data about service, quality, and cost (Table 40.1). Individual health care organizations developed their own systems for reporting the quality of the services they provided. Some of these were in the form of report cards or instrument panels. At the same time, others followed the use of new standards that were developed for reporting, including HEDIS. Other organizations followed guidelines such as those from AHCPR, but regulatory and accreditation agencies such as HCFA and JCAHO developed more rigorous and outcome-based reporting requirements (Huber & Oermann, 1998).

One of the important areas for concern in developing a health care organization's outcomes reporting method is the use of comparative data. If the information provided is to be useful to clients, employers, and insurers, then the information must be not only valid and reliable but

Research Note

Source: Murray, M.E., & Darmody, J.V. (2004) Clinical and fiscal outcomes of utilization review. *Outcomes Management, 8*(1), 19-25.

Purpose

Concurrent utilization review (UR) is used as both a quality-improvement mechanism and a cost-containment strategy. UR seeks to control length of stay (LOS) and the use of services by eliminating what is inappropriate or unnecessary. The process is that hospital staff (usually RNs) communicate clinical information about patients to payers who review the planned care and determine whether the care is appropriate, medically necessary, and allowable and approved for reimbursement. The purpose of this study was to examine the impact of denials of reimbursement on the patients' clinical outcomes and the hospital's finances. The site was a 500-bed tertiary-care academic medical center with greater than 1,000 concurrent reviews per month. Data were collected over 12 months from concurrent UR denials (n = 102) and related hospital billing records. The hospital had a nurse case management (NCM) program, and the UR process was conducted by 18 NCMs, 9 social workers, 8 case manager associates, and 2 other RNs. The staff member who conducted the UR was interviewed by audiotape as soon as possible after the denial notification. The 102 cases of denial were in 26 different clinical services, with the most (n = 21) in psychiatry.

Discussion

For clinical outcomes, in 94.9% (n = 94) of the cases a denial of reimbursement did not change the plan of care. In 29% (n = 29) of these 94 cases, denial was received after discharge. Plans of care were changed (n = 9) by making arrangements or early discharge. Billing records were examined 6 months post discharge. Only 10% of the 102 cases denied were identified as uncompensated care, and only 3 patients whose care was denied paid hospital charges out of pocket. Overall, there was a low denial rate. However, there is a high investment of RN time on both ends of the UR process. This generates additional paperwork, documentation, and costs. Physicians made most patient resource decisions yet were little involved in UR.

Application to Practice

Denials of reimbursement had little impact on clinical or financial outcomes in one hospital with a mature case management program. Benefits of UR are decreased LOS, reduced inappropriate care, and creation of provider awareness of the oversight process. However, UR is costly ($166,000 annually with an average cost per review of $11 in one study) and criticized for perceived holding back on treatment. Other strategies, such as replacing case-by-case review with targeted reviews, need to be evaluated for the evidence base and for conserving scarce resources.

---

also clear as to the outcomes that are measured. Nelson and colleagues (1995) recommended that instrument panel data collection systems be developed that would feed information into report cards. The instrument panel data would both identify performance variation within a system and provide a balanced view of outcomes, including clinical outcomes, functional health status, client satisfaction, and cost information for external health care purchasers.

The development and elaboration of performance management data systems for nursing is a current trend to watch. No consensus has been reached about the structure and content of nursing-sensitive systems. Gregg (2002) suggested a performance management data system (PMDS) designed to fit a nursing service organization's needs. The PMDS-related models in the literature include a clinical value compass, the spider diagram nursing quality report card, the dashboard, ANA Report Card, and the NMMDS. Report cards and dashboards refer to the final reports generated from PDMSs. These are data report tools for rapid analysis of nursing service performance.

Table 40.1

Quality Health Care Initiatives	
Organization	Initiative
American Nurses Association (ANA)	Nursing Report Card for Acute Care Settings
National Committee for Quality Assurance (NCQA)	HEDIS—Health Plan Employer Data and Information Set
Joint Commission on Accreditation of Healthcare Organizations (JCAHO)	ORYX—Integrates use of outcomes and performance measures into the accreditation process
Health Care Financing Administration (HCFA)	OASIS—Outcome and Assessment Information Set

Gregg's (2002) PDMS used general systems theory concepts of input, throughput and output to address the relationships between nursing services and the external environment. PDMS models are predicted to become more highly developed and widespread.

Balanced scorecards and dashboard approaches are gaining in popularity. The balanced scorecard uses four areas for data evaluation: internal business processes, learning and growth, customer, and financial. Some research is beginning to look at whether or not this is a feasible approach (Hall et al., 2003). Dashboard approaches seek to identify the key factors for which a nurse manager needs to frequently monitor data in order to manage quality and costs. Each approach struggles with issues of what is the minimum number of data elements needed versus how comprehensive and inclusive to be and what elements are needed in the dataset. Issues of feasibility, practicality, collectability, and comprehensiveness will be part of this unfolding area of nursing administration.

Work also continues in the nursing profession to describe and classify nursing-sensitive outcomes. Some of the efforts in this field have included the following:

- *The Omaha System:* This system includes standardized classifications for various conditions, interventions, and ratings of client problems.

- *The Nursing Intervention Classification (NIC) and Nursing-Sensitive Outcomes Classification (NOC)* (Johnson et al., 2000): This work identifies outcomes that are sensitive to nursing interventions and can be included in nursing clinical data sets in various settings.

- The *American Nurses Association's* efforts to identify quality indicators and measurement tools (NDNQI): These efforts are aimed at measuring the quality of nursing care in acute care settings.

As the health care spotlight has shined on quality-of-care initiatives, indicators and outcomes have received much attention. More needs to be done to determine the amount and effectiveness of nursing interventions in achieving desired outcomes and reflecting quality of care and system performance.

Summary

- Nurses always have had an outcomes focus.
- Consumers, employers, and payers are demanding outcomes evidence.
- An outcome is the result obtained from efforts to accomplish a goal.
- Indicators are valid and reliable performance measures.
- Outcomes measurement involves determining indicators, collecting and analyzing data, and taking action.

- Outcomes management is a multidisciplinary process of managing outcomes for performance.
- The lack of documentation of effectiveness plus variations in practice have triggered the demand for outcomes.
- Outcomes measures developed over the twentieth century.
- Nursing-sensitive outcomes have become more fully developed since the 1970s.
- Outcomes measurement continues to be important in nursing and health care.
- Nurse leaders and managers play a role in defining, measuring, and managing outcomes.
- Standardized report cards are being developed and used.

Study Questions

1. Are outcomes more important than processes? Why or why not?
2. Do outcomes equal quality? Discuss the rationale for why or why not.
3. What are the key indicators and outcomes for nursing?
4. Why are outcomes measures not defined consistently across organizations?

5. How do you know whether an outcome is sensitive to nursing?
6. Should nurses ignore outcomes not sensitive to nursing?
7. How do nurses determine nursing-sensitive indicators?

CASE STUDY

Nurse Gloria Davis was reviewing her population profile and related population-based data. Clearly, StayAtHome Home Health Agency served primarily the elderly. More than 78% of the agency's revenue was derived from Medicare. Also, the population of the eight contiguous counties and the county in which StayAtHome is located contained a high percentage of residents aged 65 and older, with a growing percentage of that group aged 80 and older.

Clinical management of the agency's clients necessitated a delicate balance of cost-versus-quality decisions. Hospitalizations were increasing, which potentially signaled the failure of home care. The data indicated a need to review client health care information to analyze the risk for nonelective hospitalizations in frail older adults. Nurse Davis implemented a chart review of the

CRITICAL THINKING EXERCISE

Nurse Maria Garcia works for a managed care type of health maintenance organization (HMO). The nurses at the HMO have noticed a problem with women's health care. Little concern or counseling regarding menopause and health care is being provided. Nurse Garcia sees menopause counseling as a prime opportunity for nurses to deliver needed preventive and wellness care to adult women and their families. Furthermore, the National Committee for Quality Assurance (NCQA) that accredits managed care organizations is projected to include menopause counseling in its upcoming HEDIS data set. It already has developed a national database of standardized performance and accreditation information for benchmarking.

Nurse Garcia wants to take the lead in developing a menopause counseling program. However, several questions have arisen: How much will this cost? Which personnel should do this? What should be included in the program? What groups should be targeted?

1. What is the problem?
2. Why is it a problem?
3. What are the key issues?
4. What should Nurse Garcia do first?
5. How should Nurse Garcia handle this situation?
6. What outcomes should be used for this new program?
7. What outcomes measures might be useful?

last year's records. In reviewing the data, patterns began to emerge. Six specific risk factors appeared: diagnosis of congestive heart failure, diabetes, or anemia; taking multiple medications (polypharmacy); low body mass index; and emergency department visits in the last year. Almost half of the group with any risk factor had congestive heart failure or heart disease. On average, clients had five active medication prescriptions. Many had poor physical functioning, were obese, and had poor general health and vitality scores.

Nurse Davis determined that profiles of vulnerable and at-risk elderly could be created. After doing so, she set a plan to develop nursing care interventions targeted to chronic illnesses and poor physical functioning in the elderly. The outcomes would be measured in 6 and 12 months. The creative use of patient education, monitoring reminders, nutrition and exercise coaching, and efforts to supplement social support networks interventions were developed as strategies to be delivered with each home visit to at-risk clients. In addition to checklists, intervention plans, and documentation forms, an "early alert" mechanism was developed to identify and intervene if the home care agency staff person felt that the client's status was deteriorating in any way. "Early alert" led to an intensive care team review and further planning and intervention. At 6 months, outcomes were noted to have dropped from 1 in 5 at-risk clients being hospitalized (20%) to 1 in 10 (10%).

REFERENCES

Agency for Healthcare Research and Quality (AHRQ). (2004). *Outcomes research fact sheet.* Washington, DC: AHRQ. Retrieved January 11, 2005, from *www.ahrq.gov/clinic/outfact.htm*

American Nurses Association (ANA). (1996). *Nursing quality indicators: Definitions and implications.* Washington, DC: American Nurses Publishing.

American Nurses Association (ANA). (2004). *National database of nursing quality indicators.* Silver Spring, MD: ANA. Retrieved July 21, 2004, from *www.nursingworld.org/quality*

Aydelotte, M. (1962). The use of patient welfare as a criterion measure. *Nursing Research, 11*(1), 10-14.

Cleary, P.D., & Edgman-Levitan, S. (1997). Healthcare quality: Incorporating consumer perspectives. *Journal of the American Medical Association, 278,* 1608-1612.

Daubert, E. (1979). Patient classification system and outcome criteria. *Nursing Outlook, 27,* 450-454.

Donabedian, A. (1985). *The methods and findings of quality assessment and monitoring: An illustrated analysis* (Vol. 3). Ann Arbor, MI: Health Administration Press.

Gregg, A.C. (2002). Performance management data systems for nursing service organizations. *Journal of Nursing Administration, 32*(2), 71-78.

Hall, L.M., Doran, D., Laschinger, H.S., Mallette, C., Pedersen, C., & O'Brien-Pallas, L. (2003). A balanced scorecard approach for nursing report card development. *Outcomes Management, 7*(1), 17-22.

Horn, B.J., & Swain, M.A. (1978). *Criterion measures of nursing care quality* (DHEW Pub. No. PHS78-3187). Hyattsville, MD: National Center for Health Services Research.

Hover, J., & Zimmer, M. (1978). Nursing quality assurance: The Wisconsin system. *Nursing Outlook, 26,* 242-248.

Huber, D., & Oermann, M. (1998). The evolution of outcomes management. In D.L. Flarey & S.S. Blancett (Eds.), *Cardiovascular outcomes: Collaborative, path-based approaches* (pp. 3-12). Gaithersburg, MD: Aspen.

Huber, D., & Oermann, M. (1999a). Do outcomes equal quality? *Outcomes Management for Nursing Practice, 3*(1), 1-3.

Huber, D., & Oermann, M. (1999b). Is the intersection clear? *Outcomes Management for Nursing Practice, 3*(3), 91.

Jennings, B.M., Staggers, N., & Brosch, L.R. (1999). A classification scheme for outcome indicators. *Image: Journal of Nursing Scholarship, 31*(4), 381-388.

Johnson, M., Maas, M., & Moorhead, S. (Eds.). (2000). *Nursing outcomes classification (NOC)* (2nd ed.). St Louis: Mosby.

Joint Commission on Accreditation of Healthcare Organizations (JCAHO). (2004a). *Glossary of terms for performance measurement.* Oakbrook Terrace, IL: JCAHO. Retrieved December 13, 2004, from *www.jcaho.org/accredited+organizations/long+term+care/oryx/glossary+of+terms/glossary.htm*

Joint Commission on Accreditation of Healthcare Organizations (JCAHO). (2004b). *Performance measurement in health care.* Oakbrook Terrace, IL: JCAHO. Retrieved July 21, 2004, from *www.jcaho.org/pms/index.htm*

Kalisch, P.A., & Kalisch, B.J. (1978). *The advance of American nursing.* Boston: Little, Brown & Co.

Kelly, K.C., Huber, D.G., Johnson, M., McCloskey, J.C., & Maas, M. (1994). The medical outcomes study: A nursing perspective. *Journal of Professional Nursing, 10*(4), 209-216.

Lalonde, B. (1986). *Quality assurance manual of the home care association of Washington.* Edmonds, WA: The Home Care Association of Washington.

Lancaster, D.R., & King, A. (1999). The spider diagram nursing quality report card: Bringing all the pieces together. *Journal of Nursing Administration, 29*(7/8), 43-48.

Lang, N.M., & Marek, K.D. (1990). The classification of patient outcomes. *Journal of Professional Nursing, 6,* 158-163.

Lohr, K.N. (1988). Outcome measurement: Concepts and questions. *Inquiry, 25*(1), 37-50.

Marek, K.D. (1989). Outcome measurement in nursing. *Journal of Nursing Quality Assurance, 4,* 1-9.

Marek, K.D. (1997). Measuring the effectiveness of nursing care. *Outcomes Management for Nursing Practice, 1*(1), 8-12.

Martin, K.S., & Sheet, N.J. (1992). *The Omaha system: Applications for community health nursing.* Philadelphia: WB Saunders.

Nadzam, D.M. (1997). Nurses and the measurement of healthcare: An overview. In *Nursing practice and outcomes measurement* (pp. 1-15). Oakbrook Terrace, IL: Joint Commission on Accreditation of Healthcare Organizations.

National Committee for Quality Assurance (NCQA). (2004). *NCQA releases HEDIS®2005; Focus in on health issues familiar to seniors, working Americans.* Washington, DC: NCQA. Retrieved July 21, 2004, from *www.ncqa.org/Communications/News/Hedis2005.htm*

Nelson, E.C., Batalden, P.B., Plume, S.K., Mihevc, N.T., & Schwartz, W.G. (1995). Report cards or instrument panels: Who needs what? *Joint Commission Journal on Quality Improvement, 21*(4), 155-166.

Oermann, M., & Huber, D. (1997). New horizons. *Outcomes Management for Nursing Practice, 1*(1), 1-2.

Oermann, M.H., & Huber, D. (1999). Patient outcomes: A measure of nursing's value. *American Journal of Nursing, 99*(9), 40-47.

Peters, D.A. (1995). Outcomes: The mainstay of a framework for quality of care. *Journal of Nursing Care Quality, 10*(1), 61-69.

Rinke, L. (1988). *Outcomes measures in home care: State of the art* (Vol. 3). New York: National League for Nursing.

Shaughnessy, P.W., Crisler, K.S., Schlenker, R.E., & Arnold, A.G. (1995). Outcome-based quality improvement in home care. *Caring, 14*(2), 44-49.

Sorgen, L.M. (1988). The development of a home care quality assurance program in Alberta. *Home Healthcare Services Quarterly, 7*(2), 13-28.

Tarlov, A.R., Ware, J., Greenfield, S., Nelson, E., Perrin, E., & Zubkoff, M. (1989). The medical outcomes study: An application of methods for monitoring the results of medical care. *Journal of the American Medical Association, 262*(7), 925-930.

Walton, M. (1986). *The Deming management method.* New York: Perigee Books.

Wennberg, J. (1990). Outcomes research, cost containment and the fear of healthcare rationing. *New England Journal of Medicine, 323,* 1202-1204.

Glossary

Accountability the liability for task performance.

Acculturation process of incorporating values, beliefs and behaviors from the host culture into an immigrant's world view.

Activity a basic unit of human behavior.

Administrative Controls measures that include adequate staffing patterns to prevent personnel from working alone and reducing waiting times, controlled access, and development of systems to alert security personnel when violence is threatened.

Administrative Law rules and regulations adopted by federal or state agencies to implement statutory law adopted by Congress or state legislatures.

All-Hazards Disaster Preparedness action plans for every type of disaster or combination of disaster events.

Audit and Feedback ongoing monitoring of critical indicators of practice and periodic reporting of the data/information back to the clinicians responsible for patient care.

Authority the right to act or command the actions of others.

Autonomy an individual's right of self-determination and freedom of decision making.

Bargaining the exchange of favors or trading activity.

Behavior Modifications changes in behavior that provide all workers with training in recognizing and managing assaults, resolving conflicts, and maintaining hazard awareness.

Benchmarking a process of measuring what exists against what is the best.

Beneficence doing good for clients and providing benefit balanced against risk.

Best Practice a service, function, or process that produces superior outcomes; the goal of best practice is to provide currency, relevancy, and usefulness for interventions in clinical practice.

Bias a mental preference or inclination.

Budget a written financial plan aimed at controlling the allocation of resources.

Burnout responses to chronic emotional stress that have three components: (1) emotional or physical exhaustion, (2) lowered job productivity, and (3) overdepersonalization.

Capital Budget tracks purchases of capital assets (i.e., buildings, land, and equipment).

Care Modality a method of organizing and delivering nursing care in order to achieve desired outcomes.

Case Management a collaborative process of assessment, planning, facilitation, and advocacy for options and services to meet an individual's health needs through communication and available resources to promote high-quality, cost-effective outcomes.

Cash Budget tracks cash receipts and cash disbursements.

Centralization the extent to which power and authority for decision making rests in top levels of the organization.

Change an alteration to make something different.

Change Agent someone who influences the change process or innovation decisions.

Change Champion practitioner who continually promotes use of evidence-based practices through education, demonstration, and encouragement of colleagues.

Charge the price asked for services or goods.

Charges dollar amount billed to a customer.

Civil Acts conduct that violates the rights of individuals by tort or by breach of contract; there may or may not be in existence statues prohibiting such conduct; persons who have committed civil wrongs are usually required to pay money damages to those who were wronged.

Climate perceptions held by individuals about a particular unit or environment.

Collective Action action, such as mass resignations, taken by employees or professional organization groups in order to bring about changes in terms of employment.

Collective Bargaining the process used by representatives of an employer and the certified representatives for a group of employees to negotiate and sign an agreement covering terms of employment.

Committee a relatively stable and formally composed group; a subset of a group.

Common Law a system of laws or principles based on court decisions and on customs and usages rather than on statutory written laws.

Community a locally based entity composed of systems of formal organizations reflecting societal institutions, informal groups, and aggregates.

Competence having the capacity to function effectively as an individual and an organization with the context of the cultural beliefs, behaviors, and needs presented by consumers and their communities.

Competitive Conflict Rules-based conflict with the goal to win or beat an opponent.

Confidentiality the prohibition of some disclosures of information gained in certain relationships without the consent of the original source of the information.

Conflict a clash or struggle that occurs when a real or perceived threat or difference exists in the desires, thoughts, attitudes, feelings, or behaviors of two or more parties.

Continuous Quality Improvement (CQI) a process of continuously improving a system by gathering data on performance and proposing changes.

Controlling comparing the results of work with predetermined standards of performance and taking corrective action when needed.

Conventional Performance Appraisal a systematic, standardized evaluation of an employee by the supervisor, aimed at judging the value of the employee's work contributions, quality of work, and potential for advancement.

Coordinating motivating and leading personnel to carry out the desired actions.

Corporate Culture a way or manner of doing business.

Cost the amount of money required to cover direct production inputs.

Costing Out Nursing Services methods to determine the actual costs of nursing services.

Criminal Acts conduct that is offensive or harmful to society as a whole and violates statues prohibiting such conduct; persons found to have committed criminal acts are typically fined or jailed.

Critical Path a written, structured care methodology used to standardize care by mapping time and activity sequence for an episode of care.

Critical Thinking a cognitive, rational-thinking process that includes knowledge acquisition, analysis, problem-solving behaviors, reflection, and intuition.

Culture shared beliefs, behaviors, actions, values, communication, perceptions, values, or tradition and customs common to a population.

Cultural Blind Spot area in one language that cannot be expressed well when translated into another language.

Cultural Competence the ability to recognize and respond to health-related beliefs and cultural values, disease incidence and prevalence, and treatment efficacy.

Cultural Relativism maintaining a sense of objectivity and holding multiple perspectives without judgment.

Damage Control an aspect of risk management that refers to the organizational actions taken in response to untoward events in an effort to mitigate damages.

Decentralization the extent to which power and authority for decision making are systematically filtered down to middle and lower levels of the organization; types of decentralization include vertical decentralization, horizontal decentralization, and selective decentralization.

Decision Making a behavior exhibited in making a selection and implementing a course of action from alternatives; may or may not be the result of an immediate problem.

Delegatee the person receiving the delegation.

Delegation the transfer of responsibility for the performance of a task from one person to a competent other.

Delegator the person making the delegation.

Dependence Aspect of Power power resides in the other's dependency on the powerful one.

Disaster an unforeseen and often sudden event that causes great damage, destruction, and human suffering

Disease Management a comprehensive, integrated approach to care and reimbursement based on the natural course of a disease.

Disruptive Conflict activity designed to attack, defeat, or eliminate an opponent through disruption.

Diversity a broad range of differences.

Division of Labor process by which work is broken up into pieces or tasks and then assigned.

Economic Evaluation evaluating both inputs and outputs and costs and consequences.

Employee Assistance Programs (EAPs) programs that provide a range of services to help employees cope with stressors that occur at home and at work.

Empowerment giving individuals the authority, responsibility, and freedom to act on what they know and instilling the confidence to do so.

Environmental Designs provisions that include signaling systems, alarm systems, monitoring systems, security devices, security escorts, lighting, and architectural and furniture modifications to improve worker safety.

Ethnicity shared origins and shared culture.

Ethnocentrism interpretation of the beliefs and behavior of others in terms of one's own cultural values and traditions; belief that one's own culture is superior.

Evidence-Based Practice the conscientious, explicit, and judicious use of research and other current best evidence with clinical expertise and patients' values in making decisions about health care; more recently, evidence-based practices are defined as those clinical and administrative practices that have been proven to consistently produce specific, intended results.

Expenses the costs of activities undertaken in an organization's operations.

Expense Budget tracks expenditure of resources or costs paid (i.e., wages, benefits, and maintenance costs).

Fidelity being loyal and faithful to commitments and accountable for responsibilities.

Financial Management a series of activities designed to allocate resources and plan for the efficient operation of an organization.

Fixed Staffing staffing that builds around a fixed projected maximum workload requirement.

Followership an interpersonal process of participation.

Functional Nursing assignment by functions or tasks.

Group any collection of interconnected individuals working together for some purpose.

Group Nursing private-duty nurses in group practice.

Hazard Prevention and Control the implementation of work practices to prevent and control identified hazards.

Health Care System all (1) structures, (2) organizations, and (3) services designed to deliver professional health and wellness to consumers.

Health Disparity population-specific difference in the presence of disease, health outcomes, or access to care.

Health Policy the entire set of public policies that are related to, or that influence, health and illness.

Horizontal Decentralization the decision-making power that flows outside the line of authority by which nonmanagement personnel are authorized to effect decision processes.

Indicators valid and reliable quantitative measures of structure, process, or outcome.

Job Conflict a perceived opposition or antagonistic process at the individual-organization level.

Justice being fair to all and giving equal treatment, including distributing benefits, risks, and costs equally.

Leadership the process of influencing people to accomplish goals.

Leadership Styles different combinations of task and relationship behaviors used to influence others to accomplish goals.

Legally Liable when the law imposes a civil obligation on a wrongdoer to compensate an injured party for the consequences of a wrongful act.

Line and Staff Positions the array of positions into direct producers and support positions.

Malpractice failure of a professional person to act as other prudent professionals with the same knowledge and education would act under similar circumstances.

Managed Care the systematic integration and coordination of the financing and delivery of health care; these activities are performed by health plans that try to provide their members with prepaid access to high-quality care at relatively low cost and usually are at least partly at risk for the cost of care; the health plans may rely on physician gatekeepers and prior authorization mechanisms to minimize unnecessary or inappropriate utilization.

Management the coordination and integration of resources through planning, organizing, coordinating, directing, and controlling to accomplish specific institutional goals and objectives.

Management Information System an integrated system for collecting, storing, retrieving, and processing a collective set of data; the data are transformed from storage into knowledge that is directly useful and applicable in the process of directing and controlling resources and their application to the achievement of specific management objectives.

Market a set of actual or potential buyers and users of goods, services, and ideas.

Market Research the systematic process for studying a marketing problem by designing a study, collecting, and analyzing the data and using information from the findings.

Market Share the percentage of the total market for a product or service that is captured by an organization or producer.

Marketing a social and managerial process in which individuals or groups obtain what they need and want by exchanging products and values with others.

Marketing Mix an individualized blend of marketing tools and tactics implemented to achieve goals.

Marketing Orientation the focusing of energy on the identification of the needs and wants of customers and on the delivery of services that create satisfaction.

Medicaid a joint federal and state program designed to pay for medical long-term care assistance for individuals and families with low incomes and limited resources.

Medicare the national health insurance program for persons age 65 and over, some disabled persons, and persons with end-stage renal disease.

Modular Nursing construction of geographic modules to facilitate team nursing.

Motivation the degree to which an individual is moved or aroused to achieve a goal or purpose.

Motivation to Work the degree to which members of an organization are willing to work.

Motives or Needs wants, drives, or impulses.

Mutuality back-and-forth sharing of power in a relationship.

Need for Achievement the strong desire to overcome challenges, to excel, to advance or succeed, and to grow.

Need for Affiliation the desire to work in a pleasant environment; the desire for friendly, close relationships.

Need for Power the need to be in control and to get others to behave contrary to what they would naturally do.

Needs basic biological, psychological, and social requirements.

Negligence failure to exercise the proper degree of care required by the circumstances.

Negotiation a process of give-and-take exchange among persons aimed at resolving problems, conflicts, or disputes.

New and Evolving Types mixed models emphasizing outcomes management and integrated professional practice.

Nonmaleficence doing no harm to clients.

Nonverbal Communication communication that uses affective or expressive behaviors rather than words.

Nursing Informatics the management and processing of nursing data, information, and knowledge to support the practice of nursing and the delivery of nursing care.

Nursing Management the coordination and integration of nursing resources by applying the management process to accomplish nursing care and service goals and objectives.

Nursing Shortage situation in which the number of nurses that employers would *like* to employ (demand) exceeds the number of nurses willing to be employed at a given salary (supply).

Nursing Unit small structure embedded within a larger macro-organization.

Objectives the financial or performance-based, short- or long-range targets that an enterprise wishes to achieve.

Occupational or Job Stress tension that is related to the demands of the role or job.

Opinion Leaders informal leaders who influence their peer groups to evaluate innovations for use in their settings.

Operating Budget the plan for the unit's or organization's daily operating revenues and expenses.

Organization a group of persons with specific responsibilities acting together for the achievement of a specific purpose determined by the organization.

Organizational Chart visual representation of the framework that demonstrates horizontal and vertical reporting relationships within an organization.

Organizational Communication the degree to which information is transmitted among the members and parts of an organization.

Organizational Conflict the struggle for scarce organizational resources.

Organizational Context the health system environment in which the proposed evidence-based practice is to be implemented.

Organizational Vision or Mission a guiding framework that describes what the organization views as its business and future direction.

Organizing mobilizing the human and material resources of the institution to achieve organizational objectives.

Outcomes the result(s) obtained from the efforts to accomplish a goal.

Outcomes Management a multidisciplinary process designed to provide quality health care, decrease fragmentation, enhance outcomes, and constrain costs.

Outcomes Measurement determining the indicators, gathering necessary data, analyzing that data, interpreting the results, making changes in nursing care, and evaluating effectiveness.

Outreach or Academic Detailing one-on-one discussions with practitioners in their setting to provide information, feedback, and rewards regarding evidence-based practice.

Peer Review the examination and evaluation of practice by the employee's associate.

People of Color a positive politically correct term of inclusivity to describe all non-white persons.

Performance Gap Assessment a data-driven strategy/intervention that demonstrates an opportunity for practice changes and improvement related to specific indicators.

Performance Measurement System an automated database that generates internal comparisons of organization performance over time.

Persuasion human communication designed to influence another to change attitudes or alter behaviors.

Philosophy an explanation of the systems of beliefs that determine how a mission or a purpose is to be achieved.

Planning determining the long- and short-term objectives and the corresponding actions that must be taken to achieve these objectives.

Policy a guideline that has been formalized.

Politics the process of influencing the allocation of scarce resources or the use of power for change.

Population a collection of individuals who have in common one or more personal or environmental characteristics.

Population-Based Care Management the integration and coordination of health services to a specified population.

Position a collection of tasks that are configured together for performance, usually by one individual.

Power the capability of acting or producing some sort of effect; the potential capacity to exert influence.

Practice Guideline a systematically developed standard, designed to assist both provider and patient in making decisions about appropriate health care for specific clinical circumstances.

Prejudice an emotional categorical mode of mental functioning involving rigid prejudgment and misjudgments of human acts.

Price dollar value of each input to the production process.

Primary Nursing 24-hour accountability by a nurse for specific clients from hospital admission through discharge.

Privacy a right of limited physical or informational inaccessibility.

Private-Duty Nursing one nurse caring for one client.

Problem a deficit or surplus of something; a situation that is perplexing.

Problem Solving the process that attempts to identify obstacles that inhibit accomplishment of a specific goal.

Procedure a description of how to carry out an activity.

Product anything that can be offered to a market to satisfy a want or need.

Production Process relationships of outputs to inputs.

Productivity output produced using a quantity of inputs.

Profession an occupational group.

Professional individual engaged in a profession.

Professionalism *individual:* extent to which the member adheres to standards and ethics and identifies with a profession; *group:* degree to which a group defines, standardizes and directs its own practice.

Proxemics nonverbal communication through the use of interpersonal space.

Pseudoteam a group of people who think they are a team but are not, characterized by confusion over purpose or a highly politicized purpose, dysfunctional and unhealthy interpersonal relationships and communication patterns, lack of clarity about goals, and no evaluation criteria.

Quality the characteristics of and the pursuit of excellence.

Quality of Health Care the degree to which health services for individuals and populations increase the likelihood of desired health outcomes.

Quality Improvement Program an umbrella program that provides a continuous, ongoing measurement and evaluation process.

Racism any type of action or attitude, individual or institutional, that prescribes and legitimizes a minority group's subordination by claiming that the minority is biogenetically or culturally inferior.

Recordkeeping and Evaluation of Programs systems designed to provide the data to track progress in reducing work-related assaults.

Recruitment the process used by organizations to replenish employees.

Reinfusion the planned and systematic process used to promote integration of the evidence-based practice into daily practice following initial pilot evaluation.

Relational Aspect of Power the idea that power is a property of a social relationship.

Research Utilization the use of research findings as a basis for practice encompassing critique, synthesis, evaluation, and dissemination of scientific knowledge.

Responsibility allocation and acceptance of a task.

Retention the ability to continue the employment of qualified individuals.

Revenues income or amounts owed for purchased services or goods.

Risk Adjustment a process in which differences among clients or variables such as age or disease severity are weighted or adjusted for in outcomes analyses.

Risk Factors for Violence things that predispose a workplace to violence, including interpersonal elements, environmental characteristics and design, and organizational culture.

Risk Management an integrated effort across all disciplines and functional areas to protect the financial assets of an organization from loss by focusing on the prevention of problems that can lead to untoward events and lawsuits and to maintain high-quality health care.

Risk Management Program an organization-wide program to identify risks, control occurrences, prevent damage, and control legal liability.

Safety and Health Training education designed to make all staff members aware of security hazards and ways to protect themselves through established policies, procedures, and training.

Sanctioning Aspect of Power the idea that power is an active, direct manipulation of another's outcomes.

Scalar Process the creation of levels of authority in a hierarchy.

Scheduling the ongoing implementation of the staffing pattern by assigning individual personnel to work specific hours and days in a specific unit or area.

Selection determination of the most qualified candidate for a job.

Selective Decentralization a concentration of power for decision making that resides in functional divisions within the organization; examples include a central sterile processing department, central pharmacy, central human relations department.

Self-Evaluation a self-assessment of employee's own perceptions regarding performance according to stated expectations.

Sentinel Event an unexpected occurrence involving death or serious physical or psychological injury.

Service any act or performance that one party can offer to another that is essentially intangible and does not result in the ownership of anything

Shared Governance an accountability-based model of shared decision making that leads to the empowerment and autonomy of professional nurses; through shared decision making, nurses at the point of service have control over their nursing practice, peer issues, education, quality, and work environment.

Sources of Violence violent acts committed by (1) criminals who have no connection with the workplace; (2) customers, clients, or patients; (3) current or former coworkers; or (4) persons not employed at the workplace but who have a personal relationship with an employee.

Span of Control the number of staff members reporting directly to a manager.

Staff Vacancy a budgeted but not filled employee position.

Staffing human resources planning to fill positions in an organization with qualified personnel.

Standards written value statements.

Statutory Laws laws enacted by the U.S. Congress, state legislatures, or local government bodies and signed (approved) as required by the President, Governor, or local equivalent such as a mayor.

Stereotype an assumption made about another person based on group membership.

Stereotypes fixed and/or distorted views, whether positive or negative, towards all members of a group of people.

Strategic Management management of an organization based on its vision or mission.

Strategic Plan document specifying the action plan for actualizing the organization's mission.

Strategic Planning a process of assessing an organization and its departments or divisions.

Strategy competitive move or business approach designed to produce a successful outcome.

Stress physical, mental, psychological, and spiritual responses to any stressor.

Stressor an experience in a person-environment relationship that is evaluated by a person as taxing or exceeding resources and threatening the sense of well-being.

Structure of an Organization the sum total of the ways that labor is divided into distinct tasks and then the way coordination is achieved among these tasks.

Supervision the provision of guidance or direction, evaluation, and follow-up by the licensed nurse for accomplishment of a nursing task or activity delegated to unlicensed assistive personnel, with initial direction and periodic inspection of the actual accomplishment of the task or activity.

Synergy a condition that exists when parts of an organization interact to produce a joint effect that is greater than the sum of the parts acting alone; the concept that the whole is greater than the sum of its parts (e.g., 1 + 1 = 3).

Systematic Reviews the structured and systematic combination of findings from research into powerful and clinically useful reports to guide practice.

Tactics choices for action that are made to implement a strategy.

Team a small number of consistent people who have complementary skills, a shared purpose that entails collective work, specific performance goals, common approaches to the work, and who hold themselves mutually accountable for outcomes.

Team Building the process of deliberately creating and unifying a group into a functioning work unit so that specific goals are accomplished.

Team Nursing care to a group of clients by a mixed-staff group.

Technoshrink diffusion of information and telecommunications technology.

Threat Assessment the evaluation of the threat itself and an evaluation of the threatener.

Threat Management the course of action to be taken after conducting a threat assessment.

Total Cost dollar value of the production process.

Total Patient Care one-shift responsibility for a client.

Total Quality Management (TQM) evaluation of all systems to improve the quality of goods or services by reducing costs in ways that ensure customer satisfaction; a process to involve all employees in the improvement of the quality of every product or service.

Transformational Leader a leader who inspires and transforms followers.

Translational Research the scientific investigation of methods and variables that influence use of evidence-based practices to improve decision making in the delivery of health care services.

Turnover the loss of an employee as a result of transfer, termination, or resignation.

Variable Staffing method that staffs units below maximum workload conditions and then supplements as needed.

Veracity telling the truth and not intentionally deceiving or misleading clients.

Verbal Communication communication through the use of words, either spoken or written.

Vertical Decentralization the distribution of power down the chain or command, or line of authority, flowing from the top of the organization to the bottom.

Violence *narrowly defined:* assault, battery, manslaughter, or homicide; *broadly defined:* ranging from verbal abuse, threats, and unwanted sexual advances to physical assault and homicide.

Violence Prevention Programs programs, available to all employees, that track progress in reducing work-related assaults, reduce severity of injuries sustained by employees, decrease the threat to worker safety, and reflect the level and nature of threat faced by employees.

Violence Prevention Written Plans plans that demonstrate management commitment by disseminating a policy that all types of violence will not be tolerated, ensure that no reprisals are taken against employees who report or experience workplace violence, encourage prompt reporting of all violent incidents, and establish a plan for maintaining security in the workplace.

Wants desires or preferences satisfied by specific goods and services and influenced by external cues.

Work Group collection of individuals who are led by a strong and focused leader.

Workplace Violence violent acts directed toward persons at work or on duty.

Worksite Analysis a common-sense look at the workplace to find existing or potential hazards for workplace violence.

Index

Note: Page numbers followed by f indicate figures; those followed by t indicate tables; those followed by b indicate boxed material.